# MEDICOLEGAL INVESTIGATION OF DEATH

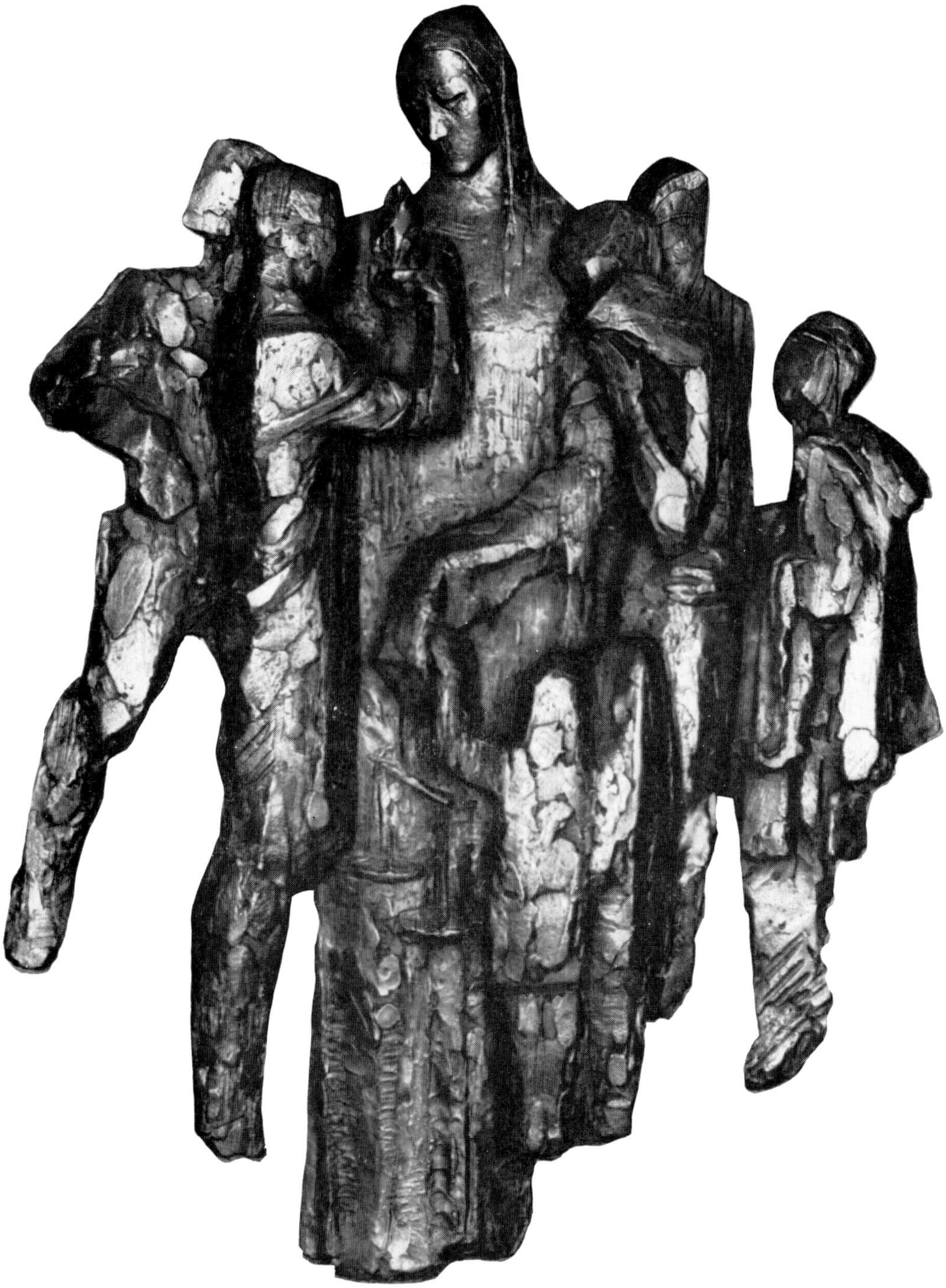

"The search for truth is the essence of forensic pathology. This truth forms an essential link between the enforcement of law and the protection of the public in the administration of justice." This illustration shows a sculpture by Una Hanbury, located in the lobby of Maryland's Medical Examiner's Building in Baltimore. The guardian figure on the left represents law. Next to it the doctor holds up the lamp of knowledge towards the symbolic figure of justice. Justice is interpreted in its aspect of love. The general public is suggested by the group of figures on the right. An inscription underneath the sculpture reads, "Wherever the art of medicine is practiced there is also a love of humanity." (Hippocrates)

# MEDICOLEGAL INVESTIGATION OF DEATH

## Guidelines for the Application of Pathology to Crime Investigation

SECOND EDITION

*Edited By*


**WERNER U. SPITZ, M.D.**

*Chief Medical Examiner*
*County of Wayne, Detroit, Michigan*
*Associate Professor of Pathology (Forensic Pathology)*
*Wayne State University, School of Medicine*
*Adjunct Professor of Chemistry*
*University of Windsor*
*Windsor, Ontario, Canada*

**RUSSELL S. FISHER, M.D.**

*Chief Medical Examiner, State of Maryland*
*Clinical Professor of Forensic Pathology*
*University of Maryland, School of Medicine*
*Associate in Forensic Pathology*
*School of Hygiene and Public Health*
*The Johns Hopkins University*
*Lecturer in Forensic Pathology*
*The Johns Hopkins University, School of Medicine*
*Baltimore, Maryland*


*With a Foreword By*


**RAMSEY CLARK**

*Former Attorney General of the United States*



CHARLES C THOMAS • PUBLISHER

*Springfield • Illinois • U.S.A.*

*Published and Distributed Throughout the World by*

CHARLES C THOMAS • PUBLISHER
Bannerstone House
301-327 East Lawrence Avenue, Springfield, Illinois, U.S.A.



ISBN 0-398-03973-9

Library of Congress Catalog Card Number: 79-20544

*With THOMAS BOOKS careful attention is given to all details of manufacturing and design. It is the Publisher's desire to present books that are satisfactory as to their physical qualities and artistic possibilities and appropriate for their particular use. THOMAS BOOKS will be true to those laws of quality that assure a good name and good will.*

**Library of Congress Cataloging in Publication Data**

Spitz, Werner U.
Medicolegal investigation of death.

Bibliography: p.
Includes index.
1. Forensic pathology. 2. Death—Causes.
I. Fisher, Russell S., 1916- joint author.
II. Title. [DNLM: 1. Forensic medicine.
W800 M489]
RA1063.4.S64 1980 614'.19 79-20544
ISBN 0-398-03973-9

*Printed in the United States of America*
*C-1*

## CONTRIBUTORS


**LESTER ADELSON, M.D.**

*Pathologist and Chief Deputy Coroner, Cuyahoga County Coroner's Office*
*Professor of Forensic Pathology*
*Case Western Reserve University, School of Medicine*
*Cleveland, Ohio*

**MICHAEL M. BADEN, M.D.**

*Chief Medical Examiner, New York, New York*
*Associate Professor of Forensic Medicine*
*New York University School of Medicine*
*Visiting Professor of Pathology*
*Albert Einstein Medical School*
*Lecturer in Pathology*
*Columbia (P&S) School of Medicine*

**JAMES C. BEYER, M.D.**

*Deputy Chief Medical Examiner, Commonwealth of Virginia*
*Lecturer in Forensic Pathology*
*Medical College of Virginia*
*Arlington, Virginia*

**JOHN I. COE, M.D.**

*Medical Examiner Hennepin County*
*Minneapolis, Minnesota*
*Professor of Pathology, Medical School*
*University of Minnesota*

**WILLIAM F. ENOS, M.D.**

*Pathologist, Northern Virginia Doctors Hospital*
*Arlington, Virginia*
*Associate Clinical Professor of Pathology*
*George Washington University, Medical School*
*Designate, Forensic Pathology, Commonwealth of Virginia*
*Lecturer in Forensic Pathology, Medical College of Virginia*

**RUSSELL S. FISHER, M.D.**

*Chief Medical Examiner, State of Maryland*
*Clinical Professor of Forensic Pathology*
*University of Maryland, School of Medicine*
*Associate in Forensic Pathology*
*School of Hygiene and Public Health*
*The Johns Hopkins University*
*Lecturer in Forensic Pathology*
*The Johns Hopkins University, School of Medicine*
*Baltimore, Maryland*

**HENRY C. FREIMUTH, Ph.D.**

*Professor and Chairman, Department of Chemistry*
*Loyola College*
*Baltimore, Maryland*
*Adjunct Associate Professor of Pharmacology and Toxicology*
*University of Maryland, School of Pharmacy*
*Associate Instructor, Training School, Maryland State Police*
*Toxicologist, Retired, Office of the Chief Medical Examiner, State of Maryland*

**CHARLES S. HIRSCH, M.D.**

*Director of Forensic Pathology*
*Hamilton County*
*Institute of Forensic Medicine,*
*Toxicology and Criminalistics*
*Cincinnati, Ohio*
*Clinical Professor of Pathology (Forensic)*
*University of Cincinnati, College of Medicine,*
*Cincinnati, Ohio*

**RICHARD LINDENBERG, M.D.**

*Director of Neuropathology and Legal Medicine*
*Maryland State Department of Health and Mental Hygiene—Retired*

**JOSEPH R. MONFORTE, Ph.D.**

*Toxicologist, County of Wayne*
*Detroit, Michigan*
*Adjunct Assistant Professor, Departments of Pharmacology and Pathology*
*Wayne State University*
*Adjunct Professor of Chemistry*
*University of Windsor*
*Windsor, Ontario, Canada*

**JOHN E. SMIALEK, M.D.**

*Deputy Chief Medical Examiner, County of Wayne*
*Detroit, Michigan*
*Clinical Assistant Professor, Department of Pathology*
*Wayne State University, School of Medicine*

**IRVIN M. SOPHER, D.D.S., M.D.**

*Chief Medical Examiner, State of West Virginia*
*Clinical Professor of Pathology*
*West Virginia University, School of Medicine*
*Charleston, West Virginia*

**WERNER U. SPITZ, M.D.**

*Chief Medical Examiner, County of Wayne*
*Detroit, Michigan*
*Associate Professor of Pathology (Forensic Pathology)*
*Wayne State University, School of Medicine*
*Adjunct Professor of Chemistry*
*University of Windsor*
*Windsor, Ontario, Canada*

**CHARLES J. STAHL, III, M.D.**

*Captain, Medical Corps, United States Navy*
*Chairman, Department of Laboratory Medicine*
*National Naval Medical Center, Bethesda, Maryland*
*Consultant in Laboratory Medicine, Bureau of Medicine and Surgery*
*Department of the Navy, Washington, D.C.*
*Professor of Pathology, School of Medicine*
*Uniformed Services University of the Health Sciences*
*Bethesda, Maryland*
*Professor of Pathology*
*Georgetown University, School of Medicine*

**JAMES TUTHILL WESTON, M.D.**

*Medical Investigator, State of New Mexico*
*Professor of Pathology*
*University of New Mexico, School of Medicine*
*Albuquerque, New Mexico*

**RUSSELL M. WILHELM**

*Firearms Examiner, Maryland State Police*
*Sergeant, Retired, Baltimore City Police Department, Crime Laboratory*

# FOREWORD

"MORDRE WOL OUT," Chaucer's Prioress tells us. But those who work in homicide investigation, forensic pathology, and criminal law know better. The true manner of death which may have been murder is not determined in tens of thousands of cases annually in our violent land. The cost to the nation in truth, justice, health, and safety is enormous.

Had Hamlet put aside indecision, sentimentality, emotion, the wan grief spent on the skull of the jester of his youth "Alas, poor Yorick! I knew him, Horatio" and obtained an autopsy on his dead father, the King of Denmark, Shakespeare's play might have turned from tragical to historical. Surely, we now see how our failures can affect history itself. The violent death of a President will always cause the deepest fears and suspicions. There will always be the allegation of gunfire from a grassy knoll.

We can determine the truth, and medical science must play a major role. The coeditor of this important volume was one of four professionals I called on as Attorney General, to review the autopsy photos and x rays of our beloved President who looked "forward to the day when America would no longer be afraid of grace and beauty." In a time of profound doubt and international concern, with the highest integrity, self-discipline, and professional skill, Dr. Fisher contributed to those most reassuring phenomena, facts linked together pointing to truth.

How many men in America can qualify for such a task? That this is the first volume in twenty-five years dealing directly and effectively with the subject of medicolegal investigation of death tells us that our neglect here is enormous. The deaths of John F. Kennedy, Medgar Evers, Malcolm X, Martin Luther King, Jr., Robert Kennedy, and Whitney Young, Jr., show how our inadequacy can alter our destiny.

About 4:45 A.M., on December 4, 1969, two young Black Panthers, Fred Hampton and Mark Clark, were killed by gunfire in the city of Chicago. The shooting occurred during the course of a police raid on Panther headquarters. There followed an official inquest, a protest inquest, three autopsies, and three grand jury investigations. Each of the autopsies was performed under conditions in a manner or reported in a way that added to speculation over the real cause of death.

A community has been left in profound doubt as to the identity of the guns from which the bullets causing death were fired, even the direction of entry and number of shots. Were the deaths accidental? Were police justified in this use of deadly force? Were the dead murdered by the police? Was Fred Hampton drugged at the time of death? That over five thousand people attended his funeral indicates the impact of our failure to establish the truth. The resulting division in the community will affect the quality of life there and, through those who live there, elsewhere for a generation or more.

Perhaps many pathologists avoid medicolegal investigation of death because its contribution to life is not clear and the happy side of the docket is with the life savers. A study of such chapters as "Investigation of Deaths from Drug Abuse," "Forensic Aspects of Alcohol," and "Aircraft Crash Investigation" immediately demonstrates the great importance of this field in life saving and social problem solving. Indeed, few in the medical profession will be more involved in the action and passion of our times than those who seek to find and demonstrate these medical facts. We can foresee the risks of willful destruction of crowded airplanes and the meaning to mass urban technological society.

With a hundred new dangerous drugs to be created by chemical science in the next five years, with a youth culture in an age of anxiety approaching incoherence, with grossly inadequate preventive research, it often will be the autopsy that tells us of the new synthetic chemicals threatening life. With this knowledge, society can endeavor to cope with one of its most difficult problems.

There are few crueler injustices directly inflicted on an individual by government than conviction of a crime one did not commit. Important chapters such as "Sudden and Unexpected Death from Natural Causes in Adults," "Trauma and Disease," and "Injury by Gunfire" show us how easy it is to misjudge the cause of death where circumstances are suspicious. It is of the utmost importance to the individual, to society, to truth, justice, and safety that we find the facts concerning death.

Because of its pathos, we too often ignore the truths disclosed in Chapter XVIII, "Investigation of Deaths in Childhood—The Battered Child." How many of our most violent criminals were the subject of physical abuse as children? Forensic pathology can give us some indication. It is important that we know. The national attitude toward violent crime could be dramatically changed by this truth.

Few professions create greater despondency about the goodness of man and the worth of life than the practice of criminal law. Not many human documents are more pessimistic than Clarence Darrow's autobiography. Few activities tend to diminish an appreciation of life more than forensic pathology as generally practiced. Neither should be. The criminal lawyer seeks justice—the forensic pathologist, truth. Noble causes. If both will abandon rhetoric, ancient dogma and fictive contentions in favor of finding and presenting fact, which is the teaching of this text, their proper purposes will be fulfilled. Practitioners will then enjoy the satisfaction of helping people.

We must have the courage, indeed the ardent desire, to know the causes of death. We cannot let the *corpus delicti* diminish our capacity for joy. We should not faint at the photos here. They are true, and while all truth may not seem beauty, all truth can strengthen our humanity. Then, however irresolute, we will find the compassion like Hamlet to hold in our hands the skull of a beloved friend, look on it and say "Here hung those lips that I have kissed I know not how oft." The great and constant need of those who investigate homicide and practice forensic pathology or criminal law is a warm humanism. A people who will not face death cannot revere life.

But these are mere musings. Study this work.

RAMSEY CLARK
Former Attorney General
of the United States

Washington, D.C.
14 July 1972

# PREFACE TO THE SECOND EDITION

WHEN THE FIRST EDITION of this text was published in 1973, we intended that it would fill an existing void for an up-to-date account of the current state of knowledge of death investigation. The need for a second printing three years later supported our original belief that such a publication did indeed meet a demand. Rather than continue with a third printing, we felt that it would be appropriate at this time to undertake a complete revision of the text and to include new developments, including primarily a considerable volume of material that had been previously omitted.

Consequently, many additions and alterations were made to nearly all of the chapters. New sections on sudden infant death syndrome and chemical considerations associated with postmortem changes were included. A new chapter dealing with methodology and interpretation of toxicological procedures was added. Furthermore, a shortcoming of the previous edition was corrected by devoting space to preparation of a medicolegal autopsy report and formulation of a medicolegal opinion, as have been found to be advantageous in the author's own experience.

Significantly more space was allotted to illustrations. We were almost tempted to include color, but in the interest of lower cost, photographs were again limited to black and white, although the emphasis on quality was continued.

In conformity with the first edition, an attempt was made to maintain the practical character of the book, and where possible, technical terminology was avoided in the interest of easier understanding for a wider spectrum of readers.

It is the editors' pleasure to acknowledge the assistance received from so many colleagues, pathologists, police officers and attorneys, who contributed by their questions and suggestions. As previously, a great debt of gratitude is owed to Mrs. Hannelore Russell-Wood (Schmidt-Orndorff) for assistance with the editorial work, preparation of the index and collating of the entire typescript. Elaine Sacra, research assistant at the Wayne County Medical Examiner's Office, helped transform a raw manuscript into a coordinated text, and Nancy Whayne prepared additional drawings. Special thanks are due to our photographers, Lester Walter and Anna Faulkner, for hours of expert labor spent in providing illustrations for the new material in this edition.

WERNER U. SPITZ, M.D.
RUSSELL S. FISHER, M.D.

November, 1978

# PREFACE TO THE FIRST EDITION

WHENEVER A NEW TEXTBOOK is to be written three basic questions should be answered by the authors: Why, who needs it? Is it needed now? Why should the authors in question, rather than others, undertake the work?

In the last thirty years there has been increasing sophistication in the training of police officers assigned to homicide investigation. To a significant degree this has been due to the philosophy developed at the Harvard Medical School in the late 1940s of teaching homicide investigators the nature of the medical aspects of injuries. This has led to the development of a sizeable corps of highly expert individuals in this field. The need for this type of information has also been greatly emphasized by the fact that throughout a large part of the United States the medical investigation of death at the scene is woefully inadequate, conducted by untrained and unskilled coroners who are frequently nonphysicians. No new textbook oriented to the homicide investigator or the novice forensic pathologist has appeared in the last two and one-half decades. It is our aim to meet the need by presenting, in readable style, an authoritative text embracing all aspects of the pathology of trauma as it is witnessed daily by law enforcement officers, interpreted by pathologists of varying experience in forensic pathology and finally used by attorneys involved in the prosecution and defense in criminal cases, as well as by those engaged in civil litigation.

Since the text is addressed to a wide range of professional disciplines, some of the chapters are inevitably directed more towards readers with medical backgrounds, whereas others are suited for general understanding. Nevertheless, the large number of illustrations and diagrams will, we hope, render the text comprehensible to all who are interested in the interpretation of forensic pathologic findings.

As it has been noted above, no up-to-date textbook covering the material contained herein is currently available. While working in the Maryland Medical Examiner's Office and its partner in teaching and research, the Maryland Medical-Legal Foundation, we have accumulated a large volume of material upon which to base the text. This material and experience also serve to answer the question: Why us? We have been concerned not only with the day-to-day investigation of sudden and violent deaths in a statewide medical examiner's system but also with teaching in medical and law schools in Baltimore and elsewhere throughout the country as well as with training of young pathologists who wish to become expert in the field. Furthermore, we have been conducting the *Frances G. Lee Seminars in Homicide Investigation* for state and other police officers for many years. It is our hope that our experiences and those of our coauthors will make a significant contribution to the improvement of the investigation of sudden and violent death, the prosecution and defense of those related to such events, and the protection of the public welfare.

W.U.S.
R.S.F.

## ACKNOWLEDGMENTS TO THE FIRST EDITION

THE IDEA OF COMPILING a book such as this was not new to us. We had been toying with this thought many times in the past. However, by insisting on the need for such a book and by impulsively establishing contact with the publishers, Col. James T. McGuire, Superintendent of the Illinois State Police, gave us the necessary impetus to go ahead with our plan. To him goes our appreciation for his insight and understanding of the need for dissemination of experience in the pathology of trauma among law enforcement personnel to help ensure a better administration of justice.

Our thanks to all those who have contributed to this book with their knowledge and experience, and who have thereby helped us make this endeavor possible.

Finally, our sincere gratitude to Hannelore Schmidt-Orndorff for her able assistance with the editorial work. Her continuous drive and suggestions have helped immensely in the task of preparing the manuscript from its inception.

The editors also wish to acknowledge the cooperation of the photographers of the Medical Examiner's Office in Baltimore—Walter C. Carden and M. Gibson Porter—for the preparation of the illustrations of the chapters contributed by the editors as well as Chapters IV, XVII, and XXI.

W.U.S.
R.S.F.

# CONTENTS

"In fine, nothing is said now
that has not been said before."

TERENCE (185-159 B.C.)

# MEDICOLEGAL INVESTIGATION OF DEATH

*Chapter I*

# HISTORY OF FORENSIC PATHOLOGY AND RELATED LABORATORY SCIENCES

RUSSELL S. FISHER

## FORENSIC SCIENCES IN ANTIQUITY

THE EARLIEST APPLICATION of forensic medicine had to do with the interdiction against suicide, which has been regarded as a crime against the public interest since before the birth of Christ. It appears that this was largely due to the fact that occasional communities, even in those days, sustained epidemics of suicides. It is probably also rooted in the primitive belief that the individual who took his own life was possessed by evil spirits and might pass them on to other members of his community. Anthropologists have reported a similar phenomenon in more modern days in certain relatively uncivilized African tribes, where the hut belonging to the victim of a suicide is burned to the ground and his family expelled from the village. It is recorded that suicide was strongly condemned in ancient Greece because the individual was regarded as a servant of the gods and self-destruction constituted an act of rebellion against the gods. It was accepted in certain instances, however, where the community had condemned an individual, as in the case of Socrates, who in turn committed suicide by drinking hemlock. A medicolegal opinion as to manner of death had to be reached in such cases in order that a decision could be rendered as to whether the penalty—usually consisting of denial of the funeral rights to those who had offended against religion—should be inflicted. In the same way, in ancient Rome, soldiers who committed suicide were treated as deserters, and criminals who committed suicide in order to escape punishment were likewise condemned.

In the tenth century suicide became a crime under the common law in England, and in 1184 the Council of Nimes made the condemnation of suicide part of the canon law of the Roman Catholic Church. The decisions as to manner of death seem to have been made mostly by an investigation of the circumstances without specific examination of the body, although historians have reported that Antistius, a physician in Rome, examined the body of Julius Caesar and reached the opinion that, of the twenty-three wounds Caesar sustained, the only mortal wound was one in the chest.[1]

In China a handbook entitled *Hsi Yuan Lu* was published in about 1250.[1] It contained guidelines for the postmortem examination of bodies, including descriptions of various wounds caused by sharp versus blunt instruments. It also offered comments on the determination of whether an individual found in the water had died of drowning or had been killed beforehand and of whether a burned individual was dead before the onset of the fire.

## THE EARLY DEVELOPMENT OF THE AUTOPSY IN FORENSIC INVESTIGATIONS IN EUROPE

The written records of the development of forensic pathology in Europe begin in 1507, when a volume subsequently known as the Bamberg Code appeared. Twenty-three years later, a more extensive penal code, known as the Constitutio Criminalis Carolina, was issued by Emperor Charles V for all the lands included in his empire. The two documents portrayed the importance of forensic pathology in requiring that medical testimony be an integral part of the proof and trials involving decisions about whether the manner of death was infanticide, homicide, abortion or poisoning. They apparently did not specify that complete autopsies were to be performed, but wounds were opened to determine their depth and direction. Thus it appears that some degree of skilled medical knowledge was required of the expert witness. Meanwhile, Andreas Vesalius, the first of the pioneers in anatomy, was dissecting cadavers and for the first time established the true facts of the anatomy of the body.

In the latter half of the sixteenth century Ambrose Paré performed official medicolegal autopsies. He reported the findings in lungs of smothered children and studied the traces left by sexual assault.[2] Fidelis and Zacchia in Italy, in the early seventeenth century, were likewise engaged in anatomical dissections and reported analyses of injuries to internal organs. Fidelis described the findings in drowned bodies that would distinguish between homicidal and accidental drowning. Zacchia's work included descriptions of bullet and stab wounds, findings in asphyxial deaths, the distinction of suicide from homicide, the differentiation of sudden death from natural causes and, in cases of infanticide, the determination of whether an infant had been born alive.

The first formal lectures in forensic pathology were held by Michaelis and Bohn at the University of Leipzig, where students were apparently instructed in the subject of violent death and simulated natural deaths. As a result of advancement of knowledge by these pioneers, the judicial authorities and the police in Europe soon began to call upon physicians to aid in the solution of fatal crimes, and most of the larger jurisdictions developed centers, commonly known as institutes of forensic medicine, where experts carried out their investigations. There was little of scene investigations by these physicians, since this chore rested principally with the police, but in instances where bodies were found in trunks or in the water it was not uncommon for the medical investigator to examine the associated evidence. Indeed, it was in this context that the recognition of the medicolegal importance of bloodstains first developed.

## THE CORONER SYSTEM IN ENGLAND

The historical developments of medicolegal investigation in America can be clearly traced back to the English coroner system, which had developed in that country some 600 years before. The *Charts of Privileges* mentioned in English historical sources include a grant of the coroner's office by King Athelstane to an English noble, identified as St. John of Beverly, in the year 925.[3] Over 200 years later, the office of the coroner is formally described when in September, 1194, the justices in eyre were required to provide that three knights and one clerk were elected in every county as *keepers of the pleas of the crown.* The appointment then included the coroner's duties. The term *coroner* is obviously a corruption of *crowner* applied to the individual charged under this law. The justices in eyre, who were apparently comparable to the travelling circuit court judges of modern day, could order the coroner to perform duties of administrative or inquisitorial nature within the region for which he had been appointed. These duties were carried out either alone or with the sheriff, but certain of them were earmarked specifically for the coroner's office, and he could perform them without being ordered to do so. Among these were holding of inquests over dead bodies and *appeals* (inspection of an individual's wounds, recording the accusation against another individual and, if the wounds appear likely to be fatal, arresting the accused individual). The coroner was also authorized by the county courts to attach or arrest witnesses or suspects and to appraise and safeguard any lands or goods that might later be forfeited by reason of guilt of the accused. Despite these descriptions of his duties, it appears that they were loosely drawn, and the coroner became concerned only with felonies that resulted in homicide or suicide or when a felony resulted in a crown plea requiring enforcement. An interesting example of the latter is *outlawry,* where, if the accused still absented himself after public demand had been made for him to appear and surrender to justice on four occasions, the justices in eyre would declare him an outlaw. Thereupon his goods and chattels were forfeited to the crown and his head could be cut off with impunity by anyone. In fact under Richard I, who reigned from 1189 to 1199, a price was paid for an outlaw's head. Blackstone has written an appropriate brief paragraph describing the coroner's duties at the time Edward I became King in 1272:

> The office and power of a Coroner are also like those of a Sheriff, either judicial or ministerial, but principally judicial . . . And consists, first, in inquiring, when any person is slain or dies suddenly, or in prison, concerning the manner of his death. And this must be upon sight of the body; for if the body be not found, the coroner cannot sit. He must also sit at the very place where death happened, and the inquiry must be made by a jury from 4, 5, or 6 of the neighboring towns over which he is to preside. If any be found guilty by this inquest of murder or other homicide, the coroner is to commit them to prison for further trial and must certify the whole of his inquisition, together with the evidence thereon, to the Court of King's Bench, or the next assizes.[4]

The sheriff had meanwhile achieved a position of honor in the community within the English judicial order. The appointments were made by the justices in eyre and were generally limited to those who had sufficiently elevated posture and considerable wealth in the community, largely in order to guarantee the financial responsibility of the sheriff. The coroner was occasionally given the authority to arrest the sheriff. He did not, however, have major responsibility for collection of the revenues in the counties in the name of the King after the twelfth century. Other than the relegation of the function of death investigation to the coroner with loss of essentially all other duties, there was little development of the coroner system in England until the middle of the nineteenth century. In 1860 the fee system was abolished and salaries were established for the county coroners. In 1877 a law was enacted requiring the inquest to be conducted whenever the coroner had reasonable cause to suspect violent or unnatural death or when the cause of death was unknown. This had the effect of granting the coroner the widest authority to investigate cases and was indeed in sharp contrast to the continental system, where investigations were commenced only by the prosecutors or police officials. Thus, the coroner system developed as a broad-spectrum investigative agency concerned with a large proportion of all deaths, including many nonviolent deaths. In 1888 the election of the coroners by freeholders was abolished and an appointee system developed under which the head of the local governmental unit appointed the coroner. There remained, however, no minimum qualifications for office. These were established in 1926, when a law was enacted requiring five years experience as a medical practitioner, barrister or solicitor if the individual was to qualify as coroner. Interestingly enough, in Northern Ireland similar legislation excluded doctors from holding the position of coroner unless they were also lawyers.

The impact of the development of institutes of forensic medicine on the continent was felt in England, and as early as 1789 Andrew Duncan, who was professor of physiology at the University of Edinburgh, began giving lectures in legal medicine and public health. In 1807 there was established at the University of Edinburgh the first chair of legal medicine in the English-speaking world. It was occupied by Andrew Duncan, Jr., for thirteen years before he moved over to the professorship of materia medica. The succession of professors to this revered chair included T. S. Traill, Douglas Maclagan, Sir Henry Littlejohn, his son Henry Harvey Littlejohn and, in the early part of the present century, Sir Sidney Smith, who served until his retirement in 1953. Other chairs of legal medicine developed in the University of Aberdeen and in England as a professorship of medical jurisprudence at Guy's Hospital Medical School in 1834. The professors of legal medicine were responsible for a series of textbooks that established legal medicine and pathology as an independent scientific pursuit. Among the more famous were those edited by Traill, Sir Sidney Smith, Douglas Kerr, father and son John Glaister, who between them held the chair of legal medicine at Glasgow for sixty-five years, and Alfred Swain Taylor, whose work *The Principles and Practice of Medical Jurisprudence* published in 1836 remains a standard textbook in many areas, even to the present day. After the beginning of the twentieth century the British Association in Forensic Medicine was established. Under their guidance new chairs of forensic medicine have been established in London, and forensic psychiatry has become an organized discipline.

In the meantime the development of good medicolegal practice came about more or less unrelated to the medical school teaching of the subject. Scotland Yard had developed into an important police investigative agency, and the coroners were accustomed to calling upon Scotland Yard to assist in their investigations. Since these included principally investigations of death, the detectives of Scotland Yard soon found themselves in need of assistance from pathologists and toxicologists and so appointed experts in these fields with the title of home office pathologist or home office analyst. The most famous medicolegal cases in England during the first quarter of the present century were indeed solved not by the professors of jurisprudence or forensic medicine but by the home office pathologists, including A. P. Luff, William Willcox and Joseph Pepper. Pepper came to the field by way of an appointment as senior pathologist at St. Mary's Hospital in London. After resigning from this position, he remained as home office pathologist, and in 1910, with the assistance of his pupil Spilsbury and the toxicologists Willcox and Luff, he brought together the many loose ends that led to the apprehension and trial of Hawley Crippen for the hyoscine murder of his wife. The body of Cora Crippen had been dissected after her death and all identifying elements removed before it was buried under the floor of the cellar in his house.

This case is of great significance because it probably represents the most important single investigation that influenced public opinion in support of forensic pathology. Until then it had been regarded with considerable disaffection, since it involved the autopsy and dependence upon science rather than detection by the lay investigators. In recent years home office pathologists have to some extent brought the two activities together. Well known in this group are Francis Camps, Keith Simpson, Donald Tear and Keith Mant, who are all vitally concerned with investigation of coroner's cases while at the same time engaged in teaching and research in the London medical school complexes.

## THE ESTABLISHMENT OF FORENSIC PATHOLOGY IN AMERICA

The early American colonists, originating in England, brought the coroner system with them in essentially the state of development it had reached by the early 1600s. Thus, there is a record of a coroner's inquest in the colony of New Plymouth, New England, in 1635; briefly, the inquiry found that John Deacon died as a result of bodily weakness caused by fasting and extreme cold.

The governor of Maryland, Leonard Calvert, appointed Thomas Baldridge of St. Mary's to be sheriff and coroner on January 29, 1637, and authorized him to, "Doe all and everything . . . the office of sheriff and coroner of any county in England doe. . . ."[5] Baldridge was soon hard at work, because on January 31, 1637, he impaneled a jury of twelve men to hold an inquest over the body of one John Bryant. Their verdict was, "John Bryant by the fall of a tree had his bloud bulke broken; and hath two scratches under his chinne on the left side; and so that by means of the fall of the said tree upon him the said John Bryant came to his death."[6] This coroner's office was one and the same as the sheriff's office, and while it did not carry any fixed stipend, it provided a substantial income because the sheriff was responsible for the collection of property taxes, poll taxes and other levies, and he usually received 10 percent of his collections. The early definition of the coroner's duties is also recorded in the Archives of Maryland, preserved by the Maryland Historical Society,[5] whereby on April 30, 1640, the governor appointed John Robinson, high constable, as coroner for St. Clements Hundred in St. Mary's County. The definition of duties included—

Upon notice or suspicion of any person that hath or shall come to his or her death entirely within the limits of that hundred to warn as many inhabitants of the said hundred as you conveniently may to view the dead body and to charge the said persons with an oath truly to inquire and true verdict to grant how the person viewed came upon his or her death according to the evidence. . . .

Autopsy examinations of bodies are recorded in Massachusetts as early as 1647, when the General Court of Massachusetts Bay concerned with the teaching of medical students authorized that "an autopsy should be made on the body of a criminal once in four years." The medicolegal application of the autopsy is recorded in Maryland on March 21, 1665, when a Mr. Francis Carpenter was brought before the Talbot County Court on suspicion of murdering one Samuell Yeoungman, a servant of his. The coroner's report absolved Mr. Carpenter, saying—

Wee of the Jury haueing viewed the Corps of Samuell Yeoungman and finding A Depression in the Cranenum in on [one] place, and another wound where all the muscle flesh was Corrupted, and withall finding Corrupt blood betweene the Dura and Piamater, and the braine and several other bruises in the head and body therefore our verdict in that for want of Looking after the abouesaid wounds, were the Cause of his death.[7]

The record does not reveal whether Mr. Carpenter may have inflicted the original wounds on the deceased's head.

The earliest teaching of jurisprudence in America would appear to have been accomplished by Benjamin Rush of Philadelphia, who included in his sixteen introductory lectures one under the title of *On the Study of Medical Jurisprudence.* He is certainly better known for his influence on the founding of medical education in Philadelphia and for membership in the Provincial Congress of 1776, whereby he was one of the signers of the Declaration of Independence in the following year. In view of twentieth-century developments it is interesting to note that as early as 1792 he wrote an article opposing capital punishment.

Perhaps the earliest formal mention of the physician in connection with the work of the coroner was in 1860 in Maryland, where the Code of Public General Laws authorized the coroner or his jury to require the attendance of a physician in cases of violent death. The choice of the physician was left to the coroner. Eight years later the legislature authorized the governor to appoint a physician as sole coroner of the city of Baltimore. In Boston in 1877 the Commonwealth adopted a statewide system requiring that the coroner be supplanted by a physician known as a medical examiner. Unfortunately, the jursisdiction of the medical examiner was confined to "dead bodies of such persons only as are supposed to have come to their death by violence."

The entry of the science of pathology as a subspecialty of medicine into the investigation of deaths began in the latter part of the nineteenth century. In 1890 in Baltimore a city ordinance authorized the Board of Health to appoint two physicians with the titles of medical examiner and assign them the duty of performing all autopsies requested by the coroner or the state's attorney of the city of Baltimore. In 1915 New York City adopted a law eliminating the coroner's office and creating a medical examiner system, authorizing investigation of deaths resulting from criminal violence, casualties or suicide, or suddenly while in apparent health, or when not attended by a physician or imprisoned or in any suspicious or unusual manner. The medical examiner was granted the authority to make a decision as to the necessity of an autopsy, and his appointment from a civil service list by the mayor provided the first civil service appointment in the annals of American medicolegal investigation. The first chief medical examiner, Dr. Charles Norris, was also given the authority to order an autopsy when in his judgement it was necessary, thus establishing the first essentials of a competent medical examiner's system, i.e. a broad spectrum of cases to be investigated and the authority to autopsy when the public interest demanded it. Further strides in the development of the New York City medical examiner's office occurred when Dr. Milton Helpern, the third chief medical examiner (Fig. I-1), convinced the city to construct the modern facility that today houses both the medical examiner's office and the institute of forensic medicine. The institute, which is the teaching arm of the New York University in that discipline, was renamed in honor of Dr. Helpern in November, 1977. This same office also justly claims to represent the cradle of forensic toxicology in North America, since it was here that Dr. Alexander Gettler firmly established the laboratory arm of the medical examiner as an integral part of the system. It should be noted that the early Massachusetts law that established the medical examiner system in name did not allow the medical examiner to perform autopsies but reserved this authority to the district attorney. It was not until 1945 that the Massachusetts law was amended to make performance of autopsies discretionary with the medical examiner. The Massachusetts system further lacked cohesion in that each medical examiner was appointed for his own district and no central facilities for the performance of toxicology or other specialized procedures were provided, such as those established in New York City when that office was created.

The latter part of the nineteenth century witnessed the emergence of the science of pathology as a subspecialty of medicine at the same time as related fields of the forensic sciences began to develop. During this period the first scientific system of identication was devised by Bertillon, and his anthropometric system was accepted until the early 1900s as the most accurate method of criminal identification. Bertillonage, as the system was known, was replaced, however, by fingerprint techniques, developed by Galton in 1892. In 1915 a simple procedure for determining the blood group of a dried blood stain was developed by Dr. Leone Lattes in Italy. In 1920 Albert Osborne published the first authoritative text on questioned documents examination.

These, as well as other scientific specialties such as chemistry, physics, biology and microscopy, developed separately, although the noted German jurist Hans Gross had published a textbook in 1893 detailing the application of information derived from these separate fields to criminal investigation. However, it was not until 1910, when Edmond Locard established the first crime laboratory in Lyon, France, that these specialties were brought together for the sole purpose of criminal investigation. The success of Locard's laboratory led to the formation of similar laboratories in different parts of Europe, and in 1923 the first complete crime laboratory in the United States was established in Los Angeles. In 1932 a laboratory organized within the Federal Bureau of Investigation made forensic sciences available on a nationwide basis for the first time in the United States. This labora-

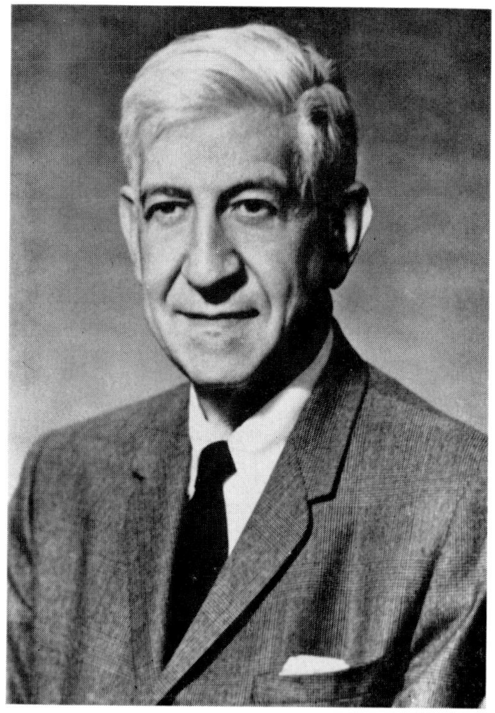

FIGURE I-1. Dr. Milton Helpern (1902-1977), New York City's third chief medical examiner, developed the institute of forensic medicine in New York City.

tory has served as the model for the formation and organization of forensic laboratories at local, state and national levels throughout the world.

In the modern, well-equipped forensic laboratory, experts from the fields of serology and immunology, ballistics, questioned documents, fingerprinting, polygraphy, analytical chemistry and geology work together for the purpose of scientific criminal investigation. Many laboratories have a toxicology unit, although in most instances toxicologists are more efficiently employed in medical examiners' or coroners' offices. In the past decade many of the sophisticated analytical techniques and instrumentation developed primarily for medicine and industry have been incorporated into forensic laboratories. Instrumentation such as gas-liquid chromatography, infrared spectroscopy, nuclear magnetic resonance and mass spectroscopy have found their fullest application in criminal investigation.

The first statewide medical examiner system was established in Maryland in 1939 and covered all but one county of the state, which came under the system two years later. This legislation is noteworthy because it adopted the New York system of investigating a broad spectrum of cases and provided for discretionary autopsies by the medical examiners. Additionally, it established centralized direction of the activities of the various deputy medical examiners in the counties, provided expert assistance in the conduct of autopsies by the chief medical examiner and his staff and made available the necessary toxicologic analyses. It established a unique method of appointment of the full-time medical examiner by a commission consisting of the professors of pathology in the two medical schools, the executive officer of the State and Baltimore City Health Departments and the superintendent of the State Police. The genesis of this type of appointment was obviously the recognition of the importance of removing the medical examiners' appointments from the political greenbag of appointments by local politicians or the governor. By thus removing the office from the political hierarchy, it set the stage for the attraction of career forensic pathologists to the positions. The commission appoints the full-time medical examiners, toxicologists and other staff members and in addition appoints deputy medical examiners in the various counties selected from a list submitted by the local medical societies. Again, the choice of this method of election was more than fortuitous. Placement of the responsibility for selection of county deputy medical examiners on the medical societies of the counties has produced, through the years, selection of men esteemed by their colleagues as discreet and competent physicians.

The teaching of forensic pathology as a subspecialty of pathology began in 1937 when Harvard Medical School established the George Burgess McGrath chair of legal medicine and appointed Dr. Alan Moritz as its first professor. With the support of the Rockefeller Foundation, Dr. Moritz established residency-type training appointments for young pathologists aiming at a career in the field. Also established was a series of seminars in which selected state police and other criminal investigators were invited to share a week of instructional activities to learn about the application of pathology and medical science to the investigation of homicide. These were begun in 1945 and were continued by the department of legal medicine until Harvard, for reasons of economy, closed the department in 1967. The seminars, entitled *The Francis G. Lee Seminars in Homicide Investigation,* have been continued under the auspices of the medical examiner's office in Maryland in conjunction with the Maryland Medical-Legal Foundation and the Department of Pathology of the University of Maryland Medical School. Numerous similar seminars have been devised in such other centers as Detroit, Richmond, Oklahoma City, Cincinnati and elsewhere. In many of the latter the instruction is aimed at physicians and attorneys as well as at police officers. The title of the original seminar owes its existence to the deep interest of Mrs. Francis Glessner Lee in the instruction of medical material to homicide

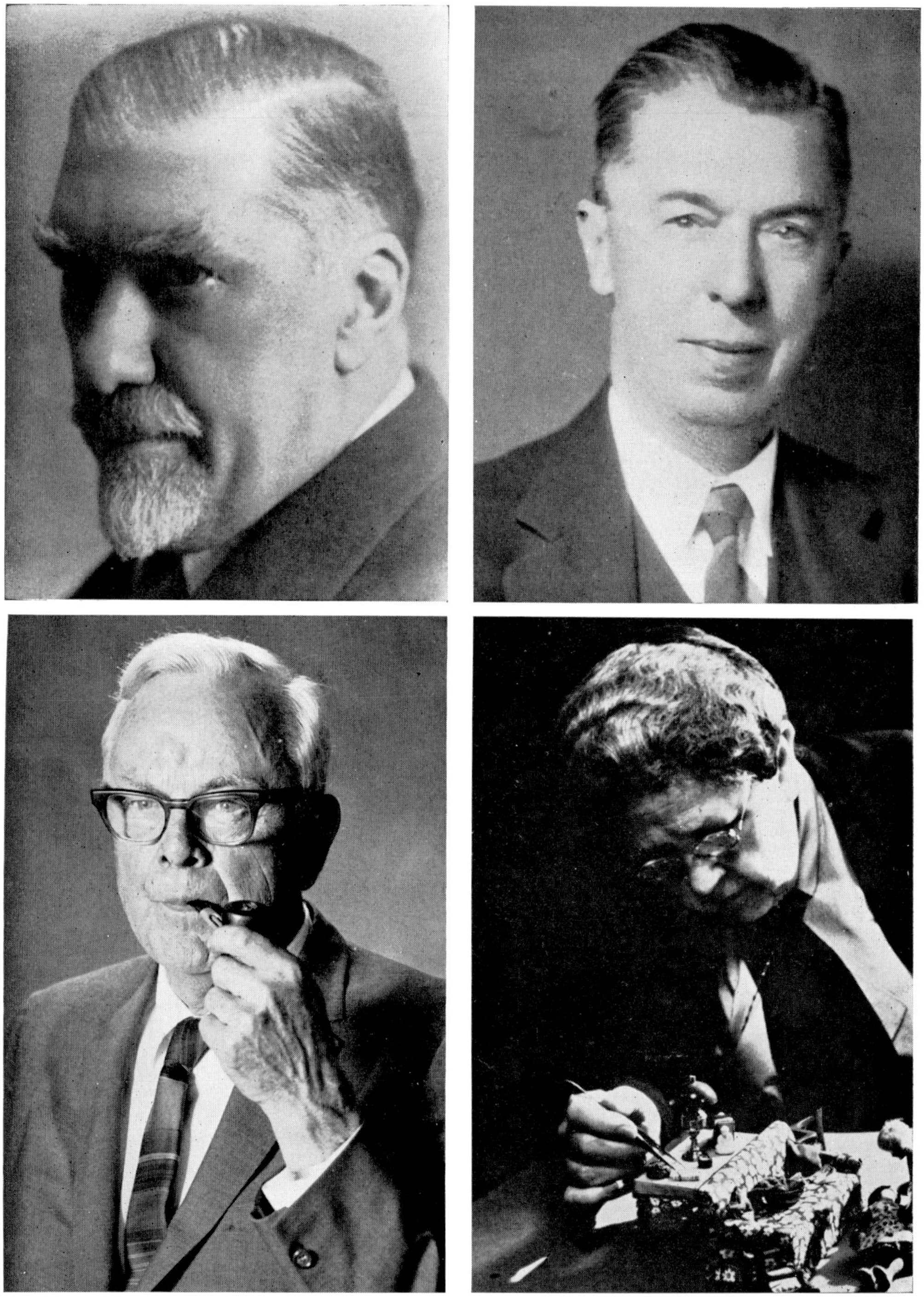

FIGURE I-2. Leaders in the development and teaching of forensic pathology in America. a: Dr. Charles Norris, the first chief medical examiner of New York City. (Courtesy Sam Shere, *Life,* © Time, Inc.) b: Dr. Alexander Gettler, first chief toxicologist of the New York City medical examiner's office. c: Dr. Alan Moritz, George Burgess McGrath Professor of Legal Medicine, at Harvard Medical School. d: Mrs. Frances G. Lee, founder of the Lee Seminars in Legal Medicine and the foremost promoter of teaching police the essentials of the medical aspects of homicide investigation.

investigators. She expressed this interest not only in assisting in the organization of the seminars but in support of the Department of Legal Medicine at Harvard from its inception until her death in 1963 (Fig. I-2).

Meanwhile, a number of large cities, the District of Columbia, as well as twenty states have amended their antiquated coroner's laws or adopted legislation providing for a medical examiner system. Several of these are in the position of having adopted enabling legislation, but due to the shortage of forensic pathologists or the failure of the legislature to provide funding, implementation of the revised coroner's laws is yet to be accomplished. In twenty-one other states either there are coroner's and medical examiner's systems in coexistence or legislation requires that the individual carrying out medicolegal investigations shall be a physician or otherwise have special knowledge or ability of the matters coming under his purview. In the remaining nine states there are no such requirements, and the individual responsible for the investigation of death is still the coroner or justice of the peace—generally an elected official whose principal qualification for the job is the ability to win the election.[8]

## REFERENCES

1. Camps, F. E. (Ed.): *Gradwohl's Legal Medicine,* 2nd ed. Baltimore, Williams & Wilkins, 1968.
2. Thorwald, J.: *The Century of the Detective.* New York, Har Brace World, 1965.
3. Wilson, E. F., and Fisher, R. S.: The medical examiner system in Maryland. *Md State Med J, 17:*51 (December), 1968.
4. Latrobe, J. H. B.: *Justices' Practice Under the Laws of Maryland,* 6th ed. Baltimore, Lucas, 1861.
5. Browne, W. H. (Ed.): *Archives of Maryland,* Vol. 3. Baltimore, Maryland Historical Society, 1885.
6. Browne, W. H. (Ed.): *Archives of Maryland,* Vol 4. Baltimore, Maryland Historical Society, 1887.
7. Pleasants, J. H. (Ed.): *Archives of Maryland,* Vol. 54. Baltimore, Maryland Historical Society, 1937.
8. Kornblum, R. N., and Fisher, R. S.: *A Compendium of State Medico-Legal Investigative Systems.* Baltimore, Maryland Medical-Legal Foundation, May 1972.

*Chapter II*

# TIME OF DEATH AND CHANGES AFTER DEATH

*Part 1*

## ANATOMICAL CONSIDERATIONS

RUSSELL S. FISHER

### DEFINITION OF DEATH

THE DETERMINATION of death created little or no problem through the centuries until the 1960s, when the advent of human organ transplantation caused minute scrutiny to be directed at the phenomenon of death itself. Black's Law Dictionary defines death as "The cessation of life; the ceasing to exist; defined by physicians as a total stoppage of the circulation of the blood, and a cessation of the animal and vital functions consequent thereupon, such as respiration, pulsation, etc." Two modern court decisions involving the definition of death depended on this definition. In Thomas *v.* Anderson a California District Court of Appeals in 1950, in ruling on the issue as to which of two persons died first, said, "In the instant case the question as to which of the two men died first was a question of fact for the determination of the trial court." They further said, "death occurs precisely when life ceases and does not occur until the heart stops beating and respiration ends. Death is not a continuous event and is an event that takes place at a precise time."[1] The other case, known as Smith *v.* Smith, was decided by the Supreme Court of Arkansas.[2] It involved a husband and wife fatally injured in an automobile accident. The husband was dead at the scene; the wife was taken to the hospital, where she remained unconscious. The allegation was put forth that she remained in coma due to brain injury; she died at the hospital seventeen days later. The petitioner argued that the deaths were simultaneous, since there was no evidence of brain activity after the accident and the physicians, although maintaining efforts to resuscitate the patient, were unsuccessful. The inference was that the resuscitative efforts were maintaining the body in a state of animation, although it could not be shown that life existed. The court dismissed this petition as a matter of law, stating that the contention according to which the wife lost her power to will at the same instant as the husband, and that her demise occurred at the same time since she never regained consciousness, was unacceptable. They requoted Black's definition and, obviously having reference to the fact that she did continue spontaneous heart action and/or respiration, simply ruled that the conditions of that definition did not exist and further stated, "Likewise we take judicial notice that one breathing, though unconscious, is not dead."

Heart transplantation, however, brought medical, ethical and legal questions into critical focus, most specifically with respect to the determination of death. The ability of medical science to maintain respiration and cardiac function for prolonged periods after the loss of all spontaneous electrical activity of the brain, spontaneous respiration or cardiac contraction has added to the difficulty of defining the point of death. The contention that death has occurred when all cerebral function has ceased and is irreversibly stopped has led to the definition of cerebral death. The criteria usually accepted in this context are (a) bilateral dilatation and fixation of the pupils, (b) the absence of all reflexes, (c) cessation of respiration without mechanical assistance, (d) cessation of spontaneous cardiac action, (e) a completely flat brain wave tracing (in the absence of barbiturate or other strong sedative effect). When all these and other related criteria, as adopted by the individual transplant teams, can be reliably shown to have existed for a period of some hours, it is customary to decide that the individual is indeed dead. If transplantation permission has been obtained, they should proceed to ready the recipient and, when all is in order, discontinue the mechanical resuscitation and cardiac activation, whereupon cessation of these vital functions occurs instantly and the person is pronounced dead.

Still another definition of death must be added to the extent that even though the person is dead, the individual muscle fibers and other cells may continue to live for a variable period of time—up to many hours. This can be readily shown by removing muscle fibers from experimental animals and stimulating the isolated fiber with electrical current. The fiber contracts just as in life. Because of this phenomenon, death of the individual as a whole has come to be known as *somatic death,* while the ultimate death of all cellular elements is similarly described as *cellular death.*

## PRONOUNCEMENT OF DEATH

In most states, although the law requires the physician last in attendance or the coroner/medical examiner to certify the cause of death, there is no statutory requirement that actual pronouncement of death be made by a member of the medical profession. Indeed, it is common practice in properly operated hospitals, nursing homes, etc., for a competent nurse to pronounce death and notify the attending physician, who may or may not choose to examine the body immediately, if at all, even though he will carry out his legal duty of furnishing a death certificate. The same philosophy is accepted in many jurisdictions whereby an ambulance attendant or police official may determine the death of an individual. This may be simply evidenced by the ambulance team deciding that it is no longer useful to render first aid or to remove the individual to a medical facility, or it may be met more squarely by the police officer in charge ordering the body not to be moved until the medical examiner or coroner reaches the scene and the homicide squad can begin their work. Obviously, one does not make such decisions lightly, and whenever there is doubt, proper resuscitative methods should be adopted.

In most cases the evidence of death is presumptive. In the immediate period after death the absence of heartbeat as noted on palpation and on listening to the heart, the absence of respiration by careful examination of the exposed chest and abdomen and such procedures as holding a cold mirror in front of the nose to detect expiration of moist air all have a respected place in the determination of death. Examination of the individual in the presence of adequate lighting is essential. If cessation of respiration is the result of electrical shock, resuscitation including both cardiac and respiratory support should be instituted immediately. These should be maintained until definite signs of death are evident. In some jurisdictions it is still mandatory that in such cases resuscitative measures be continued until livor mortis becomes manifest.

The same would be true in situations where a body is removed from the water after brief submersion. There is no absolute number of minutes as to the certainty of death after cessation of respiration. The nearest common denominator in this area is three to five minutes. Exception to such rule would be evident in situations where the body has been subjected to extreme cold, where all vital functions are retarded and the body can sustain relatively long periods of deprivation of oxygen without the occurrence of somatic death. In a case reported by Kvittingen and Naess[3] a five-year-old boy fell into a partly frozen river and recovered fully following a presumed submersion time of twenty-two minutes.

## POSTMORTEM EVENTS

### Rigidity

Immediately after death changes begin to occur in the body. Since most of these are chemical in nature and therefore are governed by the rules that govern all chemical reactions, or physical in nature and therefore are phenomena that ordinarily proceed at standard rates, it is useful to consider the various applications of the rate method to the estimation of the time of death. Rigor mortis is such a condition in which the muscles of the body become hardened as a result of chemical changes within the muscle fibers. The process is due to the appearance of lactic acid and other by-products of tissue metabolism. As the acid products accumulate in the muscle fibers, the protoplasm, which is in liquid state in life, becomes sufficiently acid that it gels, making the muscle rigid. The process begins at death, usually becomes manifest within two to four hours and advances until approximately twelve hours, when it is generally complete (Figs. II-1 and II-2). It is commonly said to begin in the muscles of the face and neck and then spread downwards over the body. This is not literally true, but the appearance of such a progression results from the fact that the shorter muscle fibers, as in the jaw and neck, develop rigidity sooner than the longer extremity muscle fibers. We do not find the sequence particularly useful in estimating the postmortem interval.

Fully developed rigor mortis persists for a variable period and then slowly disappears, with softening of the muscles occurring once again, so that the extremities, though rigid during the persistence of rigor, are again readily flexible. The time of persistence of rigidity is greatly influenced by the temperature of the body and its environment. It may disappear as soon as nine to twelve hours after death if the body is in an extremely hot environment and decomposi-

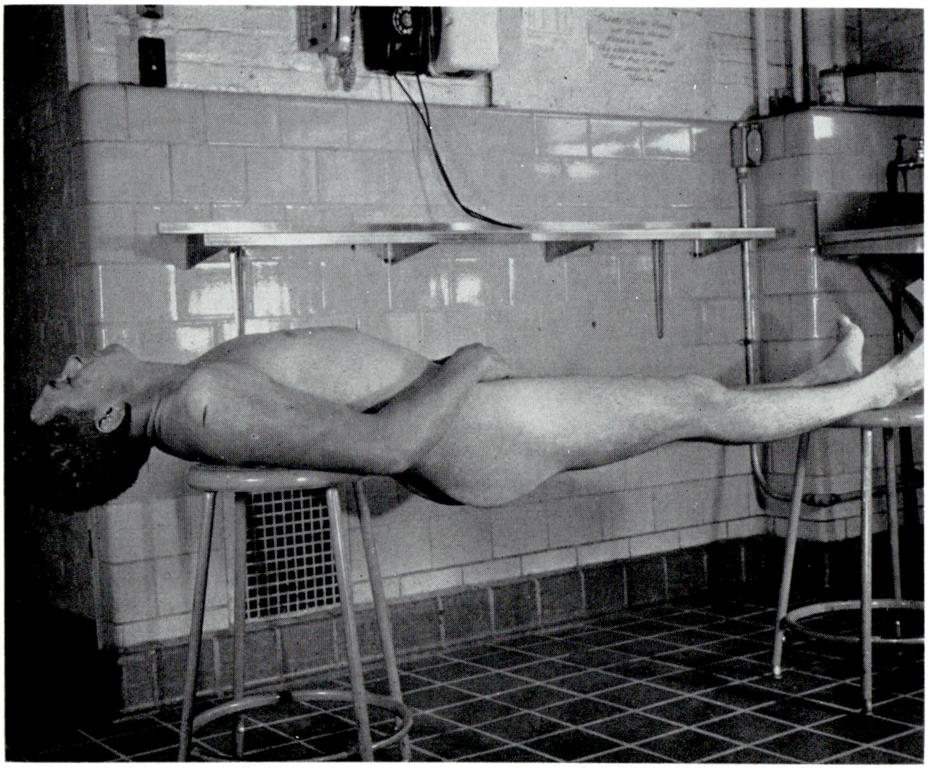

FIGURE II-1. Rigor mortis, intense enough to support the body as shown. This man had been dead for eighteen hours when the photograph was taken.

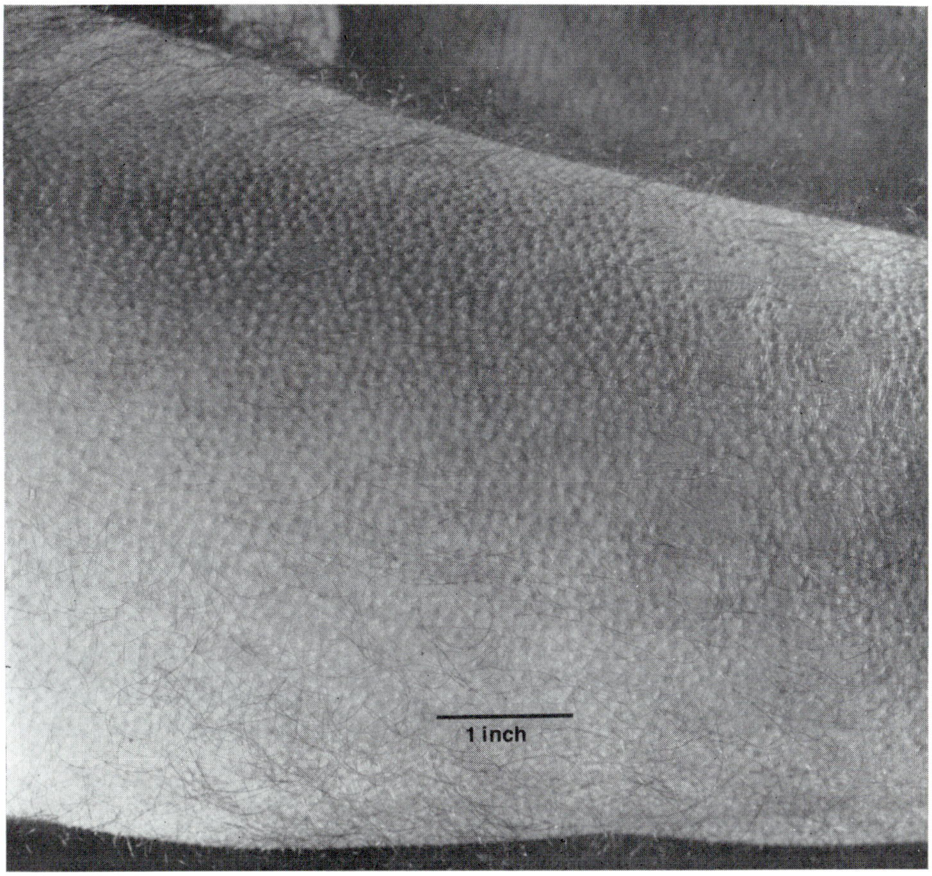


FIGURE II-2. Cutis anserina (gooseflesh) due to postmortem rigidity of short muscle fibers in the skin. This is strictly a postmortem occurrence and has no diagnostic significance.

tion begins. It also may disappear very rapidly in the presence of widespread bacterial infection, particularly with the gas gangrene bacilli, where again putrefaction begins early. The original onset of rigidity is hastened by the presence of high fever, convulsions or extreme muscle activity in the period prior to death, since all of these processes tend to diminish the residual oxygen available in the tissues and are accompanied by buildup of lactic acid in the living individual. In contrast, since the process is chemical in nature, its onset will be delayed by a very rapid cooling of the body, such as by refrigeration. Rigor is also prone to be poorly or incompletely developed in the elderly and in the very young, or in those who are severely debilitated, with consequent paucity of muscle tissue. If rigor is forcibly "broken" by manipulating the muscle groups during the developmental period, it may resume, although the resultant rigidity will be less than in other symmetrical groups that have been undisturbed. If rigor is broken once maximal development has been attained, it does not return.

As a mechanism of determining the time of somatic death, rigidity is of relatively little usefulness due to the considerable variation in onset and disappearance induced by the factors listed earlier. Of greater importance is the posture of the body maintained by the presence of rigidity but obviously not associated with the support of the body at the time of discovery. Thus, if a body is found lying on its back with feet suspended in the air, the obvious conclusion should be that the body reached full rigidity elsewhere while lying in a position where the

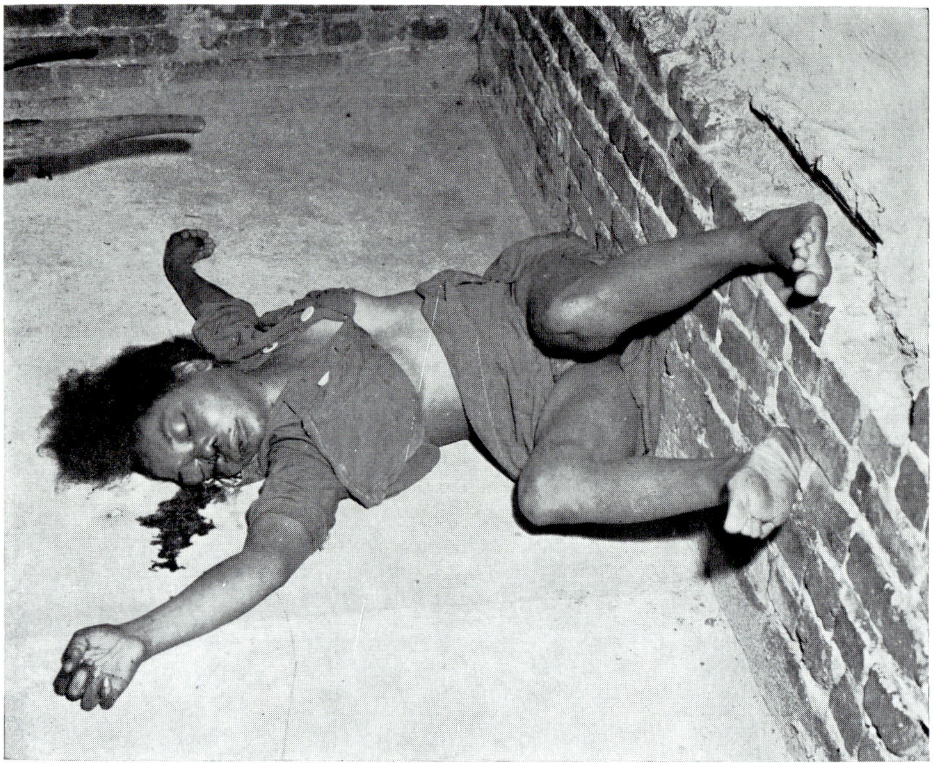

FIGURE II-3. Rigidity maintaining the legs of the victim against the brick wall. The flexed position of the legs led to the immediate conclusion that she had died elsewhere and had been moved after being dead at least six hours. Search of the area disclosed bloodstains in the home where she had been beaten. Her male friend confessed to having moved her body from the house hours later during darkness and depositing it in the court of an adjacent house in an attempt to conceal the murder.

legs were flexed or the feet suspended and that it was subsequently moved to the latter position, where the support is no longer present but rigidity holds the legs in the upright position (Fig. II-3). This example emphasizes the necessity of making observations before a body is moved in cases of possible homicide.

Finally, the old superstition concerning bodies that sit up in the coffin or in the morgue as a result of the development of rigidity should be dispelled. Rigidity refers to hardening of the muscles and not to contraction of the fibers with resultant motion of the body. There is some degree of flexion of the fingers in the postmortem interval, which results in the hand frequently being closed when the body is examined. This appears to be the result of physical contraction of the tendons that connect the muscles to the bones of the hand as they cool and is not due to rigor mortis per se.

## Livor Mortis

Livor mortis appears as a purple discoloration of the skin of the dependent parts of the dead body. It is caused by settling of the blood into the capillaries of the skin as they become dilated after circulation ceases. Since it depends on gravity, it will be absent in areas of the body where the weight produces pressure and occludes the capillaries (Fig. II-4). The usual purple color is that of the unoxygenated blood pigment hemoglobin. If a person has died of carbon monoxide poisoning, the color will be cherry red because the carboxyhemoglobin formed by the union of carbon monoxide and hemoglobin is of that hue. A second cause of pink lividity is cyanide poisoning, and still another example in which pink lividity occurs is in bodies recovered from icy waters or snow. This is believed to be due to the retention in the tissues of oxygenated hemoglobin. Sometimes lividity in parts of the body covered with moist clothes is cherry red, whereas it is the usual purple color in other areas. In severe anemia or in deaths from extensive hemorrhage, livor mortis may be so pale as to hardly be apparent.

Livor mortis formation begins immediately after death, but it may not be perceptible for as much as two hours. It is usually well developed within four hours and reaches a maximum between eight and twelve hours. During this period, if the body is turned over, the lividity that was originally dependent will shift to the newly dependent areas. However, after eight to twelve hours lividity becomes "fixed" and will remain where it originally formed. This is due to obstruction of the capillaries by gelled blood or constriction by the body fat, which, although liquid in life, congeals as the body cools. The distribution of livor mortis may thus serve as useful evidence to indicate whether a body

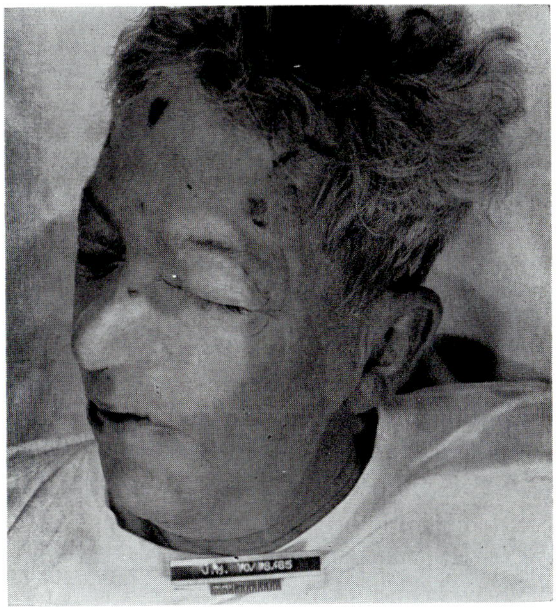

FIGURE II-4. Livor mortis. Note blanched area where face was pressed onto hard surface. This man died of heart disease. The forehead lesions are superficial abrasions sustained when he collapsed.

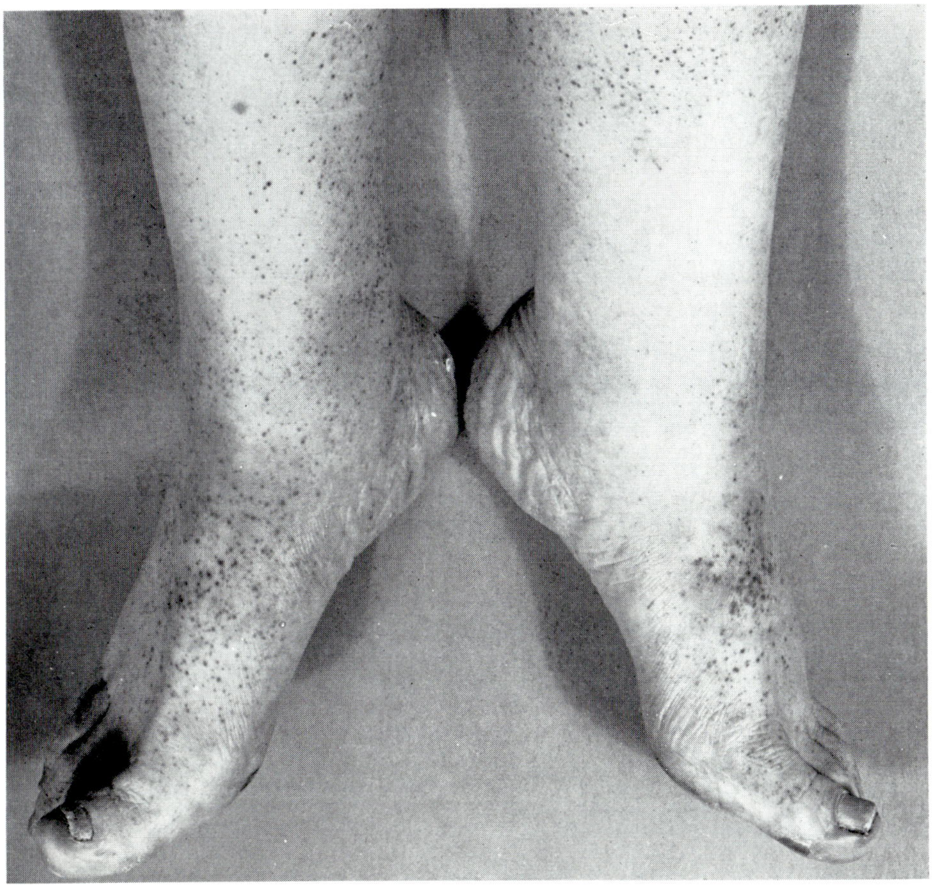

FIGURE II-5. Tardieu's spots in the feet of a hanging victim. There is also considerable swelling of the ankles as a result of hanging for several hours.

has been moved several hours after death occurred. Blanching of postmortem lividity by thumb pressure indicates that lividity is not fully fixed. In addition to lividity due purely to settlement of blood in the dependent capillaries, one occasionally sees the appearance, principally in the dependent areas, of confluent petechial hemorrhages, which may increase in size to as much as ⅛ inch in diameter. They represent actual leakage of blood through capillaries due to overcongestion and are known as Tardieu's spots, after the French medicolegist who originally described them (Fig. II-5). They are more likely to be found in cases where the mechanism of death is asphyxial, but they also occur in certain types of cerebral injury with interference with the respiratory center and in many cases of heart disease. They need not be interpreted to indicate any particular mode of death.

## Body Cooling

In the early hours after death body cooling may give some useful information in approximating the time of death. The rule of thumb most commonly applied is that the body cools 1½° F per hour. Based upon deep rectal or liver temperature of 99.6° F in the living individual, a rectal temperature of 95° F would indicate three hours postmortem interval. In our experience this is approximately correct in only about 50 percent of cases. Detailed studies of the cooling phenomenon indicate that during the first hour little cooling occurs. Thereafter the rate of cooling is influenced by a variety of factors, most importantly environmental temperature, the amount of clothing worn by the victim, the state of nutrition, the amount of wind, the contact of the body with cold or hot objects or if the body is immersed in cold water or wet from rain. Relative humidity also influences the rate of body cooling, since it controls the rate of evaporation of moisture on the body surface. Wind and low humidity tend to increase the evaporation of water, cooling the body more rapidly. Another factor making interpretations of postmortem temperature difficult is the lack of information regarding the temperature of the body at the time of death. Thus, in persons dying of pneumonia, where the temperature may be as high as 105° F, or of heatstroke, where it may reach 110° F, measurement of postmortem temperature is of little significance.

In a carefully controlled research study a series of bodies were subjected to an environment of between 59 and 68° F, and rectal temperatures were taken over a period of hours. It was demonstrated that a body temperature of 93° F was reached as early as two hours after death in some cases but in other cases as late as six hours after death. Body temperature of 79° F similarly was reached within the span of nine to twenty hours after death and body temperature of 72° F from eighteen to thirty hours after death.

## Decomposition

The time of onset and the rate of decompositional changes, like most other elements that shed some light on the time of death, are subject to enormous variation dependent upon the cir-

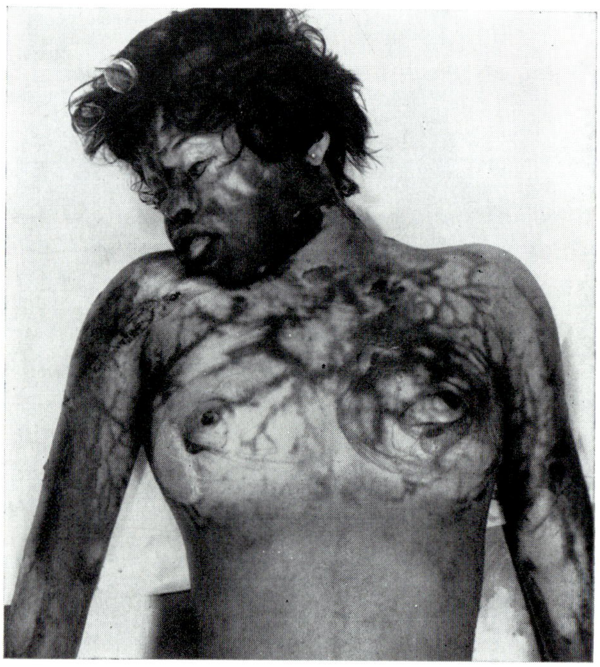

FIGURE II-6. Postmortem artifacts. Distention of tissues by gas, marbling of the skin due to hemolysis of blood in superficial vessels. Note the blister on the right breast. This is merely drainage of fluid beneath the epidermis, which detaches readily as putrefaction begins.

cumstances of the death, the temperature to which the body is subjected and preexisting conditions within the body. The two principal components of the decomposition process are autolysis and putrefaction.

Autolysis refers to the action of digestive enzymes or ferments that break down the complex protein and carbohydrate molecules in the body to simpler chemical compounds. An example of this is the digestive juices, which during life act only on food but after death will break down the tissues of the gastrointestinal tract. As a result of this activity, one occasionally finds perforations of the stomach or lower esophagus into the left pleural cavity or the abdomen within a few hours of death. Postmortem rupture of the stomach or esophagus occurs with some frequency in cases associated with high temperature, such as pneumonia, and is occasionally seen in cerebral deaths, particularly with involvement of the hypothalamic area. The mechanism in the latter condition is

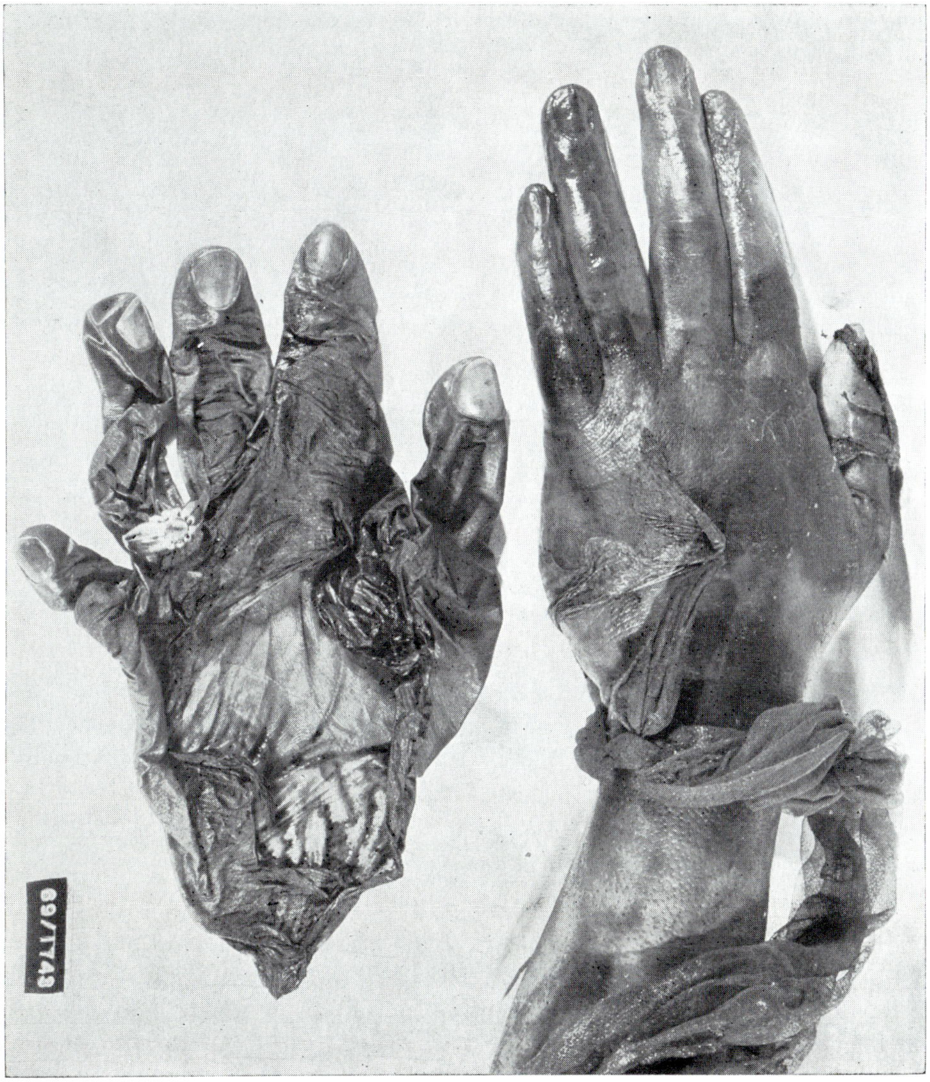

FIGURE II-7. Postmortem detachment of the skin in "glove" form. Note that the nails stay with the skin. These gloves can often yield a full set of fingerprints and should be retained until identification is certain. This was a narcotic addict (note the stocking around the wrist) whose body was found in a heated house in November. He was reported missing five days earlier.

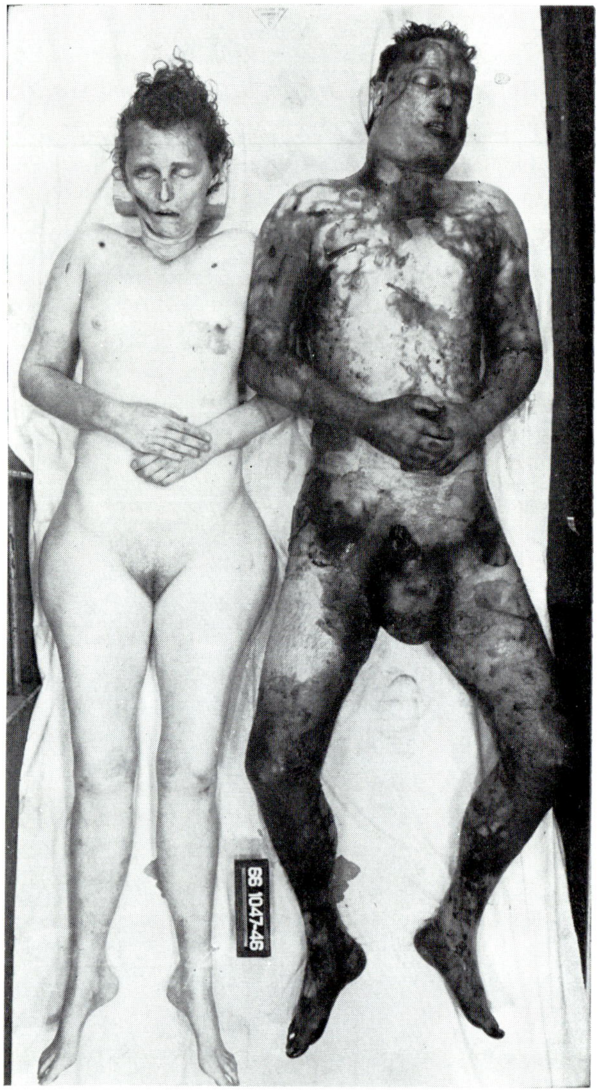


FIGURE II-8. The influence of environmental temperature on postmortem decomposition. This couple was killed at the same time by a mentally deranged son. The body of the mother was found in the cool basement, while the body of the father was discovered in a warm upstairs room. Outside temperature was 90° F, postmortem interval about forty-eight hours.

probably also a terminal rise in body temperature. Crystals of tyrosine are sometimes disseminated within the liver and on the liver surface and other abdominal organs. This results from breakdown of proteins and resembles fungal growth or foci of fat necrosis as may be seen in pancreatitis.

The other process, known as putrefaction, is due to bacterial activity throughout the body. Here there are tremendous capabilities of digestion of the tissues to a fluid consistency and the production of large amounts of foul-smelling gas. While autolysis does affect the microscopic structure of body tissues and produces limited gross changes such as the gastrointestinal perforation mentioned previously, putrefaction is the major component of decomposition. As gas is released within the blood vessels and within the tissues, the body becomes distended, the skin color changes through green to purple to black, the tongue and eyes protrude, there may be protrusion of abdominal organs through the vaginal and rectal openings and large amounts of foul-smelling bloodstained fluid exude from the body orifices. The epidermis softens and slips readily, revealing the underlying skin structures, and since most body pigment is lodged within the dermis, the remaining skin color will vary from pink to black, depending on the amount of decomposition and drying that have occurred (Fig. II-6). Exudation of bloodstained decomposition fluid from orifices and skin blisters often gives an erroneous impression of an injury sustained during life.

Skin slippage may be so complete that the entire epidermis of the hands or feet may detach in a *glove* configuration (Fig. II-7). Obese bodies tend to decompose more rapidly, but environmental temperature is the most important single factor (Fig. II-8). It is not uncommon to see advanced decomposition within twelve to eighteen hours, to the point that facial features are no longer recognizable, most of the hair slips away from the scalp and the entire body becomes swollen to two to three times normal size. External injury of the body enhances the putrefactive process by providing a portal of entry for bacteria. Also, blood provides an excellent medium for bacterial growth, which accounts for more advanced putrefaction in areas of injury. Death from sepsis is frequently followed by putrefaction to a severe degree within as little as nine to twelve hours. Conversely, at freezing or near-freezing temperatures, putrefaction may be delayed for months. A body may be submerged for the duration of the winter yet be in excellent preservation when recovered in the spring when the water warms up. However, when brought into a warm environment, such a body is prone to undergo putrefaction at an extremely rapid rate. Generally in temperate climates, according to an old rule of thumb, putrefaction proceeds at a set rate: one week in the air equals two weeks in the water or eight weeks in the soil.

Another important factor that influences the putrefactive process is invasion by insects. The time at which this occurs is determined in part by temperature and in part by accessibility of the body to flies. Flies may lay eggs between the lips and eyelids of patients *in extremis* and certainly within a few minutes after death (Fig. II-9). Certain species of blowflies actually produce live larvae so that the tiny maggots can be seen moving within a matter of an hour or so after death. For the most part, however, blowflies lay eggs that appear as yellowish white collections resembling grated cheese and are deposited in the various body openings. Even in relatively warm weather these eggs require about twenty-four hours to hatch. Thereupon the crawling larvae, commonly known as maggots, are seen. These feed on the body and grow over a period of several days, dependent again upon the temperature of the environment. The various stages of larval growth are referred to as instars. There are commonly four such instars in the development of the maggot from the time it appears until it reaches maturity and encloses itself in a brownish hard shell. At this stage the insect is said to be in pupa form. The pupa remains quiescent for several days, usually a minimum of about seven, whereupon fully developed, full-grown flies hatch from the pupa, leaving the empty shell behind. After a few hours of drying they are capable of flying and breeding. The eggs are fertilized within the female, and when deposited, the larvae are well formed within the eggs.

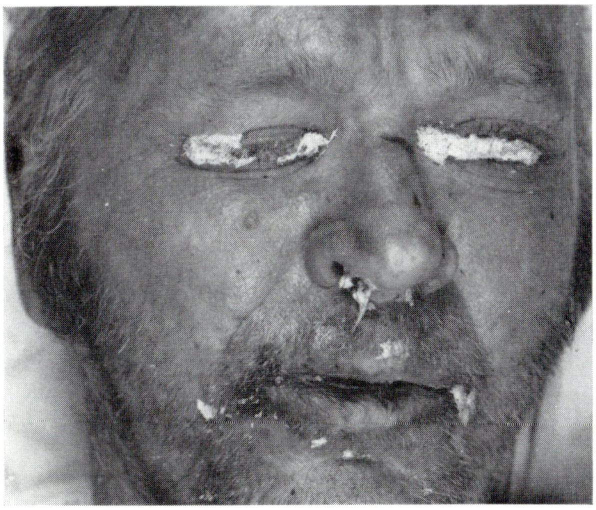

FIGURE II-9. Eggs laid by flies in the moist areas of the corners of the eyes, nares and angles of the mouth.

If blowfly invasion of the body is to be used in determining the minimum time the person has been dead it is necessary that the maggots or flies be collected and fixed in such fashion that an entomologist can study them adequately. It is also generally desirable to retain some live specimens, which the entomologist can allow to feed on appropriate material through the various instars of their growth, through the pupa stage and into the adult fly, since identification of the subspecies may be possible only on examining the adult. This is also desirable because of the varying growth rate of the larvae as influenced by temperature. Thus, the developing specimens should be subjected to similar temperature and other environmental conditions to those that were present in the body under investigation. Obviously, in collecting specimens for determination of the postmortem interval, a representative group of the largest (oldest) larvae should be collected, since only those deposited first on the body are of significance. Generally speaking, if there is no specific preservative available, the specimens may be simply dropped into boiling water for two or three minutes and then stored in refrigerated containers. The preferred preservation fluid for larvae is a solution containing 85 cc of 90% alcohol, 10 cc of 40% formalin and 5 cc of glycerin. Specimens preserved in this solution retain their shape and color indefinitely and are excellent for the various treatment procedures necessary to disclose the internal structures of the larvae.

In the case of skeletal remains where the soft

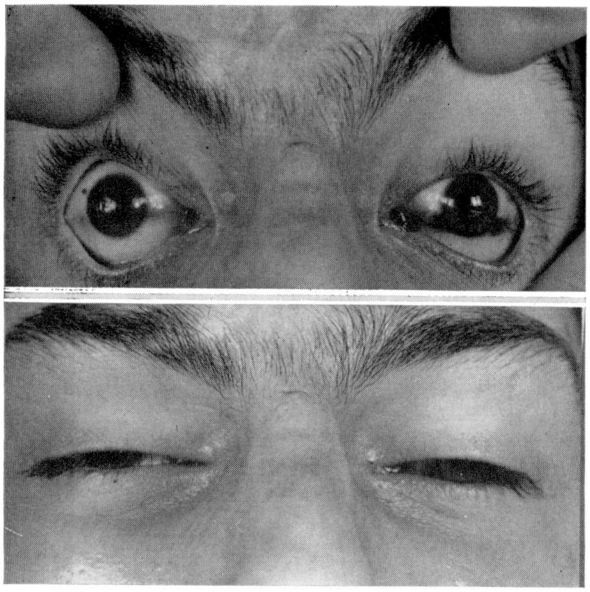

FIGURE II-10a. Drying of the conjunctivae due to partially closed eyelids occurs in the first few hours after death.

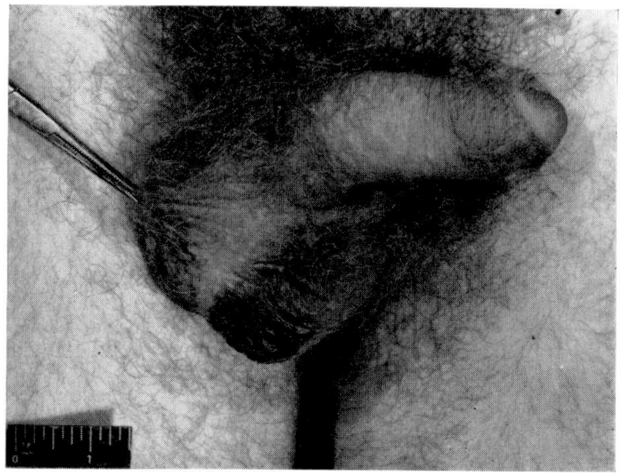

FIGURE II-10b. Drying of the scrotal skin is sometimes mistaken for bruising.

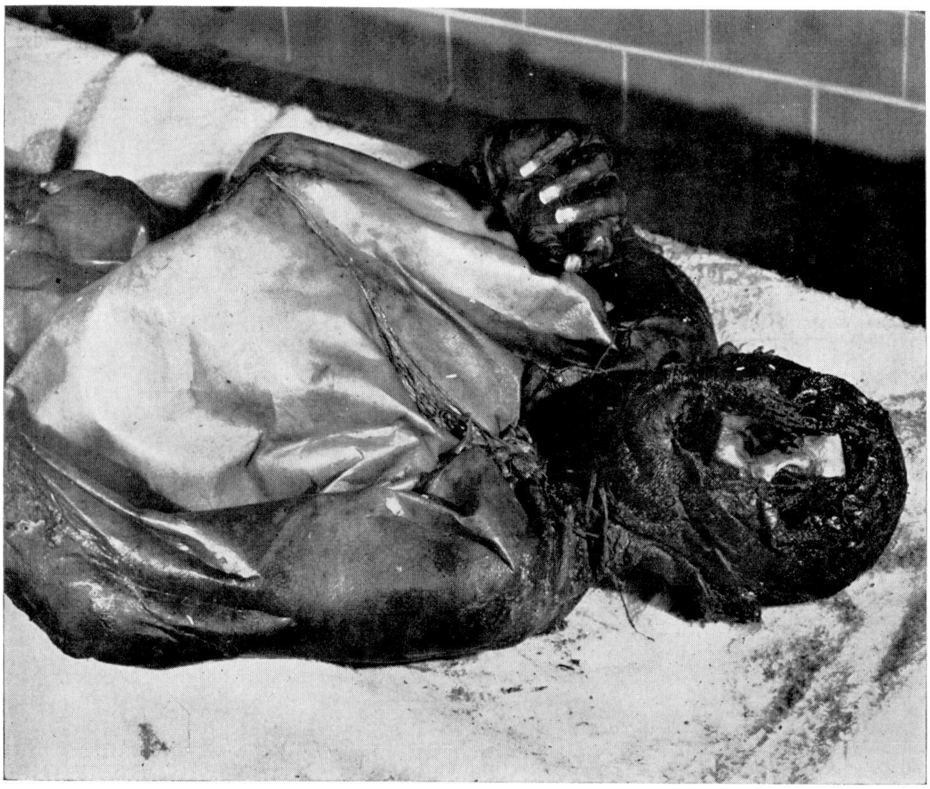

FIGURE II-11. Mummification of chest and arms. Note the parchmentlike appearance of the skin in these areas. The skull is partly exposed by maggots, the surrounding tissues decomposed and blackened. The body was found in an apartment in the middle of July. Newspapers at the door and other evidence indicated that death had occurred one week earlier.

tissues have disappeared, there are other insect invaders, including the so-called carrion beetles. Occasionally, entomologists can identify these and indicate a minimum number of months after death.

As the body dries in the hours or first few days after death (Fig. II-10), the tips of the fingers and toes and the skin of the face shrink with the apparent production of nail or hair growth. This has given rise to the erroneous lay belief that hair and nails grow after death.

In dry atmospheres the body may wither, shrivel and be converted to a leathery or parchmentlike mass of skin and tendons surrounding the bones; the internal organs are often decayed. This process is referred to as mummification (Figs. II-11 and II-12). Shrinkage of the skin due to drying may cause large splits that resemble actual injury. These are especially noted in the groin and about the neck and armpit. On the other hand, in cool, moist soil or water the soft tissues of bodies decay slowly and are converted into a peculiar grayish white cheesy state known as adipocere. This substance consists principally of hydrolyzed fat, i.e. fatty acids that infiltrate the other structures and, being acidic, inhibit putrefactive bacteria. Once adipocere is established, the body may remain in this condition for months or years. Certain molds thrive on hydrolyzed fats or adipocere, and this may cause complete obliteration of facial features. Adipocere may develop in as few as three months, but the fully developed phenomenon, where most of the body substance is converted to hydrolyzed fat, is usually not seen before five or six months after death[4] (Fig. II-13).

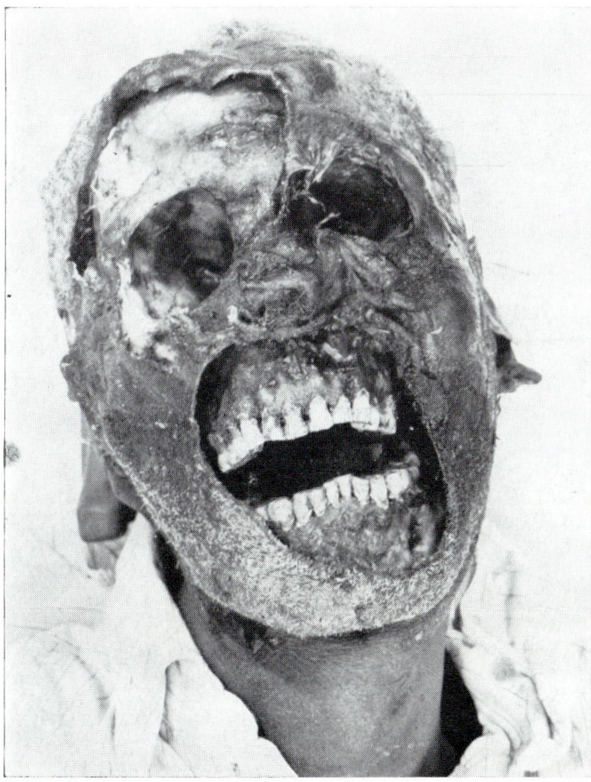

FIGURE II-12. Postmortem destruction by rats, followed by mummification. The body was found resting in a relatively dry place in winter too cold for blowfly activity. Death occurred about five weeks prior to discovery of the body.

Estimation of the time elapsed since death by the appearance of the skeletonized remains, i.e. the presence or absence of ligamentous attachments, articular cartilage and other cartilages, is extremely difficult because of the multitude of factors that influence this process. These include primarily whether the remains were buried and whether burial was underground or in a vault; if underground, the presence of subterranean streams and the type of soil must be considered. Climatic conditions, particularly temperature and humidity, and the accessibility of the remains to insects and carnivorous animals, as well as many other factors, play an important role.

The remains of a young black male were found among leaves and debris in the latter part of October in a public park in Baltimore. After the remains were identified, it was learned that the victim had been missing for exactly three months. Nearly complete skeletonization had taken place. Except for a few ligaments and cartilages, no soft tissues were found. There was no evidence of carnivorous activity.

Conversely, human remains found in northern Europe showed skeletonization similar to that in the aforementioned case after a period of approximately two to three years.

Occasionally greenish discoloration noted on the surface of certain bones is caused by contact

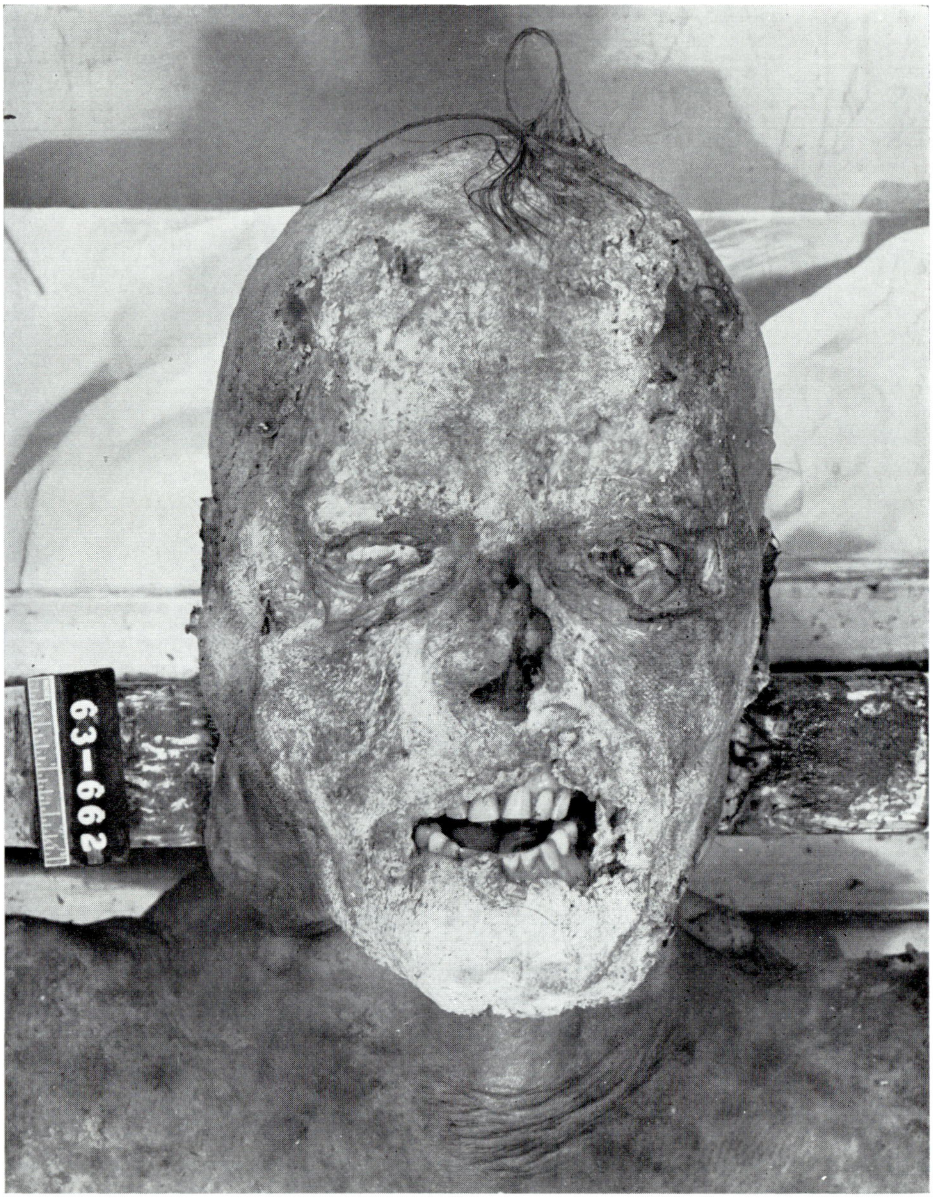


FIGURE II-13. Adipocere formation in the face and head of a seaman who had drowned six months before recovery of his body in April in the Chesapeake Bay. During winter the bay was covered with ice for two or three weeks. Water temperature when body was recovered was near 60° F. A key with the Norwegian word for cook was found in the pocket of the seaman and helped to establish identification.

with brass or copper articles such as jewelry or a belt buckle. The pale ivory color of skeletal remains is usually the result of bleaching by the sun.

### Association Factors

In addition to the bodily changes, events that occur in the environment may shed light on the time disability began or death occurred. Thus, the fact that a person is found dead in the kitchen with a partially eaten meal on the table and the electric lights on could be interpreted as evidence that disability began during the evening meal hours. Likewise, the failure to bring in the morning newspaper or milk is strongly suggestive that the routine was interrupted by the time these items are usually cared for.

In a case where the individual does not die immediately after being injured, the pathologist may be able to determine the approximate age of the wound, i.e. how long before death it was sustained, by a study of the inflammation around the wound. This in connection with other association evidence may determine the time of a fatal attack and help in establishing the opportunity for a given suspect to have committed the assault.

Another example of association evidence concerns the emptying of the stomach and passage of food along the bowel. Generally speaking, in persons without gastrointestinal disease who are not stressed emotionally, the stomach will empty a small meal or sandwich in one to two hours and a large meal in three to five hours. It becomes important, if the time of assault or death is unknown, to examine the stomach content both as to quantity and for recognizable residue of food. Then the investigator must determine when the last meal was eaten and of what it consisted. If this can be established, the pathologist may provide a useful estimate, with an accuracy of within one to two hours, as to when the fatal assault occurred. Caution must be exercised in these estimates, since any illness or emotional stress (worry, fright, etc.) may retard stomach emptying for many hours. We have not found the location of food in the small bowel or colon to be of much value in assessing the time of death.

The invasion of the body by insects was discussed earlier. It is another example of association evidence.

Finally, in the case of bodies dead for long periods outdoors, it may be useful to collect botanical specimens from beneath and near the body. Arrest of growth at identifiable stages under the body may enable a consulting botanist to give an estimate of when the body was deposited on the growing plants.

## POSTMORTEM ARTIFACTS

As a rule, an antemortem injury can be readily distinguished from one sustained after death. The application of a significant degree of mechanical violence before death characteristically results in hemorrhage. In the case of a nonpenetrating injury, such as a bruise, a crushing injury or a fracture, the extravasated blood will accumulate in the tissue spaces. If the wound involves the surface of the body, there will be both external and interstitial bleeding. It should be recognized, however, that the absence of gross bleeding does not necessarily indicate postmortem injury, nor does the presence of extravasated blood in the tissue always indicate that the wound was sustained during life. In situations where injuries are incurred that would ordinarily cause abundant bleeding but the victim goes rapidly into vascular collapse or shock, hemorrhage may be minimal. The converse is true also in that disruptive injuries received soon after death, particularly to regions of the body containing dilated blood vessels, as in the dependent areas, may result in a surprisingly copious escape of blood. Blunt impact sustained after somatic death may lacerate blood-filled vessels with resulting displacement of red cells into the tissue spaces. We have observed individuals who died with their feet in dependent positions, over the side of the bed, and where disruptions of the skin by small animals in the postmortem hours led to opening of blood vessels from which as much as a pint of blood drained out onto the floor, raising initial suspicion of antemortem injury (Fig. II-14).

All of those events that happen after death and may simulate antemortem injuries may be grouped together under the heading of postmortem artifacts. For purposes of description these may be divided into (a) postmortem injuries, (b) artifactual hemorrhages, (c) putrefactive changes, (d) injuries due to insect and terrestrial or aquatic animal life, (e) heat effects, (f) artifacts incident to embalming.

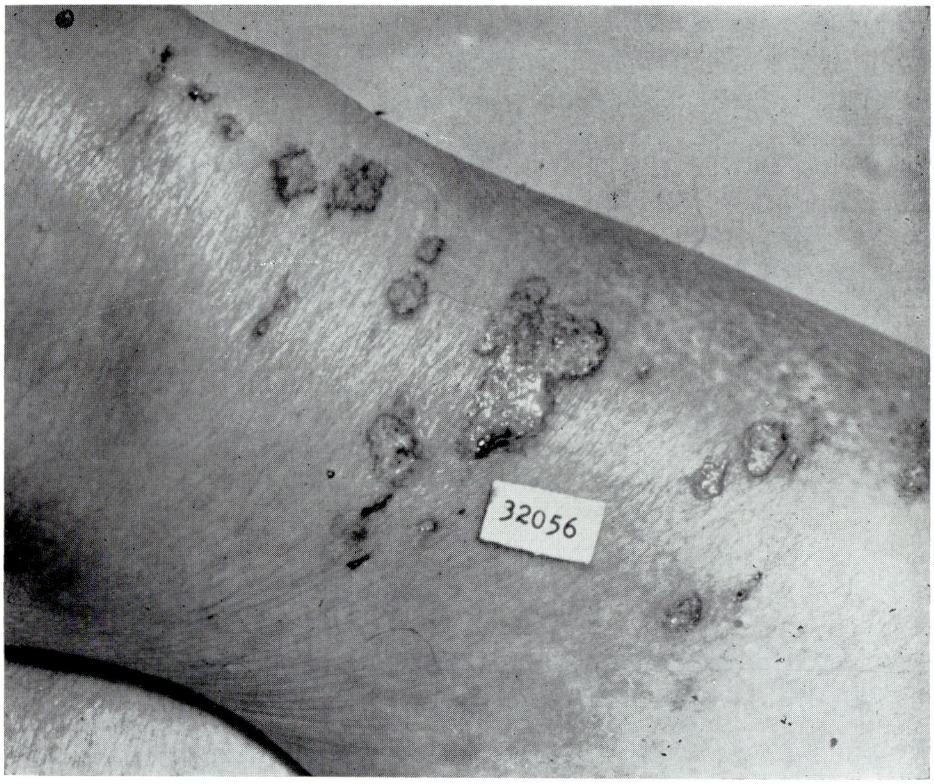


FIGURE II-14. Postmortem injury by mice closely resembling that due to roaches. The scene at first suggested violence, since there was a pool of nearly a pint of blood on the floor, which had drained out of these lesions as the deceased lay supine on her bed with the feet on the floor. She had died of chronic heart failure with marked venous hypertension.

### Postmortem Injuries

Postmortem injuries may be best exemplified by the following cases:

A seventy-seven-year-old driver of an automobile, returning from a party, was observed jumping a curb and proceeding over the median strip before striking a bar at a street corner. The vehicle was extensively damaged, and both the driver and his wife, who was a passenger in the right front seat, were dead at the scene. The autopsy showed the cause of death of the driver to be arteriosclerotic heart disease, with extensive scarring of the heart muscle due to previous infarctions. His blood alcohol was 0.02%, which confirmed the history of consumption of a small amount of beer (Fig. II-15).

A person who suffers a *blowout* of an aortic aneurysm may fall down the basement steps and sustain skull fractures. In such situations it may be difficult or impossible to determine how much, if any, of the injury was actually sustained *intra vitam*. Generally, the absence of tissue swelling due to hemorrhage and edema can be interpreted as evidence that the patient was dead or moribund and with no blood pressure at the time the injuries occurred. The opposite conclusion—that swelling is bona fide evidence of life—is subject to error also to the extent that the soft tissue around the eyes may swell remarkably if the body is prone and the face dependent (Fig. II-16). Likewise, in death by hanging, the legs and feet may show marked swelling. In open wounds, such as stab wounds or lacerations where free drainage prevents such accumulation, there is no dependable evidence to establish the ante- or postmortem occurrence of the wound unless it was sustained twenty minutes or more before death, i.e. long enough for microscopic signs of inflammation to become manifest.

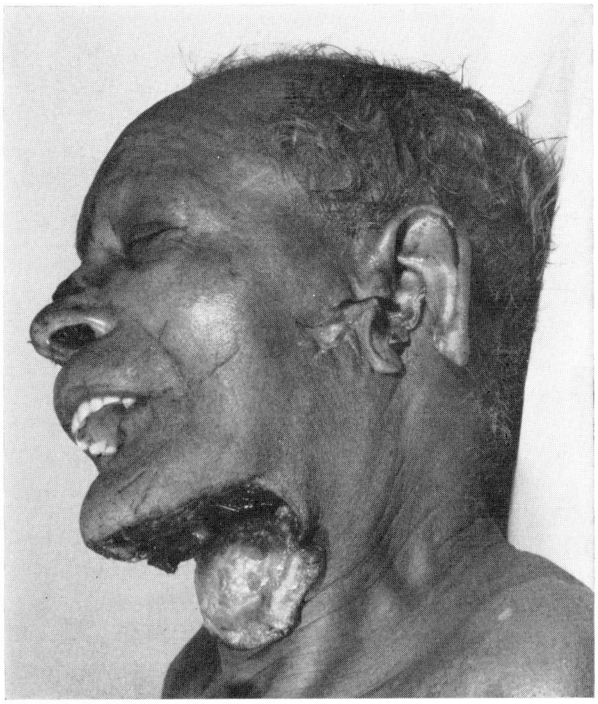

FIGURE II-15. Driver who suffered a fatal heart attack at the steering wheel of his automobile. Note the absence of hemorrhage in the injuries of the ear and chin.

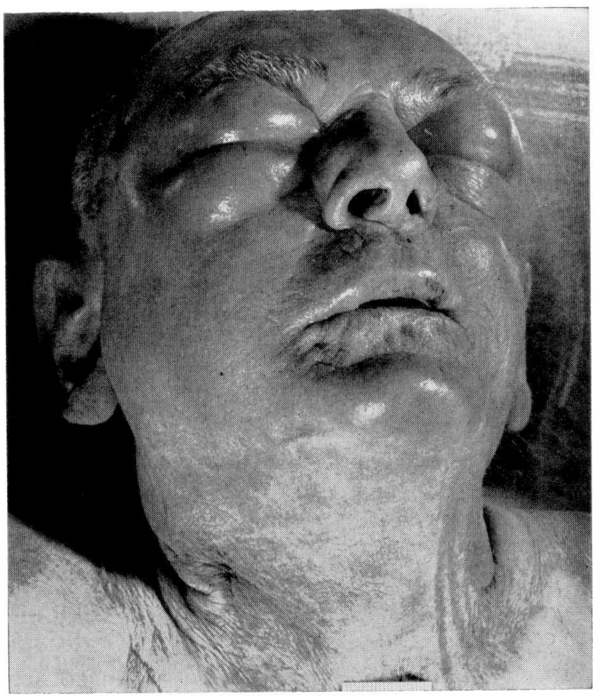

FIGURE II-16. Postmortem artifactual swelling around the eyes due to the body resting prone with the head hanging over the edge of the bed.

Postmortem injuries may show characteristic patterns that are helpful in reconstruction of the sequence. Linear fractures extending in the middle fossa of the skull are sometimes produced by the pathologist or his assistants in an attempt to complete the removal of the calvarium by use of a mallet or chisel. Such fractures may be mistaken for antemortem injuries by the inexperienced observer. The absence of hemorrhage in the fractured area and recognition of the possibility that such fractures may be artifactual should suggest to the pathologist their postmortem occurrence.

Fractures of the long bones may likewise occur in elderly or debilitated persons who have been confined to bed for a long period of time and have developed extensive osteoporosis with increased fragility of the bones. Rough handling of bodies by mortuary assistants or hospital orderlies occasionally results in fractures of ribs or the bones of the extremities. Such fractures are particularly likely to be sustained during attempts to straighten extremities contracted in a state of rigor. Again, realization by the pathologist of the possibility of such fractures and careful handling of the body to prevent such occurrence protects against misinterpretations. Of particular interest in this area are fractures of the rib cage, not infrequently accompanied by lacerations of the liver or other upper abdominal organs, incident to artificial resuscitation. Considerable hemorrhage into the surrounding tissues and the pleural and abdominal cavities as a result of forceful heart pumping incident to cardiac resuscitation is occasionally seen. Such hemorrhage testifies to the effectiveness of the cardiac massage but is apt to be misleading to the pathologist who has not been informed that the resuscitative efforts occurred. This is to be borne in mind particularly in individuals who sustained blunt injuries in such events as automobile accidents. Postmortem injuries due to resuscitation are frequently confused by the less experienced pathologist with the injuries resulting from impact on the steering wheel. Careful documentation of all resuscitative measures, an item commonly overlooked in medicolegal investigative offices where liaison with the hospital is less than optimal, is required to obviate such errors. A third area of the body where skeletal injuries are occasionally confusing includes the hyoid bone and the cartilages of the thyroid area surrounding the airway. Again, particularly in elderly people, these structures are exceedingly fragile and may be easily fractured incident to rough dissection while removing the neck organs. The key to recognition of these postmortem injuries is careful observation at the time of dissection for evidence of hemorrhages surrounding the points of fracture. In the absence of such hemorrhage, a fracture of the hyoid or thyroid cartilages must be suspected of being artifactual.

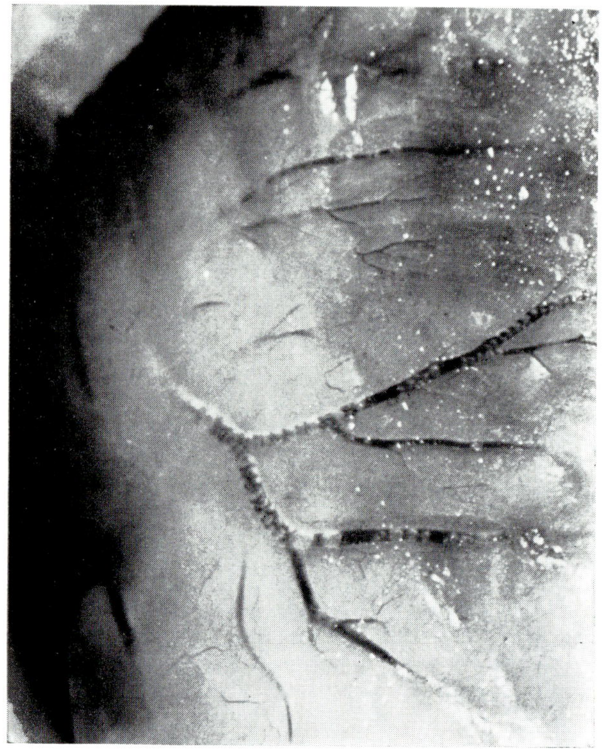

FIGURE II-17. Postmortem artifact. The air in the coronary vessels is due to moving the heart and lungs within the chest cavity after the internal mammary vessels were cut when the chest plate was removed. This should not be confused with air embolism.

### Artifactual Hemorrhage

On removal of the calvarium, large venous channels are necessarily cut, and if there is significant residual pressure in the vascular system due to congestion incident to heart failure or other causes, considerable amounts of blood escape into the layers between the skull and the brain. On occasion such blood will clot and may indeed simulate an antemortem subdural hemorrhage. If there happens to be antemortem bruising of the scalp and no adequate cause of death is readily demonstrated, the erroneous conclusion of death by head injury may result from misinterpretation of such an artifact. In the same way, during removal of the chest plate in the course of the autopsy large arteries and veins are severed, and if the chest organs are manipulated, considerable amounts of blood may escape into the pleural cavities. At the same time air may be drawn back into the vascular circulation, finding its way into coronary blood vessels and producing the false impression of air embolism (Fig. II-17).

### Putrefactive Changes

Pseudobruising due to the development of intense localized lividity of the skin because of hypostasis or due to displacement of internal pools of blood by gas pressure may simulate antemortem bruises. Likewise, internal hypostasis with hemolysis of blood cells may resemble hemorrhage, particularly in the meninges, kidneys and retroperitoneal tissues. In our experience the examination of victims of drowning presents particular difficulty in this area since, in instances in which the body is floating with the head in a downward position, suffusion of blood in the tissues of the neck may be difficult to differentiate from antemortem hemorrhage due to strangulation.

The formation of postmortem blisters with accumulation of fluid as decomposition occurs may erroneously be attributed to thermal effects with typical burn blisters (*see* Fig. II-6). In addition to softening of the skin and slipping of the epidermis seen with decomposition and with thermal exposure short of actual burning, other peculiar skin lesions of artifactual nature are occasionally encountered. Tanning of the face and skin of the neck by the coagulating action

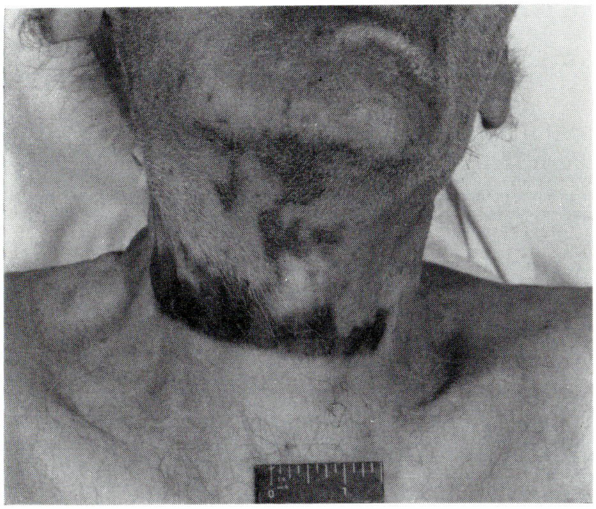

Figure II-18. Postmortem mutilation by ants restricted by the collar line could suggest strangulation.

of regurgitated gastric juices may likewise simulate antemortem burning. Similar changes occur as a result of contact of the body with gasoline. This is sometimes observed in automobile accidents or airplane crashes and is of special importance in the latter, where exposure to gasoline causes postmortem detachment of the superficial layers of the skin, leaving large areas of raw dermis. These areas turn yellow tan and leathery upon exposure to air and resemble thermal burns, which may give the false impression of fire in the crashing plane.

The postmortem purging of fluids from the nasal and oral orifices in the early stages of decomposition is easily misinterpreted as a sign of antemortem bleeding. Likewise, the development of fissures or splits in the skin as a result of putrefaction may suggest antemortem lacerations or incised wounds. It becomes particularly complicated when any degree of maggot infestation is present, since these insects have the capability of producing small round holes that may resemble those of large buckshot or bullets. Still another artifact is the development of excessive flaccidity of the vaginal orifice, together with extrusion of bloody fluid and spontaneous detachment of some of the vaginal mucous membrane, which may create the false impression of antemortem sexual attack.

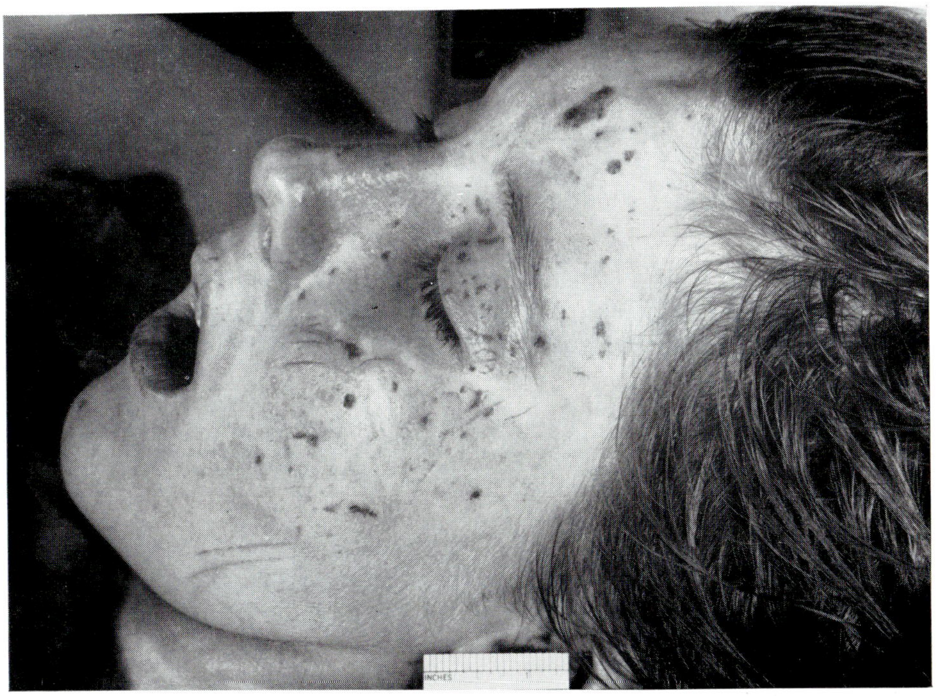

Figure II-19. Postmortem artifact. Pseudoabrasions produced by ants. The girl was dumped face down in a wooded area after being raped and strangled. The injuries of the face were first mistaken for fingernail marks. The fine linear scratches are due to twigs and undergrowth.

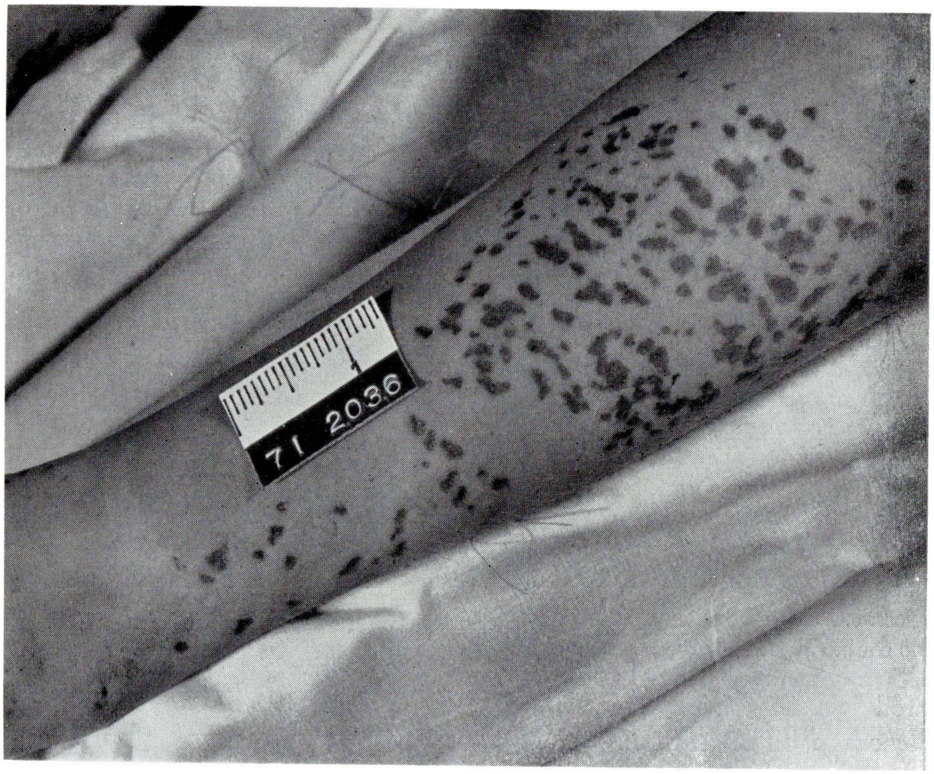


FIGURE II-20. Postmortem artifact. Skin lesions of arm caused by roaches. These are easily confused with antemortem abrasions if the roaches are not observed when the body is discovered. Note the similarity with the postmortem injuries produced by ants. The latter are somewhat smaller and more discreet.

### Injuries Due to Insect and Terrestrial or Aquatic Animal Life

Small erosions of exposed skin or of covered skin near openings in the clothing are commonly caused by ants or roaches and may give the impression of antemortem abrasions (Fig. II-18). As these postmortem insect bites become desiccated, they come to resemble brush burns in many instances (Figs. II-19 and II-20). Mice are known to attack a body and produce superficial injuries that in the early stages of decomposition resemble antemortem ulcerated skin lesions (*see* Fig II-14).

If the animals are larger, such as rats, skunks or dogs, the destruction of exposed skin areas is usually more dramatic. Often those portions most accessible from the ground, i.e. the face and neck in the recumbent body, are involved. Sometimes the false impression of knife wounds may be obtained, particularly in skeletal remains (Figs. II-21, II-22 and II-23).

Certain characteristics are useful in recognizing the postmortem small animal or aquatic animal attack. Such encroachments on the body tend to involve primarily the lips, the eyelids

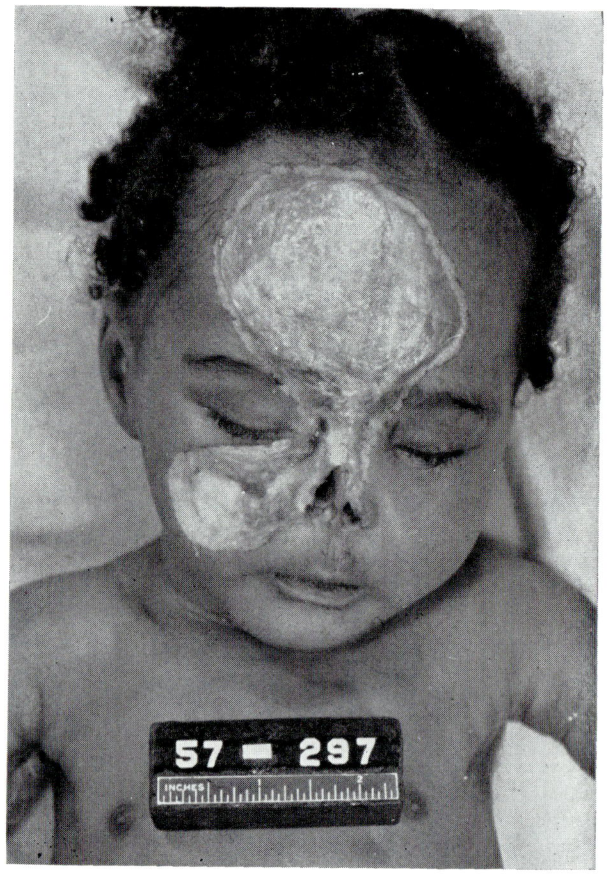


FIGURE II-21. Postmortem gnawing of flesh by rats.

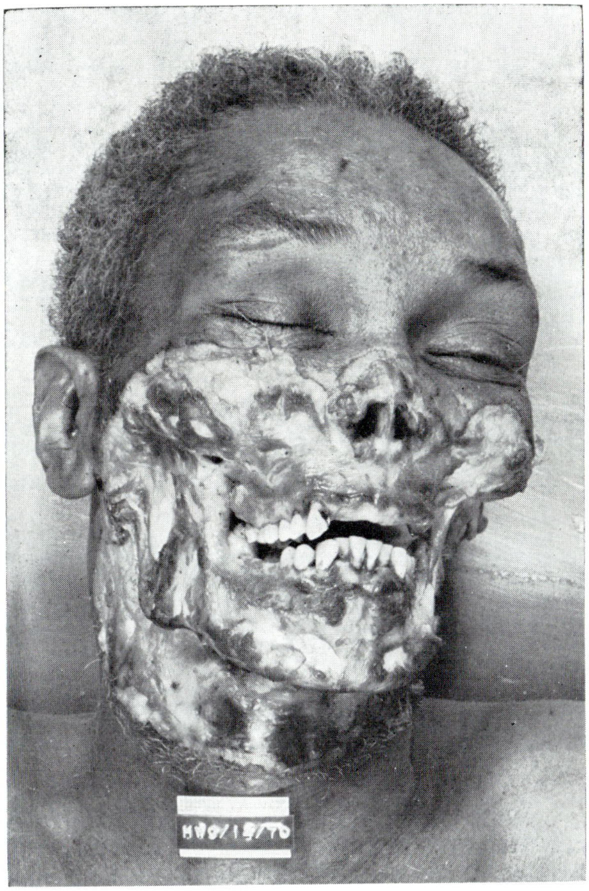

FIGURE II-22. Postmortem gnawing of flesh by small pet dog.

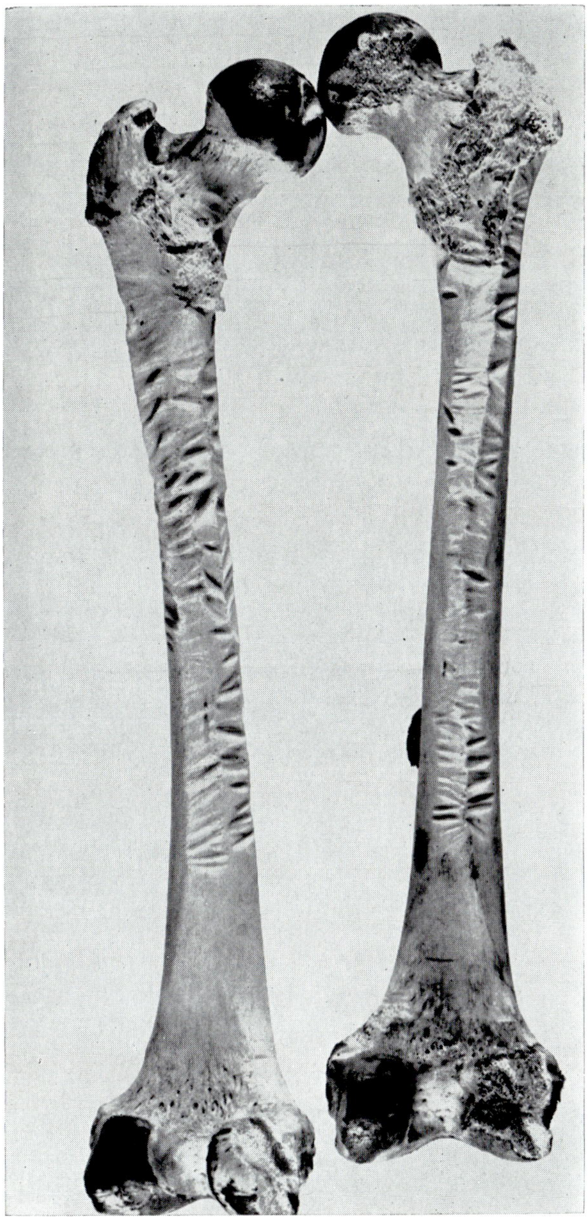

FIGURE II-23. Postmortem gnawing of human femurs, which were exposed for some months in a wooded area. The teeth marks are most likely from dogs, but smaller animals, such as opossums or skunks, may leave similar marks.

and the ears, which are the softest exposed tissues of the body. However, any animal attacking the dead body will primarily select those areas where the skin is broken; thus, it is not uncommon to find that antemortem wounds have been enlarged to a great degree by postmortem invaders.

### Heat Effects

Radiant heat reaching the body after death may cause loosening or drying and tanning of the skin. It does not cause erythema or fluid-filled blisters that can be readily confused with antemortem burns. Exposure of the body to excessive heat causes "cooking" of the muscles with considerable contraction of muscular structures, resulting in flexion of the extremities, protrusion of the tongue and other changes that should not be interpreted as indicative of the posture of the body at the time of death. Intense and protracted postmortem heating of the head not infrequently causes explosive fractures of the skull and separation of the dura mater from the skull with effusion of blood into the extradural space. As this blood is subsequently coagulated by the heat, and as the boiling juices escaping from the inside of the head through fire fractures dissect along the muscle planes of the scalp, artifacts are produced that may lead the unsuspecting pathologist to the pronouncement that death was due to head trauma and that an effort was made to conceal the homicide by setting the body on fire.

### Artifacts Incident to Embalming

The embalming process usually consists of making incisions in the axillary or supraclavicular areas through which the arterial structures may be entered. Trocars are then inserted, and embalming fluid is pumped under pressure via the arterial system until it returns on the venous side. Later in the procedure, incisions may be made in the trunk area in an effort to remove excess embalming fluid that may have accumulated. These trocar wounds have been mistaken for stab wounds and in at least one instance were so multiple that an inexperienced examiner offered the opinion that the wounds were the result of an antemortem shotgun blast. Incident to the pressure phenomenon of embalming some blood may be forced out of injured or disrupted blood vessels and may accumulate in the tissue with the appearance of an antemortem hemorrhage. Furthermore, the embalming process tends to produce transparency of the skin, and minor hemorrhages not previously visible, particularly in areas of lividity, become apparent, occasionally creating serious problems in interpretation.

### REFERENCES

1. Thomas *v.* Anderson, 215 P.2d 478.
2. Smith *v.* Smith, 217 S.W.2d 275.
3. Kvittingen, T. D., and Naess, A.: Recovery from drowning in fresh water. *Br Med J, 5341:*1315 (May), 1963.
4. Camps, F. E. (Ed.): *Gradwohl's Legal Medicine,* 2nd ed. Baltimore, Williams & Wilkins, 1968.

*Part 2*

## CHEMICAL CONSIDERATIONS

John I. Coe

Among ancillary procedures that the forensic pathologist may use, postmortem chemistry can be one of the most productive. Information derived from such studies may establish the cause of death, contribute to evaluation of autopsy findings and assist in estimating the time of death.

Historically, blood as a postmortem specimen has been most extensively studied. While some biochemical materials remain remarkably stable in the serum after death, other substances show varying degrees of change, making evaluation of possible antemortem abnormalities impossible. To overcome the inadequacies of postmortem blood studies, investigation of cerebrospinal fluid and, more recently, vitreous humor has been undertaken. The latter is more advantageous, since the eye is well protected and less subject to contamination and putrefactive changes, and postmortem biochemical changes occur more slowly there than in other sites.

The following discussion* is based on the use of chemical analyses of blood, cerebrospinal fluid, vitreous humor and urine to diagnose antemortem biochemical abnormalities in the *early postmortem period*. This period is defined as the interval between death and the onset of

* Readers interested in greater detail or complete English references are referred to the following review articles by the author:
Postmortem chemistry: Practical considerations and a review of the literature. *J Forensic Sci, 19:*13, 1974.
Postmortem chemistry of blood, cerebrospinal fluid and vitreous humor. In Wecht, C. H. (Ed.): *Legal Medicine Annual 1976.* New York, ACC, 1976, pp. 55-92.

marked intravascular hemolysis. As a consequence, the early postmortem period may last over 100 hours in bodies that are in a cool environment or be as short as four to six hours in tropical areas or in situations where a body is exposed to a high temperature for a significant period after death.

### Collection of Specimens for Analysis

Postmortem studies of glucose, pH, oxygen tension, insulin, the cardiac fraction of CPK, and certain drugs all demonstrate significant differences between specimens taken from the two sides of the heart or between intracavitary blood of the heart and samples from peripheral vessels. Therefore, if no autopsy is performed, blood should not be aspirated by blind cardiac puncture. Instead, blood samples should be obtained from the femoral or subclavian veins; this most closely resembles blood obtained from living individuals.

Collection of vitreous humor is best accomplished by inserting a number 20 needle through the outer canthus into the posterior chamber of the eye, followed by gentle aspiration with a 5 cc or 10 cc syringe. The use of vacuum tubes should be avoided, as the strong initial suction tends to pull loose retinal tissues and thus contaminate the specimen. In the adult approximately 1½ to 2 cc of crystal-clear fluid can be aspirated from each eye.

Aspirated vitreous humor is viscous and may occlude the fine tubing of automated analytical instruments in the clinical laboratory. This problem can be avoided by centrifugation of the specimen and use of the supernate for analysis.

Urine may frequently be aspirated by suprapubic puncture in a nonautopsied body. Cerebrospinal fluid is easily obtained prior to autopsy from the cisterna magna by inserting a long, large-gauge needle between the atlas and the occipital bone. Direct aspiration of cerebrospinal fluid can be done after removal of the brain from the lateral ventricles or by aspiration from the third ventricle by puncture of the hypothalamic area.

### Diabetes and Diabetic Acidosis

Blood obtained from the right side of the heart may have glucose levels frequently exceeding 1000 mg/dl due to diffusion of glucose through the inferior vena cava from the liver. While blood from peripheral vessels commonly shows serum glucose levels as low as 10 mg/dl within a few hours of death, there are numerous normal individuals in whom there is a substantial increase in postmortem glucose compared to the values existing during life. Such increases have been reported in asphyxial deaths, cerebral hemorrhage, congestive heart failure, electrocutions and following cardiopulmonary resuscitation. Routine postmortem chemical analyses in 1,000 consecutive natural deaths indicated peripheral glucose levels in excess of 500 mg/dl in 103 cases (10.3%) of nondiabetic individuals.[1] This means *the postmortem diagnosis diabetes cannot be made from examination of blood alone.*

Because of the difficulty in interpreting postmortem serum glucose values, most investigators believe that a diagnosis of diabetes can be made more easily from examination of cerebrospinal fluid or vitreous humor. In the study previously referred to there was no case in which the vitreous glucose exceeded 100 mg/dl. In over 5,000 routine analyses of the vitreous humor performed by the author, glucose values exceeding 200 mg/dl have been found only in diabetics or in the occasional hospital patient receiving prolonged intravenous infusion of glucose just prior to death. A diagnosis of acidosis can be easily established by demonstrating a significant level of ketone bodies in the vitreous humor, serum, spinal fluid or urine.

Recent work has shown that diabetic elevations of glucose in the vitreous humor remain high after embalming despite biochemical artifacts produced by the embalming process.[2]

A seventeen-year-old black, insulin-dependent woman deteriorated rapidly after she discontinued medication. Autopsy showed no cause of death, but urine gave a 3 reaction for glucose and a strongly positive test for acetone. No other chemical tests were done at that time. Eleven days later the body was exhumed and vitreous humor had a glucose of 772 mg/dl and an acetone of 17 mg/dl. The embalming fluid contained a significant amount of isopropanol but no glucose or acetone.

### Hypoglycemia

Studies on blood, cerebrospinal fluid and vitreous humor have demonstrated glycolysis in each of these media. Such glycolysis may occur very rapidly and produce a precipitous fall in the glucose level. Early workers believed that vitreous glucose values less than 25 mg/dl could be considered indicative of hypoglycemia. However, recent work has established that values of 0 for true glucose may be found as early as two hours after death in normal individuals with no antemortem evidence of hypoglycemia and no autopsy or chemical evidence of elevated insulin values.[3, 6] Consequently, *a postmortem diagnosis of antemortem hypoglycemia cannot be made with any assurance at the present time.*

It has been suggested that antemortem hypoglycemia should be diagnosable by demonstrating concomitant low values for lactic acid and glucose. This concept deserves further investigation, but at present, the rapid irregular increase in lactic acid content of blood, cerebrospinal fluid and vitreous humor has made attempts to correlate such increases with cause or manner of death impossible. Sturner[4] has found that lactic acid levels in the vitreous humor tend to be much lower in individuals dying suddenly when compared with values obtained from individuals having prolonged agonal periods.

### Nitrogen Retention and Uremia

Evidence of antemortem nitrogen retention is easily obtained by determination of urea nitrogen and/or creatinine in vitreous humor, serum or cerebrospinal fluid. Postmortem levels of either of these substances in any of the media accurately reflect the terminal antemortem blood levels in both the normal and uremic ranges. Furthermore, these substances are stable not only through the entire postmortem interval but also into the early stages of putrefaction. Moderate nitrogen retention is commonly seen in dehydration. Clinical uremia may be assumed to have existed when urea nitrogen levels exceed 150 mg/dl. Uremic levels of urea nitrogen may be demonstrated in the vitreous humor even after embalming.[2]

In contrast to urea nitrogen and creatinine, there is an increase in nonprotein nitrogen (NPN) in the serum with an increasing postmortem interval. This is caused in part by an increase in both ammonia and amino acid nitrogen in the blood after death and has been used by Schleyer as a means of estimating the postmortem interval.[5]

### Electrolyte Studies

Sodium and chloride levels begin to fall in the blood and cerebrospinal fluid immediately after death. The average rate of fall approximates 1 mEq/liter/hr in the serum postmortem, but because of great individual variations, it is impossible to determine what antemortem values might have been even when the postmortem period is known exactly.

In contrast to the levels in blood and cerebrospinal fluid, sodium and chloride remain nearly constant in the vitreous humor throughout the early postmortem period. Appreciable abnormalities in antemortem serum sodium and chloride are reflected in abnormal postmortem vitreous values, making it possible to diagnose electrolyte abnormalities that existed while the individual was alive. A study of a large number of cases[6] has demonstrated that electrolyte abnormalities tend to fall into four common patterns:

1. Hypertonic dehydration pattern. This is characterized by a concomitant increase in sodium (more than 155 mEq/liter) and chlorides (more than 135 mEq/liter) in the vitreous humor with a moderate elevation of urea nitrogen (usually between 40 and 100 mg/dl).
2. Uremic pattern. This differs from the dehydration pattern in that the vitreous urea nitrogen and creatinine levels are appreciably increased (urea nitrogen over 150 mg/dl) without a corresponding substantial increase in sodium and chloride values.
3. Low salt pattern. This pattern characteris-

tically consists of low sodium (less than 130 mEq/liter) and chlorides (less than 105 mEq/liter) in the vitreous humor, along with a relatively low potassium level (less than 15 mEq/liter). Knowledge of the potassium level is critical to separate the low salt pattern from the decomposition pattern.

4. Decomposition pattern. Like the low salt pattern, this is characterized by a low sodium and chloride level in the vitreous humor, but there is an accompanying high vitreous potassium value (more than 20 mEq/liter), which indicates a long postmortem interval and alerts the investigator that the low sodium and chloride levels are probably due to deterioration of the specimen.

Application of such data has made it possible to demonstrate evidence of hyperosmolar dehydration in cases of child neglect, homicide and certain cases of septicemia. Hyperosmolar dehydration has been described by British authors in cases of apparent sudden infant death. Decreased sodium and chloride values have been demonstrated in the chronic alcoholic and have also been found in the presence of pyloric obstruction with prolonged vomiting and in cardiac patients on prolonged Dyazide® therapy.

### Vitreous Potassium—An Indicator of the Postmortem Interval

The recognition that vitreous potassium levels go up with increasing time after death was followed by attempts to use such tests for determining the postmortem interval. It was initially believed that the method could be used with a confidence limit of plus or minus five hours and that the standard error did not increase as the death interval lengthened. However, later studies have shown that the individual variation is greater, being in the neighborhood of plus or minus ten hours the first day after death. Further, the standard error continues to increase with a longer postmortem interval, and elevated environmental temperatures severely distort the average rate of rise in vitreous potassium. For these reasons many forensic pathologists have abandoned this procedure for determining the postmortem interval.

While the margin of error is admittedly large, the test appears to be more reliable than any other chemical procedure known at the present time. Used as a routine analysis, the procedure has shown a surprisingly good correlation between the vitreous potassium level and the postmortem interval when unusual circumstances have been excluded. In several cases this procedure has given a more accurate estimation of the postmortem interval than could be obtained from a study of rigor mortis, body temperature and other physical signs commonly used to estimate the time between death and examination of the body.

During October a fifteen-year-old boy was found in a wooded area partially covered by leaves. His hands were bound behind his back, and he had been shot six times. The body was remarkably well preserved. Both the deputy medical examiner at the scene and the pathologist several hours later noticed the presence of rigor mortis involving all the large muscle groups. The excellent state of preservation and the continuing presence of rigor mortis suggested that the deceased had probably been dead less than forty-eight hours. However, vitreous potassium was determined to be 25 mEq/liter, which was more consistent with the deceased having been dead more than four days. Ultimately, investigation established that the youth had been missing for eight days prior to discovery of the body, and stomach contents at autopsy matched exactly the meal given to him by his mother only two hours prior to his disappearance.

### Dysproteinemias

Determination of postmortem serum protein levels by chemical analysis, electrophoresis and immunologic techniques revealed that they accurately reflect antemortem levels of the various fractions. Such determinations have been used to demonstrate the absence of hypogammaglobulinemia in most cases of sudden infant death syndrome. True agammaglobulinemia has been found by the author in postmortem blood samples from an individual known clinically to have this condition, as well as monoclonal elevation in the gamma globulin of a postmortem specimen from an individual dying of myeloma. Fekete[7] reports that electrophoretic curves of several clinically diagnosed gammopathies were reproduced with postmortem serum samples.

### Liver Function Studies

Evaluation of liver function from postmortem chemical tests remains limited. In jaundiced individuals postmortem serum bilirubin values accurately reflect the antemortem degree of jaundice. However, a slight increase in postmortem values makes the use of bilirubin unsatisfactory for evaluating minimal clinical jaundice in equivocal cases of liver disease.[8] Testing of urine for urobilinogen and bile is of value in questionable cases of liver disease.

As stated in the previous section, protein values after death correspond to antemortem values so that hypoproteinemia and inversion of the albumin-globulin ratio have the same significance after death as they would have had clinically before death. However, all enzymes that would be significant in demonstrating liver disease increase erratically after death and thus are uninterpretable. Wright[9] has shown that hepatic coma may be diagnosed by determination of the glutamine level in spinal fluid. Values were more than three times as high in individuals who had hepatic failure as they were in those without evidence of coma, although in the latter group some had severe fatty change or cirrhosis of the liver at autopsy.

### Cholesterol and Other Lipids

The stability of total cholesterol in the blood after death has been demonstrated.[10] In contrast, cholesterol esters decrease as postmortem time lengthens, due to the action of esterase in the serum. Other lipid substances, such as total serum fatty acids, total lipoproteins and beta lipoproteins, are all remarkably stable, with little reduction caused by autolysis.[11, 12] In general, they tend to decrease in concentration less than 0.5 percent per hour. However, interpretation of postmortem values is difficult because postmortem blood samples frequently are from individuals who are not in a fasting state at the time of death. Elevated values should be given consideration only if the stomach and at least the upper small intestinal tract are empty at the time of autopsy. Correlation of the presence of heart disease with abnormalities of lipid elements in the blood has been successful. Unsuspected familial hyperlipoproteinemias can thus be identified to the benefit of surviving relatives. Furthermore, cholesterol, being stable after death, can be used in the study of liver function and in cases of questionable thyroid disease.

In hormone studies only limited investigation of hormone levels after death has been reported. Serum cortisol is found to correspond to values obtained during life and to remain constant during the early postmortem period.[13] This has proven to be of value in excluding Addison's disease as a cause of death in individuals with hypoplastic adrenal glands or extensive adrenal hemorrhage at autopsy. In contrast to cortisol levels, the levels of epinephrine increase rapidly after death, making evaluation of postmortem specimens impossible. Thyrotoxin levels tend to decrease after death, so that one must be cautious in using them for interpretation of hypothyroidism. However, they have proven of value in diagnosing thyrotoxicosis. The levels of thyroid-stimulating hormones seem to be more stable and have helped in recognizing cases of true hypothyroidism at autopsy.[14]

Lindquist and Rammer[15] have demonstrated that postmortem serum insulin values are higher than antemortem values in healthy individuals. They also detected great variations in the concentration of insulin depending on the source of the serum. Specimens taken from the right ventricle were consistently higher in value than those from a peripheral vessel. Knowledge of postmortem insulin values enables diagnosis of fatal insulin poisoning.

Chorionic gonadotropin in postmortem blood and urine shows values corresponding to antemortem levels obtained in individuals dying of choriocarcinoma or related tumors. Levels of 17-hydroxycorticosteroids and growth hormones apparently increase after death, making interpretation unreliable.

## Enzymes

Postmortem variations occur rapidly in acid and alkaline phosphatase, amylase, transaminase, lactic dehydrogenase and total creatinine phosphokinase, so that postmortem determination of antemortem abnormalities is impossible at the present time.

Cholinesterase remains stable for prolonged periods after death.[16] This is of great significance to the forensic pathologist, who may establish the presence of organic phosphorus poisoning by a decrease in serum cholinesterase values. Enzyme studies have also proven to be of value in diagnosing death *in utero* and clinical brain death.

## Minerals

Early studies suggested that serum calcium levels remain constant during the early postmortem interval, but this has not been substantiated by more recent work. There appears to be an increase in serum calcium as the postmortem interval lengthens. While the vitreous humor calcium level is more constant than the serum level, there is no indication that any antemortem abnormality of calcium metabolism has been diagnosed after death from such vitreous studies.

Magnesium levels increase slowly in serum, cerebrospinal fluid and vitreous humor during the early postmortem period. Measurement of magnesium levels in all three media has been proposed as an aid in establishing the diagnosis of drowning or in determining the time of submersion in sea water, but this has not been supported.

Both inorganic and organic phosphorus levels increase rapidly after death, making postmortem evaluation of phosphate metabolism impossible. In contrast, sulfate levels remain constant in the early postmortem period but seldom have been used in diagnosing antemortem abnormalities.

## Blood Oxygen in Asphyxia and Sudden Cardiac Arrhythmia

Experimental work has indicated that death from asphyxia may be distinguished from sudden death caused by cardiac arrhythmia by measuring the level of oxygen tension in postmortem aortic blood. The partial pressure of oxygen ($Po_2$) in experimental animals dying from cardiac arrest exceeded 25 mm Hg for many hours after death. In animals dying of asphyxia the $Po_2$ was always less than 12 mm Hg, even in specimens obtained as early as one hour after death. Osterberg has shown that this is also true for humans in a controlled hospital environment. However, results are equivocal in routine medicolegal cases, and the difficulties in getting valid results in this procedure make it a poor test for routine work.

## Vitreous Toxicology

Vitreous humor is an excellent medium for determination of the presence of alcohol when a question may be raised about possible contamination of blood specimens or when a body has been embalmed and no blood is available for analysis. Many toxic substances diffuse into the vitreous humor and can be of use to forensic pathologists in the estimation of length of time between the administration of a drug and death.

Drugs, including digoxin, barbiturates, propoxyphene, amitryptyline, pentazocine, methadone, salicylates, ethchlorvynol and quinine, have been identified in vitreous humor. However, the variation of drug levels existing between blood and vitreous humor presents considerable difficulty in separating toxic from therapeutic levels of these drugs based on vitreous levels alone.

## REFERENCES

1. Coe, J. I.: Postmortem peripheral blood glucose and cardiopulmonary resuscitation. *Forensic Sci Gazette, 6(4)*:1, 1975.
2. Coe, J. I.: Comparative postmortem chemistries of vitreous humor before and after embalming. *J Forensic Sci, 21*:583, 1976.
3. Coe, J. I.: Postmortem chemistries on human vitreous humor. *Am J Clin Pathol, 51*:741, 1969.
4. Sturner, W. Q.: Lactic acid levels in vitreous humor. Medical Examiner's Office, Providence, Rhode Island, personal communication, 1975.
5. Schleyer, F.: Determinations of the time of death

in the early postmortem interval. In Lundquist, F.: *Methods of Forensic Science,* Vol. 2. New York, Wiley, 1963, pp. 253-293.
6. Coe, J. I.: Further thoughts and observations on postmortem chemistry. *Forensic Sci Gazette, 5(5)*:2, 1973.
7. Fekete, J. F., and Brunsdon, D. F. V.: The use of routine laboratory tests in postmortem examinations. *Can Soc Forensic Sci, 7*:238, 1974.
8. Coe, J. I.: Postmortem chemistries on blood: Particular reference to urea nitrogen, electrolytes and bilirubin. *J Forensic Sci, 19*:33, 1974.
9. Wright, Ronald: Diagnosis of hepatic coma from glutamine level in spinal fluid. Medical Examiner's Office, Miami, Florida, personal communication, 1975.
10. Glanville, J. N.: Postmortem serum cholesterol levels. *Br Med J, 2*:1852, 1960.
11. Enticknap, J. B.: Lipids in cadaver sera after fatal heart attack. *J Clin Pathol, 14*:496, 1961.
12. Enticknap, J. B.: Fatty acid content of cadaver sera in fatal ischemic heart disease. *Clin Sci, 23*:425, 1962.
13. Finlayson, N. B.: Blood cortisol in infants and adults: A postmortem study. *J Pediat, 67*:284, 1965.
14. Coe, J. I.: Postmortem values of thyroxine and thyroid stimulating hormone. *J Forensic Sci, 18*:20, 1973.
15. Lindquist, O., and Rammer, L.: Insulin in postmortem blood. *Z Rechtsmed, 75*:275, 1975.
16. Petty, C. S., Lovel, M. P., and Moore, E. J.: Organic phosphorus insecticides and postmortem blood cholinesterase levels. *J Forensic Sci, 3*: 226, 1958.

*Chapter III*

# IDENTIFICATION OF HUMAN REMAINS

Charles J. Stahl, III

Identification of a deceased person is mandatory for completion of official records, notification of next of kin, settlement of estates and insurance claims and for the establishment of the *corpus delicti* after homicide. Methods of identification that are commonly applied to physical evidence found at the scene of death include fingerprints, bloodstains, hairs, fibers and bite marks.

In the United States the medical examiner or the coroner, as the case may be in the particular jurisdiction, has the statutory authority for the performance of medicolegal autopsies as well as the responsibility for identification. Because of the lack of uniformity in the laws, it is advisable for investigators and pathologists to become familiar with the current laws in their respective jurisdictions. A recent compilation of medicolegal autopsy laws by the U.S. Department of Health, Education and Welfare is available for reference.[1]

Either the medical examiner or the coroner will often participate in the on-the-scene investigation with the law enforcement agency or will arrange to conduct an independent medicolegal investigation. The assistance of other forensic scientists, such as physical anthropologists, serologists, hair and fiber examiners, dentists and fingerprint experts, is often imperative for conclusive identification. The methods used in a given case are dependent upon records available for comparison as well as upon the completeness and the degree of preservation of the remains.

## PHYSICAL EVIDENCE

The interest of the community in the scene of death after the discovery of remains or after a mass disaster is often overwhelming. The disturbance of a scene by curiosity seekers or by poorly trained law enforcement officers may preclude not only accurate identification of the bodies but also complete collection of physical evidence. Therefore, it is recommended that personnel responsible for these medicolegal investigations have clearly defined responsibilities on the scene. Chronological records of all events should be kept. The investigators should establish a perimeter about the scene, maintain effective security within the area, utilize consecutive numbers for the remains, establish the chain of custody and provide an adequate system of communication. Identification problems anticipated in the investigation of mass disasters, particularly aircraft accidents, are discussed in Chapter XVI. Valuable additional information may be obtained from textbooks edited by Reals[2] and Stewart.[3] Examination of evidence found at the scene of a crime may assist in identification of the assailant, provided known information or materials are available for comparison.

On-the-scene investigation in the home of a woman who had been stabbed by an unknown assailant disclosed an avulsed nail (Fig. III-1). Although the nail was well groomed, visual examination did not reveal whether it was a fingernail or a toenail or whether it was from the victim or from the assailant. Since the hands and feet of the victim had not been examined during the autopsy and nail clippings were not available from a suspect, the origin of this nail was not determined. Nevertheless, evidence of this type is amenable to scientific examination. If sufficient blood had been found in the attached tissues of the nail bed, determination of the blood group might have been possible. Ground portions of nails are also suitable for serologic studies to determine the blood group.

Neutron activation analysis is now available for comparative identification of hair and nail clippings, provided hair and nail clippings from

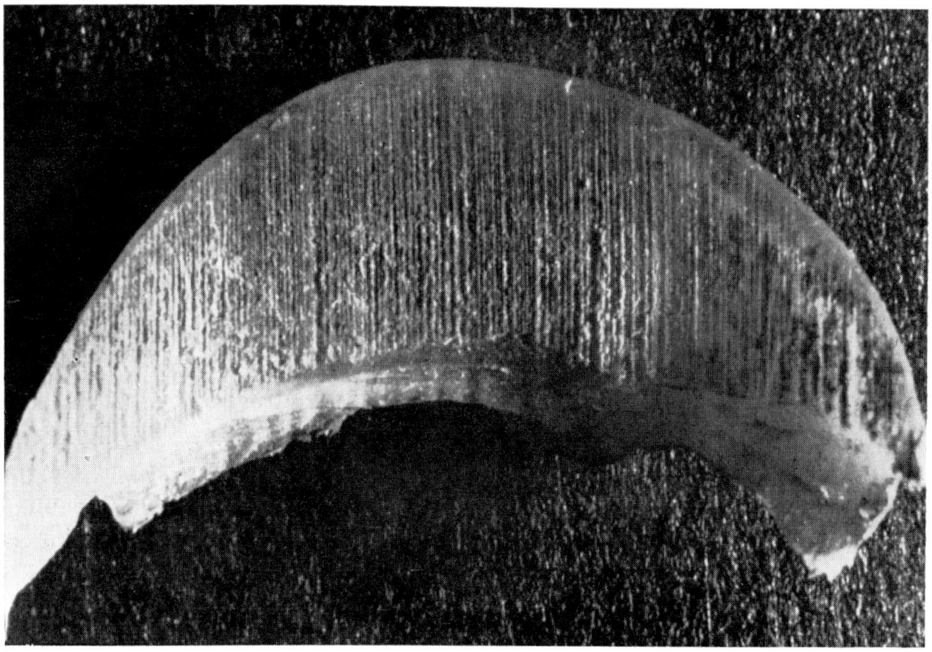

FIGURE III-1. Although the linear striations of an avulsed nail provide the basis for comparison with nails of either the victim or the assailant, identification was not possible in this case because nail clippings of the victim and of the assailant were not available for comparison.

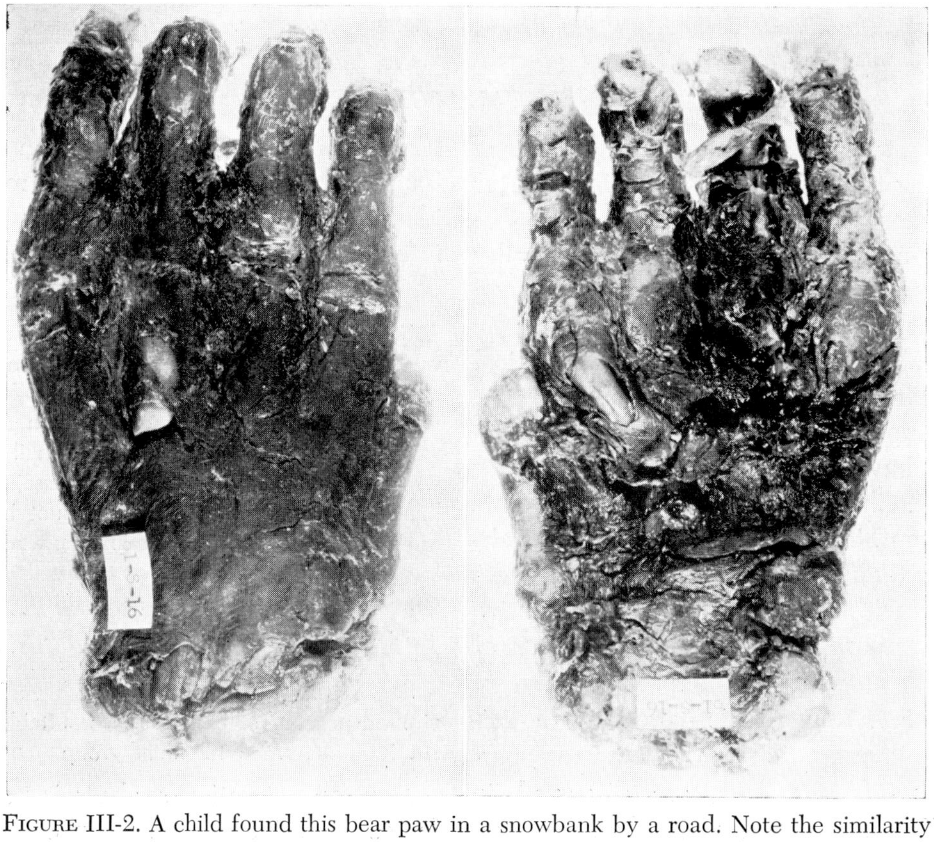

FIGURE III-2. A child found this bear paw in a snowbank by a road. Note the similarity to a decomposed human hand. Further studies were required to identify the specimen as a bear paw.

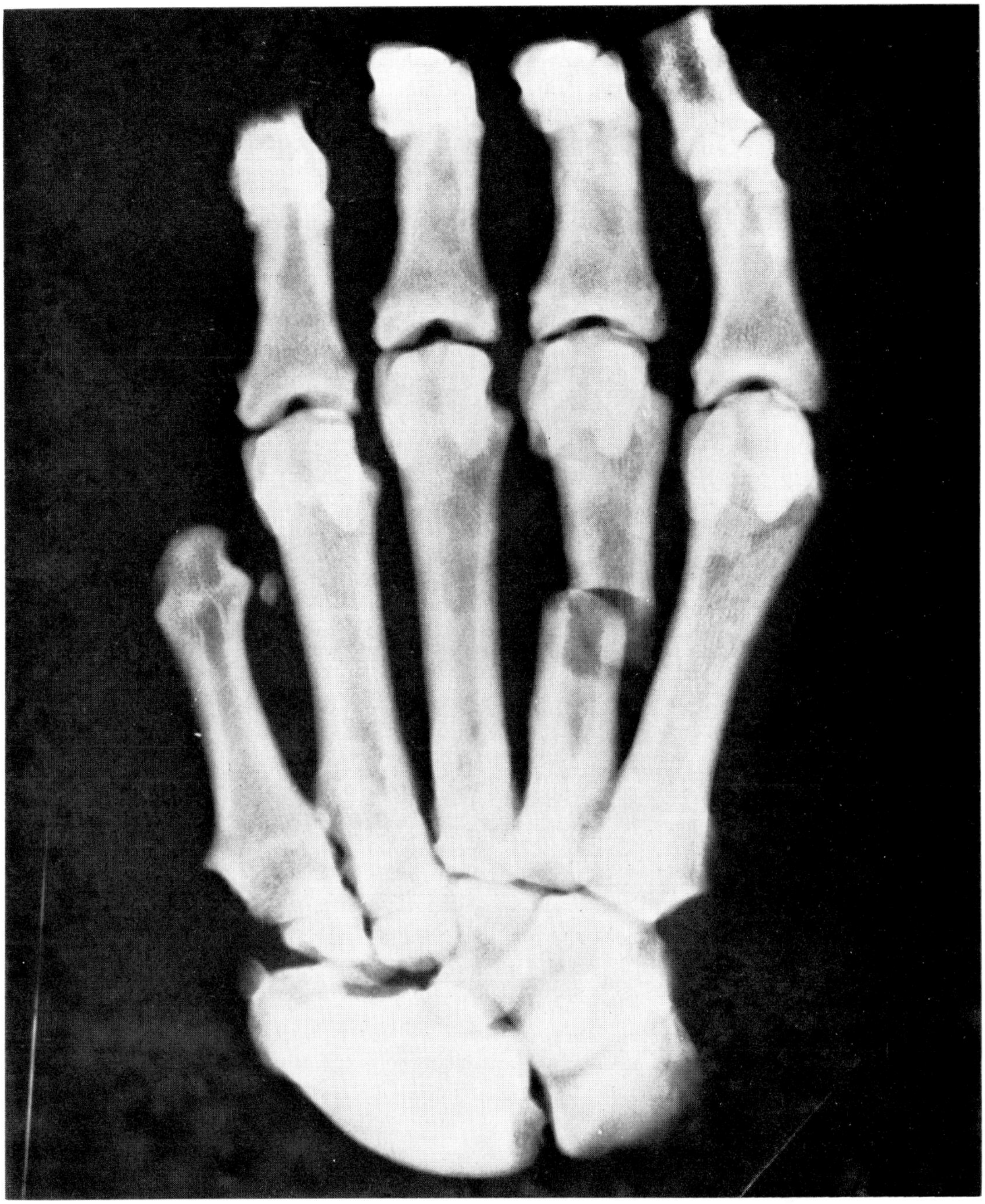

FIGURE III-3. An x ray film of the bear paw seen in Figure III-2 shows the presence of numerous sesamoid bones, as well as a fracture of one bone.

the involved persons are available for comparison.[4] Recently, comparison microscopy has been used by Thomas and Baert[5] to examine the longitudinal striations of fingernails and toenails. It is believed that the pattern of the striae resulting from parallel ridges on the nail bed becomes more prominent with advancing age but remains otherwise unchanged during the life of the person.

Before the medicolegal investigation becomes

extensive and time-consuming, it is important to determine whether or not the remains are human.

During winter an eleven-year-old child found what appeared to be a decomposing hand in a snowbank by a road in a rural area (Fig. III-2). Radiographic examination of the hand disclosed a fracture of the fourth proximal phalanx as well as numerous sesamoid bones (Fig. III-3). The presence and distribution of the metacarpal bones were not consistent with those of a human hand (Fig. III-4). Furthermore, comparison of the scale pattern of hair from the hand with that of human hair did not show similar findings (Fig. III-5). The specimen proved to be a bear paw, most likely discarded by hunters.

The discovery of unidentified bones on his property and a report of a missing person resulted in the imprisonment of a man in a foreign country. He remained in custody for nearly two years pending completion of the examination of the bones. Unfortunately, the bones had been misplaced by a clerk. The age of the missing person and the circumstances leading to the disappearance were unknown. Subsequently, the bones were found and submitted for examination, which revealed that they were not of human origin but most likely from an ungulate animal.

In some cases an extensive amount of information is obtained by examination of unknown remains, but identification is not possible because comparative data are not available.

The remains of an infant were found in a paper bag on a field. Radiologic examination of bones indicated an age of about thirty-seven weeks gestation. The white male infant had been born alive. There were no records available for comparison with the findings, and identification was not possible.

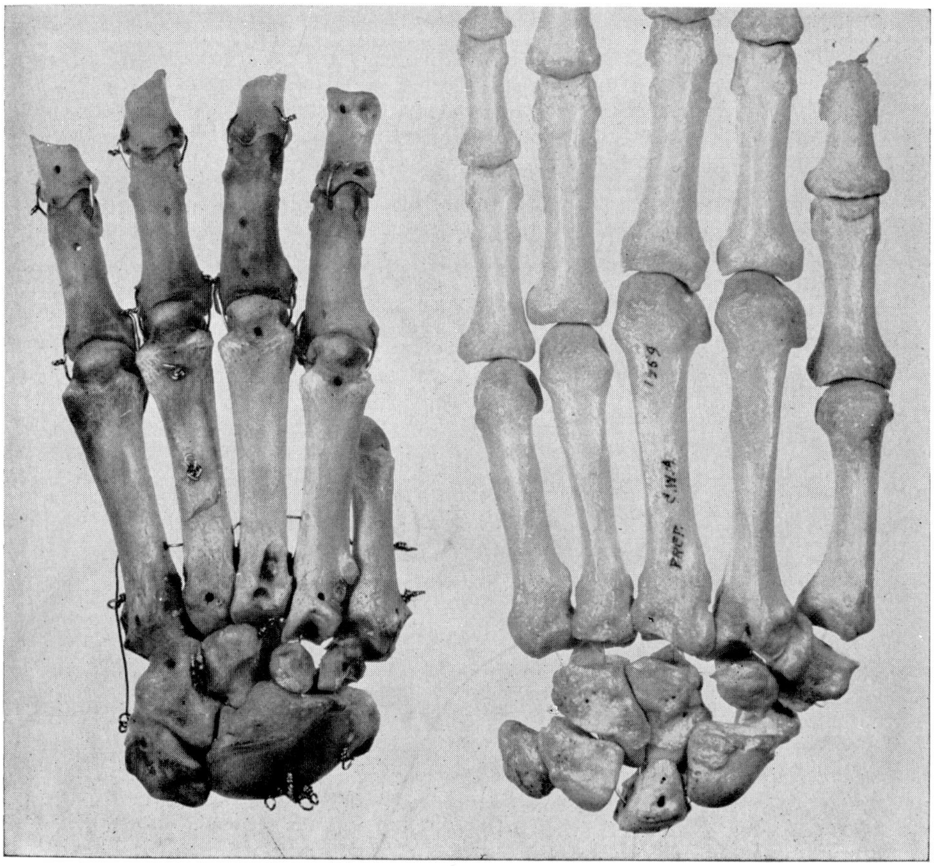

FIGURE III-4. After removal of the soft tissues from the bear paw seen in Figures III-2 and III-3, the bones were assembled in anatomic order and articulated with wire. The bones of the bear paw (left) were compared with the bones of a human hand (right). Note the fracture of one of the bones in the bear paw, as observed previously by roentgenographic examination. Differences in the bones of the wrist are also seen in this photograph.

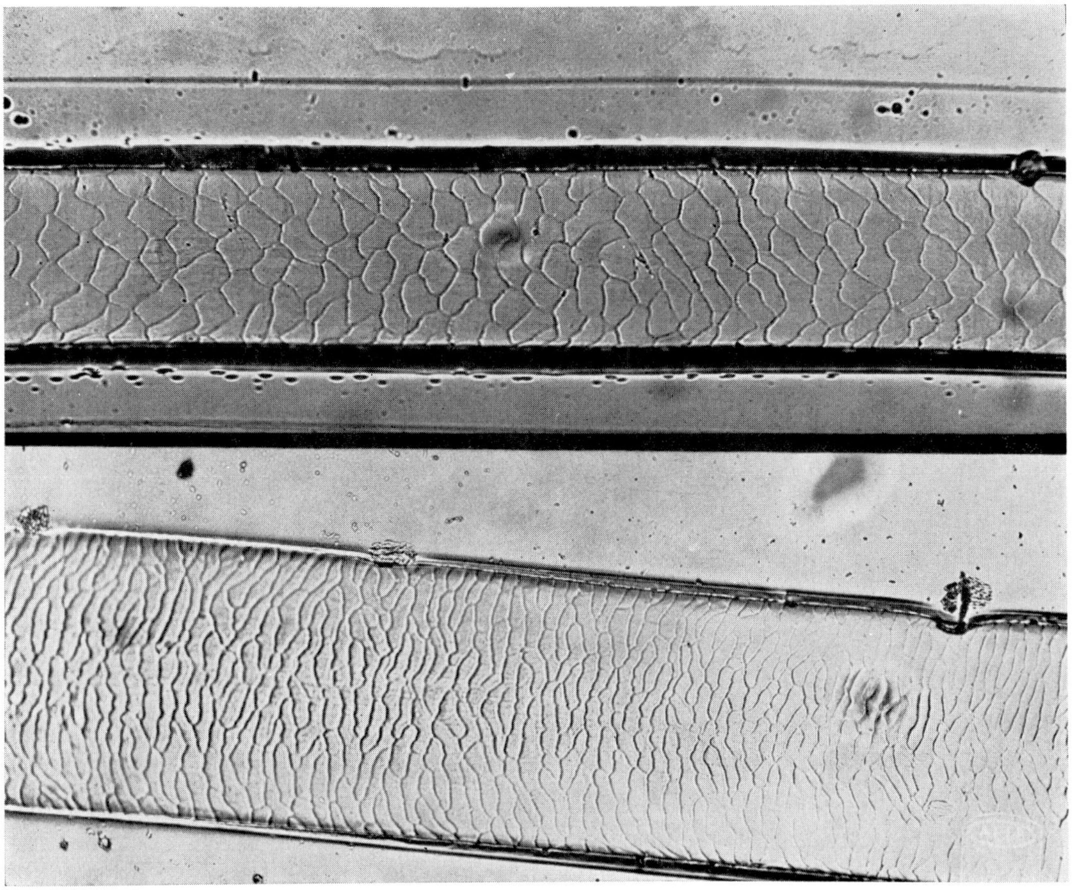

FIGURE III-5. A comparison of the scale pattern of hair from a bear paw (above) is made with the scale pattern of human hair (below). The evaluation of scale pattern, as well as cross sections of hair, is used not only to distinguish animal hair from human hair but also to determine racial groups.

A more interesting and complex case was reported by Finck[6] as follows:

The decomposed remains of a white male were found on an Indian reservation in South Dakota. Although the victim died as the result of a perforating bullet wound of the head, the other six holes on the left side of the skull were old burr holes (Fig. III-6). Extensive pathologic and anthropologic examinations were made, but conclusive identification was not possible due to the absence of appropriate records for comparison.

## METHODS OF IDENTIFICATION

As in the identification of physical evidence, identification of unknown human remains is based upon careful examination, recording of results and comparison with known information. The following records are used for comparison with the results of examinations: reports of missing persons, fingerprints, dental records, health records, x ray films, laboratory reports (such as those of blood group and type), employment records and police records (Fig. III-7).

Information often derived from the external examination of the remains includes sex, age, race, estimate of living stature and weight, color of eyes and hair, evidence of scars, birthmarks, congenital defects or prior injuries, tattoos and occupational marks or injuries (Fig. III-8). The internal examination, along with microscopic examination of selected organs, provides the basis for additional information concerning the cause of death, as well as evidence of prior

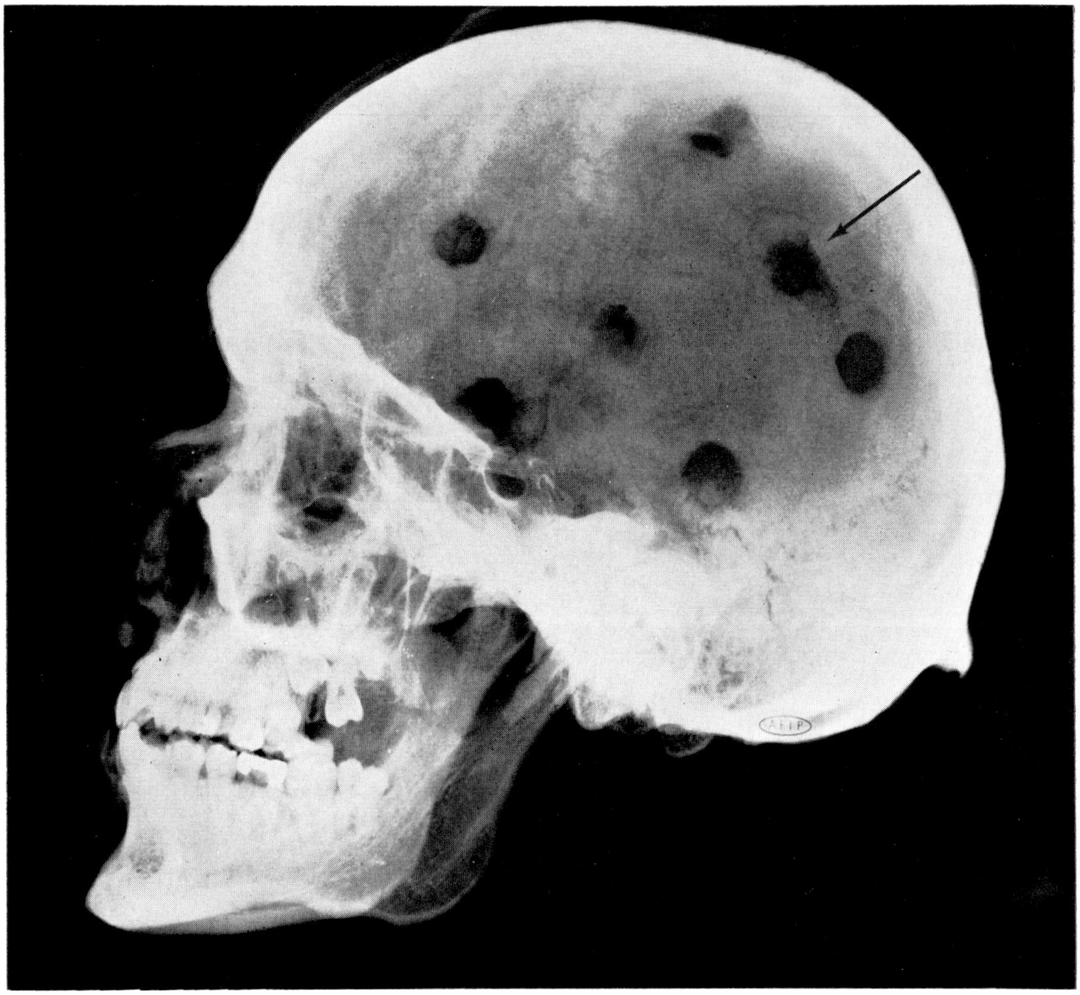

FIGURE III-6. This x ray film of the skull of an unidentified man shows the bullet hole (arrow) as well as the burr holes from previous surgical procedures. Note the fillings in the teeth.

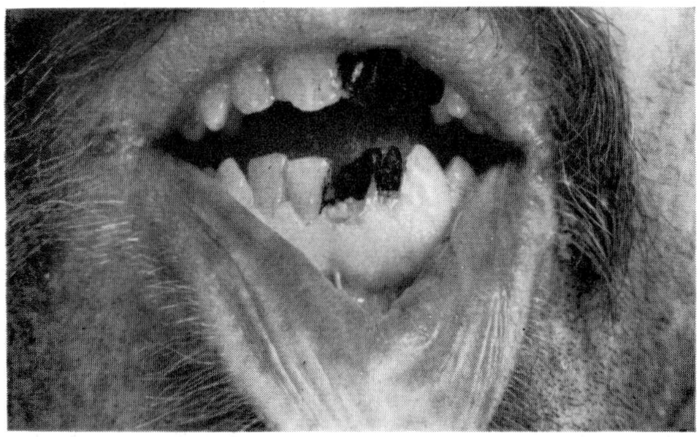

FIGURE III-7. This individual donned a large cap and scarf and blacked out some teeth so as not to be recognized during a robbery. He was shot. The officer fingerprinting the body found cellophane tape over the fingers, another attempt to conceal identity.

disease and injury, to compare with medical records. Photographs of the remains are indicated, particularly of tattoos and distinctive physical features, for comparison with photographs obtained during life. Roentgenographic examination of the remains compared with roentgenographs obtained during life is extremely useful.

### Recognition of Features

The least reliable methods of identification include personal recognition by relatives or friends and the comparative examination of clothing and personal effects. Personal recognition of a person is based upon recall from ex-

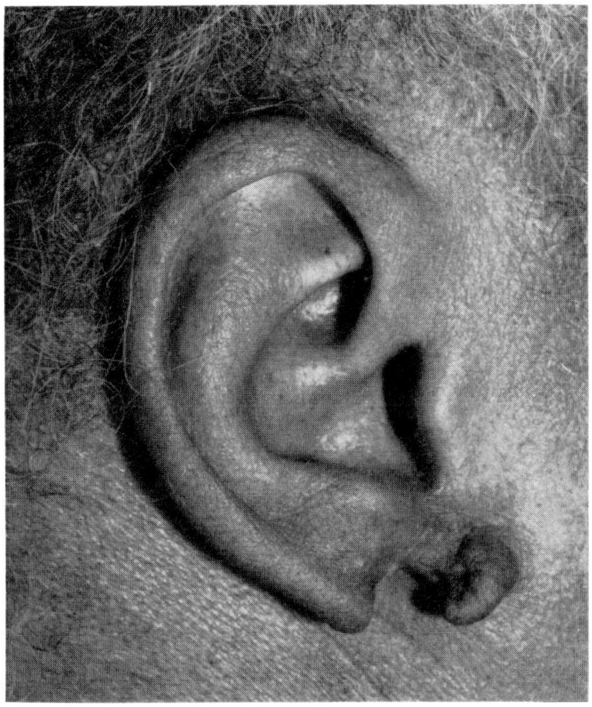

FIGURE III-8. Torn earlobe as a result of wearing a heavy earring for many years. The scarred edge of the tear formed keloid.

perience as well as upon a rapid comparative analysis of physical characteristics. Examination of unidentified remains by possible relatives or friends is often a highly emotional experience, and failure to achieve an identification under such circumstances is not uncommon; it is also possible for an erroneous identification to be made.*

Fingerprints from the deceased would provide proof of identity in questionable cases.

* In order to diminish the emotional impact of identification by direct viewing of the body, the Wayne County Medical Examiner's Office in Detroit has been using closed-circuit black and white television for this purpose. This system, acceptable to the local courts, has minimized the traumatic process of identification and increased the accuracy considerably.

In cases where identification has not been possible by usual means, it has been the practice of the Wayne County Medical Examiner's Office in Detroit to have the news media publish an artist's drawing of the deceased's face (Fig. III-9). We have resorted to these sketches because the newspapers are reluctant to publish actual photographs of dead people. The drawing is accompanied by a brief description of the individual and a public appeal. We have had satisfactory results with this procedure.—ED.

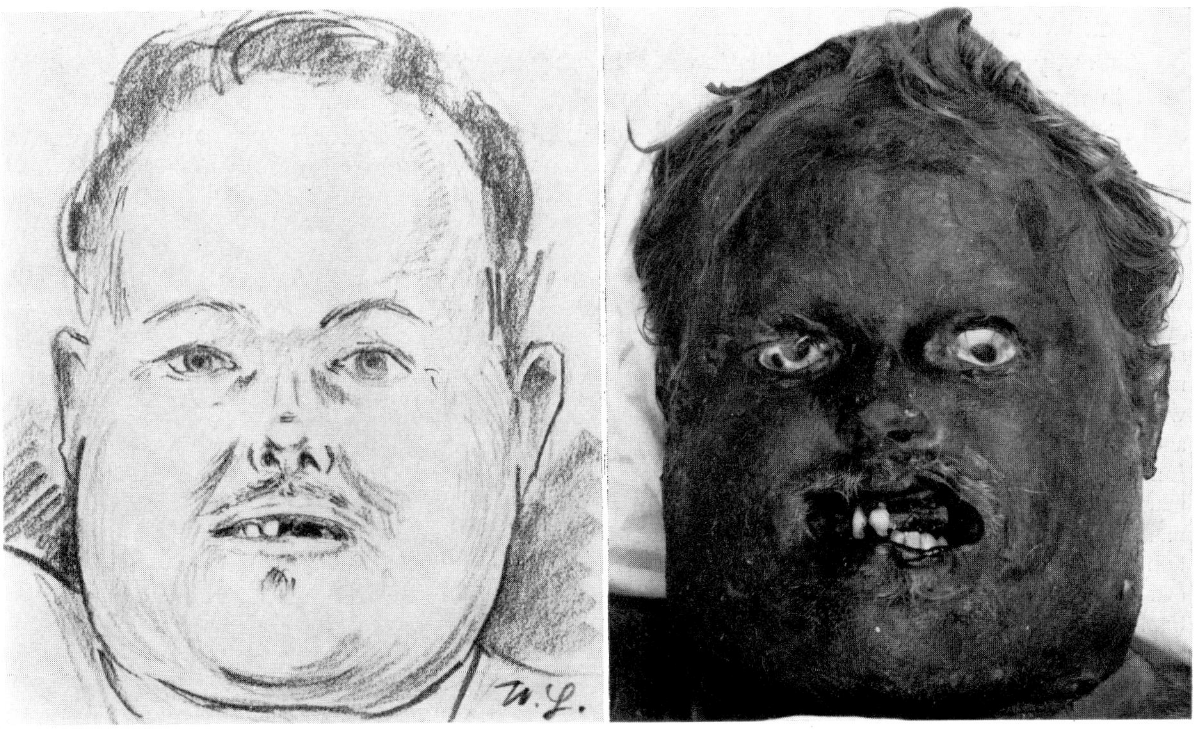

FIGURE III-9. Extremely mummified body of a thirty-four-year-old Caucasian male (right) identified through an artist's sketch published in a major Detroit morning paper (left).

Several medicolegal departments in the United States retain fingerprints in the files of all victims of homicide and many victims of suicide, even if identification has been established by other means.

The characteristic features of the external ear may serve as the basis for comparison, provided prior photographs of the person are available. Iannarelli[7] has described a system for the identification of ears, and further information regarding the comparative identification of ears is also available from physical anthropologists.

Spitz et al.[8] compared the ear and the forehead hairline of an extensively mutilated person with enlarged press photographs of a missing person. Based upon this comparison, the missing person was excluded from further consideration. Conclusive identification of the deceased was made by other means.

If latent prints are available for comparison, lip prints may also serve as a means for identification of remains.[9]

## Clothing and Personal Effects

Examination of clothing and personal effects is frequently helpful in the identification of victims in mass disasters such as fires, explosions and aircraft crashes. Based upon a careful description and examination of each article of clothing and personal items associated with a remains, a comparison is made with reports of missing persons or passenger manifests.

A young man who had been wading along the shore of a tropical island inside the reef was reported missing by two companions, and an air-sea search was begun. A denture, portions of swimming trunks and a nearly skeletal right lower extremity with canvas shoe were found. Jagged marks along the lower margins of the swimming trunks were consistent with marks made by shark teeth. The name and identification number of the victim were inside the shoe on the extremity, thus permitting the presumptive identification.

Following a fire in a house trailer, the charred remains of two men were found. The external examination revealed remnants of clothing, including laundry marks. A comparison of the identification numbers of the victims with the laundry marks, as well as differences in the color of hair, provided the presumptive identification of the men. Subsequently, conclusive identification of the victims was made by dental methods.

Clothing provides a clue to the social status and occupation of the deceased. Bullet holes, cuts or tire marks found upon examination of a victim's clothing may yield information regarding the cause and manner of death. The report of examination should include a detailed description of the size, color, condition and type of each garment and a record of laundry marks, name tags and labels (Fig. III-10). Most long-term care facilities, i.e. nursing homes, county hospitals, etc., mark patients' personal clothing with at least a name. Some maintain a ward clothing *grab bag* with all pieces marked with the hospital name and ward number. Photographs and examination for invisible laundry marks by ultraviolet light are indicated. The sex of the deceased is not always represented by the articles of clothing found on the body. Frequently people wear unisex-type clothing. Rarely there is the possibility that the death was associated with transvestism during autoerotic activities.

The requirements for the examination of personal effects are similar to those for clothing. Military identification tags and dentures are quite resistant to thermal effects. Exposure of

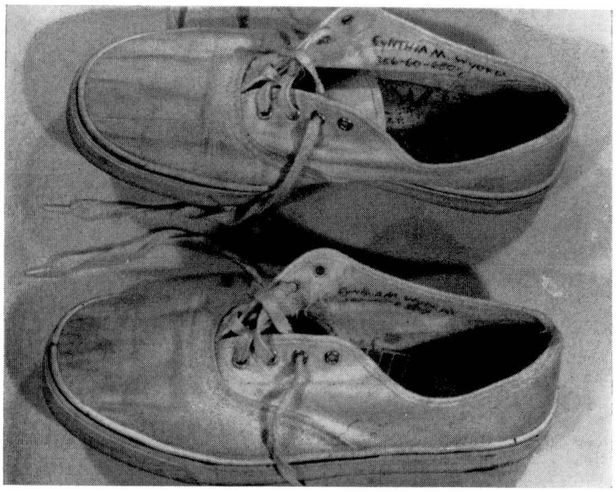

FIGURE III-10. The name and social security number in the shoes provided identification of this young woman. She had jumped off a bridge, and her markedly decomposed body was found several weeks later.

identification tags to temperatures between 1700° and 2500° F results in oxidation of the surface without significant structural change. The imprinted tags remain legible at temperatures up to 2500°F, but the metal tends to fuse above this temperature. Dental identification is discussed in Chapter IV, but recent advances in the use of dentures for identification are worthy of mention.

Although gold alloys melt and synthetic porcelain fuses at temperatures between 1600° and 2000° F, teeth of dentures are often resistant to temperatures over 2000° F (Fig. III-11). Jerman[10] has reviewed the role of dentures in identification by the military services in the United States, and he recommends the incorporation of the social security number and branch of service of the individual into the denture base of each complete or partial denture (Fig. III-12). The social security number is typed on stainless steel metal .001 in. thick in the denture base and covered with a clear resin. The application of the social security number is significant, for nearly all American adults have an assigned number. The Dental Corps of the United States Navy has promulgated the recommendation by Jerman.[11]

Wallets and keys are also helpful for identification. Membership cards, licenses and credit cards establish appropriate information for comparison with records of missing persons, provided there has been no attempt at criminal interchange of identity. The distinctive shape and markings on keys yield information about the characteristics of the locks for which they are designed. If they provide access to an automobile or a home of a missing person, presumptive evidence of identification is accomplished. Other personal effects, particularly watches, identification bracelets, rings and belt buckles are often engraved with initials, names or dates.

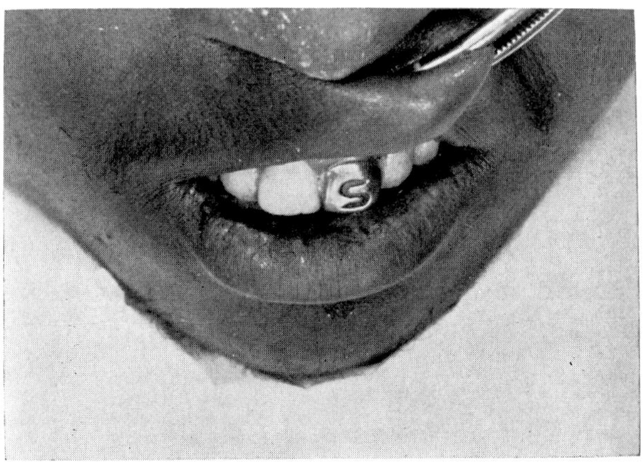

FIGURE III-11. A gold cap on a tooth, inscribed with an initial or a design, assists in identification.

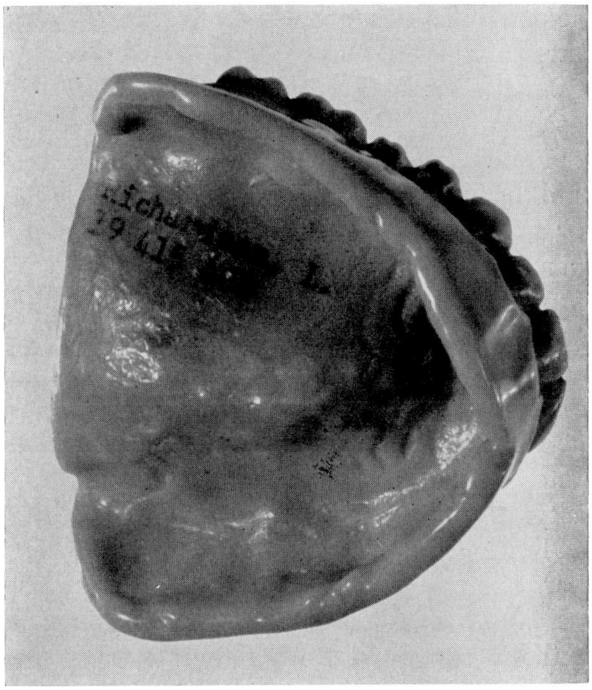

FIGURE III-12. Since dental plates are quite resistant to the effects of trauma and heat, they serve as an excellent location for the name and identification number of the owner.

### Fingerprints

The most reliable method of identification is that of fingerprinting. During the eighth and ninth centuries in China fingerprints were used in sales contracts for the identification of persons and also for the identification of immigrants and visitors.[12] Official documents dated 1691 in an English cathedral have signatures as well as thumbprints and fingerprints for identification.[13] Nevertheless, the application of fingerprinting to the identification of criminals did not occur until the latter portion of the nineteenth century, and the greatest advances in the scientific applications of fingerprints occurred in the twentieth century.

Based upon the ideas of Dr. Henry Faulds in Japan and Sir William James Herschel in India, Sir Francis Galton, a cousin of Charles Darwin, published the results of his own research, *Finger Prints,* in 1892. During the same decade Juan Vucetich, a police official in Argentina, and Inspector-General of Police Edward Richard Henry in Bengal, India, studied Galton's work independently and developed systems for the classification of fingerprints. Modifications of the Henry system are used today in the United States. Fingerprinting for identification of criminals was introduced in England and Wales in 1901 and in the United States in the following year. The rapid adoption of fingerprints as the preferred method for identification of criminals in the United States after 1903 was the result of the fallibility of other methods. A national repository for data was developed by the Identification Division of the Federal Bureau of Investigation (FBI) in 1924.

When the hands of a deceased individual are well preserved, fingerprints provide the basis for rapid, conclusive identification in the United States. The files of the Identification Division of the FBI contain fingerprint records for nearly 100 million persons. These records are supplemented by fingerprint records in the files of state and local law enforcement agencies. Attempts at obliteration of identity by mutilation of the patterns or by skin grafts have been unsuccessful. It may be difficult to obtain adequate prints if the remains have been immersed, putrefied, desiccated or charred. Under some circumstances where the skin of the fingers is wrinkled, it may be possible to obtain adequate prints by injection of warm water under the skin. Also, the flap of wrinkled skin may be cut out and dressed on the examiner's finger, then inked and printed. Dried fingertips are best soaked in warm water until soft and pliable. Other procedures are available to alleviate problems for the procurement of legible prints.[14] The Identification Division of the FBI will assist local police departments in difficult cases. Amputation of the hands of a body at the wrists and submission to the FBI will frequently provide identification in cases in which other methods have failed.

Separation of the epidermis in a manner not unlike a glove is frequently observed in victims recovered from water or exposed to severe heat. A similar phenomenon occurs in the course of putrefaction. This glovelike separation of the skin may be used to obtain fingerprints. If the areas to be fingerprinted are damaged, the internal aspect of the *glove* may be used for the same purpose, giving a mirror image of the prints. Should the *glove* be unavailable, adequate impressions may nevertheless be obtained from the denuded hand.

The fine pattern of ridges in the skin can be found also on parts of the palms of the hands as well as on the soles of the feet and on the toes. Thus, if the hospital record for an infant includes legible footprints, the comparison of toeprints, ridge details and flexion creases may also serve as the basis for identification.[15] Footprints have been filed in the records of certain military pilots of high-performance aircraft for comparison, but this practice is not widespread.

In 1879 Alphonse Bertillon, an assistant in the First Prefecture of Police in Paris, France, developed a method for identification of criminals based upon skeletal, or anthropometric, measurements. He believed that the dimensions of the human skeleton did not change during adult life and that with the use of fourteen different anthropometric measurements there was theoretically only one chance in 286 million of finding an exactly identical person. The fallibility of the system of bertillonage was discovered in 1903 when two federal prisoners named William West and Will West, respectively, were found to have not only eleven identical anthropometric measurements but also similar physical appearances. Fingerprints, however, were dissimilar and provided the basis for identification.

### Roentgenologic Examinations

Roentgenologic examinations are helpful not only in the evaluation of poorly preserved re-

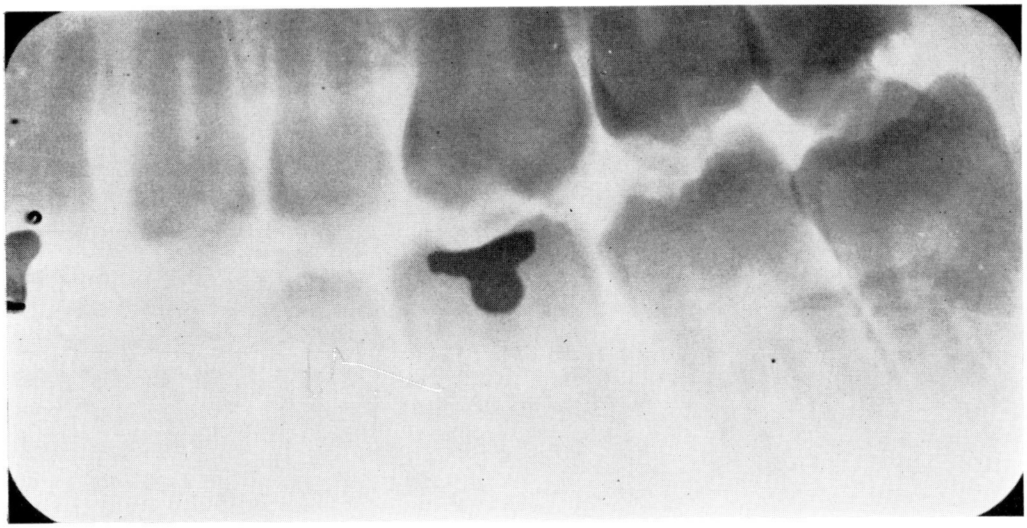

A

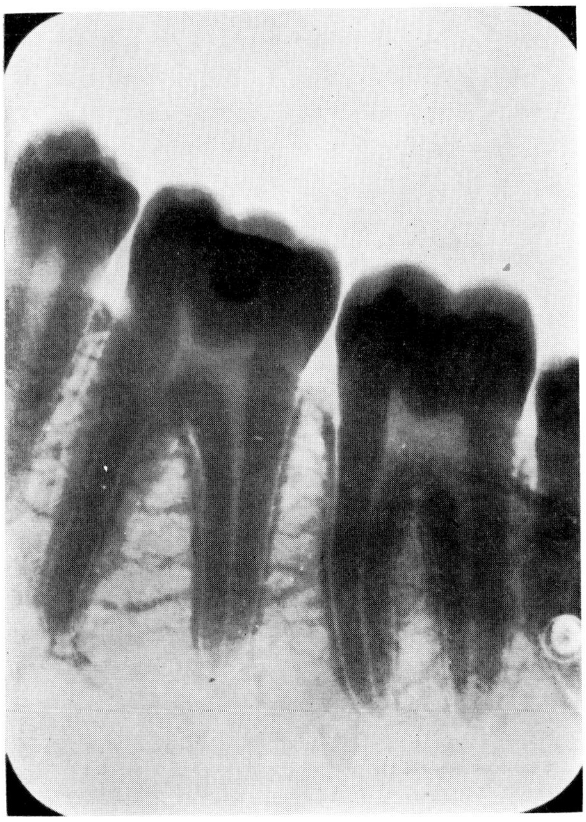

B

FIGURE III-13. The skeletal remains of a man were found in a wooded area nearly five months after he had been reported missing. He had died as the result of a perforating bullet wound of the chest, and a rifle was found between the lower extremities of the skeletal remains. Dental examination disclosed a single filling in the first lower right molar tooth, and an x ray film of the teeth (above) provided the basis for comparison with dental roentgenograms obtained during the life of the individual (below).

mains but also for the examination of clothing and personal effects. Foreign material and metallic objects not observed prior to or during the postmortem examination may be detected by x ray films. Prior to the preparation of permanent films, it is often desirable to examine remains, clothing and personal effects by fluoroscopy. If the remains are skeletonized, badly putrefied or charred, foreign bodies or metallic fragments, such as bullets, may be observed by x rays. When commingled (or mixed) bones are found, the use of ultraviolet light before roentgenographic examination may enable segregation of bones of different persons.[16] Dental roentgenograms, when compared with films obtained during life, frequently serve as the basis for identification in the absence of other dental records (Fig. III-13).

The skeletal remains of a young woman, subsequently identified as a Mongolian female, were discovered in a wooded area near an abandoned sand quarry. Although the specific cause of death was not determined, the circumstances indicated that she had been murdered. Based upon examination of the skeletal remains, including hair and teeth, and comparison with reports of missing persons and health records, her identification was confirmed. An x ray film of the pelvis of the skeleton compared with an x ray film of the pelvis of the woman obtained during life (Fig. III-14) showed

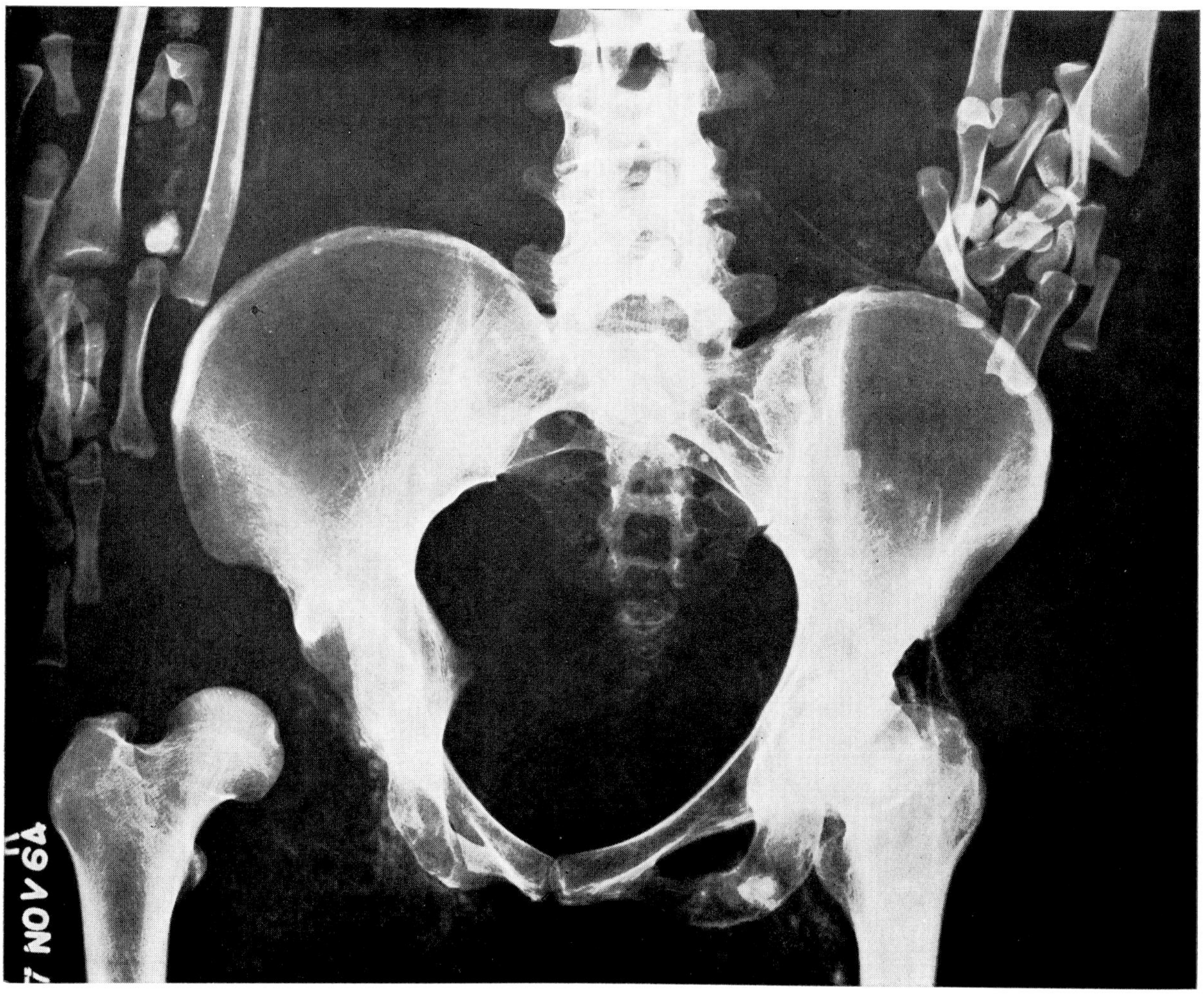


FIGURE III-14a. Roentgenograms of these pelvic skeletal remains were compared with roentgenograms taken during life of the young woman believed to be the deceased. This comparison disclosed identical features.

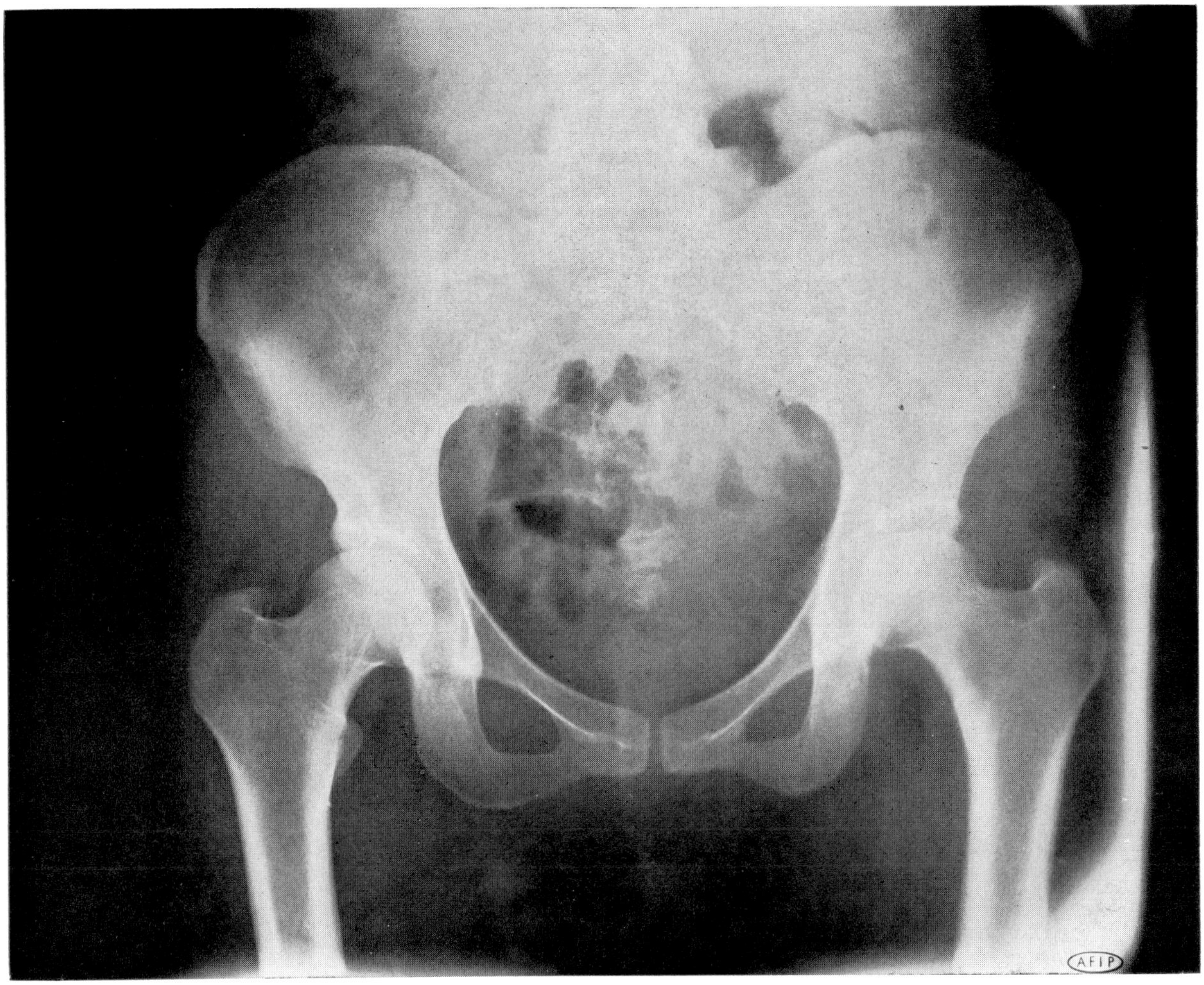


FIGURE III-14b. X ray film of the pelvis taken during life that served as the basis for comparison with postmortem films of the skeleton mentioned in Figure III-14a.

identical features. The contours of the iliac crest, the stress lines and the trabecular pattern of the femoral head and neck and the distinctive features in the spinous and transverse processes of the vertebrae served as the basis for this comparison.

During the autopsy of the victim of an aircraft accident a vascular malformation of a vertebra was found (Fig. III-15a). Roentgenographic examination of the vertebral bodies obtained at autopsy served as the basis for comparison with x ray films of the victim during life (Fig. III-15b). Microscopic examination of the vertebra confirmed the diagnosis of vascular malformation.

In children and young adults roentgenographic evaluation of the degree of ossification and fusion of epiphyses, as well as the development of teeth, serves as the basis for estimation of age. Standard tables are available for comparison with the findings.[17, 18] When previous x ray films of the skull are available for comparison with postmortem films, measurements of the skull and a detailed evaluation of the frontal sinuses, sphenoid bones and mastoid area may serve as the basis for identification in adults.[19]

A motorist and his wife saw a burning automobile parked on a dirt road in a rural area. While they were calling the fire department, they heard an explosion. Dense black smoke came from the windows of the burning vehicle. By the time firemen arrived at the scene, the interior of the vehicle had burned completely. When the blaze was extinguished, a charred body was discovered on the front seat. The exterior of the vehicle did not appear damaged except for scorch-

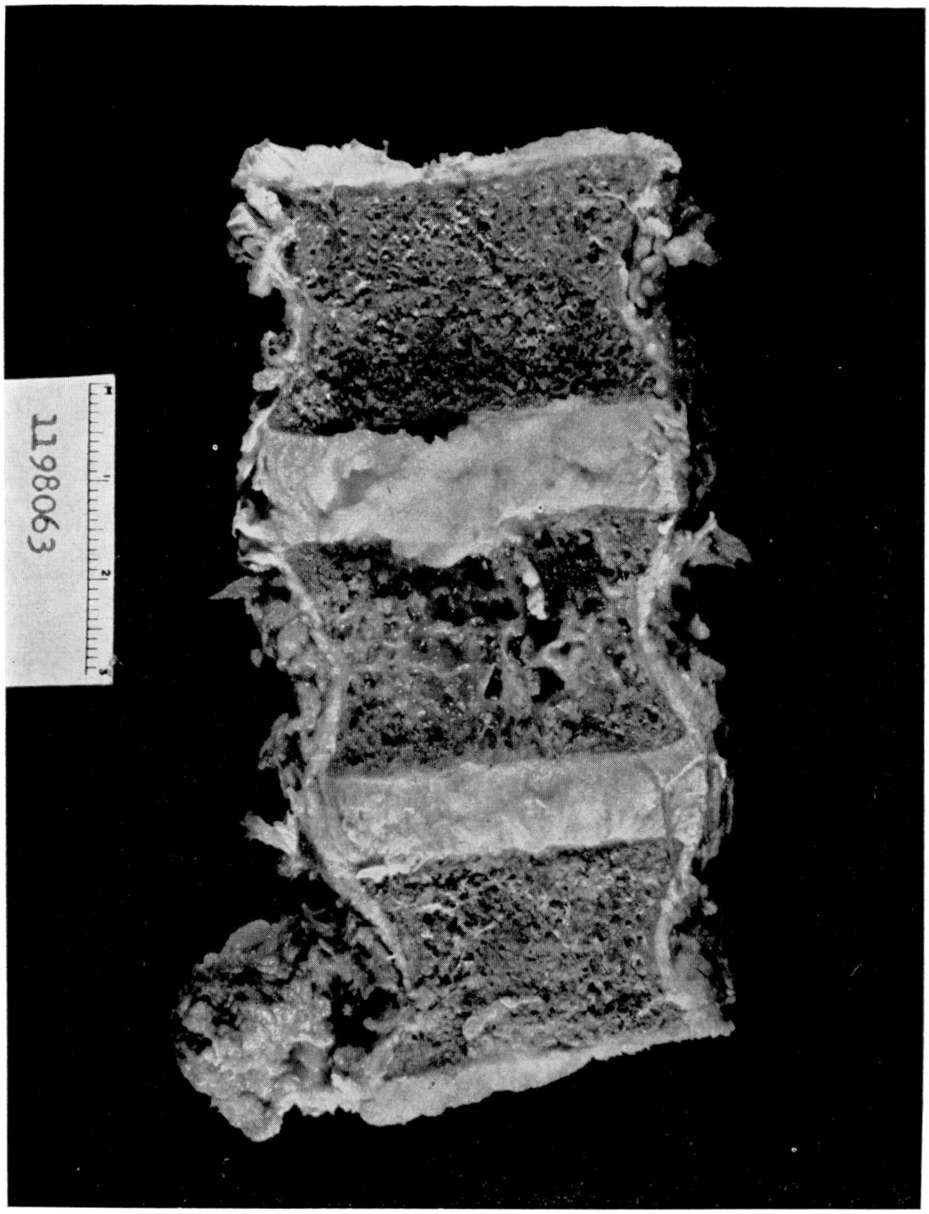

FIGURE III-15a. A vascular malformation or hemangioma is seen in the vertebra in the center of this photograph. A comparison of the pathologic findings with medical records and x ray films may serve as the basis for presumptive identification of the deceased.

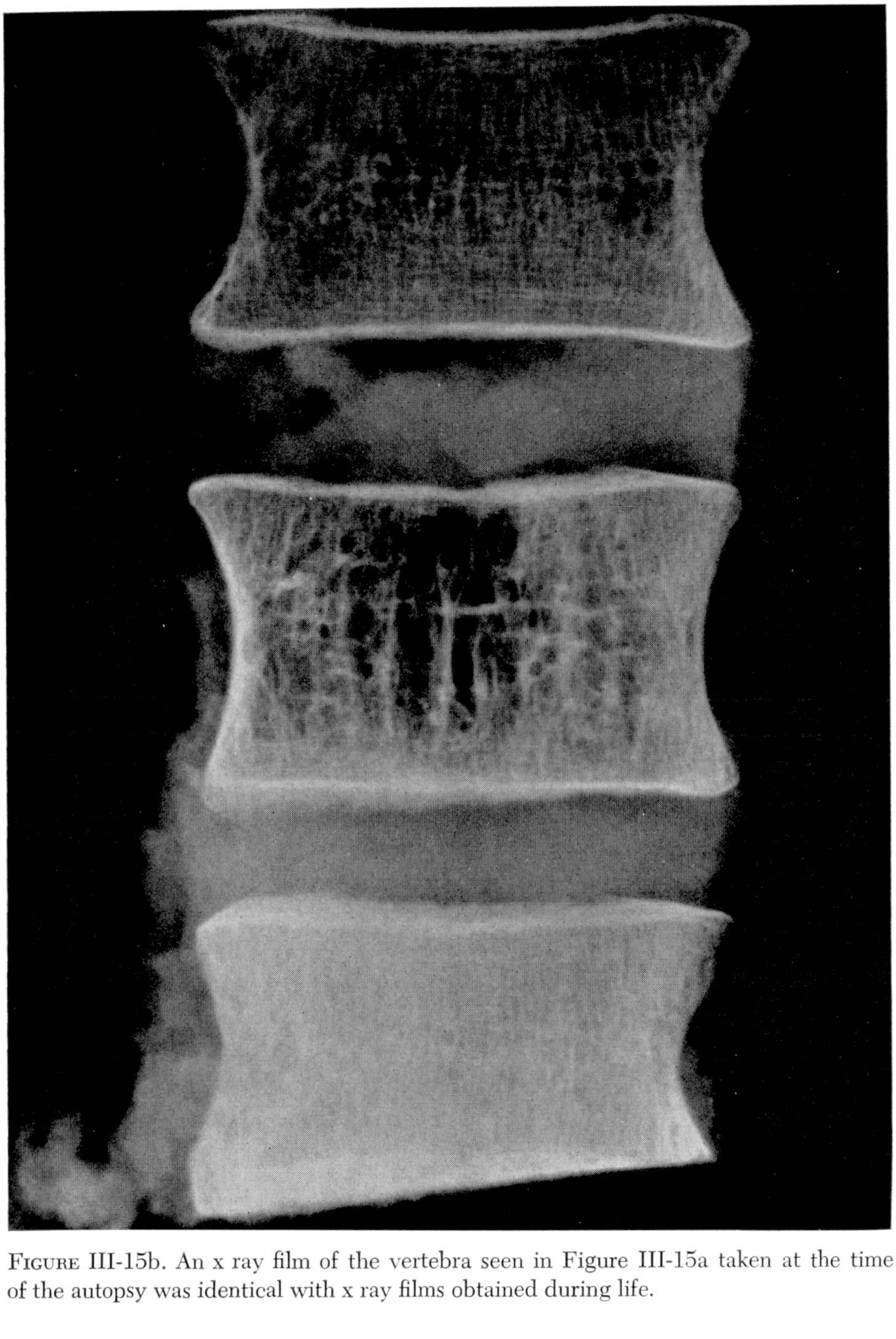

FIGURE III-15b. An x ray film of the vertebra seen in Figure III-15a taken at the time of the autopsy was identical with x ray films obtained during life.

ing of the paint on the roof and window frames. A tentative identification of the victim was made from the registration records of the vehicle. Except for charred remnants of a left shoe and fragments of cloth about the groin, no articles of clothing were observed. Near the head, spectacles and a charred one-gallon gasoline can were found. Irregular, hard globules of molten metal were noted on the body and the front floor of the vehicle. All of the instrument knobs of the vehicle had melted, including the ignition switch. Identification of the victim was made by dental and anthropologic methods as well as by comparison of the postmortem findings, the examination of the spectacles and medical records (Figs. III-16 and III-17; Tables III-I, III-II and III-III). Postmortem toxicologic studies were negative. Total body x ray films were compared with previous roentgenographs of the chest, cervical spine and skull. The films revealed similar dental restorations in the teeth, and the roentgenographic features of the maxilla, mandible and cervical spine were identical.

A review of medical records revealed that the man had received 0.25 mg of reserpine twice daily for over six months. His clinical diagnoses included arteriosclerotic cardiovascular disease, benign hypertension and mild diabetes. During the period he had been on therapy with reserpine his associates noted that he had become increasingly depressed. According to the manufacturer, mental depression is one of the adverse effects of *Rauwolfia* preparations such as reserpine, and the possibility of suicide should be given consideration. In this case the medicolegal investigation disclosed that the manner of death was suicide and that the death resulted from the extensive thermal burns.

Two boys were riding through the woods when they came upon the remains of a human body. State police

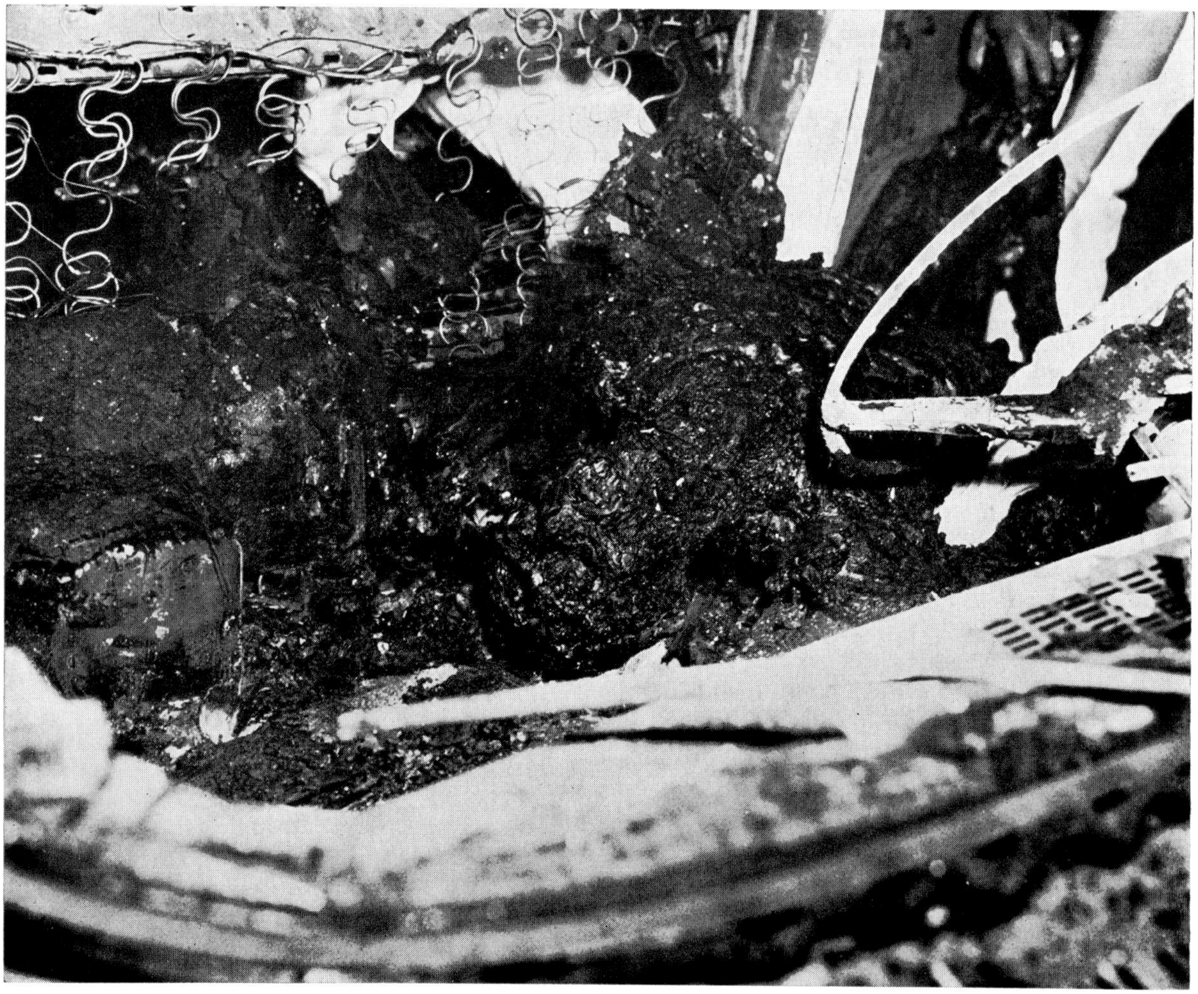

FIGURE III-16. The remains of a burned body are seen through the broken windshield of the automobile. Note the container for gasoline on the right side of the front seat.

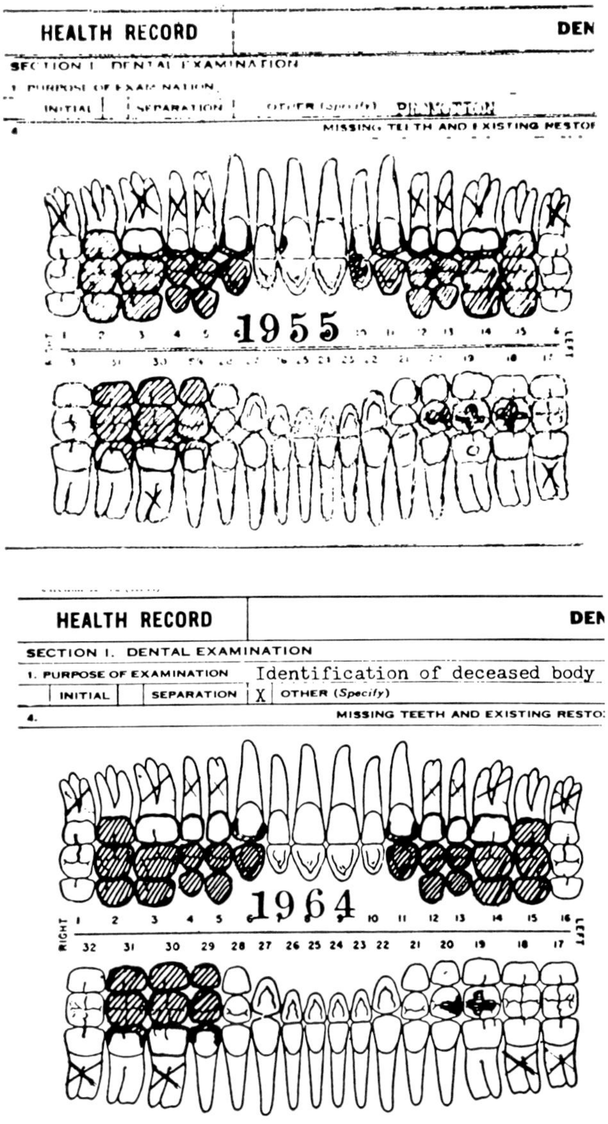


FIGURE III-17. The dental records prepared in 1955 were similar to those records prepared during the identification of the deceased man in 1964.

TABLE III-II

IDENTIFICATION OF SPECTACLES

| | | | |
|---|---|---|---|
| Spectacle Prescription: | | | |
| "OD | +2.00 − 1.50 × 110 | | |
| OS | +1.75 − 1.00 × 80 | | |
| Add | +2.25 (split between trifocal)" | | |
| Damaged Spectacle Prescription (civilian trifocals): | | | |
| OD | +2.26 = −1.50 × 104 | | |
| OS | +2.00 = −1.00 × 76 | Pd = 68/65 | |
| Add | OD INTER. +1.50 | Add N.P. | +3.25 |
| | OS +1.50 | | +3.25 |
| Frame: | | | |
| Shuron All Aluminum | Bridge | 22mm | |
| | Temple | 4½ 5¾″ | |
| | Box | 48mm | |
| Flat-Top Trifocal | Pd 68/65 | | |
| | 25mm Segment | | |
| | 7mm Inter. | | |

The prescription for the spectacles is similar to the results of the examination of the damaged spectacles. The characteristic features of the frame of the spectacles were identical; the differences in the prescription for the lenses were attributed to the effects of heat.

were notified. The right hand was missing, the lower arm of the victim had been chewed by animals and the abdominal viscera were absent (Fig. III-18). The decomposed remains were infested by maggots. Subsequent examination of the skull and the petrous portion of the temporal bones revealed that the middle ear had irregular spaces within the bone, and these spaces were surrounded by dense sclerotic bone. Identification of the victim as a 53-year-old white man (Fig. III-19) who had disappeared from a state mental institution several months prior to the discovery of his body was confirmed by the fact that he had a medical history of a chronic ear infection.

Comparison of x ray films taken during life with a postmortem film revealed the following similarities: the general configuration of the thorax and of the ribs were the same; patterns of the scapulae were the same; there were bilateral calcifications of the first costal

TABLE III-I

ESTIMATION OF LIVING STATURE BY EQUATION OF TROTTER AND GLESER

1 inch equals 2.54 centimeters

Estimated Living Stature (cm) = 2.52 $\text{Tibia}_m$ + 78.62 ± 3.37

Total Length of Right Tibia (from intercondylar eminences to tip of medial malleolus, measured parallel to shaft) = 14.5 inches = 36.83 centimeters.

Estimated Living Stature (cm) = 2.52 × 36.83 + 78.62 ± 3.37
= 92.81 + 78.62 ± 3.37
= 171.43 ± 3.37
= 168.16 to 174.70

Estimated Living Stature (inches) = 66.2 to 68.7

Estimation of living stature, based upon careful measurement of a long bone, is provided by the equation of Trotter and Gleser.

TABLE III-III

IDENTIFICATION OF UNKNOWN HUMAN REMAINS

| *Unknown* | *Known* |
|---|---|
| Male | Male |
| Caucasian | Caucasian |
| Hair: red and gray | Hair: red and gray |
| Blood Group: O | Blood Group: O |
| Rh: Positive | Rh: Unknown |
| Height: 66″ to 69″ | Height: 68½″ |
| Weight: Unknown | Weight: 130 pounds |
| Eyeglasses: Presbyopia | Eyeglasses: Presbyopia |
| Teeth: Extensive gold bridgework | Teeth: Extensive gold bridgework |
| Personal Effects: Distinctive gold ring on left hand | Personal Effects: Distinctive ring |
| Physical Defects: Enlarged right lobe, thyroid gland | Physical Defects: Enlarged right lobe, thyroid |
| Benign prostatic hypertrophy | Benign prostatic hypertrophy |
| Arteriosclerosis of aorta, internal carotid arteries, coronary arteries | Arteriosclerotic cardiovascular disease |

The identification of an unknown body is based upon comparison with information derived from the reports of missing persons, health records, dental records, fingerprint records and the autopsy. As a result of extensive burns, fingerprints were not available for comparison in this case. A comparison of the known data with the information derived from the examination is tabulated for comparison.

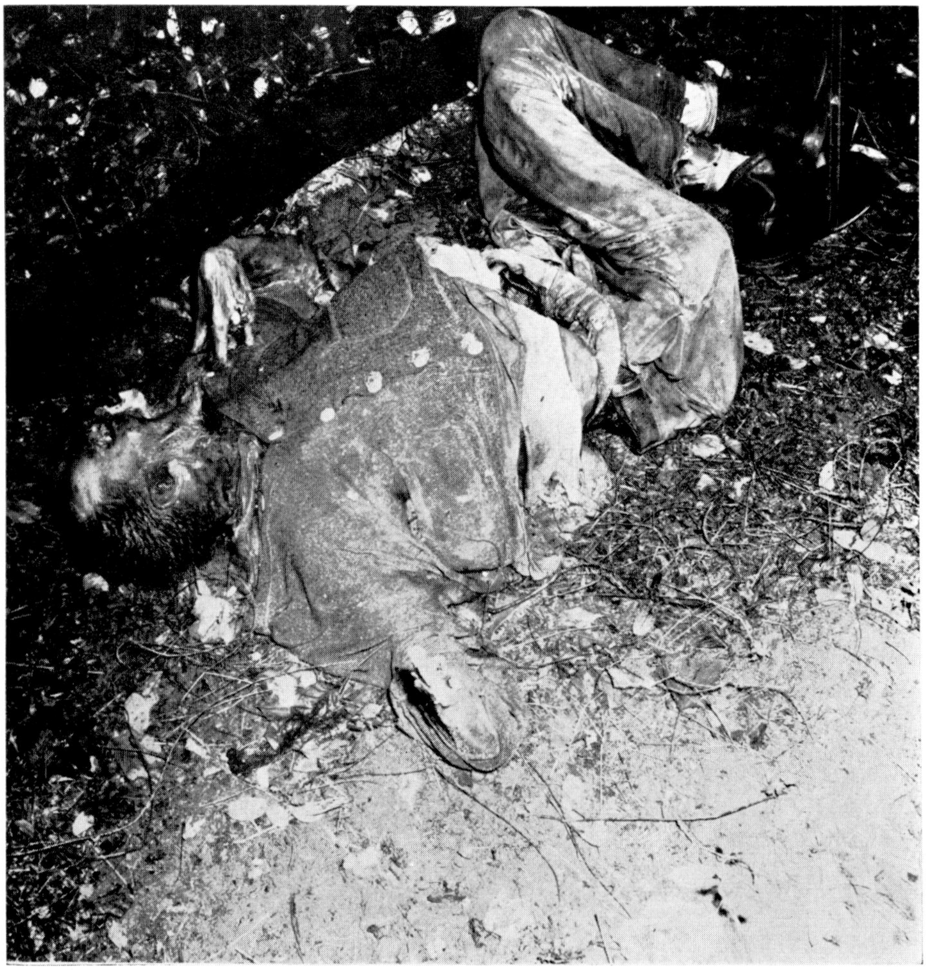

FIGURE III-18. The decomposed body of a man was found in a wooded area. The right hand was absent, and the bones of the forearm had been chewed by carnivorous animals.

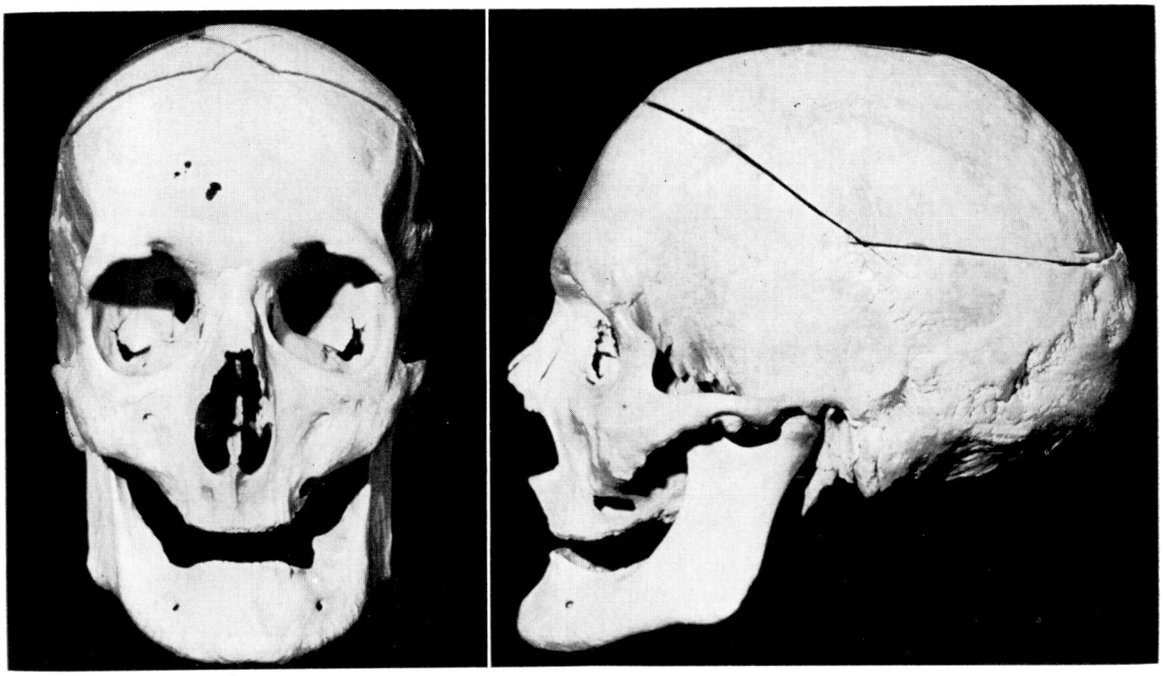

FIGURE III-19. (a): The features of the skull are consistent with those of a middle-aged or elderly Caucasian male. The cause of the erosion of bone in the frontal area is unknown. (b): The lateral view of the skull shows the prominent mastoid bone and brow ridge, the absence of teeth and of prognathism, and closure of the cranial sutures.

cartilages, and the left first costal cartilage had a beak-like configuration on both films; the lower borders of the posterior aspects of the eighth, ninth, and tenth ribs were similar. The estimate of living stature of 5′5″ to 5′8″ was based upon measurement of the right femur and the use of the formula of Trotter and Gleser.[20] The actual height of the subject was 5′5½″.

The art of mummification, developed in Egypt as early as the fourth dynasty (2613-2494 BC) and highly developed by the twenty-first dynasty (1085-935 BC), was used for the preservation of bodies prior to entombment. Gray[21] examined mummies in the museums of Great Britain and other European countries. He found that radiographic examination of these mummies was helpful not only for the estimation of age and the determination of sex but also for the evaluation of embalming techniques and paleopathology.

### Skeletal Examination

The finding of skeletal remains usually warrants consultation with a physical anthropologist. Whereas older studies of skeletal remains were mostly based on morphological traits in a descriptive manner, newer studies focus primarily on measurements and statistical evaluation. Advanced decomposition, mutilation or incineration of a body often limit the extent of the information obtained from other scientific methods of examination. It is appropriate, therefore, to derive the information required for identification from the examination of the skeleton. Human bones are remarkably resistant to the effects of time and environment. To a lesser extent they are also resistant to the effects of heat. An extremely high temperature of prolonged duration is required to completely consume the bony structures.

An incomplete skeleton, as well as the possibility of commingled bones, may limit the information derived from the examination. If commingling of bones from more than one skeleton is suspected, a shortwave ultraviolet lamp is used to segregate the bones. When the surfaces of bones are exposed to ultraviolet radiation they reflect a variety of colors. The radiated color is derived from fluorescence of organic elements in the bones, inorganic substances on the surface of the bones and, to a lesser extent, reflected light. The differences in color emissions of commingled skeletal remains serve as a basis for their separation.[16]

The skeletal remains of one person or several people after segregation should be arranged in anatomic order. It is indicated to accompany the description of the remains with appropriate photographs and diagrams of the skeleton to record the findings. Subsequently, a correlation of the findings can be made with missing persons records of alleged victims. If teeth are present with the skeletal remains, they are perhaps the most reliable means of identification, as discussed in Chapter IV, provided appropriate dental records are available for comparison.

A purse containing identification cards of a woman was found, along with ladies' clothing, in a wooded area. Investigation revealed that a female patient whose description matched that given in the identification cards had disappeared from a hospital seven months earlier. Consequently, when human bones extensively mutilated by animals were later found in the same area, tentative identification was based on these findings. Upon examination, the skeletal remains were consistent with those of a white female between the ages of forty and sixty years with an estimated living stature of 57.6″ to 63.5″. The teeth were carious. The corners of the upper and lower incisors were chipped, probably by some activity such as biting on bobby pins. Based upon the configuration of the skull, an origin in the Balkan or southeastern European areas was suggested by the consultant in physical anthropology. Hair found at the scene revealed head hair of Caucasian origin showing evidence of exposure to sun, resulting in bleaching. Hair not exposed to sunlight, found beneath the skull, matched hair samples obtained from among the victim's possessions. Hospital records listed her height as 65″ and indicated that the patient had been born in Czechoslovakia. A positive dental identification was made following comparison of teeth with a Panorex® dental roentgenograph obtained during life, revealing more than eighteen points of identity.

### *Determination of Sex*

Advanced decomposition or mutilation, as by fire, does not necessarily hamper the determination of the sex of the individual. The uterus and the prostate gland are markedly resistant to decomposition, as they are to fire, and breast

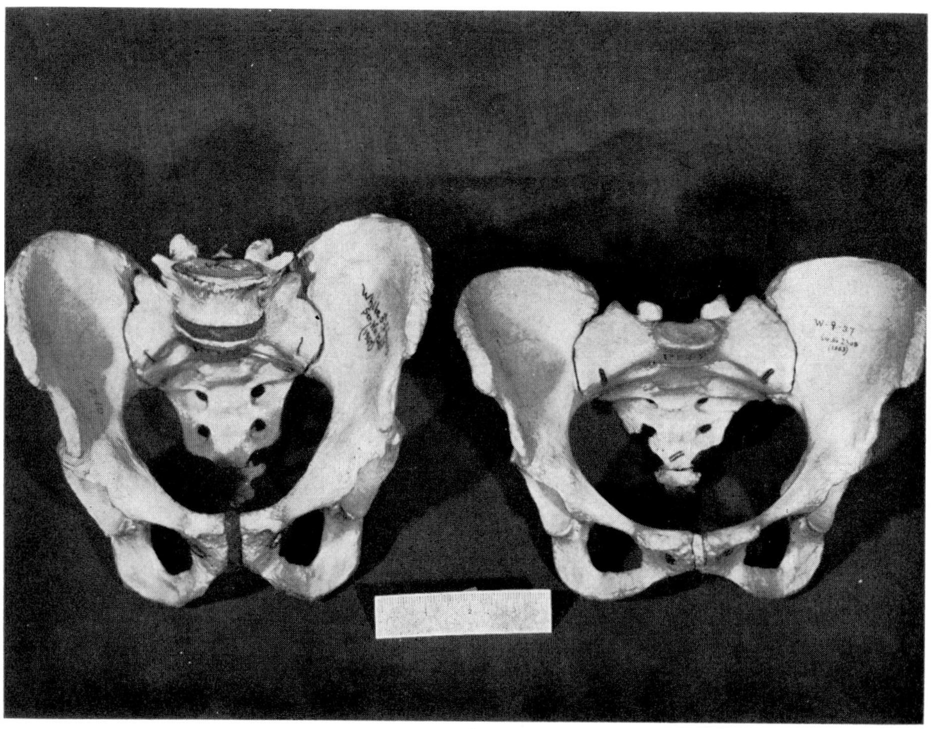

FIGURE III-20. The pelvis of a female is designed to serve as the birth canal. In the pelvis of a man (left) the inlet is narrower, and the sacrum is tilted forward. Notice the greater dimensions in the pelvis of a woman (right).

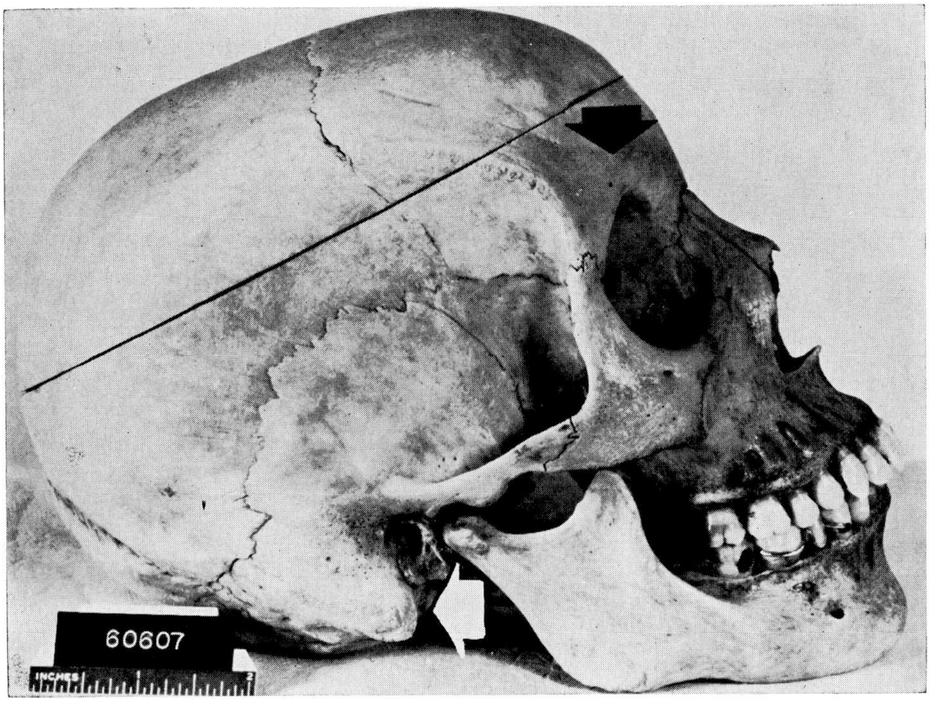


FIGURE III-21a. The features of the skull of a Negro woman shown in this lateral view include absence of brow ridges (black arrow), significant prognathism and delicate mastoid bones (white arrow).

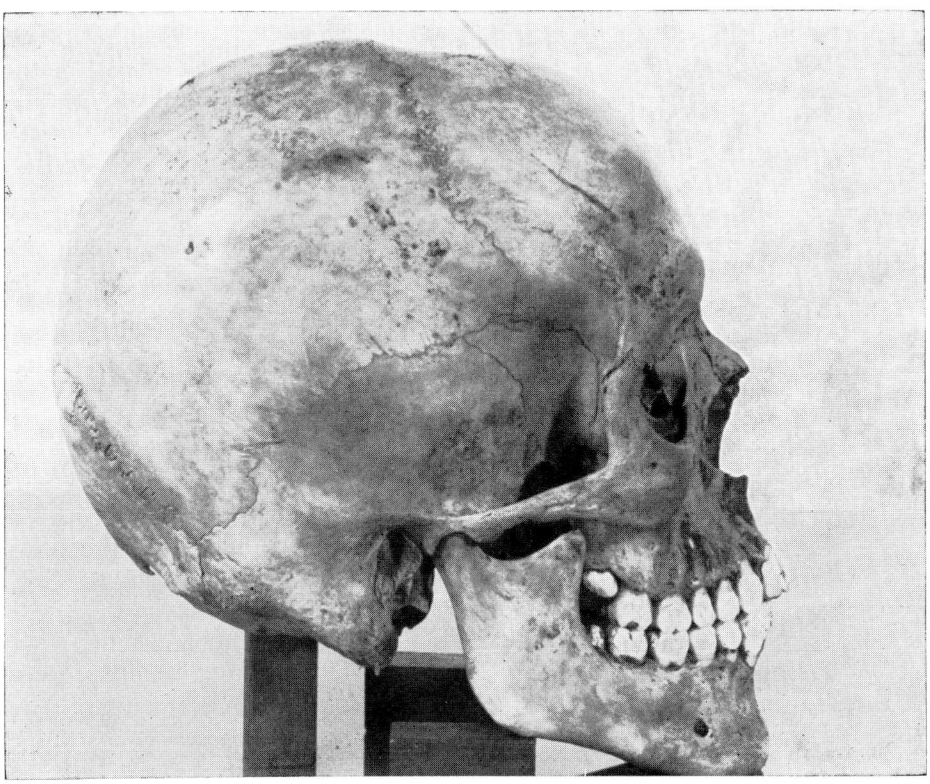

FIGURE III-21b. For comparison, the skull of a Negro man shows distinct brow ridges and more prominent mastoid bones.

tissue often persists even after charring of the body. In skeletonized remains the characteristic features of the pelvis serve as the best means for determination of sex. The sacrum in the female is flat, short and wide, compared to the curved, long and narrow sacrum in the male (Fig. III-20). The sciatic notch in the female is wide, often forming an obtuse angle, compared to the narrow sciatic notch of the male.

Examination of the pubic bones in females often reveals evidence of parturition pits indicative of prior pregnancy. It is believed that the pits are formed during the last stages of pregnancy as a result of bone resorption.

The skull is also useful for evaluation of sex, for the ridges of the brows in males are prominent compared to the absent or delicate brow ridges in females. The mastoid bone is often more massive and longer in males than in females (Fig. III-21).

### *Determination of Age*

The estimation of age usually presents no problems in persons in the early postmortem period. In assessing the age of a skeleton, however, the state of the teeth, extent of cranial and epiphyseal unions, degenerative bone and joint changes and the presence and size of ossi-

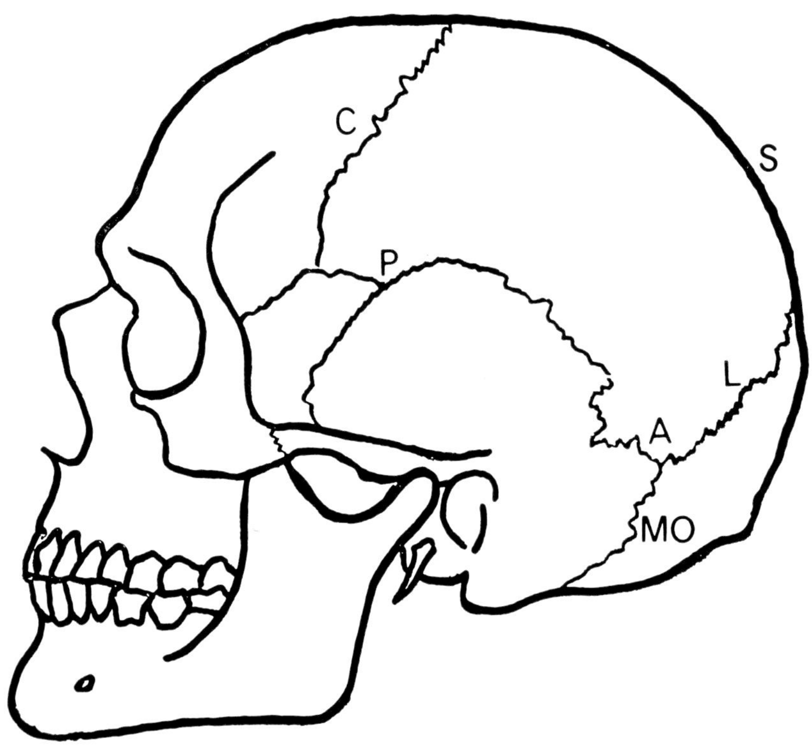


TABLE III-IV

AVERAGE AGE ESTIMATION BASED ON CLOSURE OF CRANIAL SUTURES

| | | *Age (years)* |
|---|---|---|
| Fusion of spheno-occipital synchondrosis (not shown) | | 20 |
| Commencement of closure of coronal suture | (C) | 25 |
| Vault sutures (coronal, sagittal, lambdoid) halfway closed | | 30 |
| Commencement and termination of closure of: | | |
| sagittal suture | (S) | 25-40 |
| lambdoid suture | (L) | 35-45 |
| pterion | (P) | 40-65 |
| masto-occipital suture | (MO) | 45-80 |
| asterion closed | (A) | 50 |

fication centers are helpful criteria. The latter is particularly applicable to remains of the prenatal and neonatal period.

Age estimation by the cranial sutures alone may be misleading and can be placed in rough estimates (decades) only. Suture closure begins at the inner aspect of the skull and progresses outward. It is mandatory that the skull be opened before assessing age on the basis of the closure of cranial sutures (Table III-IV).

Upon examination of the anterior surface of the pubic symphysis in adults, particularly Caucasian males (Fig. III-22), it is possible to provide an estimate of age based upon the work of McKern and Stewart,[22] who detailed the changes in shape and in the relative roughness of the surfaces. The pubic symphysis is probably the most reliable simple criterion for estimating the age of a skeleton. In correlation with other skeletal parts, when available, the pubic symphysis should facilitate ageing within five-year spans. Union of the iliac crest usually begins at about seventeen years and is completed by twenty-three years. The comparative examination of multiple bones, particularly the clavicle, sacrum and sternum, is also useful for the determination of age in adults. During infancy and childhood the teeth and the epiphyses of long bones are most useful for determination of age.

Epiphyseal union of the ankle, hip and elbow can be observed by twenty years of age, whereas the epiphyses of knee, wrist and shoulder are

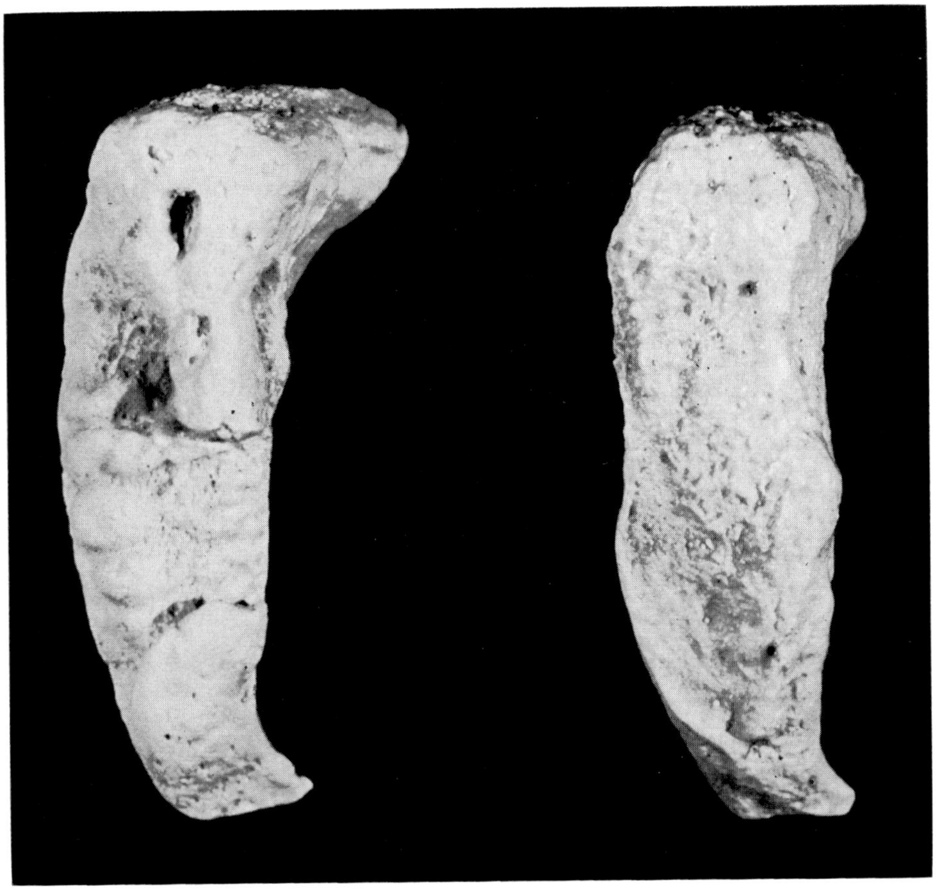

FIGURE III-22. Models of the pubic bones show two of the three symphyseal components used for estimation of skeletal age in young Caucasian American males. The model on the left shows a developmental stage of the ventral rampart. The model on the right shows a sharply defined symphyseal rim with evidence of lipping on the ventral edge. Detailed instructions for the use of these plastic models are given in the technical report by McKern and Stewart.[22]

completely fused between twenty-three and twenty-four years of age.[23] Kerley[24, 25] developed a method for the microscopic examination of the shafts of long bones for estimation of age. This method is particularly helpful when only fragments of skeletal remains are recovered. The accuracy of this method has been better than 85 percent within a plus-or-minus five-year range for more than 100 cases. Another microscopic method is based upon the gradual fatty replacement of red bone marrow with advancing age. Jaaskelainen[26] found that the proportions of red to fatty bone marrow in age groups twenty to forty years, forty to sixty-five years and sixty-five to ninety years were 0.55, 0.18 and 0.05 respectively. Bass[27] reviewed the various scientific criteria for the determination of age and sex in skeletal remains. Study of these criteria includes visual examination, measurements of bones and statistical analysis of these findings, determination of development and eruption of teeth and roentgenographic and microscopic examination. It is believed that microscopic methods will be used more frequently in the future.

### *Determination of Race*

The determination of race from a skeleton is often based upon examination of the skull and pelvis as well as upon measurements of long bones. Individual variations, and variations within races, often preclude a precise opinion concerning the race of an unknown person. American Indians and Eskimos, for example, show skeletal changes similar to those of Mongolians. The prognathism, or protrusion, of the jaw in Negroes is also observed, to a lesser extent, in Mongolian races (Fig. III-23). The shape of the orbits in Negroes tends to be somewhat square as compared to the rounded and triangular shape of orbits in Mongolian and Caucasian races. The Caucasian pelvis is relatively broader and its symphysis lower than that of the Negro. The long bones of the extremities in Negroes are straighter and slightly longer as compared to those of Caucasians.

There are frequently remnants of scalp, including hair, among skeletal remains. Hair is more resistant to the effects of putrefaction than other portions of the skin. Hair may also be used for determination of race, as will be discussed in a later section, although the characteristics are not always reliable.

### *Estimate of Living Stature*

If only bones are found, an estimate of the living stature is obtained by accurate measurement of long bones, particularly the femur and tibia, and by comparison of the measurements with the tables prepared by Trotter and Gleser.[20] An old and valuable rule of thumb for rapid estimation of the height is the length of the humerus multiplied by five. Accurate measurement of the humerus is necessary, as any error

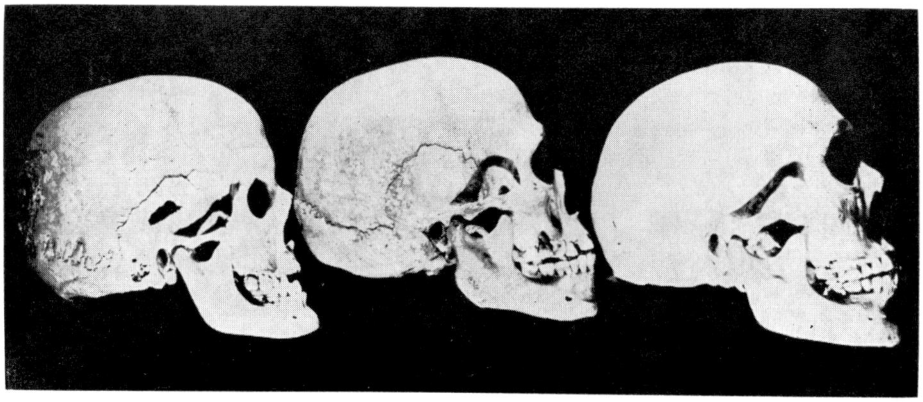

FIGURE III-23. The racial differences of the skull, particularly the degree of prognathism, are seen in these lateral views of Caucasian (left), Negro (center) and Mongolian (right) skulls.

would be compounded by five. To obtain the exact length of the humerus it is best to place one end of the bone against a wall and hold a book against the other end while making certain that the book and the wall are in perfect parallel alignment. The length of the bone can now be measured. This method has an accuracy average of $\pm 1$ in. for total body length. An experienced physical anthropologist is able to obtain many other facts by the examination of skeletal remains, including evidence of cultural effects, prior diseases and injuries, evidence of recent injury and postmortem artifacts.

### Color of Eyes and Hair

The color of the eyes in a fresh corpse is easily recognized. With the onset of putrefaction, however, the resultant cloudiness of the corneas renders this criterion of limited value. Hair is resistant to the effects of putrefaction, and the examination of hair may reveal the effects of heat, brushing, cutting, dyeing or bleaching.

### Birthmarks, Congenital Defects, Tattoos, Prior Injuries and Scars

All skin markings are of considerable importance and should be carefully measured and recorded. Tattoos may be found anywhere on the body; they are frequently related to socioeconomic status, occupation and background of the person, but they are not necessarily indicative of educational success or failure.[28] A variety of tattoo patterns are available representing amorous, pornographic, sexual, religious or violent subjects. At times a conclusive identification of the victim by tattoos of military service number, prisoner of war number or social security number is possible. A professional tattoo is generally fine and smooth in appearance. *Homemade* tattoos, characterized by porous dots and uneven color, are often made in prison (Fig. III-24). This may provide a key to identity in that fingerprints will be on records locally or with the FBI. On occasion a tattoo is indicative of homosexuality (Fig. III-25). A tattoo may also show

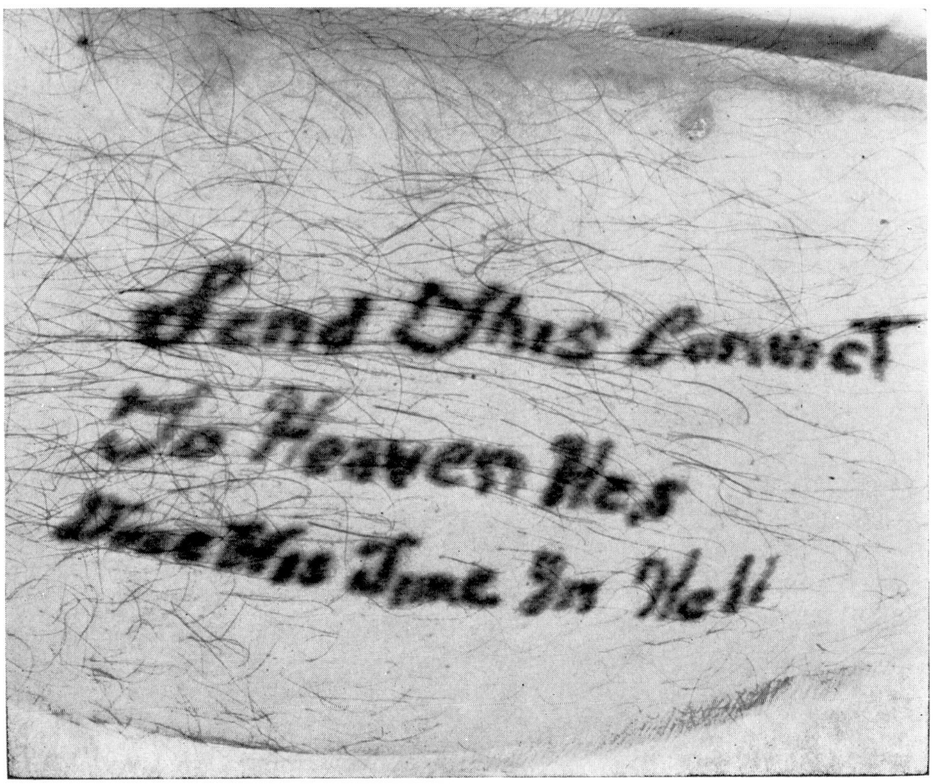


FIGURE III-24. Tattoo on the arm of a deceased man. The *homemade* nature of this tattoo and its contents suggest that it may have been made in jail.

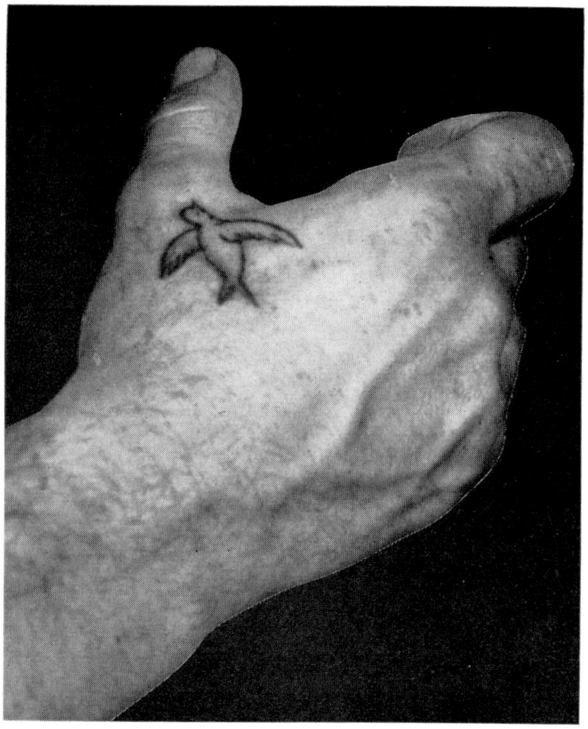

FIGURE III-25. The behavioral characteristics of a person during life are suggested, at times, by a tattoo. This tattoo of a dove, for example, suggests homosexuality.

evidence of attempted obliteration (Fig. III-26). No tattoo can be completely removed, except surgically. Nonsurgical attempts at removal of a tattoo result in infection and often large unsightly scars.

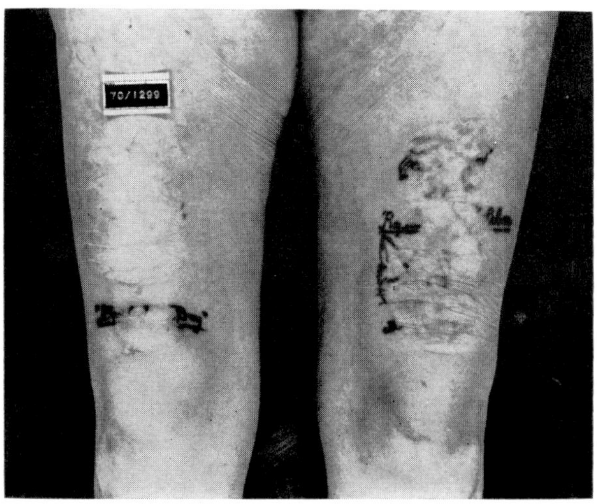


FIGURE III-26. These tattoos on the front of the thighs of a woman show attempts at obliteration.

The image of a tattoo may reflect certain personality traits of the individual, e.g. *Born to Lose* or *Here Today–Gone Tomorrow*. Accurate description of tattoos as well as photographs are indicated. Tattoos are sometimes obliterated by discoloration of the body associated with decomposition or by the effect of heat, as in a smoldering fire. Wiping of the area where a tattoo is suspected, to remove the epidermis, will disclose its presence.

The internal examination provides the basis for additional information concerning the cause of death, as well as evidence of prior disease, to compare with medical records. Evidence of the surgical removal of organs and pathologic changes in any of the organ systems are significant findings. Appropriate samples are retained for microscopic, serologic and toxicologic studies. It is a common misconception that a burned or decomposed body is not amenable to internal examination. It is often the case, however, that the internal organs are well preserved, enabling the pathologist to determine the cause of death and to obtain information about the sex and health of the individual. The absence of organs, indicative of prior surgical procedure, serves as a basis for comparison. Identification of the genital organs determines the sex of the individual.

### Serologic and Cytologic Examinations

During the past decade reagents and methods of greater sensitivity and specificity have been available to determine human blood groups. The individuality of blood provides the basis for these scientific methods. The red blood cells in human beings have many known antigens as well as other antigens that remain unrecognized. Certain antigens may be detected in all persons, or in persons of one family, or in only one race. Blood group antigens are inherited and are present not only on red blood cells but also on other cells of the body. In the ABO blood group system, antibodies in the serum are directed against antigens not present on the red blood cells. For example, persons with A antigens on the red blood cells are Group A, and they have antibodies against B antigens in the serum. In the United States the frequency of ABO blood groups, in decreasing order, is O, A, B and AB for both Caucasians and Negroes. Since the discovery of the ABO system in 1900 and the complex Rh system in 1940, numerous additional blood group systems and subgroups have been discovered, such as the Lewis, Kell, P, Vel and Duffy blood group systems. Blanc et al.[29] has applied the typing of the Gm factor to the racial origin of blood stains. Although the Gm-6 factor has not been found in Caucasians, it has been detected in a significant number of Negroes.

Provided records are available for comparison and the blood submitted for examination has not been affected by putrefactive changes, it is possible to determine whether or not the blood groups are similar by serologic methods. Although the microscopic examination of mammalian blood may not show distinctive features, it is possible to differentiate it with certainty from blood from birds, fish, reptiles and amphibious animals by the absence of nucleated red blood cells (Fig. III-27). A variety of immunologic and serologic techniques applied to blood are available for identification of the species.

Using cytologic methods it is possible to determine the sex of a person by examination of either blood or epithelial cells. The Barr body,

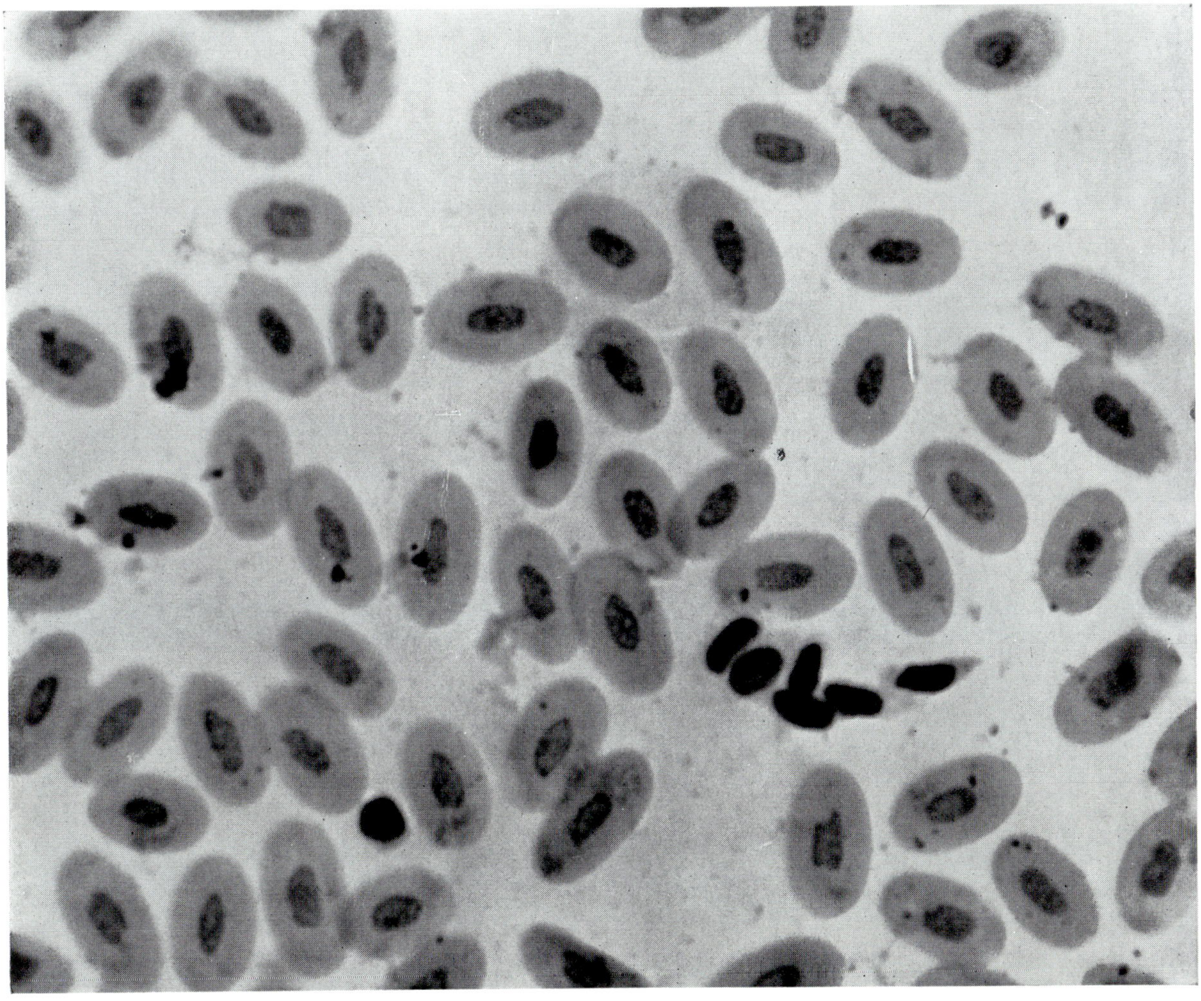

FIGURE III-27. Microscopic examination of a stained smear of blood disclosed the presence of nuclei in the red blood cells. Nucleated red blood cells are not found in adult human beings, but they are found in birds, reptiles and amphibious animals. This microscopic slide was prepared from the blood of a snake.

or sex chromatin body, is found along the inner aspect of the nuclear membrane of epithelial cells, especially those from the buccal mucosa in females (Fig. III-28). Although the sex chromatin body is reportedly present in about 50 percent of the epithelial cells in females, it is readily recognized in only about 25 percent of these cells. In males the sex chromatin body is found in less than 10 percent of the epithelial cells. Polymorphonuclear leukocytes from the peripheral blood of females show small appendages of nuclear sex chromatin with a frequency of 0.6 percent to 2 percent; similar cells in males are practically devoid of these appendages. Other methods, such as karyotyping, are available for chromosome analysis, but the sex chromatin count serves as a useful screening procedure for well-preserved blood and epithelial cells.

### Examination of Hair

The comparative examination of human hair is useful not only in the crime laboratory for evaluation of physical evidence but also in the determination of the race of unknown human remains. For this purpose, hair from the scalp is more useful than hair from the axillary, pubic or body surfaces of the person.

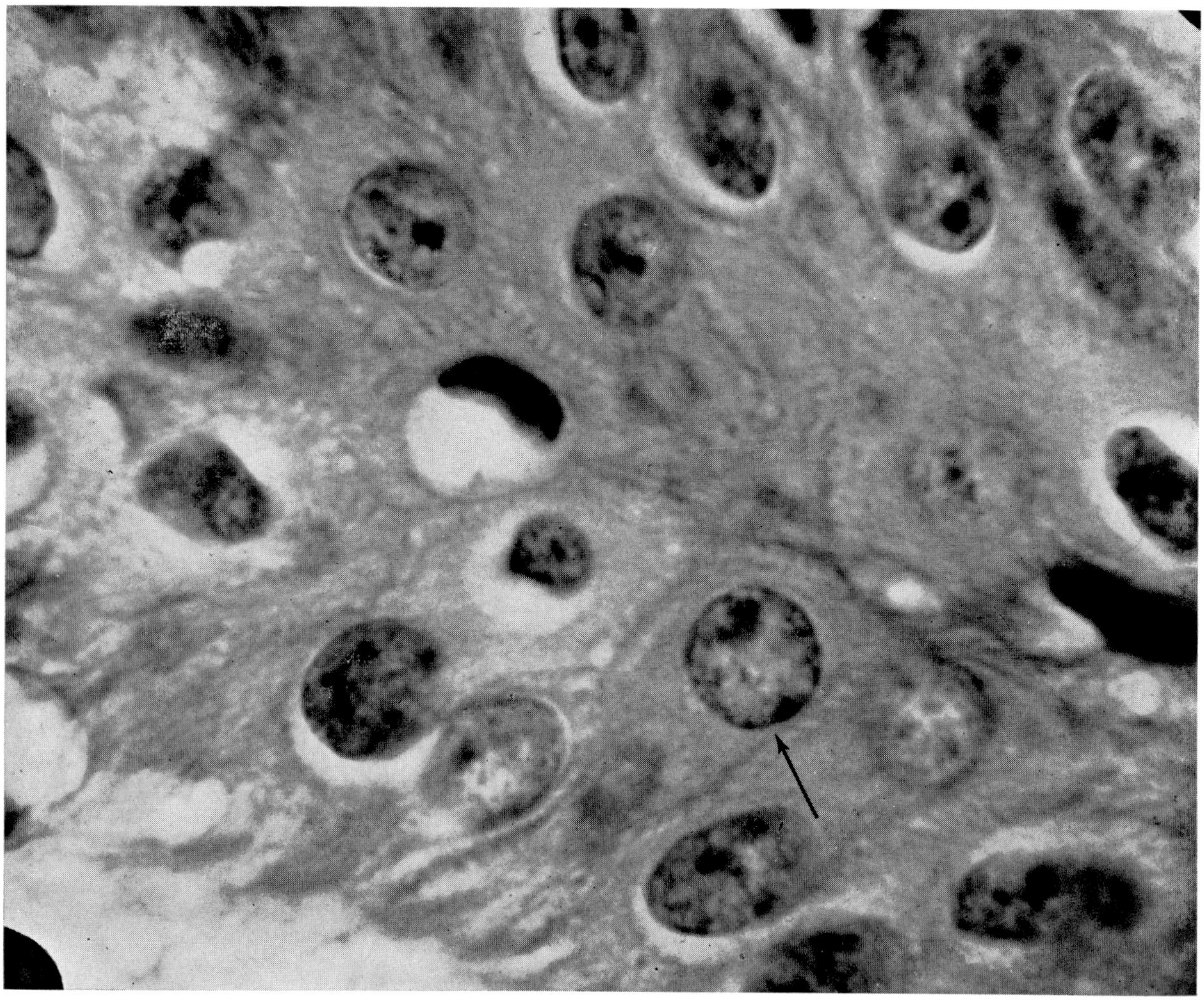

FIGURE III-28. The microscopic examination of epithelial cells in the skin or exfoliated epithelial cells from the buccal mucosa may reveal Barr bodies (arrow) on the inner surface of the nuclear membrane. In well-preserved biologic material, the finding of Barr bodies is helpful for the determination of sex.

A hair consists of a root and a shaft with a distal tip. The shaft has an outer layer of cuticle composed of microscopic scalelike plates. There is an inner cortex between the cuticle in which pigment granules are found. The central portion of the hair, known as the medulla, is not observed in all specimens. The scale pattern of hair, as well as other characteristic features, serves as the basis for distinction between animal hair and human hair. Appropriate specimens for comparison are required to achieve identification of the source of the hair.

The evaluation of the cuticular pattern is based upon microscopic examination of casts prepared from impressions of the cuticle of the hair (Fig. III-29). Unstained mounts of hair are also examined under the microscope to determine the degree of pigmentation and the size of the hair. Hair is placed on a glass slide with a drop or two of mounting medium and a coverslip.

Comparison microscopy is used for evaluation of known and unknown hairs. Although there are certain features, such as evidence of bleaching, dyeing or brushing, that may help to distinguish the hair of females from that of males, interpretations of this type are less valuable when the present hairstyles of men are considered. For the determination of race, cross sections of hair are prepared and examined under the microscope (Fig. III-30). In the crime laboratory cross sections of hair are made with a special hand microtome. For the pathologist, however, such sections can be obtained by inserting several hairs into a cut placed in a ½ in. cube of formalin-fixed liver tissue. This procedure will ensure adequate positioning of the hairs during cutting. Cryostat sections are satisfactory. Paraffin embedding can equally be used. Corresponding fixation is required for other methods of embedding such as the celloidin technique. The latter method is considered su-

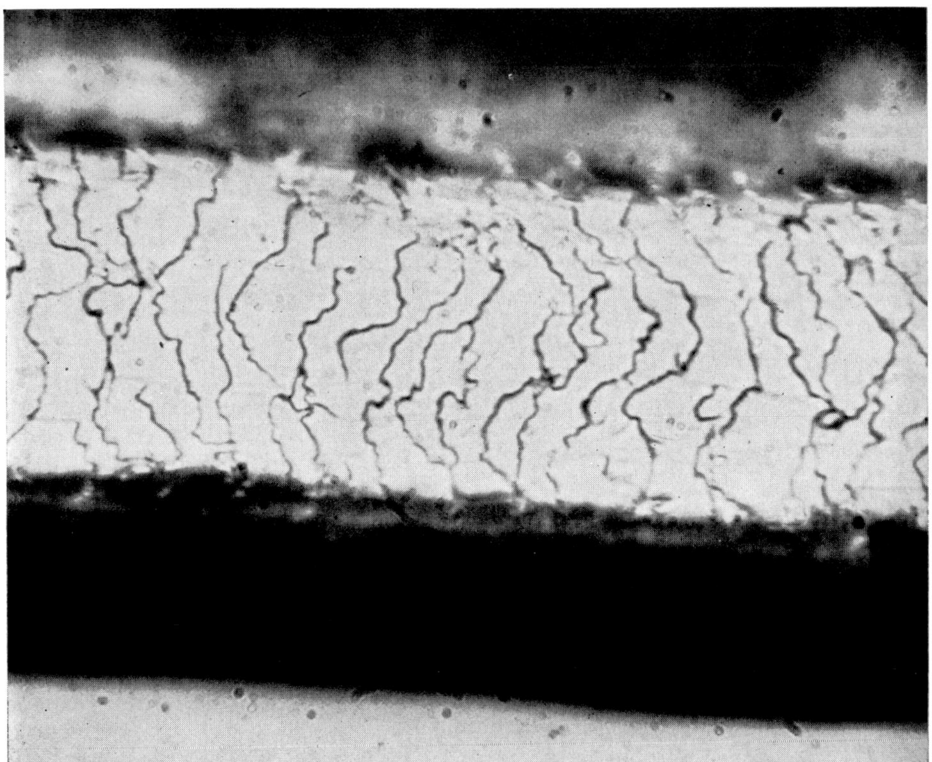

FIGURE III-29. The characteristic appearance of the cast of the scale pattern of a strand of human hair, seen in this photograph, serves as the basis for comparison with the cast of the scale pattern of hair from animals.

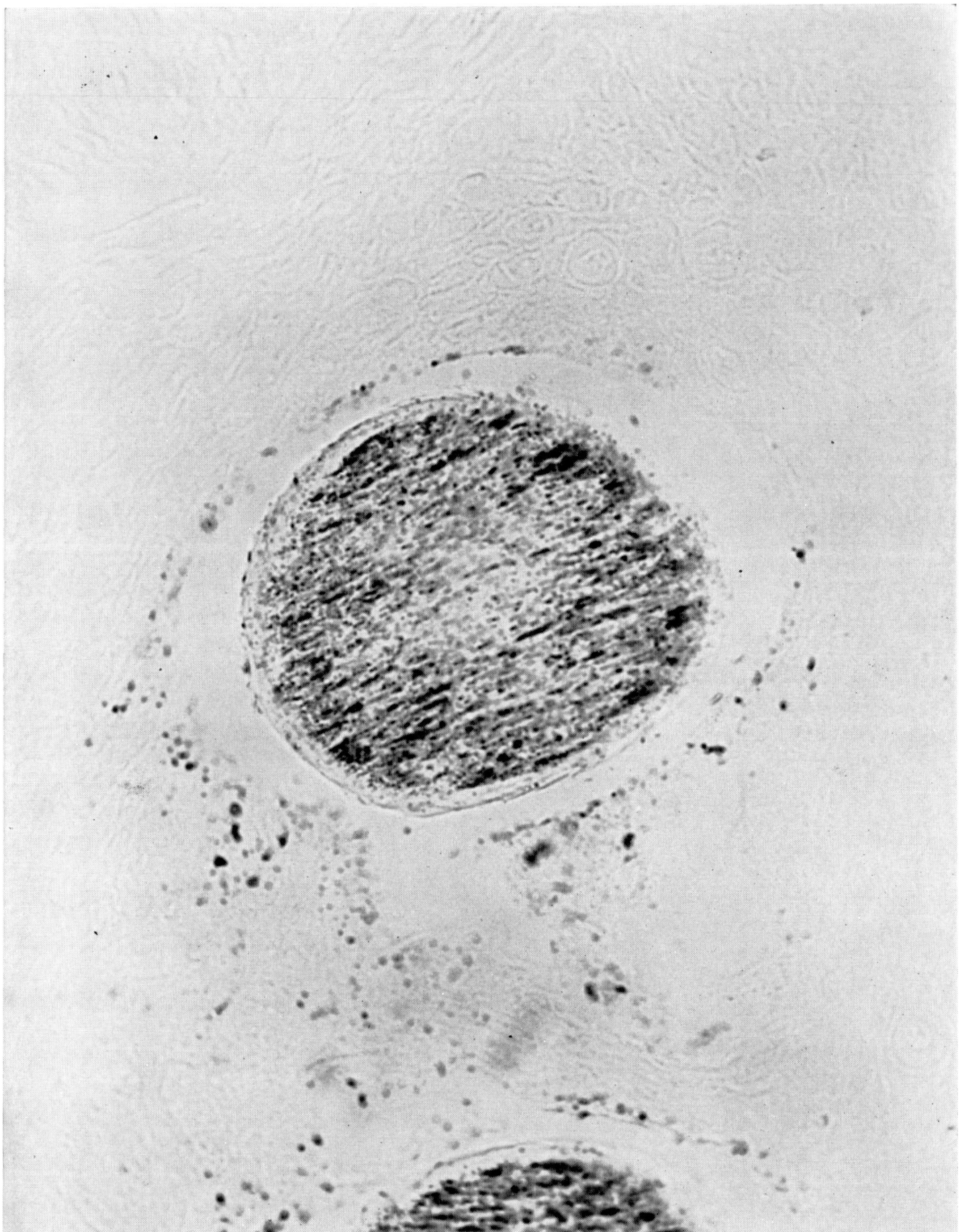

FIGURE III-30. The microscopic examination of cross sections of hair shows not only the distribution of pigment and the thickness of the cuticle but also the configuration of the hair shaft. In this case, the dense pigmentation, relatively thick cuticle and round shape of the hair in cross section are consistent with hair from a Mongolian person.

perior, but it is not always readily available.

The hair from Mongolians, including American Indians and Eskimos, is similar. The hair from Mongolians and Negroes is densely pigmented, but there is a tendency for the distribution of pigment in Mongolian hair to be more uniform. Mongolian hair is usually circular on cross section and has a uniform pigmentation and a dark medulla. Negro hair also has dense pigment with an irregular distribution. On cross section, a flattened shape is seen. Caucasian hair tends to have an oval shape with uniform distribution of fine or coarse pigment (Fig. III-31). Except for hair from infants, it is not possible to determine age with certainty. In his review Niyogi[30] provides not only the criteria for differentiating human hair from the hair of animals but also a discussion of methods of examination.

Nuclear techniques such as neutron activation analysis are useful for identification of hair. When hair is irradiated in a nuclear reactor, elements are converted to radioactive isotopes. Comparison of the radiation emitted from the hair with known standards provides a quantitative comparison.

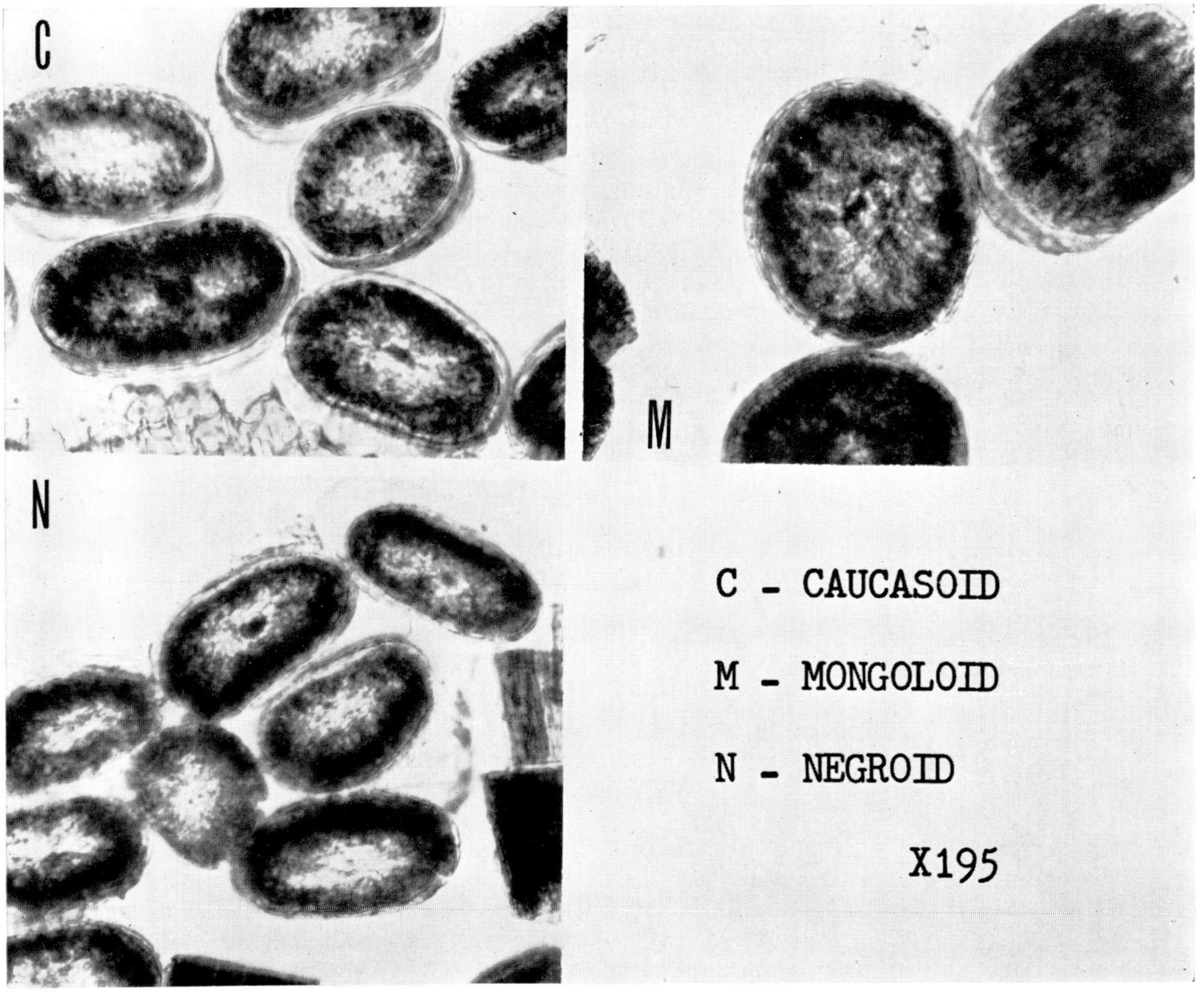


FIGURE III-31. The appearance of cross sections of hair from Caucasoid, Mongoloid and Negroid persons are seen in this photograph.

## REFERENCES


1. Health Services Administration: Dental investigation—An analysis of laws and policies of the United States, each state and jurisdiction (as of January 31, 1977). DHEW Publication No. (HSA) 78-5252. Washington, D.C., U.S. Govt. Print. Office, 1977.
2. Reals, W. J. (Ed.): *Medical Investigation of Aviation Accidents.* Chicago, Coll Am Path, 1968.
3. Stewart, T. D. (Ed.): *Personal Identification in Mass Disasters.* Washington, D.C., National Museum of Natural History, Smithsonian, 1970.
4. Guinn, V. P.: Forensic neutron activation analysis. In Stewart, T. D. (Ed.): *Personal Identification in Mass Disasters.* Washington, D.C., National Museum of Natural History, Smithsonian, 1970, pp. 25-35.
5. Thomas F., and Baert, H.: The longitudinal striation of the human nails as a means of identification. *J Forensic Med, 14:*113, 1967.
6. Finck, P. A.: Ballistic and forensic pathologic aspects of missile wounds. Conversion between Anglo-American and metric-system units. *Milit Med, 130:*545, 1965.
7. Iannarelli, A. V.: *The Iannarelli System of Ear Identification.* Police Science Series. Brooklyn, Foun Pr, 1964.
8. Spitz, W. U., Sopher, I. M., and DiMaio, V. J. M.: Medicolegal investigation of a bomb explosion in an automobile. *J Forensic Sci, 15:*537, 1970.
9. Suzuki, K., and Tsuchihashi, Y.: Personal identificaation by means of lip prints. *J Forensic Med, 17:*52, 1970.
10. Jerman, A. C.: Denture identification. *J Am Dent Assoc, 80:*1358, 1970.
11. Code 611, BUMED: Denture identification. *US Navy Med, 56:*28, 1970.
12. Kiel, F. W.: Forensic science in China: Traditional and contemporary aspects. *J Forensic Sci, 15:* 201, 1970.
13. Simpson, K. The development of scientific methods in crime investigation. *J Forensic Med, 8:*148, 1961.
14. Federal Bureau of Investigation: Problems and practices in fingerprinting the dead. Reprinted from *FBI Law Enforcement Bull,* April, 1949, as revised January, 1962.
15. Edberg, S., Mandella, A., and Hochman, C. H.: The use of footprints for identification in infanticide: Report of a case. *J Forensic Sci, 10:* 225, 1965.
16. Department of the Army: Short wave ultra-violet rays for segregation of commingled remains. In *Identification of Deceased.* Personnel, Dept. of the Army Techn. Manual 10-286. Washington, D.C. Headquarters, Dept. of the Army, January, 1964, Appendix IV.
17. Garn, S. M., Rohmann, C. G., and Silverman, F. N.: Radiographic standards for postnatal ossification and tooth calcification. *Med Radiogr Photogr, 43:*44, 1967.
18. Stewart, T. D.: Evaluation of evidence from the skeleton. In Gradwohl, R. B. H. (Ed.): *Legal Medicine.* St. Louis, Mosby, 1954, pp. 425-427.
19. Krogman, W. M.: *The Human Skeleton in Forensic Medicine.* Springfield, Thomas, 1962, pp. 277-299.
20. Trotter, M., and Gleser, G. C.: Estimation of stature from long bones of American Whites and Negroes. *Am J Phys Anthropol, 10:*463, 1952.
21. Gray, P. H. K.: Radiography of ancient Egyptian mummies. *Med Radiogr Photogr, 43:*34, 1967.
22. McKern, T., and Stewart, T. D.: Skeletal age changes in young American males. Technical Report EP-45. Natick, Massachusetts, Headquarters, Quartermaster Research and Development Command, May, 1957.
23. McKern, T.: Estimation of skeletal age: From puberty to about 30 years of age. In Stewart, T. D. (Ed.): *Personal Identification in Mass Disasters.* Washington, D.C., National Museum of Natural History, Smithsonian, 1970, pp. 41-56.
24. Kerley, E. R.: The microscopic determination of age in human bone. *Am J Phys Anthropol, 23:*149, 1965.
25. Kerley, E. R.: Age determination of bone fragments. *J Forensic Sci, 14:*59, 1969.
26. Jaaskelainen, A. J.: A method for the estimation of age in the identification of mass casualties. *J Forensic Sci, 13:*528, 1968.
27. Bass, W. M.: Recent developments in the identification of human skeletal material. *Am J Phys Anthropol, 30:*549, 1969.
28. Earls, J. H., and Hester, R.: Tattooed sailors: Some sociopsychological correlates. *Milit Med, 132:* 48, 1967.
29. Blanc, M., Gortz, R., and Ducos, J.: The value of Gm typing for determining the racial origin of blood stains. *J Forensic Sci, 16:*176, 1971.
30. Niyogi, S. K.: A study of human hairs in forensic work. A review. *J Forensic Med, 9:*27, 1962.

*Chapter IV*

# FORENSIC ODONTOLOGY

IRVIN M. SOPHER

THIS CHAPTER IS DESIGNED to serve as a primer of forensic odontology for the pathologist or physician as well as for law enforcement personnel. It is hoped that police personnel will gain insight into what can be expected from the examination of oral structures in the medicolegal setting. For the physician, a glossary of applicable dental terminology is provided to enable him to understand the language of dentistry so that he may individually solve the routine dental identification problems that arise in the realm of forensic pathology. With a basic understanding of dental nomenclature, materials and techniques, the pathologist or physician can easily qualify himself to handle uncomplicated dental identification cases. It is also intended that this chapter shall represent a comprehensive review of forensic odontology for the forensic pathologist.

## HISTORICAL BACKGROUND

Historically, the earliest recorded case of dental identification dates to the fifteenth century. Through the ages before the existence of dentistry per se as a science, cases are on record of personal identification based upon the mere presence or absence of teeth, the general condition of the teeth, peculiar alignment of the dentition and the presence of restorations or dentures. Paul Revere, the *Minute Man* dentist, utilized dental identification in the recognition of the remains of Dr. Joseph Warren, a patriot killed at Bunker Hill. A classic in the history of forensic odontology was the Parkman-Webster case in 1849. Professor Webster of the Harvard Medical School murdered his friend Dr. Parkman and incinerated the body. Charred jaw bones and dental structures retrieved from Webster's laboratory furnace were identified by Parkman's dentist as being those of the murdered man. The dentist's testimony led to the conviction. The exhumed body of John Wilkes Booth, Lincoln's assassin, was identified by *a gold-plugged tooth on the right side of his jaw.*[1] Several other cases of odontological identification are recorded for the 1870-1890 era, including the fraud-murder Goss-Udderzook case.[2] The Bazar de la Charité and the Iroquois Fires[3, 4] represent early examples of mass tragedies wherein identification of remains was accomplished by dental means. In 1934 the dental identification of the lye-corroded buried body of a member of the John Dillinger gang received much acclaim.[5] The positive identification of the remains of Hitler was based upon dental comparison.[6]

Forensic odontology cases of recent interest include the Baptist Church Cellar case, wherein identification of the dismembered buried victim was made on the basis of root tips within the maxilla.[7] Identification by intact dentures found amid human remains submerged in a sulfuric acid tank was described in the Haigh Bath Murder.[8] The identities of the victims of the double murder Ruxton case were accomplished despite the postmortem extraction of teeth by the physician-murderer. Dental fragments served to identify the murdered and burned body in the Carron case, and dental evidence was the means of identification ten years after death of the partially burned remains in the Australian Pyjama Girl case.[9]

The ubiquitous availability of mass dental care in the civilized countries of today, in conjunction with the maintenance of dental records including dental x rays, has served to enhance the specificity of the dental examination as a tool in identification. The continued rapid growth of the field of forensic pathology in this country further emphasizes the need for dissemination of information concerning forensic odontology. Such knowledge applies not only to the routinely encountered identification of single unknown bodies, but is especially pertinent to the prospect of inevitable mass disasters involving aircraft of increasing size and capacity.

The importance of dental identification in 116 air disaster victims of 4 air crashes has been stressed by Stevens and Tarlton.[10] Other reports that illustrate the value of positive identification in air disasters solely by dental means report identifications ranging from 15 to 66 percent of victims.[11–14] The combination of dental data with other modes of identification elevates these percentages further.

## GENERAL CONSIDERATIONS OF DENTAL IDENTIFICATION

The accurate identification of human remains is a public duty justified by social, legal and insurance considerations. The principles of general identification are discussed in Chapter III; however, the point that bears repetition is that fingerprints and dental means represent the most scientifically reliable methods of identification. In general, the greater the degree of tissue destruction, the greater the importance of dental characteristics in effecting proper identification.

Upon exposure to physical injury and putrefactive changes, the human dentition, the enamel of which is the hardest substance of the body, outlasts all other tissues. The preservation of teeth in ancient human relics buried for centuries attests to this fact. The materials used in dental restorations (fillings, etc.) are also extremely resistant to destruction by chemical and physical elements.

The adult dentition is comprised of thirty-two teeth; each tooth possesses five surfaces visible on oral examination. The innumerable combinations of missing teeth, filling materials, carious lesions and prostheses involving these 160 surfaces form the basis for dental identification. Specific morphologic patterns of individual restorations (fillings and crowns) further enhance characterization. When one considers the additional identifying features incorporated within root canals, periapical and surrounding bone and soft tissues, it can be realized how specific the oral structures can be in terms of identification. A computer has shown that there are more than 2.5 billion different possibilities in charting the human mouth. The concept that no two dentitions are alike is a basic premise of dental identification.

Dental identification assumes a paramount role in the identification of remains wherein postmortem changes, traumatic tissue injury and/or lack of a previous fingerprint record for comparison invalidate the employment of the visual or fingerprint methods. In such circumstances dental identification becomes of primary importance. One must realize that it is hazardous to accept only visual identification in cases where physical features are severely impaired. Numerous instances are on record where subsequent dental examination revealed visual misidentification.[11, 15, 16, 17]

## THE DENTAL IDENTIFICATION

The fundamental principles of dental identification are those of comparison (when antemortem records of the proposed deceased are available) and exclusion (when antemortem records of other persons only are available). Effectual identification necessitates a list of the possible persons involved so that the appropriate antemortem record can be located. The availability and accuracy of this record determine the success of the identification. Unfortunately, all too often dentists maintain poor records, resulting in confusion and inconsistencies.

All available antemortem material (charts, x rays and dental casts, if present) should be requested from the attending dentist. In some instances the deceased may have received care from numerous dentists over a period of years. Obviously, the more recent the antemortem record, the more reliable the data. Antemortem dental x rays are of immense value for comparison, especially as an adjunct to a poor dental chart. In addition, the x ray discloses very specific morphologic patterns of the individual restorations as well as information regarding areas of the teeth and jaw tissues not accessible to visual examination (root canal treatment, buried root tips, jaw bone pattern).[19] If antemortem records are not available, as much dental information as possible must be obtained by interrogation of relatives and friends of the suspected deceased. This may frequently prove unreliable;[16] however, certain noticed dental peculiarities or restorations (gaps between teeth, broken teeth, gold crowns) may stand the test of comparison and, if specific enough, may enable an identification to be made. Such information is better than none at all and may aid in the corroboration of identification by other means such as jewelry or medical data.

The nature and idiosyncrasies of the dental work observed may suggest the economic status of the patient or the place where the dental work was done.[20]

A human skeleton containing a .38 caliber bullet, numerous shotgun pellets and several fractured ribs was found in an isolated wooded area. Death was believed due to a shotgun wound of the chest. The dentition was recovered intact. Dental examination disclosed several restorations, many of which were of gold foil material. In addition, evidence of a left mandibular abscess was noted upon examination of the jaws (Figs. IV-1 and IV-2).

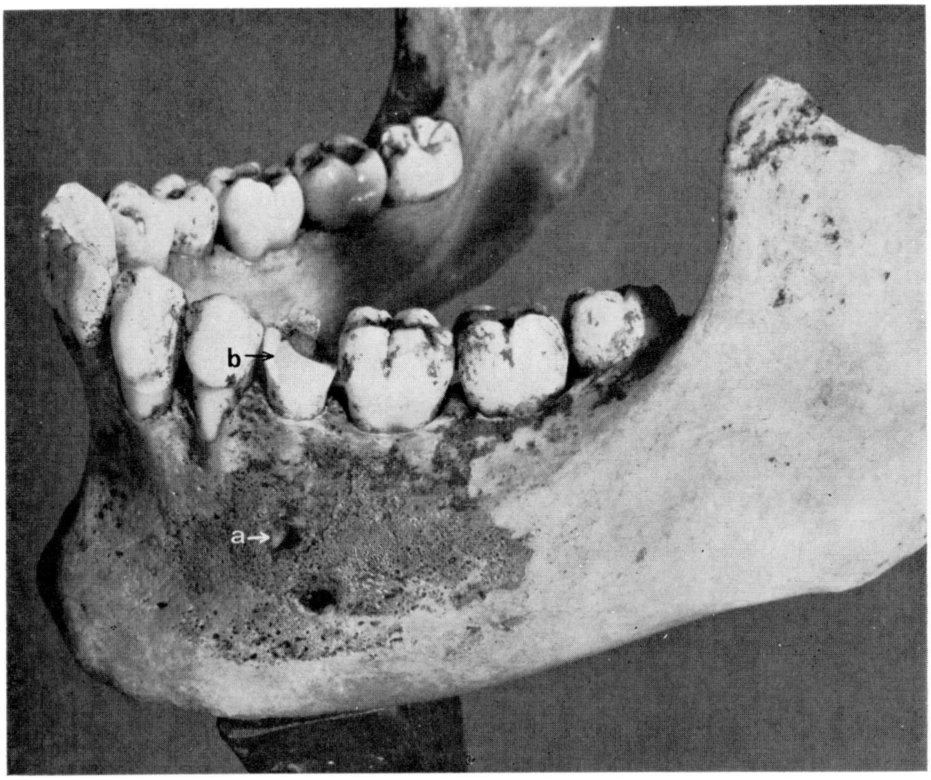


FIGURE IV-1. The lateral plate of the left mandibular bicuspid area discloses roughening and discoloration consistent with reactive periostitis with a central perforation (a) contiguous with the root tip of the carious second bicuspid. The perforation is secondary to a periapical abscess, which resulted from carious involvement of the pulp. Recent fracture of the enamel of the buccal cusp of the bicuspid is seen at (b). Notice the unstained (from foodstuffs, etc.) underlying dentin, indicating that the fracture probably occurred postmortem.

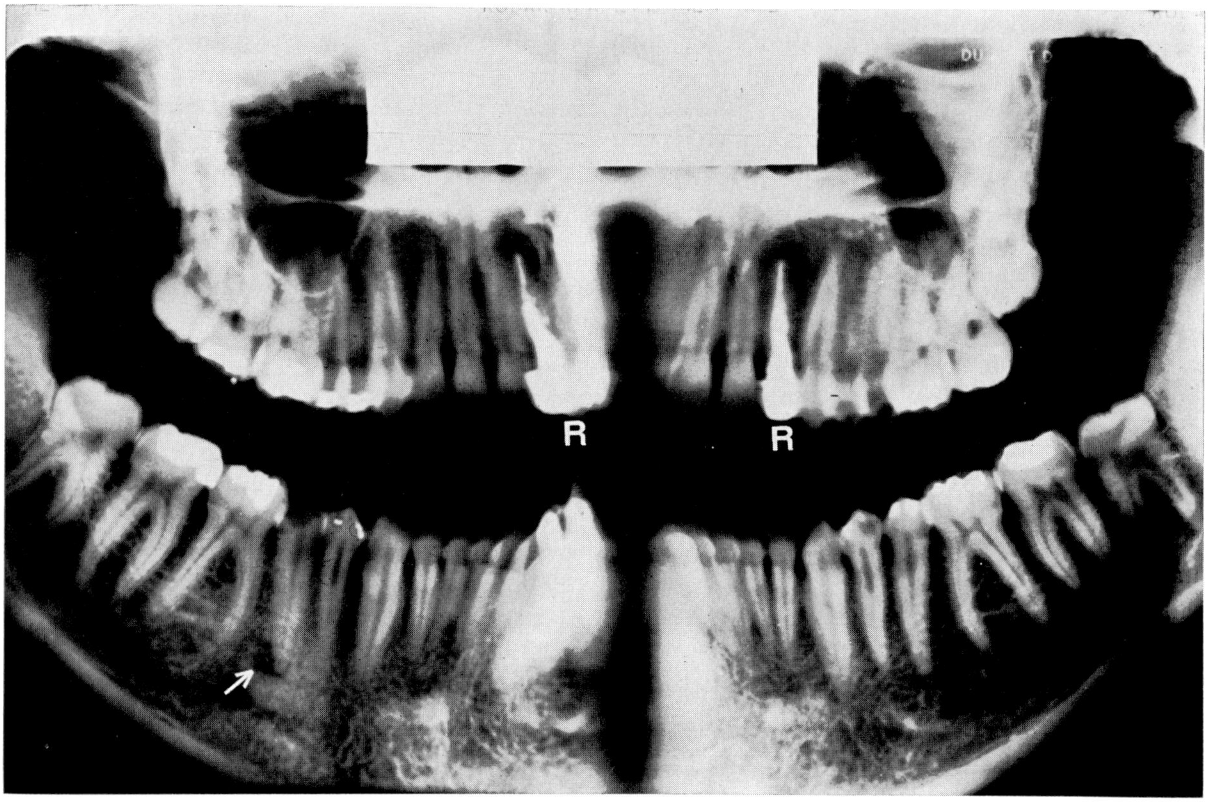


FIGURE IV-2. Postmortem Panorex® radiograph of the jaws. The x ray is read as though one were inside the mouth looking out. The arrow indicates the abscess radiolucency of the lower left second bicuspid. Note the individual morphology of the various metallic restorations. Such points of comparison are not visible on the gross oral examination. Two root canal treatments of the maxillary dentition are present (R).

The neatness of the restorations in general and especially the presence of gold foil as a filling material strongly suggested that the work may have been performed at a dental school, more specifically the local University of Maryland School of Dentistry. (Gold foil is a superior restorative material but is expensive and extremely time consuming to insert. It is generally found in two populations: in the well-to-do person who can afford the care and in the indigent, where the work is obtained in dental schools, thus enabling dental students to gain skills in the handling of gold foil material.) To establish identification we were prepared to examine the dental school patient records of all black males from age eighteen to twenty-six, the latter figures suggested by anthropological data retrieved from the skeleton. Fortunately, we were spared such a search, for at this time the wife of the deceased, having read about the finding of the skeleton in the newspaper, reminded police of an earlier report regarding her missing husband filed three months previously. Interrogation of the wife revealed that her husband had received treatment at the dental school and had complained of a sore jaw with extreme swelling when last seen three months earlier. The dental school records under the husband's name disclosed a perfect comparison with the skeletal findings.

The pathological bone findings in this case indicated a mandibular abscess, which corroborated the history, but this was not necessary for identification.

In terms of probability, the more dental work performed in a given individual, the greater the number of surfaces altered and hence the higher the available points of comparison. Indeed, children with few or no fillings may represent difficult identification problems.[17] On the other hand, even a single filling, if specific enough in location, morphology and material, may be sufficient to establish identity.[21] At the other extreme of age, elderly individuals with upper and lower dentures also may present an identification dilemma. Even complete dentures, however, may retain the *signatures* of the attending dentist and his laboratory. This is especially true of older dentists who still personally construct their own denture cases. These dentists often can recognize their work at a glance, much like other artisans with their handicrafts.

In the course of draining a reservoir, a 1949 Nash automobile containing a human skeleton was discovered settled within the muddy silt of the lake bed. An elderly gentleman, upon seeing the photo of the scene in a newspaper, recognized the car and license plate as belonging to his missing brother, who had mysteriously disappeared twenty years earlier.

Fortunately, the attending dentist of the deceased was alive and located. This older dentist specialized in the construction of dentures and had personally made the dentures of the deceased in his own laboratory. The missing man was a very close friend of the dentist, and, despite the fact that his records had been destroyed many years ago, the dentist was able to draw and describe the exact details of the prosthetic devices. The partial dentures were recovered several days later in the muddy lake bed; they exactly matched the previous descriptions given by the dentist and were subsequently also identified by him.

Even with the construction of dentures in commercial laboratories, the mold, shape and type of teeth, as well as the nature of the base material used, may be on record and thus enable positive identification to be made. Haines[11] discusses the problem of denture identification in detail. Often, the family may have an old *spare* denture of the deceased on hand that can be used for comparison of the alveolar ridge contour and palatal soft tissue configuration. Retained impression casts of the ridges may also be useful in these instances. The mandatory incorporation into denture plates of a means of identification would represent a large step forward in solving the problem of identification among denture wearers.

Any deviation from normal may represent a vital finding regarding specificity in a dental comparison. Such findings include unusual spaces between teeth, retained deciduous teeth, malposition or malrotation of teeth and any pathological conditions of the oral tissues. The commonly found mandibular or palatal tori (bony exostoses) should also be mentioned in this regard. The finding of Dilantin®-induced hyperplasia of the gums may not only aid in identification but may also suggest the cause of death, namely an epileptic seizure. Heavy metal poisoning, such as lead poisoning, may cause pigmentation of the gums and thereby suggest a cause of death and/or be of occupational significance regarding identification. The commonly seen linear defects in the enamel of the front teeth may relate to long-term febrile illnesses in childhood and may prove to corroborate other points of identification. The type of occlusion (the relationship between the teeth of both jaws when in opposition) should be noted. The reference here is whether the upper anteriors overlap the lower anteriors, whether the closed bite is edge to edge or whether the lower jaw protrudes. The following incident illustrates the value of a rare pathological finding as a means of identification of a charred body:

On a cold winter evening, a fire occurred in an abandoned downtown Baltimore warehouse that was a known habitat for homeless, wandering alcoholics. The Arson Squad discovered the charred body of a white male within the ruins. The dental structures of the deceased were intact; however, a period of five weeks elapsed before a lead developed that eventually solved the identity. The wife of the deceased had heard from a local *wino* that her husband had died in the above incident. She contacted the Medical Examiner's Office where the autopsy was performed and stated that her husband had received care at a local state hospital. She also said that as the result of such treatment he had suffered a peculiar condition wherein every time he would blow his nose, *air would whistle through an opening in his upper jaw.* The upper jaw was then dissected, and a healed oroantral fistula was noted of the right posterior maxillary region. The state hospital dental records later confirmed this and other points of comparison.

## THE POSTMORTEM DENTAL EXAMINATION

The postmortem oral examination should include not only the oral cavity of the victim but, when applicable, the surrounding scene as well. Especially in cases of conflagration or injuries, only remnants of the dental arches may remain scattered amid rubble and debris. This material should be carefully sifted for dental fragments. It is important to have a forensic pathologist or dentist available from the outset of the discovery of the remains to aid in the search for such objects. Police and fire department personnel are not expected to recognize dental remains. In decomposed bodies or skeletal remains the teeth commonly loosen from their bony sockets (especially single-rooted anterior teeth) and are found in the surrounding soil. Such displaced teeth should be saved, labelled as to body and/or location at site and later secured into the intraoral position using adhesive cement.

The finding of an open socket within the jaws of the deceased need not be confusing. Most open alveoli are the result of postmortem tooth loss. In recently recovered remains postmortem tooth loss discloses a clean socket devoid of blood clot. In skeletons, in which postmortem loss of teeth is common, the bony rim of the alveolus is sharp and feathered; however, one cannot eliminate the possibility that extraction or tooth loss occurred within several days before death.

In contrast, extraction or tooth loss in a living person is followed by the formation of a blood clot within the alveolus. Subsequent fibrous tissue obliteration of the clot and reparative bone resorption of the alveolar rim result in a smooth, rounded socket rim. Within five or six months following tooth loss, new bone

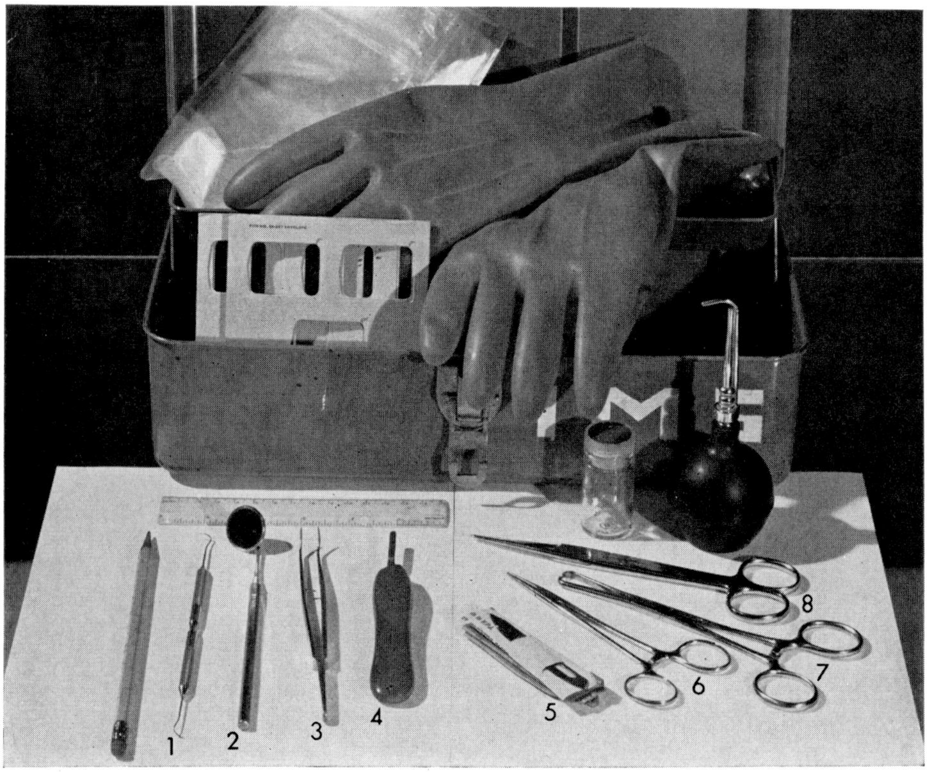


FIGURE IV-3. The basic dental examination kit should include (1) dental explorer, (2) dental mirror, (3) tissue forceps, (4) heavy-duty autopsy scalpel handle, (5) autopsy scalpel blades, (6) tissue clamp, (7) tongue clamp and (8) tissue scissors. A ruler and pencil should also be available. The rubber air or water irrigating syringe is optional. Rubber autopsy gloves and polyethylene specimen bags are seen in the box with a cardboard dental x ray folder. For examinations performed outside of the autopsy room, gauze sponges (for tooth cleansing), a source of illumination (flashlight or battery-operated headlamp) and the dental examination form should be included.

formation fills in the socket; however, the alveolar outline may still be visible on x ray examination. Within six months to one year, complete remodeling of the extraction site results in new bone obliteration of the alveolus and slight depression of the bone outline.

The antemortem loss of teeth due to trauma at or near the time of death is frequently associated with fracture of the thin bony plate surrounding the alveolus.

Dental examination in mass disaster victims often by necessity must be accomplished under less than ideal conditions. This includes the accident site and/or temporary mortuary, where lighting may be less than optimal. The fact that the bodies are so often severely disfigured, making funeral viewing impossible, enables the examiner to dissect and remove the facial and jaw musculature at will in order to gain proper exposure. The cheek soft tissues should be trimmed away, and the *tight* jaws should be pried open. The latter is best accomplished by inserting a large rongeur or instrument handle in the space behind the last molars and levering the jaws into the open position. A mouth prop may then be inserted. Care must be exercised not to fracture or loosen the dentition. In some cases it is advantageous to remove the jaws in their entirety. This is best performed as outlined in Chapter XXIV.

The instrumentation that should be incorporated into the basic dental examination kit is shown in Figure IV-3. This kit is inexpensive and can be purchased at any dental supply house. The postmortem dental examination form is seen in Figure IV-4.

Ideally, the examination should be performed by two persons thoroughly familiar with dental terminology, one actually performing the examination and one recording the data. The recorder should view the actual teeth in order to record the basic morphological pattern of the restorations or cavities. The examiner should also review the completed chart. The use of two persons not only saves time but enables more accurate records. The time factor is especially important in mass disasters, where anxious

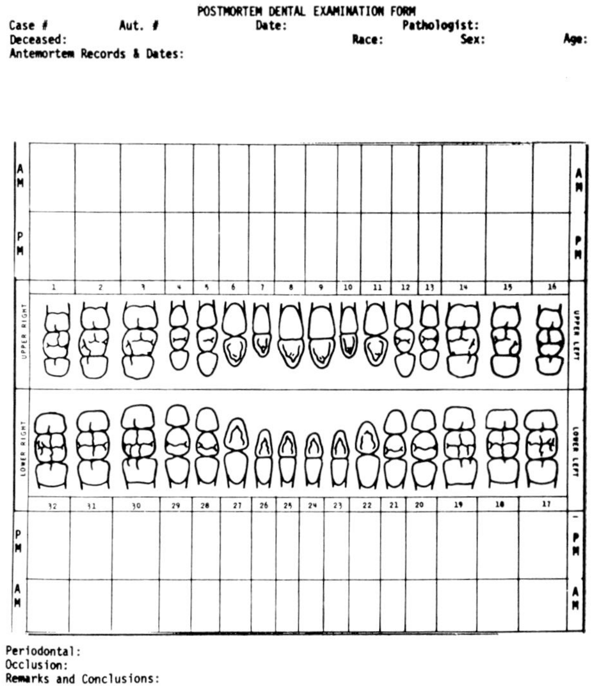
POSTMORTEM DENTAL EXAMINATION FORM

Case # Aut. # Date: Pathologist:

Deceased: Race: Sex: Age:

Antemortem Records & Dates:

AM

PM

1 2 3 4 5 6 7 8 9 10 11 12 13 14 15 16

UPPER RIGHT UPPER LEFT

LOWER RIGHT LOWER LEFT

32 31 30 29 28 27 26 25 24 23 22 21 20 19 18 17

PM

AM

Periodontal:

Occlusion:

Remarks and Conclusions:

FIGURE IV-4. Postmortem dental examination form. AM—antemortem data; PM—postmortem charting.

families and news media are pressing for identification. Local dental societies or dental schools are usually more than willing to assist in times of mass disasters. Advanced dental school students are helpful as recorders.

The postmortem dental charting should include the following:

1. Missing, unerupted or extracted teeth; supernumerary teeth.
2. Restorations and prostheses (surfaces, morphology, configuration and material).
3. Decay (surfaces and configuration) and broken teeth.
4. Malposition, overlapping, crowding and spacing.
5. Malrotation (abnormal rotation of teeth).
6. Peculiar shapes of teeth (e.g. peg-shaped lateral incisors).
7. Root canal therapy on x ray examination.
8. Bone pattern on x ray examination.
9. Complete dentures (type, shade and material).
10. Relationship of the bite.
11. Oral pathology (tori, gingival hyperplasia, etc.).

Most routine dental identifications are accomplished on the basis of the first three items listed and can easily be performed by the pathologist.

Once the examination is completed, the process of comparison with available antemortem records begins. Where an antemortem record is unavailable, the postmortem chart of the deceased can be used to exclude his identity upon comparison with the available antemortem records of others. In mass disasters the process of matching becomes quite tedious. The easiest cases should be matched first. Both ante- and postmortem records should be initially separated into categories based upon the presence of bridgework, partial dentures and gold crowns. These less common restorative procedures will enable rapid elimination of certain persons. Complete upper and lower denture cases should be placed in another separate category. It is important to obtain the latest antemortem record available, since the deceased may have received the services of several dentists. In such cases, if only the earlier record is obtained, havoc may result with the comparison procedure. The time-consuming comparisons involve those victims having only the common silver (amalgam) fillings and missing teeth. Postmortem dental x rays may be needed to increase points of comparison. Although useful, postmortem x rays are generally not necessary. When needed, the use of the Panorex® x ray technique (*see* Fig. IV-2) enables rapid full-mouth x ray examination as well as an easily read panoramic view of the dentition. It also represents an excellent pictorial dental record easily understood by laymen, an asset in medicolegal jury cases. Panorex® equipment is available in most dental schools and in the offices of some dental practitioners. Autopsy room x ray equipment can also be adapted for the taking of intraoral dental radiographs. Dental x ray film can be obtained from any dental supply house.

The ideal cases for comparison are those wherein the dental arches are recovered intact in their entirety and where accurate up-to-date antemortem records are available. Given time, these cases become rather straightforward identifications. The problem cases arise when only portions of the dentition remain and poor or no antemortem records can be located.

In dealing with mass disasters the construction of an identification elimination chart as devised by Delaney in the Noronic fire[16, 22] is of immense value in facilitating the organization of identification data. The handling of the identification of victims in the Noronic disaster should be familiar to all persons who may become involved in mass identification.

In cases where identification remains undetermined for any reason, the cleaned dental arches should be removed en bloc and retained in formalin solution. They can then be retrieved months or years later if subsequent information becomes available. Removal of these portions of the jaws is easier, less expensive, less time consuming and quite superior to the construction of plaster casts from dental impressions.

## AGE DETERMINATION BASED UPON DENTAL DATA

The small variation in tooth formation and eruption among individuals has placed the dental estimation of chronological age as the primary method of age determination from birth to fourteen years of age. During this age range tooth formation exhibits less variability when compared with chronological age than other anthropological methods. Such determinations are based upon the degree of formation of root and crown structures, the stage of eruption and the intermixture of primary and adult dentitions. Dental x rays are necessary for evaluation of root formation and the developmental status of unerupted teeth; however, less precise but approximate determination of age can be accomplished by utilization of the eruption pattern alone. The eruption and calcification chart as mentioned by Gustafson[18] should be utilized by those performing age determinations in this age group. Schour and Massler[23] represent another popular reference regarding such data, including a pictorial chart of dental develop-

TABLE IV-I
CHRONOLOGY OF THE HUMAN DENTITION*

| | Tooth | *Maxillary* | | *Mandibular* | |
|---|---|---|---|---|---|
| | | *Eruption* | *R.C.*† | *Eruption* | *R.C.*† |
| Deciduous dentition *(baby teeth)* | central incisor | 7½ mo. | 1½ yr. | 6 mo. | 1½ yr. |
| | lateral incisor | 9 mo. | 2 yr. | 7 mo. | 1½ yr. |
| | cuspid | 18 mo. | 3¼ yr. | 16 mo. | 3¼ yr. |
| | first molar | 14 mo. | 2½ yr. | 12 mo. | 2¼ yr. |
| | second molar | 24 mo. | 3 yr. | 20 mo. | 3 yr. |
| Permanent dentition | central incisor | 7- 8 yr. | 10 yr. | 6- 7 yr. | 9 yr. |
| | lateral incisor | 8- 9 yr. | 11 yr. | 7- 8 yr. | 10 yr. |
| | cuspid | 11-12 yr. | 13-15 yr. | 9-10 yr. | 12-14 yr. |
| | first bicuspid | 10-11 yr. | 12-13 yr. | 10-12 yr. | 12-13 yr. |
| | second bicuspid | 10-12 yr. | 12-14 yr. | 11-12 yr. | 13-14 yr. |
| | first molar | 6- 7 yr. | 9-10 yr. | 6- 7 yr. | 9-10 yr. |
| | second molar | 12-13 yr. | 14-16 yr. | 11-13 yr. | 14-15 yr. |
| | third molar | 17-21 yr. | 18-25 yr. | 17-21 yr. | 18-25 yr. |

* From Logan, W. H., and Kronfeld, R.; slightly modified by McCall, J. O., and Schour, I.: *J Am Dent Assoc., 32*:139, 1936.

† Root completed; x-ray examination necessary.

ment. The work by Garn et al.[24] is a more recent critique of earlier tooth formation age values, revealing increasing variability of tooth formation than that previously recorded. A table depicting the chronology of the dentition is provided in Table IV-I.

From the chronological age of fourteen to twenty years, dental age estimation is based upon the stage of development of the third molar (wisdom tooth) and the root formation of the second molar. X ray examination is necessary, of course, to evaluate the crown and root calcification status of these teeth. There is much variation in these phenomena; hence, accuracy of dental age estimation during this interval diminishes, so that a variability of about plus or minus three years may exist. The presence of fully erupted third molars usually indicates that an individual is at least seventeen years of age. If the third molar is erupted but root formation is incomplete, the age is less than twenty-two to twenty-four years of age.

In some individuals, due to inadequate jaw space, the third molars may never erupt into the oral cavity. This is particularly true of the mandibular third molars. Such *trapped* teeth are referred to as impacted teeth, and the presence of impacted teeth should not be interpreted as being representative of a person less than seventeen years of age. In case of unerupted third molars, x rays of the third molar areas are necessary to evaluate the calcification status of these teeth; hence, only then can dental age be estimated.

A skeleton was found in an abandoned warehouse. The scene investigation (belt around neck suspended from a rafter) suggested that the manner of death was

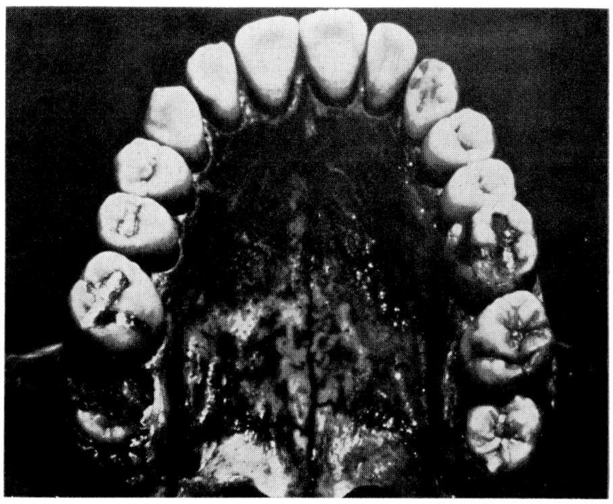

FIGURE IV-5. The unerupted maxillary third molars are evident. Note that there are only two molars on the right side and three molars on the left. The right first molar has been extracted several years earlier, and the second and third molars have drifted mesially, thus eliminating the first molar space.

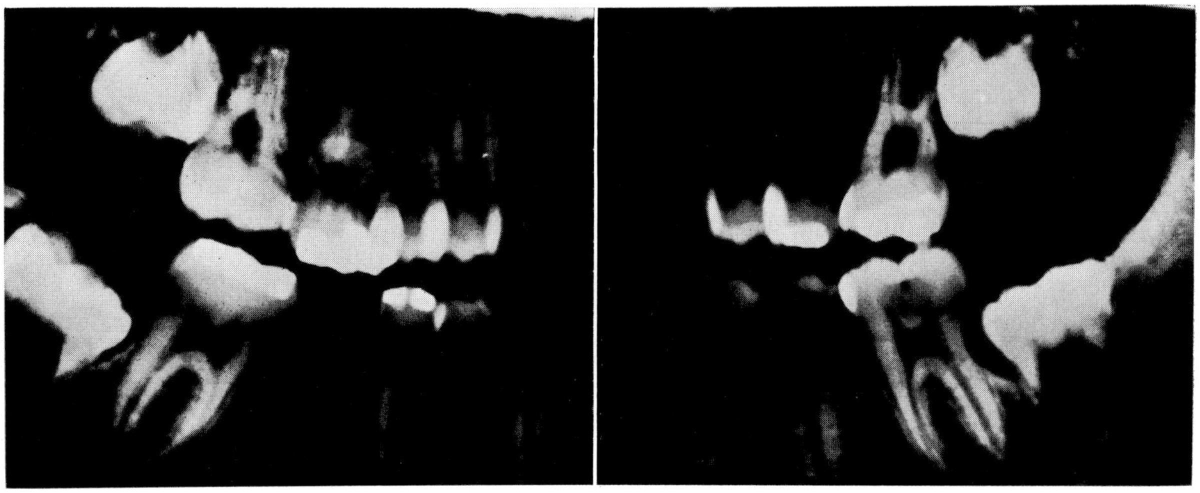

FIGURES IV-6 and IV-7. Postmortem radiographs of the third molar regions show a stage of root calcification compatible with a person of estimated fifteen and one-half years of age.

suicide. A general anthropologic survey of the skeleton indicated that the bones in question were from a black female in her late teens. The dentition was intact and served as the mode of identification as well as to further estimate the age.

The third molars were still partially encased in the respective jawbones in an unerupted state (Fig. IV-5). Roentgenographic examination of the third molars indicated root formation comparable to that expected for a person of approximately fifteen and one half years of age plus or minus one year (Figs. IV-6 and IV-7). Further examination of the teeth revealed that the nature and neatness of the restorations were indicative of their placement by a conscientious dentist, with a suggestion that the work may have been done by a young dentist working in a public school clinic. A tentative identification was subsequently established by correlating the estimated age, sex, race, interval since death and nature of the clothing with a listing of the Missing Persons Bureau. This tentative identification was verified by comparison with the antemortem dental records located at the clinic where the girl attended school. Had the Missing Persons Bureau not led us to the putative identity in this case, we had proposed to investigate the nearby neighborhoods for school clinics on the assumption that the girl probably had lived in the area where the body was discovered. Once the case was completed, the relative locations of the home, warehouse and the school clinic were noted to be within a six-block radius of one another. The adolescent had passed her sixteenth birthday on the day prior to her disappearance and was extremely dejected at not receiving any presents. She was additionally depressed by her recent rejection by a boyfriend.

Age determination on the basis of teeth becomes exceedingly difficult beyond the age of twenty years. Gustafson devised a method based upon chronological age and its morphological changes in the tooth and its supporting structures.[18] These detailed micromethods employ the expertise of a well-trained dental histologist and are not relevant to the purpose of this chapter. In a similar context, the designation of sex and race based upon dental characteristics is quite complex, often disputable and unreliable, and should be relegated to the anthropologist or forensic odontology expert.

## OCCUPATIONAL AND SOCIAL STIGMATA OF TEETH

A person's occupation or oral habits frequently leave telltale signs upon the dentition. Carpenters, upholsterers and electricians comprise the *nail holders* and may notch the upper incisors due to the gripping of nails between the front teeth. Dressmakers and tailors also have similar smaller pin notches. Many women open bobby pins with their teeth, leading to broad notches in the upper central incisors. Wind instrument musicians may have broad areas of attrition of the anterior teeth due to clenching of the instrument mouthpiece. Long-time inveterate pipe smokers often develop diamond-shaped or irregular gaps in the closed bite spanning several teeth located at the angles of the mouth. A black-brown nicotine stain is found adjacent to the gingival margins on the lingual and interproximal surfaces of teeth of heavy cigarette and pipe smokers. In general, the presence of poor oral hygiene, characterized by few restorations, many decayed teeth and signs of inflammation of the gums, connotes an individual of low economic status. The finding of many previously extracted teeth without replacement by bridgework or partial dentures also correlates with persons of lower social standards.

## BITE MARKS

On occasion, bite marks have played a decisive role in criminal identification. The substance bitten may be the body (as in sexual crimes), foodstuffs or other materials. Numerous instances of bite mark identification are recorded.[5, 9, 25–29] The interpretation and correlation of bite marks found at the scene of a crime or on a victim with the dental pattern obtained from the suspected criminal require the attention of a skilled dental expert. The techniques of obtaining proper impressions, the preparation of casts and the actual comparison of bite patterns does not fall within the realm of the pathologist. Even experts in the field of bite mark comparison admit that numerous limitations exist in the interpretation of such data.

Gustafson[18] presents a broad, detailed description of the methods and problems involved, and an excellent discussion of comparison techniques involving bite marks is afforded by Furness.[26]

Upon discovery of a possible bite mark injury, the pathologist or official investigating the crime should contact the dental consultant so as to establish a further course of action. This must be done as soon as possible and prior to any manipulation of the tissue. Handling of the body and autopsy introduce artifacts. Postmortem changes may lead to shrinkage or bloating of the tissues, loss of tooth indentations and diffusion of hemorrhage under the skin so as to distort the original tooth pattern.

Similarly, foodstuffs (cheese, fruit, butter) alter their form upon drying or with temperature change. Foodstuffs should be wrapped in paper, soaked in formalin and delivered immediately to the crime laboratory, where impressions can be made.

Swabbing of the skin or other specimen for possible salivary secretor substance retrieval should be done early in the bite mark examination. Approximately 80 percent of persons are *secretors,* and the basic A, B and H blood group antigenic complexes are present in the various body fluids of such persons, including the saliva. The detection of salivary secretor substances may serve to further implicate or eliminate a particular suspect in a given case. The test for secretory antigens is usually performed by the serology section of the police crime laboratory and should be implemented as soon as possible to minimize changes resulting from autolysis. Such changes set in quite rapidly due to proteolytic enzymes present in saliva.

Accurate documentation of a bite mark is of great significance. Photography of the injury prior to excision, with a millimeter rule included in the picture, is recommended for possible later use as evidence. Ultraviolet or infrared illumination may be utilized to demonstrate faint areas of bruising not readily recognized under ordinary light. After registration and adequate documentation of a bite mark has been completed, a section of bruised skin from the injury should be excised for subsequent microscopic examination to ascertain the timing of the injury relative to the time of death.

*Registration of the dentition of the victim* may be of significance in instances where the anatomical position of the bite mark on the victim is consistent with self-biting. Such a procedure may be required to dismiss any possibility that the deceased had bitten himself or herself. In cases where the suspected assailant is believed to have been bitten by the deceased, the registration of the victim's dentition may be necessary to relate the assailant to the crime.

In a situation where an animal attacks and kills a person, the bites are usually easily distinguished from human bite injuries due to differences in arch alignment and specific tooth morphology. Dog bites, perhaps the most common nonhuman bite, are characterized by a narrow anterior dental arch and consist of deep tooth wounds over a small area. The dog has small central and broad lateral incisors compared with the broad central and narrow lateral incisors of the human. The dog or other carnivorous mammal is more apt to cause laceration and avulsion of tissue during violent biting than is the human (*see* Fig. VII-47), although portions of breasts or ears may be completely bitten off in human bite attacks. Cat bites are small and round, with pointed cuspid tooth impressions due to the conical shape of those teeth. Claw scratches are also often noted in feline bites.

## DENTAL TERMINOLOGY

Dental nomenclature is presented to narrow the communication gap that exists between the physician and dentist.

1. *Anterior teeth:* From cuspid to cuspid, inclusive (cuspids, lateral and central incisors).
2. *Posterior teeth:* All bicuspid and molar teeth.
3. *Mesial, distal, occlusal, buccal, lingual:* Tooth surfaces visible in the mouth (*see* item 10).
4. *Caries:* Cavity due to erosion of tooth structure by bacterial acid formation.
5. *Preparation:* The change in tooth structure performed by the dentist to remove decay and alter the tooth in order to retain the filling material or crown in adherence to laws of stress and strain.
6. *Restoration:* Substance used to repair teeth and restore structure and function of teeth. The damaged tooth is *prepared* (as in item 5) prior to the use of the following restorations:
    a. *Amalgam:* Silver filling; an alloy composed primarily of silver and tin mixed with mercury; used predominantly on posterior teeth and represents the most common restoration encountered in the mouth.
    b. *Gold inlay:* A cast gold restoration made from an impression of the preparation and cemented in place; used on anterior and posterior teeth; expensive. Designates high quality dental care or work performed in a dental school.
    c. *Gold foil:* A cohesive gold restoration wedged and molded into the preparation; used on anterior or posterior teeth; very expensive. Implies high quality dental care or work done in a dental school.
    d. *Silicate:* An esthetic silica cement used on anterior teeth appearing the same shade as the surrounding tooth structure.
    e. *Acrylic:* A polymerizing plastic resin used on anterior teeth cosmetically blending with tooth color.
    f. *Temporary cements:* White-gray substances placed in incompleted restorations; used on all teeth.
    g. *Crown:* A cap. A complete or partial coverage of a single tooth by a gold construction that fits over the prepared tooth as a glove fits a hand. Crowns may have superficial outer layers of porcelain or plastic, partial or total, so as to appear as normal tooth color. Used on all teeth.
7. *Prosthesis:* An appliance utilized in the replacement of or substitution for missing teeth.
    a. *Fixed prosthesis:* A bridge; nonremovable. A bridge is a fixed, cemented device used to span a gap in the dentition; usually formed by crowns at either side of the gap (the abutment teeth) with a pontic section(s) replacing the missing tooth or teeth. A bridge may span as many as five or six teeth (Fig. IV-8).

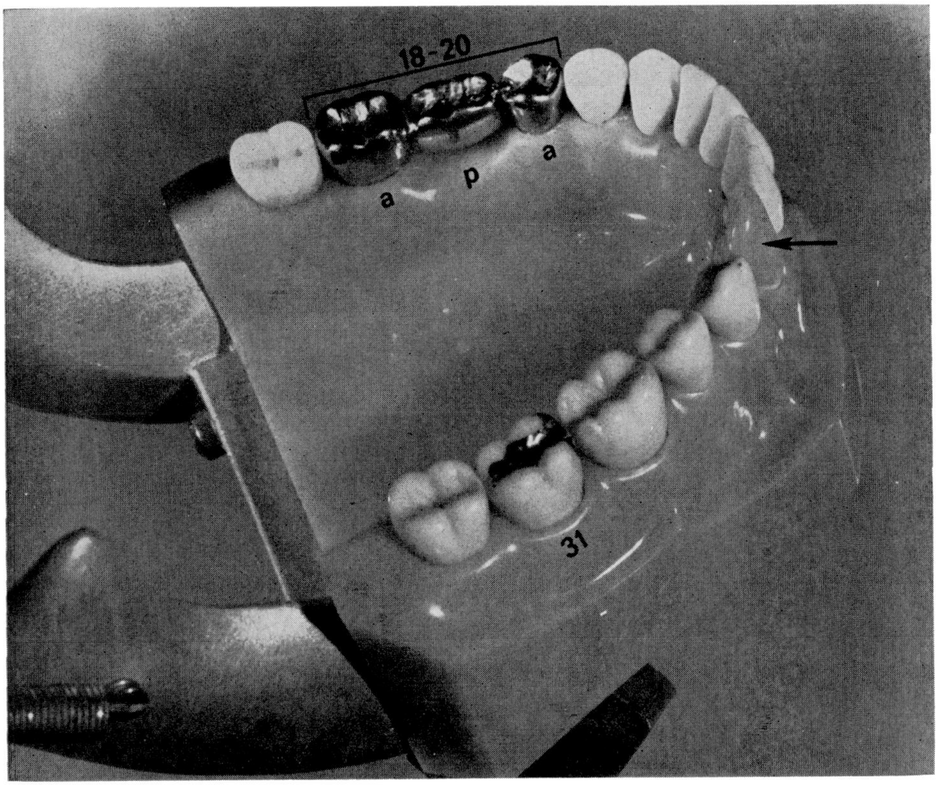


FIGURE IV-8. A three-unit bridge involving the lower left second and first molars and the second bicuspid is shown. The tooth replaced by the pontic (p) is the first molar (#19). The abutment teeth (a) fitted with complete gold crowns are the second molar (#18) and second bicuspid (#20). The arrow depicts a single full crown restoration of porcelain. The lower right second molar (#31) contains a mesio-occlusal (MO) restoration.

b. *Removable prosthesis:* 1. False teeth, complete denture; with plastic pink base and embedded teeth of acrylic or porcelain. Usually seen as complete pair, i.e. upper and lower; 2. Partial denture; false teeth replacing only a segment or segments of the missing dentition of a dental arch. Attaches to remaining teeth by clasps and hooks. Contains a gold, stainless steel or pink acrylic base.

8. *Root canal (endodontia):* Cleansing and removal of the pulpal tissue with filling of the pulp chamber and root canals by silver points or cementlike substance. Can only be noticed by x ray, as such treatment is performed within the tooth and then covered by a restoration (*see* Fig. IV-2). Of great significance in identification, as these are uncommon procedures. May be performed on anterior or posterior teeth.

9. *Dentition numbering systems:* Various dentists utilize many different numbering systems for the dentition, and the physician should not be confused by the variety of systems employed. A commonly used numbering system is the Universal System wherein the right upper third molar is #1 and the left upper third molar #16. The lower left third molar is #17, and the right lower third molar is #32 (Figs. IV-9 and IV-10). If difficulty arises, one can always recite the actual tooth, i.e. right upper second bicuspid (rather than #4), in discussing a case. Most patient dental charts depict the numbering system used by the

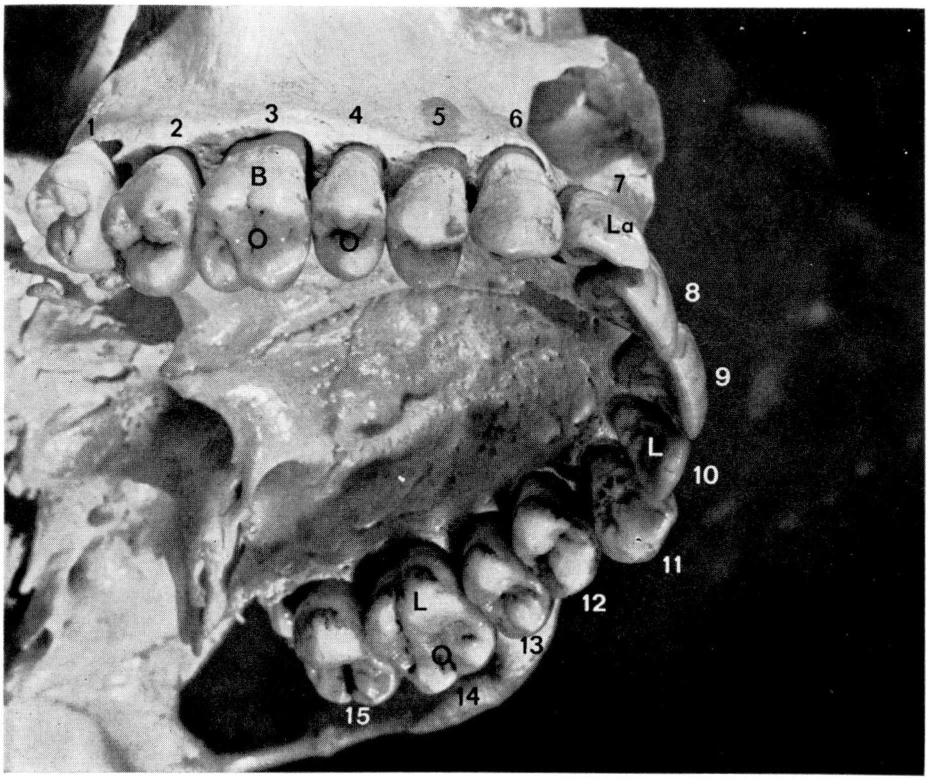


FIGURE IV-9

dentist in the tooth diagram section of the chart.

10. *Tooth surface nomenclature:* As mentioned earlier, each tooth presents five surfaces upon intraoral visual examination. These surfaces are named in the following manner (Fig. IV-11):
   a. The *occlusal* (O) surface is the surface that contacts the opposing tooth when the jaws are in occlusion (closed). It can be regarded as the chewing surface of the tooth. On anterior teeth, this surface is referred to as the incisal surface or edge.
   b, c. The two surfaces in direct contact with the adjacent neighboring teeth are known as the proximal surfaces and are called the *mesial* (M) and *distal* (D) surfaces. These surfaces are named according to their relationship with the anterior midline of the jaw. The mesial surface is the surface of the tooth directed towards the midline. The distal surface faces away from the midline. These surfaces roughly correspond in familiar anatomical nomenclature to medial and lateral, respectively.
   d, e. The two remaining surfaces are those that face the cheek (posterior teeth) or lips (anterior teeth) and the tongue. The surface of the posterior teeth directed toward the cheek is the *buccal* surface (B). This corresponds to the labial surface of anterior teeth. The inward-directed surface of all teeth is the *lingual* (L) surface.

In practical use, the letters M, O, D, B, L refer to mesial, occlusal, distal, buccal and lingual respectively. The filling materials used on any given tooth are described according to the altered tooth surfaces involved. For example, a single surface occlusal silver filling on a molar would be called *an occlusal (O) amalgam on tooth*

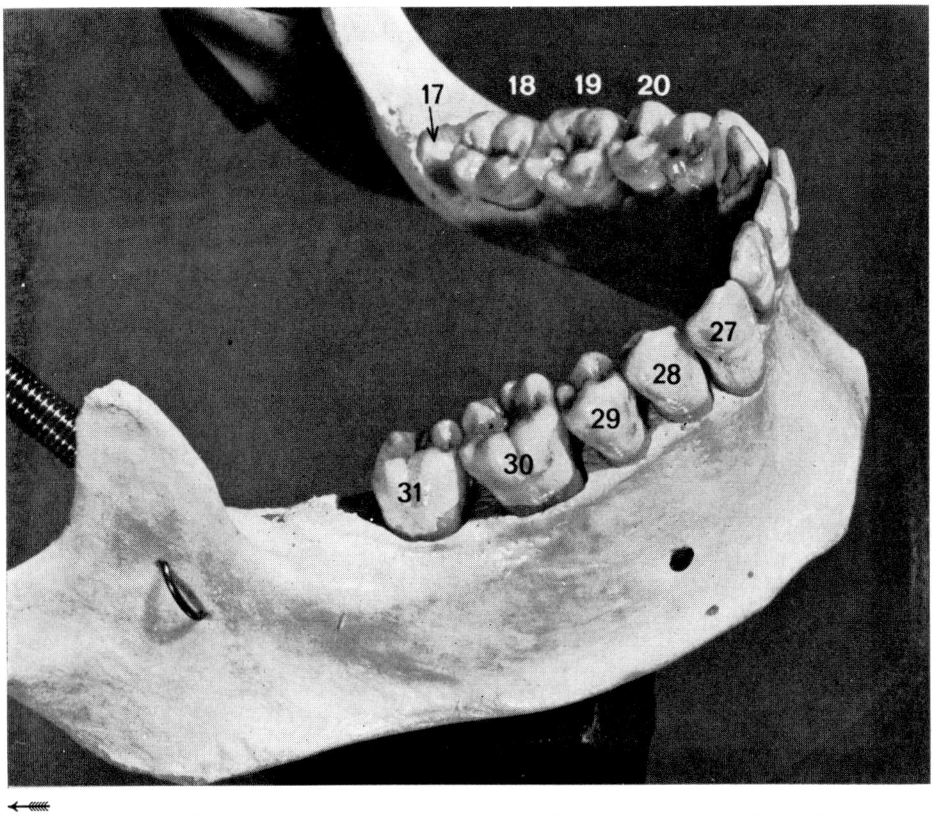


FIGURES IV-9 and IV-10. A commonly used numbering system as it applies to the dental arches:

| Right Lower | Right Upper | | Left Upper | Left Lower |
|---|---|---|---|---|
| #32 | #1 | third molars | #16 | #17 |
| 31 | 2 | second molars | 15 | 18 |
| 30 | 3 | first molars | 14 | 19 |
| 29 | 4 | second bicuspids | 13 | 20 |
| 28 | 5 | first bicuspids | 12 | 21 |
| 27 | 6 | cuspids | 11 | 22 |
| 26 | 7 | lateral incisors | 10 | 23 |
| 25 | 8 | central incisors | 9 | 24 |

Also designated are several tooth surfaces: O—occlusal, B—buccal, L—lingual, La—labial.

# . . . . . More complexly, a two-surface restoration would be a mesio-occlusal (MO), disto-occlusal (DO), occluso-buccal (OB) or occluso-lingual (OL) restoration, depending upon the surfaces involved. One can even have more extensive fillings involving three or even all five surfaces. Such an example would be *an MOD amalgam on tooth #* . . . ., which designates a continuous silver restoration involving the mesio-occluso-distal surfaces of the particular tooth. A MODBL restoration would, similarly, represent a mesio-occluso-distal restoration with continuous buccal and lingual extensions. The restoration of a tooth, then, is designated by surface(s) and type of material. A *distal (D) silicate* would refer to a silicate restoration on the distal surface of the particular tooth. A *buccal (B) amalgam* would refer to a single surface amalgam restoration on the buccal surface.

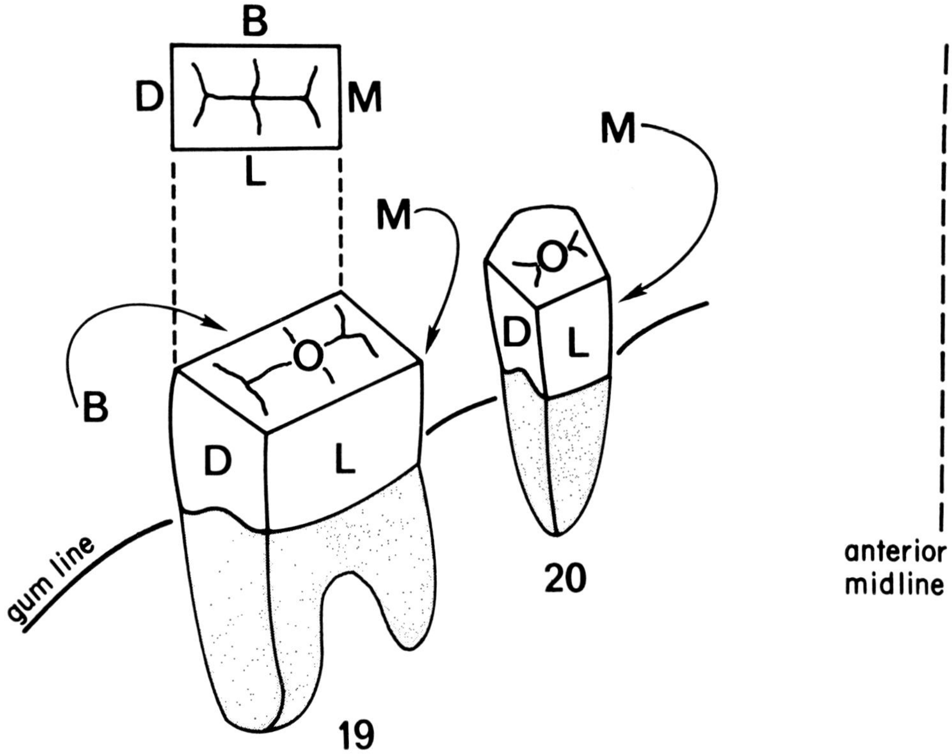


FIGURE IV-11. A diagram of the lower left molar area illustrates the various tooth surfaces. The view is from the lingual aspect, and a schematic separation is interposed between the first molar (#19) and the second bicuspid (#20). O—occlusal, B—buccal, L—lingual, M—mesial, D—distal.

## REFERENCES

1. Personal and General: Identified by tooth. John Wilkes Booth's body recognized three years after death. *Am Dent J, 2:*477, 1903.
2. Identification by the teeth. *Dent Advertiser, 22:*15, 1891.
3. Amoëdo, O.: The rôle of the dentists in the identification of the victims of the catastrophe of the Bazar de la Charité, Paris, 4th of May, 1897. *Dent Cosmos, 39:*905, 1897.
4. Editorial: The Iroquois Fire. *Am Dent J, 3:*139, 1904.
5. Verne, D.: Bridging the gap. *Cleve Dent Soc Bull V,* 1950, p. 16.
6. Bezymenski, L.: *The Death of Adolph Hitler.* New York, Har Brace World, 1968.
7. Fry, W. K.: The Baptist church cellar case. *Br Dent J, 75:*154, 1943.
8. Simpson, K.: "Rex vs. John George Haigh": The acid-bath murder. *Med Leg J, 18:*38, 1950.
9. Cleland, J. B.: Teeth and bites in history, literature, forensic medicine and otherwise. *Aust Dent J, 48:*107, 1944.
10. Stevens, P. J., and Tarlton, S. W.: Identification of mass casualities: Experience in four civil air disasters. *Med Sci Law, 3:*154, 1963.
11. Haines, D. H.: Dental identification in the Stockport air disaster. *Br Dent J, 123:*336, 1967.
12. Stevens, P. J., and Tarlton, S. W.: Medical investigation in fatal aircraft accidents. *Br Dent J, 120:* 263, 1966.
13. van Wyk, C. W., Kemp, V. D., and Burkofzer, H.: The role of identification in the Windhoek aircrash. *Med Leg J, 37:*79, 1969.
14. Keiser-Nielsen, S.: Forensic odontology—Cases and comments. In Wecht, C. H. (Ed.): *Legal Medicine Annual 1970.* New York, Appleton, 1970, p. 31.
15. Rosenbluth, E. S.: A legal identification. *Dent Cosmos, 44:*1029, 1902.
16. Grant, E. A., Pendergast, W. K., and White, E. A.:

Dental identification in the Noronic disaster. *J Can Dent Assoc, 18:*3, 1952.

17. Knott, N. J.: Identification by the teeth of casualties in the Aberfan disaster. *Br Dent J, 122:*144, 1967.
18. Gustafson, G.: *Forensic Odontology.* London, Staples Press, 1966, pp. 30, 111, 118-131, 140-165.
19. Luntz, L. L.: Dental radiography and photography in identification. *Dent Radiogr Photogr, 40:* 83, 1967.
20. Rogers, A. P.: Identification by dental means. *J Am Dent Assoc, 23:*181, 1936.
21. Gustafson, G., and Johanson, G.: The values of certain characteristics in dental identification. *Acta Odontol Scand, 21:*367, 1963.
22. Singleton, A. C.: The roentgenological identification of victims of the Noronic disaster. *Am J Roentgenol Radium Ther Nucl Med, 66:*375, 1951.
23. Schour, I., and Massler, M.: The development of the human dentition. *J Am Dent Assoc, 38:*1153, 1941.
24. Garn, S. M., Lewis, A. B., and Polacheck, D. L.: Variability of tooth formation. *J Dent Res, 38:* 135, 1959.
25. Simpson, K.: Dental evidence in the reconstruction of crime. *Br Dent J, 91:*229, 1951.
26. Furness, J.: A new method for the identification of teeth marks in cases of assault and homicide. *Br Dent J, 124:*261, 1968.
27. Sopher, I. M.: *Forensic Dentistry.* Springfield, Thomas, 1976, Chapter IX.
28. Layton, J. J.: Identification from a bite mark in cheese. *J Forensic Sci Soc, 6:*76, 1966.
29. Furuhata, T., and Yamamoto, K.: *Forensic Odontology.* Springfield, Thomas, 1967, pp. 99-102.

*Chapter V*

# SUDDEN AND UNEXPECTED DEATH FROM NATURAL CAUSES IN ADULTS

LESTER ADELSON AND CHARLES S. HIRSCH

EVERY UNEXPECTED death has an actual or potential medicolegal aspect, and in most countries such deaths come under the scrutiny of a medicolegal investigative official, who may be called a coroner, medical examiner, medical referee or by some other title. He has the responsibility for establishing the *cause* and *manner* of death in these unanticipated fatalities and also in those in which violence of some type is known or alleged to have played a part.

That sudden, unexpected and violent deaths are uniquely important to society is indicated immediately by the fact that they fall under the jurisdiction of a special *medicolegal* government official. Medical interest lies in accurate establishment of the nature of the fatal disease or injury and correlation of this information with the circumstances surrounding death. Legal importance derives from the availability and utilization of precise and objective medical data for the administration of justice, whether it be a civil action for wrongful death, workmen's compensation, insurance benefits under an accidental death policy and the like, or a criminal prosecution for some degree of homicide.

This chapter deals with several medicolegal problems that arise when death occurs suddenly or unexpectedly solely from *natural causes in an adult.* Reference will be made to traumatic situations and incidents for purposes of illustration, but the emphasis here is on those deaths that result entirely from disease.

## UNEXPLAINED DEATHS

Clinically *unexplained* deaths fall into two categories: (a) those that occur in patients who have been studied extensively during prolonged, complex illnesses without a satisfactory diagnosis having been established; (b) those that follow an illness of such brief duration that there has been little or no opportunity for medical observation or studies to provide a reasonable explanation for what has occurred.

The more *unexpected* the death, the more likely it is to be *unexplained.* Ample experience has taught that it is more difficult to make a correct diagnosis in persons taken acutely ill who die shortly after admission to the hospital than in persons dying under almost any other circumstances. A meager or absent history combined with a hasty, incomplete physical examination and insufficient time to carry out informative tests in a dying, uncooperative patient often lead to deductions that are, at best, haphazard speculations.

## INCIDENCE OF SUDDEN AND UNEXPECTED NATURAL DEATHS

Sudden deaths in adults from presumably natural causes occur more frequently than is commonly supposed. Numerically they constitute a significant fraction of the total mortality in any sizeable community. Where sound laws govern the administration of the Coroner's or Medical Examiner's Office, this governmental agency investigates between 15 percent and 25 percent of *all* deaths within its jurisdictional area. Approximately 60 to 70 percent of *these* deaths result from natural causes (Figs. V-1 and V-2).

Although no age group is exempt, sudden and unexpected deaths from disease are relatively uncommon between ages one and thirty and after age seventy. The most common causes

**TYPES OF CASES RECEIVED BY THE CORONER'S OFFICE**
**COUNTY OF CUYAHOGA**

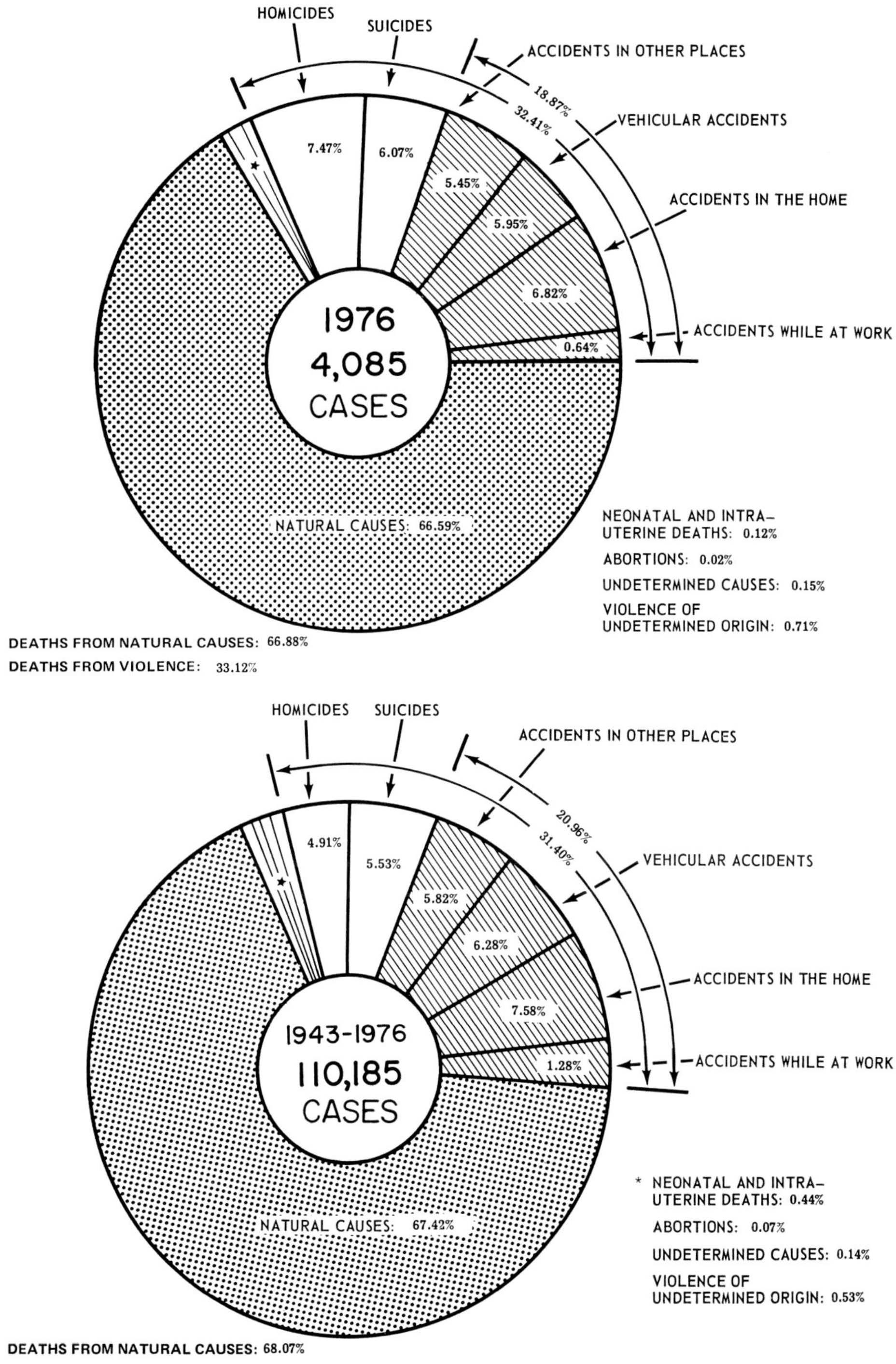


FIGURES V-1 and V-2. Graphic illustrations of types of deaths processed by a large metropolitan medicolegal investigative office (Cleveland, Ohio) on annual (1976) and long-term (1943-1976, inclusive) bases.

of these deaths are clinically silent, degenerative diseases *(vide infra)*. Such pathologic entities are infrequent in early life, and the victim in the older age group has usually given some overt indication of the disease which ultimately proves fatal to him.

Men outnumber women by far as the victims of this type of demise,[1] and the economically depressed are more likely to succumb in this fashion than the prosperous.

## CAUSE, MANNER AND MECHANISM OF DEATH

Before proceeding further, it is essential that several terms that will come up repeatedly in this discussion be strictly defined in order to eliminate semantic confusion.

The *cause of death* is the disease or injury responsible for initiating the train of events, brief or prolonged, that produced the fatal end result.

The *manner of death* is the fashion in which the *cause of death* came into being. If death results solely from disease, the *manner of death* is *natural (natural causes)*. If death is caused solely by injury or is hastened as the result of injury in a person rendered vulnerable by preexisting natural disease, the manner of death is *violent* or *unnatural*.

Violence may be *accidental, homicidal, suicidal* or of *undetermined origin*, depending on the circumstances surrounding the traumatic incident. Thus, the *cause of death* of a person who died as the result of a bullet passing through his head is a gunshot wound of the head with perforations of the skull and brain. The *manner of death* is *homicide* if the gun was fired by some other person who intended to harm or kill the victim, *accident* if the gun was fired inadvertently by the victim or by someone else without intent to do harm ("I didn't know it was loaded."), *suicide* if the victim deliberately and intentionally pulled the trigger in the purposeful attempt to end his own life and *undetermined in origin* if the circumstances surrounding the fatal shooting cannot be established with reasonable certainty.

The *mechanism of death* is the physiologic derangement or biochemical disturbance produced by the *cause of death* which is incompatible with life. It includes such phenomena as asystole and ventricular fibrillation, hemorrhagic shock, severe metabolic acidosis and alkalosis, sepsis, toxemia, respiratory depression or paralysis and the like.

## MEDICOLEGAL MASQUERADES

One basis for the deep interest of the law in sudden and unexpected death derives from the fact that one type *(manner)* of death frequently masquerades as another. This is especially true when the entire fatal episode transpired so quickly that it was not possible to establish either the cause or the manner of death with sufficient certainty or precision to allay suspicion and to eliminate violence as a factor.

Deaths from natural causes often occur so rapidly or in such fashion or under such circumstances as to suggest erroneously that violence has somehow been involved. Unless one establishes clearly and unequivocally the true manner of such a death, the police may be put into the impossible position of trying to find a nonexistent murderer, or the deceased may be unfairly stigmatized as having committed suicide with its attendant sequelae (e.g. voiding of life insurance policies, withholding of religious burial rites, etc.), or a double indemnity accidental death benefit on a life insurance policy of workmen's compensation may be wrongly awarded.

A married couple was heard arguing and scuffling in their apartment about the wife's excessive drinking. A door slammed, and the husband was seen leaving the house. Several hours later neighbors found the woman dead in a pool of blood. Her face, arms and trunk bore multiple recent and fading bruises.

The husband was found and immediately taken into custody by the police on suspicion of homicide. Autopsy revealed no internal evidence of injury. The blood at the scene was the result of massive bleeding (hematemesis) from ruptured esophageal varices, secondary to portal cirrhosis arising on the basis of her prolonged alcoholism. This death, which had presented itself originally as a homicidal assault, was thus demonstrated as having arisen from a totally different, noncriminal causation. The husband was released immediately.

In another case the driver of a speeding auto that ran into a tree was dead when he was removed from the wreckage. External and internal examination revealed severe injuries of the chest and abdomen including multiple bilateral comminuted rib fractures, a fractured sternum, and lacerations of the heart, lungs and liver, accompanied by *no internal bleeding.* Severe coronary atherosclerosis and a healed myocardial infarct were also present. It was concluded that death had occurred as a result of natural (coronary) disease prior to the violent impact, and that *death had caused the accident.*

The converse of the preceding proposition is equally true. Persons may be murdered, commit suicide or die as a result of accidental injuries in such fashion or under such circumstances that casual observation or superficial study creates the mistaken impression that they succumbed to natural disease. This erroneous conclusion becomes even more plausible where the decedent has a history of some disease with lethal potentialities. *The presence of previously diagnosed, far-advanced natural disease affords no guarantee that violence played no part in the death.*

When a physician is called to the scene of death of a stranger or even of one of his patients, he should approach the body and his responsibilities with a healthy suspicion that the obvious or the expected may not have happened. Too often there is a naive presumption of natural death.

Rapid or delayed deaths can result from violence which produces little or no external evidence of injury. The variety of such concealed or latent traumata is quite broad.

Fatal electric shock can occur with only a minute (and readily overlooked) electrical burn to indicate the nature of the agent responsible for death. Indeed, when death is caused by passage of a low voltage current (110 v, AC) entering and leaving the body through wide, moist surface areas, there may be no visible cutaneous injuries whatsoever, despite the fact that the electrical disturbance was sufficiently potent to cause ventricular fibrillation or respiratory paralysis.

Fatal blunt head trauma can occur with no externally visible injury of the scalp, especially when the decedent has a full head of hair or was wearing a hat. Likewise, blunt force applied over a broad area of the trunk can create lifetaking intra-abdominal and intrathoracic injuries without the telltale presence of external bruises or abrasions. Many deaths from poison provide the most striking examples of fatal (chemical) violence that kills without creating external or internal gross or microscopic evidence of injury.

A fifty-seven-year-old woman with known disseminated cancer following radical amputation of her breast who had been progressing slowly downhill was *unexpectedly* found dead one morning. Autopsy revealed that the cancer had spread to her lungs, liver, hilar lymph nodes and thoracic vertebrae. Chemical analyses of her blood and viscera demonstrated massive quantities of glutethimide (Doriden®). Interrogation of the family revealed that a suicide note had been disposed of in an attempt to conceal the true nature of her death.

In summary, then, there are two equally faulty opposing approaches to the general problem of sudden and unexpected deaths insofar as their manner is concerned. The first is the erroneous assumption that all such deaths are the result of disease, and the other is based on the fallacious presumption that they always result from violence. Both generalities are dangerous and disturbing.

That one type of violent death may masquerade as another (e.g. homicide simulating accident, suicide suggesting homicide) is axiomatic to all who have had even a modicum of experience in the field of medicolegal investigation. However, the present consideration of sudden and unexpected death is limited to those deaths resulting from natural causes, and the challenging facets of those produced by violence is not germane to the present discussion.

## COEXISTENCE OF TRAUMA AND DISEASE—CONSEQUENCE OR COINCIDENCE?

The victim of sudden natural death may sustain noncontributory injury incident to an agonal episode in which he collapsed and fell without being able to protect himself. If the fall takes place on the pavement, an uncarpeted floor or some other hard surface, contusions, abrasions and lacerations may be sustained that suggest that trauma is somehow involved in the death. This is especially true if the decedent fell down a flight of stairs or from an elevated object. Complete *external* and *internal* examination are essential to disclose the role, if any, played by trauma in such a death.

On the other hand, natural diseases do create situations that can lead to fatal injury. Epileptics can drown as a result of a seizure; the patient with Ménière's disease (paroxysmal labyrinthine vertigo) can fall from a height during an episode of nausea and dizziness; and the cardiac patient can incur fatal injury from an auto accident that resulted from his losing consciousness during the attack of Stokes-Adams syndrome as he drove along the highway.

The potential interplay of trauma and natural disease in causing or contributing to death can give rise to even more complex and perplexing situations. If the victim of injury dies shortly after being hurt or even at some considerably later time, and if postmortem examination indicates that death was caused by injury, there is no problem as to the *manner* of death. However, knotty questions may arise where there is a symptom-free interval between apparent recovery from trauma and death from well-documented natural disease. If justice is to be done, the causal or contributory effect of the injury to death must be accurately evaluated. For example, granted that the victim died of a myocardial infarct secondary to arteriosclerotic heart disease, what weight, if any, should be given to the leg fractured at work two weeks prior to the fatal episode? Deaths due to intracerebral hemorrhage at some time following head injury[2] may present difficult problems in medicolegal interpretation. Such questions require circumspect and objective assessment of all data before one can offer a sound and fair opinion as to the causal or contributory responsibility of trauma to death.

## CIRCUMSTANCES SURROUNDING SUDDEN AND UNEXPECTED NATURAL DEATHS

Sudden and unexpected deaths occur in persons with varying medical backgrounds, including those in whom a diagnosis of potentially lethal disease has never been made. Generally, with the exceptions noted in the following section, these victims have harbored some preexisting chronic disease of which neither they nor their friends were aware. Such lack of awareness can result from absence of significant preceding symptomatology or because clear-cut manifestations of illness have been ignored, minimized, misinterpreted or rationalized.

At the opposite extreme are unexpected deaths occurring in the course of well-documented chronic diseases that have either progressed rapidly to a stage incompatible with life or have triggered the development of quickly fatal sequelae or complications.

### *Sudden* Death and *Unexpected* Death

The terms *sudden* and *unexpected* have different meanings for different people.[3] *Sudden* death is usually both *quick* and *unexpected.* How soon must the victim die after the appearance of the unexpected illness for his death to be truly sudden? While no definite or categorical answer can be given to this question, it is fair to say that while death need not be instantaneous, it cannot be long delayed. Death from peritonitis complicating a perforated peptic ulcer forty-eight hours after the onset of acute abdominal pain in a previously *healthy* adult might well be considered *sudden and unexpected* by his family and friends. The physicians in attendance would probably not consider such a death as either sudden or unexpected.

The death of a forty-eight-year-old man with a reliable history of hypertension and arteriosclerotic heart disease who collapses and dies instantaneously while playing golf is only *relatively* unexpected. His cardiovascular disease renders him vulnerable to sudden death at any moment. Such *relatively* expected or *predictable* deaths, to phrase it differently, resulting from these varieties of chronic disease that seem to offer no immediate threat to the patient's life, comprise the common category of unexpected death.

From the medicolegal point of view, the *unexpected* aspect of death is more significant than its *rapidity*. It is the *dramatic intrusion of the unexpected that is so often responsible for arousing the suspicion of violence.* Many deaths that occur while the patient is under medical observation and care—indeed, while he is confined to the hospital—are *sudden* but hardly *unexpected.* The slowly deteriorating victim of a previously diagnosed carcinoma of the lung who dies immediately following massive bleeding from the air passages is a case in point. This spectacular termination of the patient's life is an anticipated manifestation of the natural course of the disease, and its occurrence occasions little surprise among those familiar with the behavior of this frequently encountered cancer. The medicolegal officer has little or no official interest in this type of death, despite its suddenness, if the decedent has been under the care of a physician who can (and will) sign the death certificate.

Absence of medical attention or failure of the physician to establish the correct diagnosis and prognosis of a potentially fatal illness help create situations where the abrupt appearance of death may be considered as totally *unexpected.* The forensic pathologist occasionally encounters *sudden and unexpected* deaths resulting from large intracranial tumors in persons who have been under observation and treatment for psychoneurosis, hysteria or psychosis. Here, the attending physician has ascribed the presence of such symptoms as headache, vomiting and emotional lability to some unresolved conflict when they were actually produced by the tumor of the brain or its surrounding membranes.

In this context the *either/or fallacy* of diagnosis deserves brief comment. In making his diagnosis on the basis of history, clinical observation and laboratory studies, the physician is strongly inclined to ascribe subjective and objective abnormalities either to *this* disease or to *that* disease. However, there are very few diseases whose presences are mutually exclusive, and in many instances two separate and distinct clinical entities are present in the same patient and perhaps in the same organ. Neurotic and psychotic patients are not immune to serious organic disease, and many sudden and unexpected deaths in these unfortunate individuals are the result of the families and physicians being misled by the *psychiatric* background and *emotionally disturbed* aspects of the overall presenting clinical picture.

A high threshold for pain and discomfort combined with self-neglect can help create the impression that a particular death was *sudden and unexpected.* In forensic pathologic practice it is not unusual to discover that the man who collapsed and died suddenly in a barroom while ordering a drink and complaining of a bad cold was the victim of full-blown lobar pneumonia. The extent, severity and stage of the disease readily demonstrable at the autopsy table indicate that there must have been ample warning symptomatically to alert the patient to the fact that he was seriously ill. However, as a result of stoicism, acute and chronic alcoholism, psychosis or some other factor that led to minimizing or ignoring what undoubtedly was unmistakable evidence of serious disease, he collapsed and died *unexpectedly.*

The forensic pathologist who is intimately concerned with the anatomic investigation of sudden, unexpected and violent death is confronted repeatedly by instances of far-advanced disease that inevitably must have produced prominent and even disabling subjective and objective phenomena (e.g. high fever, jaundice, accumulation of large amounts of fluids in the abdominal cavity, vomiting, coughing of blood) and yet never induced the victim to seek readily available medical attention. These types of sudden death are completely different from that produced by massive pulmonary embolism secondary to *silent* thromboses of the legs and pelvis where there have been no warnings of impending disaster.

Faulty self-diagnosis arising from misinterpretation or rationalization of symptoms is an additional mechanism that leads to the occurrence of *unexpected* deaths. Thus, proprietary gastric antacids are found frequently in the pockets of persons who have died suddenly from arteriosclerotic heart disease. Interrogation of the family and associates of the victim elicits a history of *acid stomach* or *heartburn* for which the antacid was self-prescribed and administered. That death was due to a heart attack and that the "stomach trouble" was cardiac in origin comes as a complete surprise to all.

## ESTABLISHMENT OF THE CAUSE OF DEATH

Two different sources and types of information, utilized individually or in concert, are available to the medicolegal investigator. In every instance he should acquire all available *anamnestic* data from witnesses to the terminal episode or illness, together with whatever medical background information can be obtained from family, friends, persons and institutions that have furnished medical care to the decedent in the past. Reliable witnesses, lay or professional, who can (and will) relate their observations of the victim from the time he became ill until he died are extremely valuable to the investigator of any sudden and unexpected death. Such details as the absence or presence of probable precipitating factors (severe physical exertion, emotional strain, engagement in an altercation, sexual intercourse, etc.) take on considerable weight under these circumstances. The speed with which death occurs following the onset of the terminal episode may also have diagnostic significance.

Absence of witnesses to the dying episode places a heavier burden on the investigating officials. (*"He was all right when I saw him last night, and I found him dead this afternoon."*) Unreliable, mendacious and dishonest witnesses provide only misleading and frustrating data. In the latter instances the decedent's personal effects and investigation of the scene of death provide the only reliable source of *historical* data.

### The Role of the Laboratory

Laboratory observations provide the second source of information utilized in establishing the cause of death. They include *complete* gross and microscopic anatomic study of the victim, together with whatever additional studies (bacteriological, virological, biochemical or toxicological) the immediate situation requires.

Ideally, complete autopsy, with indicated histologic and other diagnostic measures, should be carried out in *all* sudden and unexpected deaths. However, from the standpoint of day-to-day practicality, such a sweeping and nonselective approach may not be feasible because sufficient funds are not available for personnel to perform necessary laboratory and clerical work.

Autopsy can reasonably be omitted where there are sufficient reliable data to provide a valid explanation as to what disease is responsible for the sudden and unexpected demise and where the circumstances surrounding death point unmistakably to a natural cause. A verified history of recent headache, dizziness and stiff neck followed by coma and rapid death (in the absence of any history of trauma) in a person with known hypertension indicates that a spontaneous intracranial hemorrhage probably occurred. Profuse vomiting of blood followed by hypovolemic shock and death in the presence of previously diagnosed portal cirrhosis points strongly to the common terminating mechanism of ruptured esophageal varices.

In summary, if the details of the dying episode are accurately observed and truthfully reported by rational and sober witnesses, *and* if the underlying disease has been soundly diagnosed and documented, death may be certified without autopsy as having probably resulted from the known natural disease process, *provided that there is no history or evidence of injury that may have caused, hastened or contributed to death.* If there is any question whatsoever about whether recent or remote trauma (accidental, occupational, willful or otherwise) played any part in the death, the performance of a complete autopsy is practically mandatory.

The practice of doing *partial* autopsies is mentioned only to be condemned or discouraged. Such incomplete studies may necessitate the complicated, expensive procedure of exhumation and the performance of second and even third autopsies with all their attendant limitations. More important, repeated autopsies are rarely as rewarding or informative as a searching and complete initial examination.

### Arriving at the *Cause of Death*

Determination of the cause of death following autopsy is an interpretive, two-step intellectual procedure deriving from and depending upon sound evaluation of anamnestic data, circumstances surrounding death, morphologic evidence of disease (and injury) and the results of additional laboratory studies.

The first step requires recognition of the structural organic changes or chemical abnormalities responsible for cessation of vital function. The second step is based on understanding the mechanism by which the anatomical (and chemical) deviations from normal actually cause death, i.e. how they create or initiate the train of functional disturbances that are sufficiently potent to lead either to cardiac standstill or respiratory arrest, the two ultimate lethal processes. The responsible physiologic disturbances range in complexity from those that are overwhelmingly obvious to others that are complicated and subtle.

Sudden deaths *must* be studied from the perspective of disordered physiology as well as from the standpoint of morbid anatomy. The postmortem findings in a person who died instantaneously or extremely rapidly from natural causes may not be significantly different from those observed in persons of similar age and anatomic status who died directly from violence. In other words, although anatomic evidence of a disease capable of causing death is present, we know that persons with similar and perhaps even more severe anatomic abnormalities can carry on quite satisfactorily. Death must thus be viewed as having resulted from cessation of physiologic function rather than purely as a consequence of an anatomic state.

### The Certainty of the Cause of Death

Victims of sudden and unexpected natural death fall into several different categories with respect to the degree of certainty with which the cause of death can be established.[4]

In the first category the structural abnormalities establish beyond any doubt the identity of the disease that caused death. It is readily apparent that the lesion or lesions observed are incompatible with life and that they are antemortem in origin. Into this group fall such self-evident entities as massive pulmonary thromboembolism, ruptured myocardial infarct and spontaneous intracerebral hemorrhage.

The second category includes fatalities in which postmortem examination discloses the cause of death with a degree of probability amounting *almost* to certainty. The anatomic changes observed are not necessarily incompatible with life, but the entire investigation reveals no other reasonable explanation for death, and the location, nature, severity and extent of the anatomic changes are *adequate* to account for death. This group of deaths includes such diseases as grossly recognizable lobar pneumonia and advanced, chronic heart disease.

In the third category the cause of death is established primarily by anamnestic facts that are confirmed or supported by positive and negative anatomic and chemical findings. Thus, a known epileptic who is found dead and in whom no gross or microscopic evidence of other significant natural disease or trauma is observed may be considered as having died of epilepsy, provided that indicated chemical studies are negative. From the standpoint of the pathologist, the evidence on which the cause of death is based in this category is less satisfactory than it is in the preceding two groups, inasmuch as the critical facts upon which the diagnosis rests are not of his own acquisition.

Deaths falling into the fourth category are those in which neither the anamnestic data nor laboratory studies, anatomic and otherwise, individually or in combination provide sufficient evidence for one to do more than merely speculate as to the cause of death. Such fatalities, in which the autopsy and other laboratory findings are limited to trivial or equivocal changes and do not reveal a valid cause for death, are a source of perplexity to the pathologist who earnestly seeks to establish the real reason for death. Mild degrees of natural disease should not be implicated as causal or contributory.

A striking example of this puzzling group of fatalities is found in *bangungut,* a name derived from the Tagalog word for nightmare. This name is applied to rapid and unexpected death that takes place during sleep in previously healthy, well-developed, nonobese Filipino men in their third and fourth decades. It is rare in Chinese and Japanese and in those past forty-five. The entire course of the "illness" is extremely brief and characteristically follows a well-defined pattern with remarkably stereotyped clinicopathologic manifestations.

Shortly after having eaten a typical heavy Filipino meal followed by no complaints of discomfort, the victim goes to sleep. Within a few hours he appears to be experiencing violent and terrifying dreams from which he cannot be awakened. This phase is manifested by agitation, groaning, yelling, thrashing about and the coughing up of frothy fluid. Death follows soon.

Postmortem findings are nonspecific, indicating only acute cardiorespiratory failure of undetermined etiology. No satisfactory theory or hypothesis has been put forward that explains the selectivity of bangungut for males of a particular racial and age group. Histories of exposure to toxic substances are uniformly negative, and no ill effects are observed in others who partook of the same food. The cause of this dramatic and mysterious entity is still an open question.[5]

Because many nonmedical persons believe that the cause of death is *always* revealed by autopsy, the pathologist may be pressed into making positive or dogmatic statements despite the absence of sound objective data to support his opinion. In such instances he should admit his inability to comply with what appears to be a perfectly reasonable request.

However, even in these frustrating instances, the negative anatomic and chemical examination has considerable value in excluding injuries or *poisons* that may have been alleged to have caused or played some part in the death. The possible presence and participation of infectious, cancerous, occupational and other diseases are also eliminated from consideration. The result is that although the pathologist *cannot* establish the cause of death, he *can* rule out many situations and factors that have been conjectured erroneously as having some etiologic role or importance in the death.

Deaths whose causation remains unexplained after complete anatomic and other laboratory studies make up a small percentage of the forensic pathologist's case load. They are examples of functional failure of a vital tissue or an organ without corresponding or recognizable structural abnormality.

### Instantaneous Physiologic Death

An unusual type of death that formerly fell into the preceding category is the so-called *instantaneous physiologic death,*[3, 6, 7] *death from inhibition,*[8] *death from primary shock* or syncope with *instantaneous exitus.*[4]

Deaths from inhibition are defined as sudden

deaths that occur within seconds or a minute or two (no more!) after minor trauma or peripheral stimulation of relatively simple and ordinarily innocuous nature. Investigation of the circumstances surrounding death discloses that peripheral irritation or stimulation has probably initiated a fatal cardiovascular inhibitory reflex. Neither the pathologist nor the toxicologist can, by the methods available to him today, establish either the extent or the nature of the responsible changes, even though the changes result in death.

An eight-year-old boy collapsed and died in a public playground *immediately* after having been struck on the front of the chest by a ball, batted by a playmate. The incident occurred in full view of the playground supervisor and other spectators. Complete gross and microscopic anatomic studies were negative for disease, congenital malformation or trauma. Only the nonspecific changes of acute circulatory failure were present.

The syndrome is thus characterized by fulminant circulatory failure following either reflex (vagocardiac) slowing or stoppage of the heart, reflex vasodilation with profound fall in blood pressure, or a combination of both mechanisms. The myocardium and its neuromuscular control are extremely complicated and sensitive structures; they can, under unique circumstances, be thrown into lethal malfunction by mechanical stimuli that are not sufficiently forceful to produce a wound.

A variety of incidents have been incriminated as precipitating factors for death from inhibition, e.g. a blow to the larynx or solar plexus, a kick in the scrotum, pressure on the carotid sinus, canalization of the cervix, etc. Death from inhibition is thus *accidental,* inasmuch as it is initiated by *microtrauma,* defined as an injury so slight that it does not produce a wound. It is described here because failure to entertain it as a possibility when anatomic and chemical studies are negative may lead either to the cause of death being ascribed wrongly to some natural disease entity or to the matter being left entirely open.

The diagnosis of death from inhibition is made only by exclusion and is completely dependent on the availability of accurate observation by reliable witnesses concerning the circumstances of death and the fatal incident. After serious natural disease has been eliminated by complete autopsy and when the toxicologic analyses are noncontributory, then and then only may the probability of this type of death be fairly considered, *provided* that there is a sound history and description of a valid precipitating incident.

## SPECIFIC CAUSES OF SUDDEN AND UNEXPECTED NATURAL DEATH

Sudden and unexpected natural deaths are caused by diseases originating in almost every organ system. Speaking generally, any illness capable of causing death may, on occasion, do so unexpectedly. The responsible diseases range from acute fulminating infections that carry off hitherto healthy adults within a few hours of their onset to prolonged chronic disorders that have undergone abrupt functional or anatomic changes, transforming them from latent, relatively benign processes into those that are rapidly lethal. The relative frequencies of the multiform causes of sudden death in a community depend in part on the composition of the population at risk and in part on the general disease pattern in that area.

### Cardiovascular Disease

Sudden deaths resulting from diseases of the heart and of the cardiovascular system generally are more numerous than sudden deaths resulting from diseases in all other organ systems combined.[3] The most vulnerable structure in the entire cardiovascular circuit is the *artery.* Thrombotic or embolic occlusion, arteriosclerotic narrowing or rupture can lead to sudden and unexpected death, depending on the size and location of the involved vessel. Thus, thrombosis or arteriosclerotic narrowing of a coronary artery, embolic occlusion of a major pulmonary artery or rupture of an intracerebral artery are among the most frequently encountered causal factors in the adult *sudden death syndrome.*

Organic heart disease, most often of the acquired type and occasionally of the congenital variety, is the single most common cause of sudden and unexpected death in adults.

Although some persons with severe cardiac damage or malformation survive much longer than an apparently sound prognosis would indicate possible, nevertheless a significantly damaged heart is liable to sudden and unexpectedly lethal failure at any moment. This statement holds true not only for the heart actively involved by an acute disease but also for the heart permanently injured by a disease process whose active phase has long since subsided. Even the heart that has been subjected to reparative surgery is vulnerable to this type of precipitate failure.

This damage can involve any part of the heart: pericardium, valves, myocardium, coronary vasculature or any combination of these anatomic components; and the heart may have been performing adequately under ordinary and perhaps even under extraordinary conditions. Frequently at autopsy no *new* or recent organic changes can be identified that indicate or explain why death occurred at this time or under the specific circumstances surrounding the fatal episode. Although excessive somatic, visceral and emotional stress can place an intolerable burden on a damaged heart and throw it into irreversible failure, nevertheless most sudden and unexpected deaths from heart disease occur while the victim is at rest or is engaged in an activity that he has performed repeatedly and uneventfully in the recent past.

### *Arteriosclerotic Heart Disease*

While any type of heart disease renders the subject vulnerable to sudden death, the frequency with which the different etiologic varieties are encountered in day-to-day experience is a function of the incidence of the different types of heart disease in the community. In Europe and North America the cardiac abnormality most often responsible for sudden and unexpected death is arteriosclerotic heart disease (synonyms: coronary sclerotic heart disease, ischemic heart disease).[1, 3, 9] Indeed, the large majority of instantaneous and rapid deaths in adults are caused directly by this disease process. Thus, in a study of approximately 500 white males who died within less than one hour of the onset of their terminal episode, 91 percent succumbed to this all-too-common abnormality of their cardiovascular system.[10]

MORBID ANATOMIC-CLINICAL INCONGRUITIES IN ARTERIOSCLEROTIC HEART DISEASE. Although the common denominator in death (and clinical illness and disability) from ischemic heart disease is coronary arterial luminal narrowing or occlusion, the anatomic abnormalities responsible for (or observed in) sudden death are varied. The fact that cessation of cardiac activity can result from (or with) any one of several different morphologic changes is perplexing and thought provoking. When the attempt is made to correlate morbid coronary arterial and myocardial anatomy with sudden cessation of cardiac function, several problems are encountered. Other than the self-evident situation presented by a ruptured myocardial infarct, the question of sudden death due to coronary disease is often an enigma.

The puzzle is not simplified by the observation that severe coronary disease is often present in persons dying from other, unrelated causes. Many victims of immediately fatal violence have more severe coronary sclerotic disease than that observed in individuals whose death is attributed to this cause. Conversely, it is not rare to find that the victim of sudden death from stenosing coronary atherosclerosis presents only a few scattered foci or perhaps only a solitary site of significant luminal narrowing.[11]

The importance of hemorrhage into a coronary atheroma as the factor responsible for initiating the terminal lethal mechanism is debatable. Some authors[12] emphasize that this complication of atherosclerosis frequently precipitates fatal attacks. Others minimize the significance of these hemorrhages and consider them incidental findings in persons dying of coronary disease or other causes. Master[13] states that bleeding into atheromas plays no part in the development of fatal coronary thrombogenesis.

Tearing of the coronary arterial intima, which allows contact between the bloodstream and internal structure of the artery, including atheromatous material, has also been implicated as a cause of thrombosis.[14]

Most pathologists and clinicians readily accept recent thrombotic occlusion of a major coronary artery as a cause of sudden death, presumably mediated by an intolerable arrhythmia or total cessation of cardiac action. Absence of demonstrable myocardial infarction in these instances stems from the brief interval between vascular occlusion and death. However, many hearts do survive a major occlusion and the ensuing infarct. If one inculpates injury current created by anoxic or damaged myocardium as the lethal pathogenetic mechanism, it is difficult to explain why such an injury current is sufficiently potent to throw one heart into fatal fibrillation and yet is inadequate to create a similar disturbance and end result in a second heart with equal or greater injury.

The riddle of coronary cardiac death is carried a step further when no recent vascular occlusive lesion is found in a person suddenly dying from stenosing coronary atherosclerosis, an anatomic state of affairs that is twice as common as the demonstration of new vascular or parenchymal heart damage.[11,15] In this regard, Spain and Bradess[16] noted a positive relationship between survival time and incidence of recent coronary thrombi. Only 17.5 percent of 80 subjects who survived less than one hour following the onset of their attack had recent thrombi. On the contrary, 36.4 percent of 22 subjects who survived from one to eight hours and 57 percent of 100 persons who survived longer than eight hours had recent thrombi. The authors suggest that coronary thrombi do not usually trigger the onset of the fatal attack but develop as secondary phenomena incident to the attack.

Many techniques have been used in an attempt to demonstrate myocardial injury before the appearance of changes that require a survival interval of several hours prior to their recognition by traditional light microscopy. These techniques include macroscopic color changes that delineate zones of diminished myocardial dehydrogenase activity, electron microscopy, a variety of histochemical procedures and determination of potassium/sodium ratios in samples of myocardium.[17] Intervals of more than six to eight hours between death and autopsy vitiate electron microscopy and enzymatic reactions, rendering these techniques ineffective in routine forensic practice. However, alteration of K/Na ratio is believed to be independent of autolysis; with more widespread trial, this method may prove to be the most practical tool for demonstrating early myocardial injury.

Fatal Physiologic Consequences of Coronary Atherosclerosis. Cardiac stoppage as a consequence of stenosing coronary atherosclerosis and its sequelae may result from (a) muscle destruction and dysfunction from repeated episodes of myocardial infarction, chronic widespread anoxia or both and (b) reduction in coronary flow with insufficient circulation to the myocardium to maintain the heartbeat.

Beck[18] proposed a third mechanism: an unstable electrical condition in the myocardium that precipitates ventricular fibrillation. He hypothesized that electrical instability arises from varying degrees of oxygenation in different zones of the myocardium as a consequence of nonuniform coronary narrowing. Such lethal electrical discharges are not injury currents in the usual sense because they do not arise from recognizable new myocardial injury.

The hypothesis that myocardial hypoxia can generate a lethal electrical disturbance furnishes a plausible solution for an otherwise difficult problem. Support for this theory is furnished by the observations of Chiang et al.[19,20] who found that 38 of 45 victims of sudden coronary death had prior documentation of arrhythmias or conduction abnormalities. In this study 10 of 165 persons over age thirty who had premature ventricular systoles died suddenly (a projected rate of 61 per 1000), whereas 35 of 3459 individuals without the finding died suddenly (a rate of 10 per 1000). The authors suggest that ectopic ventricular impulses may arise as a consequence of abnormal action potential differences between ischemic and normal myocardium.

Additional corroboration comes from the studies of Hinkle and his coworkers,[21] who monitored the electrocardiograms of 300 ambulatory, ostensibly healthy men and women between ages twenty and sixty during an entire day. The subjects performed such varied activities as changes in position, Valsalva's maneuver, climbing stairs, brief walks out-of-doors and the Master test. They also ate a large meal and were subjected to three hours of moderately challenging and anxiety-producing psychological tests and interviews. Electrocardiographic changes in S-T segments and T waves were common, and a variety of ectopic rhythms and conduction disturbances were noted. Most men in their fifties had at least a few ventricular premature contractions per hour, and they increased in frequency with anxiety and eating, sometimes appearing in pairs or bursts. The authors suggest that ordinary events of daily life may initiate serious episodes of arrhythmia or even ventricular fibrillation in persons with damaged hearts.

Regardless of the character of the varying mechanisms that precipitate sudden death, all interfere with cardiac contraction and lead to actual or functional asystole with resultant cerebral anoxia.

Some Clinical and Anatomic Features of Sudden Coronary Deaths. The figures and trends derived from the study of large numbers of sudden deaths from coronary disease, investigated in different areas by different observers, are in close agreement, indicating basic similarities in epidemiologic and anatomic features.[11, 22–25] The subjects' ages range from the third through the ninth decades, and the majority are white males, in excess of their representation in the general population. Occupation is without etiologic importance in rendering the victim vulnerable to this type of exitus. All trades and professions are represented in study populations, with the more humble callings predominating.[13] However, Kuller and others[1] pose an interesting question regarding frequency of medically unattended and sudden deaths in lower, compared with upper, socioeconomic classes. They point out that medical examiner and coroner case study populations are biased in favor of persons in the lower social strata. Many of these individuals commonly receive medical care in hospitals and clinics that do not certify deaths in patients who die at home or in places other than the medical institution itself. Accordingly, these deaths must be certified by the local medicolegal authority. Conversely, out-of-hospital deaths in more affluent persons are much more likely to be certified by their private attending physicians.

The proportion of hearts with recent coronary thrombi, with or without accompanying recent myocardial infarcts, ranges from 27 percent[26] to 33 percent.[11] The remaining two-thirds of the victims have no *new* anatomic disease. Recent coronary thrombi are found more frequently in the younger age group. The frequency of healed infarcts and above-normal heart weight increases progressively with age.[11]

When death is accompanied (or precipitated) by a recent thrombotic occlusion, acute myocardial infarct or both, 70 percent of the victims voice or exhibit some indication that they are ill, e.g. chest pain, dyspnea, nausea and vomiting, profuse perspiration, "dizzy feelings," etc. When death occurs in the absence of *new* recognizable anatomic changes in either the vessel or the myocardium, subjective complaints or objective manifestations of illness are present only half as frequently. In Wikland's[27] study of 2678 deaths from arteriosclerotic heart disease that occurred outside the hospital, previous symptoms were absent in 37 percent of men below age fifty and in about 20 percent of older persons of both sexes. Observations by Gordon and Kannel[9] on premature mortality from coronary heart disease in Framingham provide comparable data.

Ruptured Myocardial Infarcts. The one

form of sudden death from coronary disease whose mode and mechanism are self-evident is that resulting from a ruptured myocardial infarct, a catastrophic complication seen more often in women than in men and increasing in frequency with age.[27] When the rupture involves the interventricular septum or a papillary muscle, death usually follows within a few hours as a result of acute myocardial failure. When the rupture traverses the left ventricular wall and communicates with the pericardial space, death takes place within minutes from rapid accumulation of blood within the sac *(pericardial tamponade)*.

Rupture is favored by elevated intraventricular pressure resulting from physical activity, hypertension or a valvular lesion. The entire thickness of the ventricular wall is usually involved by the infarct *(transmural)*, and the infarct generally has evoked a marked acute inflammatory infiltrate.

A surprising feature of some ruptured myocardial infarcts is that they are occasionally observed in persons who have been carrying on normal or only slightly restricted activity for several days prior to their sudden fatal collapse. Thus, a major transmural infarct may elicit neither sufficient symptoms nor physical signs to indicate the presence of severe myocardial injury. Ruptured myocardial infarcts have been found relatively frequently in ambulatory institutionalized psychotic patients.[28] This prevalence is reasonably explained by postulating that mental illness may either make the patient oblivious of his bodily symptoms or interfere with his ability to communicate. Moreover, *objective* signs of serious illness may be overlooked in a large mental hospital with limited medical personnel. Nonetheless, the same apparently paradoxical situation occurs in nonpsychotic persons. While absence of pain and other symptoms may result from a high pain threshold *(silent infarct)*, it is difficult to understand the failure of massive acute disease to evoke shock and other clinical phenomena characteristically associated with severe myocardial damage. This is yet an additional example of the great discrepancy that may exist between the gravity of an organic lesion and the comparatively trivial clinical manifestations associated with it.

Sudden Deaths from Nonarteriosclerotic Coronary Disease. Nonarteriosclerotic coronary arterial diseases that lead to significant alteration or diminution in myocardial blood supply can also cause sudden death. Thus, such diverse disorders of the coronary arteries as rheumatic arteritis, dissecting hematomas *(aneurysms)*,[35] hypersensitivity angiitis, thromboangiitis obliterans and congenital anomalies[36] can be responsible for precipitating sudden exitus. However, all these different etiologic varieties of coronary artery disease combined contribute but a minute fraction of the total number of sudden deaths arising from disease in the coronary vasculature.

A Final Look and a Caveat Concerning Sudden Death from Coronary Disease. Because the majority of victims of sudden coronary death do *not* present a fresh thrombus or a recent myocardial infarct at autopsy *(vide supra)*, correlation of the morbid anatomy with the suddenness of the death must be based on hypotheses and mechanisms not ordinarily encountered or required in hospital postmortem work. Here the patient who died from coronary disease who is studied at the autopsy table has usually been under medical observation and care for days or weeks. The problems confronting the forensic pathologist in his investigations of sudden and unexpected deaths from coronary disease (or other causes, for that matter) necessitate standards of judgement and evaluation that are not part of the day-to-day responsibility of the hospital pathologist.

Demonstration of severe, stenosing coronary atherosclerosis does not establish, in and of itself, that this disease is the cause of death. Death should not be ascribed to coronary atherosclerosis until anatomic study is completed and results of toxicological analyses are available.

Autopsy of an elderly vagrant found dead in an alley revealed severe coronary atherosclerosis with a healed myocardial infarct, which had given rise to a large left ventricular aneurysm. Injuries were absent, and other anatomic findings were without lethal potentialities. Routine blood and urine alcohol determinations disclosed fatal concentrations of methyl alcohol.

### *Valvular Heart Disease*

Much of what has been said about sudden death from coronary disease is applicable to sudden deaths resulting from chronic valvular lesions, which are usually rheumatic. Syphilitic damage of the aortic valve and congenital valvular deformities are responsible for only occasional victims in this category of unexpected fatalities.

In most instances a diagnosis of organic heart disease has been made previously, and many of the subjects had been able to carry on active existences with minimal or only slight physical limitations. Then, after having been well tolerated for many years, the valvular deformity suddenly gives rise to acute cardiac failure. The fatal collapse may occur while the decedent is at rest or, more often, while he is engaged in comparatively mild physical activity.

The valvular deformity is readily apparent at autopsy and is usually accompanied by greater or lesser degrees of myocardial hypertrophy and changes indicative of acute terminal cardiac insufficiency. No *new* lesions or anatomic changes are ordinarily present to explain why death occurred at this time and under the circumstances immediately present.

CALCIFIC AORTIC STENOSIS. Calcific aortic stenosis is among the more frequently encountered valvular lesions responsible for causing sudden death. The controversy about its origin, rheumatic or nonrheumatic, has not been resolved and is not germane to the present discussion of its rapidly lethal propensities.

Anatomically the valve presents fusion of the cusps accompanied by deposition of abundant calcium in the scarred structure. The free margins of the valve are thickened, rolled and eburnated, and its aperture is rigid and seriously narrowed. Left ventricular hypertrophy, created by the constant stress of ejecting blood through the narrowed orifice, is complicated by impaired filling of the coronary arteries whose ostia lie in the aortic sinuses behind the rigid cusps. The situation is thus doubly dangerous as a result of diminished coronary blood flow in the face of an overworked, increased myocardial mass.

It has been estimated that when the valve opening reaches a critical area, usually approximately 7 $mm^2$, the left ventricle is unable to maintain an adequate output and acute cardiac failure ensues.[29] The cardiac morphology in persons dying suddenly from calcific aortic stenosis is similar to that observed in persons who expire with chronic congestive failure caused by the same valvular deformity.

Two features of calcific aortic stenosis deserve brief comment. One is prolonged survival, which is possible even with severe damage to the valve. In one report 11 of 49 persons with advanced calcific and stenotic changes in their aortic valve were more than seventy-five years of age when they died.[30] The other noteworthy aspect is the extreme degree of myocardial hypertrophy that is frequently present. Heart weights of 700-800 gm are common in persons who die suddenly from calcific aortic stenosis.

Sudden deaths from congenital aortic stenosis[31] and muscular subaortic stenosis[32] have been reported but are uncommon.

LUETIC AORTIC VALVULAR DISEASE. Syphilitic aortic valvular damage that leads to insufficiency and regurgitation can also cause sudden death. The strain on the left ventricle with this type of valvular damage is even greater than that produced by stenosis, and the extent of the myocardial hypertrophy can reach truly enormous proportions, with the heart attaining weight in excess of 1 kg. Here, too, coronary filling is compromised as a result of diastolic reflux, and the coronary ostia are frequently narrowed as a consequence of luetic mesaortitis with scarring.

OTHER VARIETIES OF RAPIDLY FATAL CARDIAC VALVULAR DISEASES. Rheumatic mitral stenosis is encountered occasionally as the cause of sudden death. It may be accompanied by a damaged aortic valve, or it may be the sole valvular abnormality. When mitral stenosis is complicated by the formation of a left atrial thrombus, sudden death may result from coronary embolism or from *ball valve* action of the thrombus.

Bacterial endocarditis, usually of the subacute type and most often superimposed on chronic rheumatic or congenital heart disease, is observed from time to time as a cause of sudden and unexpected death. When one visualizes the active valvular inflammatory changes and the distant sites of embolic damage and associates these anatomic phenomena with the toxicity and malaise that are so characteristic of this infectious disease, it is difficult to understand how the decedent was able to carry on and why he did not seek medical attention.

CARDIAC HYPERTROPHY. Acute central cardiac failure can occur as a result of hypertensive left ventricular myocardial hypertrophy, or the enlargement may be predominantly right-sided as a consequence of long-standing bilateral pulmonary disease with resultant persistent elevation in the pulmonary arterial circuit *(chronic cor pulmonale)*. Severe thoracic kyphoscoliosis can produce similar chronic right ventricular strain and hypertrophy.

Cardiac enlargement involving mainly the left ventricle is found most often in persons who have exhibited systemic arterial hypertension of the so-called *essential* type. Sudden death from hypertensive heart disease is seen more commonly in blacks than whites.[1] The degree of cardiac enlargement observed in these instances is usually less than that found in victims of sudden death caused by cardiac valvular disease.

As with so many other instances of acute central cardiac failure, there is often no reasonable anatomic explanation for sudden, fatal cardiac dysfunction. Many of these individuals have at least a moderate degree of coronary atherosclerosis or myocardial arteriolar sclerosis, the deleterious effect of which is magnified by myocardial hypertrophy.

In the absence of a reliable history of a pressor episode precipitated by physical exertion or emotion, initiation of the terminal cardiac insufficiency remains an unsolved problem.

### *Myocardial Disease*

The burden on the myocardium that ultimately leads to decompensation is usually imposed from without, e.g. valvular or coronary disease, hypertension or chronic lung disease. Occasionally, intrinsic myocardial disease precipitates acute, irreversible lethal cardiac failure.

MYOCARDITIS. The most common fatal primary myocardial disorder is an inflammatory process, which may be acute, subacute or chronic. Myocarditis can occur as a complication of many infectious processes brought on by a wide variety of etiologic agents: bacteria, viruses, fungi, protozoa and even helminths. It can also occur as a result of local allergic reactions. The histologic response may be specific (the Aschoff nodule of acute rheumatic myocarditis) or nonspecific. The inflammatory process may be clinically apparent during the height of the primary disease, or it may first make itself manifest during the convalescent phase. It may be a complication of an obvious, grave systemic disease, follow what appears to be a mild respiratory infection or be of unascertainable origin.

Clinically the diagnosis of myocarditis is usually made in the presence of such symptoms as chest pain, dyspnea and signs of cardiac failure, with confirmatory changes in the electrocardiogram. In the presence of a fulminating, complex primary infection, evidence of myocardial damage is often obscured. If the myocardial lesions are focal or primarily interstitial and do not involve the conduction apparatus, clinical recognition may be difficult.

Sudden and unexpected myocardial failure characterized by acute circulatory collapse and irreversible shock can occur readily in the absence of obvious indications of disease in this vital issue. The lethal mechanism is usually initiated by damage to the conduction system or the establishment of ectopic foci of myocardial irritability, which in turn give rise to a fatal arrhythmia.

Grossly the heart may appear normal. Occasionally a hint of disease is suggested by flabbiness to palpation or the presence of myocardial petechiae. The diagnosis of myocarditis is made on the basis of microscopic study of the myocardium, which reveals cellular infiltration of various types and of varying degrees of severity, occasionally accompanied by myocardial fiber degeneration and necrosis and by interstitial edema.

In general it may be said that myocarditis is more frequently diagnosed by the pathologist than by the clinician. In no other cause of sudden death is the necessity of microscopic study so important in establishing the presence of a fatal lesion in the absence of gross abnormalities as it is in myocarditis.

However, a postmortem diagnosis of death from myocarditis should be approached with caution in the absence of antecedent clinical documentation of illness. Just as the presence of severe stenosing coronary atherosclerosis does not categorically establish that it was responsible for death, so a finding of focal or diffuse myocarditis does not exclude the participation of other diseases, injuries or toxins. Myocardial foci of lymphocytic infiltration are observed occasionally in random histologic sections of hearts obtained from individuals whose death is clearly unrelated to myocarditis, e.g. immediately fatal gunshot wound of the head. Accordingly, myocarditis should be regarded as the cause of death only after complete anatomic and indicated chemical studies exclude alternative causes.

Sarcoid Heart Disease. Myocardial sarcoidosis can cause sudden and unexpected death.[33] Porter[34] reported that 22 of 33 cases of sarcoid myocarditis terminated in this fashion and that one-fourth of the victims had had no premonitory symptoms. Almost all victims of myocardial sarcoidosis have similar granulomata in other organs.

Variation in myocardial localization of the granulomata accounts for differences in the clinical picture. Several types of arrhythmias and electrocardiographic findings have been described, including different degrees of heart block and conduction delay, paroxysmal atrial and ventricular tachycardias, and S-T segment and T wave changes.

Clinically, symptomatic patients may present angina pectoris, palpitation or Stokes-Adams syndrome. As with other forms of myocardial disease, sudden expiration has been ascribed to interference with conduction or the initiation of intolerable arrhythmias.

Miscellaneous Cardiac Disorders. Other forms of myocardial disease are encountered infrequently as a cause of sudden death. Into this category fall such entities as myocardial amyloidosis, primary cardiac tumors and asymmetrical hypertrophy of the heart.[32, 35] This heterogeneous group of lesions furnishes a minor fraction of sudden deaths arising from a primary myocardial basis.

### *Emotional Factors and Acute Fatal Cardiac Failure*

That an episode of emotional stress, whether it be anger, fear, joy or apprehension, can precipitate acute failure in persons with organic heart disease, especially of the coronary atherosclerotic type, is common knowledge. The work load on the heart is significantly augmented as the physiological result of emotional excitement and upheaval with its attendant phenomena of increased heart rate, greater force of heartbeat, elevation in systolic pressure and central shifting of venous blood.[3] This additional burden can overtax the limits of tolerance of a damaged, laboring heart.

Such a pressor episode does *not* cause permanent anatomic damage in a normal heart, and the healthy organ may show only a transient dilatation, which disappears with recovery following rest. However, it has been suggested that disturbed physiological mechanisms can produce fatal acute cardiac disturbance even in persons with normal hearts. Some authors[36] have pointed out that such common lay terms as *scared to death* and *frightened to death* can be literally true when the immediate response to unusual and extraordinary fright is overwhelming. Sudden release of epinephrine incident to extreme terror in a person with an anatomically normal heart can initiate runs of ventricular tachycardia, which can progress to ventricular fibrillation and death. At this stage of our knowledge no dogmatic stand can be taken on this aspect of sudden cardiac death.

## Hemorrhage

Escape of blood through a defect or rent in the wall of a diseased blood vessel (hemorrhage) is a frequent mechanism of sudden, rapid death. The interval from onset of symptoms to exitus usually ranges from a few minutes to several hours. The underlying disease processes vary widely in etiology, and the primary sites of damage are located in the head, chest and abdomen. Arteries are more commonly involved, but fatal venous bleeding is not rare.

### *Lethal Mechanisms in Hemorrhage*

Hemorrhage can produce several different physiologic disturbances, any one of which can be fatal:

1. Rapid loss of about one-third of the circulating blood volume in the average, healthy adult results in irreversible hypovolemic shock *(exsanguination)*. During the course of the bleeding, progressively increasing disproportion between the capacity of the circulatory apparatus and the volume of circulating blood initiates such compensatory mechanisms as hemodilution, vasoconstriction and tachycardia in an effort to maintain equilibrium. If blood loss continues, compensation ultimately breaks down, and blood pressure falls to shock levels, with resultant cerebral ischemia and death from cerebral anoxia.
2. Hemorrhage can kill quickly by creating increased pressure in or on a vital organ to the extent that its functional capacity is fatally compromised. This is the lethal process in hemopericardium *(pericardial tamponade)* and in spontaneous subarachnoid or intracerebral hemorrhage.
3. Sufficient bleeding into the trachea or bronchi can result in rapid death from asphyxia, the blood acting as a mechanical barrier to respiratory exchange. This type of hemorrhage is a common terminating mechanism in bronchogenic carcinoma and pulmonary tuberculosis.

When fatal hemorrhage involves the respiratory or gastrointestinal tracts, there is usually obvious clinical evidence of the terminal event in the form of hemoptysis, hematemesis or melena. If fatal bleeding takes place in some other site, no external manifestations may be present, and correct antemortem diagnosis must be based on proper evaluation of clinical and laboratory findings.

Deaths from hemorrhage are among the most readily diagnosed conditions encountered at autopsy. The presence of large quantities of blood in a body cavity, in the retroperitoneal space or within the substance of an organ usually permits the pathologist to make a prompt identification of the underlying disease and the site of the fatal vascular defect.

Cerebrovascular Diseases. Although fatal hemorrhages occur in many different, widely scattered sites, several areas are especially vulnerable to this common lethal mechanism. Chief among these is the central nervous system.

Spontaneous intracranial hemorrhages fall into several fairly well-defined categories:

*Intracerebral hemorrhage (apoplexy)*, usually attributable to a combination of arterial hypertension and arteriosclerosis, is the cerebrovascular catastrophe encountered most frequently in middle-aged and older persons. The usual source of hemorrhage is rupture of a lenticulostriate branch of the middle cerebral artery with subsequent bleeding into the basal ganglia and adjacent structures. Occasionally the pons or cerebellum is the primary site of bleeding.

Progressive extravasation of blood into the cerebral parenchyma leads to mounting intracranial pressure, brain swelling and herniations with resultant cardiorespiratory failure. Rupture of the intracerebral hematoma into a cerebral ventricle or through the cortex permits escape of blood into the subarachnoid space. If the arachnoid is torn by the explosive force of the hemorrhage, blood enters the subdural space, thus simulating a traumatic lesion from which the spontaneous hemorrhage must be differentiated.

*Spontaneous subarachnoid hemorrhages* account for approximately 4 to 5 percent of all rapid and unexpected natural deaths. The source of bleeding is generally perforation or rupture of a saccular *berry* aneurysm, located almost always at the bifurcation of one of the constituent vessels of the circle of Willis or of one of its major branches, which permits blood to accumulate rapidly on the undersurface of the brain. As bleeding continues, blood advances along the fissures, into the major cisterns and thence into the fourth ventricle. Aneurysms frequently rupture into the cerebral parenchyma or into the subdural space. In fact, subdural and/or intracerebral hemorrhage without concomitant subarachnoid bleeding may be produced by a ruptured aneurysm.[37]

Estimates of the rapidity with which death ensues following rupture of berry aneurysms depend upon the source of the study population. Study of patients dying in hospitals tends to exclude sudden death, and persons surviving longer than one day are less likely to be autopsied at a medicolegal facility. Germane to the present context is Freytag's[37] analysis of 250 consecutive deaths due to ruptured intracranial aneurysms. These individuals were autopsied at the Office of the Chief Medical Examiner of Maryland; 60 percent had *no survival*, and an additional 29 percent lived less than one day. The longest survival in her study was seven weeks. Some individuals survive their initial bleeding episode only to die with a recurrence. Former bleeding, which in most instances was asymptomatic leakage, from a fatally ruptured aneurysm is common.

Spontaneous subarachnoid hemorrhages, unlike the intracerebral variety, do not require the presence of associated hypertension for their occurrence. The preexisting vascular defect responsible for their genesis ruptures readily under normotensive conditions. Nevertheless, 25 percent of patients with ruptured cerebral aneurysms are hypertensive.[38]

Postmortem search for the offending aneurysm should be made while the brain is fresh, i.e. prior to fixation in formalin. Otherwise the extravasated blood that surrounds the vessels congeals and makes the task of demonstrating the vascular defect extremely difficult. Multiple aneurysms are present in approximately 12 percent of persons dying from spontaneous subarachnoid hemorrhages.[37]

The origin of the aneurysm has been ascribed to a focal congenital defect in the muscularis of the vessel with subsequent overstretching and degeneration of the internal elastic lamina. There is no evidence that small vessels arising from apices of primitive vascular forks, vestiges of embryonic capillaries or inflammatory processes play a part in the genesis of the ordinary subarachnoid saccular aneurysm.[39] Although there is still some disagreement as to whether or not the aneurysm is actually present at birth *(congenital)* or whether only the original muscular defect and weakness are congenital with later appearance of a true aneurysmal sac *(developmental)*, it is probable that postnatal circumstances enhance the production of saccular dilatation and the probability of its rupture.

Grossly the aneurysms are eccentric or rounded evaginations measuring from 1 to 2 mm to several centimeters in maximum dimension. Histologically the wall reveals absence of normal layering with degenerative changes in media and intima. Stehbens[39] states that the architectural differences between the uninvolved portion of the arterial wall and the aneurysm can probably be explained by the expansion that takes place in forming the saccular outpouching. Phagocytosed blood pigment is frequently visible in the adventitial portion of the aneurysm wall, indicating previous leakage. The presence of arteriosclerotic changes in the aneurysmal wall does not imply an arteriosclerotic origin of the lesion but rather degeneration superimposed on the congenital lesion or organization of mural thrombi.

Other Causes of Fatal Spontaneous Intracranial Bleeding. In addition to the common type of berry aneurysm responsible for the great majority of spontaneous subarachnoid hemorrhages, other varieties of cerebrovascular malformation can also lead to fatal bleeding into the subarachnoid space. Angiomas and arteriovenous malformations are said to account for about 9 percent of all spontaneous subarachnoid bleeding.[38]

*Arteriovenous aneurysms* (a poor name) are clearly the result of maldevelopment secondary to faulty differentiation of intercommunicating embryonal arterial and venous channels. These lesions are, in reality, enlarged arterial and venous pathways with one or more arteriovenous anastomoses, located usually on the surface of the cerebral hemispheres. Occasionally they extend into the subjacent cerebral parenchyma in wedge-shaped fashion. The neighboring or intervening brain tissue frequently presents anomalous neural development, necrosis or gliosis secondary to compression by the angioma or to circulatory deprivation as a result of the blood being drawn away by the arteriovenous shunt.[38]

*Mycotic aneurysms,* which develop following lodgement of septic emboli at points of bifurcation in the circle of Willis or distally in its major branches, can be responsible for fatal cerebrovascular rupture. Infected vegetations from heart valves damaged by congenital or acquired disease (subacute bacterial endocarditis) are the usual source of the bacteria-containing thrombotic masses that produce a localized destructive, suppurative arteritis, which ultimately goes on to complete mural destruction.

Fusiform arteriosclerotic cerebral aneurysms are almost always associated with gross, generalized cerebral atherosclerosis and are readily differentiated from other types of aneurysms. Luetic cerebral aneurysms are rare.

C.V.A. AND C.V.E. At this juncture a caveat is in order against use of the term *cerebrovascular accident (C.V.A.)* when referring to cerebral hemorrhage, thrombosis or embolism. This is a particularly unfortunate appellation because the word *accident* carries with it the implication of mishap, misadventure or negligence and can lead to serious misunderstanding on the part of lay relatives and friends of the decedent. If a catchall phrase is used for this group of cerebrovascular catastrophes, the term *cerebrovascular episode (C.V.E.)* is preferable. Best of all is use of the specific diagnostic term that accurately describes the lesion: cerebral hemorrhage, thrombosis or embolism. Cerebral thrombosis or embolism frequently causes sudden incapacitation but seldom results in sudden death.

### Diseases of the Aorta

Inasmuch as the aorta carries more blood at higher pressure than any other vessel, exsanguinating hemorrhage occurs more often from mural disease in this major conduit than in any other vascular channel. Occasionally, spontaneous perforation of a major branch of the aorta (splenic artery, iliac artery, etc.) damaged by disease is the source of fatal blood loss.

ARTERIOSCLEROTIC ANEURYSM OF THE AORTA. Progressive arteriosclerotic degeneration of the aorta with weakness and thinning of the wall leads to formation of fusiform or saccular aneurysms. These can rupture and result in massive hemorrhage, which usually proves fatal within a few hours following onset of symptoms. Because most arteriosclerotic aneurysms of the aorta are located in its abdominal portion, bleeding is usually retroperitoneal, with comparatively slight extravasation of blood into the peritoneal cavity. Occasionally the defect in the aneurysm is located on its anterior surface and communicates directly with the peritoneal cavity. In these instances the fatal course is usually more rapid because bleeding proceeds more quickly into the peritoneal cavity than into the retroperitoneal space.

In addition to the two foregoing sites, arteriosclerotic abdominal aortic aneurysms may rupture into other structures. Communication of the rent in the aortic wall with the inferior vena caval lumen can cause death from acute heart failure as a consequence of sudden creation of a major arteriovenous fistula. Intraduodenal rupture has also been reported, with the clinical picture simulating bleeding peptic ulcer.

DISSECTING ANEURYSM OF THE AORTA. Intramural bleeding within the aorta with formation of a dissecting medial hematoma is responsible for a modest number of rapid deaths, the bulk of the victims of this lesion dying more than four hours following the onset of symptoms.[40] The ages of the victims range from the second decade through senility.

The anatomic basis for medial dissection is a mucinous, cystic condition of the aortic media, probably congenital in origin, or degeneration of the media as a component of systemic connective tissue disorders. Syphilis and arteriosclerosis play no etiologic role in the production of this vascular lesion. Many victims of dissecting aneurysm are hypertensive, but its importance in the pathogenesis of the lesion is not yet completely understood.

Intramural aortic bleeding is apparently initiated by rupture of vasa vasorum with hemorrhagic extravasation into the abnormal, weakened media. Continuing bleeding leads to progressive medial splitting, with eventual extension of the dissection to the intima, which it tears. The full head of intra-aortic pressure is now transmitted to the site of medial dissection, with rapid extension of the medial splitting, which frequently involves major branches of the parent vessel. Exit of the medial hematoma through the adventitia leads to death from pericardial tamponade or exsanguination. Occasionally the dissecting hemorrhage finds its way back into the lumen of the aorta by creating a second intimal tear, and the patient may survive with the formation of a double-barreled aorta only to die months or years later from delayed rupture of the diseased vessel.

Syphilitic Aneurysm of the Aorta. Spirochetal invasion of the aortic media during the secondary stage of syphilis, with subsequent damage to elastic and muscular tissue in this area, is the foundation for the development of a fusiform or a saccular aneurysm years later. The weakening of the vessel wall as a consequence of the inflammatory destruction of those elements that confer strength and elasticity leads to mural thinning and outpouching in the thoracic area. Subjected to the constant recurring physiologic stress of systolic pressure, the weakened area becomes thinner and thinner until it can no longer withstand the demand imposed on it and it ruptures, with resultant rapidly fatal hemorrhage. Bleeding is usually internal, with the blood accumulating in one of the pleural cavities (usually the left) or in the pericardial sac. If the aneurysm ruptures into the lung or a major bronchus, death is accompanied by massive hemoptysis, and when the aortic defect communicates with the thoracic esophagus, hematemesis is a prominent feature of the terminal episode. Rapidly lethal extracardiac shunts can be produced by rupture of syphilitic aortic aneurysms into the superior vena cava or pulmonary artery.[15]

Diagnosis of the luetic origin of the aneurysm is based on its location in the thoracic aorta (arteriosclerotic aneurysms of the aorta are rare above the level of the diaphragm) and the gross and microscopic stigmata of syphilis. Longitudinal intimal striations and wrinkling *(tree barking)* seen with the naked eye point to the syphilitic etiology of the lesion, and this impression is confirmed by the histopathologic criteria of the disease, which include destruction of the medial elastic fibers, with scarring and vascularization, and endarteritis obliterans of the adventitial vasa vasorum accompanied by perivascular infiltration with lymphocytes and plasma cells.

### *Gastrointestinal Bleeding*

Peptic ulcers of the stomach and duodenum and esophageal varices are the two most frequent sources of fatal acute gastrointestinal hemorrhage. In the former two the hemorrhage is arterial and originates from a vessel that has been encroached upon and eroded by the progressively enlarging ulcer. The eroded artery may be visible to the naked eye in the base of the ulcer.

Fatal *venous* bleeding in the gastrointestinal tract is most often the result of long-standing cirrhosis with portal hypertension and formation of esophageal varices. Postmortem demonstration of the source of esophageal bleeding is usually difficult because the formerly distended venous channels are now empty and collapsed. The presence of large quantities of blood in the stomach and intestine together with a granular or *hobnailed* liver point to this diagnosis in the absence of other lesions capable of producing significant bleeding into the upper digestive tract. In addition to portal cirrhosis, other diseases that create portal hypertension give rise to esophageal varices and can terminate in similar fashion.

All other causes of unexpected, fatal acute gastrointestinal hemorrhage constitute but a small fraction of deaths from this mechanism. They include such diseases as ulcerating benign and malignant gastric and intestinal tumors and the Mallory-Weiss syndrome, the latter referring to hemorrhage from gastroesophageal lacerations induced by violent vomiting.

### *Respiratory Tract Bleeding*

Bleeding originating in the respiratory tract, including the pharynx, can lead to death in one of two ways. The hemorrhage may be sufficiently voluminous to result in exsanguination and fatal hypovolemic shock, a sequence of events that occurs when the source of the bleeding is a comparatively large artery whose wall has been destroyed by some extravascular disease. The latter may be primarily infectious (e.g. tuberculosis, lung abscess, bronchiectasis) or neoplastic (e.g. bronchogenic or other type of respiratory tract carcinoma).

Respiratory tract bleeding can be fatal even though the quantity of blood lost is far too small to cause hemorrhagic shock. Even moderate degrees of bleeding into the tracheobronchial tree can lead to speedy asphyxia as a result of the intraluminal blood being churned into a thick froth by the respiratory efforts of the victim. Bloody froth of this type is an effective barrier to the passage of air into and out of the trachea and its branches, and the victim literally *drowns in his own blood.*

### *Miscellaneous Intraperitoneal Hemorrhages*

Implantation of the fertilized ovum in some site other than the endometrial cavity, usually the uterine tube, results in the development of an ectopic (i.e. extrauterine) pregnancy, thus providing the basis for potentially exsanguinating intraperitoneal hemorrhage. Progressive growth of the fetus and other products of conception eventually leads to tubal stretching and rupture, with resultant brisk intra-abdominal bleeding, which is usually fatal if surgical intervention is not instituted promptly. At autopsy the characteristic findings include massive hemoperitoneum and a uterine tube showing evidence of intraluminal and intramural hemorrhage, chorionic villi and a fetus of six to twelve weeks gestational age.

Other infrequent causes of fatal intra-abdominal bleeding include such entities as spontaneous rupture of a large cavernous hemangioma *(cavernoma)* of the liver or of a hepatoma *(hepatocellular carcinoma).*

Spontaneous rupture of a spleen enlarged as a result of infectious mononucleosis, typhoid fever or malaria can also precipitate lethal intraperitoneal hemorrhage.

## Pulmonary Embolism

Acute thromboembolic occlusion of one or more major pulmonary arteries has long been recognized and feared as a cause of sudden death in patients confined to bed. The preceding thrombogenesis responsible for the fatal embolus is usually initiated by a combination of bed rest or immobilization of a limb in a cast, with consequent slowing or stagnation of the circulation and changes in the blood composition, which favor the development of a phlebothrombotic process in the major veins of the legs or pelvis.

Similar phlebothrombotic activity, which can be the source of suddenly fatal pulmonary embolism, occurs also in ambulatory, apparently healthy persons in the prime of life. Breckenridge and Ratnoff[41] reported 27 sudden deaths in such persons, with the victims ranging in age from fifteen to forty-five. None had a history or anatomic evidence of recent trauma, surgical procedures or associated serious disease. Several of the victims were young women in the first trimester of pregnancy. The study period covered by the report preceded the introduction of oral contraceptives. A second study of similarly caused sudden deaths in the same community covering the years *following* the appearance of oral contraceptives failed to demonstrate an increased incidence of acutely fatal pulmonary embolism in women in their childbearing years.[42]

The mechanism by which pulmonary emboli produce sudden death depends, in part, on the size of the occluding clot (or the diameter of the occluded vessel). When the offending mass of blood clot is sufficiently large to obstruct the bifurcation of the pulmonary artery or one of its major branches, the right side of the heart undergoes immediate acute dilatation and failure *(acute cor pulmonale).*

When sudden death closely follows the obstruction of smaller radicles of the pulmonary arteries, a more complex group of physiologic disturbances has been described. Generalized pulmonary vasospasm, triggered by impaction of the embolus (or emboli) and mediated reflexly by the autonomic nervous system, leads to sudden sharp increase in blood pressure in the lesser circuit with simultaneous marked dilatation and overdistension of the right ventricle. Associated with the cardiopulmonary dysfunction is systemic shock with peripheral hypotension and interference with coronary filling and coronary flow. The entire complex of cardiopulmonary vascular disturbance results in immediate cessation of vital function.

### *Other Types of Embolism*

Nonpulmonary thrombotic emboli are rarely, if ever, *suddenly* fatal. Occlusion of a major cerebral artery by an embolus arising from a mural thrombus in the left atrium or left ventricle or from a vegetation on the mitral or aortic valves usually leads to a relatively prolonged clinical course before death supervenes, the interval from embolism to exitus ranging from hours to days. *Saddle emboli* lodged at the bifurcation of the aorta or occlusive emboli in the major branches of the aorta (superior mesenteric, carotid, femoral) usually create recognizable syndromes that do not fall into the category of sudden and unexpected death.

## Central Nervous System Causes of Sudden and Unexpected Death

Cerebral parenchymal and meningeal diseases of widely varying etiologies (infectious, neoplastic or idiopathic) can cause sudden and unexpected death. (Unexpected, rapid deaths from cerebrovascular catastrophes have been discussed earlier in this chapter.) The mechanism of death (central cardiorespiratory failure or paralysis) may be evoked by direct damage to the cerebral vital centers by the disease process itself; or it may arise secondary to increased intracranial pressure produced by space-occupying lesions, by cerebral edema and swelling or by a combination of both.

Invasion of and damage to vital areas within the brain by a virus occasionally produces quickly fatal encephalomyelitis. Rupture of a brain abscess is frequently followed by speedily lethal diffuse, purulent meningitis or ependymitis. Syphilis in the form of acute luetic meningitis, acute luetic cerebral arteritis or general paresis is yet an additional possible cause of sudden and unexpected death.

### *Intracranial Tumors*

The majority of primary intracranial tumors, whether cerebral or meningeal in origin, usually give rise to progressively increasing signs and symptoms, which frequently extend over periods of months or years. The disabling character of the clinical response in such instances is ordinarily severe enough to induce the patient to seek medical aid, and when death supervenes under these circumstances, it is usually not of the sudden, unexpected or unattended type that falls within the jurisdiction of the medicolegal functionary. Nonetheless, sudden and unexpected deaths from intracranial tumors are not rare in forensic pathologic practice.[43] Such deaths can be precipitated by any one of several different mechanisms.

Gliomas that infiltrate and replace cerebral tissue in *silent* areas of the brain can attain comparatively large dimensions without producing symptoms of sufficient magnitude, significance or clarity to justify or stimulate clinical study and are thus ignored by the patient. Their early manifestations may appear in the emotional or psychic spheres and be regarded erroneously as indicating mental or emotional instability or functional psychosis. Meningeal tumors pressing on silent areas can enlarge slowly for many years without producing noteworthy subjective or objective changes because of compensatory cerebral mechanisms.

Distinctive clinical phenomena often appear first when the tumor has created a critical level of increased intracranial pressure. This point may be reached either as a result of a sudden increase in the volume of the intracranial contents that does not allow time for compensatory mechanisms to go into operation or because gradual enlargement of the tumor has taxed the compensatory mechanisms beyond their limits. In either event, death may ensue very quickly.

Abrupt, sudden increase in volume of the intracranial contents can come about either as a result of edema in and around the tumor or from sudden hemorrhage into the tumor, the latter event occurring most often with glioblastoma multiforme. This malignant glioma characteristically contains many atypical blood vessels, which may rupture spontaneously or following minor trauma. Moreover, this tumor has a tendency to replace cerebral parenchyma as it grows, thus delaying the appearance of significantly increased intracranial pressure until the neoplasm is quite large.

Sudden swelling of a cystic tumor or pressure from a neoplasm in the region of the hypothalamus, aqueduct of Sylvius or fourth ventricle can cause sudden death from central disruption of autonomic control of cardiorespiratory function.

In addition to killing suddenly as a *direct* result of their internal expansion and encroachment, intracranial tumors may be responsible for sudden (violent) death *indirectly* by precipitating fatal traumatic incidents as a consequence of ataxia, dizziness, mental confusion or seizures, which often precede diagnostic clinical symptoms from intracerebral new growths.

Metastatic brain tumors are, on rare occasion, responsible for the types of situations just described. The most frequent primary sites for these tumors are lung and breast.

### *Epilepsy*

Epilepsy, regardless of etiology, can cause sudden and unexplained death in several different ways, including initiation of fatal mishaps during a seizure in which loss of consciousness or of muscular control permits the occurrence of traumatic incidents (e.g. drowning, motor vehicle accidents) or results in obstruction of the respiratory tract due either to aspiration of gastric contents or to the position of the individual following the attack. Epileptics with significant stenosing coronary atherosclerosis can die suddenly of acute coronary insufficiency as a result of severe muscular exertion, hypoxia and hypertension precipitated by a violent seizure.

Epilepsy in and of itself can be responsible for sudden and unexpected death, sometimes with a single tonic convulsion.[44, 45] Seizures limited to the autonomic nervous system without motor involvement *(paroxysmal autonomic dysfunction)* have been invoked as the mechanism of death in some epileptics found dead in bed without evidence of a major convulsion having taken place. Absence of tongue biting or fecal and urinary incontinence does not exclude the occurrence of epileptic convulsions, a fact well and amply documented by witnessed fatal seizures. Cardiac and respiratory exhaustion can follow in the wake of prolonged and repeated epileptic convulsions *(status epilepticus).*

Although death may occur during the first major epileptic convulsion, a sound diagnosis of epilepsy as a cause of death cannot be based solely on the presence of some type of convulsive phenomena during the agonal period. Such indications of cerebral irritability are nonspecific and occur with many different lethal processes.

Gross and microscopic examination of the brain in known epileptics frequently shows no characteristic changes or lesions that permit the pathologist to make an objective diagnosis of epilepsy. Many victims of epilepsy have anatomically normal brains. If death is to be ascribed to this disease, there should be a history of convulsions *(fits, fainting spells)*, ideally supported by abnormal electroencephalographic tracings. In many instances it is quite difficult to obtain the details of previous convulsive episodes because the family desires to avoid the social stigma that is often associated with the diagnosis of epilepsy. In the absence of witnesses to the terminal episode, the verdict of *death from epilepsy* should be based on a reliable history and the performance of a complete autopsy that discloses no other anatomic or chemical cause of death.

## Respiratory Tract Disease

Sudden and unexpected deaths occur with a variety of acute and chronic pulmonary disorders and as a result of several different lethal mechanisms. Reference has already been made to exsanguinating and asphyxiating pulmonary hemorrhages, pulmonary embolism and acute failure of chronic cor pulmonale.

### *Lobar and Bronchopneumonia*

Lobar pneumonia and extensive confluent bronchopneumonia accounts for the single largest group of victims dying unexpectedly from *acute* pulmonary disease. The pneumonia may be *primary*, or it may be associated with and follow a severe viral disease such as Asian influenza.[46] Again, the observer is impressed with the striking discrepancy between the *classical* textbook description of the clinical manifestations demonstrated by the patient with grave pneumonia, e.g. shock, prostration, marked dyspnea and the like, and the fact that many persons with extensive pneumonia are able to be up and about and to carry on in some fashion up to the moment of collapse and death. These persons are frequently chronic alcoholics.

### *Pulmonary Tuberculosis*

Pulmonary tuberculosis is an example of a *chronic* infectious pulmonary disease that is encountered occasionally as a cause of sudden and unexpected death. The lethal mechanism may be hemorrhage *(vide supra)* or toxicity. Once more we are confronted with the paradoxical situation where the victim has somehow managed to remain ambulatory despite the presence of far-advanced, active caseating and cavitating disease, thus creating a serious public health menace. When the cause of such a death is established by the coroner, he must immediately notify the public health authorities so that a search can be instituted promptly for contacts who may have been infected by the decedent.

### *Bronchial Asthma*

A modest proportion of all deaths from chronic bronchial asthma is provided by fatalities that occur rapidly and acutely. Sudden deaths ascribable to bronchial asthma may be the result of acute failure of a chronic cor pulmonale. However, the majority of patients who die quickly and unexpectedly from bronchial asthma usually do so during an acute asthmatic paroxysm. Such deaths are the result of widespread airway occlusion and are preceded by prominent asphyxial phenomena.

The bronchi and bronchioles become obstructed by a combination of factors, including the presence of tenacious, viscid mucoid exudate, edematous swelling of the mucosa and submucosa, and spasm of the airway musculature. These mechanically obstructive changes may be superimposed upon and complicated by chronic emphysema and right ventricular failure from chronic cor pulmonale. As the acute process progresses and becomes more widespread and increasingly severe, ventilatory capacity is reduced until oxygen intake and carbon dioxide elimination are critically compromised. Rapid asphyxial death then ensues in which respiratory acidosis plays a prominent role.

At autopsy the lungs of persons dying of an acute asthmatic paroxysm are voluminous, pale and distended and often present shallow indentations resulting from pressure of the overinflated organs against the ribs. Trachea and bronchi contain large quantities of thick, inspissated mucoid exudate, which effectively plug their lumens.

Microscopic study establishes the presence of similar material in bronchioles as well, and in all sites the mucus frequently contains a liberal admixture of eosinophilic leukocytes. Connell[47] has noted decreased numbers of mast cells in the bronchi of patients who died of asthma, suggesting that mast cell degranulation is part of the pathophysiology of asthma. Other stigmata of chronic asthma usually present include hyaline thickening of the basement membrane of the bronchial mucosa, varying degrees of bronchial and bronchiolar smooth muscle hyperplasia, hyperactivity of the mucous glands and abundant peribronchial infiltration by a pleomorphic cellular exudate in which lymphocytes and eosinophiles are prominent elements.

These gross and microscopic criteria are found in practically all cases of rapid death from uncomplicated bronchial asthma. Variations from patient to patient are usually quantitative, i.e. greater or lesser degrees of cellular exudation and infiltration or squamous metaplasia of the bronchial epithelium.

Other disease processes that produce high-grade sudden respiratory obstruction are equally capable of causing unexpected death within minutes or hours of the onset of premonitory dyspneic manifestations. Angioneurotic edema of the glottis and laryngeal diphtheria fall into this group of illnesses.

## Alimentary Tract Disease

Sequelae, complications and exacerbations of several chronic diseases in different portions of the gastrointestinal tract are occasionally responsible for unexpected and rapid rather than sudden deaths. Fatal hemorrhages originating from active chronic gastric or duodenal peptic ulcers or from ruptured esophageal varices secondary to hepatic cirrhosis have already been described. Perforation of a peptic ulcer with subsequent generalized fibrinopurulent peritonitis and shock can be a speedily fatal complication of this common disease. So, too, strangulated hernias (inguinal, femoral, umbilical or internal) whose signs and symptoms have been ignored can quickly progress to gangrene of the compromised intestine with resultant peritonitis, shock and death.

### *Acute Pancreatitis*

Although acute pancreatitis is a disease with commonly recognized lethal potentialities, it is not ordinarily considered as a cause of sudden death. However, in some instances the clinical course is truly hyperacute and fulminating, with death supervening extremely rapidly if not instantaneously. Such abbreviated terminal episodes have been ascribed to preceding alcoholic debauches,[48] but they occur also in teetotalers. The etiology and pathogenesis of the diffuse, destructive inflammatory process is not yet completely established, but the lethal mechanism is one of overwhelming shock with violently disturbed electrolyte and protein levels.

### *Fatty Liver*

An up-to-now unexplained type of sudden death is that seen in association with, and usually ascribed to, fatty metamorphosis (fatty alteration, fatty phanerosis) of the liver, a condition seen most commonly (but not exclusively) in severe chronic alcoholics. Studies of series of sudden natural deaths certified following medicolegal autopsy have consistently demonstrated that a significant fraction of the victims were young adults whose only morbid anatomic finding was a fatty or cirrhotic liver. Deaths of this type are more common in men than women, and are more frequent in lower social classes.[49]

Durlacher et al.[50] reported that 5 of 25 chronic alcoholics who died suddenly, and in whom the sole noteworthy *gross* anatomic abnormality at autopsy was fatty liver, were victims of massive pulmonary fat embolism, much more than that seen with fatal fat embolism following fractures of long bones. They concluded that sudden death in some persons with an alcoholic fatty liver was produced by extensive obstruction of the pulmonary vessels by fat globules originating in lipid-distended liver cells that had ruptured.

This explanation (hypothesis) has not been acceptable to other observers, who were unable to confirm these findings. Other possible bases for sudden death in persons with extreme fatty change in their liver have included a broad variety of metabolic and biochemical abnormalities, e.g. hypoglycemia, polyvitamin deficiencies, disturbances in blood ammonia levels, anaerobic glycolysis with excessive lactic acid production and dysfunction in porphyrin metabolism. None is as yet generally accepted as explaining the sudden death.

Mann[51] has summarized the problems raised by sudden death in persons whose sole postmortem abnormality is widespread fatty vacuolization of the hepatic cells, whether this change takes the form of one large intracellular globule of fat that displaces the nucleus to the edge of the cell or of many fine droplets that do not disturb the nuclear location. His observations indicate that in some cases the association of fatty liver and sudden death is purely fortuitous and that in others the mechanism of death is quite uncertain. He cautions that the term *acute hepatic failure* should be limited to patients dying in hepatic coma with clinical and laboratory evidence of well-defined, far-advanced liver disease and that the deaths of persons who succumb suddenly and in whom the sole abnormal finding is a fatty liver are most correctly designated as *Cause of death: undetermined. Manner of death: natural.*

## MISCELLANEOUS CAUSES OF SUDDEN, UNEXPECTED AND RAPID NATURAL DEATH

There still remains a heterogeneous group of unexpected natural deaths not readily classifiable in any of the preceding categories. Chief among these are fatalities from bacterial infections in which there exists marked virulence of the microorganism, low host resistance or various combinations of both factors. Included in this consideration are untreated or neglected infection such as supperative pyelonephritis.

Other examples of rapid deaths from infectious causes have been given earlier in this chapter, i.e. lobar pneumonia and suppurative meningitis.

### *Waterhouse-Friderichsen Syndrome*

The classic model of fulminating, fatal bacterial disease is the so-called *Waterhouse-Friderichsen syndrome,* of which Herrick said, "No other infection so quickly slays." The syndrome is characterized by bloodstream invasion by a virulent organism, most frequently the meningococcus, and bilateral adrenal hemorrhages. Intense cyanosis and cutaneous hemorrhages ranging in severity from a few scattered petechiae to large confluent, reddish purple macules are common. Hemorrhagic lesions also may be present in the oral cavity and conjunctivae.

Microscopically the dermal lesions reveal interstitial extravasation of erythrocytes or hemorrhagic foci of acute exudative inflammation. The adrenal changes vary broadly in degree from capillary engorgement through focal cortical hemorrhages to diffuse destructive hemorrhagic necrosis of cortex and medulla, converting the organs into *bags of blood.*

Clinically the patient presents a toxic, febrile illness of acute onset, soon followed by severe circulatory collapse and death. The entire course of the disease from apparent health to death may transpire in a few hours, much too short an interval for the development of a full-blown meningeal inflammatory response. The lethal mechanism is probably a combination of overwhelming bacterial toxemia and acute adrenal insufficiency, which produces profound shock.

### *Hemophilus Influenzae Type B. Epiglottitis*

Infection produced by other toxic, virulent organisms such as *Hemophilus influenzae,* Type B, can be fatal even though the bacteria remains localized and do not find their way into the bloodstream. Examination of cervical viscera is essential to disclose the acute suppurative epiglottitis and laryngitis, the most prominent anatomic manifestation of colonization by this death-dealing organism. Clinically the patient may have complained only briefly of a sore throat prior to unexpected collapse and death.

### *Metabolic and Endocrine Causes*

In the absence of anatomic abnormalities or exogenous chemical agents that can be implicated as having caused death, consideration must be given to the possibility or probability of the presence of some metabolic disturbance in body chemistry or endocrine function that can lead to sudden death. Into this group fall such entities as the two extremes of faulty blood glucose regulation, hypoglycemia from hyperinsulinism arising from a functional adenoma of the islets of Langerhans and acutely developing diabetic ketoacidosis. The former diagnosis is made in the presence of a pancreatic tumor that has the characteristic histologic appearance of an islet cell adenoma and that contains large quantities of insulin.

Death can be ascribed to diabetic acidosis when large quantities of glucose and acetone are found in the urine, vitreous humor and cerebrospinal fluid at autopsy. The usual background for this type of fatality is either lack of awareness on the part of the victim that he was suffering from diabetes mellitus or failure to realize the significance of the premonitory symptoms of impending coma.

Postmortem blood sugar levels are not sufficiently reliable to permit the establishment of a diagnosis of either of the aforementioned glucose disturbances. A study by Sturner and Gantner[52] suggests that the vitreous glucose concentration reflects the agonal blood sugar level quite accurately and may thus aid in documenting the presence or absence of either metabolic abnormality.

Pituitary insufficiency has been implicated as a cause of sudden and unexpected death in young women who have previously suffered an infarct of their adenohypophysis following postpartum hemorrhage.[53] Such sudden deaths are usually preceded by indications of anterior pituitary hypofunction in the form of failure of lactation, amenorrhea and depressed thyroid activity, and they occur under conditions of stress. The responsible mechanism is probably adrenal insufficiency secondary to decrease in ACTH secretion by the damaged hypophysis.

Toxic thyroid nodules, myxedema and adrenal insufficiency of diverse etiologic origins have also been described as causes of sudden and unexpected death.

### *Sickle Cell Disease*

Sickle cell disease is characterized clinically by chronic hemolytic anemia, episodes of abdominal and joint pain, recurrent infections and thrombotic events. Hypoxia, acidosis and dehydration can precipitate massive intravascular sickling in these patients, with resultant sudden death. The occurrence of rapidly fatal intravascular sickling following physical exertion at relatively high altitude has been reported also in military personnel with sickle trait.[54]

### *Complications of Labor and Delivery*

Occasional instances of sudden death from amniotic fluid embolism or uterine rupture were noted in Luke and Helpern's[55] study of medicolegal autopsies on young persons.

### *Senility*

Finally, death may occur suddenly and unexpectedly in persons of advanced years without the presence of any special anatomic features to furnish a sound explanation for the unanticipated exitus. Senile atrophy of the brain, brown atrophy of the heart, generalized arteriosclerosis and arteriolar sclerosis constitute the usual complex of findings that are lumped into the all-inclusive phrases *senility* or *senile marasmus*—descriptive but nonexplanatory terms for a puzzling syndrome.

## REFERENCES

1. Kuller, L., Lilienfeld, A., and Fisher, R. S.: An epidemiological study of sudden and unexpected deaths in adults. *Medicine, 46:*341, 1967.
2. Morin, M. A., and Pitts, F. W.: Delayed apoplexy following head injury. *J Neurosurg, 33:*542, 1970.

3. Burch, G. E., and DePasquale, N. P.: Sudden unexpected natural death. *Am J Med Sci, 249:*86, 1965.
4. Adelson, L.: No anatomic cause of death. *Conn State Med J, 18:*732, 1954.
5. Aponte, G. E.: Enigma of "Bangungut." *Ann Intern Med, 52:*1258, 1960.
6. Pruitt, R. D.: On sudden death. *Am Heart J, 68:* 111, 1964.
7. Weiss, S.: Instantaneous "physiologic" death. *N Engl J Med, 223:*793, 1940.
8. Kayssi, A. L.: Death from inhibition and its relation to shock. *Br Med J, 2:*131, 1948.
9. Gordon, T., and Kannel, W. B.: Premature mortality from coronary heart disease. *JAMA, 215:* 1617, 1971.
10. Spain, D. M., Bradess, V. A., and Mohr, C.: Coronary atherosclerosis as a cause of unexpected and unexplained death. *JAMA, 174:*384, 1960.
11. Adelson, L., and Hoffman, W.: Sudden death from coronary disease. *JAMA, 176:*129, 1961.
12. Paterson, J. C.: Stress, intimal hemorrhage and coronary occlusion. *J Occup Med, 3:*59, 1961.
13. Master, A. M.: Role of effort and occupation (including physicians) in coronary occlusion. *JAMA, 174:*942, 1960.
14. Friedman, M.: The coronary thrombus: Its origin and fate. *Hum Pathol, 2:*81, 1971.
15. Edward, J. E. Pathology of sudden death. *Minn Med, 48:*1519, 1965.
16. Spain, D. M., and Bradess, V. A.: Sudden death from coronary heart disease: Survival time, frequency of thrombi and cigarette smoking. *Chest, 58:*107, 1970.
17. World Health Organization: Pathological diagnosis of acute ischemic heart disease. *WHO Technical Report Series,* No. 441, 1970.
18. Beck, C. S.: Coronary heart disease: Three dominant causes of death. *Am J Surg, 95:*743, 1958.
19. Chiang, B. N., Perlman, L. V., Ostrander, L. D., Jr., et al.: Relationship of premature systoles to coronary heart disease and sudden death in the Tecumseh epidemiologic study. *Ann Intern Med, 70:*1159, 1969.
20. Chiang, B. N., Perlman, L. V., Fulton, M. et al.: Predisposing factors in sudden cardiac death. *Circulation, 41:*31, 1970.
21. Hinkle, L. E., Jr., Carver, S., Benjamin, B., et al.: Studies in the ecology of coronary artery disease. *Arch Environ Health, 9:*14, 1964.
22. Spain, D. M., and Bradess, V. A.: Relation of sex, age and physical activity to sudden death from coronary arterial occlusion. In Rosenbaum, F. F., and Belknap, E. L., *Work and the Heart,* New York, Hoeber, 1959, p. 283.
23. Furberg, C., Romo, M., Linko, E., et al.: Sudden coronary death in Scandinavia, *Acta Med Scand, 201:*553-557, 1977.
24. Lovegrove, T.: Sudden death from ischemic heart disease: A review of five hundred consecutive cases. *Med J Aust, 1(5):*128-129, 1977.
25. Prineas, R. J., and Blackburn, H. (Eds.): Sudden coronary death outside hospital. *Circulation 52(6 suppl. 3):* 1-283, 1975.
26. Rabson, S. M., and Helpern, M.: Sudden and unexpected natural death. II. Coronary artery sclerosis. *Am Heart J, 35:*635, 1948.
27. Wikland, B.: Death from ASHD outside hospitals: A study of 2678 cases in Stockholm with particular reference to sudden deaths. *Acta Med Scand, 184:*129, 1968.
28. Jetter, W. W., and White, P. D.: Rupture of heart in patients in mental institutions. *Ann Intern Med, 21:*783, 1944.
29. Glover, R. P., and Gadboys, H. L.: Practical management of aortic stenosis. *JAMA, 168:*229, 1958.
30. Anderson, M. W., Kilsey, J. R., Jr., and Edwards, J. E.: Clinical and pathological considerations in cases of calcific aortic stenosis. *JAMA, 149:*9, 1952.
31. Glew, R. H., Varghese, P. J., Krovetz, L. J., et al.: Sudden death in congenital aortic stenosis. *Am Heart J, 78:*615, 1969.
32. Teare, D.: Asymmetrical hypertrophy of the heart in young adults. *Br Heart J, 20:*1, 1958.
33. James, T. N. Sarcoid heart disease. *Circulation, 56:*320-326, 1977.
34. Porter, G. H.: Sarcoid heart disease. *N Engl J Med, 263:*1350, 1960.
35. James T. N., and Marshall, T. K.: De subitaneius mortibus. XII. Asymmetrical hypertrophy of the heart. *Circulation, 51:*1149-1166, 1975.
36. Harvey, W. P., and Levine, S. A.: Paroxysmal ventricular tachycardia due to emotion: Possible mechanism of death from fright. *JAMA, 150:* 479, 1952.
37. Freytag, E.: Fatal rupture of intracranial aneurysms. *Arch Pathol, 81:*418, 1966.
38. Pool, J. L.: Diagnosis and recent advance in treatment of subarachnoid hemorrhage. *JAMA, 187:* 404, 1964.
39. Stehbens, W. E.: Histopathology of cerebral aneurysms. *Arch Neurol, 8:*272, 1963.
40. Hume, D. M., and Porter, R. R.: Acute dissecting aortic aneurysms. *Surgery, 53:*122, 1963.
41. Breckenridge, R. T., and Ratnoff, O. D.: Pulmonary embolism and unexpected death in supposedly normal individuals. *N Engl J Med, 270:*298, 1964.
42. Zimmerman, T. S., Adelson, L., and Ratnoff, O. D.:

Pulmonary embolism and unexpected death in supposedly normal persons—a second look. *N Engl J Med, 283:*1504, 1970.
43. Bailey, O. T.: Unexpected death due to intracranial tumors. *N Engl J Med, 241:*988, 1949.
44. Freytag, E., and Lindenberg, R.: 294 medicolegal autopsies on epileptics—Cerebral findings. *Arch Pathol, 78:*274, 1964.
45. Hirsch, C. S., and Martin, D. L.: Unexpected death in young epileptics. *Neurology, 21:*682-690, 1971.
46. Oseasohn, R., Adelson, L., and Kaji, M.: Clinicopathologic study of thirty-three fatal cases of Asian influenza. *N Engl J Med, 260:*509, 1959.
47. Connell, J. T.: Asthmatic deaths: Role of the mast cell. *JAMA, 215:*769, 1971.
48. Berman, L. G., Dunn, E., and Straehley, C. J.: Survey of pancreatitis. *Gastroenterology, 40:*94, 1961.
49. Kramer, K., Kuller, L., and Fisher, R. S.: The increasing mortality attributed to cirrhosis and fatty liver in Baltimore (1957-66). *Ann Intern Med, 69:*273, 1968.
50. Durlacher, S. H., Meier, J. R., Fisher, R. S., and Levitt, W. V., Jr.: Sudden death due to pulmonary fat embolism in persons with alcoholic fatty liver. (Abstract) *Am J Pathol, 30:*633, 1954.
51. Mann, G. T.: Sudden death with fatty liver. *Medico-Legal Bulletin,* No. 138. Richmond, Virginia, Office of the Chief Medical Examiner, October, 1964.
52. Sturner, W. Q., and Gantner, G. E.: Postmortem vitreous glucose determinations. *J Forensic Sci, 9:*485, 1964.
53. Israel, S. L., and Conston, A. S.: Unrecognized pituitary necrosis (Sheehan's syndrome). *JAMA, 148:*189, 1952.
54. Jones, S. R., Binder, R. A., Donowho, E. M., Jr.: Sudden death in sickle-cell trait. *N Engl J Med, 282:*323, 1970.
55. Luke, J. L., and Helpern, M.: Sudden unexpected death from natural causes in young adults. *Arch Pathol, 85:*10, 1968.

*Chapter VI*

# TRAUMA AND DISEASE

Russell S. Fisher

A significant percentage of all deaths that occur following a traumatic episode will raise problems of interpretation because of the concurrent presence of a disease process. The combination of trauma and disease obviously raises the following questions: (a) Was the traumatic event wholely and solely responsible for the death? (b) Did it contribute to the death to a greater or lesser degree? (c) Was the death in fact due solely to disease, and should the trauma be excluded as a factor in causation of the death? Because of the differing statutory provisions applicable to criminal and civil litigation in tort action and in workmen's compensation cases, the problem can be best considered separately under these three categories.

## TRAUMA AND DISEASE IN CRIMINAL CASES

In most states there is a statutory provision that the death of the victim of an assault must occur within a year and a day of the assault if action on a charge of homicide is to be brought against the assailant.

In any situation in which an individual is accused of causing the death of another and the investigation and autopsy findings indicate that there is a combination of injury and disease responsible for the death, the pathologist must analyze the situation carefully and show in his report and opinion the relative role of the two events in causing the death. This is perhaps best approached by dividing the medical situation into one of three categories: (a) where preexisting disease is complicated by intentional or negligent injury on the part of the accused and leads to death; (b) where death is due to medical complications of ordinarily nonfatal injuries, but where the complications are one of the natural consequences of the injury; (c) injury followed by complications classified as therapeutic misadventure, i.e. accident, and where the misadventure appears to be the proximate cause of the death.

In considering the *preexisting disease complicated by intentional or negligent injury*, the classical situation is portrayed by the following case:

An elderly man who had recently recovered from a severe heart attack was assaulted by a number of young men attempting to rob him. In the course of the robbery he was restrained bodily, thrown to the ground and his clothing was torn. He was then left collapsed at the scene. Within a few minutes, although he was able to get up and make his way back to his home, he collapsed and died. The autopsy revealed no significant injuries, but there was a severe degree of arteriosclerotic heart disease with large old scars in the heart muscle. The medical opinion was that his death was due to heart disease but that the stress incident to fear and physical resistance to his assailants was sufficient to precipitate an acute episode of dysfunction of the cardiac electrical system with resulting acute heart failure and death. The assailants were apprehended and tried on a murder count. The medical opinion that the death was indeed precipitated by the events associated with the robbery led to the conclusion that the assault was truly a contributing cause to the death, and the defendants were convicted.

Such convictions usually are at the manslaughter level, but in the instant case first degree murder was held because the death was precipitated by acts incident to the felonious assault and robbery. The pathologist's opinion was reached by first posing the question, Was injury or stress truly a contributing cause to the death? Since the answer was affirmative, the second question was posed: Was the injury likely to have been fatal even without disease? Here the answer was negative, but prosecution followed because the pathologist's opinion, based on his findings and the clear-cut history of assault and prompt onset of cardiac failure was that the man would, to a high degree of medical certainty, not have died at this time in the absence of the assault. Had the cardiac failure been delayed several hours or days, it is unlikely that the pathologist's opinion would have been sufficiently strong to justify homicide prosecution.

There are numerous precedent cases in the legal records. One that illustrates the problem well is that of *State v. O'Brien* rendered by the Supreme Court of Iowa on October 13, 1890.[1]

"Appellant was indicted and tried for the crime of murder and was found guilty of manslaughter. He was adjudged to be imprisoned for two years of hard labor in the penitentiary at Anamosa and to pay the cost, and from that judgement he appeals.

"The State claims and the evidence tends to show that the material facts of the case are substantially as follows: Prior to the 15th day of July 1888, the defendant entertained ill will toward one Henry Stokem on the alleged ground that the latter had accused him of throwing cream cans into the well of a Mr. Lida. He threatened Stokem with physical violence to different persons and seemed to be seeking an encounter with him. Both were boys about seventeen years of age and were about the same size and weight, but Stokem had been affected for some time by heart trouble and was not strong. During the evening of the day named, defendant, accompanied by Warren and Willie Murphy, met Stokem on the Highway and assaulted him, knocking him down, holding and choking him after he was down and kicking him himself or causing him to be kicked by Warren Murphy. After Stokem was released he was chased for a considerable distance. Stokem was much excited by the encounter and lost health and strength rapidly from that time until the 28th day of July, 1888 when he died from the effects of the injury caused by the defendant. It is admitted by defendant that he encountered Stokem at the time and place claimed by the State and that he then struck him; but that he claims that no one was present but himself and Stokem and that all he did was done in self-defense. He denies that the death of Stokem was a result of injuries received in that encounter and claims that it was due to causes for which he was not responsible."

"*The Court said:* It is suggested that the verdict is not supported by the evidence and that it is not shown that the death of Stokem resulted from injuries inflicted by defendant. The evidence shows that the decedent had not been in good health for several months. About three weeks before the assault in question, he consulted a physician who found his heart in a diseased condition and treated him for heart difficulty. He improved steadily under that treatment until the assault was made. If this testimony at the preliminary examination and his dying declaration were correct, he was choked and kicked and otherwise grossly maltreated by defendant. It was certain that he was greatly excited by the encounter. Immediately after it occurred, he applied at a house in the vicinity for shelter stating that he was afraid to go home, on account of the defendant and the Murphy boys. A witness said of his appearance at that time, "He acted just scared to death, his face was pale as death; his lips were swollen, his hat was torn and had mud on both sides." His health failed rapidly from that time. The witness that saw him a day after the assault described his appearance and condition as follows: "I discovered he was in pretty bad shape; he was pale, haggard, almost impossible for him to breathe. I thought he would reel right over on the stoop there. His shoulder blades worked like a bellows. His voice was weak, his lips dark blue." The medical testimony shows that his condition and failing health after the assault and his death were natural and probable results of his physical condition on the night of July 15th and of great excitement and physical exertion. It was the province of the jury to determine whether the wrong of the defendant caused or contributed to his death. The fact that he was afflicted with a disease which might have proved fatal would not justify the wrongful acts of defendant, not constitute defense in law. Nor would ignorance on part of defendant of the deceased physical condition of Stokem excuse his acts. We think the evidence sufficient to sustain the verdict and find no error prejudicial to the defendant of which he can complain. The judgement of the district court is affirmed."

The situation is readily summarized by the simple statement that the defendant is responsible for the natural consequences of his acts, even though he may not at the time have known of the illness of his victim or that the consequences would be as severe as they eventually turned out to be.

*Death due to medical complications of ordinarily nonfatal injuries* includes the common situations where an individual sustains what appear at the outset to be relatively minor injuries, but where such complications as blood clot formation in the leg veins with detachment of thrombi and fatal pulmonary embolism occurs. A similar situation involves such complications of a relatively minor penetrating injury as gas gangrene or tetanus bacillus invasion, with systemic poisoning and death of the injured party.

Here again the legal principles are well-established that where the defendant inflicts an injury which brings on a diseased condition from which the injured person dies, the defendant is guilty of homicide. The pathologist in reaching opinions concerning the manner of death must of course evaluate the complications. He should be of the opinion that the complications which were fatal are in fact to be ascribed to the original injury and would *not,* with a reasonable degree of medical certainty, have developed independently of the primary injury for which the accused is responsible.

*Injury followed by therapeutic misadventure or medical mismanagement* and death also involves the medical judgement of the pathologist, because the legal principles call for substantial opinions concerning the inherent danger of the original wound and the relative importance of the improper medical treatment in the eventual death of the victim. Again the legal precedents go back many years and have been stated in the following language in two appellate court decisions. In *Parsons v. State of Alabama* (1852)[2] the Court said—

> "If a wound is inflicted not dangerous in itself and the death which ensues was evidently occasioned by the grossly erroneous treatment of it, the original author will not be accountable, but if the wound was mortal or dangerous the person who inflicted it cannot shelter himself under the plea of erroneous treatment."

In *State v. Karsunky* (1938)[3] the Supreme Court of the state of Washington held—

> "If one unlawfully inflicts upon the person of another a wound calculated to endanger or destroy life, it would not be a defense to a charge of unlawful homicide, where death ensues, to show that the wounded person might have recovered if the wound had been more skillfully treated. Even unskillful or negligent treatment of the wound on the part of the wounded person or his physicians, which may have aggravated the wound and contributed to the death, does not relieve the assailant from liability. He must, as we said in State v. Baruth, 47 Wash. 283, 91 P. 977, 983, . . . show that the negligent and unskillful treatment was the sole cause of death, before he can escape the consequences of his unlawful act on this ground."

During a street fight a boy of nineteen was stabbed in the abdomen. The wound penetrated into the stomach but did not cause major hemorrhage. The boy was promptly taken to the hospital, where surgical exploration was carried out. Before surgery, a blood specimen was taken for typing and crossmatching, and two pints of blood were ordered. The surgeon found little or no soilage of the peritoneal cavity, and the stomach and abdominal wall wounds were readily sutured. The two pints of blood were administered. After surgery the boy's father inquired of the surgeon what was the chance of his son recovering. The surgeon replied, "Ten to one, he will be home in fine shape in two weeks or less." Unfortunately, the victim's kidneys shut down, and he died ten days later. Investigation showed that renal failure was caused by mismatched blood transfusion of the two pints given during surgery. The technician who had *set up* the blood had placed the tube drawn from the injured boy in a rack in the blood bank when he was interrupted by the telephone. Upon returning to type the boy's blood, he picked up a different tube. From there on the crossmatching was done impeccably. Unfortunately, the second tube he picked up was from a person of another blood group—with the resultant mismatch.

The medical examiner in testimony explained the above-stated facts to the Court, who promptly overturned the murder indictment against the individual who had inflicted the stab wound. The assailant was, however, convicted of assault with a deadly weapon and assault with intent to murder and was sentenced to six years in prison.

In assessing this type of situation it is useful to ask the question, Is there cause for action on a criminal negligence basis against those making the medical mistake? If the answer is affirmative, the assailant's contribution is probably nonactionable. If the answer is negative, the assailant must be charged and the pathologist must be prepared to give a full explanation of the misadventure to the court or jury who, under instruction, based on precedent decisions, will, it is hoped, reach a just decision. The difficulties that confront the pathologist are evident and sometimes overwhelming, since the opinions he renders in criminal actions, to be acceptable in court, must be to a reasonable medical certainty or beyond a reasonable medical doubt.

## TRAUMA AND DISEASE IN CIVIL LITIGATION

In tort actions in general the quality of proof upon which the jury or judge must reach a decision (unlike the criminal case, where reasonable medical certainty prevails) is by a preponderance of the evidence. Factors that further complicate the matter are those elements of negligence on the part of the injured party. Although there may be exceptions, the general principle is that, in the causation of an accidental injury or death, negligence on the part of the victim that contributes to the causation of his injuries constitutes a bar to recovery. That is to say, there is no comparative negligence under which the defendant would be held responsible merely because the degree of negligence he evidenced was greater than that of the plaintiff, who was also negligent. This principle holds with regard to causation of the primary injury or death but not to negligence occurring in the treatment of the injured condition. Where there is negligence on the part of an individual in obtaining proper medical care or negligence on the part of those rendering medical care, the doctrine is better described as avoidable consequence, and such negligence is not a bar to recovery. It will influence the amount of damages assigned, since the defendant will be responsible only for that portion of the total damages or disability which can properly be ascribed to his negligence in causing the original injury, as distinct from those portions of disability or damage resulting from the negligence of the plaintiff in caring for the original injuries. The picture is also clouded by the particular statutory provisions having to do with the responsibility for proof; thus, in Massachusetts, Maryland and many other states the burden of proving lack of care on the part of the plaintiff rests on the defendant. In Maine, on the other hand, the burden is upon the plaintiff to show affirmatively that no lack of ordinary care on his part contributed to cause his injuries. William Prosser states the principle clearly in his *Law of Torts:* "Thus concerning the plaintiff injured in an automobile collision, his contributory negligent driving before the collision will prevent any recovery at all, but his failure to support proper medical care for his broken leg will bar only his damages for the subsequent aggravated condition of the leg."[4] It is to be emphasized that these complexities of the legal situation must be understood by the physician who is to evaluate the consequences of a given injury, and he must seek every assistance possible by collection of complete medical history, not only concerning the events of the injury but also concerning the preceding health condition of the victim and the course of events subsequent to the time of injury. To render opinions with less than this information is not only foolhardy on the part of the physician but is dangerous to the administration of justice.

## TRAUMA AND DISEASE IN WORKMEN'S COMPENSATION CASES

While the relative importance of trauma and disease in causing disability or death in the workmen's compensation situation is rarely a matter of police interest insofar as a crime is concerned, the majority of deaths occurring at work become the subject of investigation by the medical examiner or coroner, who in turn is frequently dependent upon police investigation of the nature of the accident. This is required in order that he may evaluate the medical aspects of the case and document the facts for the workmen's compensation commissioner or similar official, who must ultimately decide if an award is due the injured or deceased employee or his dependents. The quality of proof required for such awards is generally of a lower order than that commonly classed as preponderance of evidence. Indeed, in many states it appears that any reasonable medical sequence that connects a disability or death with an event at work is legally adequate grounds to support an award. This concept is inherent in the philosophy of workmen's compensation, since it was devised as a means of relief for injured employees. They would otherwise have, as their only alternative, to bring action in tort accusing the employer of negligence and hoping therefore to gain recompense. Furthermore the maximum amounts of award allowed under workmen's compensation are generally smaller than might occur as a result of tort action and are limited by law. Therefore, the courts have agreed that interpretation of the law must be made broadly in favor of the employee where a reasonable doubt exists.

The laws generally provide that compensation shall be paid for the *disability or death of an employee resulting from an accidental personal injury, arising out of and in the course of his employment, without regard to fault, except where injury is caused by the willful intention of the injured to bring about the injury or death of himself or another, or where injury results solely from the intoxication of the injured employee while on duty.* Accidental is defined in a variety of ways but generally includes any fortuitous, casual and unexpected happening that causes personal disability or death; thus, heatstroke or heat prostration may be an accident within the definition.

Some most unusual consequences develop in the application of the definition, as in a situation where a number of employees drank from a common water bucket that was filled at a nearby spring by the water boy assigned to the crew.[5] The spring was contaminated with the typhoid fever bacillus, and a number of the employees contracted typhoid fever. The Appellate Court, in ruling in their favor, stated that the accidental nature of an injury is not lost by calling consequential injury a disease or by the fact that a dangerous substance was taken into the body by ingestion rather than by external wounding. The Court specifically stated that there need not be an external wound or violence to create liability under the law.

In acquiring a history of a given event from which an injury derives, it is of utmost importance that a careful and detailed inquiry be made and recorded. The inquiries made at the time of the original event are much more apt to be accurate than subsequent reconstructions, colored not infrequently by the desire on the part of the individual to receive compensation.

This is illustrated by a famous Maryland case involving injury in 1950, entitled *Kelly Springfield Tire Company and Liberty Mutual Insurance Company v. Louis E. Daniels.*[6] The Appellate Court upset a lower court holding that a herniated intervertebral disc was an accident.

The testimony that was offered indicated that the patient sustained a pain while lifting a bag to attach it to a filling machine. It was stated that the bag was not unusually heavy, that Daniels did not lift the entire bag and that his part weighed only about 40 lb. Furthermore he testified this was his usual job for some months, and during the previous five months he had lifted many equally heavy bags. He further indicated that he did not fall or slip and that nothing fell on him or struck him. Specifically he noted nothing different than usual in his work except for the onset of pain. The Court said that in Maryland the sudden unexpected rupture of some portion of internal structure of the body or failure of some essential function of the body is held to be an accidental injury only when it results from some unusual strain or exertion of the employee or some unusual condition in his employment. The Court further pointed out that Maryland's view on this may not be as wide as elsewhere in the United States.

In the interpretation of *resulting from,* it is obvious that many times the connection of a given medical event, such as a heart attack or rupture of an intervertebral disc, with an unusual stress or strain or some other event of work becomes a matter of opinion. Here the experience of the physician is of greatest importance in assessing the situation.

An instance involving a death following surgical repair of a ruptured intervertebral disc serves to illustrate the problem.

The individual in question had sustained a ruptured disc while at work and was admitted to the hospital for surgical treatment thereof. The operation was performed successfully, but seventeen hours after the operation, the patient developed delirium tremens and died. The opinion was offered that death was due to alcoholism, but this was disputed by the appellee. It was further contended that the anesthesia may have played some role in precipitating the delirium tremens and that the abstinence from alcohol necessary for the anesthesia and surgical treatment in and of itself arose because of the injury and did precipitate the onset of the fatal delirium. The Court, in discussing whether this was a probability sufficient to be the basis of an award or a mere possibility, stated that "A sequence of events plus proof of possible causal relationship may amount to proof of probable causal relationship in the absence of evidence of any other equally probable cause." The death benefit was awarded.[7]

The heart-attack-at-work situation is one of the most frequent and difficult problems in the compensation area. There is a general tendency of the public, and especially the affected individual or his protestors, to blame any heart attack having onset at work, or even occurring hours after an individual had experienced some minor stress at work, on the occupational activity. Our procedure in analyzing these cases is to try to separate them clinically into those that are coronary occlusion and myocardial infarction and those that are cardiac rhythm disturbances.

In the case of occlusive coronary artery disease, unless the onset is anginal and manifests itself while the stress is occurring, we are extremely dubious of any affirmative relationship between the two conditions. Masters[8] and others have published extensively in this field and have shown that the onset of occlusive episodes is equally distributed between time spent in various levels of activity and in rest. Thus, if one assumes eight hours of sleep daily, one-third of occlusive episodes occur during this period. This, coupled with the fact there is no firmly established pathologic sequence from stress without physical injury to vascular occlusive disease, is the basis for our conclusion.

In cases where fatal arrhythmia occurs during a stress episode, we subscribe to a *precipitating cause* relationship. It has been amply demonstrated that sudden fright or other emotional or physical stress is capable of increasing cardiac rate and aggravating conduction defects in individuals with preexisting arrhythmias or with a particular tendency to bring on such an arrhythmic episode. Perhaps the best example of this is the *Master's test*. Individuals with normal electrocardiograph readings but suspected coronary disease climb steps rapidly or run on a treadmill, with resultant appearance of EKG abnormalities immediately following the exercise. In the course of a fatal arrhythmia that occurs during unusual physical or emotional stress, or within minutes thereafter, it is a reasonable medical conclusion that the stress precipitated the arrhythmia, which then caused the death. Such a conclusion is only justified when autopsy or clinical evidence of heart disease is established. We do not believe this process occurs in the absence of advanced preexisting coronary, hypertensive or certain other cardiac diseases.

An obese middle-aged fireman known to have hypertension died of an arrhythmia within a short time of fighting a brush fire. At autopsy the heart was enlarged to approximately 150 percent of the normal size and showed moderate coronary artery sclerosis. The opinion was that death was due to *hypertensive heart disease with fatal arrhythmia precipitated by the stress of fighting a brush fire.* Compensation was awarded. Eventual analysis under a *subsequent injury procedure* led to the partition of 75 percent of his death due to preexisting disease and 25 percent due to work-related factors. Had his collapse and death been delayed more than an hour or so after return to the firehouse our opinion would have been different, since individuals with the same disease may die spontaneously without stress.

## REFERENCES

1. State v. O'Brien, 81 Iowa 88.
2. Parsons v. State, 21 Ala. 300.
3. State v. Karsunky, 84 P.2d 39.
4. Prosser, William L.: *Handbook of Torts.* St. Paul, Minnesota, West Pub, 1955, p. 287.
5. Union Mining Co. v. Blank, 28 A. 568.
6. Kelley Springfield Tire Co. and Liberty Mutual Insurance Co. v. Daniels, 85 A.2d, 795.
7. Paul Construction Co. and New Amsterdam Casualty Co. v. Powell, 88 A.2d 837.
8. Master, A. M., and Rosenfeld, I.: Two-step exercise test: Current status after twenty-five years. *Med Conc Cardiovasc Dis, 36:*19, 1967.

*Chapter VII*

# BLUNT FORCE INJURY

WERNER U. SPITZ

A SHARP OBJECT cuts and divides the tissues as it penetrates, but a wound produced by blunt impact tears, shears and crushes. Falls, collisions or blows with a blunt instrument, such as a hammer, brick, bat, fist or pipe, typically result in blunt force injury. Extensive bleeding into the adjacent soft tissues is the rule. Hemorrhage of similar magnitude is practically never seen in the margins of cuts and stab wounds.

The cutaneous manifestations of blunt trauma differ depending on the force and nature of the impact. Three basic lesions are recognized: (a) contusion, (b) abrasion, (c) laceration.

## CONTUSION

A contusion (bruise) signifies hemorrhage into the skin, the tissues under the skin or both. It is usually the result of a blow or squeeze that crushes the soft tissues and ruptures blood vessels but does not break the skin. The *black eye* following a fistfight, the scalp hemorrhage from a fall and the *black and blue* mark appearing after an arm is squeezed too tightly are some examples.

Some bruises are patterned, and their recognition may help to reconstruct the circumstances of injury in order to differentiate the more likely

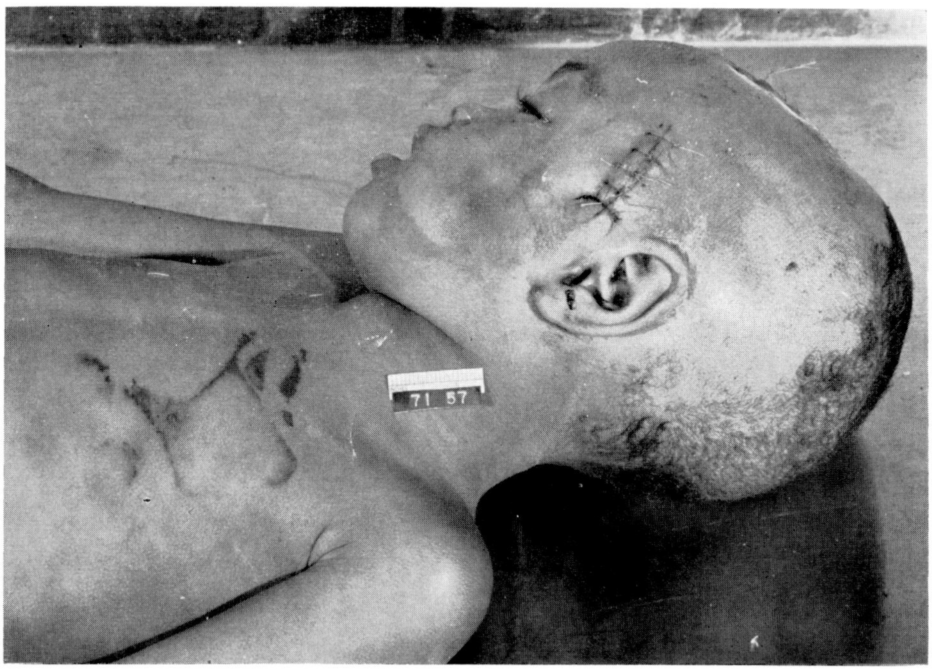


FIGURE VII-1. This three-year-old girl was unconscious when brought to the hospital by her father. She had allegedly fallen down several steps. At autopsy scattered facial bruises, a skull fracture with associated brain injury, severely contused buttocks and the injury to the chest shown in the photograph were noted. Battering was suspected, especially since the pattern of the chest injury was inconsistent with a fall. Detailed questioning of the father resulted in his admission that he had beaten the child with a belt; the imprint was caused by the buckle.

of two or more implements or to implicate a category of agents (Figs. VII-1, VII-2 and VII-3). The imprint of the steering column on the chest of a driver or tire marks on a pedestrian run over by an automobile are familiar examples.

Less well known are the two parallel linear hemorrhages that frequently result from a blow with a rod, a stick or a whip. The intervening skin remains apparently unchanged because the blood is displaced to the sides by the pressure of the implement (Fig. VII-4). Horseshoe-shaped, double-lined bruises are often seen in battered children and are caused by whipping with a looped rope or extension cord.

Bruising of soft tissues is sometimes confined to deep structures, especially if sustained by a blow with a wide and smooth object. Such hemorrhage may gravitate along fascial planes to adjoining areas, giving the impression that the injury occurred at the place at which the hemorrhage is apparent. The actual site of injury must at all times be ascertained at autopsy. A fractured jaw is frequently followed by gravity shifting of the hemorrhage into the neck, simulating direct trauma. A fractured pelvis may result in hemorrhage into the thighs by dissection of the blood along the femoral sheath.

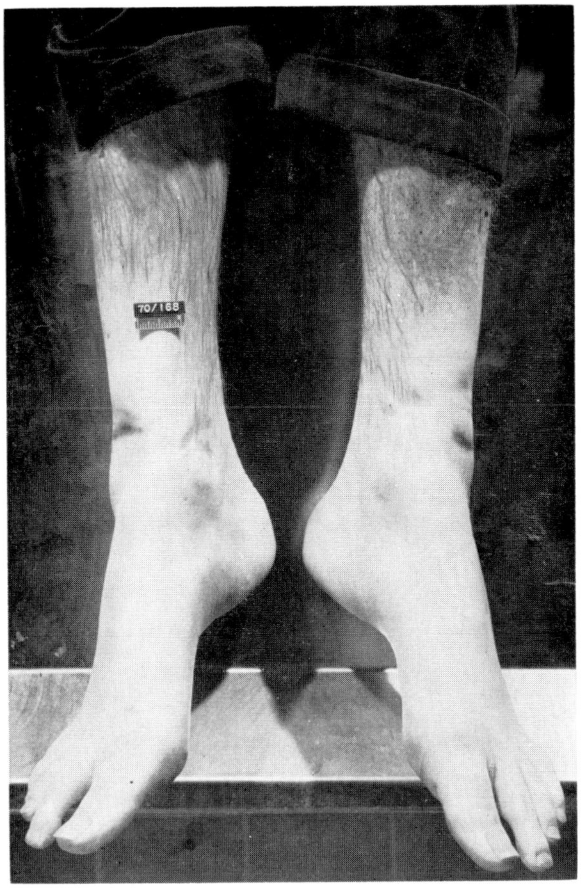

FIGURE VII-3. Circumferential contusions of the ankles indicative of binding. This man, a narcotics pusher, was executed by dissatisfied customers.

Hemorrhages in the soft tissues around the eyes and in the eyelids (so-called spectacle hematomas) commonly suggest a fracture of the base of the skull. Less frequent and not associated with any fractures, these hemorrhages may also follow blunt impact to the forehead that jolts the eyeballs out of their sockets, with resultant tears of small orbital blood vessels. The latter hemorrhages may not become apparent unless the body lies face down and the blood is allowed to seep downward (Fig. VII-5).

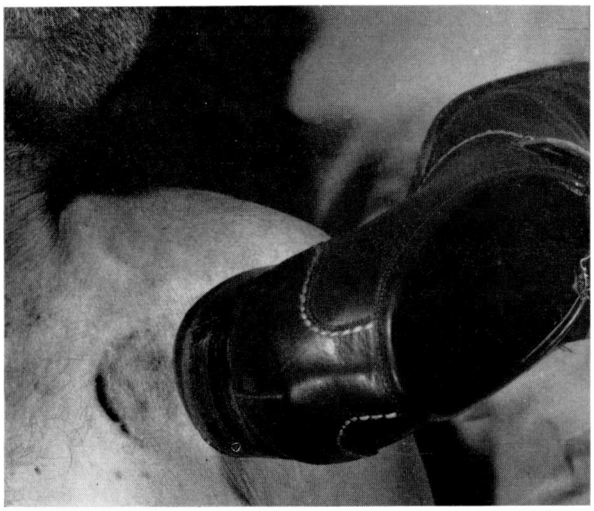

FIGURE VII-2. Semicircular abrasion and contusion produced by the heel of a shoe. This man was stamped to death. He died of asphyxia due to edema of the larynx, which resulted from a similar impact on the neck.

In an individual who survives an injury, a deep bruise may not become apparent on the body surface until several days after the injury. If death occurs before the bluish purple discoloration in the skin has had time to become manifest, only incision of the area will disclose the presence of the injury.

Hemorrhages are sometimes seen in areas of

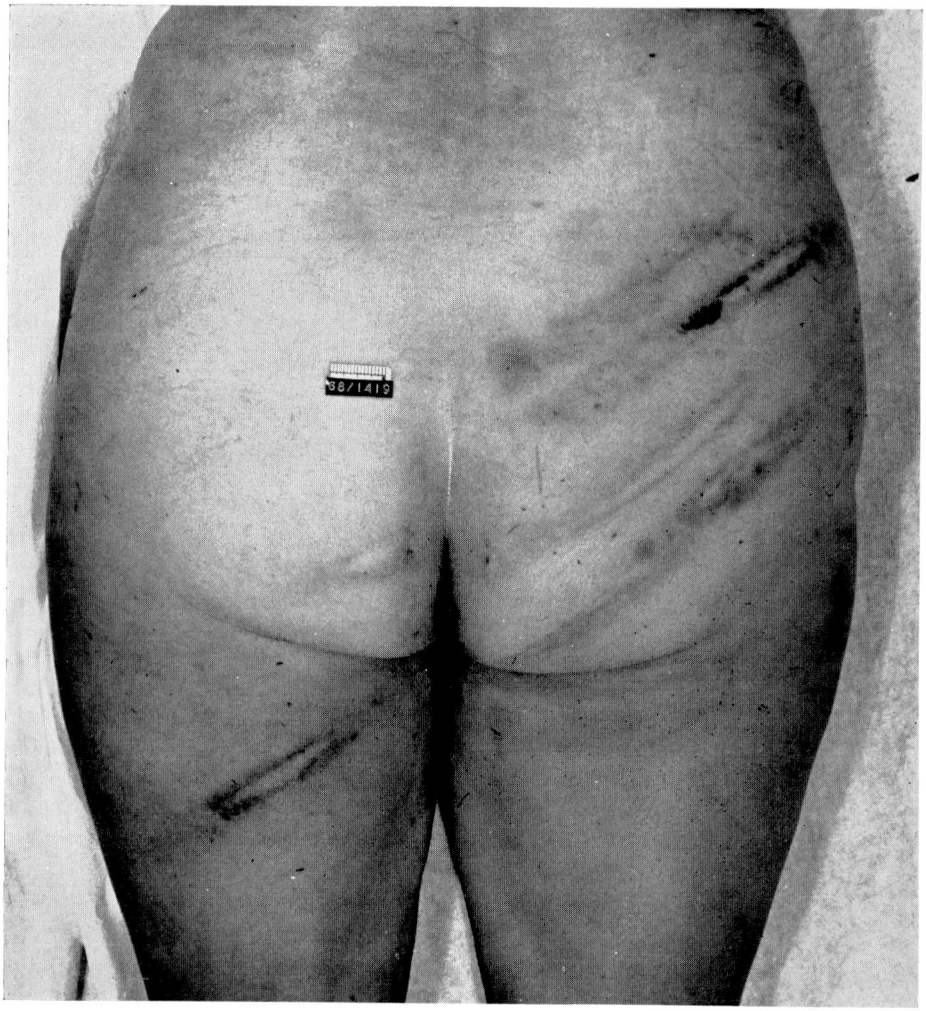


FIGURE VII-4. These injuries were inflicted with a nightstick. Note the two parallel linear hemorrhages for each impact.

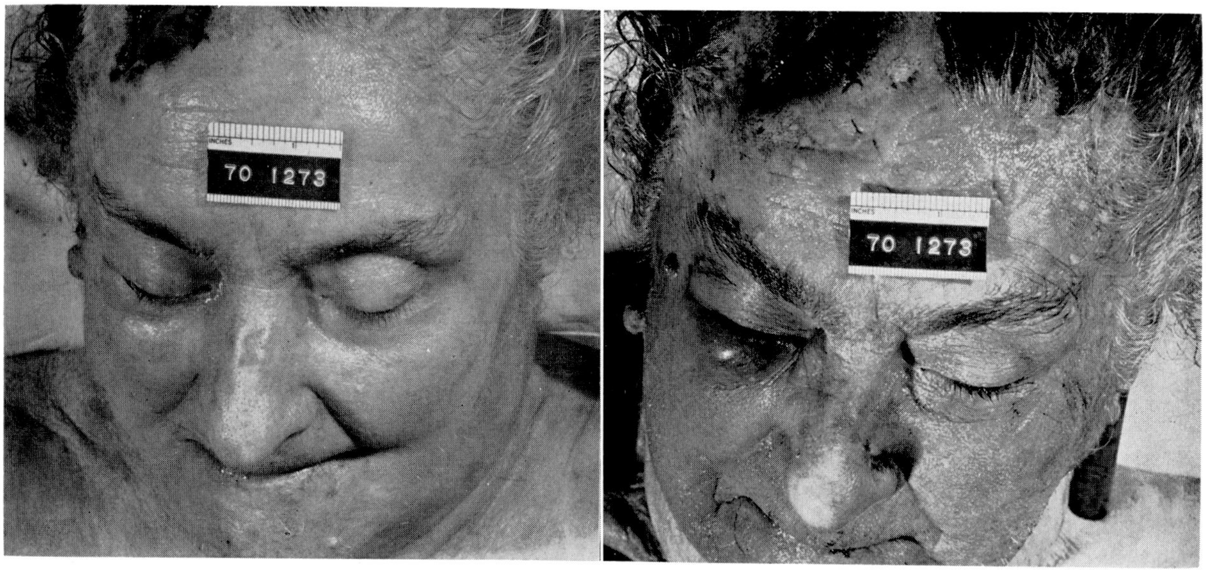


FIGURE VII-5. (a): Elderly woman who fell from a first floor window, striking the right side of the forehead. No periocular hemorrhage was noted when the body was first viewed six hours postmortem. (b): Same woman as in Figure VII-5a after the body lay face down overnight. Note the hemorrhage in the right lower eyelid. No intracranial injury was noted at autopsy. The dusky color of the face is due to postmortem lividity.

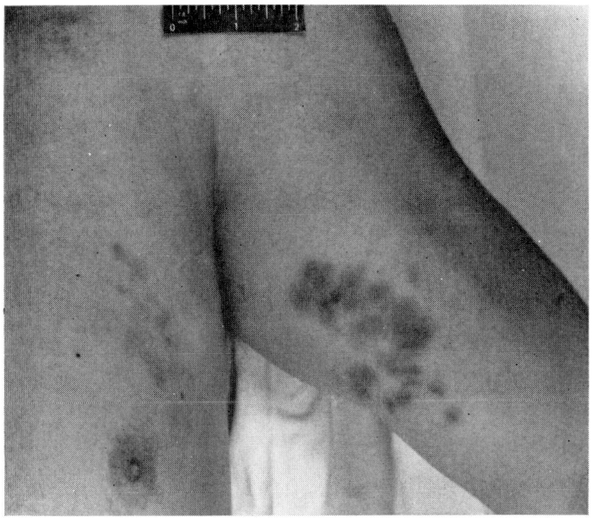

FIGURE VII-6. Artifactual hemorrhages on the inner aspect of the arm produced by seepage of blood from small veins torn when the body was lifted.

lividity on the arms or shoulders of obese individuals without evidence of trauma elsewhere on the body. These hemorrhages are produced by tearing of small veins in the skin when the body is lifted for removal from the scene of death (Fig. VII-6).

The color of a bruise changes from light bluish red to dark purple, green, yellow and brown. This change proceeds from the periphery of the bruise toward its center and vice versa; it may be used as a guide to the age of the injury. Often a bruise has a doughnutlike configuration, with the center a lighter shade. This results from outward pressure of extravasated blood by the impact. In broad terms it may be said that the light bluish red discoloration of a bruise usually becomes noticeable after a few hours; until that time slight swelling may be all that is evi-

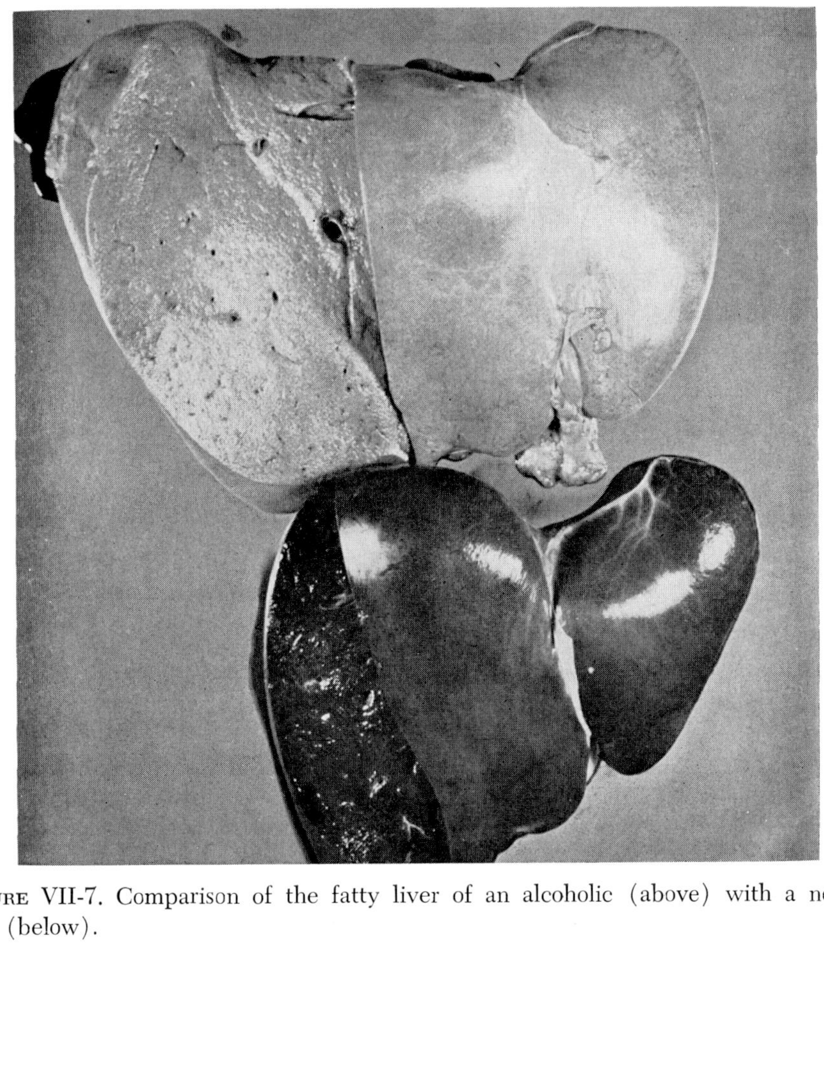

FIGURE VII-7. Comparison of the fatty liver of an alcoholic (above) with a normal liver (below).

dent externally. The change to dark purple occurs roughly within a week, at the end of which greenish yellow and later brown discoloration appear. Disappearance of a bruise may be expected within two weeks to one month. This, however, depends on numerous factors, including among others the extent of the bruise, its depth and the efficiency of the local circulation.

Microscopic examination for the aging of a bruise is considerably more reliable and should be employed whenever more accurate evaluation is desired. Hemosiderin within the macrophages may be seen as early as twenty-four hours after injury. Hematoidin is also intracellular but does not appear before several days or a week. Hematoidin is deposited as amorphous yellow granules or sheaves of crystals. Unlike hemosiderin, it does not react with potassium ferrocyanide and hydrochloric acid (Prussian blue reaction) but gives the Gmelin reaction for bile.

Numerous bruises of different ages and consequently of various colors located particularly over joints and other frequently traumatized areas of the body are often encountered in chronic alcoholics. The head is also commonly involved, and subdural hemorrhage may well be the underlying cause of death.

A frequent concomitant finding in the chronic alcoholic is atrophy of the brain. The increased subdural space that results from brain atrophy causes excessive exposure of the *bridging veins* between the dura and the arachnoid membrane on the brain surface. These vessels are the common origin of subdural bleeding. Their increased exposure renders them especially vulnerable to minimal trauma of the head. Fatal subdural bleeding may take hours to develop before intracranial pressure rises sufficiently to compress the vital centers. It is, therefore, not uncommon to find an alcoholic dead in his bed following a head injury that he sustained

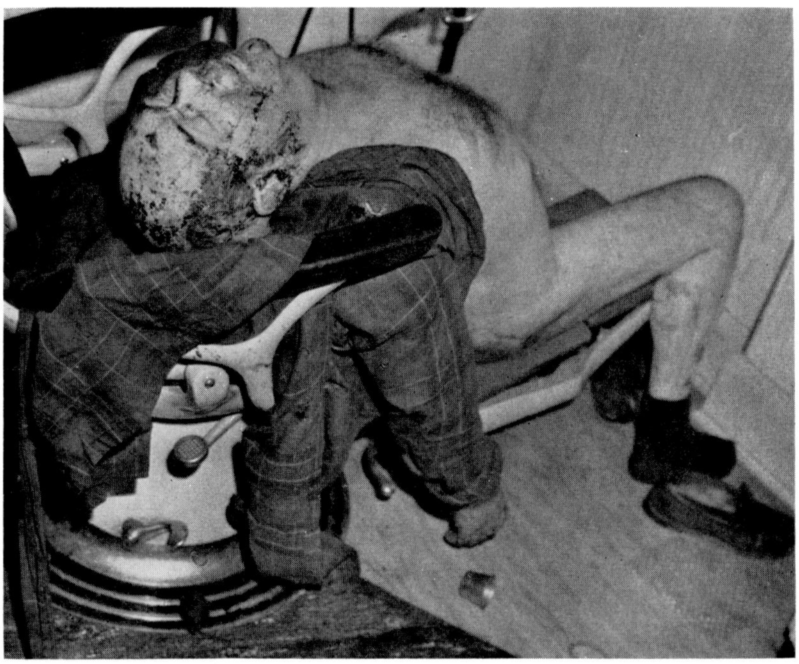

FIGURE VII-8. Middle-aged dentist, known chronic alcoholic, found as shown. He lived at the same address. Empty whiskey bottles were found in the wastepaper basket and elsewhere in the house. Blood was present in the sink, on the floor and smeared on the walls. Homicide was suspected, but the only injury was a superficial tear of the scalp, sustained when his head struck some apparatus. From this injury he bled to death. Autopsy showed advanced cirrhosis of the liver. The blood alcohol was 0.20%.

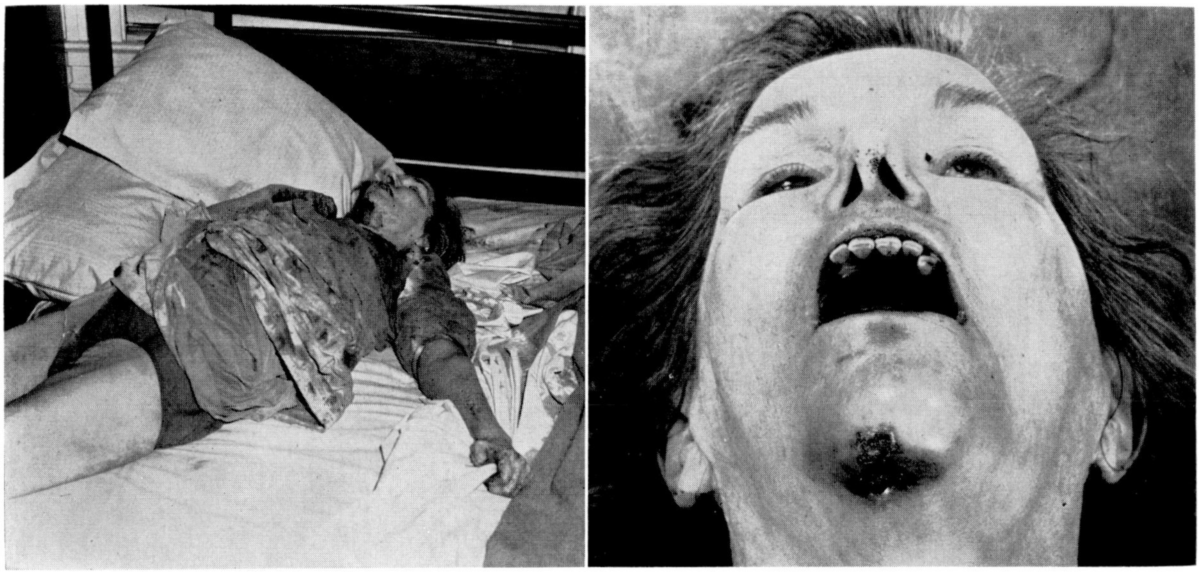

FIGURE VII-9. Elderly woman who was found dead in her apartment. Her clothes were soaked in blood, and bloodstains and smears were present throughout the room and on the walls. There was a bloody screwdriver on the windowsill. The window was slightly raised, and the lower part of the frame was likewise smeared with blood. Postmortem examination showed far-advanced nutritional changes of the liver resulting from chronic alcoholism. The only injury of the deceased was a laceration of the chin. This was initially believed to be a stab wound inflicted with the screwdriver. Postmortem examination, however, showed this injury to be a superficial tear due to a fall. The woman apparently used the screwdriver to pry open the window in search of help. Her blood alcohol was 0.32%.

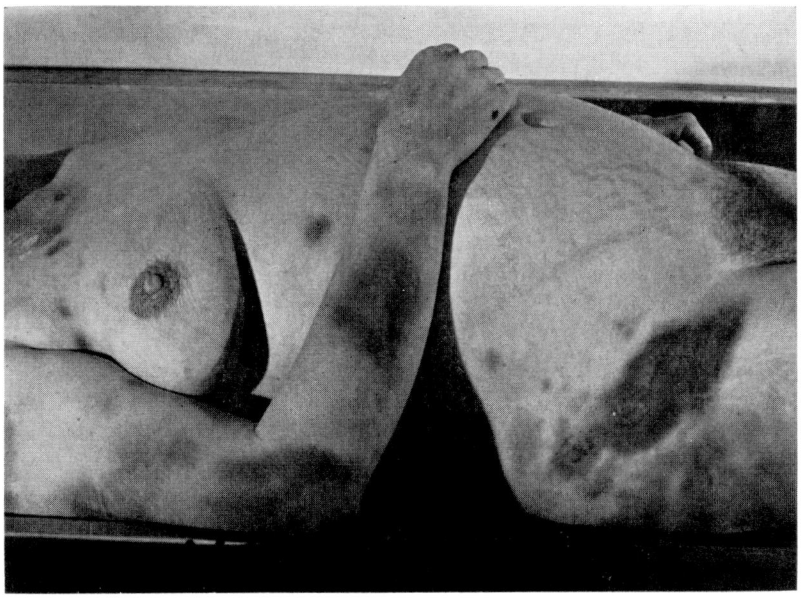

FIGURE VII-10. Chronic alcoholic with cirrhosis of liver showing numerous bruises of various ages over the entire body. Death was due to subdural hemorrhage.

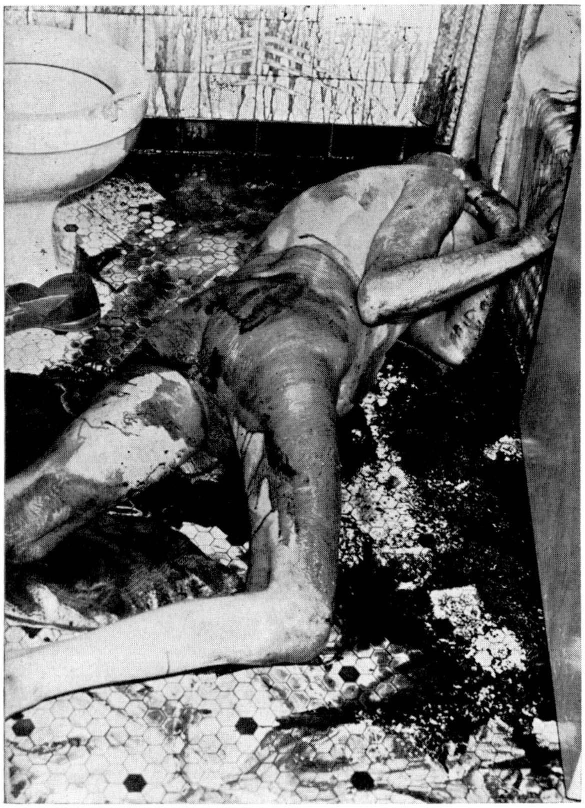

FIGURE VII-11. This seventy-one-year-old man with history of hypertension and arteriosclerotic heart disease fell, striking his head on the bathtub. He sustained a superficial ¼ in. laceration above the eyebrow and a ½ in. laceration at the outer angle of the eye. No other injuries. A heart attack apparently caused the fall, and the subsequent confusion and excitement explain the findings at the scene. Note the extensive blood loss. No blood alcohol.

the preceding day. Such a death may appear to be due to natural causes if no autopsy is performed.

At autopsy many chronic alcoholics are found to have fatty alteration of the liver and/or cirrhosis, either of which may be associated with faulty blood clotting (Fig. VII-7). This in turn leads to easy bruising and extensive hemorrhage from minor trauma. Pools of blood, blood-soaked clothes and walls smeared with blood frequently suggest murder; yet without doubt, the explanation of these scenes is the terminal confusion of the alcoholic victim (Figs. VII-8 and VII-9).

The widespread injuries of the chronic alcoholic also frequently result in the mistaken assumption of a homicide, although the different ages of the bruises are indicative of long-standing repetitive trauma (Fig. VII-10). Certain diseases of the blood are associated with defective clotting, so that a small injury causes profuse bleeding even to the extent of exsanguination.

One relatively common injury notorious for extensive bleeding in the absence of underlying disease is a tear of the eyebrow such as that frequently sustained by boxers. The origin of such bleeding is from small arteries that are crushed on the bony ridge above the eye socket. Commonly, medical attention is required to halt such bleeding, and many boxing matches have been stopped for just this reason. It should be mentioned in this regard that superficial face and scalp wounds generally tend to bleed more profusely than similar injuries elsewhere (Fig. VII-11).

Elderly people often get superficial hemorrhages in the skin following trivial injury, especially on the forearms, due to a particular age-linked fragility of the small blood vessels. While technically these are contusions, for practical purposes they may be considered spontaneous bleedings.

## ABRASION

An abrasion is due to scraping of the skin with removal of its superficial layers. Small flaps of the uppermost layer of the skin may remain attached to the end of the abraded area, indicating the direction in which the scraping occurred (Fig. VII-12). Drying of the area causes the initial pale yellow-brown color to change to dark brown, even black. Abrasions may thus be overlooked on first inspection of a body recovered from water until drying of the skin renders the injury noticeable.

Depending on the mechanism of the abrasion, it may be called a *graze,* such as when a bullet sideswipes the body, a *scratch* when caused by a sharp edge or fingernails, or a *brush burn* if caused by the frictional force of rubbing against a surface, as in dragging over the ground (Fig. VII-13).

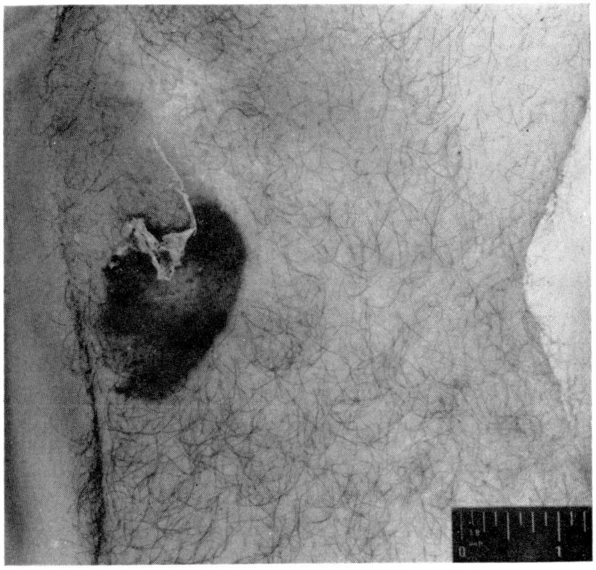

FIGURE VII-12. Scrape of the knee. The underlying tissues have become dark brown after drying. Flaps of epidermis are attached to the terminal end of the wound, indicating the direction in which the scraping occurred.

A scratch, especially when dry and dark brown, may resemble a burn. A linear scratch may simulate an injury caused by the edge of a hot knife blade. Microscopic examination is sometimes required to establish the true nature of the injury.

Rope burns are caused by friction of the rope against the skin. While considerable heat may be generated as a result of such friction, causing a second degree burn to develop, it is more likely that the friction will cause blisters by expressing tissue fluids into the upper layers of the skin. A rope burn would thus be another variety of abrasion (Fig. VII-14).

Ordinary abrasions are also caused by handcuffs, binding and tying. In all such cases it is important to incise the skin directly under the restraints in search of hemorrhage. Where wrists or ankles have been restrained, incision should

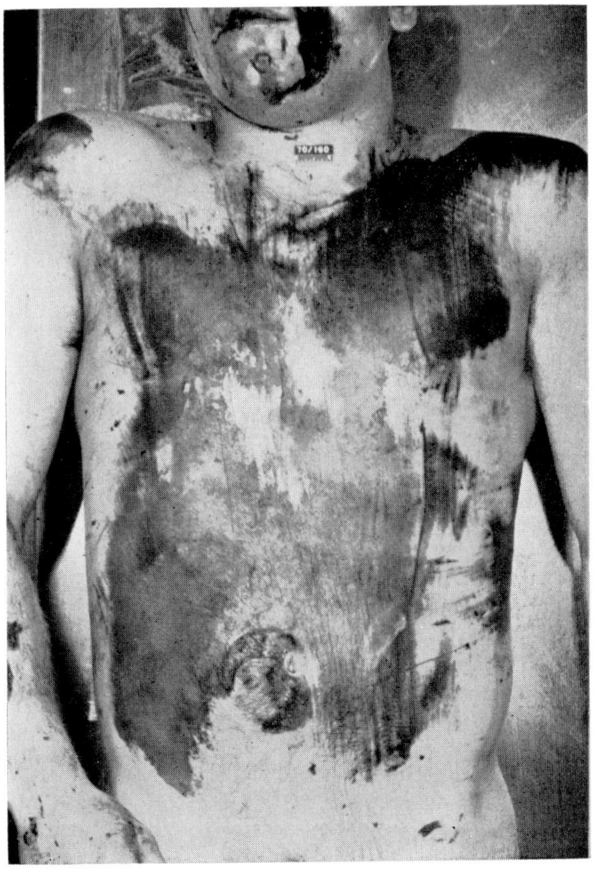

FIGURE VII-13. Driver of an automobile, involved in a collision, who was thrown out of his car and received brush burn injuries by scraping along the road surface.

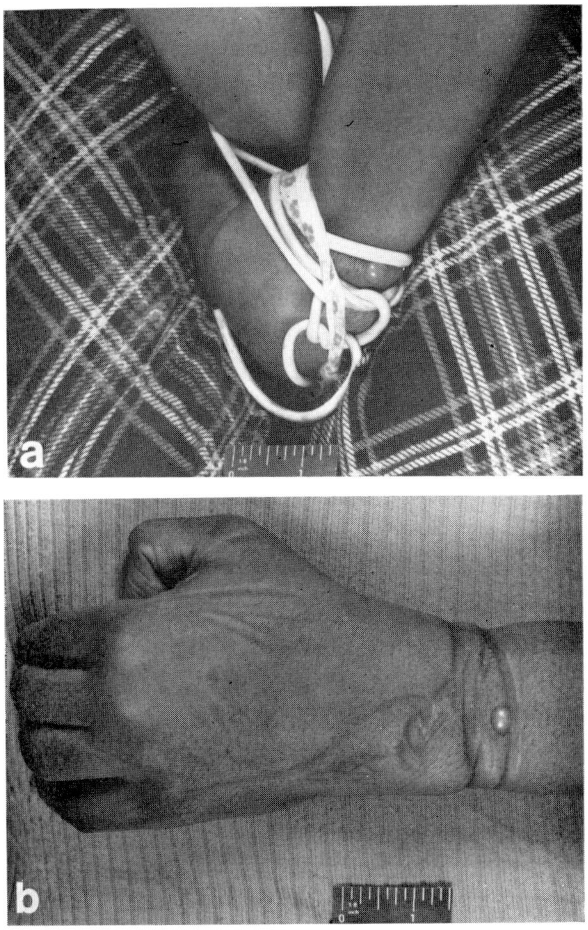



FIGURE VII-14. (a): Individual tied with clothesline. (b): Rope burns with blister formation.

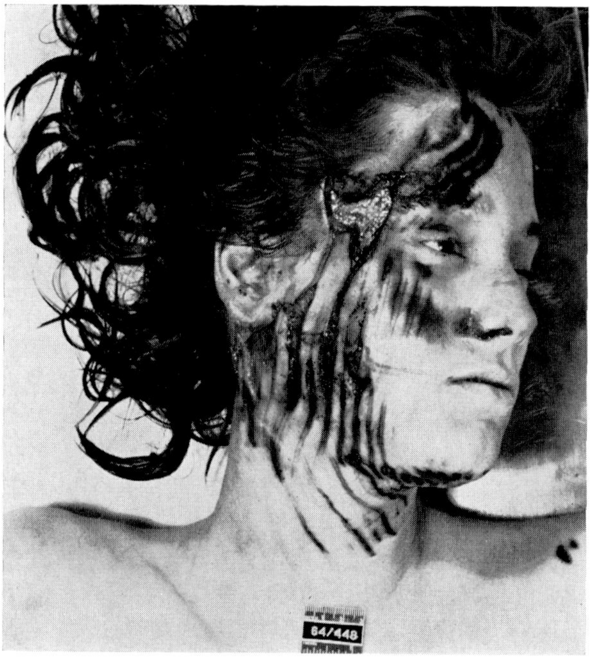

FIGURE VII-15. Fourteen-year-old spectator at a stadium stampeded to death when the moving stairway on which she was standing came to a sudden halt and she was thrown to the ground. The face and neck show the imprint of the escalator tread.

be made over the bony prominences rather than on the front or back surfaces. The presence of hemorrhage indicates that the victim was alive when tied. Conversely, the absence of hemorrhage does not imply that the individual was dead when bound. Certain types of ligatures are more apt to cause hemorrhage than others. A clothesline or electric wire is more likely to bruise the tissue than wide tape or a towel.

It is frequently difficult to distinguish between an abrasion sustained during life and one that occurred after death. Bleeding does not usually occur, due to the superficial nature of an abrasion, unless the scraping action responsible for the injury is associated with a direct, forceful impact in the same area. Brush burns, for instance, sustained by scraping along a road surface and extending over vast areas of the body, usually show no trace of underlying bleeding. If there is hemorrhage in the adjacent tissues, the injury was sustained during life. Confusion may arise, however, if the injury is located in a dependent area of the body in

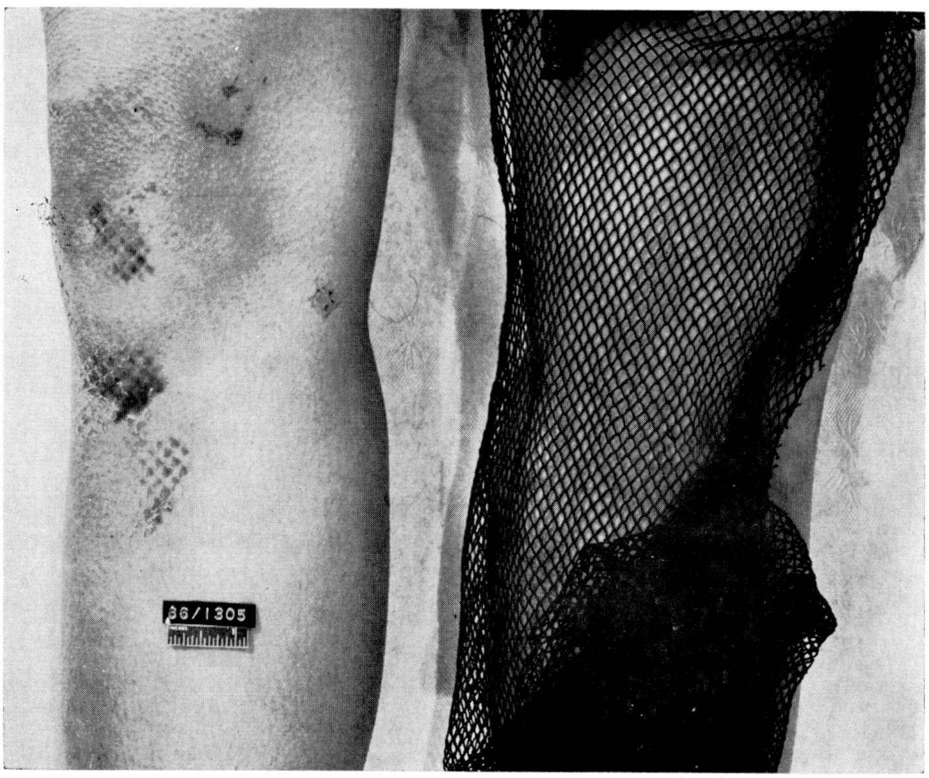

FIGURE VII-16. This young woman was a pedestrian who was struck by an automobile and survived three days in a hospital. At autopsy it was first thought that she had been run over by a motorcycle because of the peculiarly patterned abrasions on her knee and leg. Investigation revealed that the pattern was due to the imprint of her stocking.

which postmortem lividity will develop. Under such circumstances blood loss is likely to occur from vessels torn after death. It may be difficult to distinguish this type of *bleeding* from genuine antemortem injury.

Healing begins within several hours, and the reaction of the body generally permits a rough appraisal of the age of the lesion. A fresh abrasion usually oozes tissue fluid for a day or two before it is gradually covered by a crust or scab under which the healing proceeds until complete. Individual red blood cells may be entrapped within the scab. The duration of the healing process depends on the extent of the injury, secondary infection and repeated trauma to the same area.

Abrasions are often characteristically patterned, thereby providing information regarding the nature of the force. A fall to the ground or

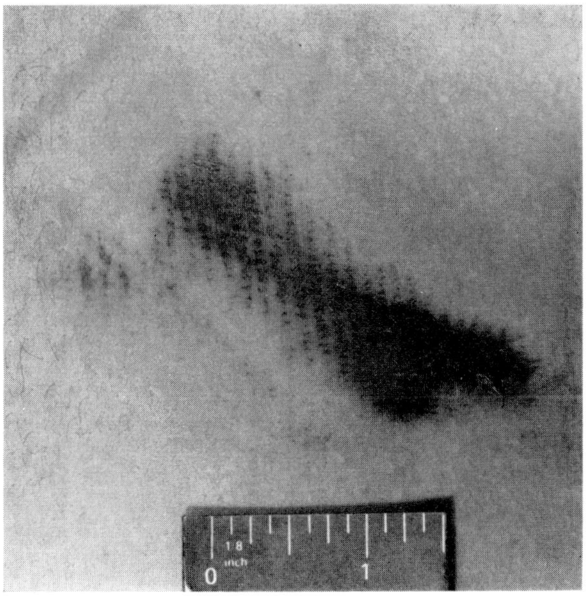

FIGURE XII-17. Abrasion showing the weave of the victim's clothing.

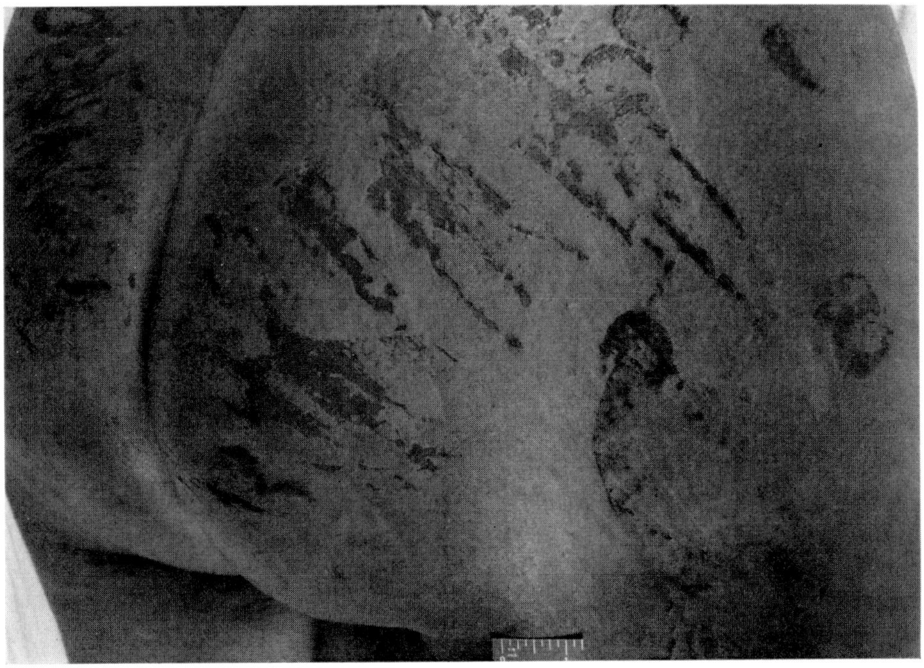

FIGURE VII-18. Sadomasochistic murder. Parallel and circular abrasions, produced with the handle and the head of a hammer, respectively. Death was caused by several impacts to the head.

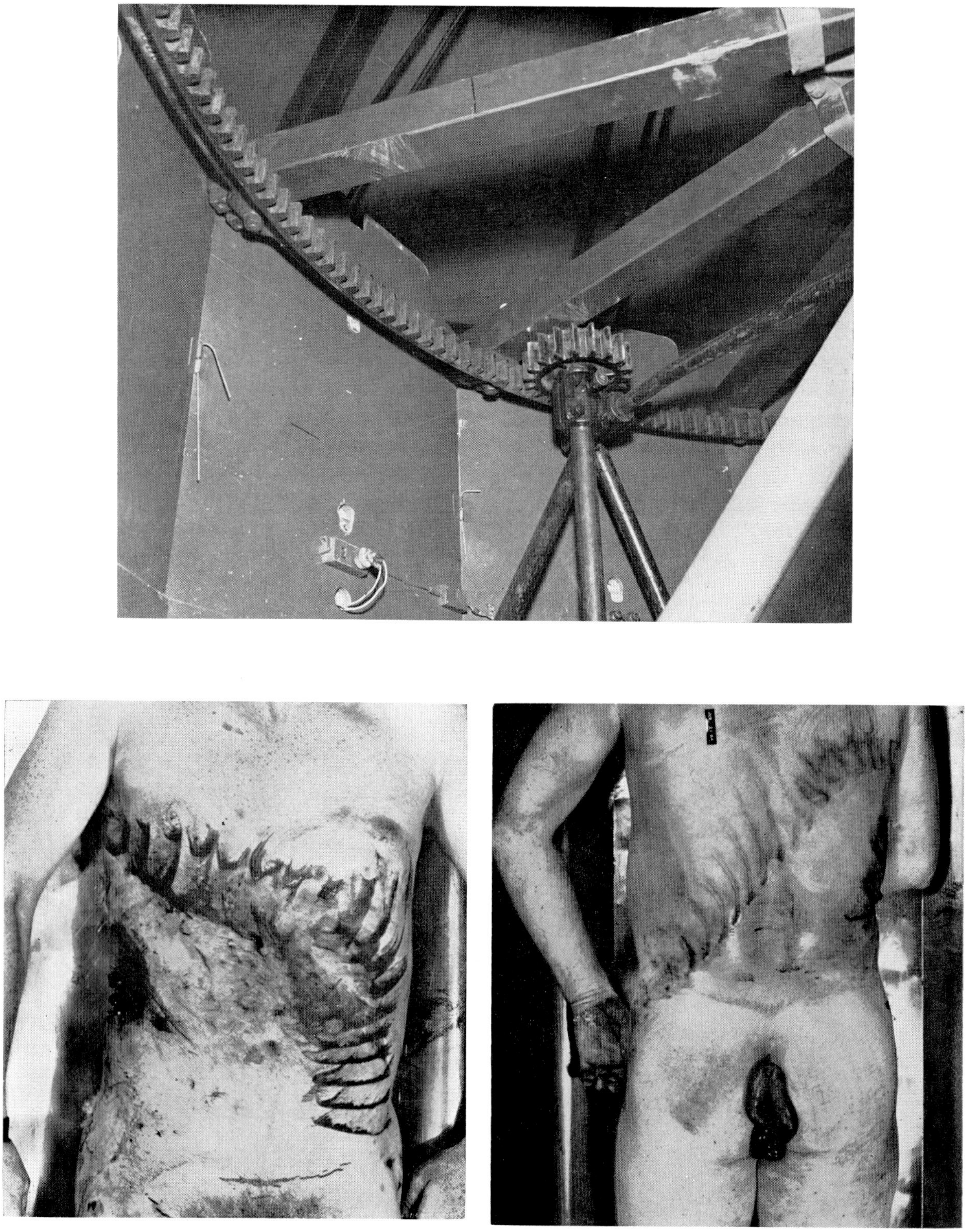

FIGURE VII-19. (a): Gears of a merry-go-round. The clothes of operator were caught in the gears, pulling him in. (b): Imprint of the gears on the skin. Just above the pubic hair and in the right groin are superficial tears of the skin, which are due to overstretching. (c): Rear view of the individual shown in Figure VII-19b. Bowel prolapse due to the immense pressure on the abdomen.

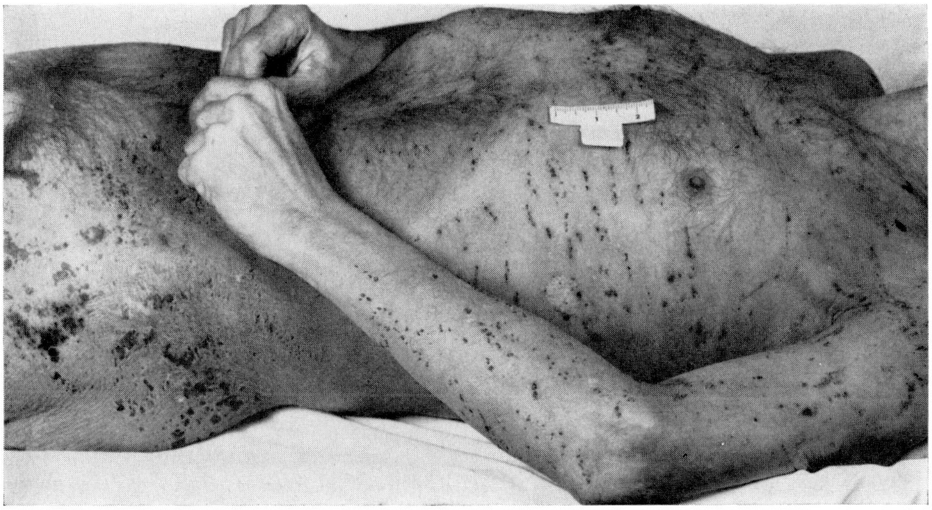

FIGURE VII-20. The body of this fifty-six-year-old flea-infested derelict shows scattered abrasions, the pattern of which indicates they were produced by scratching. The abrasions on the chest area are horizontal, along the ribs; on the arms they are vertical; and on the hips the scratching motion was circular.

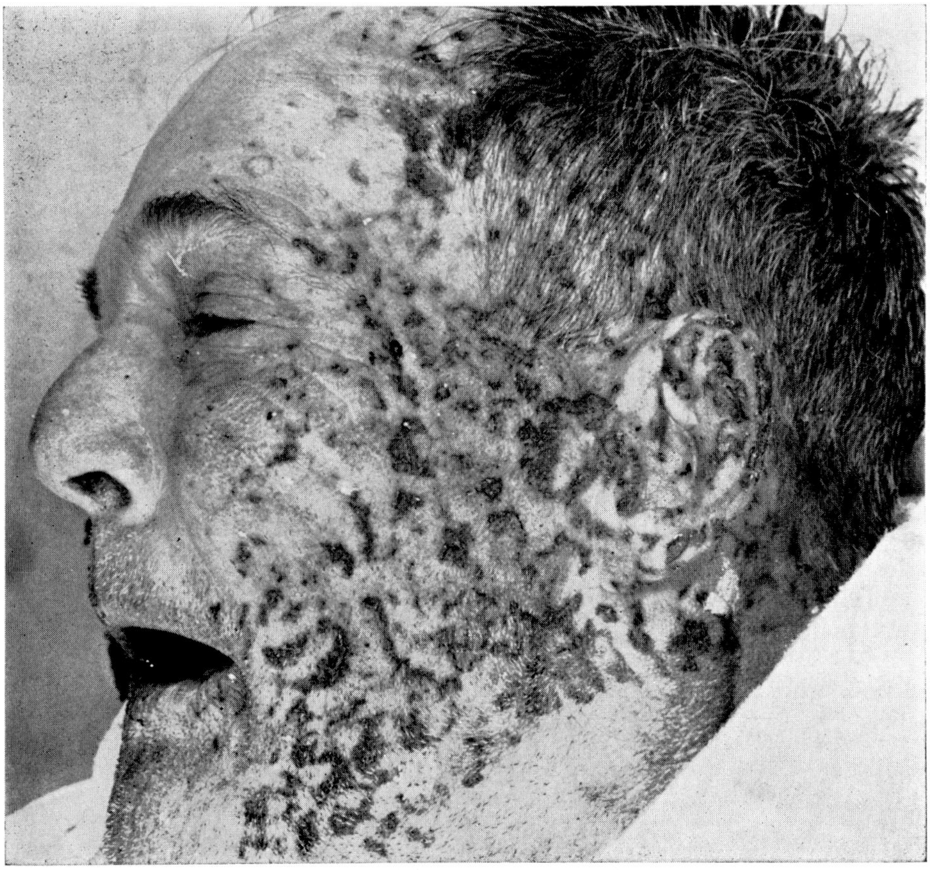

FIGURE VII-21. Patterned abrasions from falling on gravel.

a hard blow to the body with a flat object may cause an abrasion patterned after the weave of the clothing. This is especially true with coarse material. An impact with a textured object, such as a rough board or a threaded pipe, may also cause a patterned injury (Figs. VII-15 to VII-20).

An elderly man was found lying on a sidewalk. He was taken to a hospital and pronounced dead on arrival. At autopsy the cause of death was determined as an acute myocardial infarction. The cause of certain injuries on the left side of the face, however, was not resolved. On-the-scene investigation showed the pattern compatible with striking gravel at the time of collapse (Fig. VII-21).

## LACERATION

A laceration is a tear produced by blunt trauma. The force and its direction determine the appearance, depth and associated injuries, such as fractures. Undermining of the edges of a laceration indicates the direction in which the impact occurred. Equal undermining on all sides of a laceration is evidence of a perpendicular impact.

Two types of lacerations are most common: (a) those due to a perpendicular blow with a relatively broad object, such as a hammer or a bottle, or as is frequently sustained when

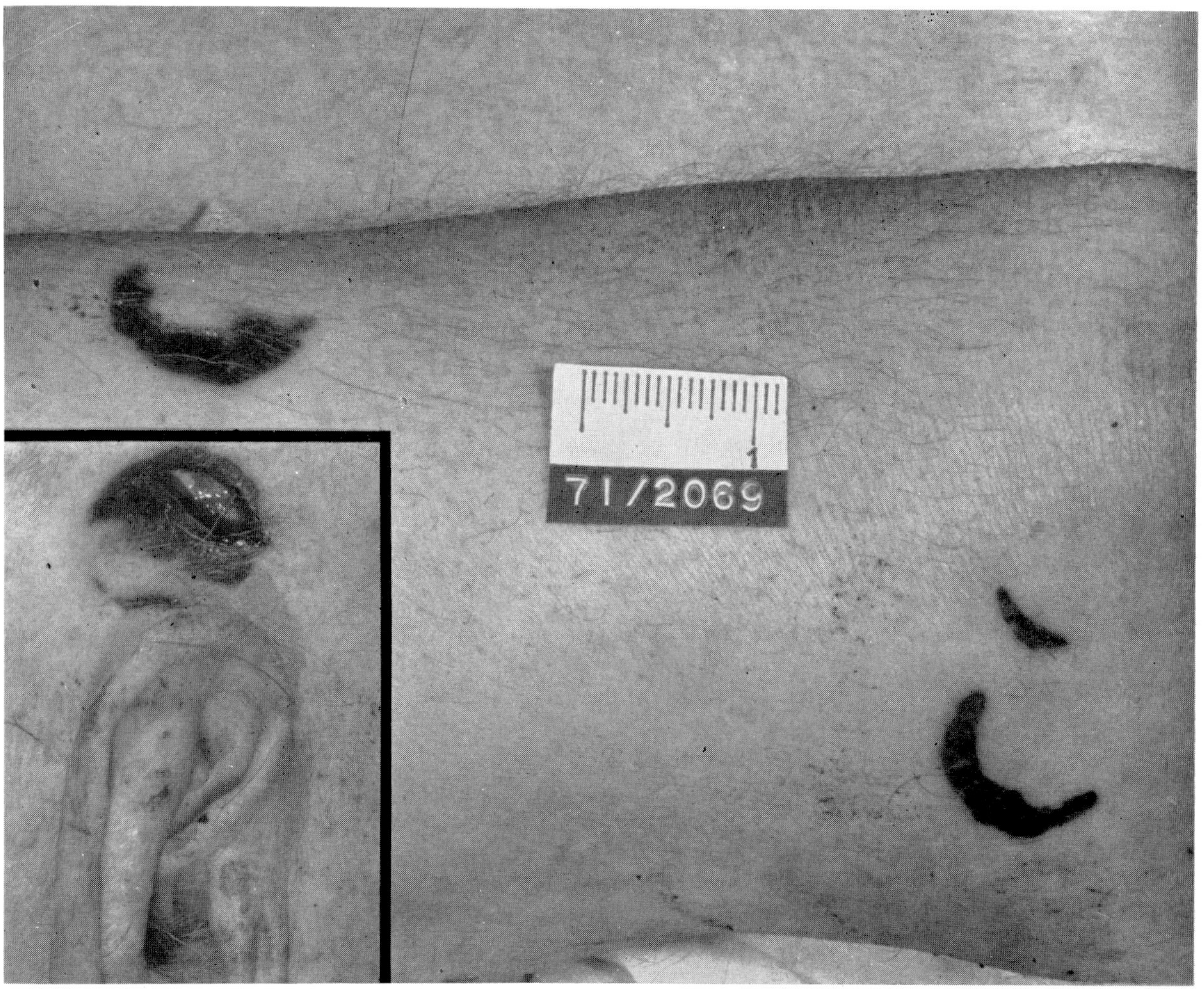


FIGURE VII-22. Crescent-shaped injuries on a leg produced by the flat end of a hammer. Insert: same individual, showing circular injury above right ear.

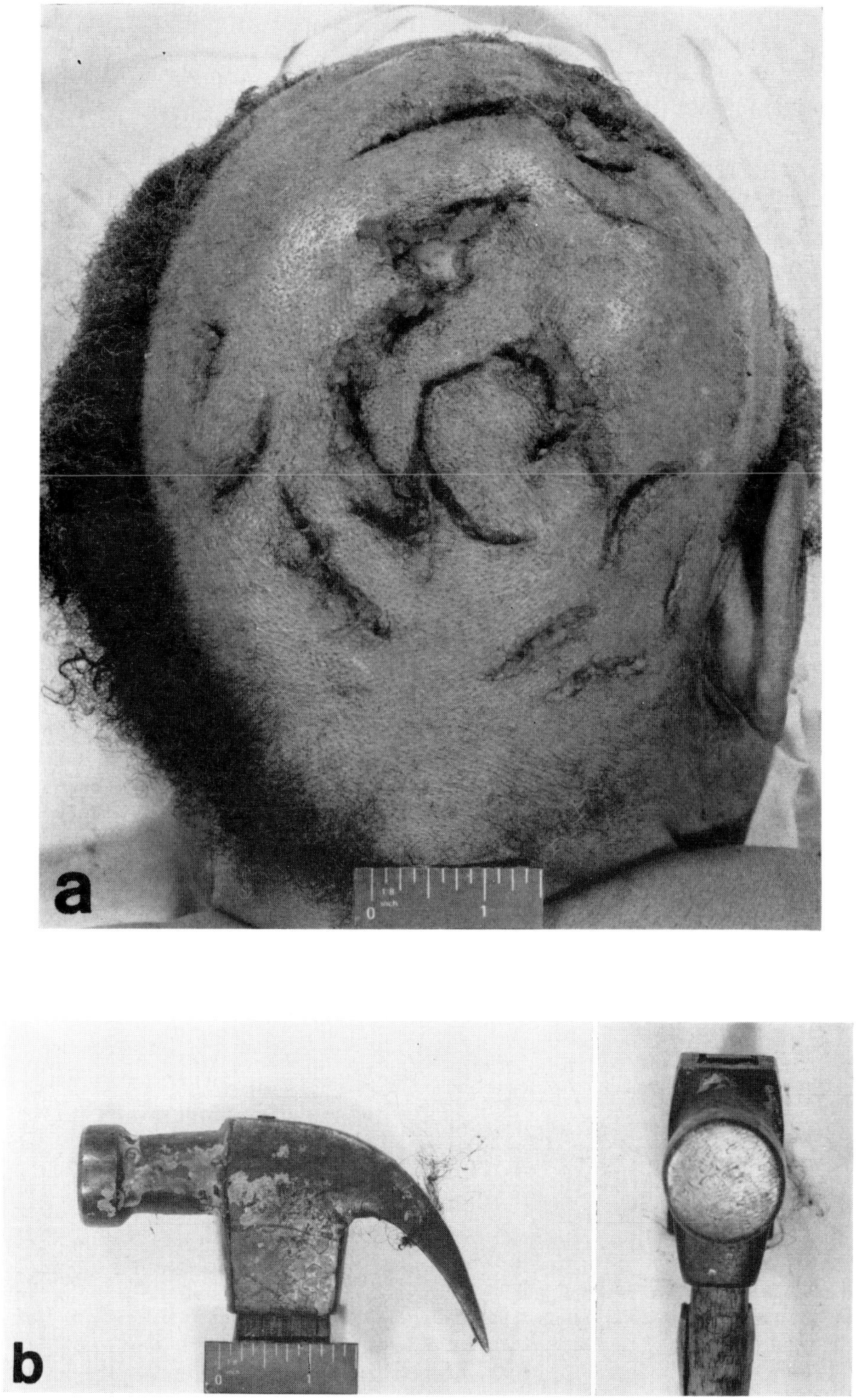

FIGURE VII-23. (a): Semicircular tears of the scalp due to beating with the round end of a claw hammer. (b): The hair on the hammer is from the victim. Completion of the circular pattern of the scalp wounds accurately reflects the diameter of the round end of the hammer.

falling to the ground (Figs. VII-22 to VII-29); (b) those due to a glancing blow, which if superficial may tear only the skin, or if deeper may separate the skin and subcutaneous tissues from the underlying muscle fascia and create a gaping and profusely bleeding wound (Fig. VII-30).

The edges of a laceration, particularly one over a bony area such as the skull, are characteristically undermined due to the crushing and tearing force of the impact. Between the opposing sides run multiple delicate threads of tissue *(tissue bridges)* consisting of nerve, elastic and connective tissue fibers and blood vessels. The wound edges are commonly abraded, and the abraded area corresponds to that of the impacting surface. Whereas injuries on the face caused by blows may involve any area, those sustained by falling are generally located on the protuberant parts, i.e. over the bony prominences. Thus, in a fall, the eye and eyelids are mostly spared, while the skin over the outer and upper rims of the eye socket is commonly abraded or torn, depending on the severity of the impact. The skin over the cheekbones and the lower jaw is also commonly injured in a fall. A fall from an upright position usually results in extensive tears.

In the case of a fall on the back of the head, the abraded scalp surface will be circular and will completely circumscribe the laceration. By contrast, a blow with a blunt, narrow object, such as the edge of an angle iron or a crowbar, will probably produce a linear tear whose finely abraded edges may be difficult to perceive and which shows insignificant undermining (Figs. VII-31, VII-32 and VII-33).

Foreign bodies, such as fragments of glass, chips of paint or gravel, are sometimes found in a laceration. Particularly when there is doubt regarding the cause of a tear, a search for foreign material in the depth of the wound may give the answer.

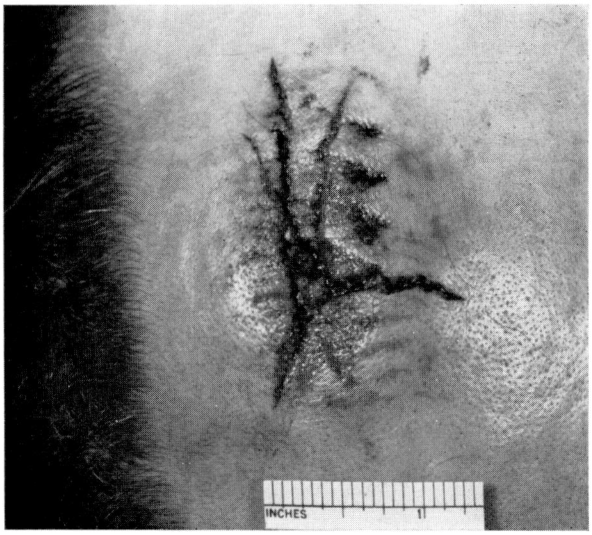

FIGURE VII-25. Middle-aged man involved in a domestic quarrel during which he was struck on the head with a Chianti bottle. The patterned abrasions surrounding the laceration corresponded with the thatch of the bottle basket.

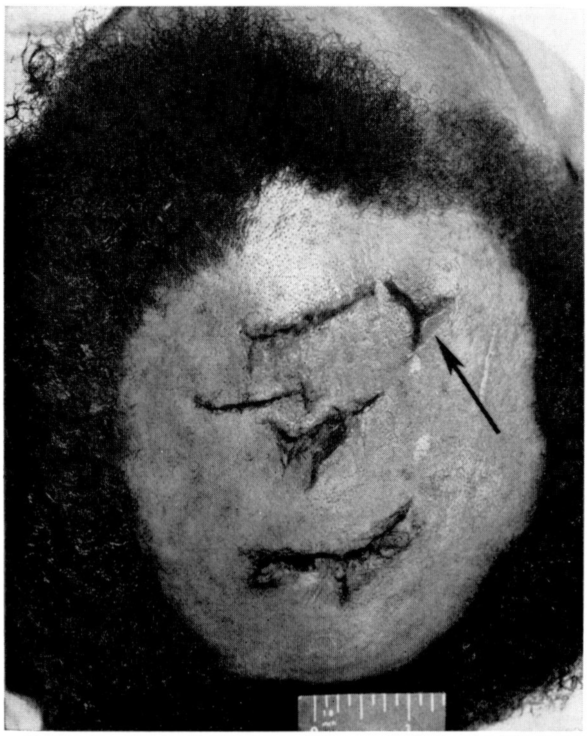
FIGURE VII-24. Multiple irregular and ragged lacerations of the scalp caused by pistol-whipping. The triangular-shaped wound (arrow) was caused by a pointed corner of the weapon, which produced the center of the wound; the three tears radiating from this center were caused by splitting of the skin. The four parallel horizontal injuries were probably produced by the blunt edge of the pistol butt. Death was due to a close-range shot of the head.

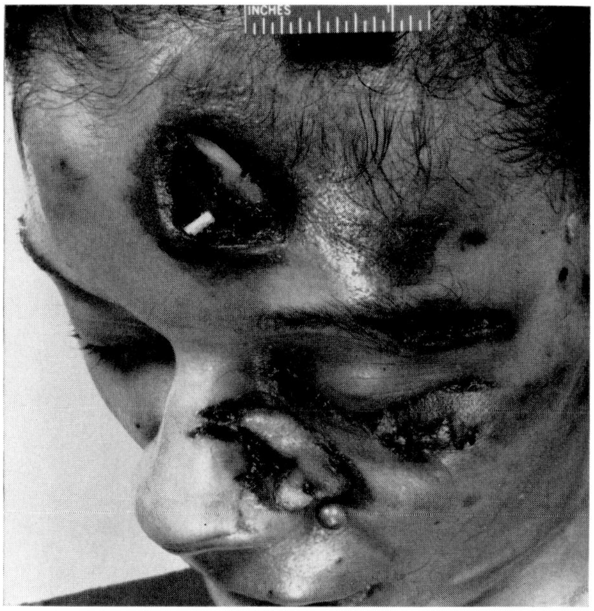


Figure VII-26. Middle-aged woman who was found in the basement of an abandoned house. She had been raped and beaten. A lamp and a broken bottle caused her injuries. The tear on her forehead is propped open to show undermining. The margins of the wound are abraded and the edges ragged. This wound was probably made with the heavy lamp base. The cut on the left side of the nose was produced by the jagged ends of the broken bottle; it shows no marginal abrasion, no undermining and smooth edges. The tear in the left eyebrow, the abrasion immediately above it and the abrasion and tear below the eye were sustained when she fell. (Compare the latter injury with Figs. VII-27 and VII-30.)

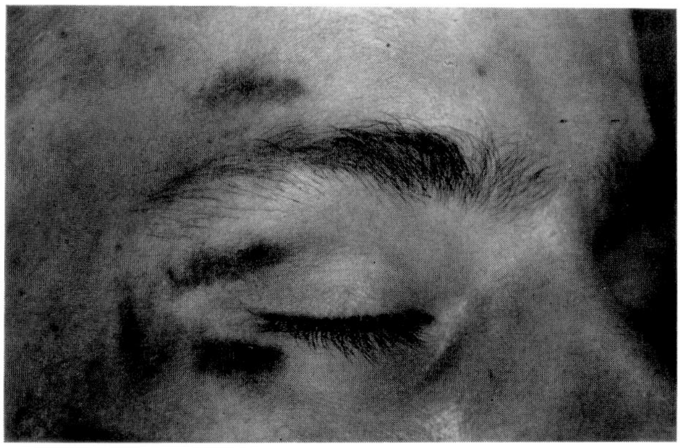

Figure VII-27. Injury sustained in a fall: superficial abrasion above the right eyebrow outlines the rim of the eye socket.

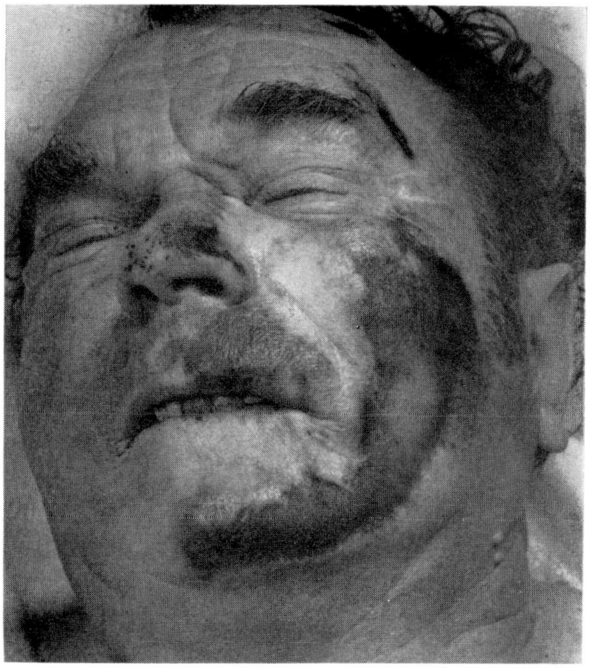

Figure VII-28. Fall on the left side of the face onto a concrete surface. The protruberant parts in the areas of impact, i.e. the chin, the entire left side of the lower jaw, the left cheek and the left side of the nose and lip, are abraded. Two smaller scraped areas are also seen on the left side of the forehead. The pale area within the abrasion on the cheek is due to the abundance of soft tissues in that location and lack of underlying bone.

However severe a blunt impact may be, external evidence of injury is frequently minimal or absent, even in the presence of massive internal injuries. A sudden sharp turn of a bicycle's handlebars to avoid a crash is frequently associated with a blow to the abdomen by the handlebar. This may tear the liver or the spleen and cause massive internal bleeding. A kick or a punch in the upper abdomen may injure the pancreas[1] and cause death within a few days from the resultant inflammation. Similar force may rupture a loop of bowel and cause death from peritonitis. Injury to the abdominal wall is seldom visible in any of these examples. The lack of external evidence of trauma in the case of injury to the pancreas may make a causal relationship between the blow and the death

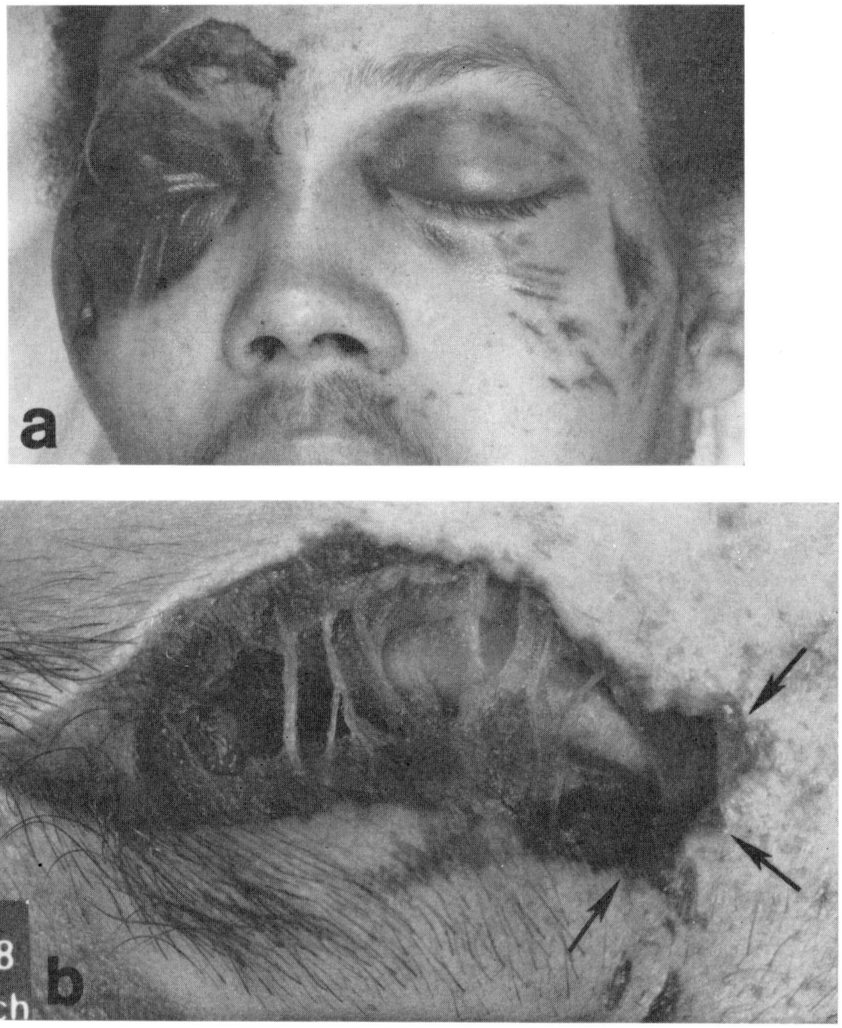


FIGURE VII-29. (a): Multiple injuries of various shapes and severity; some suggest a pattern, others are irregular and nondescript. The black eye was caused by blood that seeped under the skin to the eyelids. (b): The tear above the eyebrow (magnified) was caused by a blow above and to the right of the bridge of the nose, at which place the wound edges are typically abraded (arrows). From this area of impact, the skin split with jagged, nonabraded edges connected by fine strands of tissue.

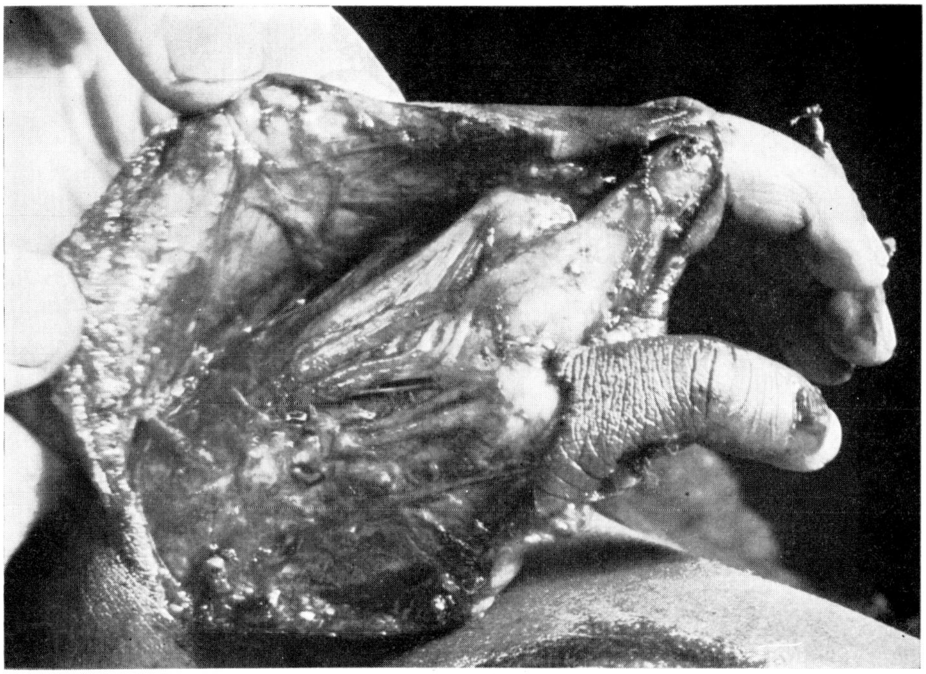

FIGURE VII-30. Tangential blow of the hand sustained by a pedestrian who was struck by an automobile. Note the vast tear and separation of the skin and underlying fat tissue from the tendons.

difficult to prove, particularly in the absence of witnesses and since pancreatitis is well known to occur spontaneously, especially in chronic alcoholics. Tears of the liver caused by flat impact to the right upper part of the abdomen are commonly located close to the ligaments of the liver, because fixation of any part of an organ makes the site more vulnerable to blunt trauma.

Tangential or glancing blunt force to the right upper quadrant of the abdomen sometimes separates the liver capsule from the underlying liver tissue. Bleeding beneath the capsule, so-called subcapsular hemorrhage, occurs and, if profuse, may rupture into the abdominal cavity. Subcapsular liver hemorrhage in newborns was relatively common before improved obstetrical care appreciably reduced its occurrence. The mechanism of this injury is believed to be the compressive and shearing forces exerted on the newborn's abdomen during passage through the birth canal. Death resulted in some cases two

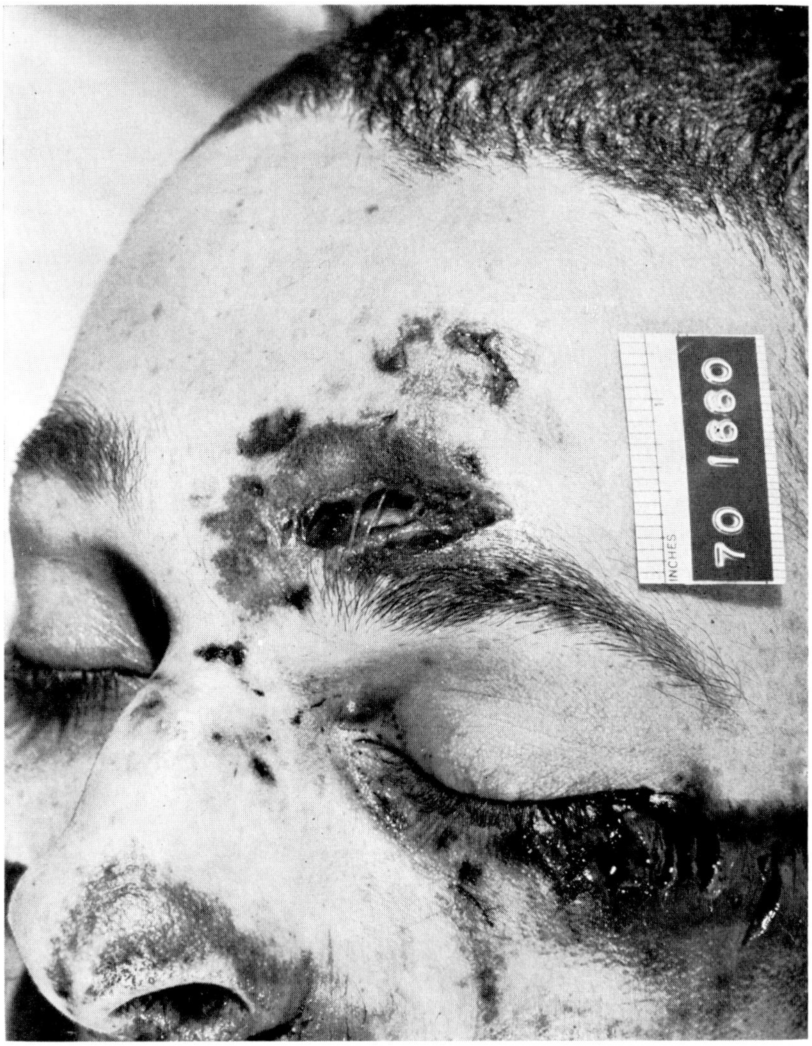


FIGURE VII-31. Young man shot in the back of the head while fleeing after he attempted a liquor store holdup. He fell on the pavement. The injuries shown were sustained in the fall and involved the facial prominences. Note the delicate tissue bridges, the undermining and the marginal abrasion of the laceration above the eyebrow. The protected orbital contents are not damaged.

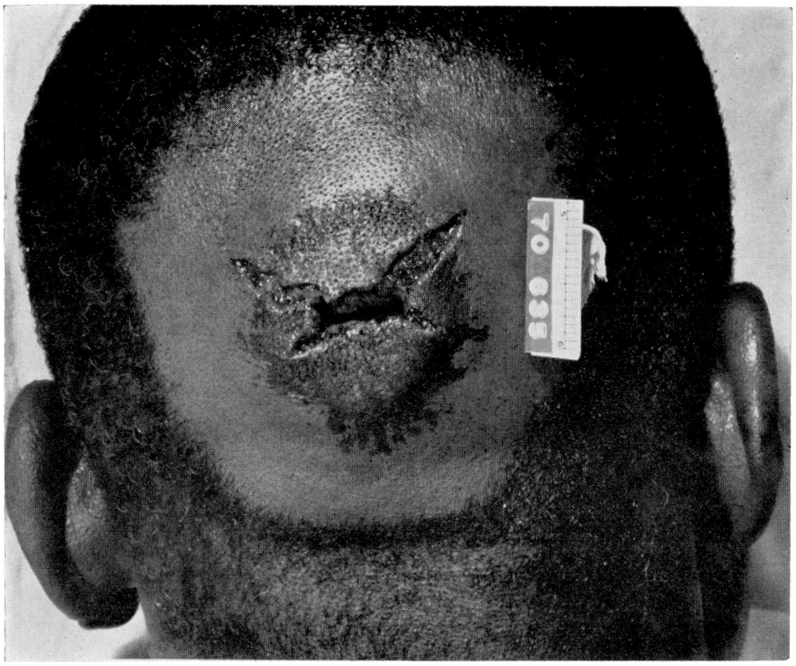

FIGURE VII-32. Star-shaped tear of the scalp due to a fall on the pavement while intoxicated. The tear is surrounded by a circular abrasion. Separation of the edges of the wound disclosed multiple soft tissue bridges and extensive undermining.

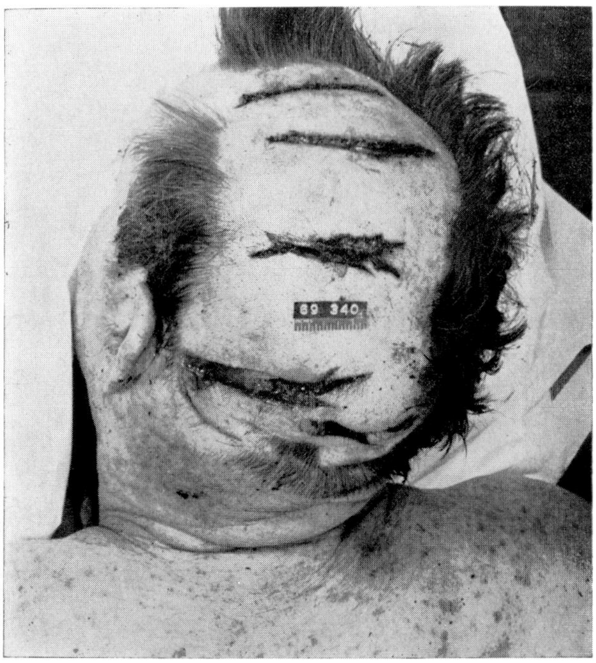


FIGURE VII-33. Night watchman struck with a crowbar during a robbery. Note the linear shape of the injuries and the V-shaped extension from each end. These tears result from bursting of the skin due to pressure between the implement and the underlying bone. The injuries show fine marginal abrasions.

or three days after delivery due to massive intra-abdominal bleeding. Potter[2] describes a similar injury in newborns if the upper abdomen is grasped too firmly during delivery and Stahl, of the Armed Forces Institute of Pathology, relates having seen several battered child cases with laceration of the liver believed to be due to the same mechanism. Tearing of the liver in an infant is sometimes associated with dislocation or other whiplash-type injuries of the upper cervical spine. This, in our estimation, is caused by violent shaking of the child while it is being firmly grasped around its middle.

Blunt trauma can be fatal with neither external nor internal evidence of injury. Thus, a sudden forceful impact to the chest in the area of the heart may cause instantaneous cardiac arrest *without* demonstrable damage to the chest wall or an internal organ. Arrhythmia of the heartbeat is believed to be the mechanism of this phenomenon. In the same fashion a heart that has stopped beating may be reactivated by sharp blows to the chest, as is sometimes practiced in external cardiac massage.

## SKELETAL INJURIES

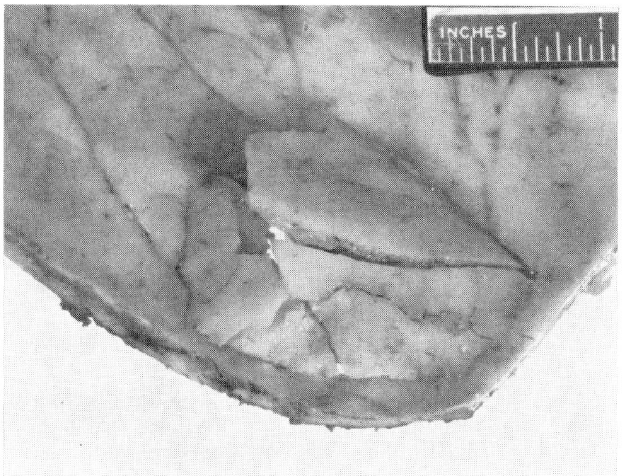


FIGURE VII-34. Internal view of a depressed skull fracture caused by a fall on a sharp corner of a piece of furniture. Note the inward displacement of the bone fragments.

Just as certain external and internal bodily injuries often permit conclusions regarding the type of violence involved, similar information may frequently be derived from the appearance of skeletal injuries. The skull is especially helpful in this regard. Although fractures are normally avoided by the shape of the skull, its bony elasticity and its construction in a number of elastic arches, when fractures do occur, the fracture lines usually conform to certain characteristic patterns. For example, a fall on a sharp corner of a piece of furniture, a blow by a hammer or impact with the pointed edge of a rock will probably cause a depressed fracture in which the bone fragments are pushed inward. Rarely only the inner bony layer beneath the

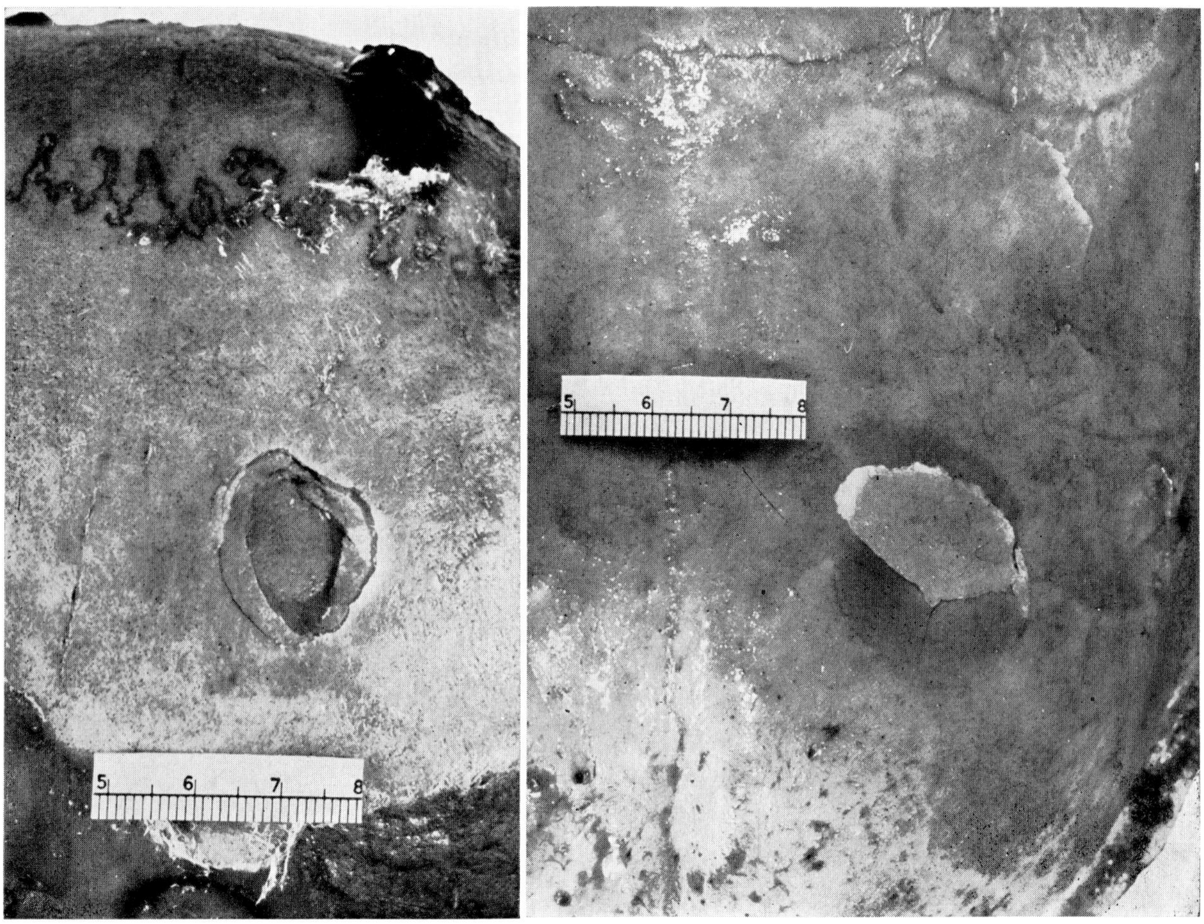


FIGURE VII-35. External view (left) and internal view (right) of an experimentally produced depressed fracture of the skull using a ball peen hammer.

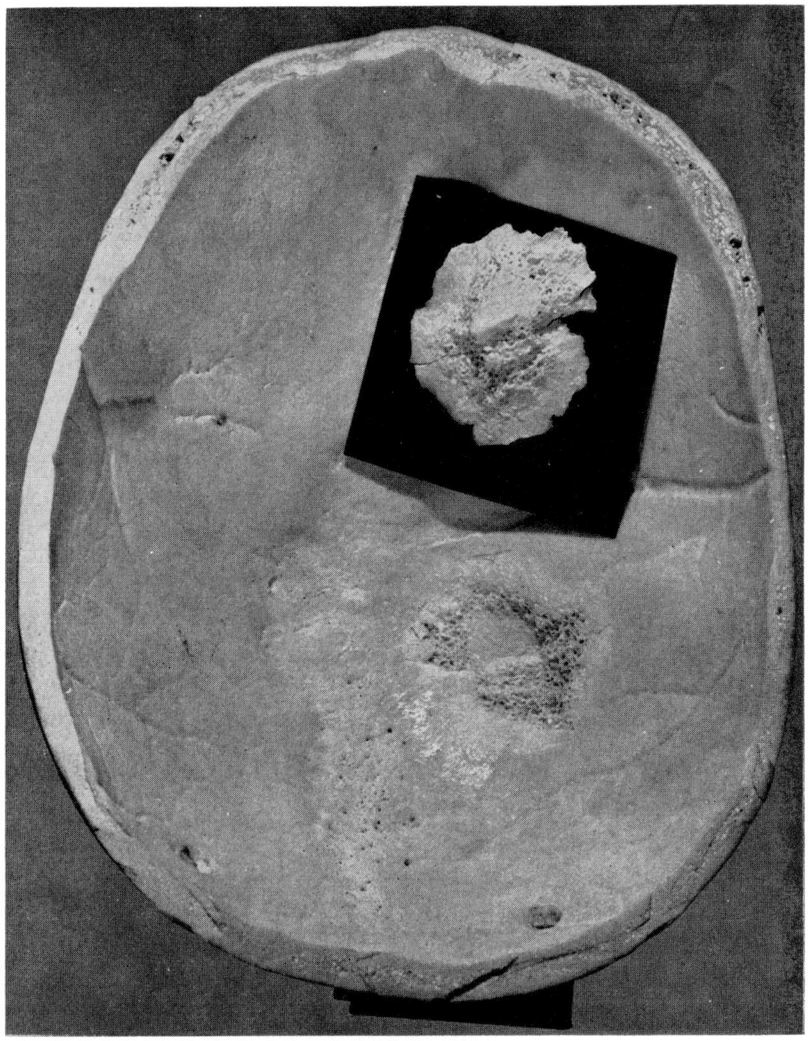

FIGURE VII-36. Experimental fracture of the skull produced by a blow with the flat end of a small hammer. The outer table of the bone is intact, while a *plug* is broken out of the inner surface.

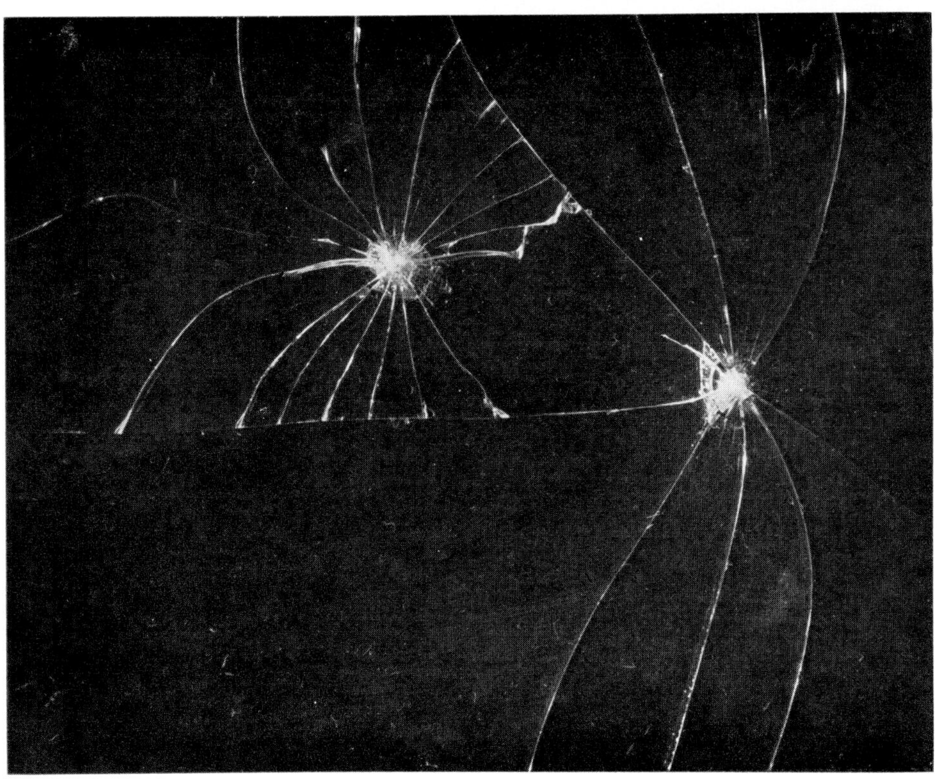

FIGURE VII-37. Piece of glass showing two impact sites with radiating cracks. The pattern of the cracks indicates that the blow on the right was made first, because the cracks radiating from the blow on the left are arrested by those already present.

site of impact may fracture, leaving the outer table intact (Figs. VII-34, VII-35 and VII-36). Commonly the fracture site resembles the radial pattern of a spider web. In the case where the outer table is left intact, the mechanism is thought to be in the manner of transmission of the force. (This mechanism can be compared to the breaking of a plaster ceiling when the floor above is hit with the end of a broomstick.)

By contrast, a fall on a flat surface resulting in a fractured skull shows one or several fracture lines radiating from the point of impact, but depression of bone fragments is practically never seen. The scalp indicates the site of impact by an extensive hematoma, and hemorrhage may sometimes be noted in the underlying spongy layer of the bone. In the case of a blow and subsequent fall, the fracture lines resulting from

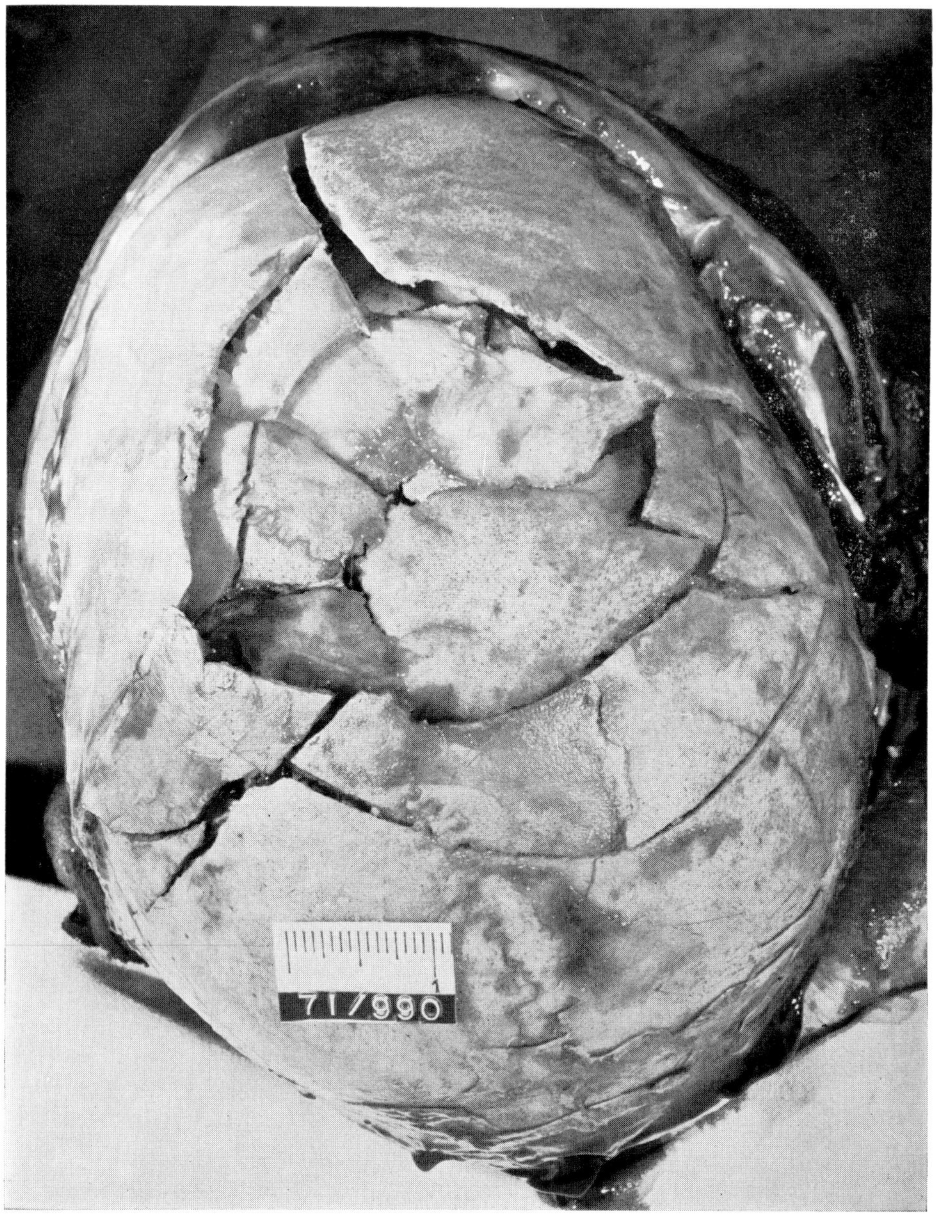


FIGURE VII-38a. Forty-three-year-old construction worker who was struck on the head by a falling brick. The top of the skull was extensively fractured. Note the depressed center of the fracture (site of actual impact) and the concentric ripples.

the fall are arrested by those produced by the blow. The same holds true of two blows, and it may be possible to determine which of the two was inflicted first. Cracks in a window serve to illustrate this sequence (Fig. VII-37). In general it may be said that an injury to the head sustained as a result of a fall is more commonly located in the level of the *brim of the hat*, while an injury resulting from a blow is mostly situated above this level. Rarely, particularly in cases of beating, the fracture fragments are many, with marked displacement, so that evaluation and interpretation of the injuries is impossible without prior replacement of the broken pieces. This is best done by drilling small holes in adjacent pieces of bones and wiring them together in an attempt to *reconstruct* the skull (*see* Chapter XXIV).

The changes in the skull will complement the finding of contusions in the brain (as described in Chapter XVII) and will greatly facilitate the interpretation of the injuries when evaluated jointly. A fall on the back of the head or a blow to the top of the head frequently causes independent fractures of the roofs of the orbits, particularly in elderly individuals. These fractures may be comminuted and sometimes depressed, but they are not usually evident unless the overlying dura mater is stripped. They are believed to result from the *contrecoup* of the orbital lobes of the brain on these paper-thin bony surfaces (Fig. VII-38). Orbital roof fractures may also be seen as a result of sudden violent increase in intracranial pressure, particularly in suicidal gunshot wounds of the head where the weapon is fired in contact with the skin. The sudden release of gases in the skull appears to be the major cause of these fractures, but considerable controversy still persists regarding this mechanism.

In the individual who survives the injury for several hours or longer, hemorrhages associated

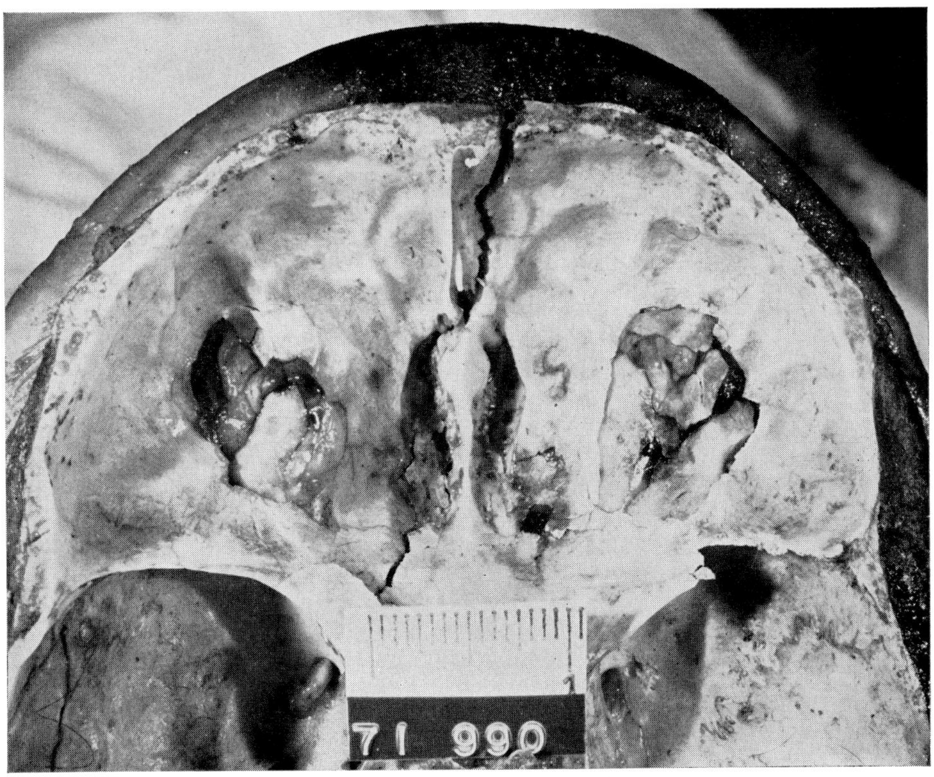


FIGURE VII-38b. Front half of the base of the skull of the same individual, showing bilateral fractures of the orbital roofs as a result of impacts transmitted by way of the frontal lobes of the brain.

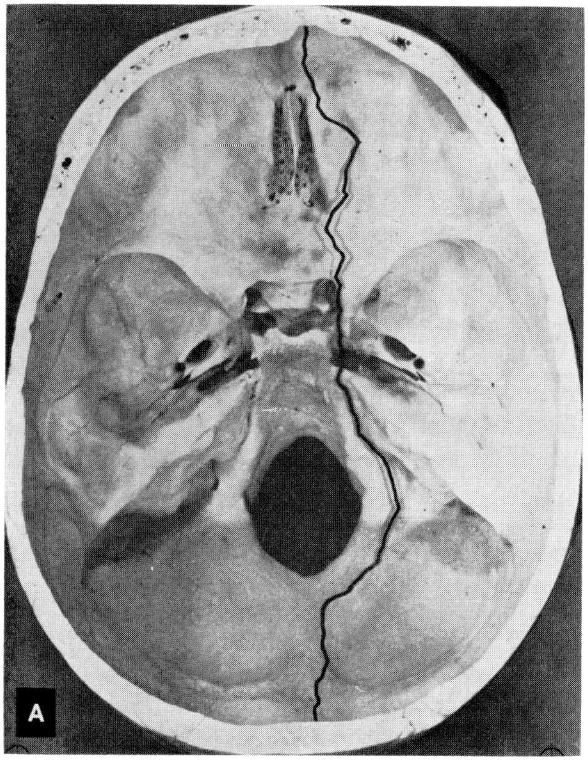


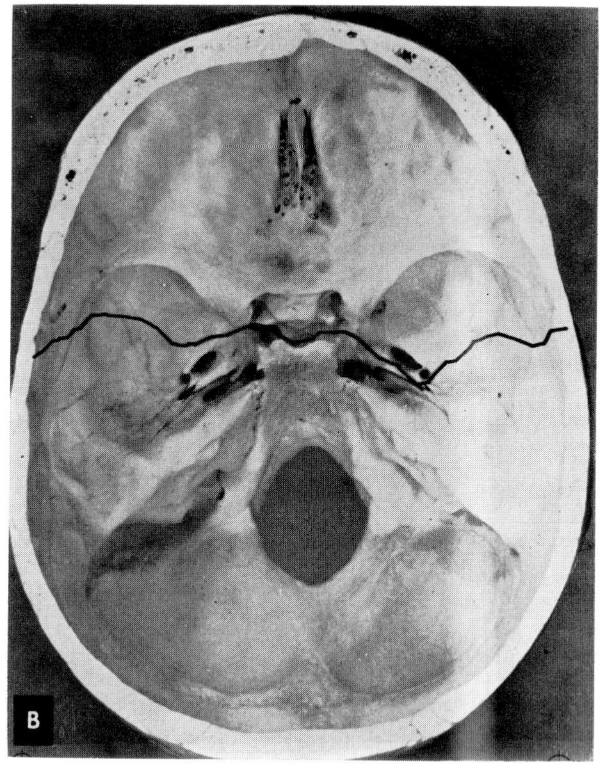


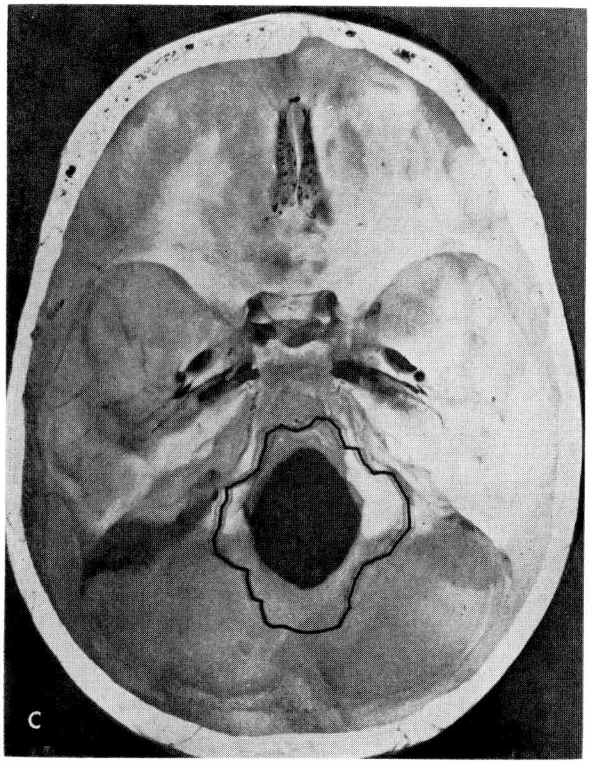


FIGURE VII-39. (a): Longitudinal fracture of the base of the skull, dividing it into two halves. (b): Transverse, so-called hinge fracture of the base of the skull. (c): Ring fracture of the base of the skull.

with orbital roof fractures are often seen in the soft tissues of the eye sockets and in the eyelids. This must not be interpreted as evidence of direct impact to the eyes.

Three principal types of fractures of the base of the skull are generally recognized, depending on the direction of the impacting force:

1. Longitudinal (front-to-back) fracture, which divides the base of the skull into two halves (right and left). This may occur as a result of blunt impact either on the face and forehead, on the back of the head or in front-to-back (and vice versa) compression of the head, as when the head is run over by an automobile (Fig. VII-39a).
2. Transverse (or side-to-side) fracture, which divides the base of the skull into a front and rear half. This type of fracture occurs from impact on either side of the head or as a result of side-to-side compression of the head, as when the head is run over by an automobile (Fig. VII-39b). Thus, in general, fracture lines of the base of the skull run in the same direction as the force. In children and young persons in whom the sutures between the skull bones are still open, fractures need not occur in the manner described, since separation of the sutures and considerable displacement of the bones commonly takes place.
3. Ring fracture of the base of the skull separating the rim of the foramen magnum from the remainder of the base. This type of fracture occurs in a fall from a height if the victim lands on his feet or buttocks, thus driving the vertebral column into the skull (Fig. VII-39c). The mechanism of this fracture may be compared to tightening a hammer handle by banging the opposite end of the handle on the floor.

In a fall from a height the leg bones, in par-

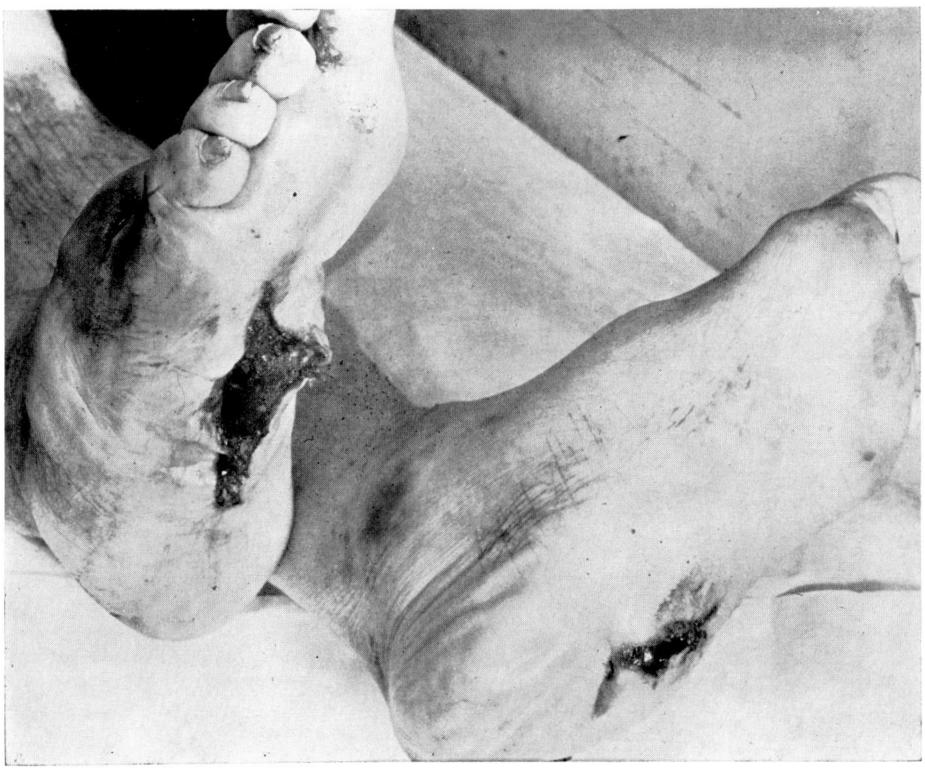

FIGURE VII-40. Middle-aged window washer fell on his feet from the tenth floor of an office building. The tibiae were driven through the feet into the soles of the shoes. A ring fracture of the base of the skull was likewise present.

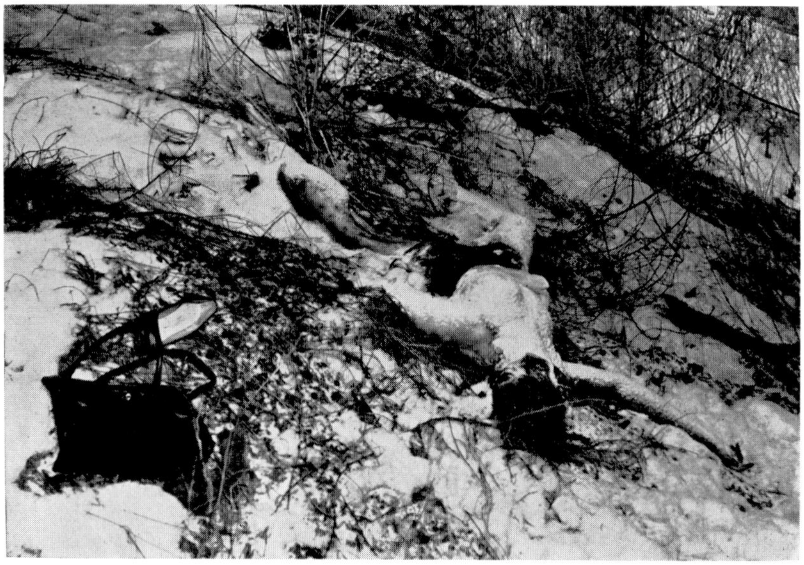

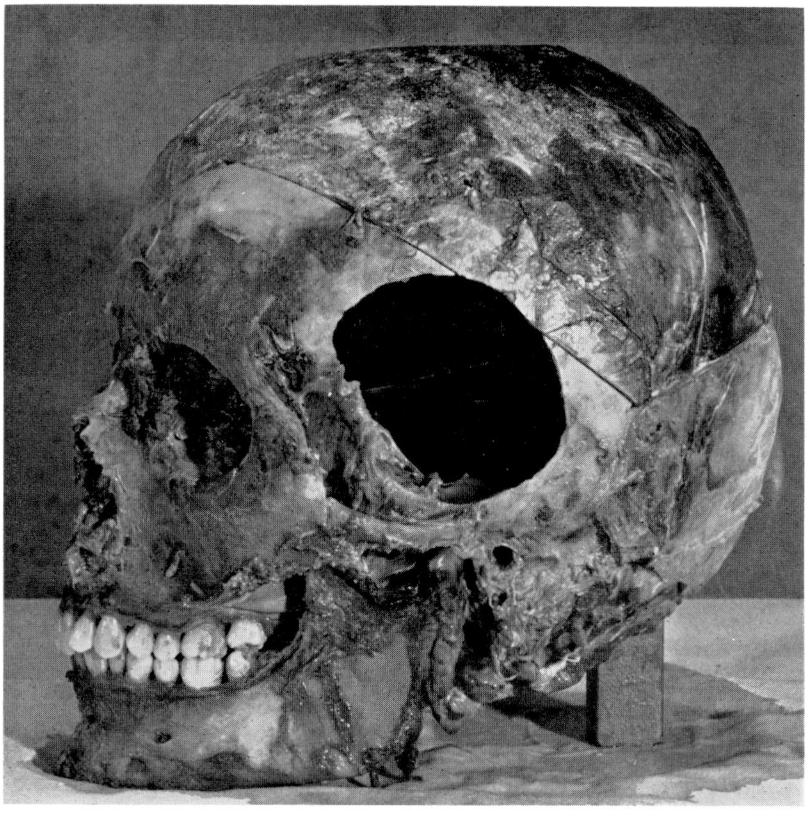

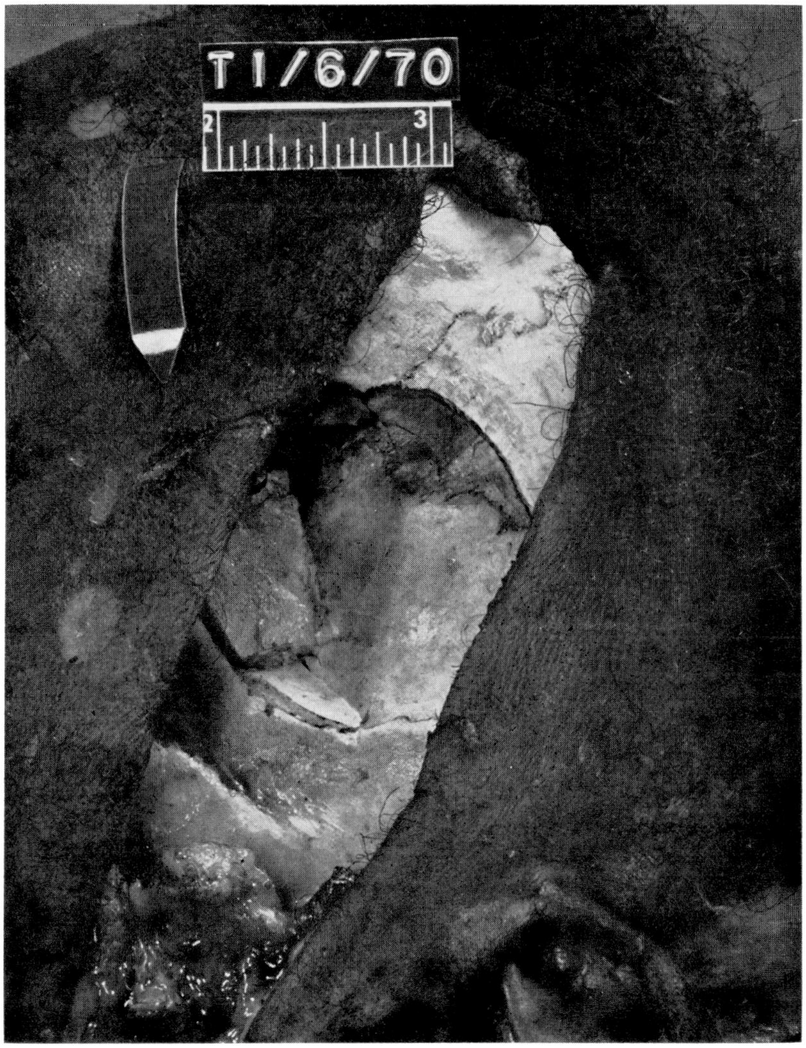


FIGURE VII-41. (a): Partly decomposed and frozen body of a young woman found in the rear of an abandoned brick factory three months after she had been reported missing. (b): Circular fracture of the left temple. The bone fragments were pushed inward. Very little bleeding was noted in the remaining soft tissues surrounding the defect in the bone. An important aspect of the investigation pertained to the instrument that had been used to inflict this injury. (c): Experimentally produced fracture of the left temple to provide a clue regarding the implement that had been used in the attack on the young woman. This circular fracture was produced by a forceful impact with the corner of a brick. The point of impact in the skin, which shifted to the left following an incision of the area, is indicated by the arrow. There was no perforation of the skin, and had this person been alive, the amount of external bleeding would probably have been minimal or absent altogether.

ticular the tibias, are sometimes driven through the soles of the feet (Fig. VII-40). Severing of the major blood vessels near their junction with the heart and small horizontal tears of the inner lining of the carotid arteries may sometimes be found. The heart may be driven through the pericardial sac and the diaphragm. In a young man who had jumped from the roof of a thirteen-floor apartment building, landing on his feet, the intact heart was found among intestinal loops deep within the pelvis. It had been torn from its pedicle about 1½ in. above the aortic valve. Bursting of the heart and exposure of its ventricles is also known to occur in this type of fall.

Spasic et al.[3] described ring fractures of the base of the skull due to a forceful blow on the chin in motor vehicle accidents. The authors believe these fractures result from forces transmitted into the back of the skull by way of the mandibular joints.

Bleeding from the ears, nose or mouth following head injury suggests a fracture of the base of the skull. Brain tissue may sometimes exude through these apertures, a sight unfamiliar to the inexperienced examiner, particularly if no other external evidence of injury is noted. A fracture of the base of the skull involving the sella turcica provides direct communication between the cranial cavity and the airway via the sphenoid sinus, which represents the roof of the nasopharynx. This permits the passage of blood from the base of the skull into the airways of the lungs. Areas of inhaled blood in the lungs are commonly seen, and their presence indicates that death was not instantaneous. Respiration must have continued briefly for even a small quantity of blood to be inhaled.

Numerous other fractures that are characteristic with respect to the mechanism of injury are well documented, particularly in the orthopedic and surgical literature. Colles' fracture (fracture of the distal end of the radius) occurs frequently. It is almost invariably caused by a fall on the outstretched hand. Another common bony injury is fracture of the calcaneus. It is generally due to a fall from height, with the person striking one or both heels. The height does not need to be great, and in older individuals such an injury may occur in a fall from four or five feet. In falls from a greater distance other skeletal injuries, particularly compression fractures of the vertebrae, are frequently associated. A fall into a manhole because a cover tipped over when stepped upon may result in severe injuries to the perineum and scrotum as well as fractures of the pelvis and tearing of the urethra.

The common skeletal changes of the battered or maltreated child and certain bony injuries incurred in motor vehicle accidents may serve as additional examples of this point.

Fractures whose mechanism is difficult to interpret are sometimes encountered.

The partly decomposed and frozen body of a young woman was found in a field in the rear of an abandoned brick factory about three months after she had disappeared. A perfectly circular depressed fracture two inches in diameter was found in the left temple. The overlying skin was mostly absent due to postmortem mutilation by animals. At autopsy the pathologist was unable to determine what could have caused the fracture. The police had evolved the theory that the murder had taken place in a different location, since no evidence of bleeding could be detected where the body was found. Experimentation showed that an identical fracture could be produced by a blow with the corner of a brick. The impact did not break the skin, indicating that bleeding had not necessarily occurred if indeed a brick had been used (Fig. VII-41).

## Fat Embolism

An infrequent cause of death complicating injury is fat embolism, which signifies the presence of fat droplets in the bloodstream. It occurs in all varieties of blunt force injury, and the most important causative injuries are (a) fractures of bones and (b) crushing and tearing injuries of the subcutaneous fat tissue. Many studies indicate that the incidence of fat embolism following fracture of bones is nearly 100 percent. Thus, it is obvious that most cases of posttraumatic fat embolism are not fatal. The presence of fat droplets in the bloodstream indicates that the injury leading to fat embolism was sustained during life. Estimates of the amount of embolic fat necessary to produce death in adults range from 12 to 120 ml.

Shrinkage of tissues, as in postmortem charring of the body, may cause fat to be moved into the blood vessels and produce a picture identical with fat embolism. In a decomposed body large pools of liquefied fat derived from fat cells in the tissues may be found in the blood. The presence of fat in the bloodstream is also frequently associated with surgical procedures, particularly orthopedic surgery and operations involving adipose tissue. A further source of fat embolism is fractures of the ribs and sternum, which may occur during resuscitative efforts. In these cases bone marrow and fat are dislodged from the marrow cavities and trapped in the lungs. With the current emphasis on cardiopulmonary resuscitation, this is probably the most common cause of pulmonary fat embolism seen at autopsy. Quantitatively, such fat in the bloodstream cannot be equated with pulmonary fat emboli that cause death. Fat droplets in the blood may be seen in certain nontraumatic conditions, such as diabetes mellitus, sickle cell crisis, pancreatitis, a variety of infectious diseases, following blood transfusion, in carbon tetrachloride and phosphorus poisoning and in fatty alteration of the liver as seen in chronic alcoholics.

There is much controversy regarding the origin of embolic fat, and two main views currently prevail:

1. The classical mechanical theory holds that fat embolism of the lungs follows the entrance of crushed fat, bone marrow and even bone spicules into traumatized vascular channels at the site of injury.
2. According to the physicochemical theory, most of the intravascular fat in the lungs is derived from lipids normally present in the plasma. Following trauma, an alteration of the normal plasma colloidal dispersion of chylomicrons brings about the coalescence of chylomicrons to form larger fat droplets. The high cholesterol content of some embolic fat globules, as described by LeQuire et al.,[6] substantiates the assumption that this circulating fat is not solely derived from stationary depot fat.

During the past decade much research has been directed toward the resolution of this controversy, and, while the argument remains unresolved, important information has been gained concerning the changes that occur in the physical properties and coagulation of blood following trauma. Indeed, an attractive theory postulates that the shock state following trauma results in certain physical-chemical changes in the blood, which are further influenced by the sudden mobilization of storage fat for energy purposes to combat the shock state. This mobilized fat acts as a trigger to disturb the equilibrium of the fat normally suspended in the circulating blood, leading to formation of large globules of visible fat.

Very few expulsive heartbeats are required to move a droplet of fat from anywhere in the body into the pulmonary circulation. The presence of intravascular fat globules in the lungs does not necessarily preclude *instantaneous* death, considering that the heart may continue to function for some time after respiration and other vital signs have ceased. Obviously, fat embolism cannot be expected if the heart is severed from the great vessels. Systemic fat embolism develops when fat globules are forced through the lung capillaries and arteriovenous anastomoses into the pulmonary veins. The pulmonary vascular tree is an efficient filter. One or two days after an injury, systemic fat embolism usually becomes apparent. This gives rise to a fairly characteristic clinical picture. Coma and death may occur suddenly due to involvement of the vital centers in the brain or following embolization to the myocardium and damage to the conduction system. The question of whether death can result from fat embolism in the lungs has not been conclusively resolved. Some suggest this is quite unlikely.[4,5,7] In our opinion, fatal pulmonary fat embolism alone is uncommon. Indeed, one study indicates that the incidence of pulmonary fat embolism associated with clinical symptoms with recovery was 99.2 percent.[8] However, the large amount of fat dispersed in the lungs in some cases of crushing injuries and the massive pulmonary edema seen in such cases would certainly tend to support the conclusion that pulmonary fat embolism that precipitates pulmonary edema may well play an important role in the *wet lung syndrome.* This has been characterized as playing an important role in death from shock following trauma.

On rare occasions fat embolism has been demonstrated in *decompression sickness* (caisson disease), in too rapid ascent to high altitudes without a functional pressurized cabin or under simulated flight conditions in decompression chambers.[9] In divers fat embolism has also been documented in conjunction with the general picture of caisson disease. In both instances death due to systemic fat embolism may occur within a few hours.

The salient gross anatomical findings in death from systemic fat embolism are pinpoint hemor-

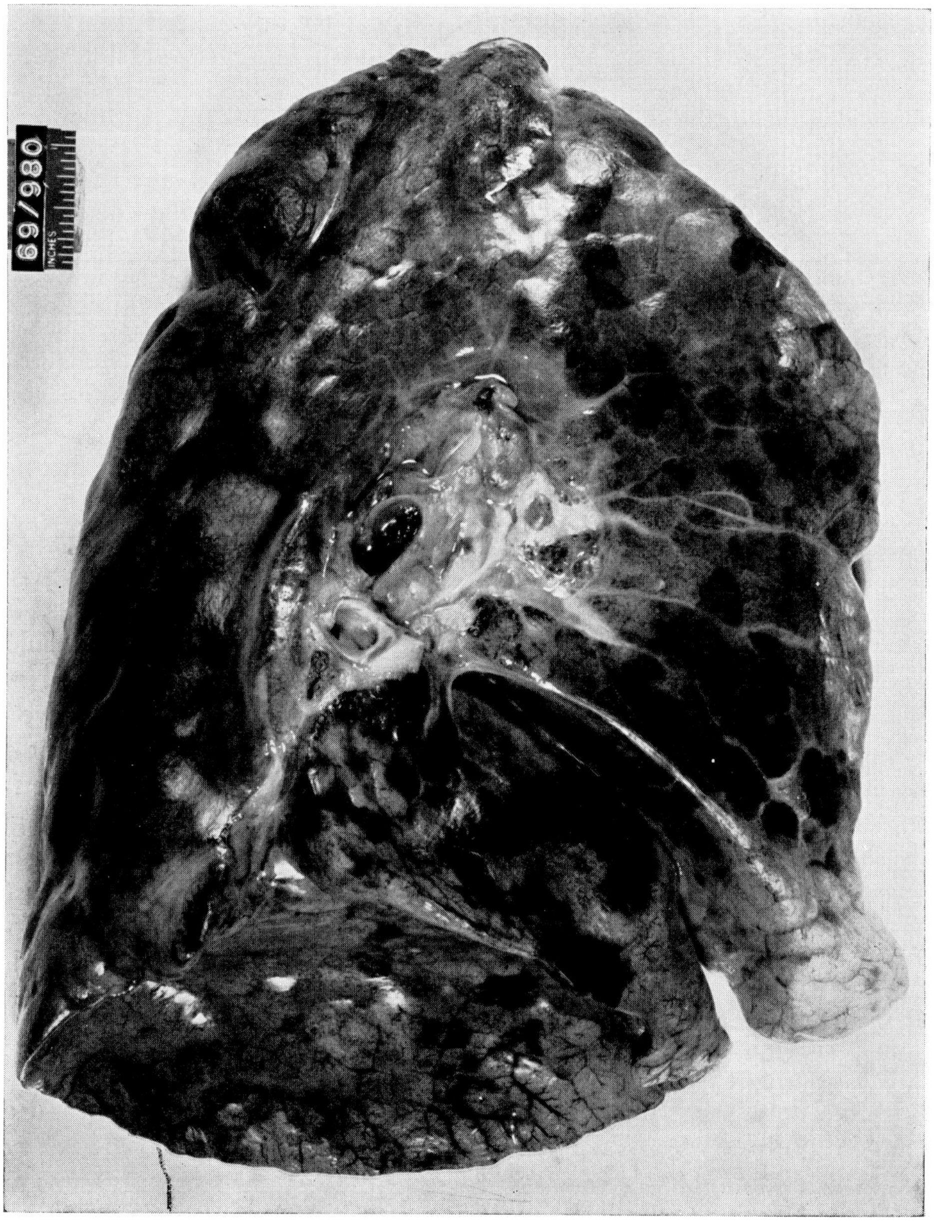

FIGURE VII-42. Lung: Foci of aspirated blood. The blood came from the mouth.

rhages in the skin and conjunctivae. In the skin the purpura is conspicuous on the shoulders, particularly about the armpits. In the brain punctuate hemorrhages are scattered throughout the white matter. In the lungs the findings are nonspecific and consist essentially of edema and congestion. Individual pinpoint hemorrhages may be noted on the surface of the kidneys and throughout the cortex. Microscopically, fat embolism is readily demonstrated in frozen sections stained with any of the conventional fat stains. In hematoxylin-eosin-stained paraffin sections fat embolism may still be recognized as small hollow intravascular spaces. These are especially prominent in the alveolar capillaries of the lungs and in the renal glomeruli.

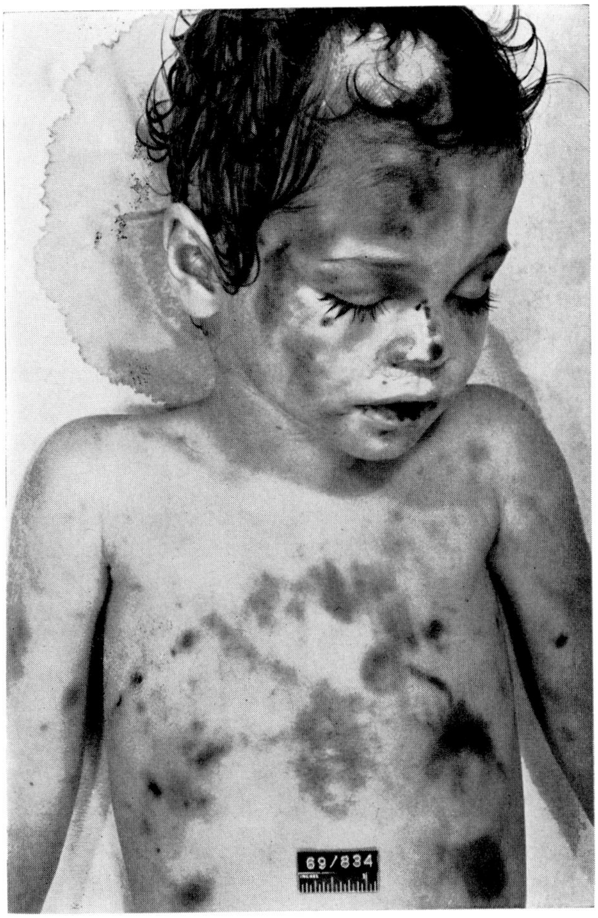


FIGURE VII-43. Three-year-old child who was brought to the hospital unconscious following an alleged fall in the bathroom, with his head striking the tub. Intensive care measures were instituted. Oxygen was given, and external cardiac massage as well as artificial respiration were carried out. The injuries suggested a battered child. Subsequent investigation, which extended to two hospitals, the ambulance crew that transported the child, and the parents, indicated that the history of a fall as given by the parents was correct. The child had struck the right side of his forehead and right temple. All remaining injuries had resulted from the resuscitative efforts.

### Injuries by Resuscitation

Fractures of the sternum and ribs are commonly seen following attempted resuscitation by means of external cardiac massage. The sternum fractures through the middle of the sternal body or at the junction of the body and manubrium. Hemorrhage often infiltrates the

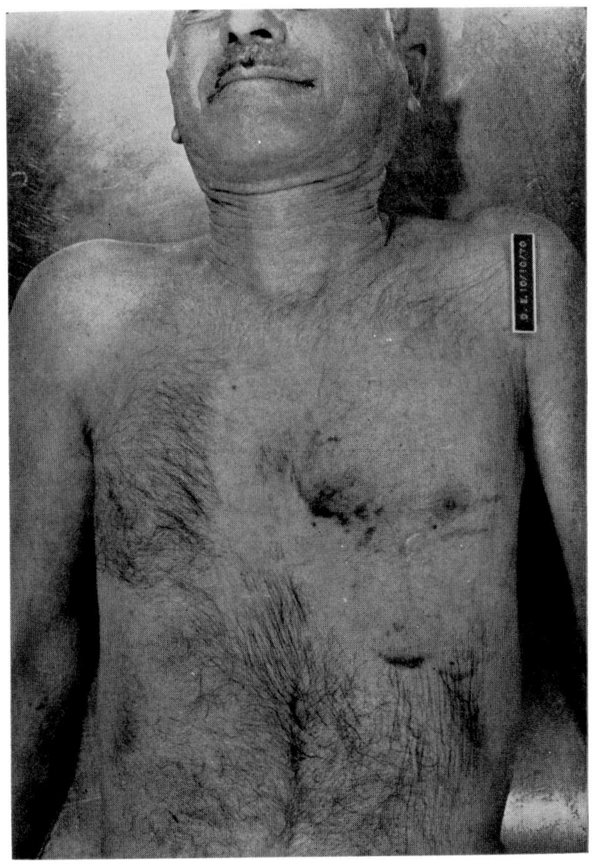

FIGURE VII-44. Elderly man who collapsed in a supermarket. Abrasions and contusions of the left chest wall are due to external cardiac massage. Underlying fractures of ribs and sternum were noted at autopsy. The cause of death was a fresh myocardial infarction. In a traumatic death it might have been difficult to ascertain the origin of these injuries.

soft tissues in the area of the fracture, as manipulation of the heart may either produce some pumping action or reactivate the spontaneous beat for a short while. The fractures may be associated with tears of the lungs and release of free air into the tissues. Hemorrhages in the lungs are frequently associated with remote parenchymal and subpleural hexagonal foci of aspirated blood. These hemorrhages are due to displacement by respiratory movements of blood in the bronchial tree from the areas of hemorrhage to distant locations (Fig. VII-42). Hemorrhages in the heart muscle, bleeding into the pleural cavities and tears of the liver are also often seen as complications of the resuscitative effort. The latter results from direct manipulation of the liver area as well as by a push-and-pull effect on the liver ligaments and the diaphragm. The spleen may be lacerated due to the same mechanism, but this does not occur as commonly. The heart sac may contain abundant blood as a result of intracardiac injections. At autopsy several ounces of blood may be found in the pericardial cavity if a branch of a coronary artery was punctured accidentally. Distinguishing between injuries due to resuscitation and those resulting from an assault may sometimes be difficult in the absence of a detailed account from the ambulance or rescue squad as well as the hospital emergency room or intensive care unit, particularly since both sets of injuries commonly occur a short while prior to death (Figs. VII-43, VII-44 and VII-45).

Compression of the chest, as occurs when the victim is run over by an automobile, usually causes extensive damage to all structures involved. In children, however, the ribs may not be fractured due to their marked elasticity. The heart is commonly torn as a result of compression because the blood it contains is incompressible. It is believed that the heart is especially prone to rupture when it is full, as at the end of the diastolic phase. Bursting of the heart may result from a violent blow on the chest, as in an automobile accident with impact of the

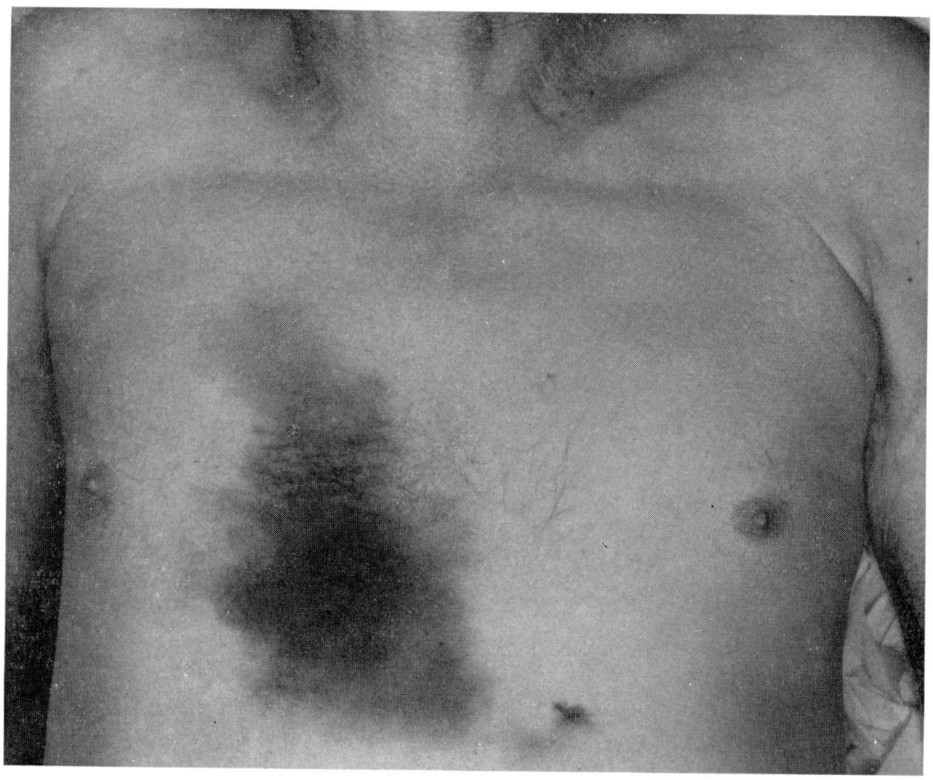

Figure VII-45. Bruising of the chest wall due to external cardiac massage.

driver on the steering column. The latter type of injury is relatively rare and is generally attributed to the pendulumlike suspension of the heart.

Tears of the heart more commonly involve the right ventricle. The right ventricle is thinner than the left and is located anteriorly, immediately under the sternum. The left ventricle more often ruptures spontaneously due to an acute myocardial infarction. A tear of the heart wall causes bleeding into the pericardial sac. The amount of blood in the pericardial sac required to bring the heart to a standstill depends on the rapidity with which the blood accumulates. The amount of blood found in the pericardial sac in fatal stabbings or shootings is usually 10 to 12 oz. (approximately 280 to 340 cc), but considerably more blood may accumulate, depending on the length of survival.

Certain abdominal injuries have been described earlier in this chapter. Other aspects of this type of trauma include bursting of hollow abdominal organs as a result of blunt impact. As in the case of the heart, a filled stomach is more likely to rupture due to the hydrostatic effect. Of particular importance is rupture of the stomach or the small intestine due to an unexpected forceful blow. The unexpectedness of such a blow is associated with relaxed abdominal wall musculature. The abdominal skin and the abdominal wall usually show no evidence of injury. The colon bursts very infrequently. The urinary bladder is more commonly torn as the result of piercing by a sharp fragment of fractured pelvic bone rather than by an explosive type of bursting as in the case of the gut.

## INJURIES FROM BITING

Injuries due to biting are rare. Human bites seldom cause tearing of the skin and far more frequently result in the production of semicircular or crescentic patterned abrasions with associated extensive hemorrhages beneath the skin. Injuries from biting generally have sexual overtones. They are usually located on or about the genitalia and/or female breasts. Bites inflicted upon an assailant in self-defense may occasionally be observed. Identification of a suspect by comparing his bite pattern with marks left on the victim may be performed but not without caution and awareness of the limitations of the methods (Fig. VII-46). The skin may become twisted or distorted during the act of biting, with subsequent distortion of the pattern. Emphasis should also be placed on possible changes in the teeth occurring between the time of commission of the assault and apprehension of the suspect. Extraction of one or more teeth must be considered. Expert dental consultation is advisable.[10]

Animal bites may be recognizable by their patterns (Fig. VII-47). The number and depth of the individual injuries, reflecting the number and length of the teeth, and the distance between adjacent injuries, particularly those made by the incisors and canines, may permit identification of the species. An attacking dog usually tears his prey extensively. Due to the length and sharpness of a dog's canines, individual

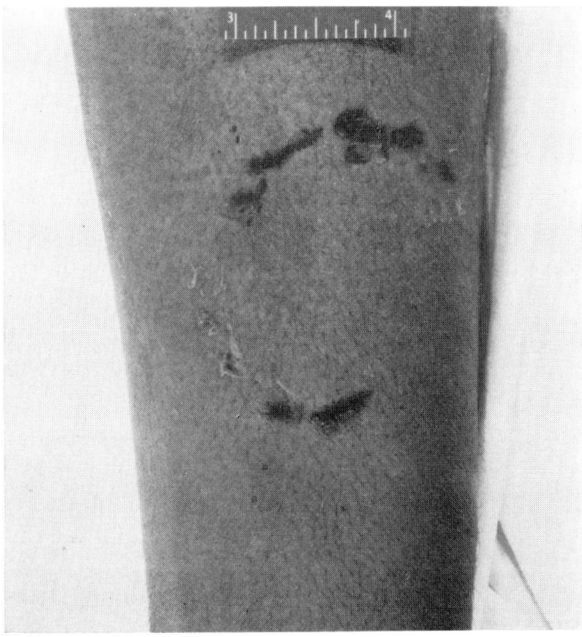

FIGURE VII-46. Arm of a man who had been bitten during an argument. The imprint on the skin depicts an incomplete denture, although the assailant had all his teeth.

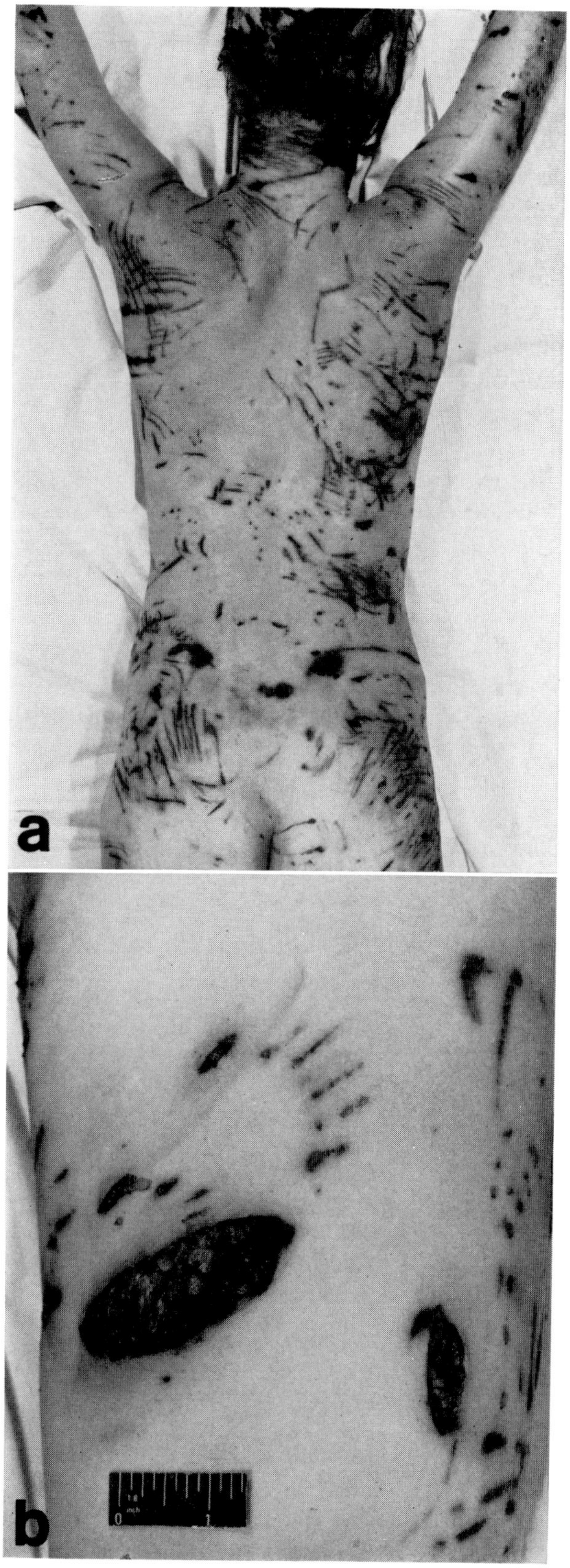


punctures may closely resemble stab wounds.

Postmortem mutilation of the human body by animals has been mentioned in Chapters II and III. It should be added that such mutilation may proceed to dismemberment if dogs or some other meat-eating animals are involved. Both ante- and postmortem injuries by wolves and bears have been reported.

## REFERENCES

1. Spitz, W. U.: Hemorrhagic pancreatitis following a kick in the abdomen. *J Forensic Med, 12:*105, 1965.
2. Potter, E. L.: *Pathology of the Fetus and the Newborn.* Chicago, Year Bk Med, 1953, p. 336.
3. Spasic, P., and Rezic, A.: Ein Beitrag zur Kenntnis des Entstehungsmechanismus der Schädelbasisringbrüche. *Z Rechtsmed, 67:*324, 1970.
4. Sevitt, S.: In Clark, R. (Ed.): *Modern Trends in Accident Surgery and Medicine.* London, Butterworth, 1959, p. 110.
5. Sevitt, S.: *Fat Embolism.* London, Butterworth, 1962.
6. LeQuire, V. S., Shapiro, J. L., LeQuire, C. B., Coob, C. A., Jr., and Fleet, W. F., Jr.: A study on the pathogenesis of fat embolism based on human necropsy material and animal experiments. *Am J Pathol, 35:*999, 1959.
7. Simpson, K.: Fat embolism. *J Forensic Med, 6:*19, 1959.
8. Wilson, J. V., and Salisbury, C. V.: Fat embolism in war surgery. *Brit J Surg, 31:*384, 1944.
9. Mason, J. K.: *Aviation Accident Pathology.* London, Butterworth, 1962, p. 165.
10. Gustafson, G.: *Forensic Odontology.* New York, Am Elsevier, 1966, pp. 161-165.

←

FIGURE VII-47. Sixteen-year-old girl who was attacked and killed by a mixed German shepherd dog. (a): The patterned injuries on her back and buttocks are bite marks. (b): The parallel vertical scratches were produced by the teeth of the upper jaw. Some of the deeper injuries resemble stab wounds.

*Chapter VIII*

# SHARP FORCE INJURY

WERNER U. SPITZ

## CUTTINGS AND STABBINGS

IN THE UNITED STATES cuttings and stabbings are second only to gunfire as a cause of homicidal death. Information of great importance in the reconstruction of a given case may be derived from precise examination of a cut or a stab wound.

**A cut (or incised wound)** results whenever a sharp-edged object is drawn over the skin with sufficient pressure to produce an injury that is longer than it is deep (Fig. VIII-1). For example, a sharp knife, a razor blade or a piece of glass or china could cause a typical cut. The wound edges may be straight or jagged, depending on the shape of the cutting instrument, but they are never abraded or undermined. The two latter points are most helpful in distinguishing an injury caused by a sharp object from one caused by blunt impact as from a hammer or a stone. Blunt force produces a tear or laceration. Another differential feature of a laceration from an injury produced by a sharp object is the absence of small, thin, delicate *bridges* of soft tissue between the sides of the stab wound or cut. A sharp object cuts and divides as it penetrates, whereas in a blunt impact the injury results from crushing and tearing of the tissues, frequently sparing small blood vessels, nerves and strands of connective tissue (Fig. VIII-2).

**A stab wound** results from penetration of a pointed instrument into the depths of the body, causing a wound that is deeper than its length on the skin. The thrust of a knife, for instance, produces such an injury. As in a cut, the edges of a stab wound are sharp, straight and not undermined. The lack of crushing and tearing of tissues associated with sharp force injury is the reason why the skin in the vicinity of a stab wound is usually devoid of bruising. If bruising is noted in proximity of a stab wound, it is most likely caused by the impact of the fist that held the weapon (Figs. VIII-3 and VIII-4).

Abrasion of the edges of a stab wound is usually absent, except when the handle or the hilt of the knife abuts the skin. Abrasion or bruising of the edges of a stab wound consequently suggests that the blade had been completely inserted, particularly if coarse fabric of clothing intervened between the handle of the weapon and the skin. It is imperative in such cases that the suspected knife, if available, be examined by the pathologist who performs the autopsy and that a decision be made regarding the compatibility of the shape of the abrasion around

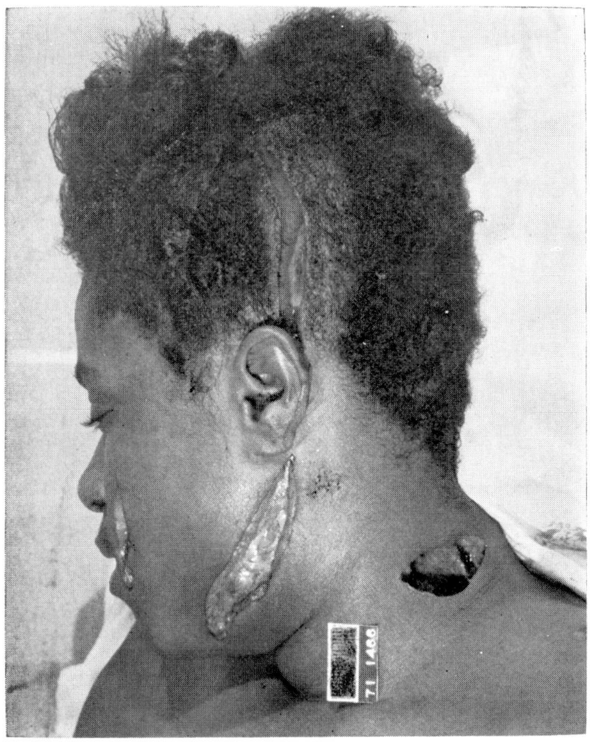

FIGURE VIII-1. Homicidal cuts of scalp and face: A cut is longer than it is deep. The injury of the neck is a stab wound.

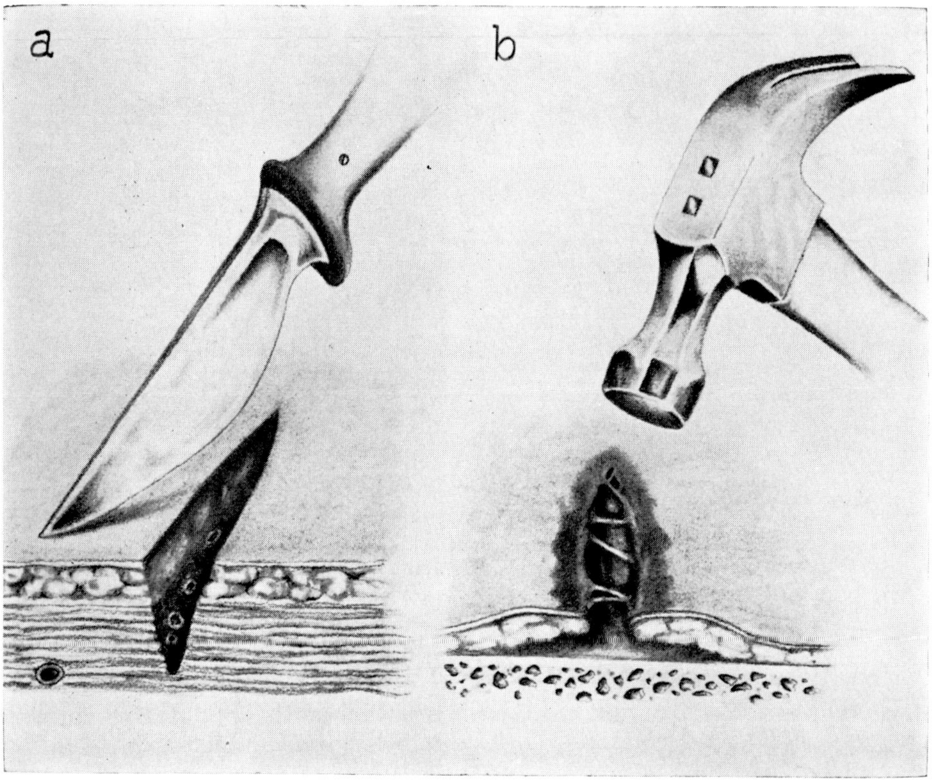


FIGURE VIII-2. Distinction of sharp from blunt force injury. Note the straight, *clean*, nonabraded edges of the cut (a) compared to the abraded and irregular undermined margins of the laceration (b), as well as the thin and delicate bridges of soft tissue within the latter type of wound.

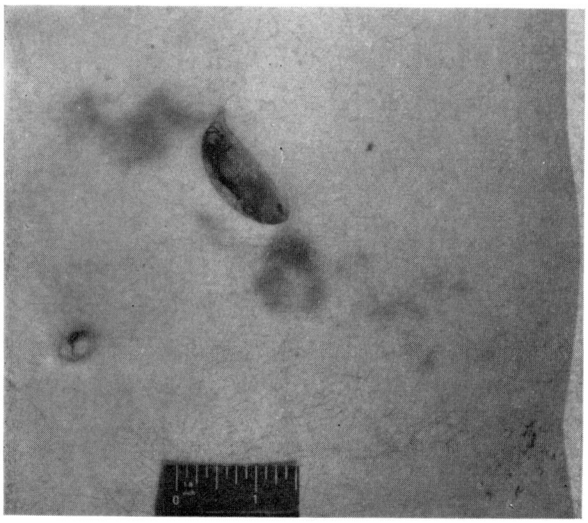

FIGURE VIII-3. Considerable bruising of the skin adjacent to a stab wound of the abdomen. The bruising was produced by the impact of the assailant's fist against the somewhat obese abdominal wall.

the stab wound with the handle of the knife in question (Fig. VIII-5). It must be noted that unless the blade penetrates the body at a 90° angle, all sides of the hilt may not be equally imprinted on the skin. Consequently, if the blade strikes in a downward direction, the hilt mark is accentuated above the stab wound; but if the blade is directed upward, the mark is below the stab wound. The same is true if the weapon is thrust sideways (Figs. VIII-6, VIII-7 and VIII-8).

The examination of a cut or a stab wound frequently permits conclusions regarding the manner in which the injury was inflicted. A stab wound generally suggests homicidal assault by virtue of its appearance and depth. The amount of blood lost at the scene is often minimal, since bleeding may be mostly internal. Multiple stab

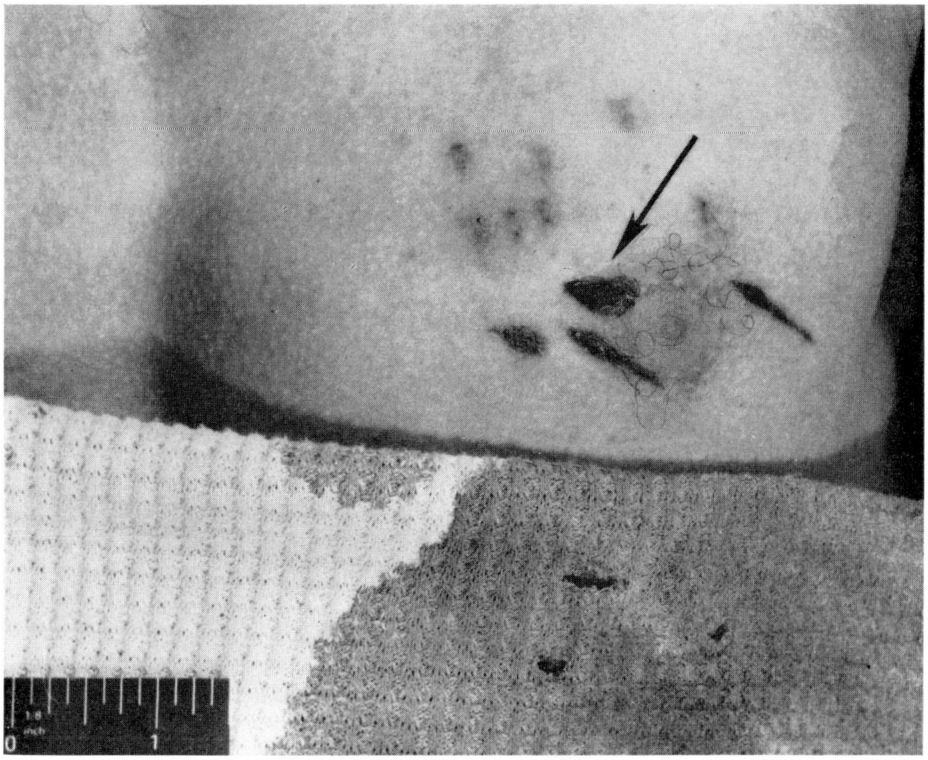


FIGURE VIII-4. Stab wound (arrow) and three superficial cuts around the left nipple. The bruises above and to the right of the nipple depict the weaving pattern of the T-shirt and were probably caused by the assailant's fist in the process of stabbing.

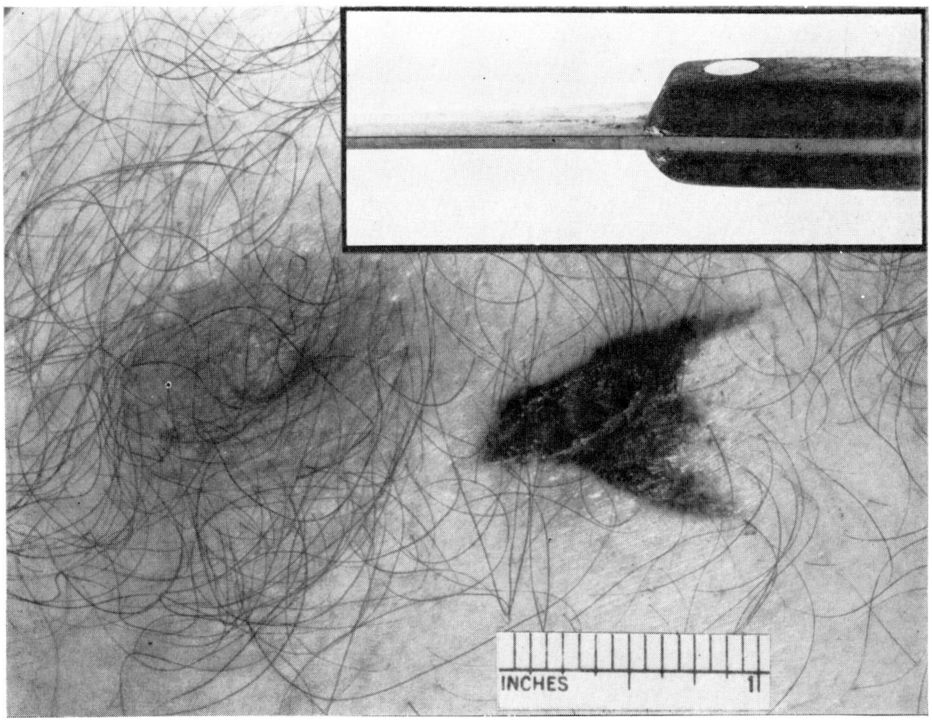


FIGURE VIII-5. Stab wound of chest. The dovetaillike abrasion of the margins was caused by the scraping action of the hilt of the knife (insert) and consequently suggests that the blade had been completely inserted.

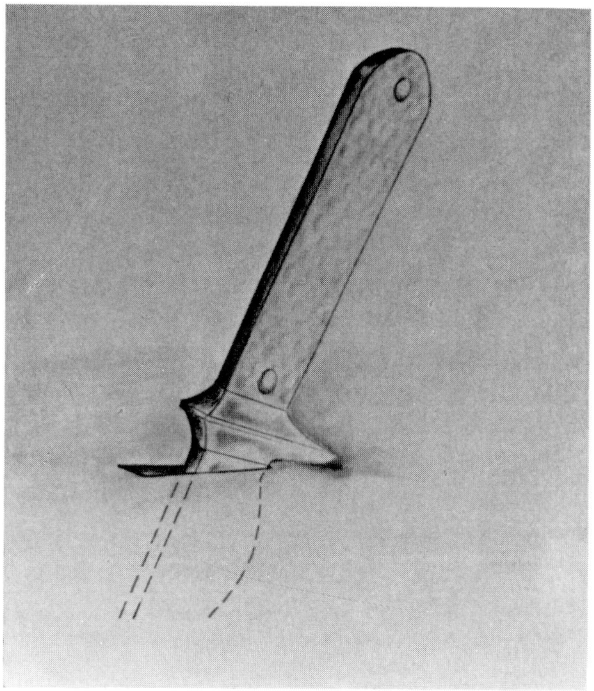

FIGURE VIII-6. Only the lower part of the hilt is imprinted on the skin if the knife slants in the manner shown.

wounds, most or all of which penetrate into internal organs, are usually indicative of homicide (Fig. VIII-9).

Cuts or slashes on the upper extremities, especially the forearms and the hands, are referred to as *defense wounds* and are sustained when the victim raises his arms or grabs at the knife in an effort to protect his face or chest by warding off the assailant's weapon (Figs. VIII-10 to VIII-14).

Defense wounds may occasionally be found on the shins and feet if the victim was lying on the ground and used his legs to defend himself. Such injuries on the lower extremities are more common if the victim is a female, and they suggest sexual assault (Fig. VIII-15). Under such circumstances, vaginal, oral and rectal smears should be prepared to determine the presence of spermatozoa, and swabs from these areas should be subjected to acid phosphatase determination.

Besides the cuts on the extremities sustained

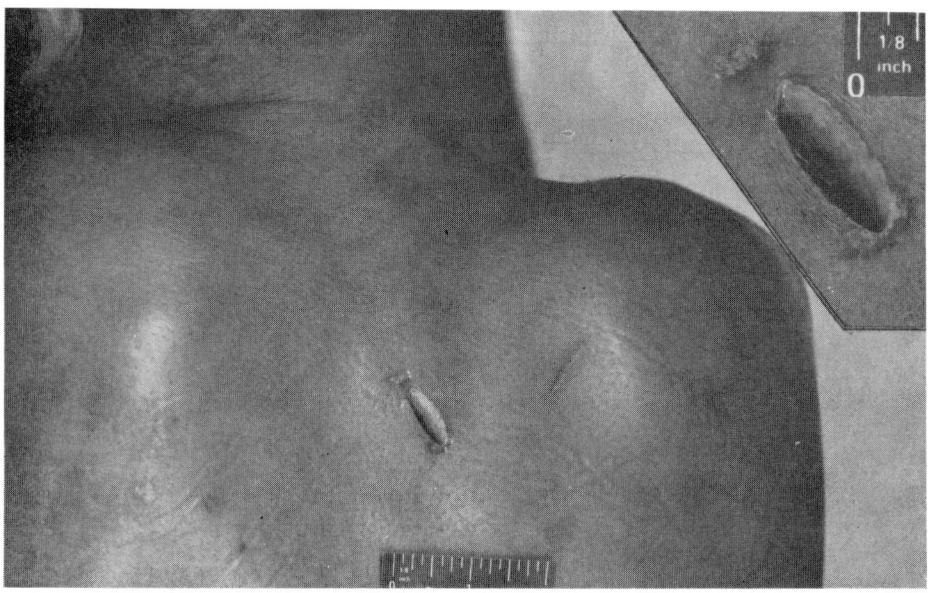


FIGURE VIII-7. This stab wound was probably caused by a daggerlike knife having a plate at the junction of the blade and the handle. Because of the downward slant of the knife during stabbing, only the upper edge of this plate was imprinted on the skin.

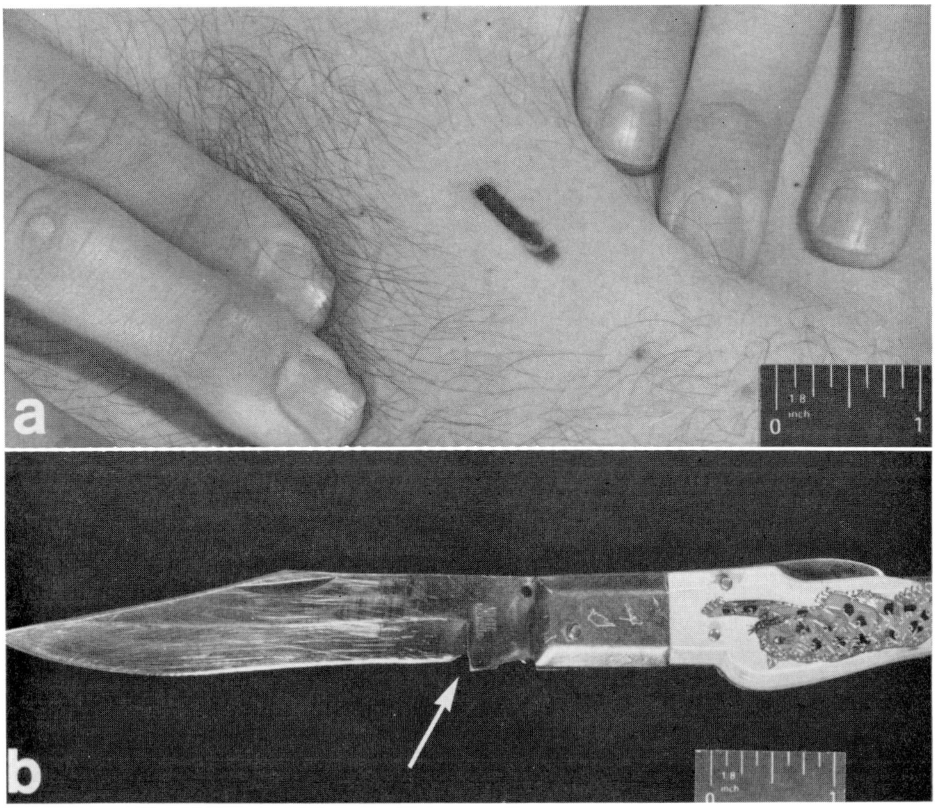


FIGURE VIII-8. (a): Stab wound of the chest. The edges of the injury are approximated to overcome distortion produced by the inherent elasticity of the skin. The upper end of the wound corresponds to the width of the blade. (b): The lower end of the wound shows an abrasion produced by the protruding portion of the blade near the hinge (arrow).

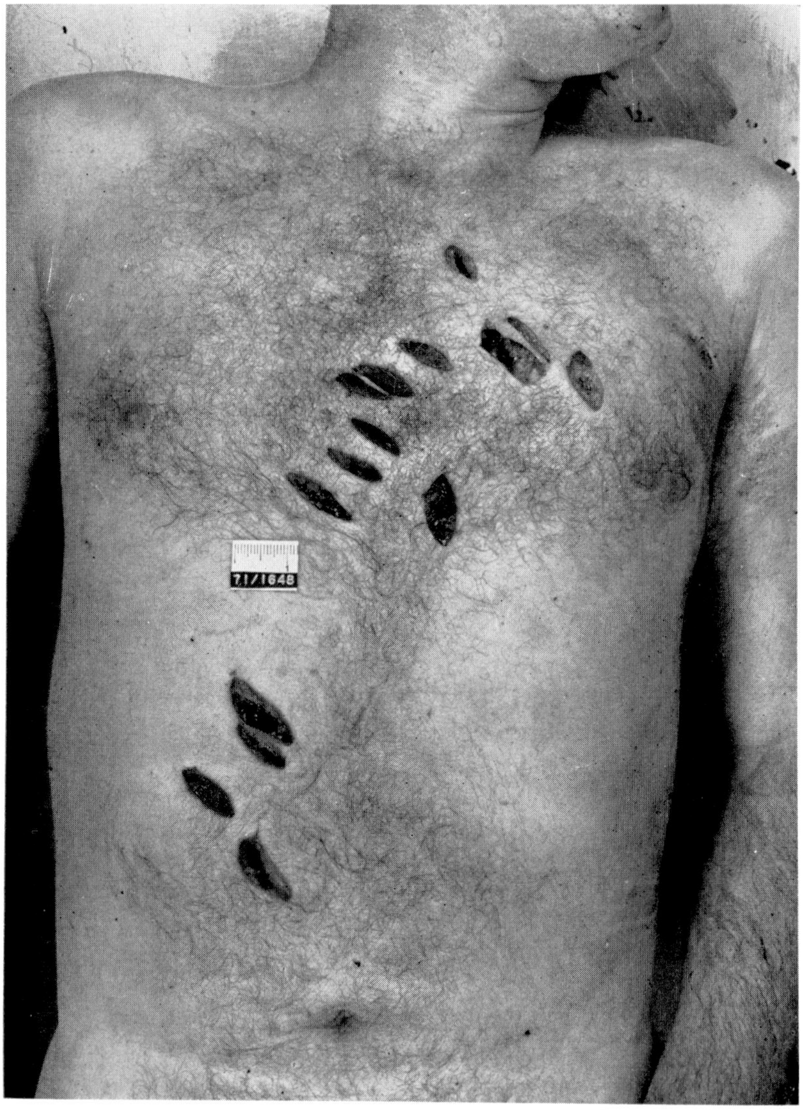


FIGURE VIII-9. Homicidal stab wounds of chest and abdomen, all penetrating the inner organs.

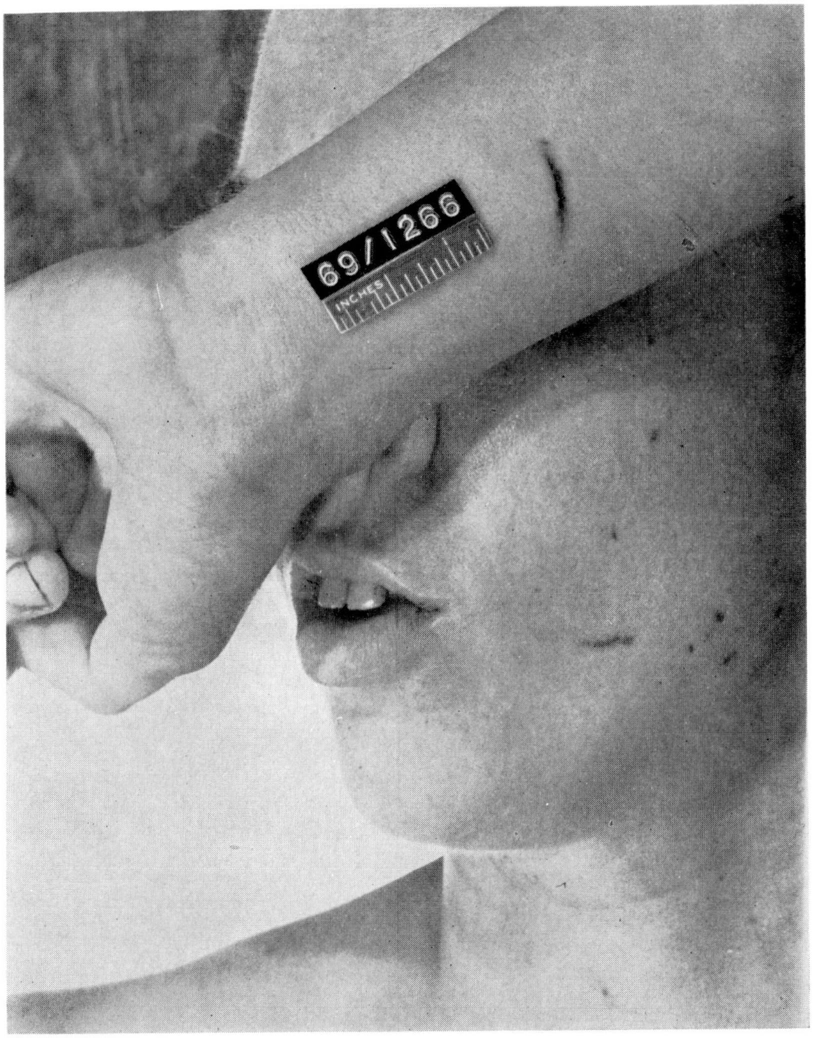


FIGURE VIII-10. Superficial defense-type cut of the right arm and scratches on the face. The injuries indicate that an altercation had taken place. Note the location of the defense wound on the arm. Death was due to a stab wound of the chest.

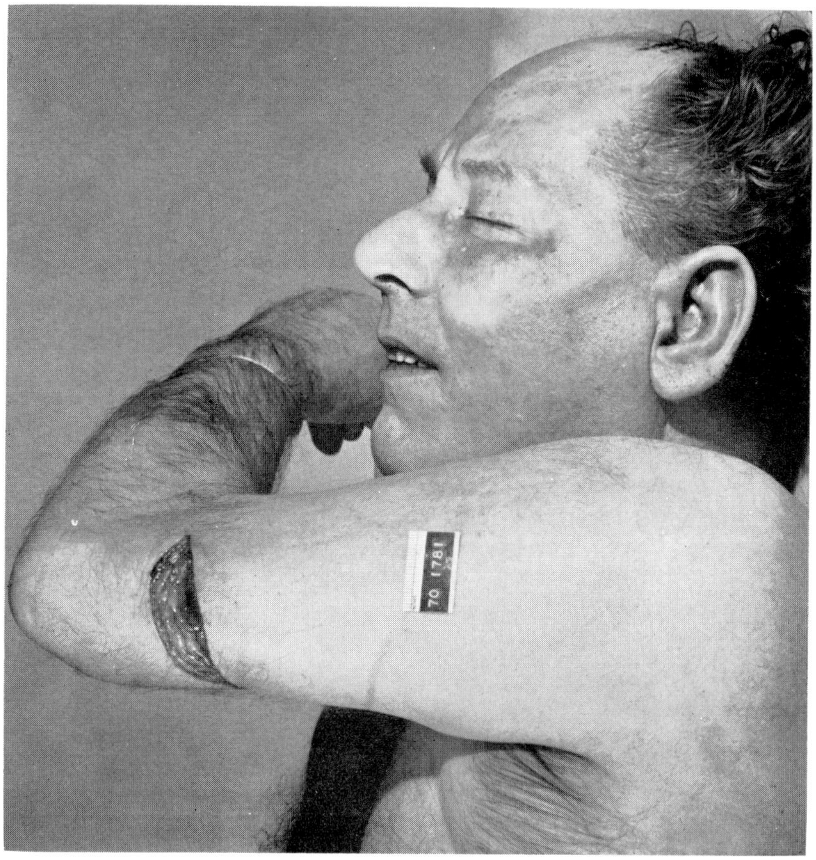

FIGURE VIII-11. Defense wound on the arm. This was the most likely position of the arm when the victim attempted to ward off the knife to protect his face. The cause of death was a stab wound of the chest.

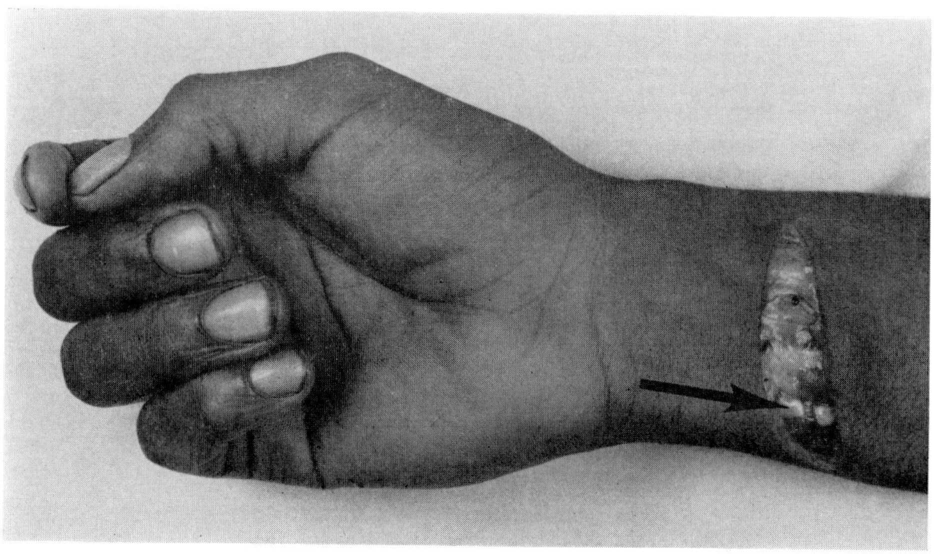

FIGURE VIII-12. Defense cut of the wrist. Note that one of the tendons is severed (arrow). Severed tendons or major nerves may be disabling, causing loss of function of certain muscles. It is essential that such injuries be correctly noted and evaluated.

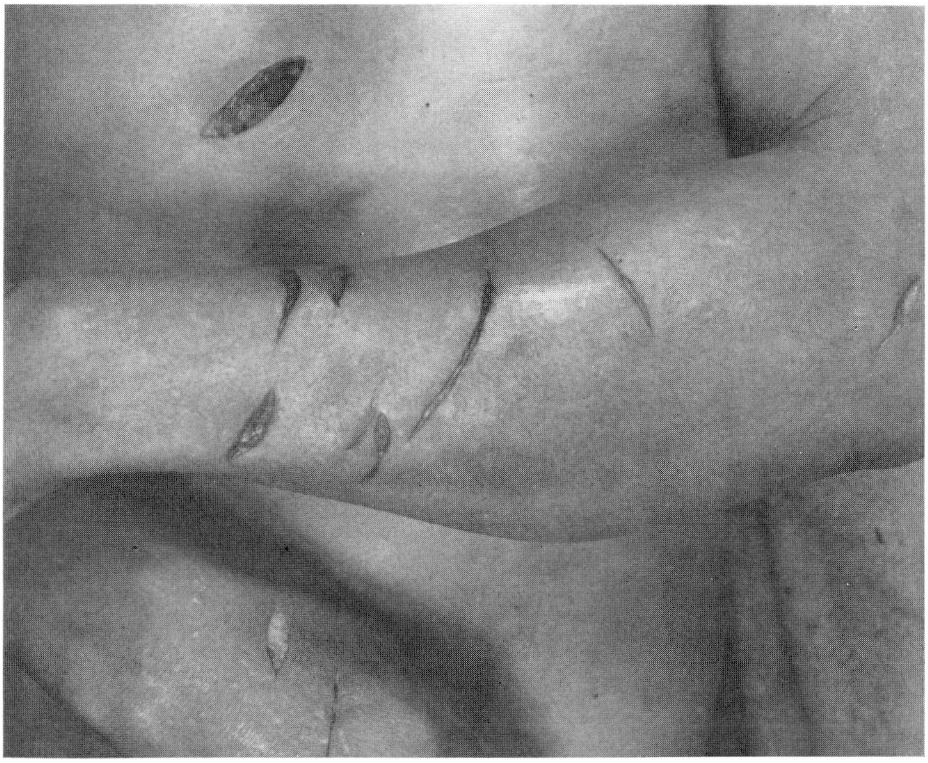

FIGURE VIII-13. Multiple superficial cuts on the forearm sustained in an effort to protect the chest. The victim was stabbed only once, in the center of the chest.

in attempted self-defense, certain other injuries on the body of the decedent invariably indicate that a struggle has taken place (Figs. VIII-16 to VIII-21).

Fingernail marks and abrasions that are produced by the tugging and rubbing of clothing occur in many instances of hand-to-hand combat and most commonly in stabbing cases. The recognition of these injuries is indispensable for reconstruction of the circumstances surrounding the death. For example, in the case of a struggle for the weapon, fingernail marks, bruises and scrapes on the victim's body lend support to the defendant's statement that he stabbed the deceased in self-defense.

Fingernail marks are most often located on the hands and wrists and less frequently on the face, neck and chest. They usually consist of superficial, semicircular and irregularly shaped defects of the outermost layers of the skin. Fingernail marks often resemble scratches and, in fact, are frequently referred to as such. When very fresh and moist they may be barely recognizable. Upon drying, however, they become dark brown or even black. Occasionally, if the assailant's nails were long, the fingernail marks may resemble small cuts and penetrate the entire thickness of the skin. The extent of injury to the soft tissues under fingernail marks varies from slight bleeding, limited to the area of injury on the skin surface, to extensive hemorrhage.

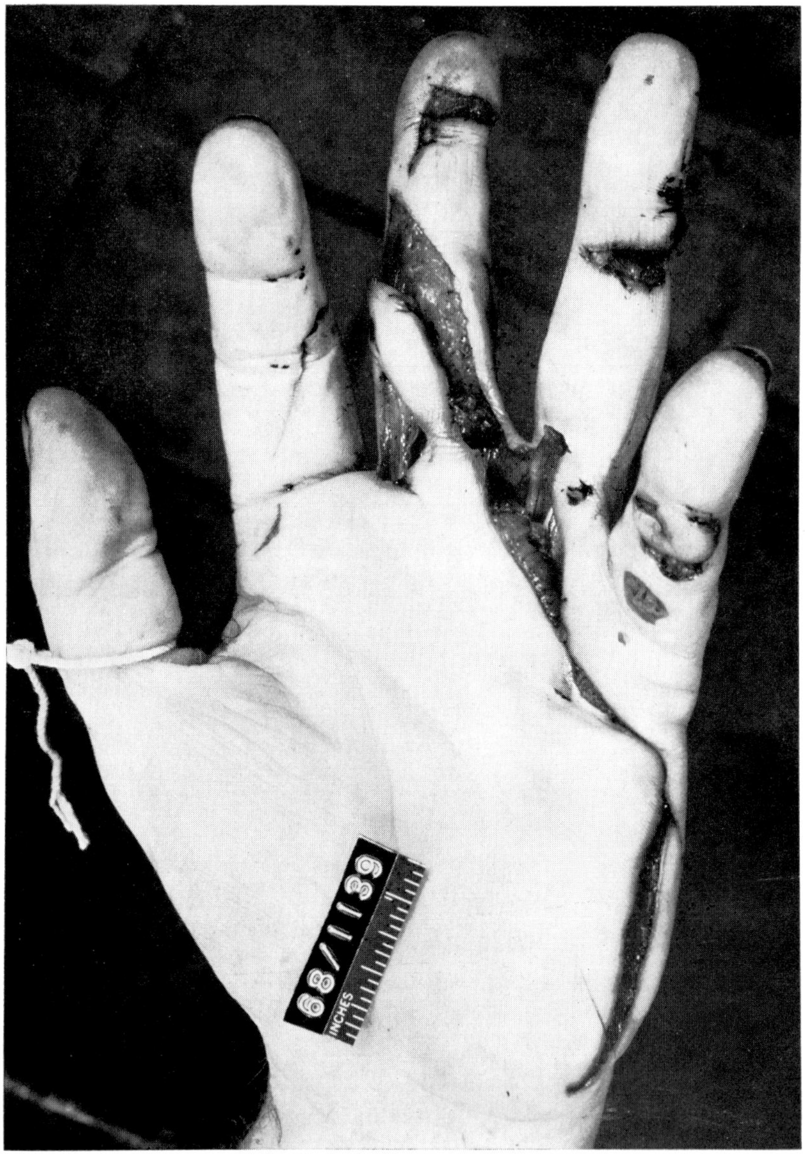


FIGURE VIII-14. Defense wounds sustained in an attempt to grab the knife. Tendons and major blood vessels are severed. The distribution of the injuries indicates that the victim repeatedly tried to hold the weapon.

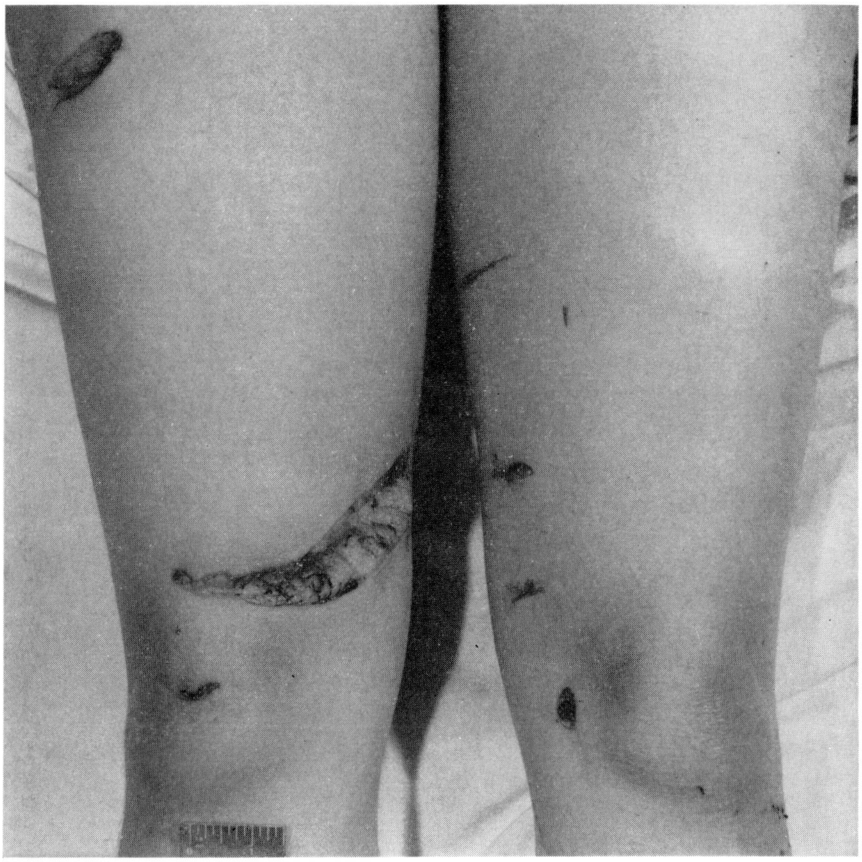

FIGURE VIII-15. Defense wounds on the knees and legs suggest that the victim was lying on the ground during the attack. Injuries in these locations tend to produce suspicion of a sexual motive for the killing.

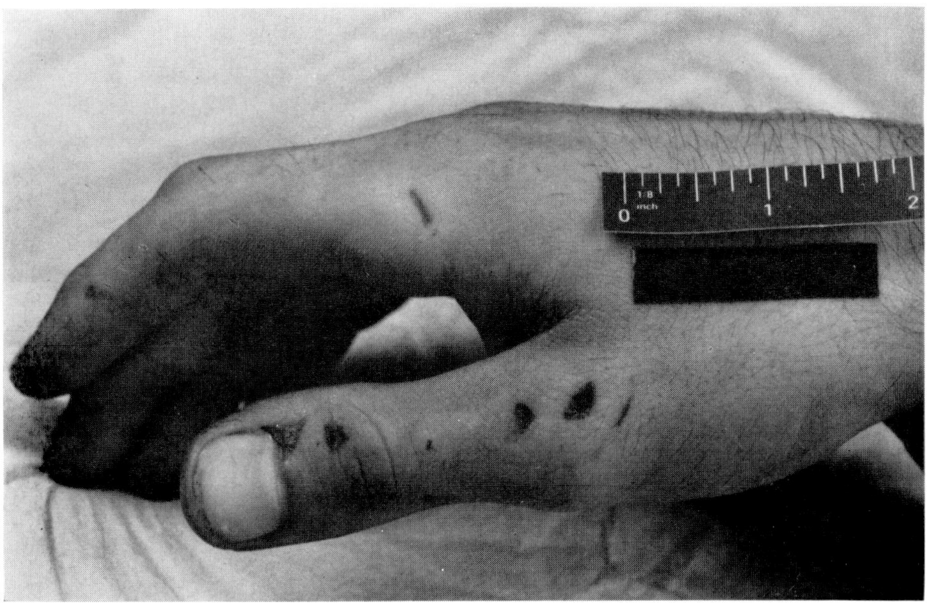


FIGURE VIII-16. Linear, slightly curved and irregularly-shaped fingernail marks.

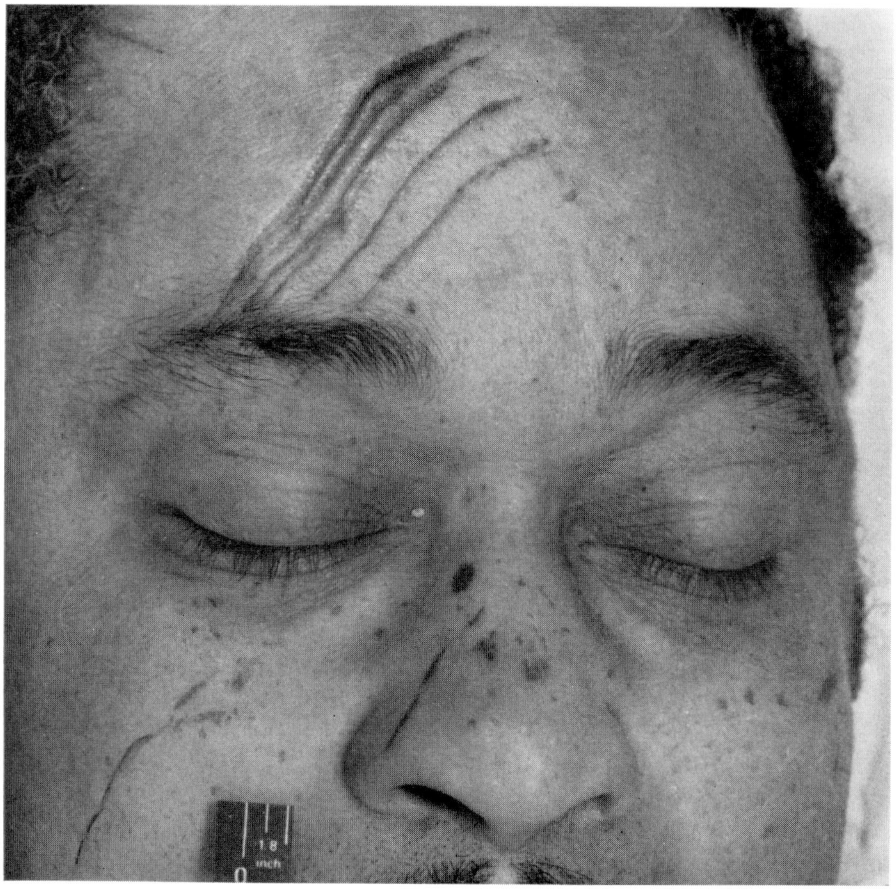

FIGURE VIII-17. Different injuries produced by fingernails during an altercation. Note the semicircular impressions on the right cheek. The cause of death was multiple stab wounds.

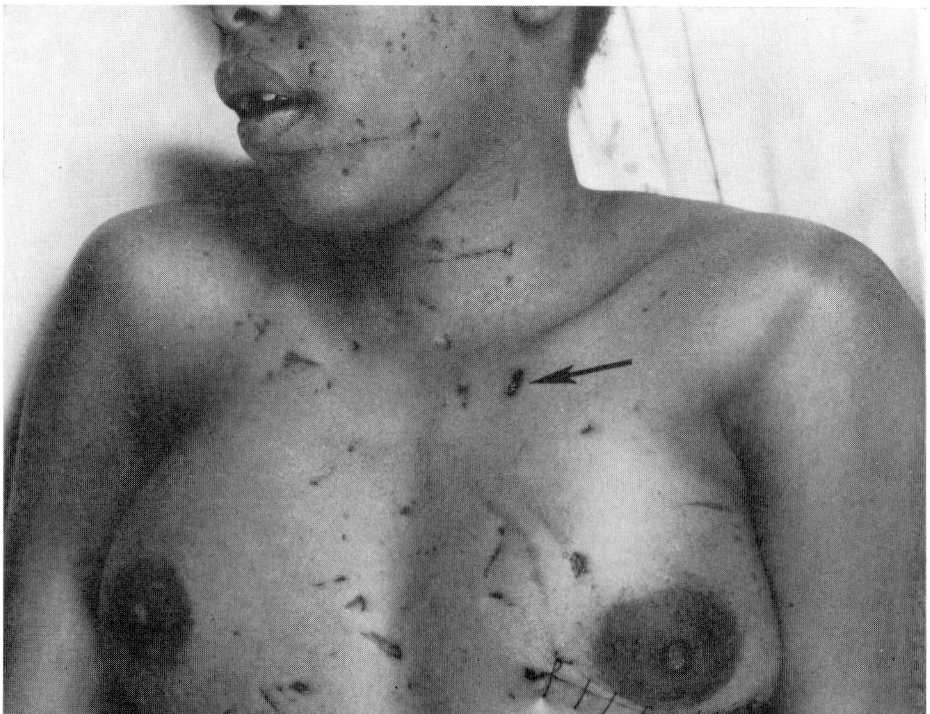

FIGURE VIII-18. Stab wound of the chest (arrow). Multiple fingernail marks as seen here suggest attack by someone of equal or less strength than the victim. Beneath the left nipple is a sutured surgical wound made in a hospital attempt at resuscitation.

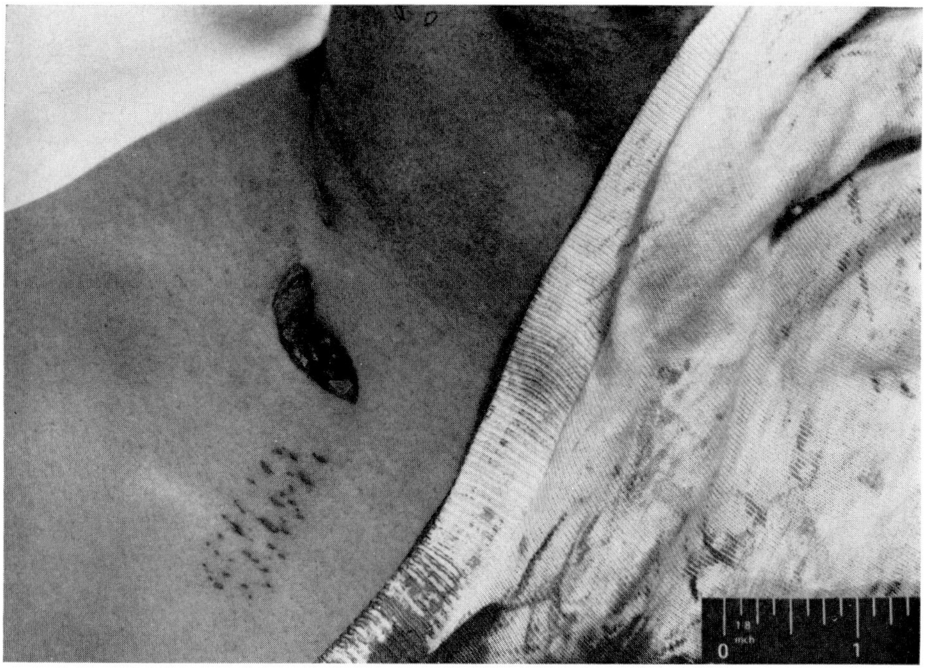

FIGURE VIII-19. The patterned abrasions below the stab wound were caused by pull and pressure of the ribbed neck of the T-shirt.

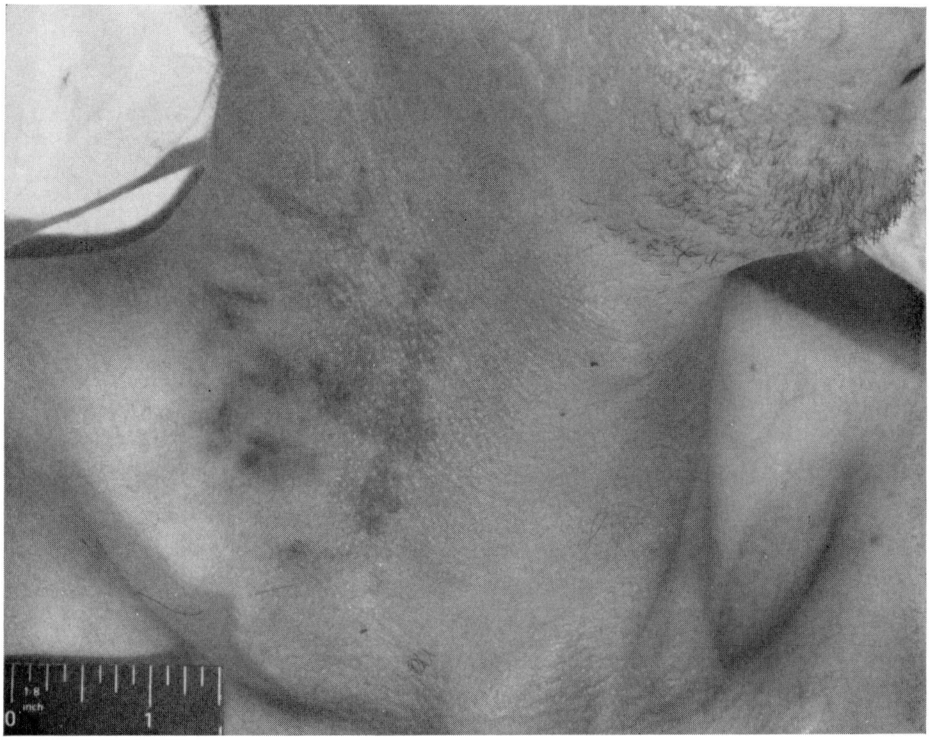

FIGURE VIII-20. Bruises on the neck caused in a struggle over a knife. The deceased was initially the assailant.

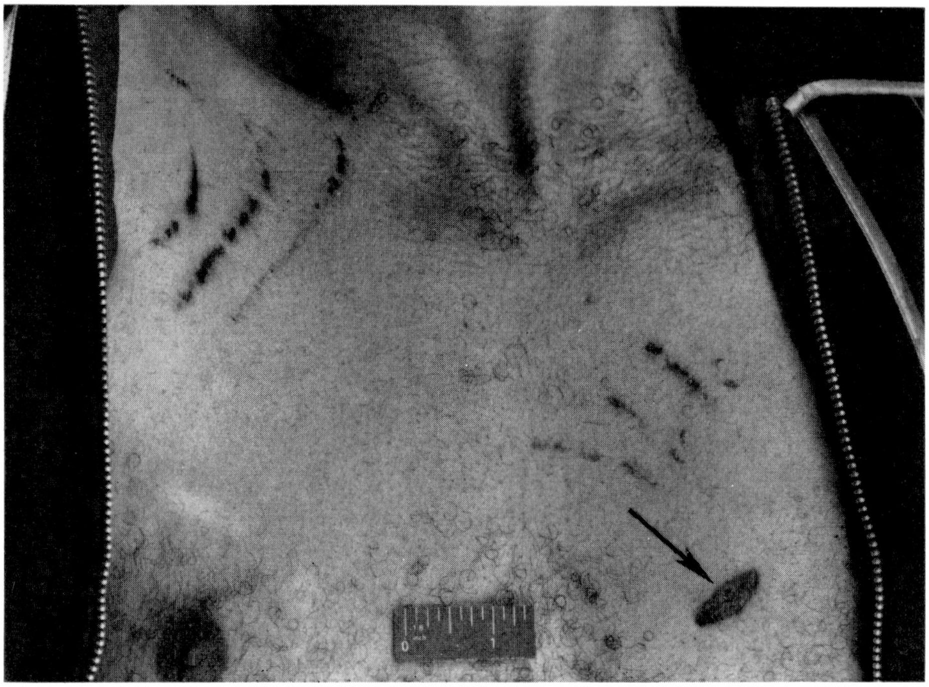

FIGURE VIII-21. The patterned abrasions on both sides of the chest were caused by the zipper teeth of the jacket.

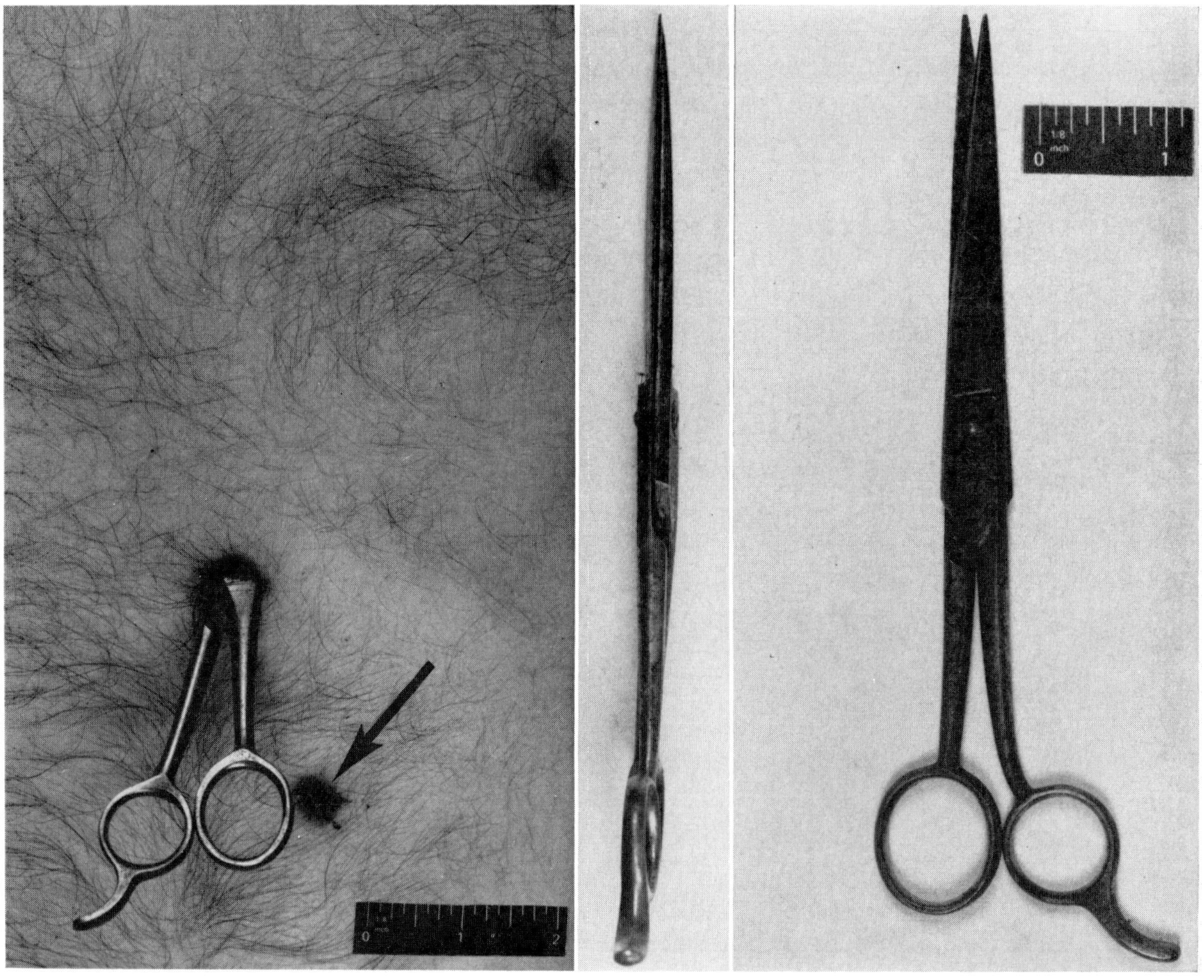

FIGURE VIII-22. This elderly barber died of a self-inflicted stab wound of the chest. The shears penetrated the heart, whereas in the lower wound (arrow) the skin is barely perforated. This shallow wound is probably the result of hesitation and, along with the undisturbed scene, recent depression and history of suicide attempts, substantiates the conclusion of death by suicide. No other injuries were noted on the body. The edges of both injuries are abraded and may be mistaken for bullet wounds.

Self-inflicted stab wounds are distinctly uncommon. When present, they are usually multiple and superficial, although one or possibly two of the injuries may penetrate a vital organ or involve major blood vessels and result in death by blood loss (Fig. VIII-22). Suicidal stabbings are frequently accompanied by cuts in other locations, particularly on the wrists and the throat, less commonly in the bend of the elbows and the ankles.

The appearance of suicidal cuts is usually characteristic: they are multiple parallel cuts of variable depth whose edges commonly reveal several sharp angles as if resulting from *sawing* of the skin with repeated tentative incisions at the same location. Frequently numerous superficial parallel cuts resembling scratches are noted, indicating repeated trials before the buildup of sufficient courage for the final deep gash that severs major blood vessels or exposes the trachea or larynx (Figs. VIII-23 and VIII-24). Such superficial cuts or evidence of *sawing* are referred to as *hesitation wounds* or *hesitation marks.* These cuts are mostly straight because sharp knives and razor blades are used. Suicidal cuts made with a straight razor are unusual, except among some older individuals, due to the decreased popularity of this kind of shaving device. Occasionally, suicidal cuts are jagged and irregular, as when they are made with a piece of broken glass.

Hesitation wounds on the wrists are usually horizontal. Vertical cuts are distinctly rare.

The appearance of suicidal cuts may be misleading. Frequently they appear considerably deeper than they are, and because estimation of the amount of blood at the scene is commonly deceiving, dissection of the wounds to ascertain their depth should be performed (Fig. VIII-25). Death may have been due to a cause other than exsanguination (Figs. VIII-26 and VIII-27).

Horizontal linear scars are sometimes seen on the wrists or the bend of the elbows in sudden unexpected deaths. Such scars may be of particular significance if no immediate cause of death can be determined at autopsy. Under such circumstances suspicion of drug overdose is indicated, and a thorough investigation of the scene and the circumstances, in conjunction with toxicological analyses of tissues from the body, should be carried out. Attempts at suicide are frequently repeated until successful, and a

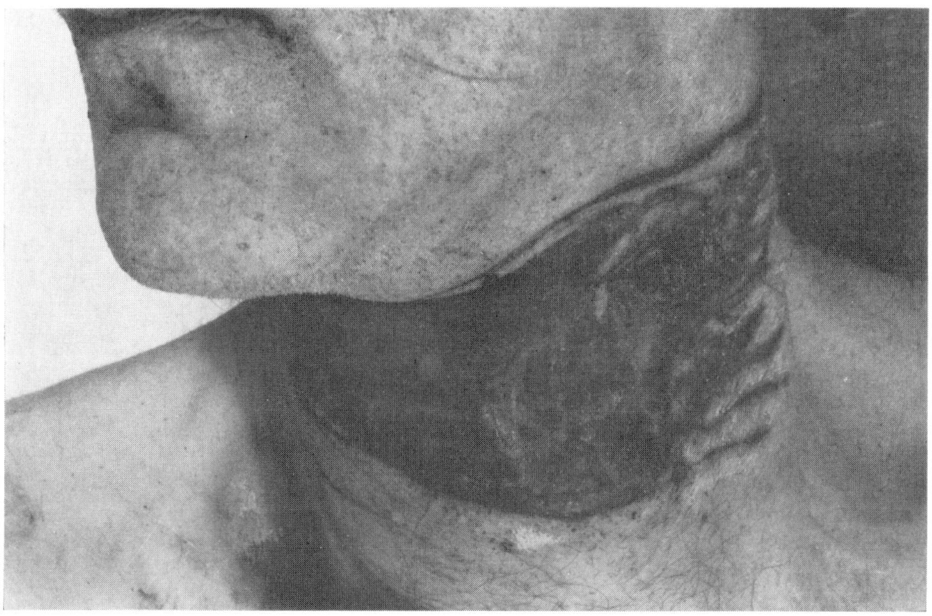

FIGURE VIII-23. Suicide by multiple cuts of throat, showing the typical *sawing* effect. Only a single cut was deep and involved the airway, causing inhalation of blood and death by suffocation.

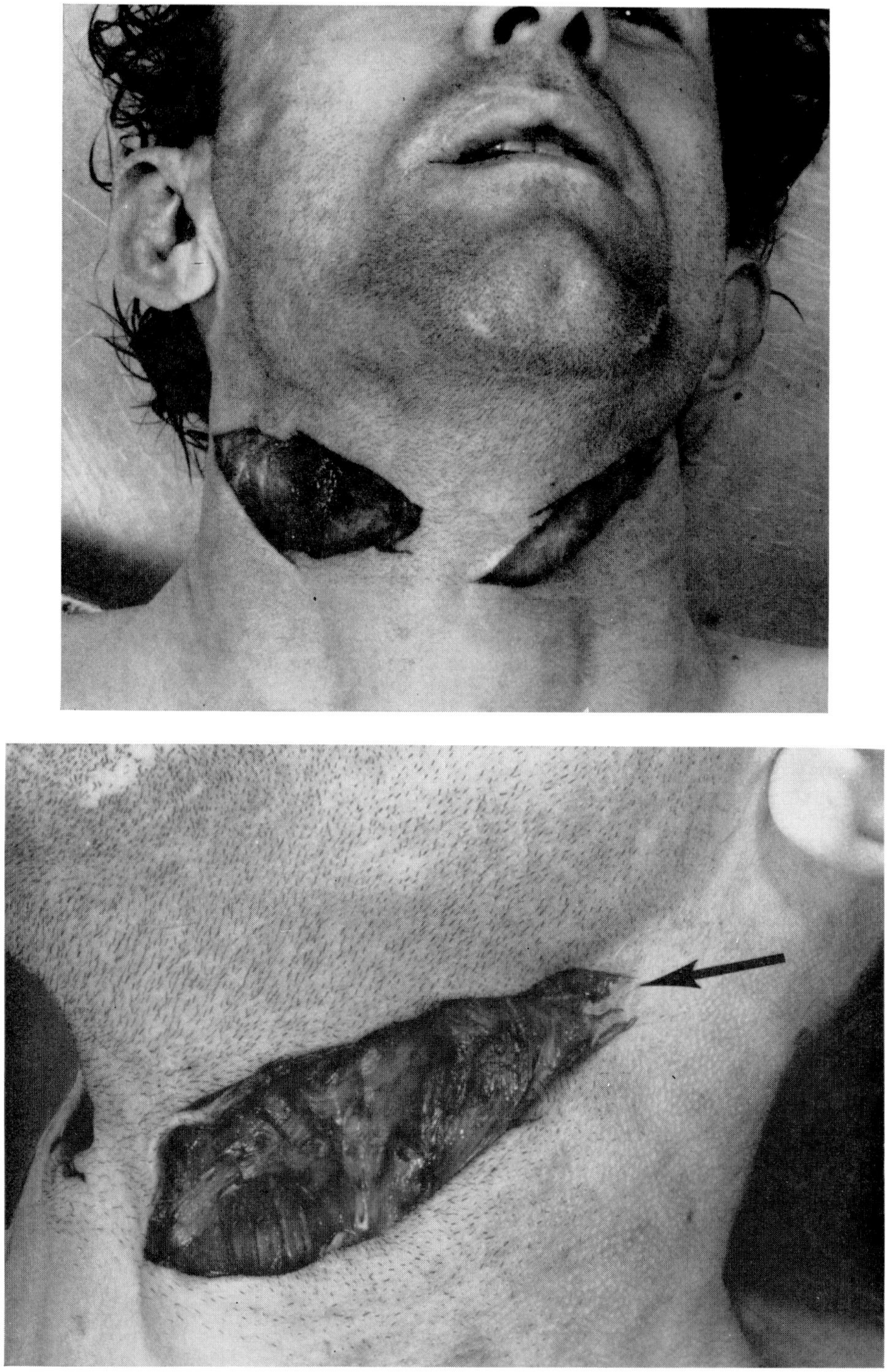

FIGURE VIII-24. Hesitation cuts are visible at the end of a fatal suicidal wound of the neck (arrow).

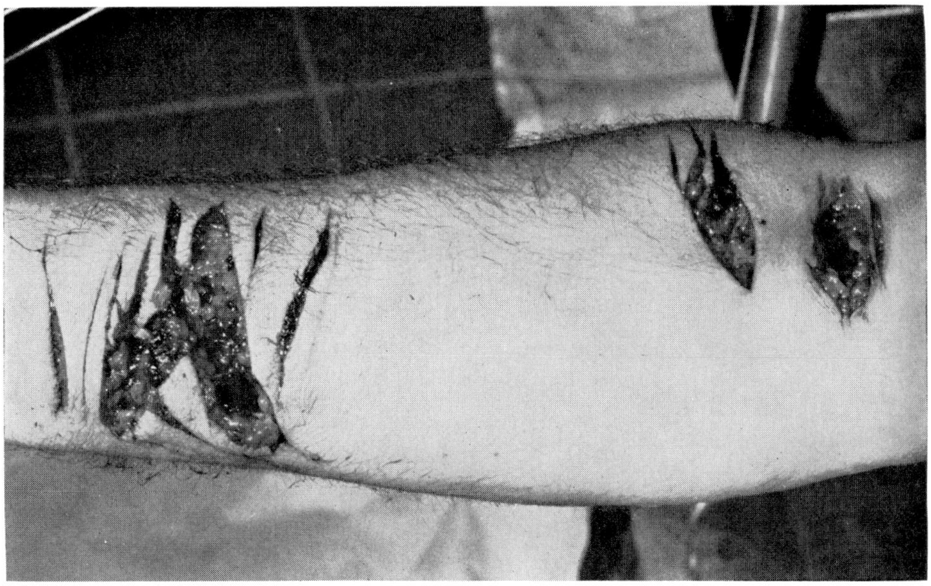

FIGURE VIII-25. Multiple hesitation cuts of forearm produced by razor blade; although they mostly appear to be deep, autopsy showed that none extend beyond the fat layer under the skin and no major blood vessels were involved. This individual stabbed himself with a pair of scissors in the chest and right temple and used a razor blade to slash his throat. Only the combined bleeding resulted in sufficient blood loss to cause death. He was still alive when found and only said, "God will hate me for this."

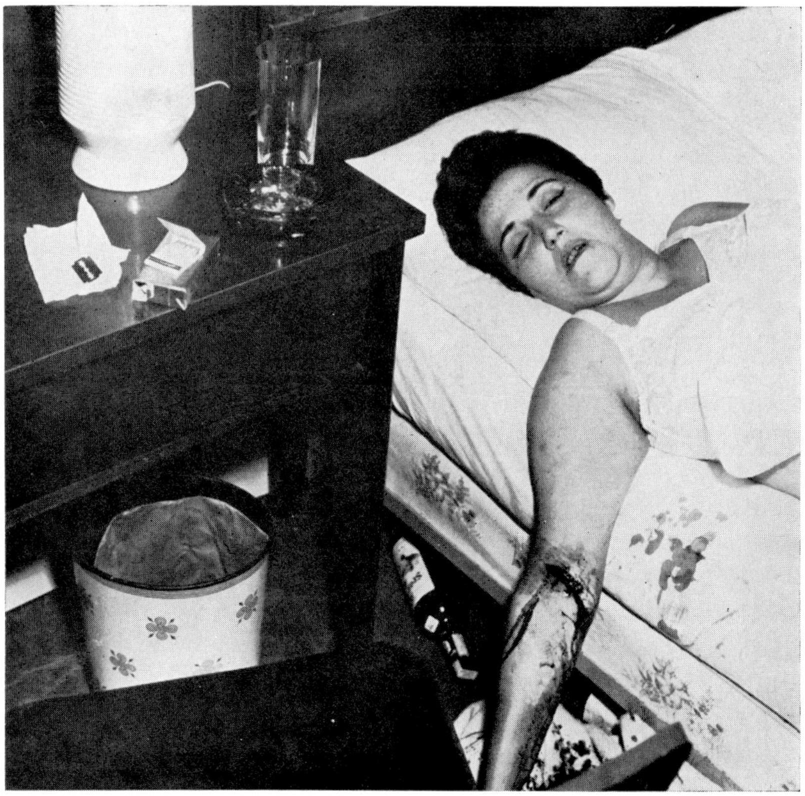

FIGURE VIII-26. Thirty-two-year-old woman found dead in a motel room. She had checked into the motel twenty-four hours earlier with a male companion. There was very little blood at the scene. Autopsy showed only one severed medium-sized superficial vein. The cause of death was acute alcoholic intoxication, with a blood alcohol level of 0.45%. A blanket was neatly folded under the arm, apparently to absorb the expected bleeding, and the bloodstained razor blade was placed on a handkerchief on the dresser.

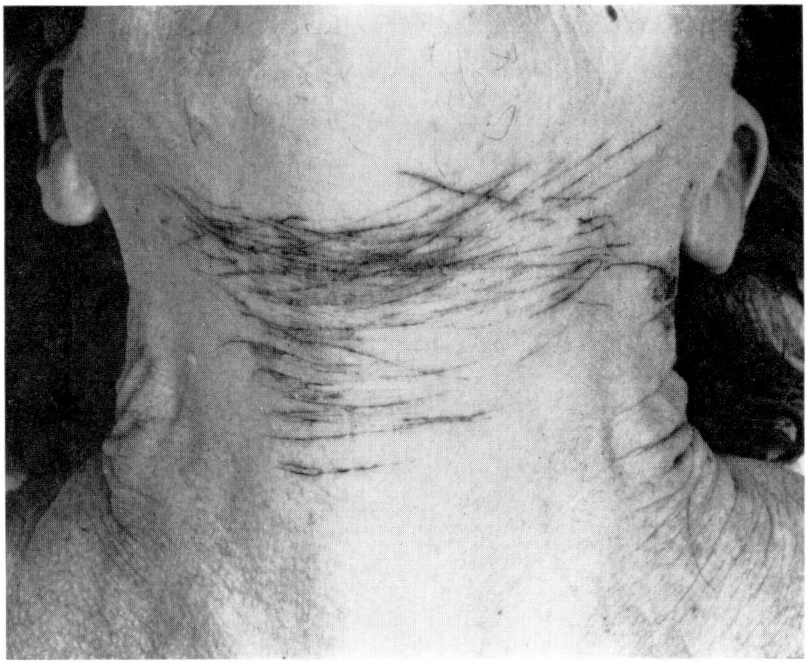

FIGURE VIII-27. Attempted suicide of a seventy-five-year-old woman. Numerous superficial parallel cuts of the throat inflicted with a razor blade. The injuries resemble linear scratches. Death was due to natural causes (arteriosclerotic heart disease), apparently associated with the emotional stress of the attempt to terminate her life.

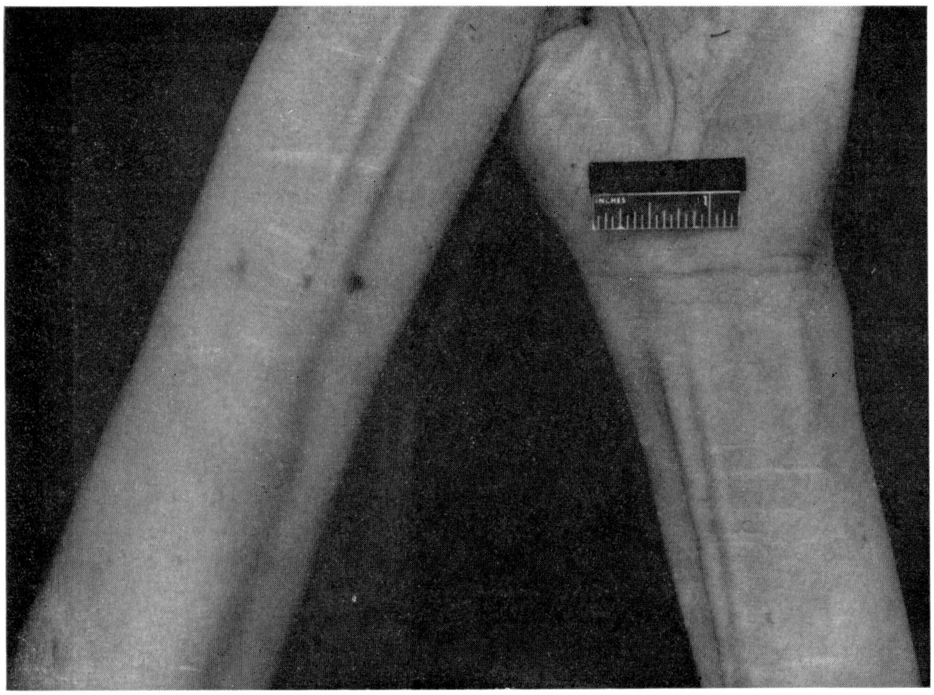

FIGURE VIII-28. Multiple horizontal scars on wrists and forearms indicative of suicide attempt(s) in the past. Cause of death was overdose of barbiturates.

variety of means may be employed by the same individual (Figs. VIII-28 and VIII-29).

A twenty-seven-year-old male with a history of repeated episodes of depression jumped out of a fifth-floor window after razor blade cuts of his wrists and throat failed to produce the desired effect.

In another case a forty-two-year-old woman was found with her head submerged in the bloody water of her bathtub. Her wrists, ankles and neck showed hesitation wounds. There was a star-shaped bullet wound on her forehead (the weapon had been fired with the muzzle in contact with the skin), and at autopsy a .38 caliber bullet was recovered from the brain. In addition, she had consumed a large number of sleeping pills.

Narcotic addicts sometimes simulate suicide attempts for the purpose of drawing attention to themselves. A young individual with multiple superficial, horizontal and parallel scars on the wrists may have died of a heroin overdose (Fig. VIII-30).

Deep and extremely mutilating, widely gaping cuts such as slash wounds are rare in suicides, in contradistinction to cases of homicide, where such injuries are not uncommon. The sweeping manner and the malicious intent with which these injuries are inflicted are usually self-evident.

While it is not usually possible to establish whether such cuts run from right to left or vice versa, a superficial extension is sometimes noted at the terminal end of the wound. Most homicidal throat slashings are produced with the assailant in back of the victim (Fig. VIII-31). Homicidal cuts of the throat are often single and deep, indicating determination. Exceptions to this are sometimes noted if the assailant is markedly intoxicated or demented (Fig. VIII-32).

Superficial injuries such as cuts and localized burning or beating are sometimes used as a means of torture to extract information. The cause of death is usually readily recognizable in these cases. An *execution-style* gunshot wound inflicted at contact or close range in the back of the head is common. Such deaths are mostly associated with the illicit drug traffic.

Simple background information, including a study of the circumstances and the scene where the body was found, is essential in all these situations because the injuries themselves may be most confusing. The cuts on the neck shown in Fig. VIII-33 would well be interpreted as hesitation cuts, and the picture could have been further complicated by other indications of suicide, as, for example, a contact shot of the temple or a fall from a height.

### Identification of the Weapon

It is relatively common that an assailant is apprehended while in possession of the sus-

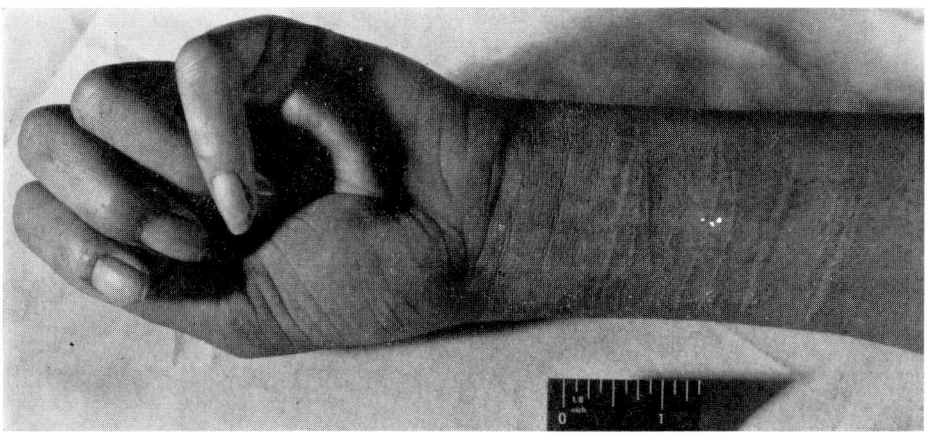

FIGURE VIII-29. Linear, mostly horizontal and parallel scars on the wrist due to previous suicide attempts. The wounds were surgically sutured, which is indicative of their severity. Suicidal cuts that are survived are more commonly superficial, requiring no surgical attention.

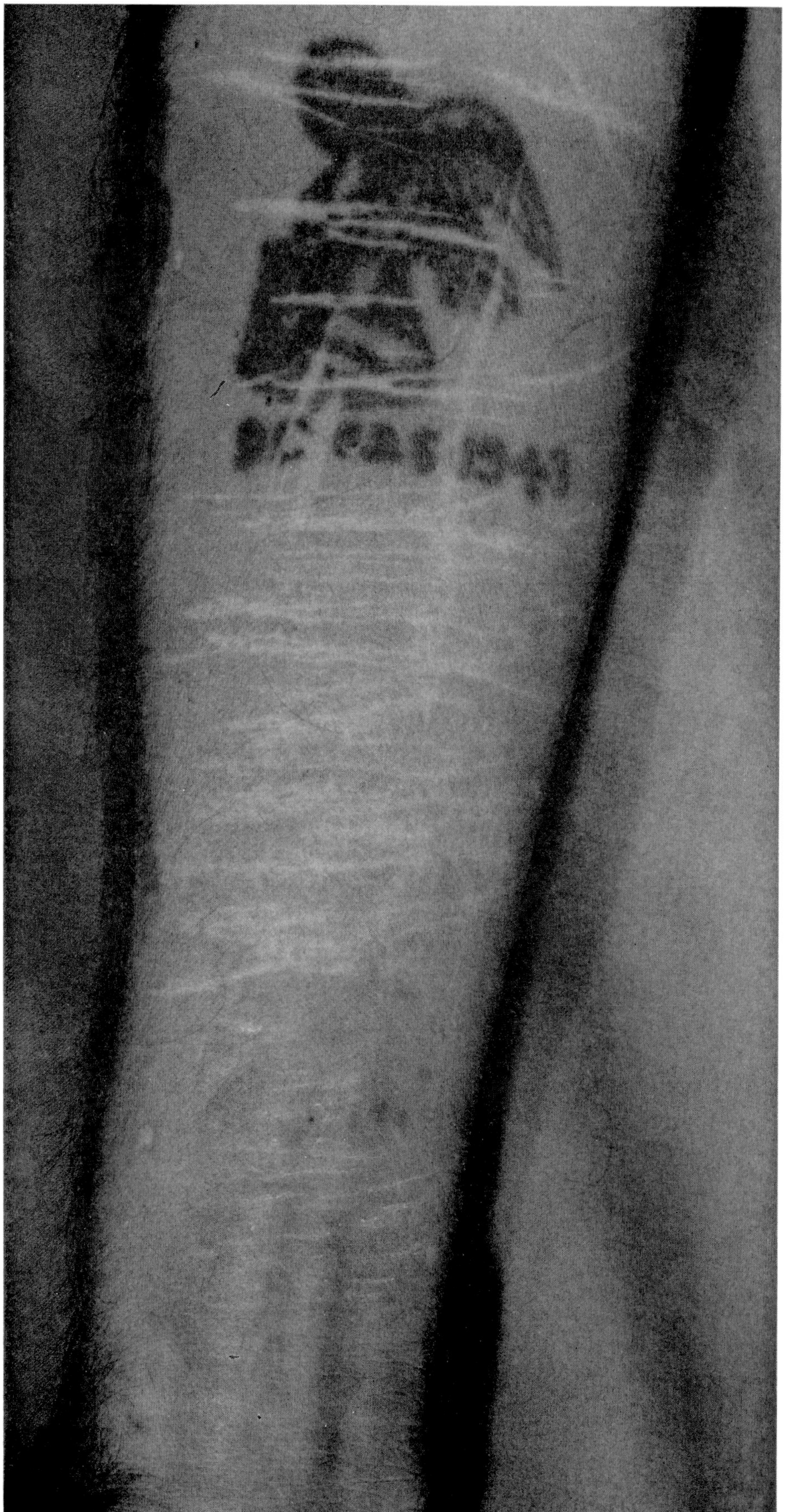

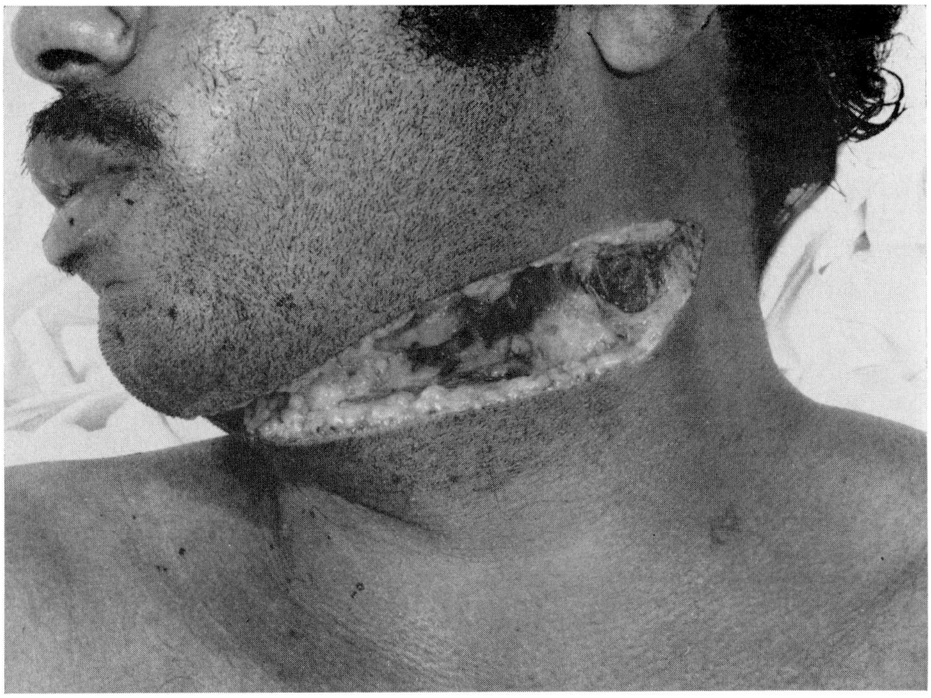

FIGURE VIII-31. Homicidal slashing of the throat.

pected weapon. Only rarely is the knife left in the victim. Sometimes the blade breaks and is lodged within the wound track. In a large number of cases, however, identification of the weapon is based on the postmortem examination of the wounds.

A stab wound inflicted with a pair of scissors, a screwdriver or another elongated, relatively dull and thick object can be distinguished from one produced by a knife. The edges of a knife wound are sharp and nonabraded, whereas the edges of a scissors or screwdriver wound become abraded as they are scraped by the dull surface of the weapon (Figs. VIII-34 and VIII-35).

The pattern or distribution of wounds may also suggest a specific type of instrument. In the case of stab wounds inflicted with a two-pronged fork, such as a barbeque or a meat fork, the distance between each of the two punctures in the skin must be carefully measured. The distance between the punctures varies depend-

---

←

FIGURE VIII-30. Narcotic addict with multiple discrete linear scars of the forearm resulting from superficial cuts. This had occurred two years before death from a drug overdose. This number of scars is distinctly unusual: two or three delicate, often faint lines are far more common.

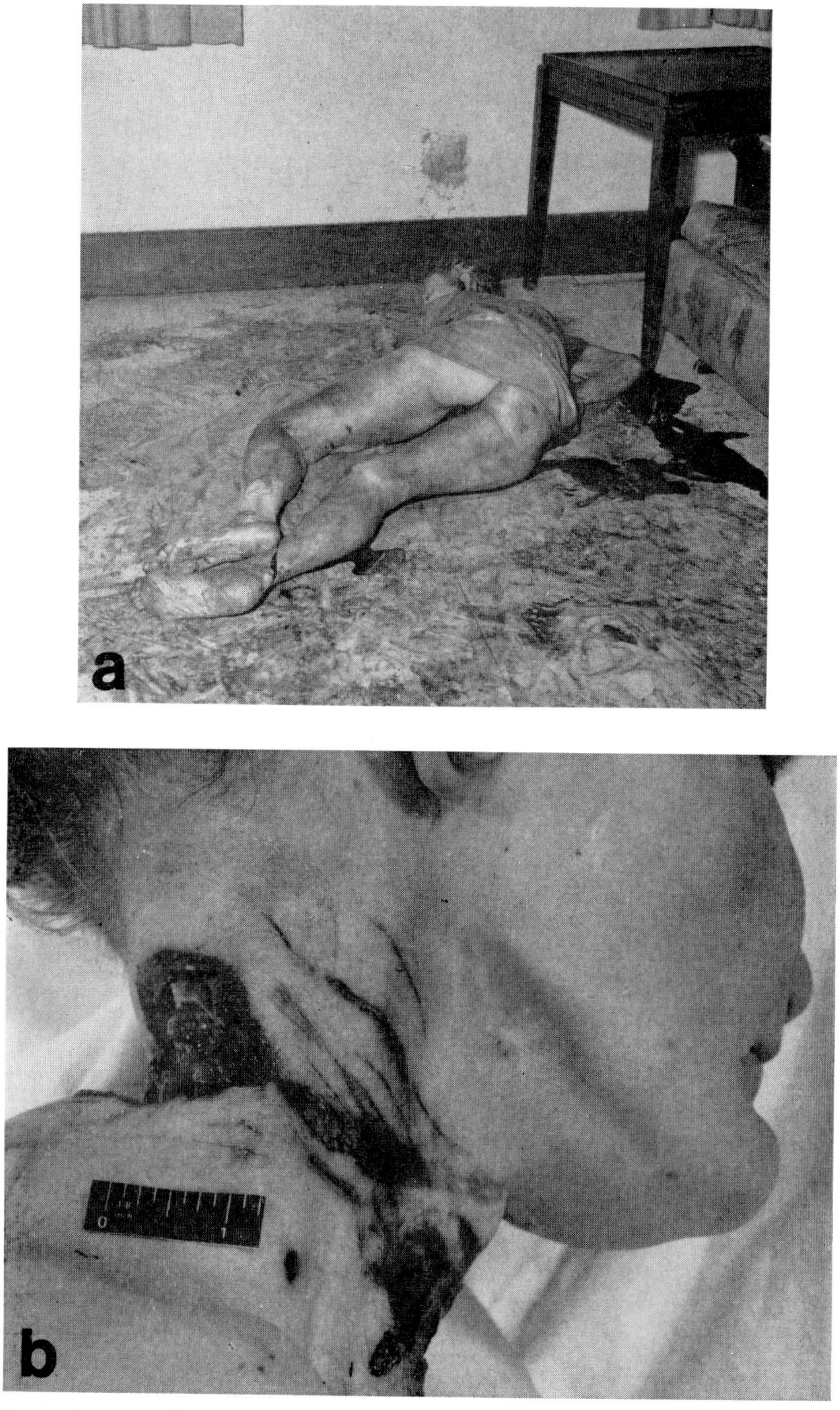


FIGURE VIII-32. This murder occurred in a nursing home for the mentally ill. A violent struggle, as evidenced by the blood smeared on the floor, wall and furniture, preceded the killing.

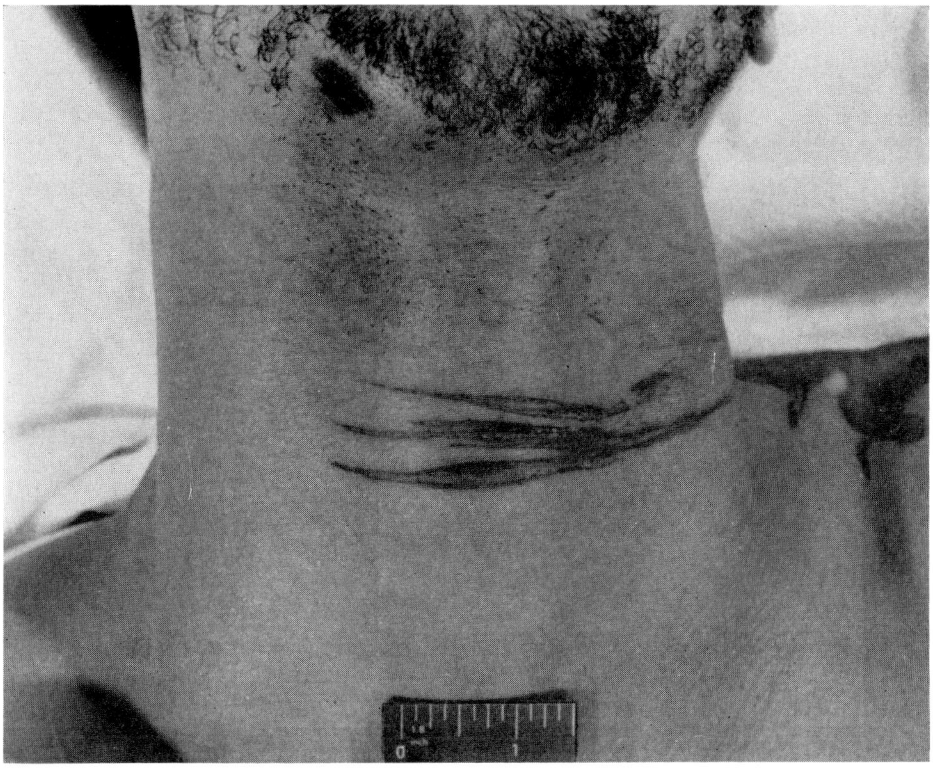

FIGURE VIII-33. Superficial cuts of the neck, apparently inflicted to extract information from a narcotic pusher, whose dismembered body was found wrapped in plastic bags in a city dumpster. Death was due to multiple hammer blows on the head.

ing on the angle of stabbing. The edges of these wounds are abraded (Figs. VIII-36, VIII-37 and VIII-38).

The most consistent feature of stab wounds caused by open scissors is a pair of wounds with one wound always above and somewhat oblique to the other. As in the case of wounds produced with a two-pronged fork, the distance between each of the two wounds differs with the angle of stabbing. Obviously, the distance between the scissor blades is variable unless the scissors are locked into position. The edges of the wounds are scraped because of the width of the blades (Figs. VIII-39 and VIII-40).

Cuts made by broken glass sometimes resemble knife wounds. This may be further com-

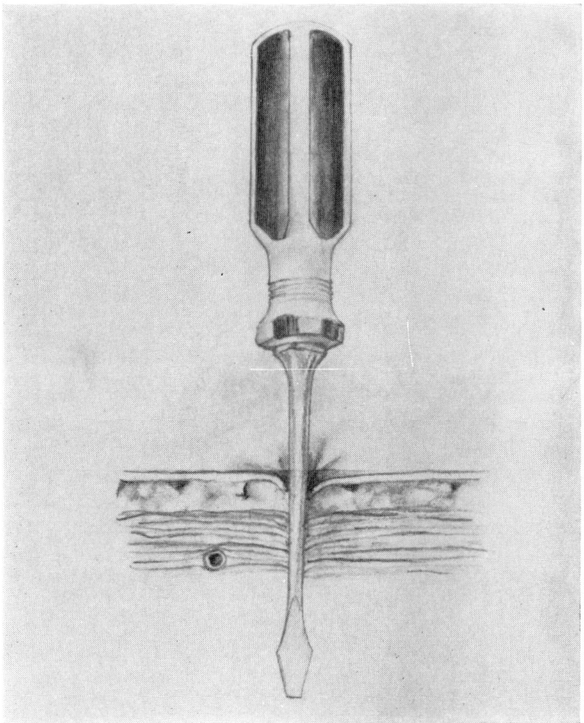

FIGURE VIII-34. Scraping of the edges of the stab wound along the surface of a blunt implement produces marginal abrasion of the injury.

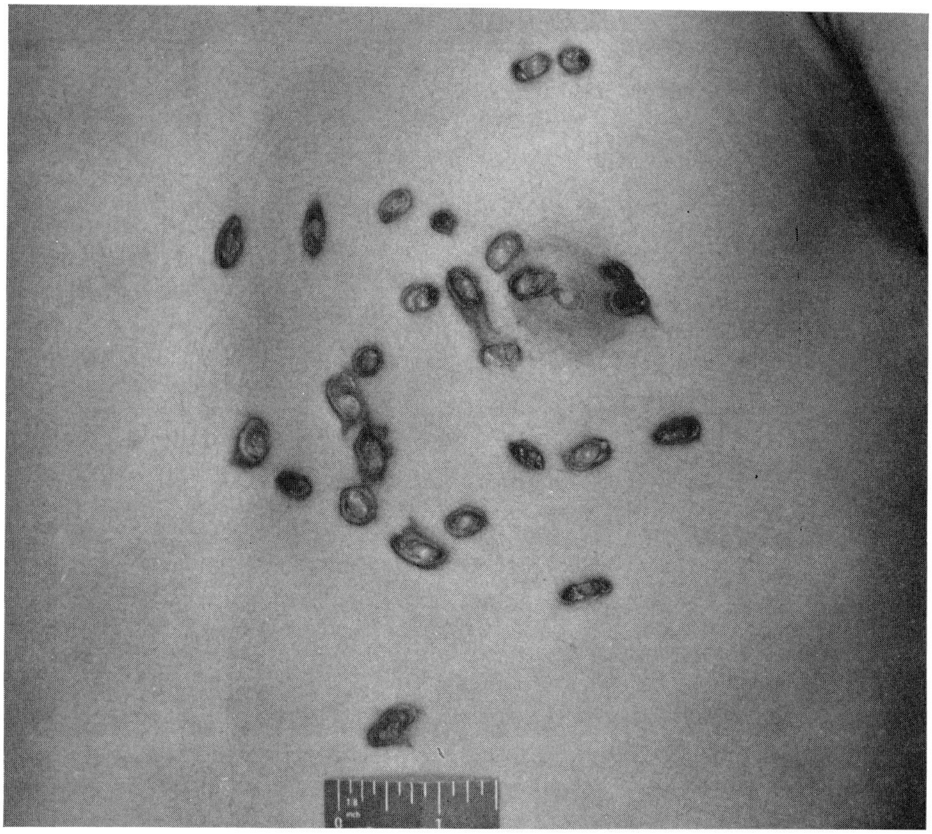

FIGURE VIII-35. Multiple stab wounds made by a screwdriver, all centered around the left nipple. Each wound has abraded edges, which are dark due to drying. The large number of stab wounds in this case represents considerable "overkill," suggestive of a crime of passion. If the victim is male, a homosexual motive may be considered.

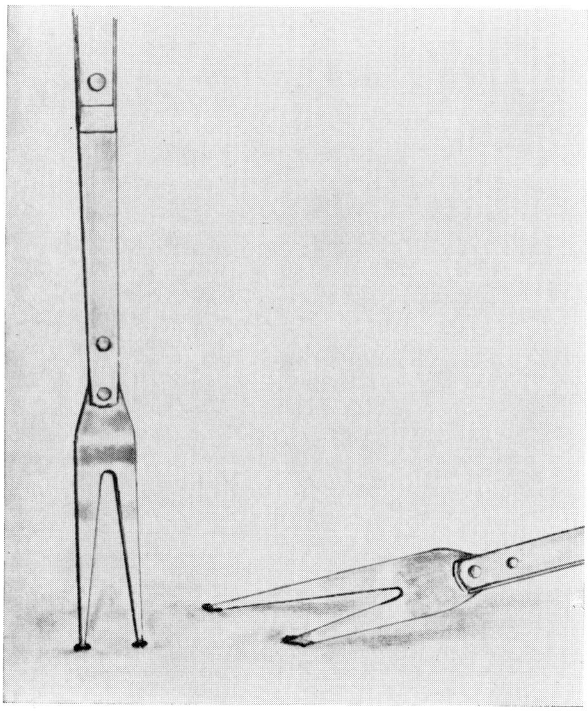

FIGURE VIII-36. Stab wounds by a meat or barbeque fork are paired, and their edges are abraded. The distance of each injury from the other differs, depending on the angle of stabbing.

pounded by the fact that small scratches from thin glass splinters may suggest fingernail marks. Wounds suspected of being caused by glass, and the intact surrounding areas and clothes, should be carefully inspected for splinters and larger fragments of glass. If found, such pieces should be kept for possible later use as evidence.

Wounds produced by broken glass are irregular and jagged, their edges sharp and not abraded (Fig. VIII-41). Their depths may vary, but they rarely penetrate a body cavity. Another injury of characteristic configuration is the wound resulting from a blow of a *chopping instrument.* Meat cleavers, axes and machetes fall into this category. Their use results in a

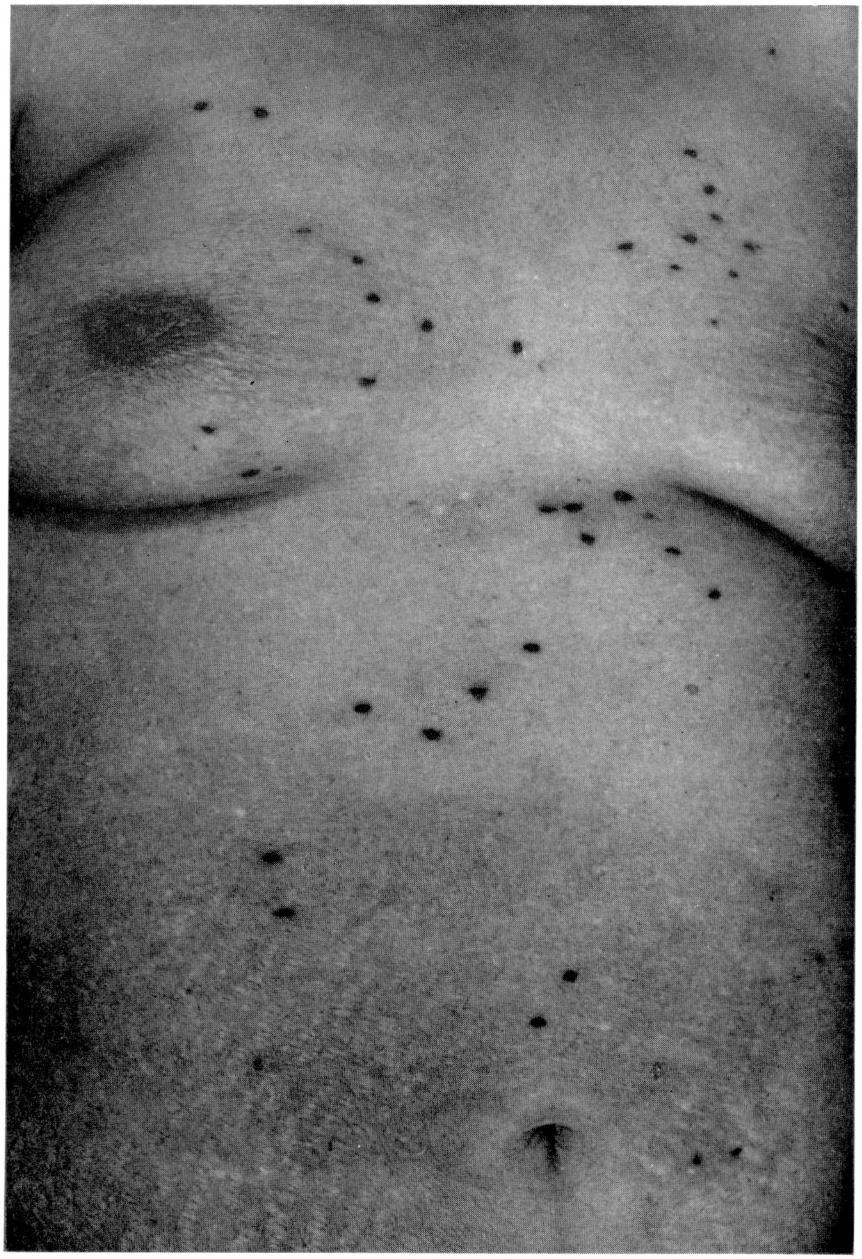

FIGURE VIII-37. Multiple paired punctures produced with a barbecue fork.

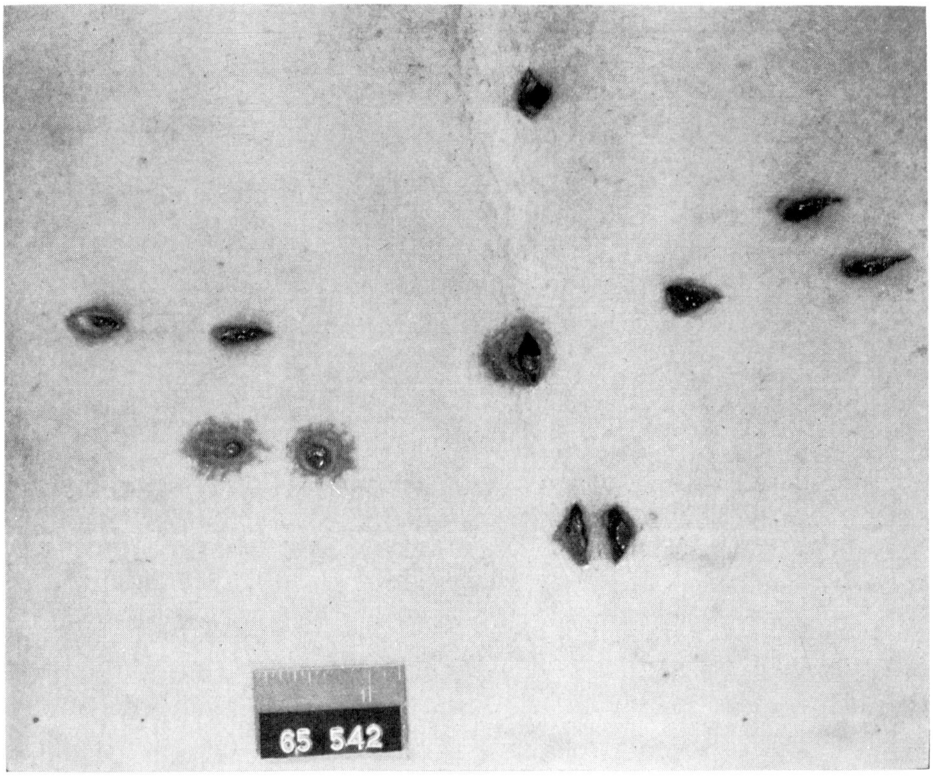


FIGURE VIII-38. Multiple stab wounds of the back in an elderly woman, inflicted during a robbery. The weapon was probably a carving fork, as suggested by the grouping in pairs of many of the injuries and their depths.

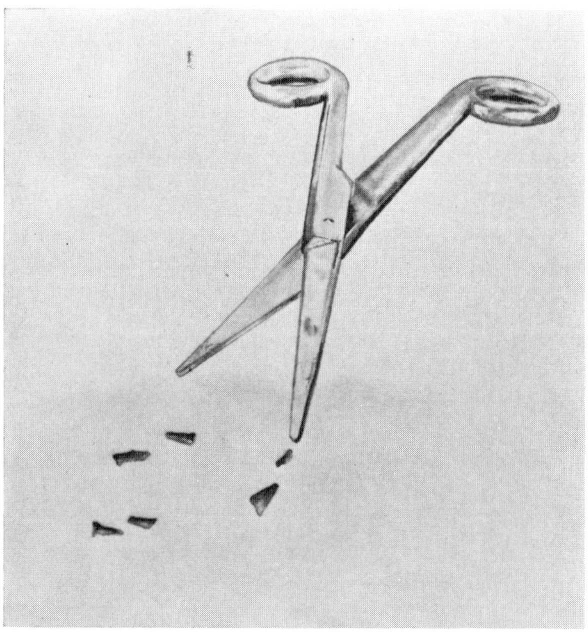

FIGURE VIII-39. Characteristic stab wounds with scissors are paired, abraded injuries. Each wound is oblique and somewhat above the other.

gaping wound of malicious appearance (Figs. VIII-42, VIII-43 and VIII-44), often showing fine abrasion of the edges and commonly associated with typical chopping injuries of underlying bones.

Due to its rigidity, bone maintains the dimensions and shape of a stab wound far better than skin or other soft tissue. In fact, it is often possible to determine the type of weapon used to inflict an injury by examining the wound in the bone. This is especially true of the skull (Fig. VIII-45).

A homicidal stab wound is rarely inflicted without some cutting taking place at the same time. The knife may be pulled upward or downward during insertion or withdrawal, thereby causing an injury that is longer than the widest part of the blade (Figs. VIII-46 and VIII-47).

The width of the back of the blade, however, i.e. its thickness, is *retained* in the stab wound. Realignment of the wound edges, at the same

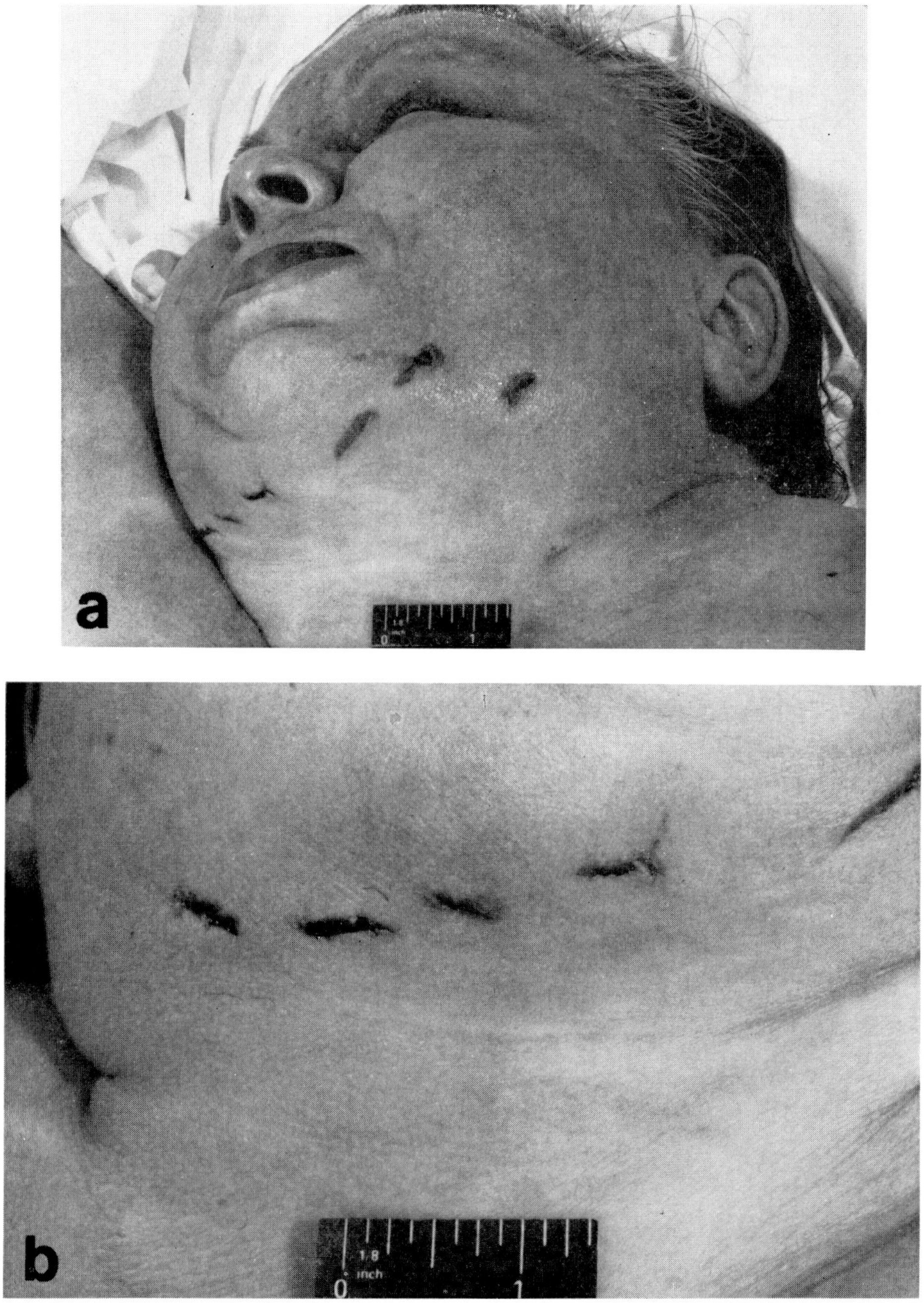


FIGURE VIII-40. (a): Stab wounds of the lower jaw inflicted with a pair of semiopened pointed scissors. (b): The wounds are jagged and slightly abraded. In addition to being arranged in pairs, one wound is always above and somewhat oblique to the other.

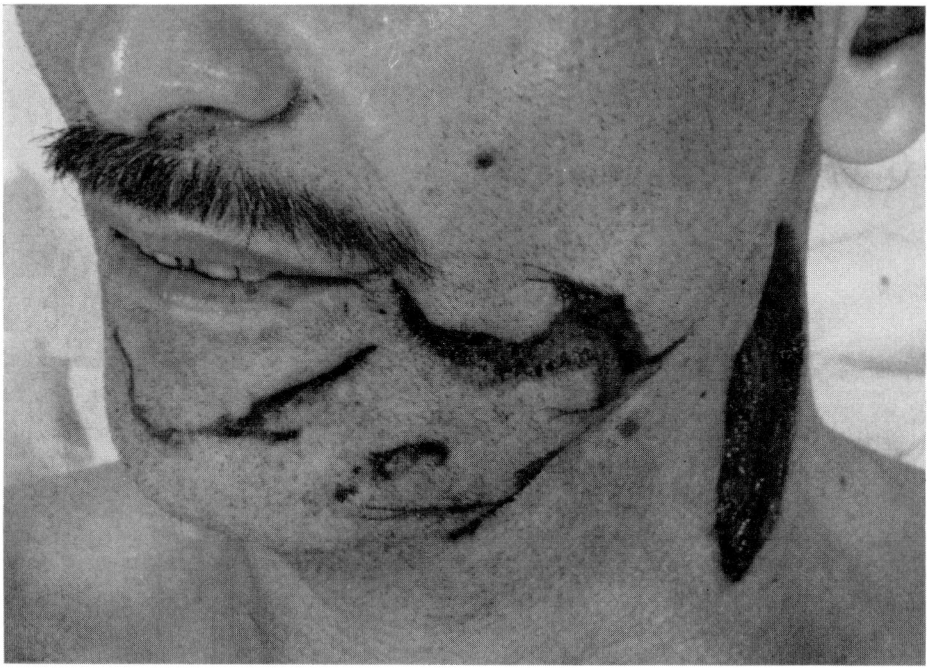

FIGURE VIII-41. Irregular jagged cuts produced with a broken wine bottle.

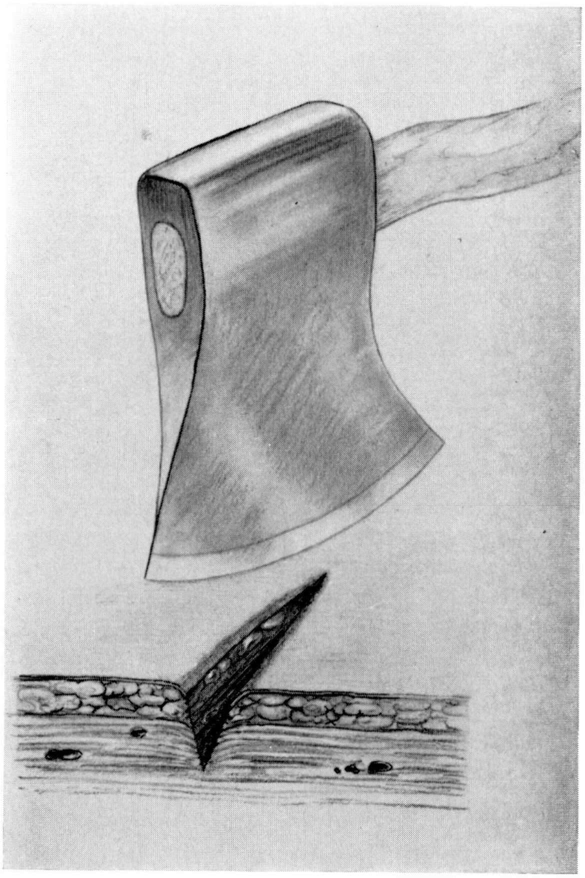

FIGURE VIII-42. A blow with an axe causes a sharp cut with fine abrasion of the wound edges due to the thickness of the blade.

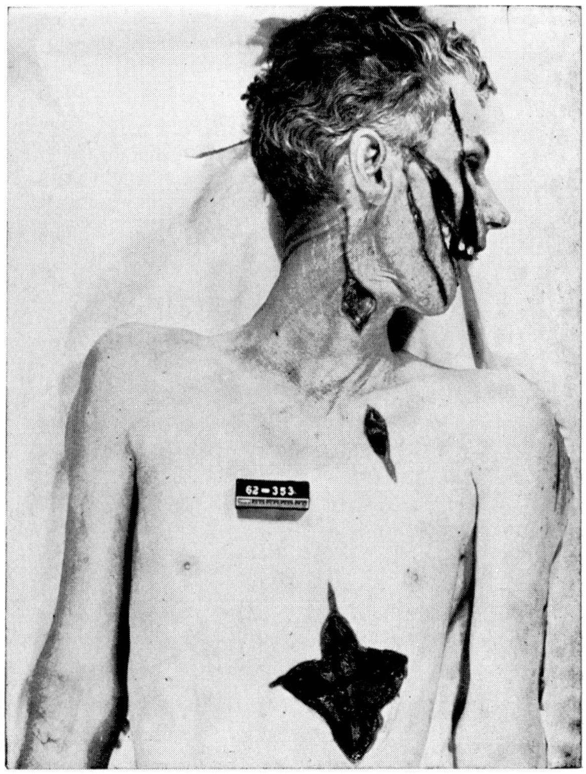

FIGURE VIII-43. Homicidal injuries produced by a meat cleaver. Note the size and the depth of the injuries. The finely abraded margins of the chest wounds are due to the wedgelike thickness of the blade of this particular type of weapon.

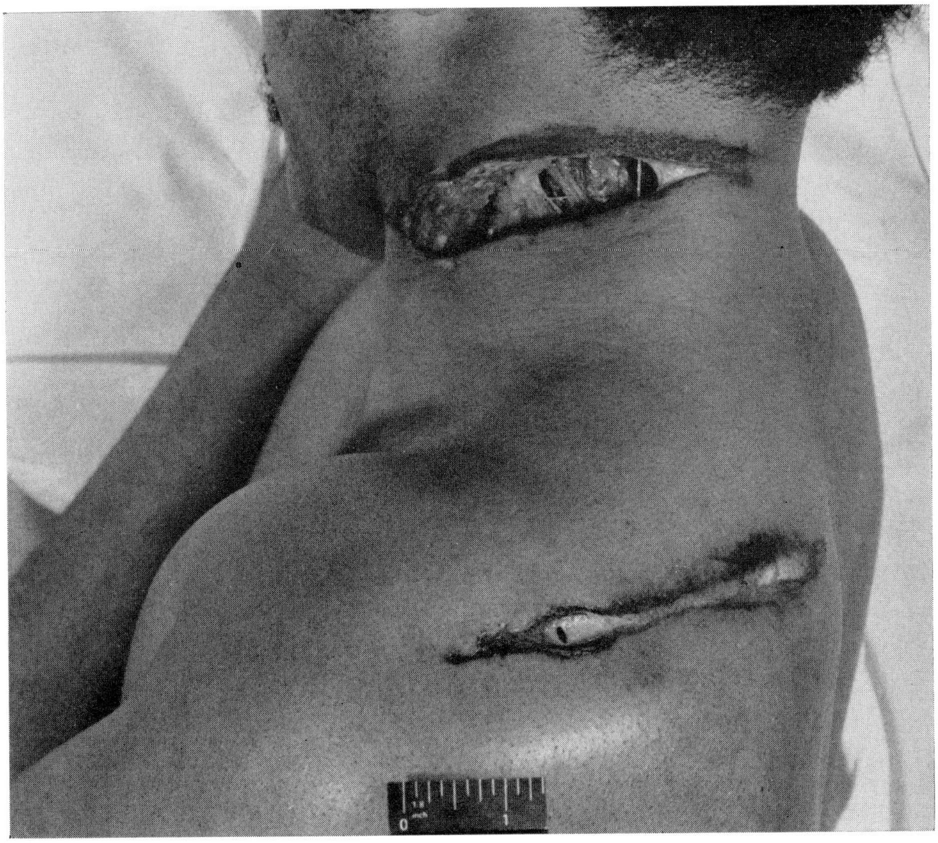

FIGURE VIII-44. This man was struck by the propeller of a small plane as he was attempting to start the engine. The wound edges are sharp, as in a cut, but are abraded due to the thickness of the blades. Injuries such as these are commonly referred to as *chop wounds.*

time exerting slight twisting of the same, will usually allow fairly accurate assessment of the thickness of the blade, thereby permitting distinction of one knife from another provided the blades are of sufficiently different thickness (Fig. VIII-48).

Stab wounds and cuts will either remain slit shaped with two acute angles or will gape open, depending on their location and their orientation with respect to the so-called *cleavage lines of Langer.* These are lines of tension that are determined by the direction of the elastic and collagenous fibers in the skin. Their locations and pathways are well established (Fig. VIII-49).

The cleavage lines correspond to the creases of the body surface. Surgeons are well aware of the directions of the cleavage lines in the various regions of the body, because an incision parallel to the lines heals with a fine linear scar, whereas an incision across the lines may result in considerable deformity and an unsightly scar.

A stab wound that severs the elastic fibers by cutting through the cleavage lines transversely will gape, whereas one that runs parallel to them will remain slit or wedge shaped and will represent with considerable accuracy the dimensions of the blade with which it was inflicted. In attempting to *restore* a given knife wound it is therefore often necessary to return the skin surrounding the injury to its position before the skin was divided. The edges of the wound may be manually approximated, or they may be held together with transparent adhesive tape (Figs. VIII-50 to VIII-53). The new dimensions of the stab wound should be measured for the record, and the *restored* injury should be photographed, whenever possible, for later use

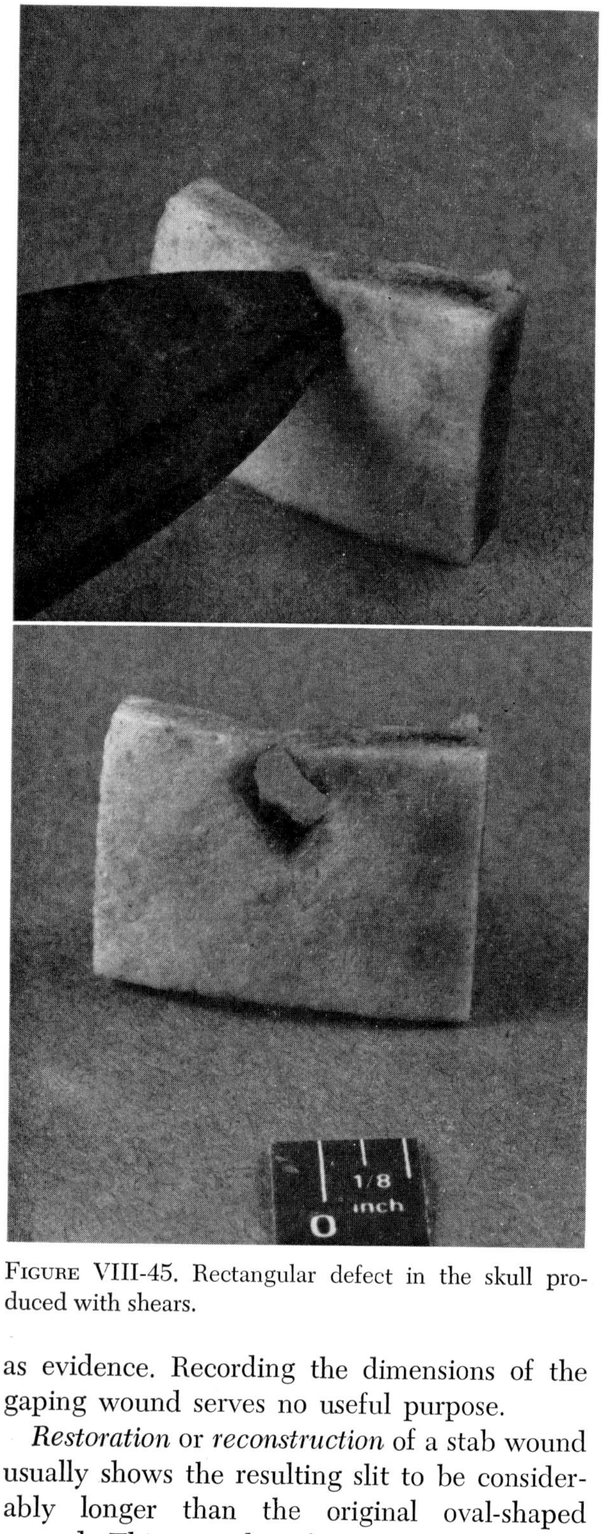


FIGURE VIII-45. Rectangular defect in the skull produced with shears.

as evidence. Recording the dimensions of the gaping wound serves no useful purpose.

*Restoration* or *reconstruction* of a stab wound usually shows the resulting slit to be considerably longer than the original oval-shaped wound. This may be of great significance to counter a possible later claim that the suggested knife could not have produced a stab wound of such small dimensions.

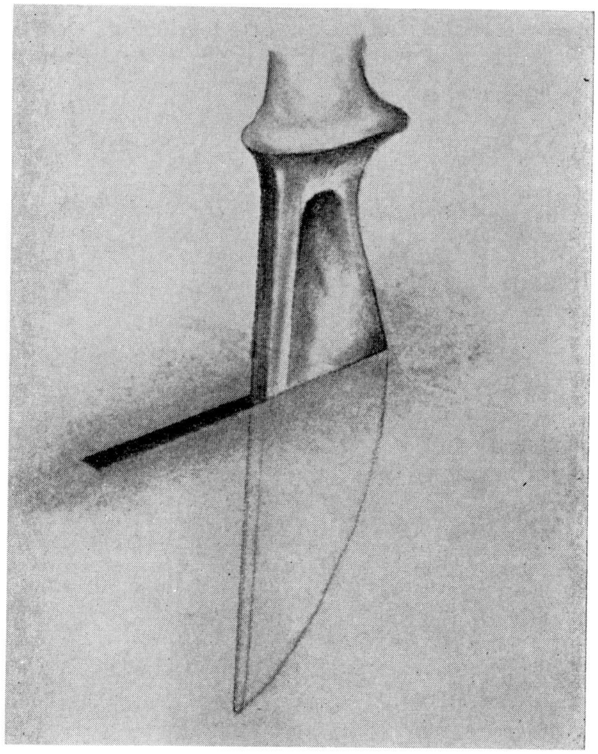

FIGURE VIII-46. Stab wounds are often a combination of stabbing and some cutting. The length of the wound in the skin is therefore not necessarily indicative of the width of the blade that caused the injury.

Thick, relatively blunt-edged blades such as bayonets may cause cross-shaped wounds,[1] because cutting and tearing of the skin occur simultaneously and at right angles to each other.[2]

Strangely shaped stab wounds such as *A*- or *V*-shaped wounds are sometimes seen. These are commonly interpreted as resulting from two distinct stabbings in the same location. Experimentation, however, indicates that stabbing, followed by simultaneous twisting and cutting, gives rise to an atypical injury as shown in Figures VIII-54, VIII-55 and VIII-56. During the process of stabbing there is considerable relative movement between the individuals involved in the struggle. Following a thrust of the knife, the victim may fall, causing the blade to be twisted in his body, or the assailant may twist the blade during withdrawal, cutting the skin at the same time. Countless possibilities exist, all capable of causing atypically shaped

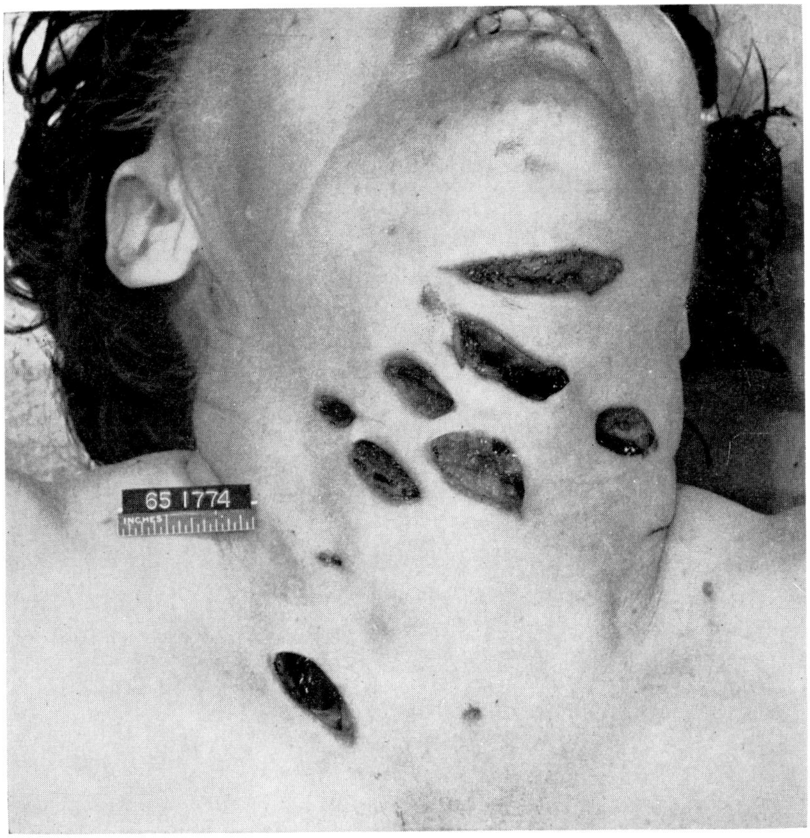


Figure VIII-47. Homicide: Multiple variously sized stab wounds of the neck produced with the same knife.

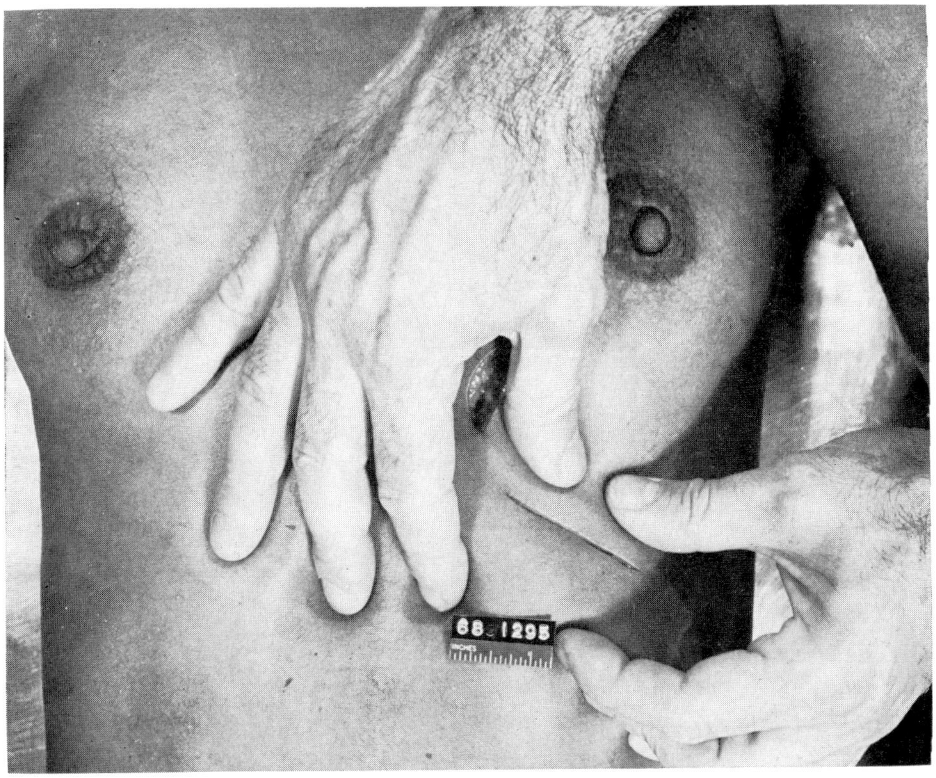


Figure VIII-48. Two gaping stab wounds of the chest caused by the same knife, each of different length. Both wounds represent a combination of stabbing and some cutting. Twisting of the edges of the lower wound while at the same time approximating the edges reestablishes anatomical relationships that existed before the injury and permits assessment of the thickness of the blade. The dimensions of the gaping wound before such *restoration* are useless.

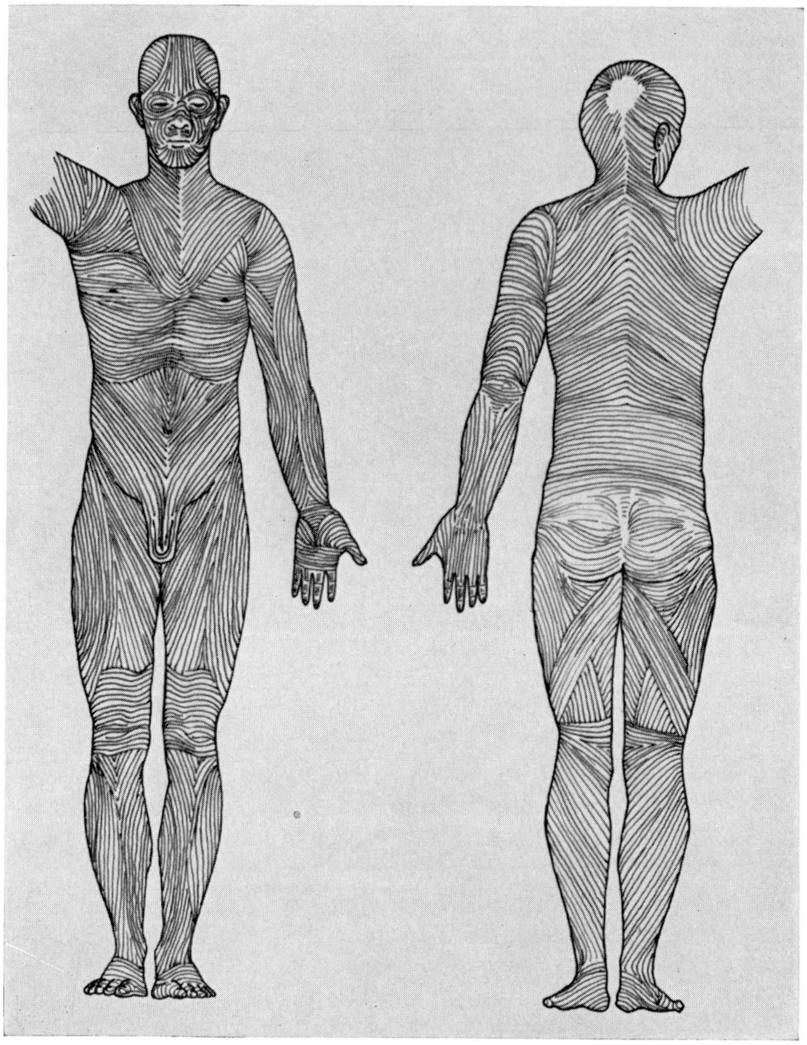

FIGURE VIII-49. Lines of cleavage (Langer).

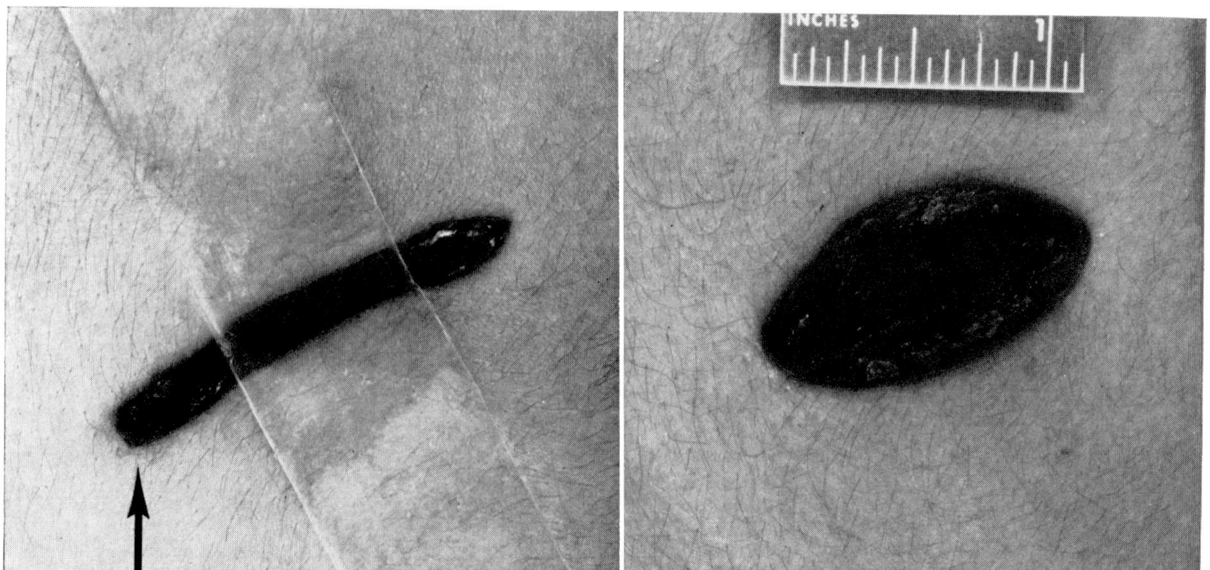


FIGURE VIII-50. Stab wound of the chest: On the right the injury is gaping and boat-shaped; on the left it is *reconstructed* with adhesive tape, indicating the thickness of the blade (arrow). The wound on the left is considerably longer.

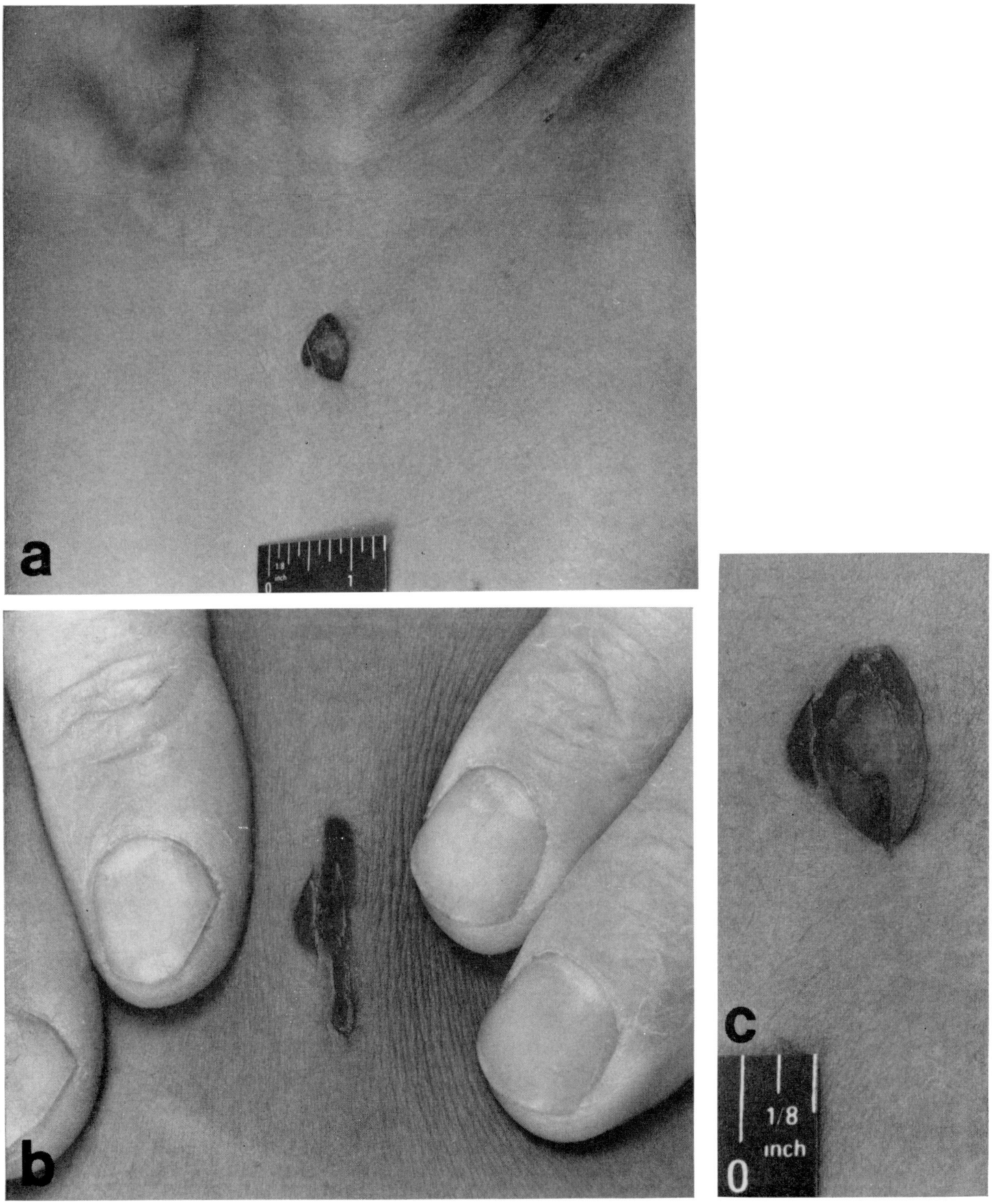


FIGURE VIII-51. (a): Stab wound of the chest produced with a pocket knife. A half-moon-shaped hilt mark can be seen on the left side of the injury. (b): After approximation of the edges, the wound appears significantly longer, and (c) the *back of the blade* may be recognized at the upper end. (Parts b and c are reproduced in the same scale.)

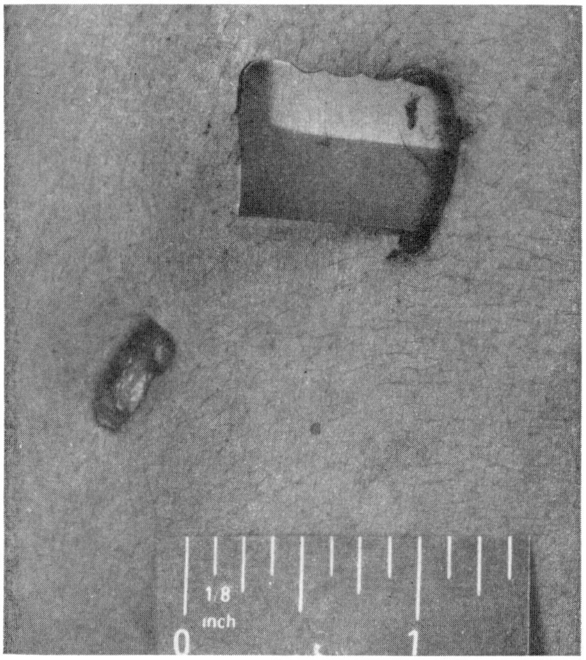


FIGURE VIII-52a. The dimensions of the uppermost stab wound are maintained by the serrated blade, whereas the edges of the lower stab wound have collapsed due to the elastic nature of the skin. A stab wound or cut produced by a serrated blade cannot be distinguished from an injury produced by a nonserrated one. Scalloped edges of a stab wound are due to twisting of the knife or movement of the victim rather than to the shape of the cutting edge. The combination of vibration and extraordinary sharp serrated blades of electric knives account for their more devastating and deeper cuts than those produced with ordinary knives.

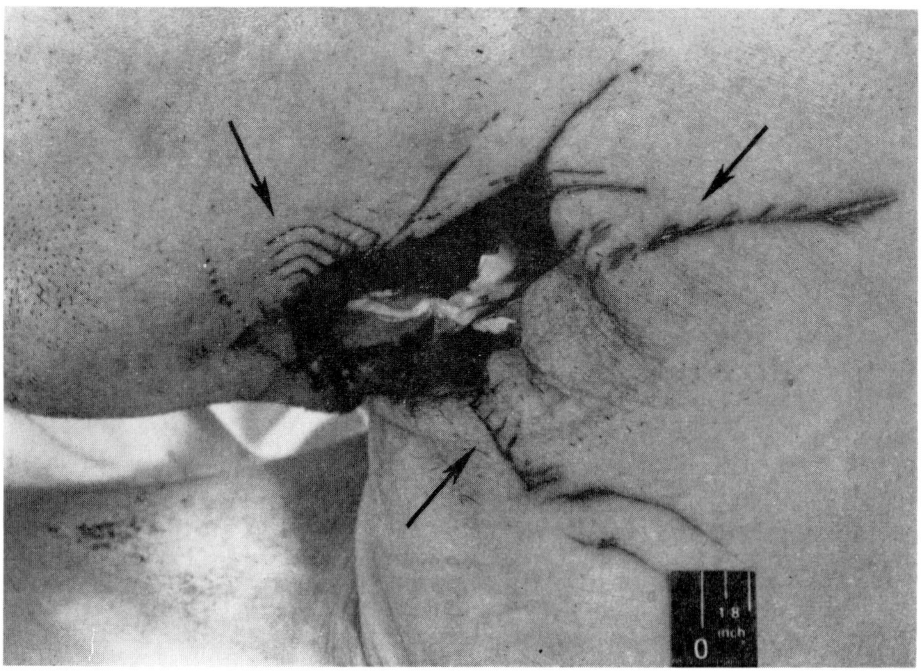


FIGURE VIII-52b. Homicidal slashing of the throat with a serrated knife. The patterned parallel scratches (arrows) were produced by the high points of the serrated edge and permit identification of the type of weapon used in the murder.

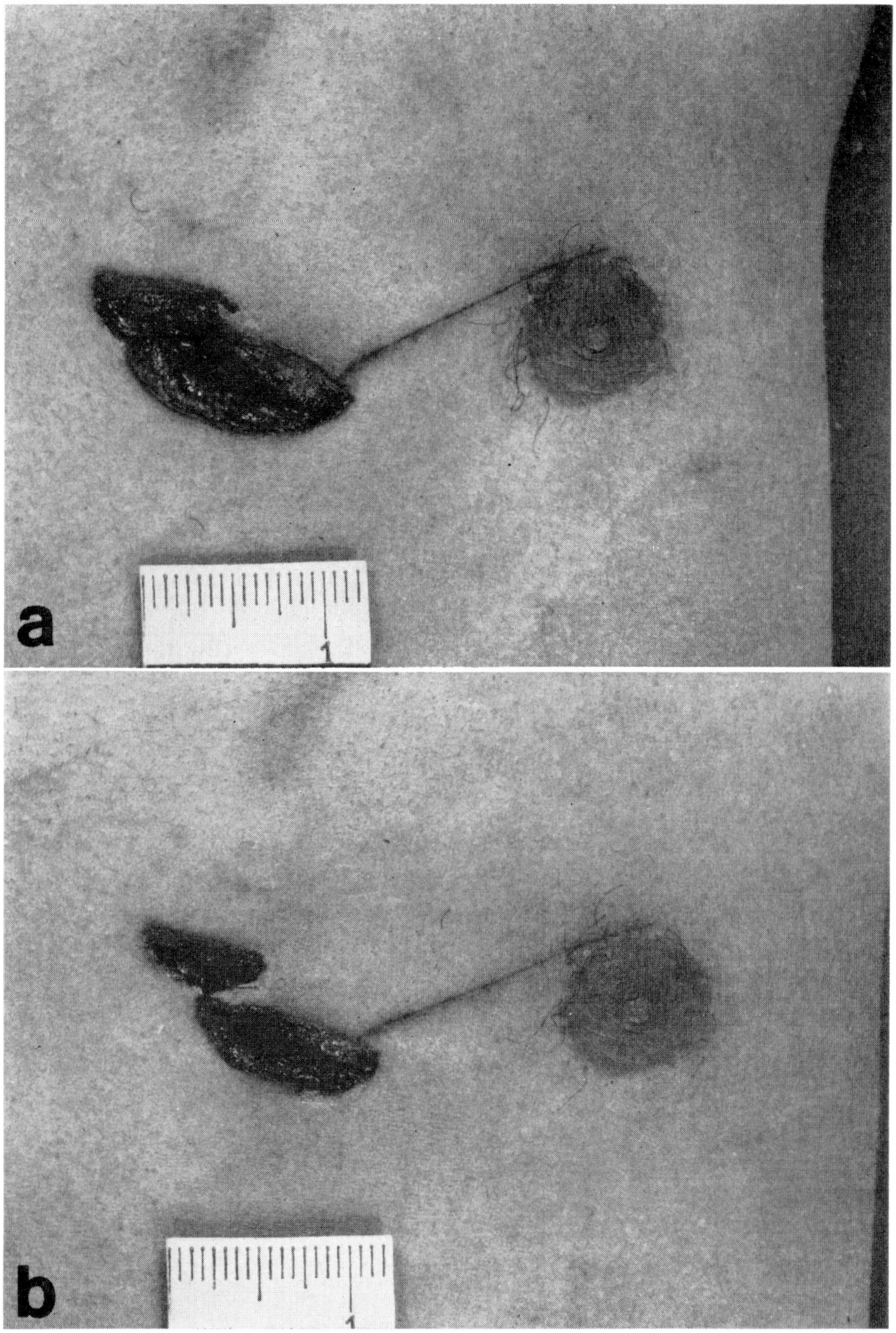


FIGURE VIII-53. An attempt at reconstruction should be a part of the examination of every stab wound. The injury above (a) was recognized as consisting of two distinct stab wounds after separation by a suture placed between them (b). The linear scratch extending to the nipple was made by the tip of the blade at the time of stabbing or withdrawal of the knife.

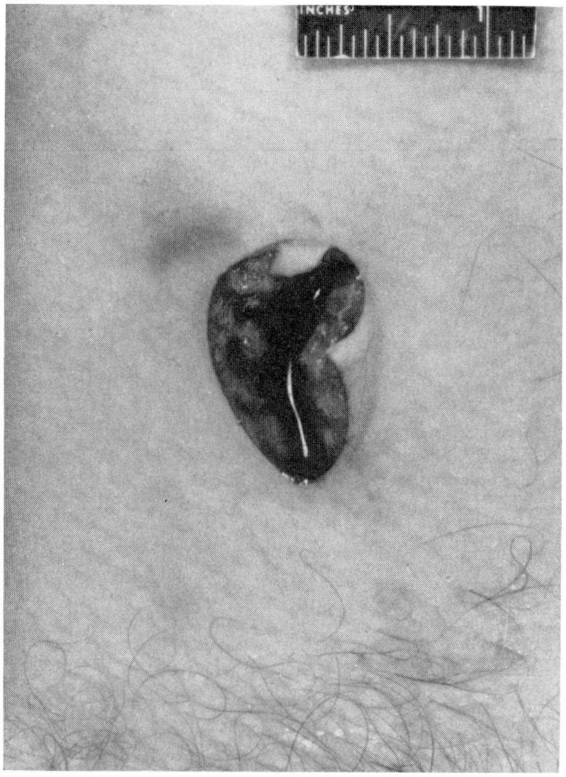


stab wounds, the interpretation of which is frequently difficult and may be quite confusing.

Stab wounds resembling small caliber bullet wounds are sometimes encountered if ice picks or similar instruments are used (Figs. VIII-57 and VIII-58). A small pocket knife may cause a similar injury (Fig. VIII-59). By contrast, a bullet wound of exit in the skin may resemble a knife wound quite closely if the bullet is fragmented or flattened by prior impact on bone. Fragments of a bone shattered by a bullet may also leave the body, producing wounds that suggest stabbing.

The wedgelike configuration of a knife wound is often clearly visible in serosal planes and

FIGURE VIII-54. Stab wound of the right lower quadrant of the abdomen produced by a butcher knife. This is a single wound; its bizarre shape resulted from twisting of the blade when the victim fell or when the knife was being withdrawn.

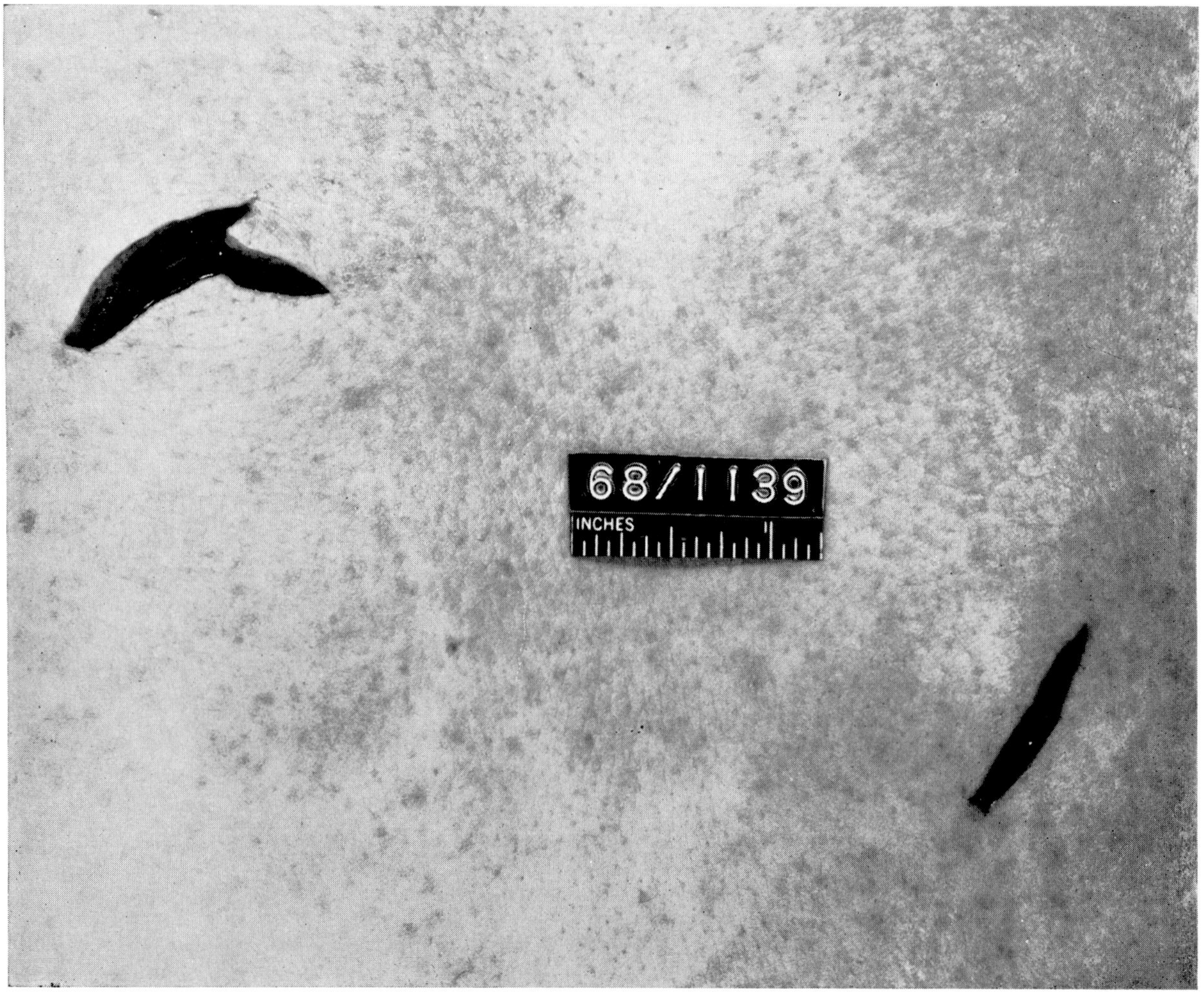


FIGURE VIII-55. Two stab wounds of the back, both produced by the same knife. The wound on the left shows a similar effect to the wound shown in Figure VIII-54.

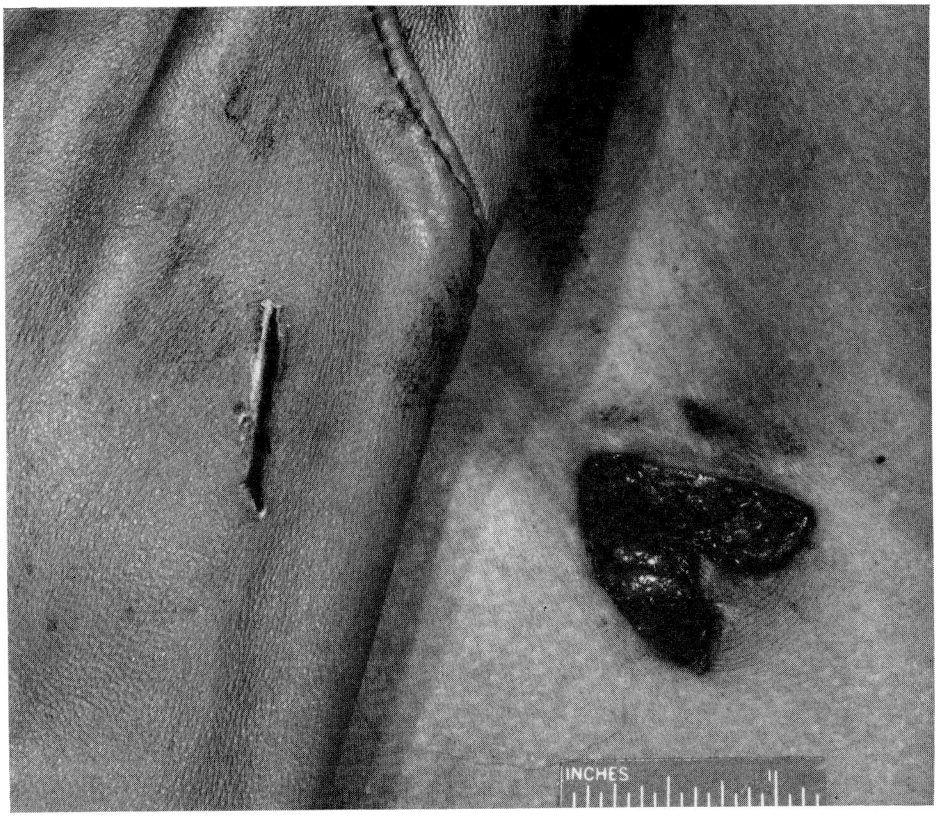


FIGURE VIII-56. Stab wound below the right clavicle. The jacket worn by the deceased shows a single slit, while the skin suggests two stab wounds. Twisting of the knife during the stabbing while the loose jacket followed suit produced this peculiar injury.

muscle fasciae. The pleural surface, the liver capsule and the pericardial sac are common examples. Accurate measurement of the dimensions of injuries in these locations will often be useful in efforts to ascertain the shape of the instrument in question and may actually reflect the thickness of a given blade with considerable accuracy.

The depth of a stab wound does not depend on the length of the blade alone. Actually, the depth of a knife wound frequently exceeds the length of the blade that caused it. This is primarily due to indentation or *give* of the body surface as a result of the thrust of the fist holding the knife. While this indentation is most pronounced in wounds of the abdomen, its presence in stab wounds of the chest and back are no exceptions, since even the rib cage is amenable to considerable caving in, particularly in young individuals. Expansion and retraction of the chest during breathing must also be taken into account. As to the force required for a certain depth of penetration, the pointedness of the blade and whether the wound track passes through bone must be considered. The type of bone involved and its thickness are equally important factors, as are the age and stature of the individual concerned. We have seen stab wounds of 6 in. and 7 in. depth produced with a 4-in. pocket knife.

Injection into the stab wound of dyes or radiopaque material to enable demonstration of the wound track by x rays has been attempted and claimed by some to be advantageous.[3] In

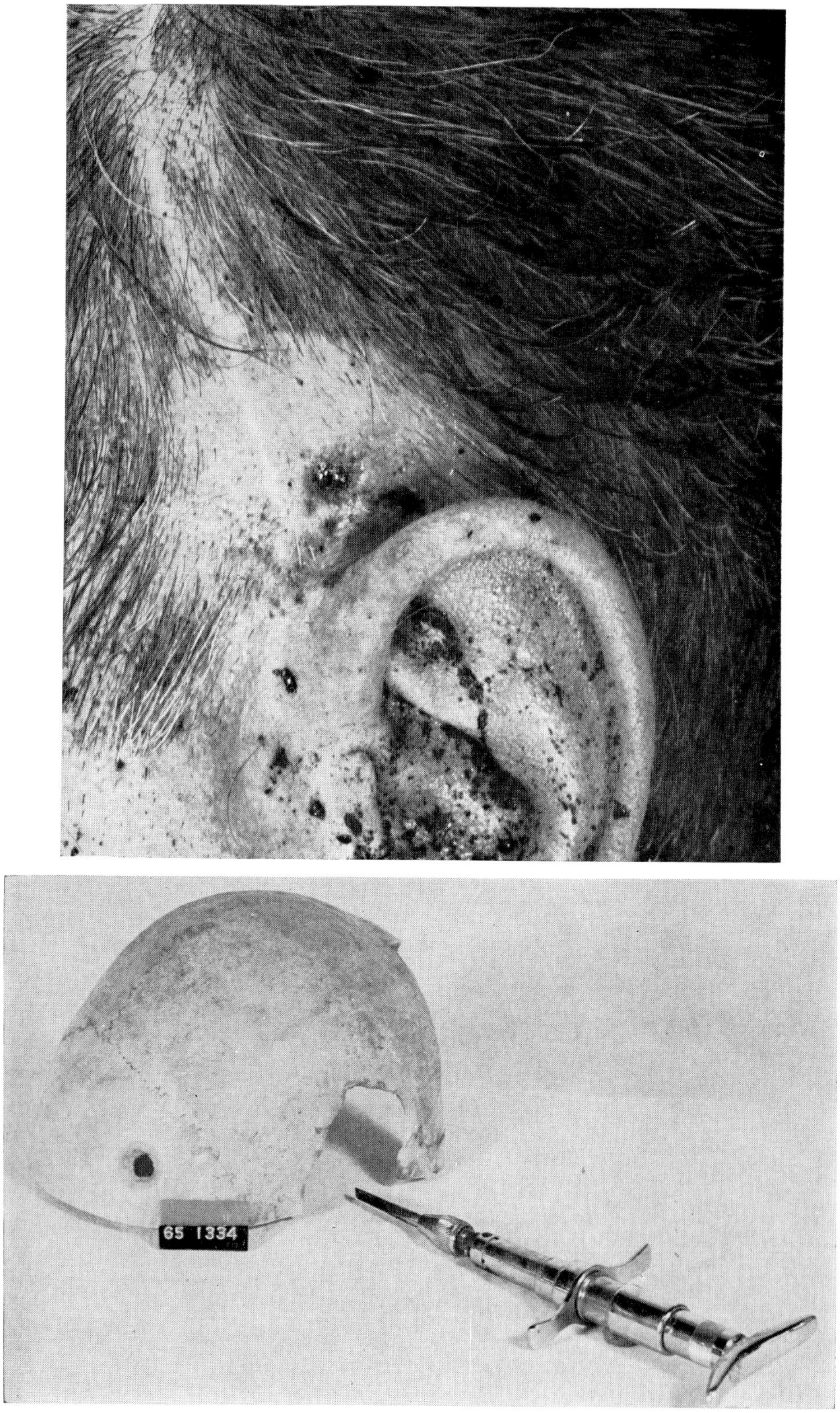


FIGURE VIII-57. Dentist with a gunshotlike self-inflicted stab wound of the left temple produced by a dental tool. The instrument was stabbed into a defect in the skull produced surgically during treatment of injuries sustained in an automobile accident fifteen years earlier.

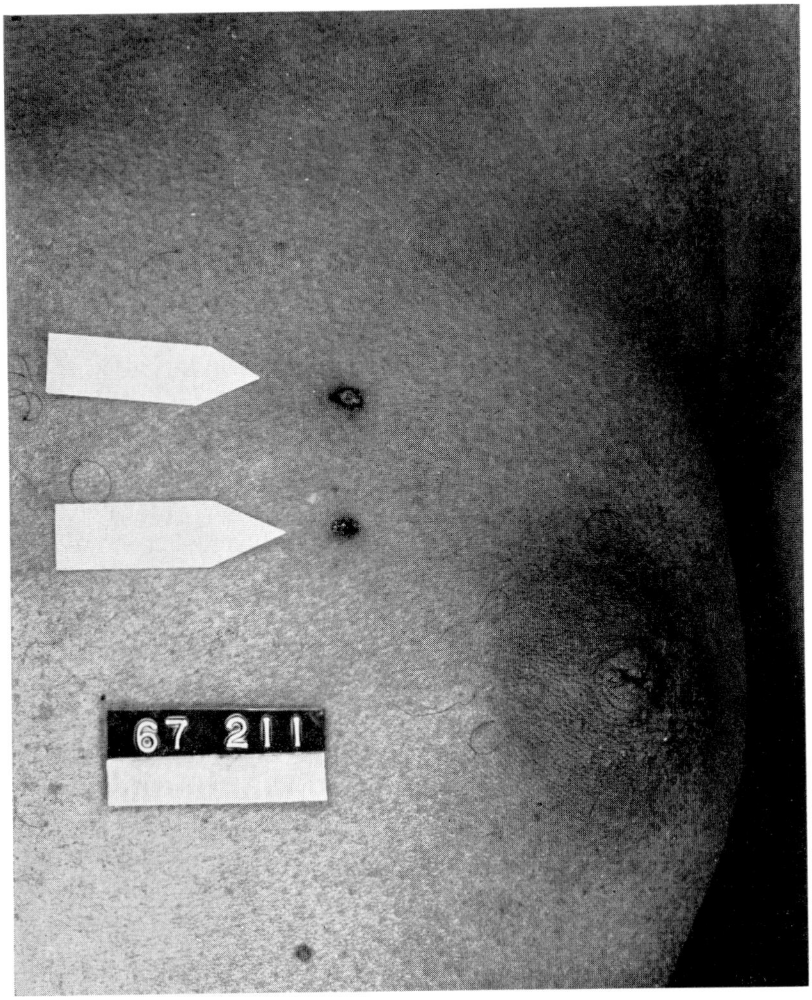


FIGURE VIII-58. Homicidal stabbing with an ice pick, resembling small caliber bullet wounds.

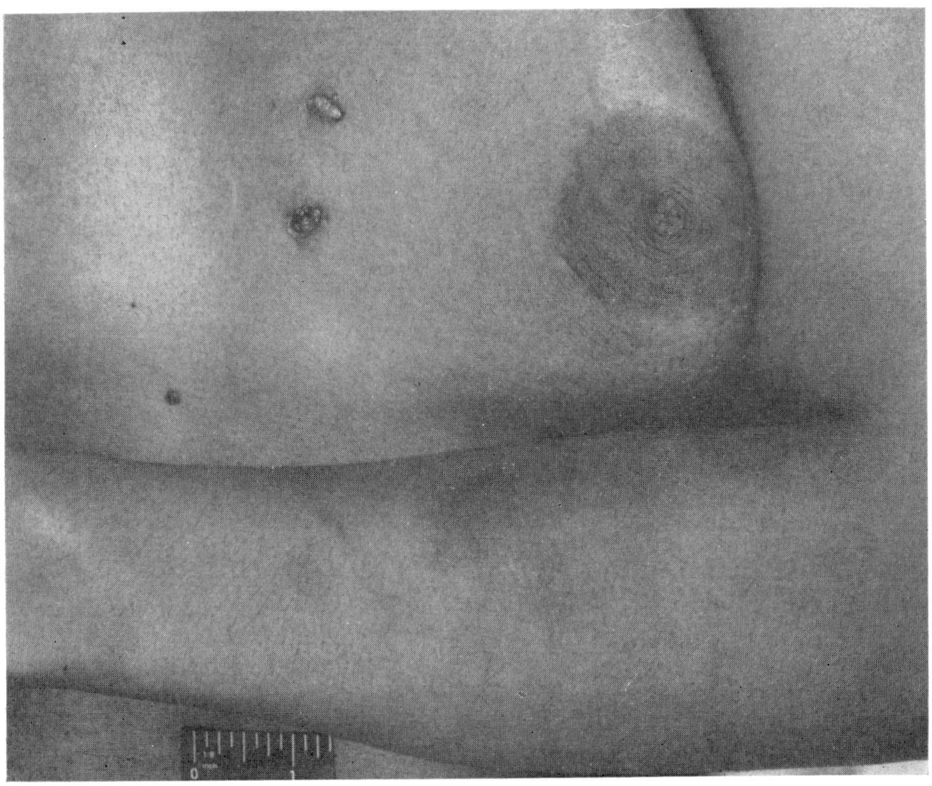

FIGURE VIII-59. Two stab wounds in the chest made by a small pocketknife. The initial police report was of a shooting.

our experience this procedure is seldom successful and frequently gives rise to false results. We do not use it.

### *Establishing the Direction of a Wound*

The direction of a knife wound can only be determined at autopsy by meticulous dissection along the track of hemorrhage. The indiscriminate and random probing of a knife wound is contraindicated and is commonly misleading. Probes should only be passed under direct vision, and probing prior to opening the body may invalidate the results by producing artifacts. After withdrawal of the weapon, the wound tends to close by expansion of the tissues along the blade's pathway. The probe may then easily pass between the fascial planes or within the musculature, producing a false track.

Excision of a stab wound and its surrounding skin with preservation of the specimen by freezing or by tacking it to a board and chemically fixing it for later use as evidence is both impractical and profitless. Removal of a flap of skin from the body alters tone and pliability of the specimen, and fixation adds a further artifact. Photographs, particularly close-ups, and an adequate description of the injury with respect to its location in relation to certain body landmarks and including its dimensions before and after restoration will usually suffice.

The clothing in a case of cutting or stabbing should be thoroughly examined, and unusual findings associated with the injury should be recorded. It is best to preserve the clothing, preferably each item in a separate plastic bag, appropriately labeled for later examination at the crime laboratory and possibly for submission in evidence. It is imperative, therefore, that the clothing be removed from the victim without cutting or tearing. The shape of a cut in the material may often aid in explaining the mechanism by which an injury was sustained, and not infrequently it will complement the results of examination of the wound with respect to the shape of the blade that caused it. Leather and certain synthetics maintain the shape of a cut relatively accurately.

Suicides commonly remove their clothing or expose the area to be injured, probably to enable better localization of the desired site.

## Complications of Cutting and Stabbing Injuries

The main factors that complicate cutting and stabbing injuries and that frequently lead to the death of the victim are (a) exsanguination, (b) air embolism, (c) asphyxia due to blood inhalation, (d) pneumothorax, (e) infection.

*Exsanguination* is by far the most common cause of death from cutting and stabbing. Bleeding is mainly into the body cavities, since the outer parts of the wound track frequently close after withdrawal of the weapon. The amount of blood at the scene of injury may be minimal unless the extremities, the head or the neck are involved.

Physical activity of varying duration and intensity may be expected in fatal stabbing cases, even if the heart, the major blood vessels or the lungs are involved.[4] A review of the subject illustrates dramatically the amount of activity that an individual may exhibit following fatal wounding:

A thirty-seven-year-old man was stabbed in the chest with a butcher knife. Following the injury he got into his automobile and drove four city blocks; he then lost control of the vehicle and crashed into a parked car. He proceeded to the hospital and died in the emergency room about twenty minutes after the injury. At autopsy there was a ¼ in. slitlike cut in the right ventricle of the heart. There were 1½ quarts (approximately 1400 cc) of blood present in the left pleural cavity and in the pericardial sac.

A twenty-three-year-old man who was stabbed with a kitchen knife walked and staggered a distance of 358 ft. and died at the hospital a few minutes after arrival there. The wound track penetrated the left ventricle of the heart and the aorta to a width of ¾ in. and caused internal bleeding of nearly 2 quarts (1900 cc).

A twenty-five-year-old man was stabbed with a kitchen knife, the wound causing severance of his left subclavian artery and vein. Following the injury the victim ran four city blocks and collapsed. He died at the hospital one hour later. The total blood loss was estimated at about 3 quarts (2800 cc).

Disability of victims of fatal gunshot injuries

appears to be more rapid than in those fatally wounded by sharp instruments.

*Air embolism* is usually the result of a cut or stab wound of the neck that exposes and penetrates one of the larger veins. Due to the negative pressure in veins, air is *sucked* into the vessels. When mixed with blood, air causes foam to be formed, which produces a *valve lock* in the heart. Death from massive air embolism is usually sudden and rapid. The injured individual makes one or two gasps and collapses.

*Asphyxia due to blood inhalation* may follow a cut or a stab wound in the neck area, exposing the trachea or larynx. This mode of death is usually quite rapid and is often associated with choking and sometimes convulsions resulting from anoxia due to the blood obstructing the air passages.

*Pneumothorax*, or air in the pleural cavity, usually results from a stab wound accompanied by bleeding into the pleural space. The term *hemopneumothorax* would consequently be more applicable. Death due to pneumothorax may occur several hours after the injury.

*Infection* of a stab wound or a cut is a late complication that may take days or weeks to develop. It is a rare cause of death, except in stab wounds of the abdomen in which the intestines are perforated, releasing bowel contents into the peritoneal cavity.

### Dismemberment

Disposal of a homicide victim by dismemberment of the body is rare, but individual cases are on record in most major medicolegal departments. Postmortem dismemberment is usually readily recognizable as such. The edges of postmortem injuries are dry and lack evidence of bleeding. The joints may be disarticulated without fracture, or the presence of fractures may suggest the application of crude force, possibly the use of an axe or similar implement. The recognition of postmortem mutilation may be of importance in the interpretation of certain murders committed by sexual perverts and other mentally deranged individuals (Fig. VIII-60). Postmortem dismemberment is sometimes performed for the sole reason of easier disposal of the body (Fig. VIII-61).

The beaten and mutilated bodies of four boys aged

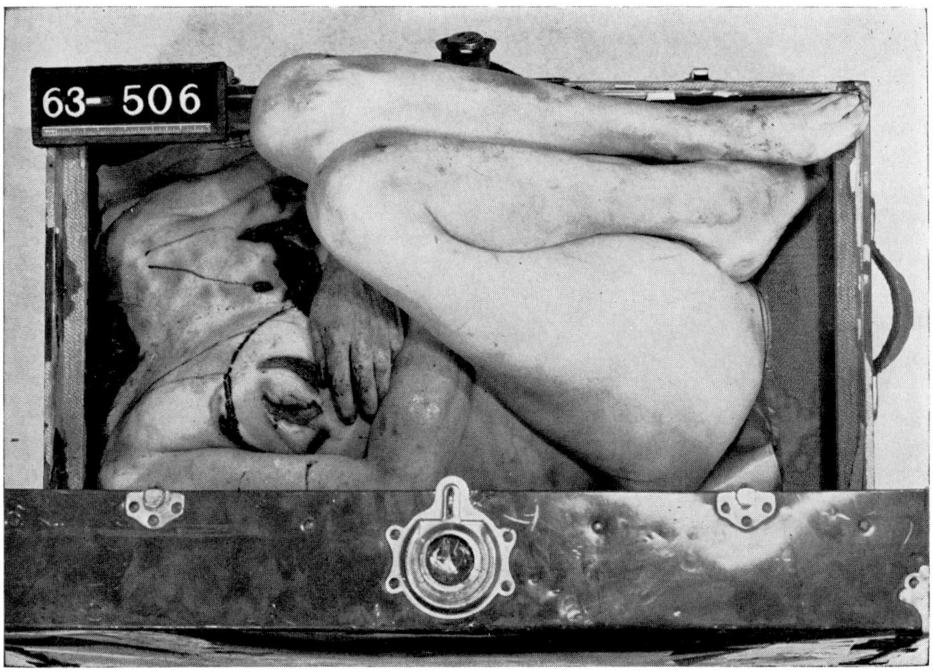


FIGURE VIII-60. Decapitated and mutilated female body found in a trunk. The lack of hemorrhage in the margins of the cuts indicates postmortem infliction.

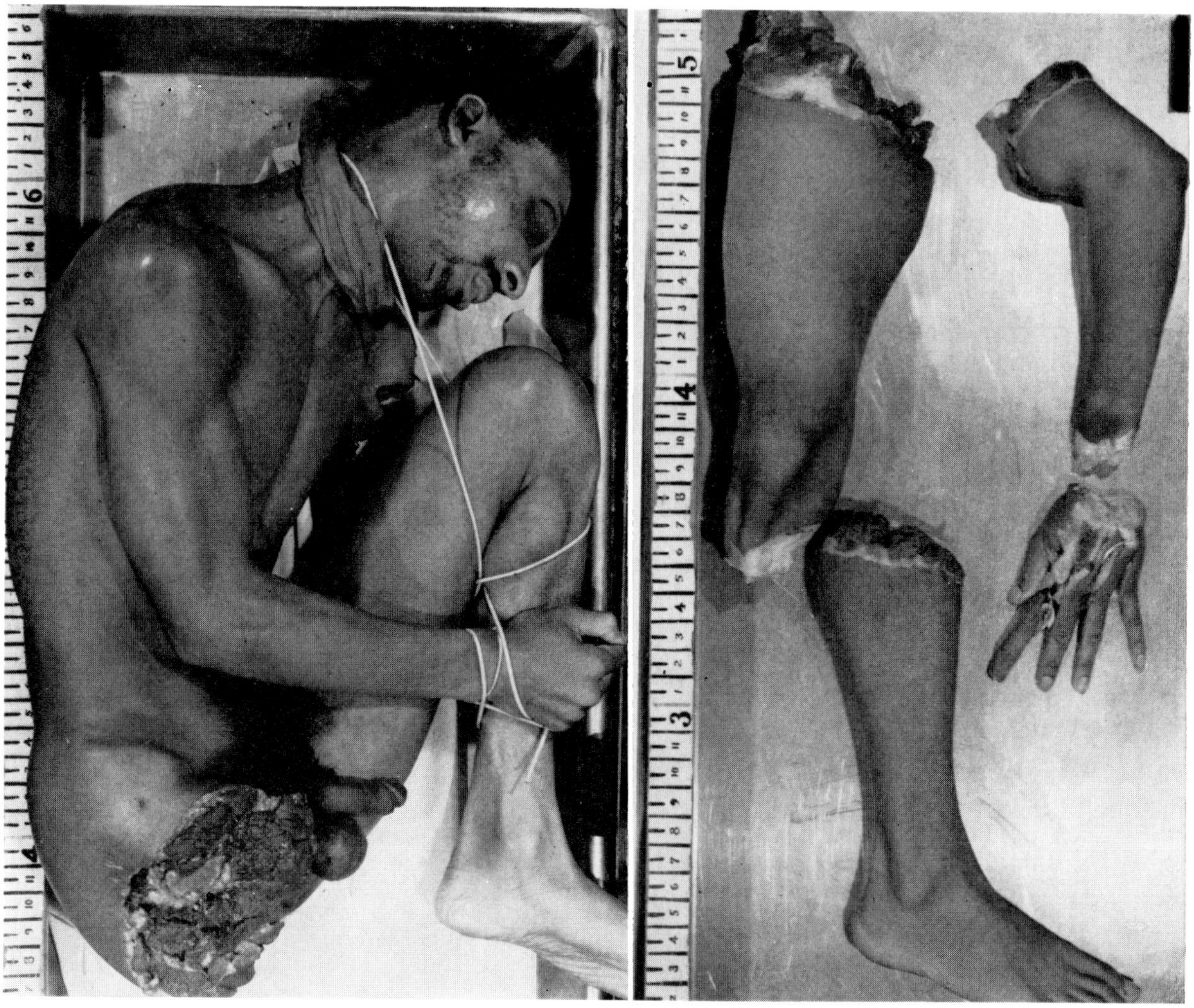

FIGURE VIII-61. The bodies of two narcotic pushers were found wrapped in plastic bags in a dumpster located in a suburban development. One of the bodies was partly dismembered and tied after death, probably for easier disposal. No hemorrhage is seen in the areas of dismemberment.

five to twelve were found in a public park. An eighteen-year-old youth was arrested. He confessed to the killings by beating and stangulation and admitted postmortem dismemberment and cannibalism. Three of the bodies showed amputation of the penis; the latter were found in the lunch box of the suspect at the time of his arrest. The hands and the hearts were found separately; both had small portions missing. Upon questioning, the suspect said he had eaten the missing parts, as well as a portion of a brain. A dull knife and a saw blade were used for the dismemberment (Fig. VIII-62).

### Other Sharp Force Injuries

Other sharp force injuries include those produced by the propeller of a boat or ship and may resemble large cuts or chopping wounds. The question of ante- or postmortem infliction of such wounds in a body recovered from water is often difficult due to *leaching* of blood from the tissues as described in Chapter XIII. Bloody infiltration of tissues at the site of an injury is probably the most valuable criterion that the injury was sustained during life. The nature of the injuries, their extent and locations may suggest ante- versus postmortem occurrence and exclude homicide with subsequent disposal of the body to simulate drowning.

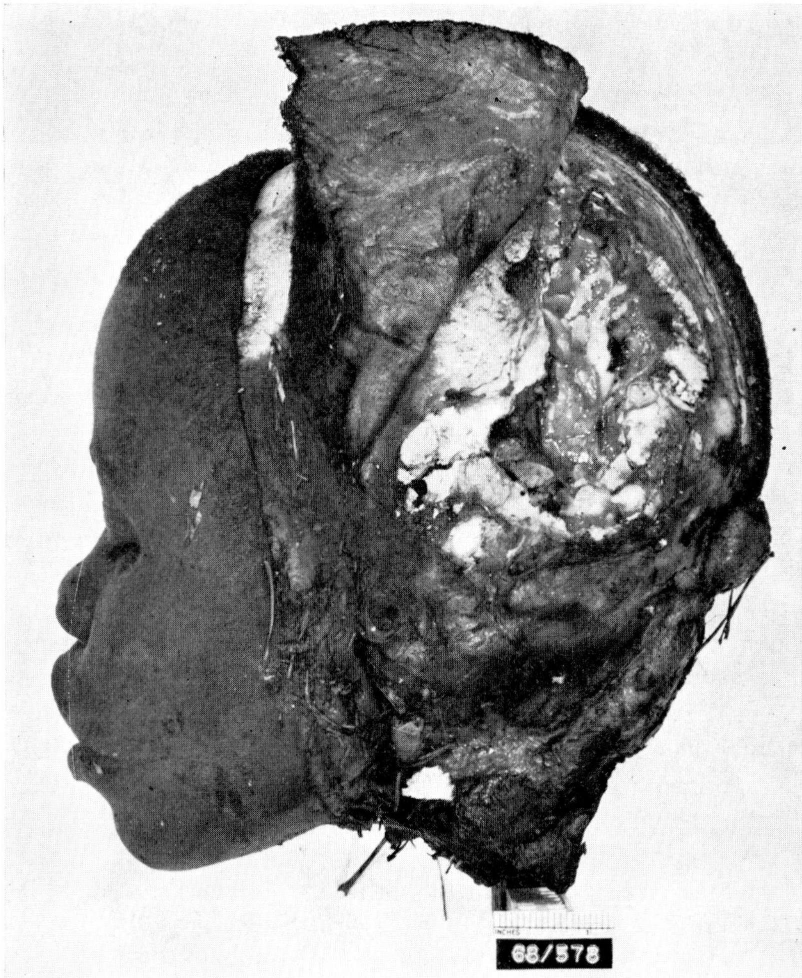


FIGURE VIII-62. The mutilated head of one of the four boys found in a public park. No hemorrhage is seen in the reflected flap of scalp and in the brain.

## REFERENCES


1. Hofman-Haberda: *Lehrbuch der Gerichtlichen Medizin.* Wien, Berlin, Urban & Schwarzenberg, 1927, pp. 305, 311.
2. Rabinowitsch, A.: Medico-legal conclusions on the form of the knife used, based on the shape of stab wounds produced. *J Forensic Med, 6:*160, 1959.
3. Mueller, B.: *Gerichtliche Medizin.* Berlin, Springer, 1953, p. 275.
4. Spitz, W. U., Petty, C. S., and Fisher, R. S.: Physical activity until collapse following fatal injury by firearms and sharp pointed weapons. *J Forensic Sci, 6:*290, 1961.

*Chapter IX*

# GENERAL CONSIDERATIONS OF FIREARMS IDENTIFICATION AND BALLISTICS

RUSSELL M. WILHELM

A FIREARM IS DEFINED as any instrument or device with which it is possible to propel a projectile by means of the expansive force of the gases generated by the combustion of an explosive substance.

It has been stated that the evolution of rifling can be followed by tracing the development of weapons, and this is true in United States' own history. The British arms, as brought to the United States with the landing of the first settlers, were large, bulky and inaccurate muskets. However, the rifle hanging over the fireplace was the family defense and frequently the only means of procuring food. Necessity thus created a desire for more accuracy and longer range. This led to much experimenting in blacksmith shops. Eliphalet Remington was a good example of this. From his first crude handwrought rifle grew one of the largest arms companies in the world, REMINGTON of Illion, New York.

It was between 1728 and 1840 that the American rifle was developed and became generally known as the Kentucky rifle, although Lancaster, Pennsylvania, was the center of manufacture. These rifles were generally between .40 and .45 caliber, with approximately 40 inch barrels. When these were loaded, the bullet was patched. Patching was used in an effort to create a tight gas fit rather than using an oversize bullet.

During this era another major improvement also developed. The accepted flintlock was fast being replaced with a new percussion type of ignition, which made its appearance in the early 1800s. However, during this same period the propellant remained unchanged—namely *black powder*. Black powder is a mixture of potassium nitrate, charcoal and sulphur. Although it was already known to the ancient Chinese, its invention is generally credited to the English scientist Roger Bacon in 1249. Its application to the propulsion of missiles in the early 1300s is credited to Bernard Schwarz, a German monk. This continued to be the propellant until the turn of the nineteenth century, when smokeless powder was developed.

The next major step was the development and patent by Smith and Wesson, in 1854, of the first American cartridge in which the bullet, powder charge and primer were all contained in a single unit as they are today.

In summation it might be noted that firearms originally fired round balls from smooth bore arms. The transition to modern rifling was motivated by the desire for higher sectional density or greater shocking power with less resistance to the air through which the projectile must travel (more weight to the bullet). It was found that if a bullet were spinning at a high rate of speed, it would tend to stay nose-on and maintain a true course. This is referred to as having gyrostatic stability and may be described as being similar to the spinning of a top. Thus, the factors of rate of twist, bullet weight and velocity are computed or mated to best obtain this stabilizing influence.

The science of firearms identification is based on the premise that it is humanly impossible to make any two articles absolutely identical. When they are viewed under the comparison microscope, this premise is verified. Even the surfaces of pieces of metal that are made by consecutive cuts on the same machine are microscopically different; the edge of the cutter becomes blunted during every cut, so there are minute variations in the marks left on the surfaces.

Similarly, surfaces that are finished by grinding or hand filing present an appearance not unlike that of a ploughed field when viewed under a microscope. These surfaces are covered with minute furrows or cuts that have been left by the file or grinder.

Since part of the science is based upon variations of the inner surface striations of the barrel, it is important to know the cause of their being (Fig. IX-1). All barrels are originally a solid steel bar. First a hole is drilled through the entire length, and then an oil drill or hone is worked through to smooth this opening. This is the bore diameter or basically the caliber. The next step is the rifling. Various methods have been used to accomplish this. Now obsolete but popular a few years ago was the hook cutter and scrape cutter method. Presently most popular is the broaching technique (Fig. IX-2). However, all of the techniques accomplish the same purpose by basically the same method. In rifling, the instrument used is moved in a spiraling motion through the bore, removing metal in elongated strips, which upon completion become the *grooves*. The strips left standing are the *lands*. These lands bite into the bullet as it passes through the bore and give the bullet its spiraling motion.

The breech block and recoil plate are parts of a firearm that are located at the breech end of the weapon. They withstand the rearward thrust exerted by the cartridge at the time of explosion. Both are either machine or hand filed. Consequently, they have striations that leave their imprint upon cartridge cases fired in weapons of which they are a part.

It has been recognized that a bullet fired through the barrel of a rifled arm contains numerous characteristics by which it can be identified. These characteristics can be divided into two groups: (a) class characterstics, (b) individual or accidental characteristics.

### Class Characteristics

The number of land and groove impressions

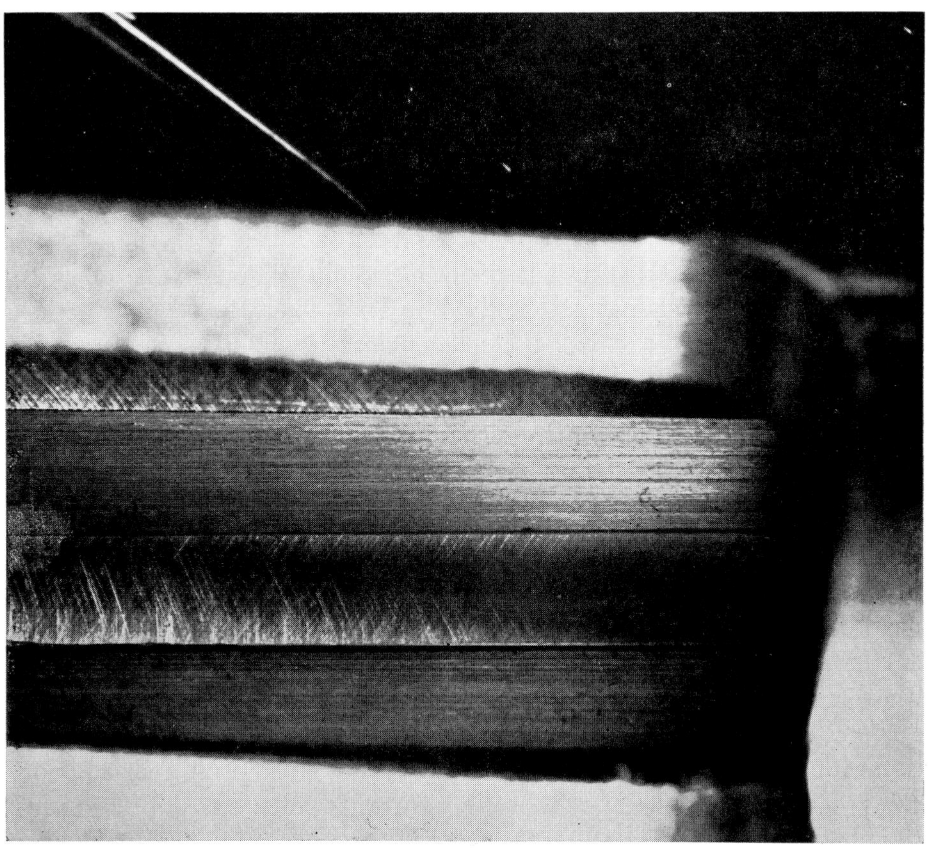

FIGURE IX-1. Sectional view of a .38 Special Smith & Wesson revolver barrel, showing lands and grooves and fine imperfections created in manufacture.

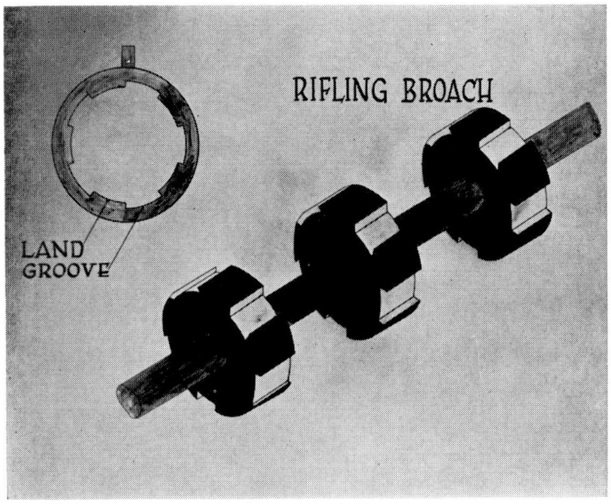


FIGURE IX-2. Rifling broach and cross section of a barrel.

and their approximate dimensions are termed class characteristics. We find this basic in our preliminary examinations. A Smith and Wesson revolver of .32 caliber is designed and built to certain specifications. It has five lands and five grooves, with the direction of twist to the right. The widths of the lands and grooves are equidistant, being .095 in. each. The Colt revolver in .32 caliber is differently constructed. It has six lands and six grooves, with the direction of twist to the left. The widths of the lands and grooves in the Colt measure approximately .048 in. and .108 in., respectively (Fig. IX-3). Consequently, a .32 caliber bullet having six land and six groove impressions with a twist to the left cannot have been fired by a Smith and Wesson revolver of the same caliber. However, should the bullet submitted in evidence and the suspect weapon have compatible class characteristics, individual or accidental characteristics must be considered.

### Individual or Accidental Characteristics

The fine striae created by the broach or hone finishing of the barrel or other surfaces of the weapon are referred to as individual or accidental characteristics. Minute chips of steel break from the broach in the process of rifling, scarring the bore with microscopic fine striae. The bullet in its travel through the barrel takes on this signature, which in effect is a summation of all accidental marks.

When a microscopic comparison is required, the suspect weapon must be fired and the bullet recovered unmarked by anything other than the bore through which it has travelled. Therefore, we fire a test bullet from the weapon in question into either a recovery box filled with raw cotton or a water recovery tank. The test bullet is retrieved, and this bullet is now mounted in juxtaposition to the evidence bullet under the comparison microscope.

### Comparison Microscope

The comparison microscope is so constructed that, by means of two separate microscope tubes joined by a bridge with prisms mounted over these tubes, the two images will be transmitted to the center of the bridge (Fig. IX-4). There, by means of another prism, both objects are brought together in a central eyepiece in which the left and right images are separated by a dividing line.

Mounted beneath each tube are movable stages, each separately manipulated by mechanical rack and pinion gears. These are moved and rotated, with the class characteristics of each bullet in as near alignment as practicable. Then a search is made with the intent to match the accidental striations produced by the rifling tool. The final conclusion rests on the number and significance of these fine scratch marks (Fig. IX-5). It should be pointed out in this regard that in the case of jacketed bullets, the pressure of the charge may only expand the base of the bullet, leaving the markings there while failing to produce a consistent continuation of the striations on the rest of the bullet.

In brief, the striations that are left on the bullet as a result of its passing through the bore are the major characteristics used for the examination. Also, the cartridge case in its rearward thrust takes on the signature of the breech face or recoil plate. These markings on the head of the cartridge case may be used for the purpose of comparison with the cartridge case of a test-fired bullet. Similarly, the extractor and ejector

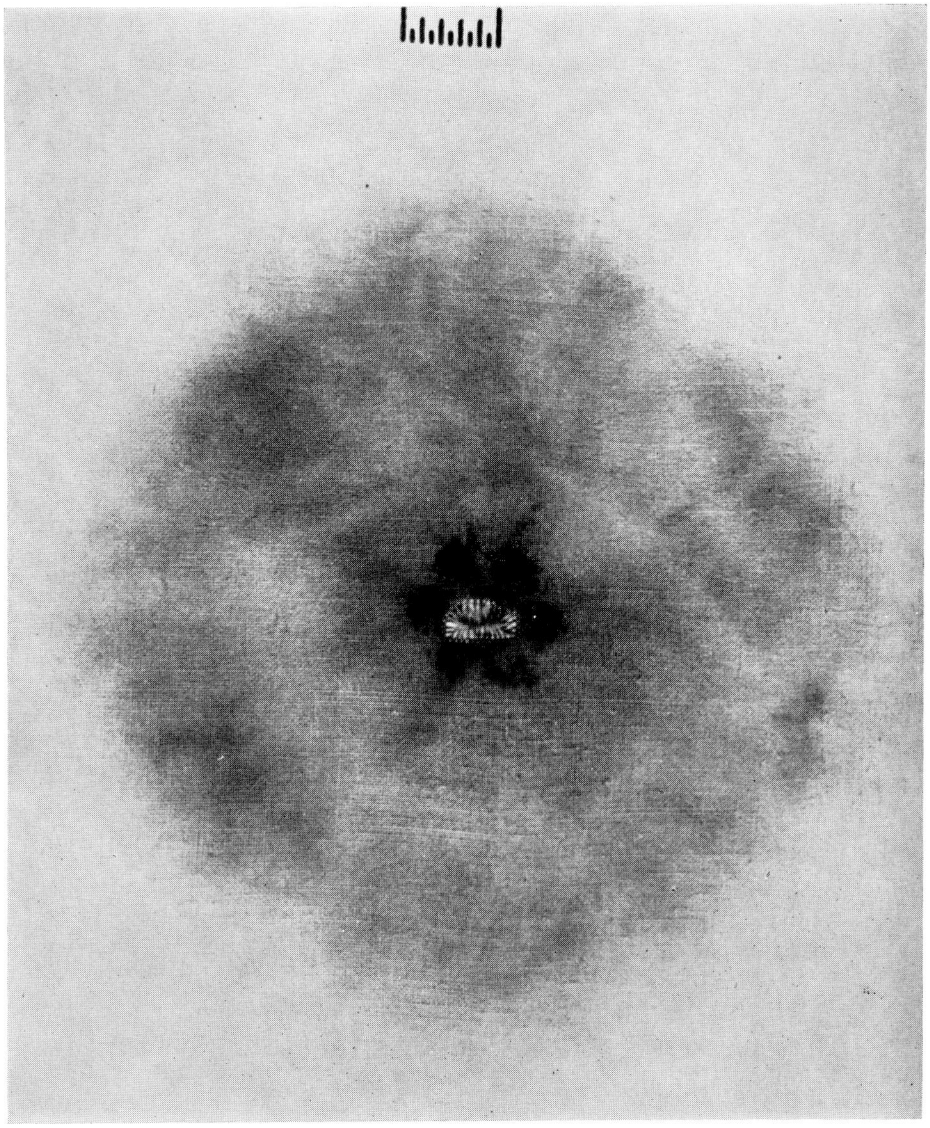

FIGURE IX-3. Close-range shot with deposits of gunsmoke. The distribution of the powder residue around the bullet hole indicates the bore pattern of the weapon by showing the number of land and groove impressions. The direction of twist cannot be determined by the pattern.

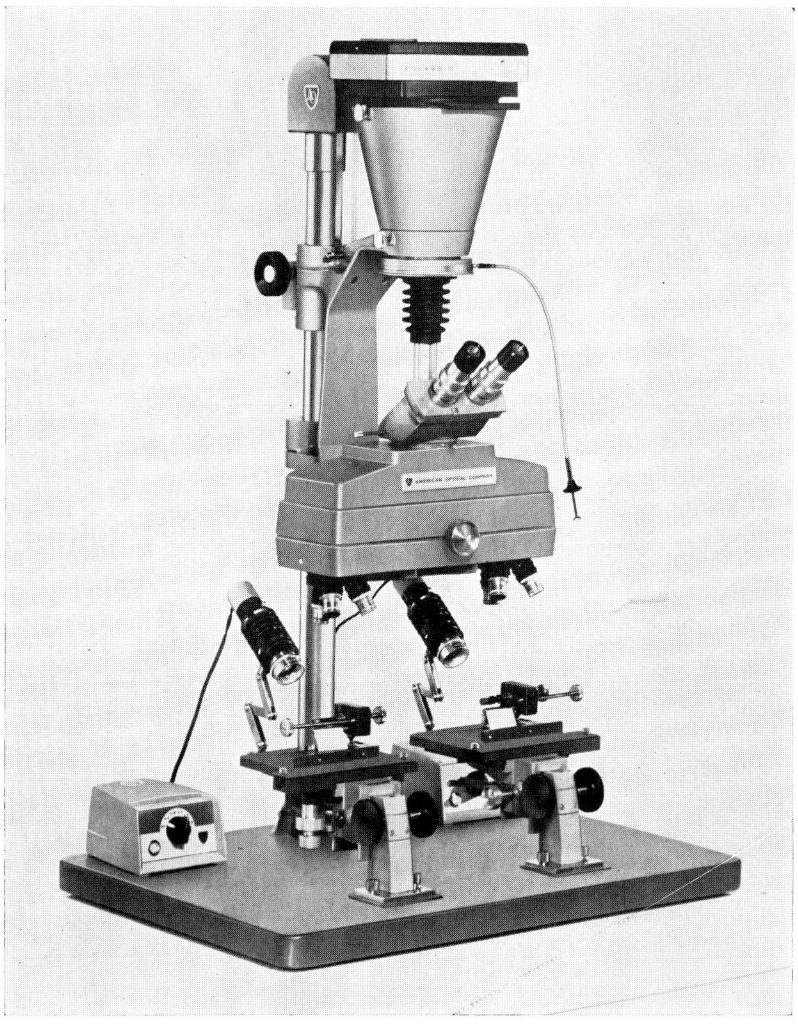

FIGURE IX-4. Comparison microscope. (Courtesy American Optical Company.)

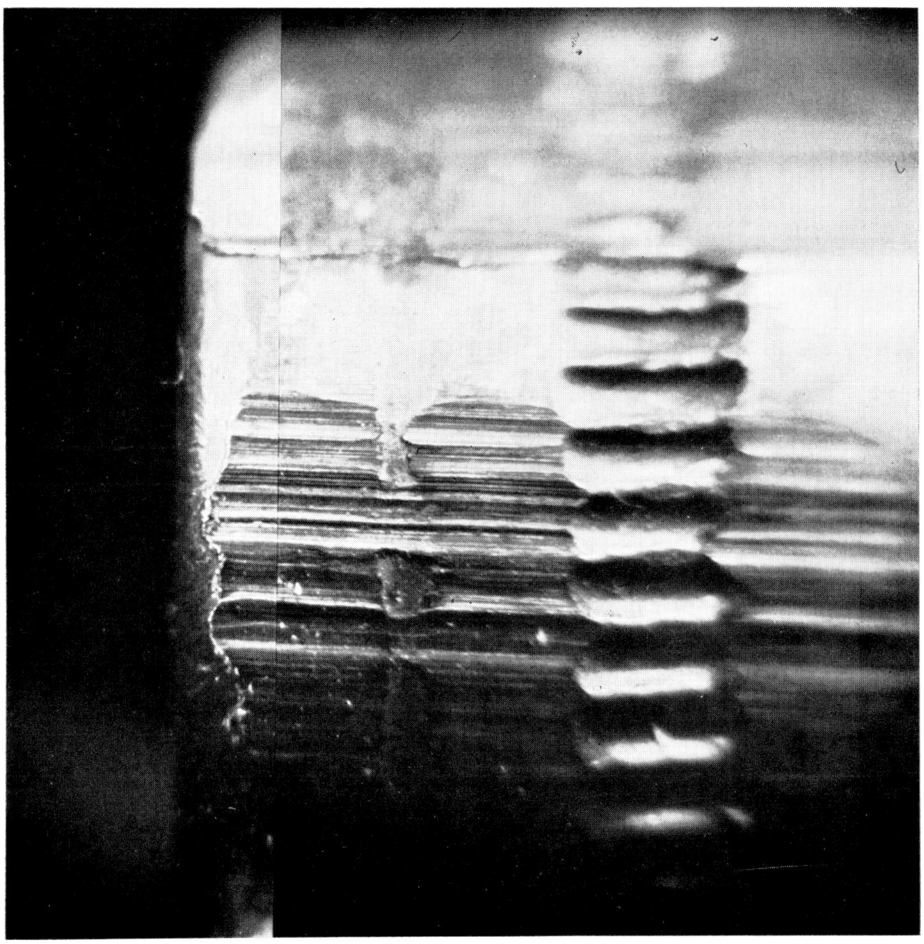

FIGURE IX-5. Coinciding of striations as viewed under the comparison microscope, with an evidence bullet on the left and a test-fired bullet on the right.

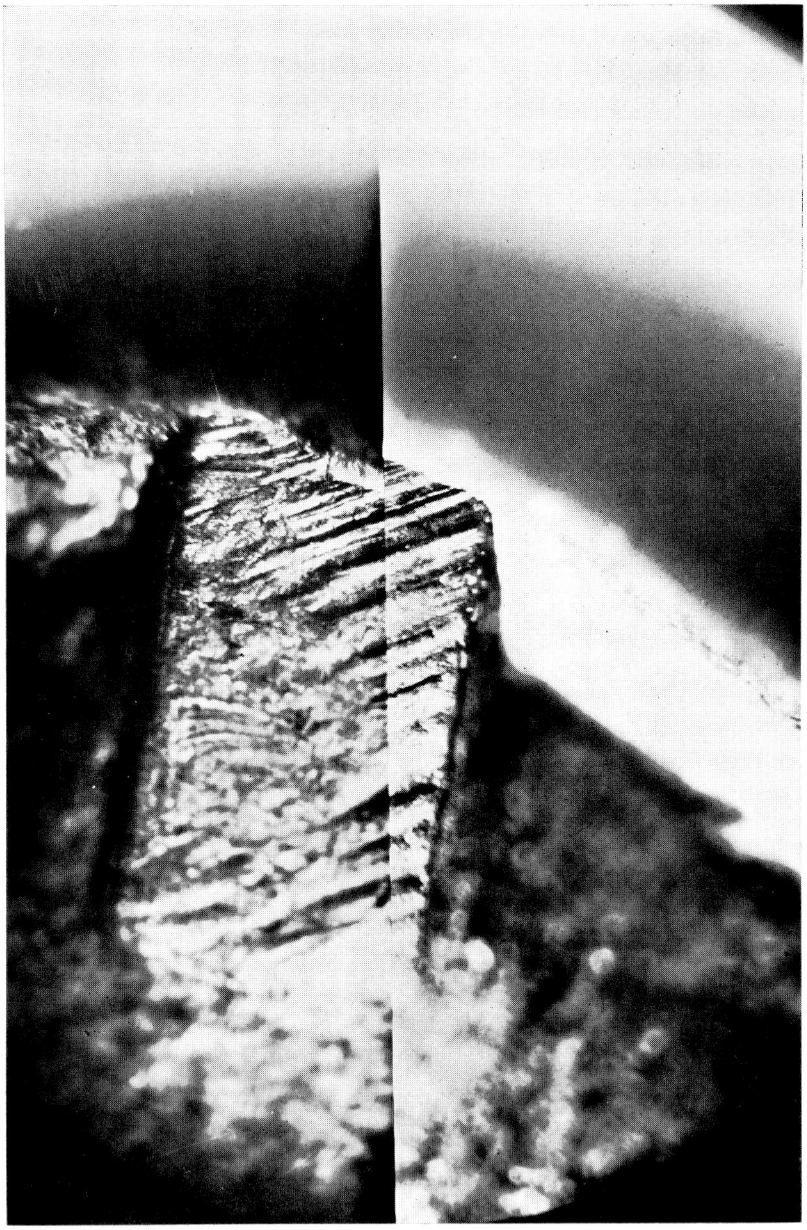

FIGURE IX-6. Alignment of striations of firing pin impression as seen under the comparison microscope. On the left a .22 caliber rimfire cartridge case submitted in evidence. On the right the test-fired cartridge case.

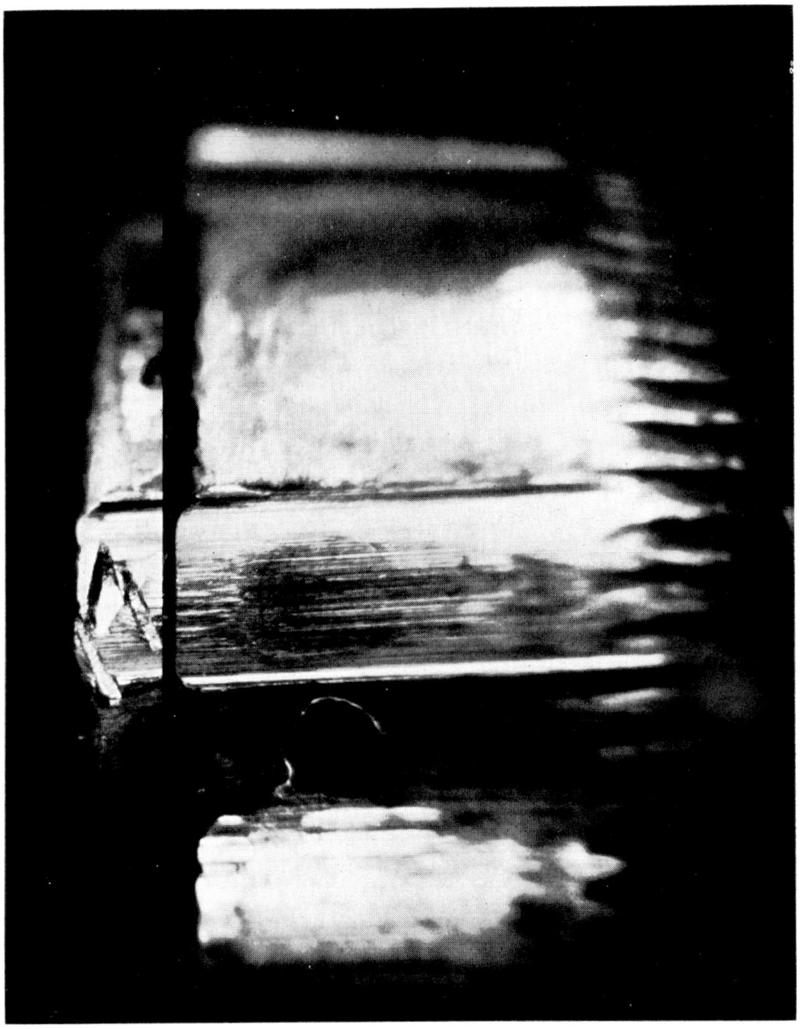

FIGURE IX-7. Alignment of fine markings is rendered impossible due to mutilation of the bullet in question (left) by handling with an instrument.

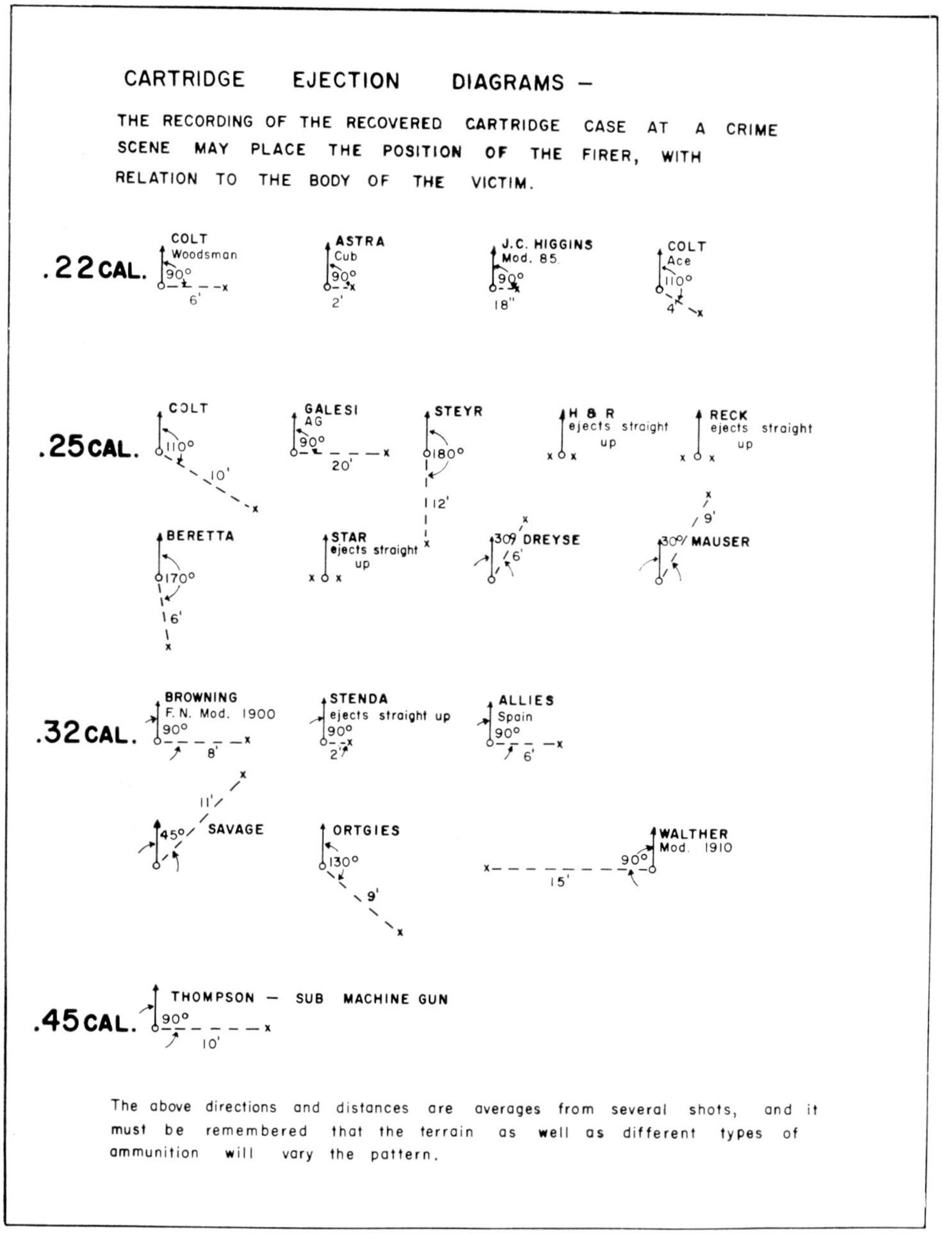


FIGURE IX-8. Ejection patterns of various firearms.

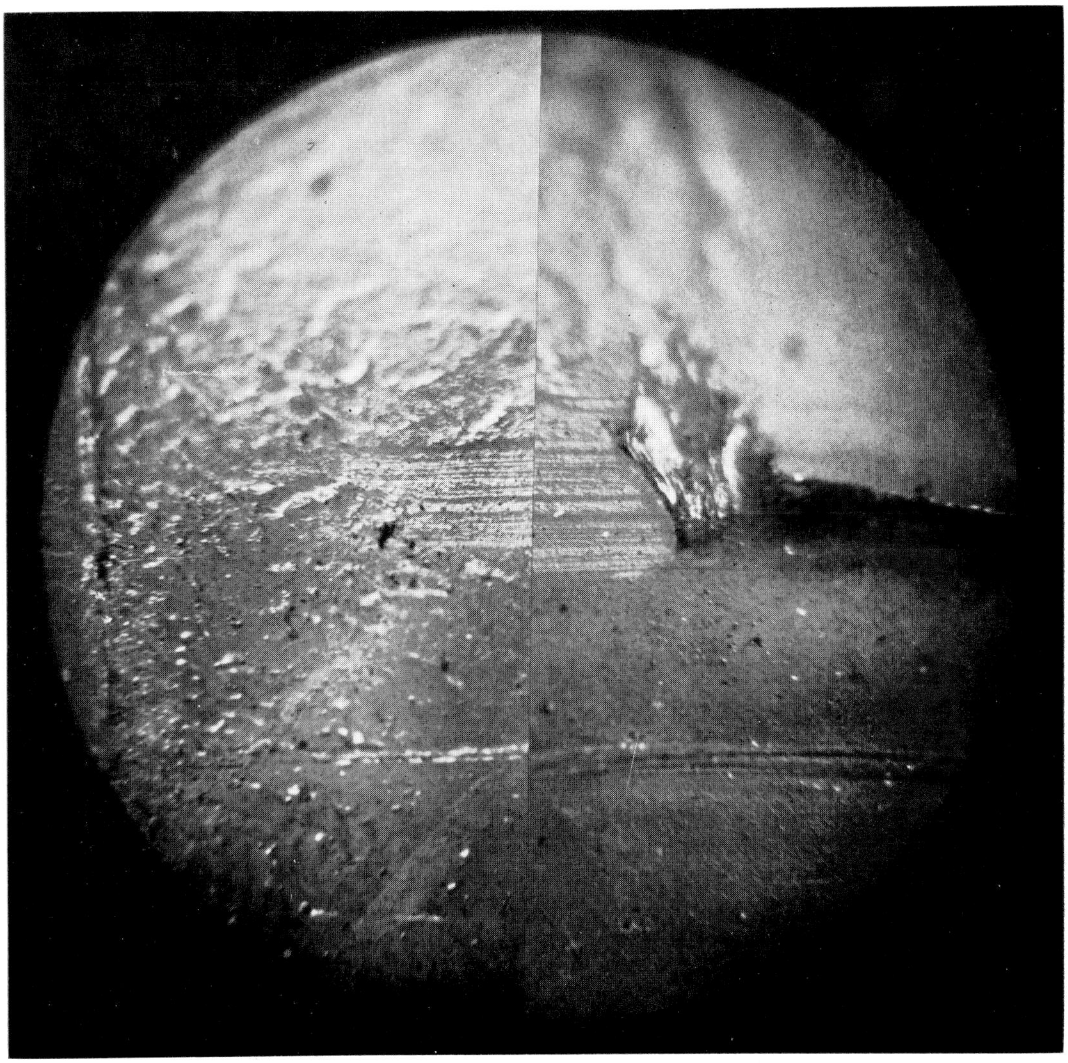

FIGURE IX-9. Striations on plastic shot pouch match those on test-fired pouch under the comparison microscope.

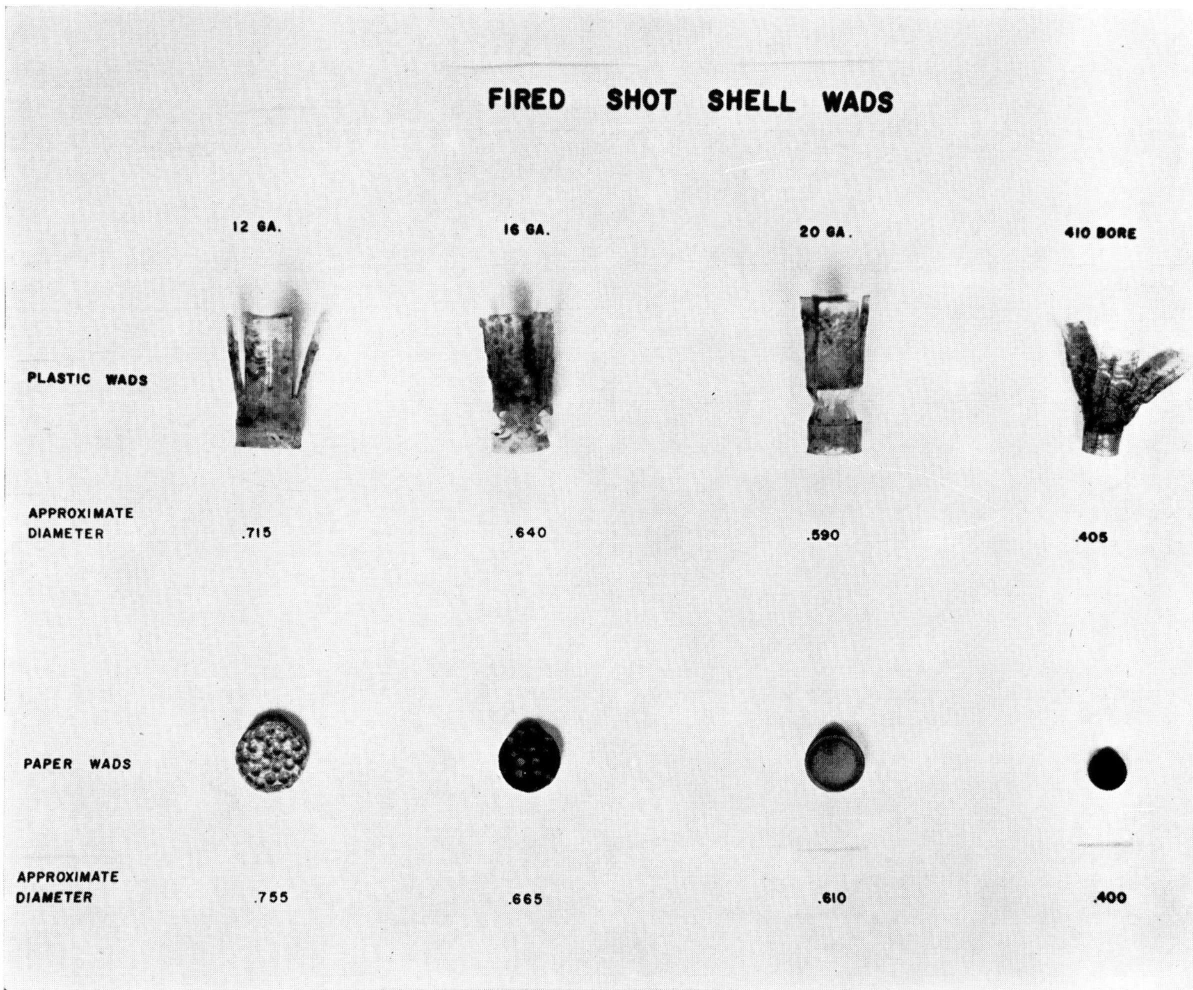


FIGURE IX-10. Various fired shot shell wads and their approximate diameter.

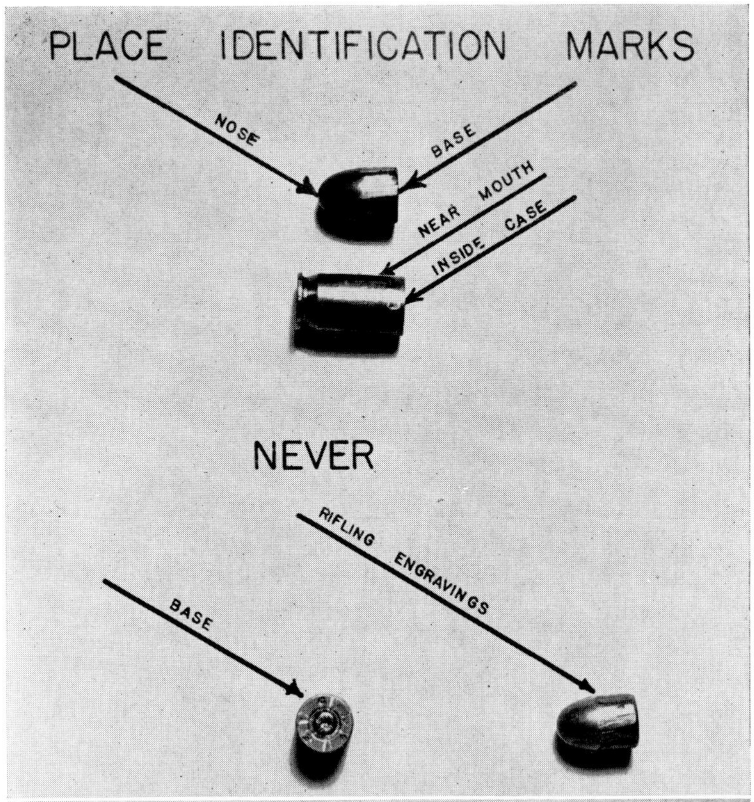


FIGURE IX-11a. Proper and improper marking placed on bullets and cartridge cases for the purpose of identification.

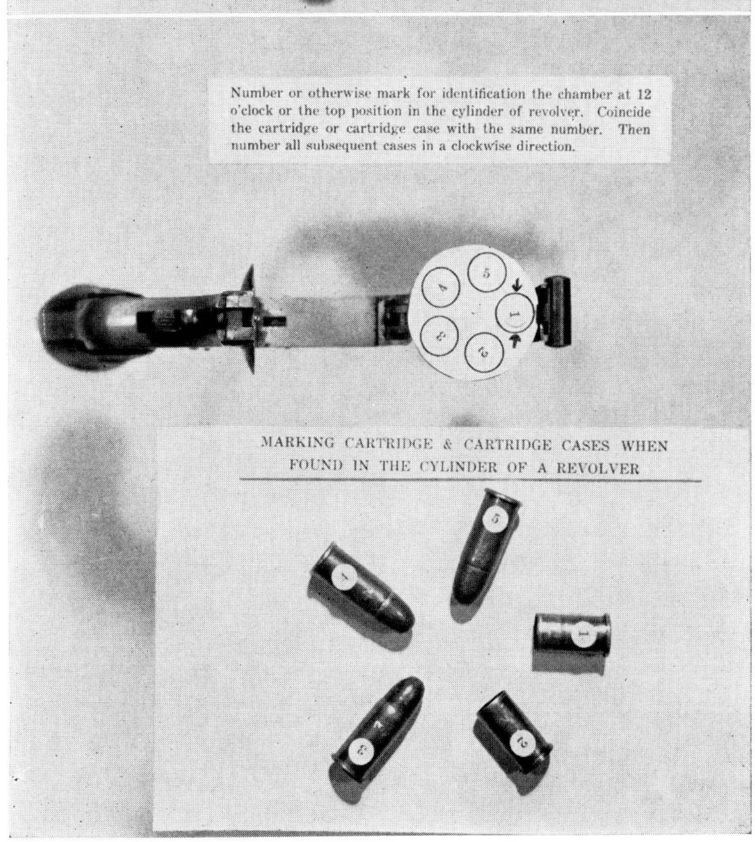


FIGURE IX-11b. In cases of defective revolvers with misalignment of the cylinder and barrel, this method of marking removed cartridges or cases will reconstruct the *shaving* of a bullet's side that results from the bullet improperly entering the throat of the barrel.

leave their markings on the rim or the area close to the rim of the cartridge case (Fig. IX-6). Any foreign marks overlapping or interfering with these signatures may eliminate matching possibilities (Fig. IX-7). By the same token, objects inserted into the barrel of a weapon may cause enough discrepancies between the evidence bullet or bullets and the test shots fired by the examiner to preclude the possibility of a match. Fingerprint examiners must be cautioned not to lift or hold firearms by the insertion of instruments into the muzzle of the weapon.

It is important that the investigator at the scene of a shooting note the location of cartridge cases, since their position may determine the location of the weapon at the time of discharge. Semiautomatic firearms eject the cartridge cases at specific angles (Fig. IX-8). While the absence of cartridge cases does not preclude the use of automatic firearms, it suggests that a revolver may have been used.

Shotgun shells also have evidence value that can be of significance to the examiner. In addition to the firing pin signature, extractor and ejector marks, there exists a possibility of matching striations on the plastic shot pouch (Fig. IX-9). It is also noted in Figure IX-10 that the gauge of the shotgun from which the shot was fired may be ascertained.

It follows that evidence must be marked properly for subsequent identification. When presented in court, all persons in whose custody this evidence has been *must,* as a matter of record, be able to establish their part in this custodial chain (Fig. IX-11).

### Approximation of Distance

Another problem also presented involves the distance from the muzzle to the target. With handguns and rifles, distance determinations are dependent upon the spread and amount of gun smoke deposited on the target. Therefore, test patterns from various distances must be made to correlate the evidence pattern with the comparable test. Even at the same distance, variations of ammunition will create discrepancies of pattern. This holds true for all firearms. In the case of shotguns an observation of shot dispersion as seen from the shot pattern is correlated to the size of the shot pattern on the victim's clothing or body (Fig. IX-12). This enables the examiner to give a close approximation of the distance at the time of the shooting.

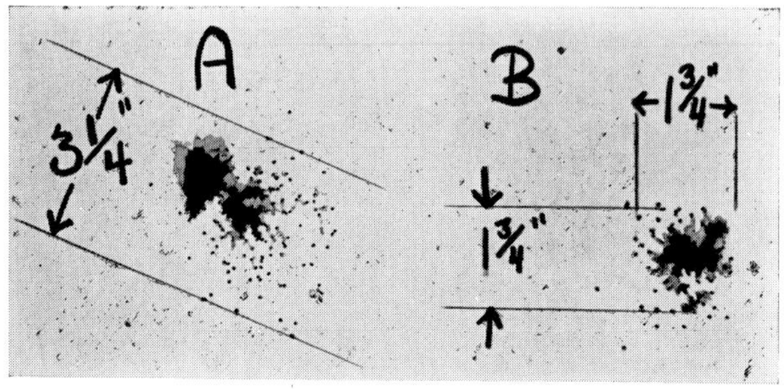


FIGURE IX-12. Pattern variations produced by different types of ammunition fired from the same distance (5 yd.) with the same shotgun (Remington, 12 gauge, model 11, full choke). (A): Remington-Peters shurshot, power piston. (B): Remington-Peters, target load.

The evaluation of distances with particular reference to wound patterns is discussed in Chapter X.

### Terminology

The following terminology is derived from Colonel Townsend Whelen's book *Small Arms Design and Ballistics.*[1] These are concise and informative definitions of commonly used terms.

*Shotgun:* A shoulder arm having a barrel that is smooth bored and is intended for the firing of a charge composed of one or more round balls or pellets of shot.

*Pistol:* A hand arm having a short barrel, usually not over 10 in. long, with a grip designed so that it can be held and fired with one hand with the arm extended. While revolvers are often included in the general classification of pistols, we prefer here to define a pistol as a hand arm in which the cartridge is loaded directly into the chamber of the barrel to distinguish it from a revolver, in which the cartridge is loaded into a cylinder in the rear of the breech of the barrel. Pistols may be single-shot or repeating.

*Single-shot:* Applies to a gun, rifle, or pistol that loads with only one cartridge. To fire a second time, the breech mechanism or action must be opened, the fired case or shell extracted and another inserted in the chamber.

*Double-barrel:* Applies to a small arm having two barrels placed either side-by-side or superimposed, each having its own firing mechanism.

*Repeating:* A small arm with magazine or recess in the breech action or under the barrel or stock and after firing; it requires hand action of the operator to eject the fired case and chamber a new cartridge.

*Semiautomatic:* Operated by the ammunition it uses automatically but requires releasing and depressing the trigger for each succeeding shot.

*Automatic:* A repeating firearm that utilizes the power of the recoil of the cartridge or a portion of the expanding gases to complete the cycle of ejecting the fired case and chambering another cartridge. An automatic arm will continue to fire with rapidity as long as the trigger is depressed or until the magazine is empty.

*Carbine:* A short-barreled musket or rifle having a barrel length generally not longer than 22 in.

*Caliber:* In the United States and all English-speaking countries the diameter of the bore of rifled small arms is designated in hundredths or thousandths of an inch. Thus, we have rifles, carbines, pistols and revolvers of .22, .25, .30, .32, .38 and .45 caliber or .220, .257, .357, and .405 caliber. On the continent of Europe and elsewhere the calibers of such weapons are designated in millimeters, as 6.5 mm, 7 mm, 8 mm and 9 mm. As an example of the equivalences, 6.35 mm equals .25 caliber, 7.65 mm equals .32 caliber and 9 mm equals .38 caliber.

*Extractor:* That mechanism in a firearm by which a cartridge or fired case is withdrawn from the chamber.

*Ejector:* In a firearm, the mechanism that throws the cartridge or fired case from the firearm.

## REFERENCE

1. Whelen, T.: *Small Arms Design and Ballistics.* Georgetown, South Carolina, Samworth Small Arms Technical Publishing Co., 1955.

*Chapter X*

# INJURY BY GUNFIRE

## General Introduction

FIREARMS ARE INVOLVED in approximately two-thirds of all homicides in the United States. Handguns, i.e. automatic pistols and revolvers, are used in the majority of cases. Rifles and shotguns are used far less commonly. The Federal Bureau of Investigation (FBI) reported that, in 1976, handguns were used in 49 percent of all murders committed in the United States, whereas rifles and shotguns were used in 6 percent and 9 percent, respectively.[1] During the same period cutting or stabbing was the cause of death in 18 percent of all murders in the United States.

Complete and accurate interpretation of firearm wounds is mandatory for effective prosecution. Because of the many characteristics that injuries by handguns have in common with injuries by rifle fire, these will be considered together. They will be referred to as gunshot wounds. Shotgun wounds are discussed separately.

*Part 1*

## GUNSHOT WOUNDS

WERNER U. SPITZ

The following are essentials derived from the external examination of a gunshot wound: (a) range of fire, (b) direction of fire.

### RANGE OF FIRE

Only test firing of the gun in question with the type of ammunition that was used in a specific case enables reliable determination of the range of fire. Nevertheless, certain general criteria exist that allow an estimation of the target-to-muzzle distance by examination of a bullet wound.

When a firearm is discharged, smoke containing abundant soot and gunpowder is ejected from the muzzle in addition to the bullet (Fig. X-1). These deposits of soot and gunpower on the target that occur around the bullet hole on close-range firing are referred to as smudging and tattooing or stippling, respectively. It is the pattern and the density of these deposits on the target which permit assessment of the distance from which the gun was fired (Fig. X-2).

Painstaking examination of the victim's clothes is imperative to ascertain the presence of gunpowder and soot around a bullet hole. When the clothes are of a light color, soiling by soot and gunpowder may be easily recognized. However, when the clothes are dark or blood soaked, identification of powder residue may not be as simple. Chemical identification of gunpowder residue has proven valuable for clothing items and occasionally for skin, when grains seen on the target are not readily identifiable as gunpowder by naked-eye examination or by using a large,

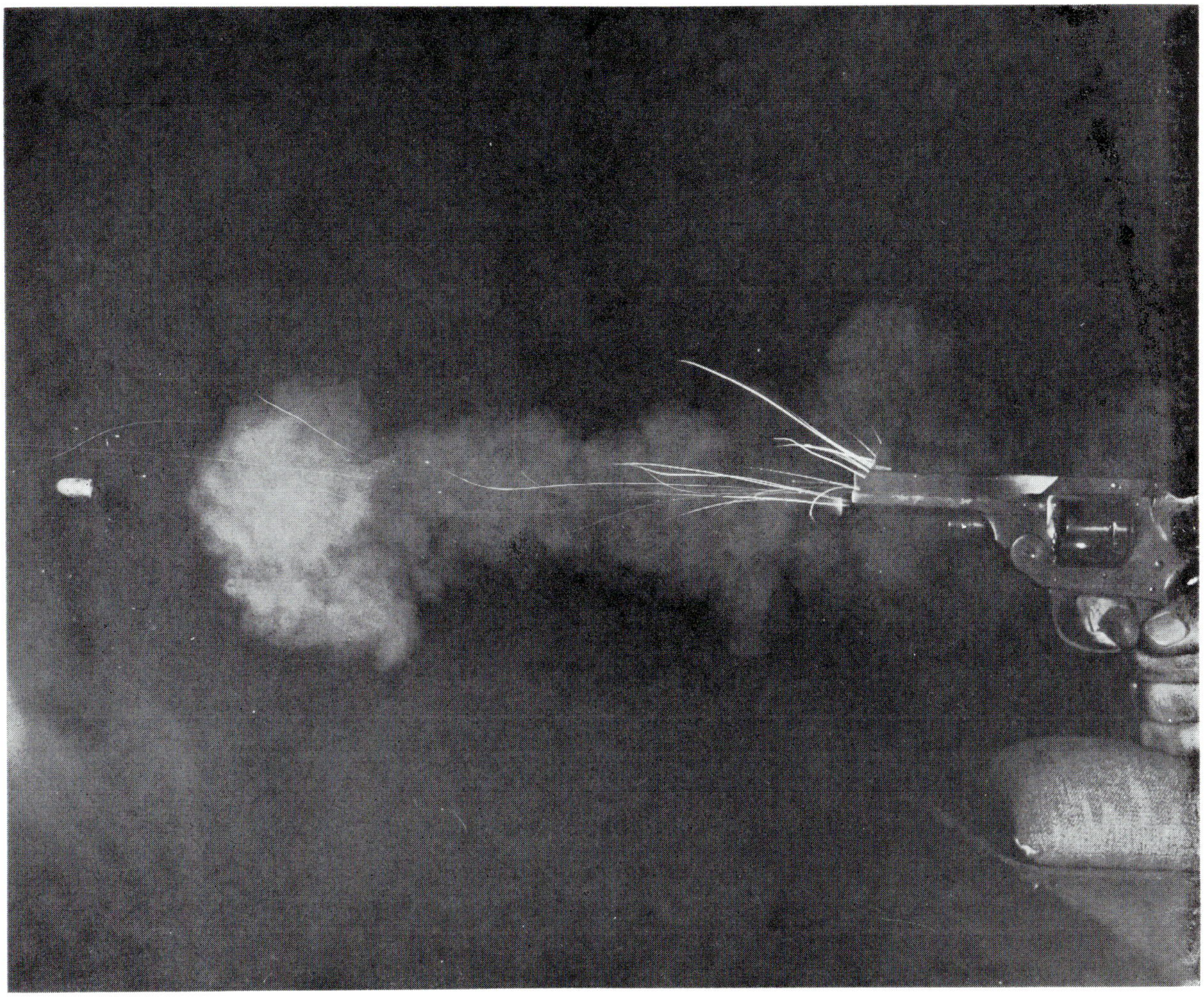

FIGURE X-1. Gunsmoke ejected from the muzzle of a revolver at the time of discharge. The volume of gas created is equal to the weight of gunpowder burnt. The light streaks are glowing particles of gunpowder. The bullet is seen on the left side of the photograph. (The author gratefully acknowledges the cooperation of Donald M. Flohr of the H. P. White Laboratories, Bel Air, Maryland, for the preparation of this photograph.)

preferably illuminated, magnifying lens.

Reliable chemical identification of grains of gunpowder is feasible by thin-layer chromatography. Recently, energy-dispersive x ray and flameless atomic absorption spectroscopy have been found to be advantageous for this purpose.[2]

The terminology most often used to describe the ranges of fire is as follows: (a) contact shot, when the weapon is fired with the muzzle in actual contact with the body, (b) close-range shot, (c) distant shot.

### Shot Fired With the Muzzle in Actual Contact With the Body

When a gun is fired with the muzzle against a clothed part of the body, the bullet hole in the cloth touching the muzzle is sometimes surrounded by a flat ring corresponding to the profile of the muzzle. This is due to distortion of the fabric as a result of the heat of combustion that develops in the barrel while simultaneously being pressed upon by the weapon. It is an *ironinglike* effect. The loose fibers of fabric in

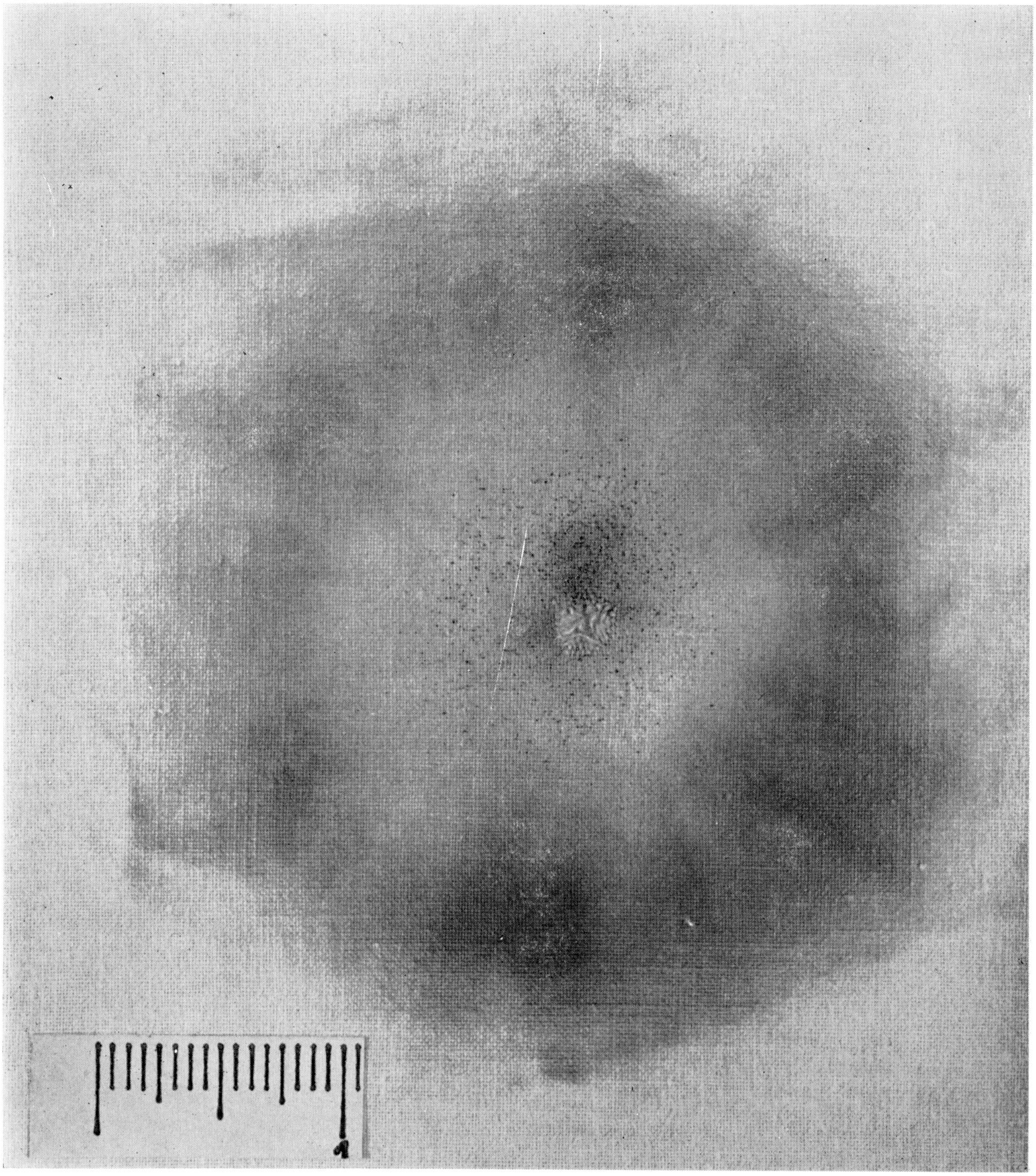

FIGURE X-2a. Test shot on a piece of cloth from a distance of 1 in. The weapon was a .22 caliber Colt Woodsman Automatic; the ammunition .22 caliber Western Super X-Long Rifle. Note the densely scattered gunpowder particles around the bullet hole, while the soot is spread over a 3½ to 4 in. diameter.

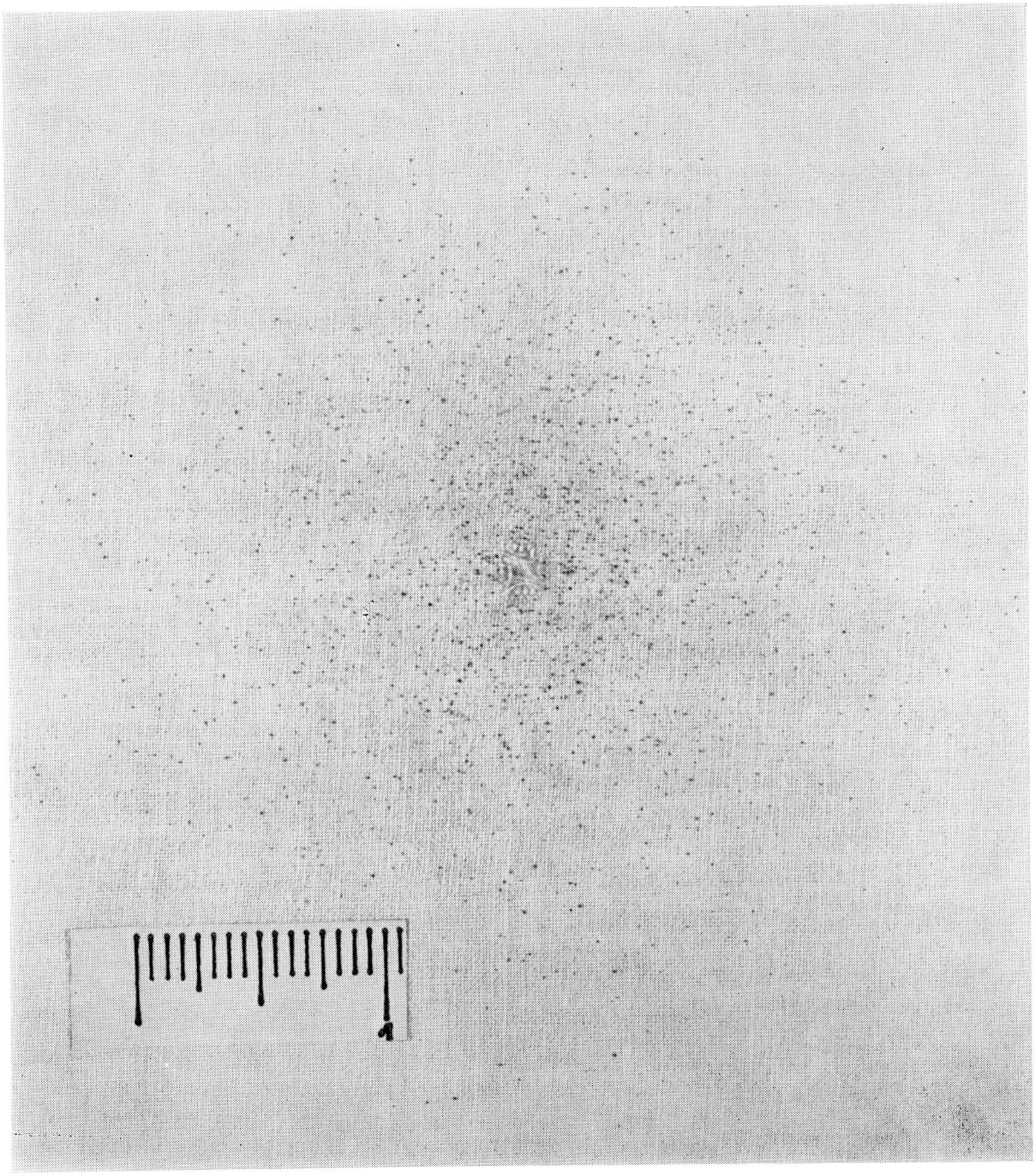

FIGURE X-2b. Using the same weapon and the same ammunition at 6 in. muzzle-to-target distance, practically no soot reaches the target. The gunpowder particles are spread over a 3 to 4 in. diameter.

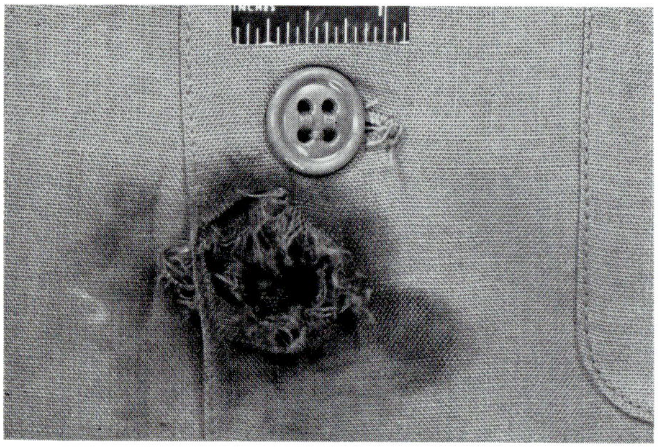

FIGURE X-3. Suicidal shot of the upper abdomen. Deposit of soot around a near-contact bullet hole in the shirt. The fibers of the fabric are mostly turned outward by the expanding gases returning through the hole.

the center of the bullet hole are often turned outward, away from the body, as a result of the expanding gases returning through the defect. Commonly, these fibers are blackened by gunsmoke. In the case of synthetic fabrics, melting of the end of these fibers may sometimes be observed. Soot in varying amounts is also deposited on the edges of the bullet hole, depending on how tightly the gun was held against the body (Fig. X-3).

Although deposits of gunsmoke on the clothing frequently remain unrecognized if the clothes are blood soaked, the inside of the garment may show abundant deposits of gunsmoke even if none were noted on the outside. This results from spreading of the smoke by the muzzle blast between the skin and the clothing and is observed especially if the shot passed through several layers of fabric. It is also commonly seen if the shot was fired through a pocket. Each layer is blackened individually on both sides of the fabric, while the wound in the skin may be devoid of gunpowder or soot.

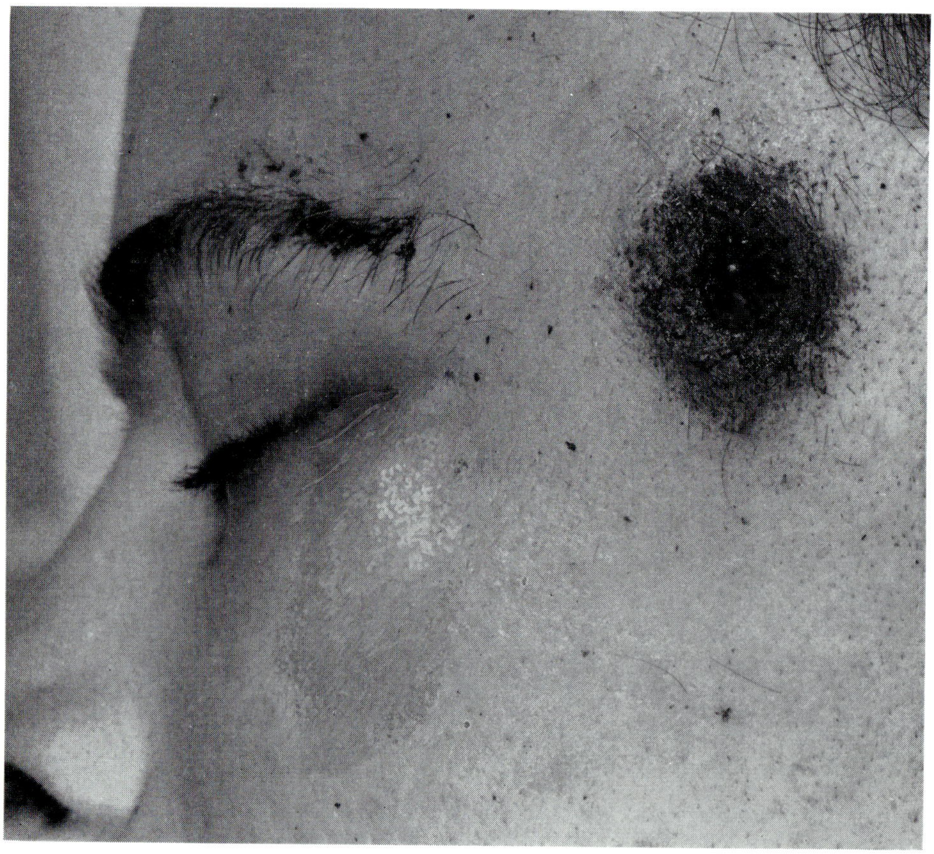

FIGURE X-4. Homicidal shot of the left temple. A small amount of soot is deposited on the edges of this loose-contact gunshot wound.

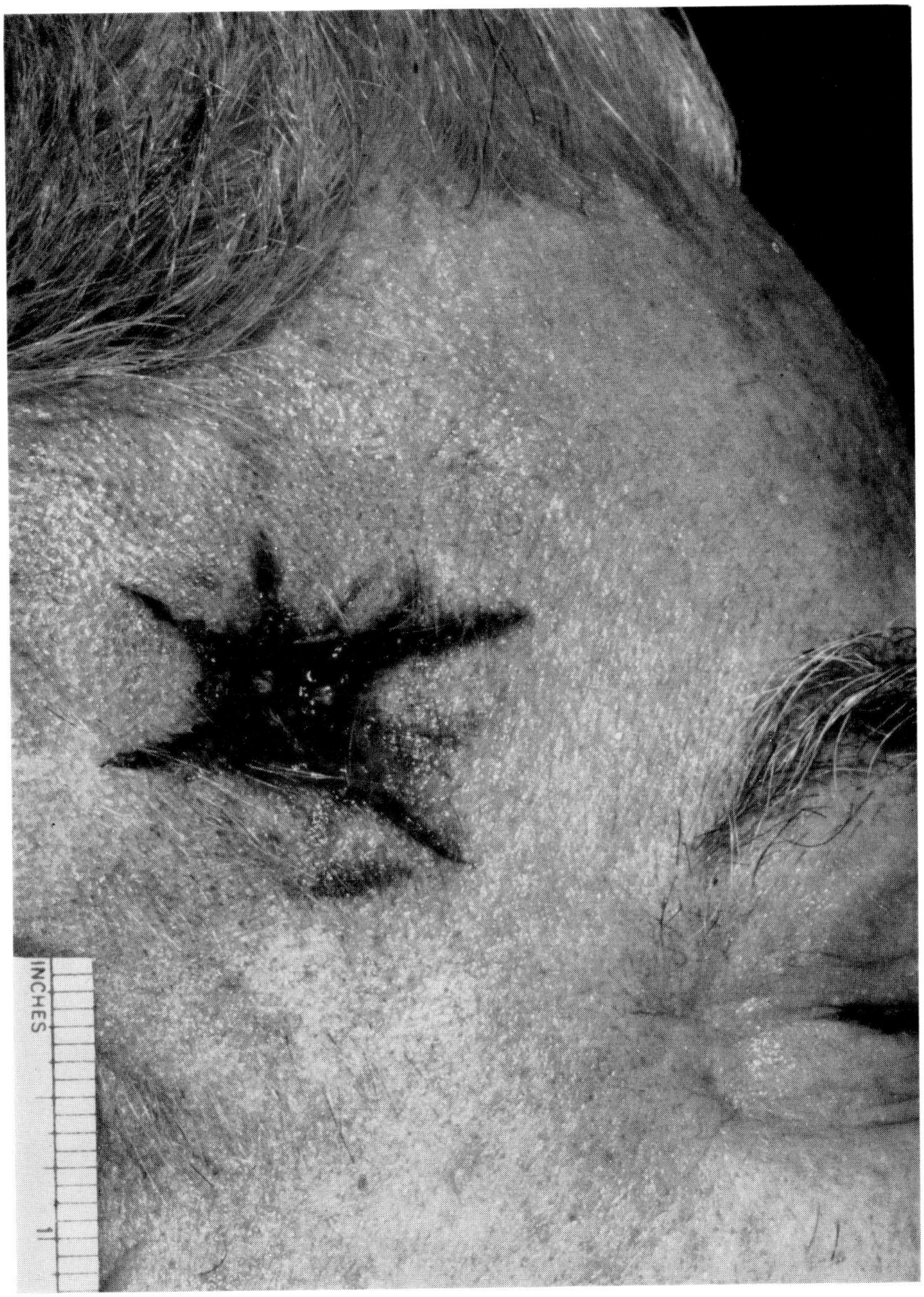


FIGURE X-5. Suicidal gunshot of the right temple. The gun was evidently held in tight contact with the skin, as evidenced by the star-shaped wound and the absence of gunsmoke on the wound margins. The small horizontal abrasion under the bullet wound probably represents a partial imprint of the muzzle.

In the absence of intervening clothing between the muzzle and the skin, the gunsmoke is propelled into the wound; however, a small amount of smoke may be deposited on the wound edges, particularly if contact with the muzzle was loose (Fig. X-4).

Careful handling and layerwise dissection of such an injury are required to reveal the fine granules of burned and unburned gunpowder and deposits of black soot in the depth of the wound. In the absence of such deposits the wound may be mistaken for a distant shot. This may mean the difference between a self-inflicted bullet wound and involvement of another party. In the case of a contact shot of the head with a revolver or a semiautomatic pistol, the wound is frequently star shaped due to tears that radiate from the sides of the wound. These tears are caused by the blast effect that follows the sudden release of gases into a confined area, between the skin and the underlying bone (Figs. X-5 and X-6). A pocket under the skin containing blood mixed with gunpowder is formed by separation of the tissues.

Soot may also be deposited on the bone around the bullet hole (Fig. X-7). An ideal procedure to document this soot is to incise the periosteum around the defect at twelve, three, six and nine o'clock, then raise the periosteum using dissecting forceps. If the surface is soiled with blood, pressing a dry paper towel to the area usually reveals the blackened edges of the hole in the bone when the paper is gently peeled back. The deposit of soot must not be mistaken for lead rubbed off on the bone during the passage of the bullet. Close examination of the defect in the bone usually shows the soot distributed circumferentially, in contrast to a localized area occupied by the lead (Fig. X-8); in addition, the metallic sheen of a fragment of lead is usually recognizable. Even in cases of prolonged survival, deposits of soot on the

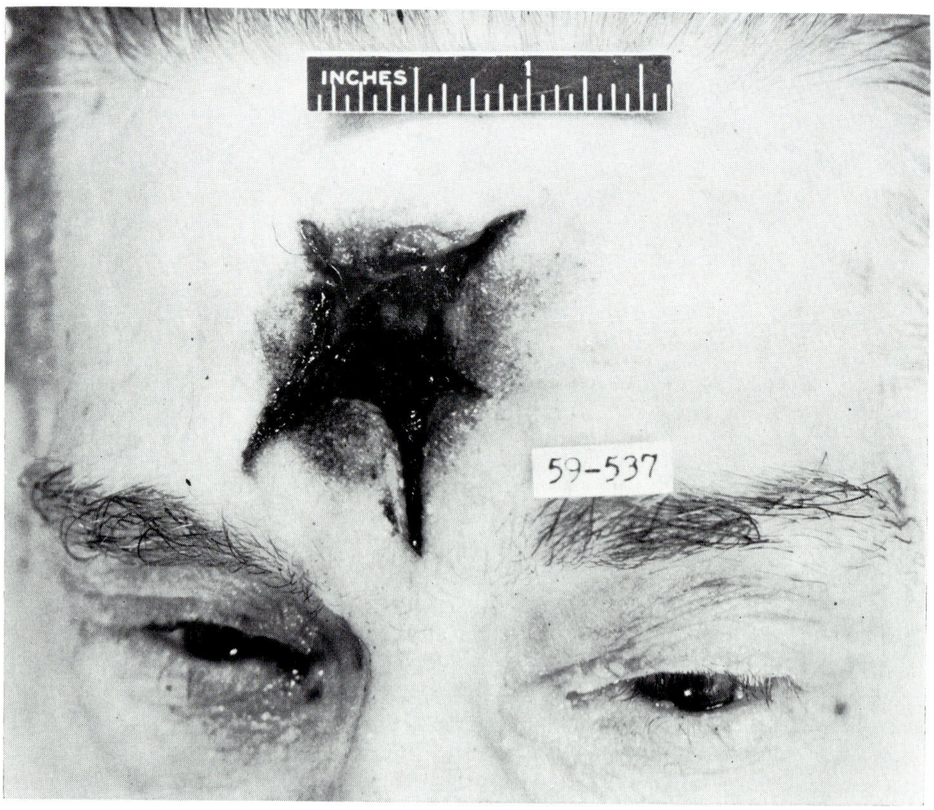


FIGURE X-6. Suicidal bullet wound of the forehead. This shot was fired with the muzzle pressed against the skin. The abraded ring around the wound is due to impact of the muzzle on the skin by the recoil of the weapon.

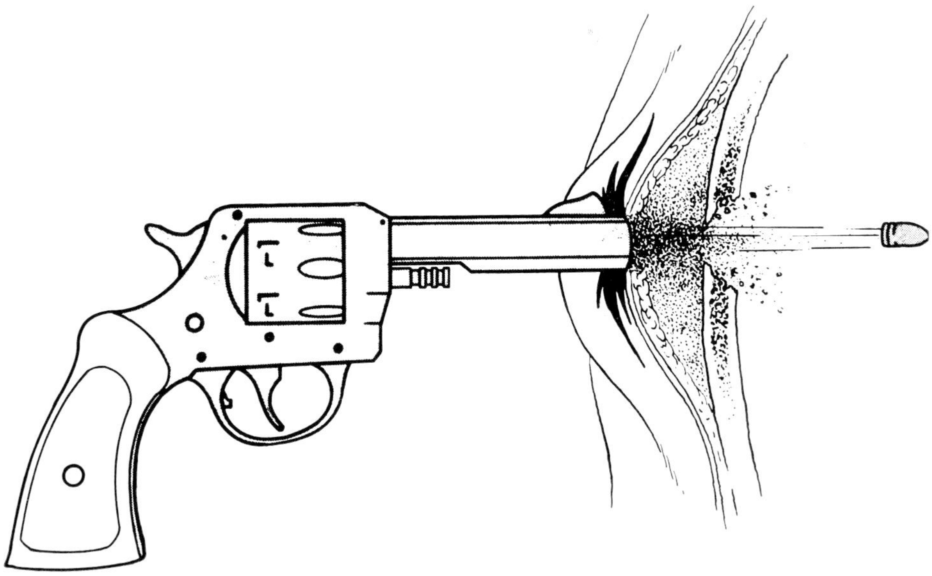

FIGURE X-7. Diagram showing the mechanism of a shot fired with the muzzle in tight contact with the skin. The *pocket* between the skin and the bone is filled with soot and gunpowder. No gunsmoke is deposited on the skin around the wound. The wound edges are split by the force of the expanding gases.

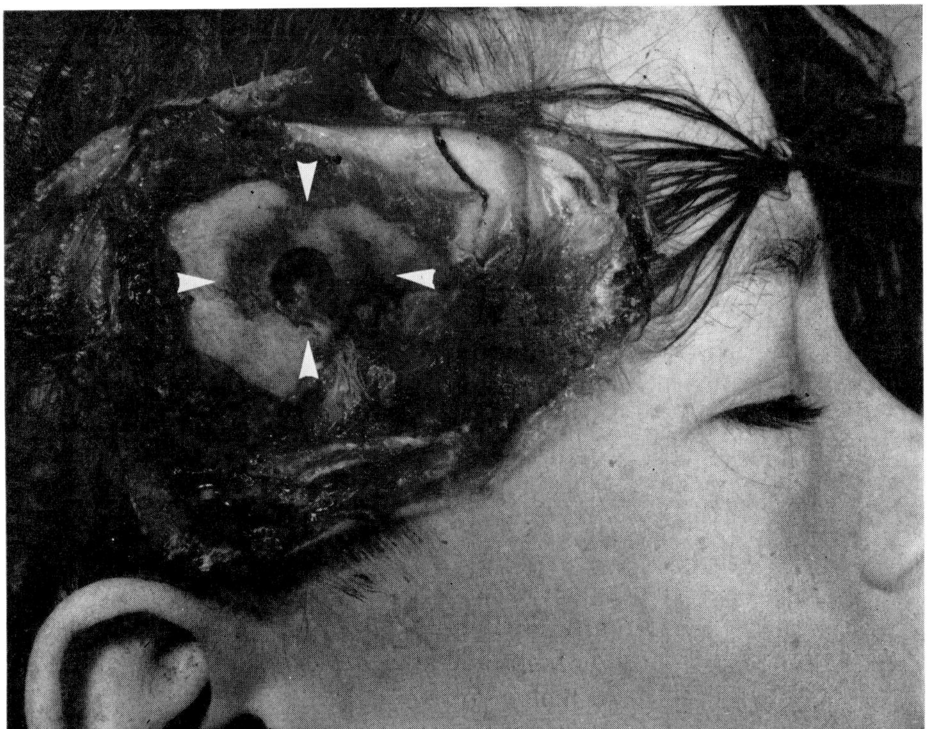

FIGURE X-8. Soot is frequently deposited on the bone underlying a contact bullet wound. The presence of this soot can usually only be demonstrated after careful removal of the area's soft tissues. Particular care must be taken in stripping the periosteum in the immediate vicinity of the bullet hole. Gunsmoke is often deposited on the bone after the periosteum has been elevated by the gas pressure.

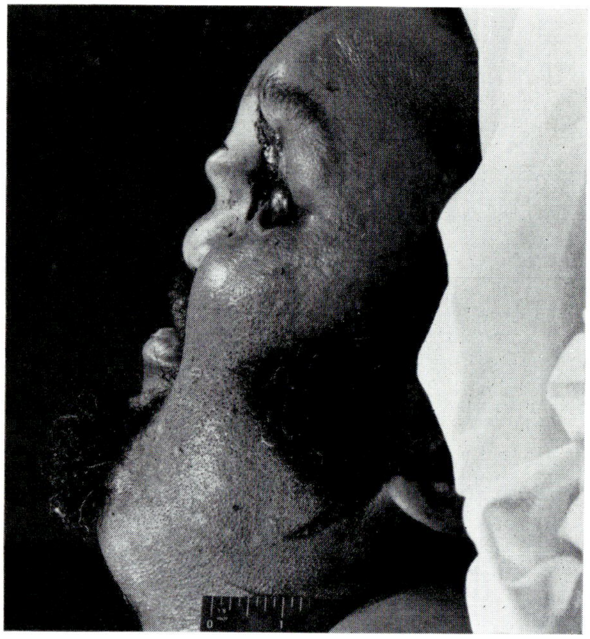

FIGURE X-9. High-powered rifle shot into the mouth. A gaping exit wound was situated at the back of the head. The facial skeleton is caved in. Tears are noted at the inner angles of the eyes and ears due to overstretching as a result of an intense increase in pressure within the skull.

bone may be identified for a considerable time. We have observed this in a young woman who survived three months after she shot herself in the temple. Frequently, soot is pushed deeper into the wound track, and a faint gray or black discoloration may be noted on the inner surface of the skull around the bullet hole and on the dura mater.

Fragments of bone no larger than ⅛ to ¼ in. in diameter derived from the bullet hole in the skull are sometimes carried by the missile deep into the brain tissue. Such fragments may be of great significance in cases where a contact shot is suspected yet no soot was noted on the skin or adjacent tissues. The fragments should be rinsed under cold water to remove blood and to disclose the presence or absence of soot deposits. Small pieces of fabric from the victim's clothing are occasionally carried into the wound by the bullet, regardless of the range of fire. Such fabric, if dark or blood soiled, may resemble soot, and its presence in a wound has led to the mistaken diagnosis of a contact shot.

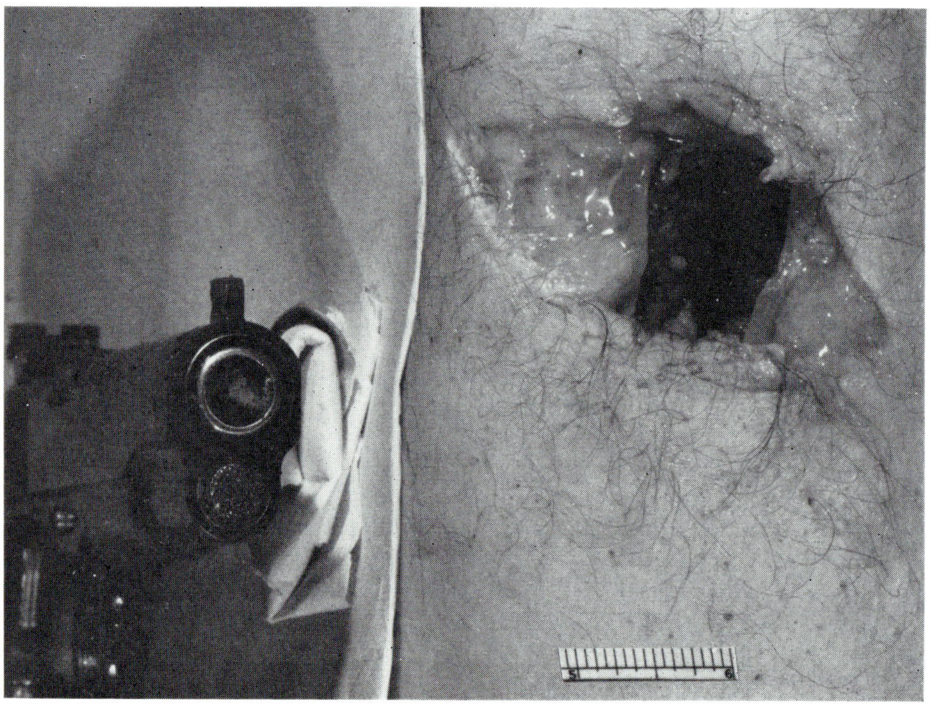

FIGURE X-10. This injury was produced with a .45 caliber blank cartridge when the weapon was held in contact with the skin. Fat tissue was noted in the barrel of the pistol.

Microscopic examination of suspicious fragments is sometimes required to ascertain their true nature.

Fracture lines often radiate from the circular defect caused by the bullet, particularly if a caliber larger than .22 has been used. Undoubtedly the mechanism of these fractures is the tremendous sudden expansion resulting from the muzzle blast. Independent fractures of the orbital roofs due to the same mechanism are also observed with some frequency in contact shots of the head, particularly in elderly individuals in whom these plates are thin and fragile. The dura mater over the orbits is usually intact.

Fractures of the orbital roofs were described in the autopsy of President Abraham Lincoln, although the shot was not fired at contact. Lincoln was shot in the back of the head at close range with a Derringer pistol firing a ball ½ in. in diameter. It appears likely that the caliber of the missile or possibly the increase of intracranial pressure resulting from hemorrhage and brain swelling was responsible for the orbital roof fractures in this case. A comprehensive discussion of the medical aspects of the assassination of Abraham Lincoln was published by Gilmore.[3]

In the case of a high-powered rifle, the amount of gas generated by the blast is so large that a shot fired in contact with the head causes massive destruction. Facial features are frequently

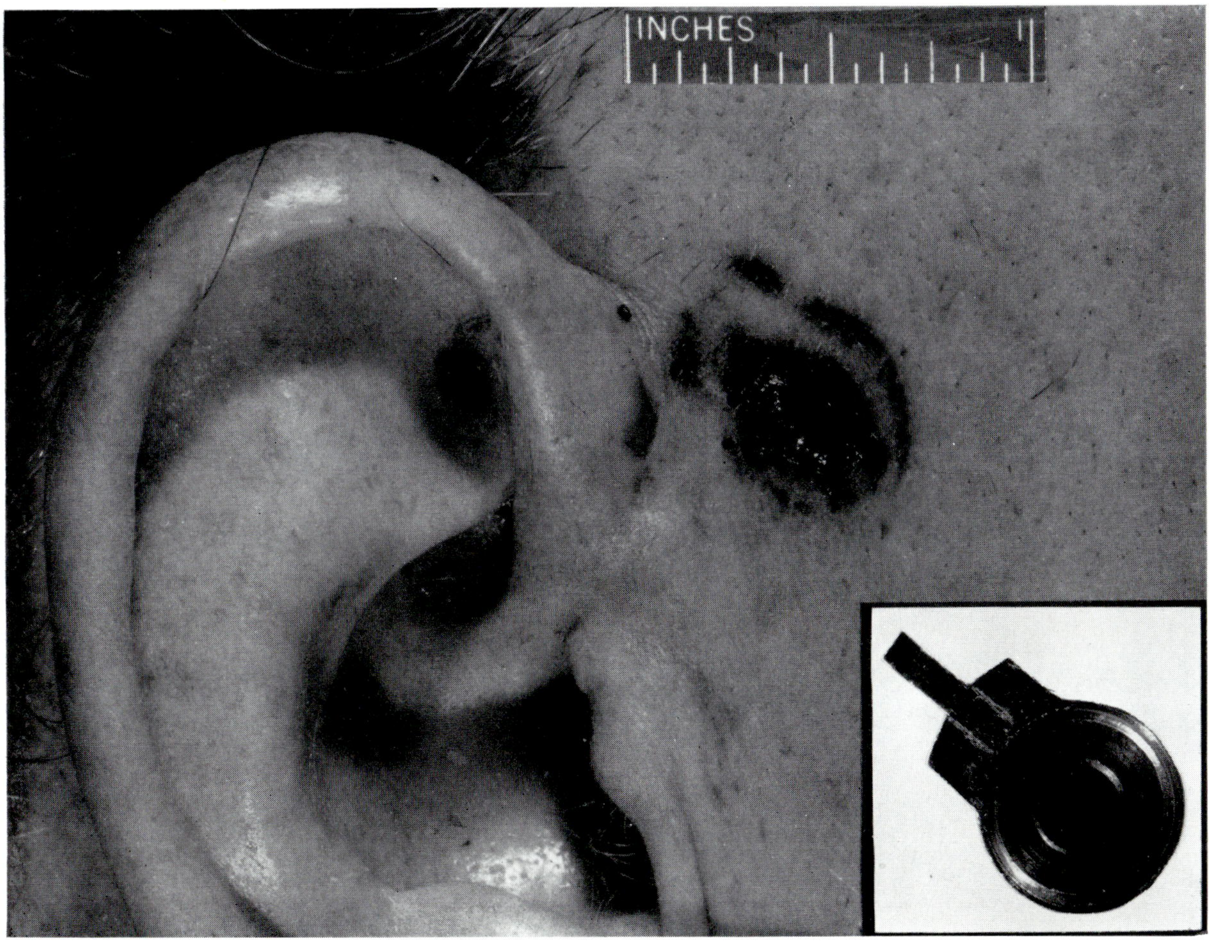


FIGURE X-11. Suicidal shot of the right temple. The patterned abrasion around the bullet wound corresponds to the contour of the muzzle profile shown in the insert. The weapon was a .22 caliber Ruger semiautomatic pistol.

distorted beyond recognition. Discharge of a high-powered rifle into the mouth or below the chin is associated with tremendous overexpansion of the tissues of the entire head. This causes tears of the skin in front of the ears and along the creases on either side of the mouth and nose as well as the inner angles of the eyes. The presence of such tears suggests the location of the entrance wound. Destruction is often so intense that identification of the entrance wound may be possible only by finding the muzzle imprint on the skin, with underlying soot and gunpowder (Fig. X-9). The presence of gunsmoke may be further compounded by widespread tissue scattering. Restoration of the skull by replacement of the bone fragments to determine the direction of the shot by direction of the bevelling is helpful and is performed as outlined in Chapter XXIV.

The muzzle blast of a gun fired in contact with a body and the negative pressure in the barrel following discharge may cause blood, hair and fragments of tissue and fabric to be found several inches back inside the barrel (Fig. X-10). An imprint of the muzzle profile on the skin around a bullet wound or adjacent to it is due to the recoil of the gun, but the muzzle blast must also be considered in this regard (Figs. X-11 and X-12). An imprint of the muzzle on the skin is not limited to contact bullet wounds of the head area; the same imprint may be observed in contact shots in other parts of the body (Fig. X-13).

Near-contact between the muzzle and the skin will provide for the escape of the gases when the gun is fired, with resulting dispersion of the muzzle blast. The characteristic features of such a shot fired in near-contact are consequently somewhat modified. The blast effect is not as pronounced as in the case of tight contact, and splitting of the wound edges does not occur. Fractures of the skull radiating from the bullet hole are observed only rarely under such circumstances. The bright yellow flame, which extends 2 to 2½ in. from the muzzle at the time of discharge, scorches the clothing and adjacent skin and singes the hair. Soot is deposited on

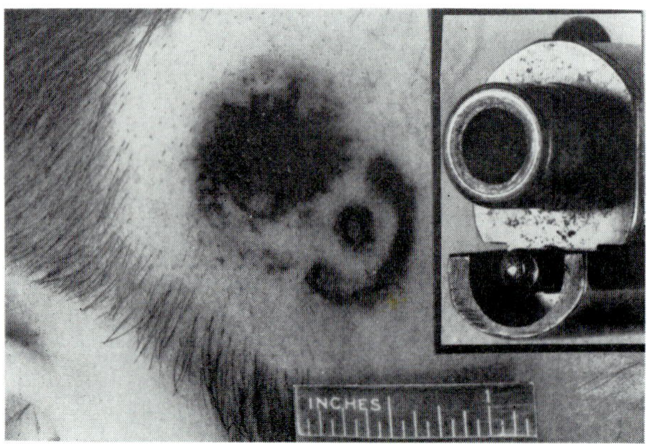


FIGURE X-12. Suicidal shot of the right temple. The gun was held in contact with the skin. The patterned injury adjacent to the bullet wound is the imprint of the housing frame and recoil spring guide of the pistol.

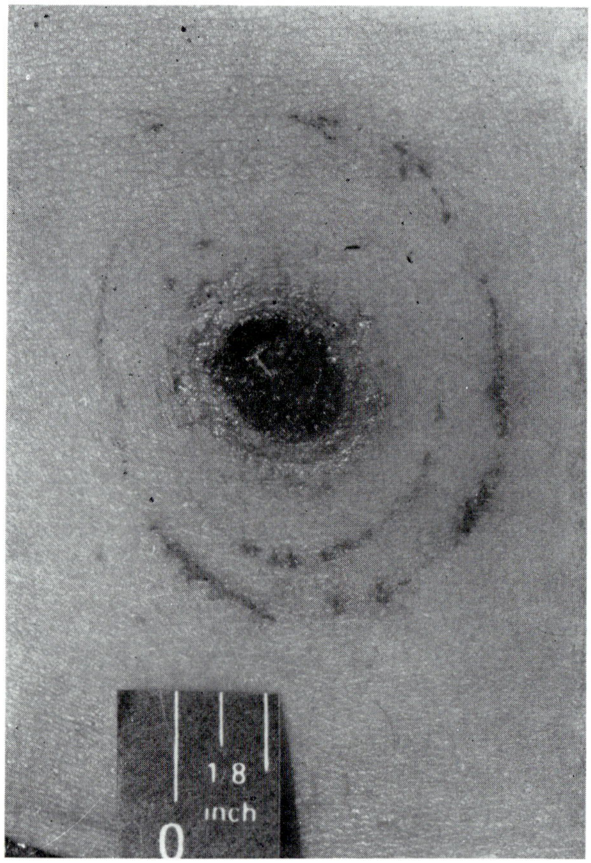


FIGURE X-13. Imprint of a .22 caliber rifle muzzle on the abdominal skin in a suicide. The absence of soot on the surface suggests this was a *pressure contact shot*. The edges of the bullet wound are not torn because of ample space for gas expansion in the abdominal cavity.

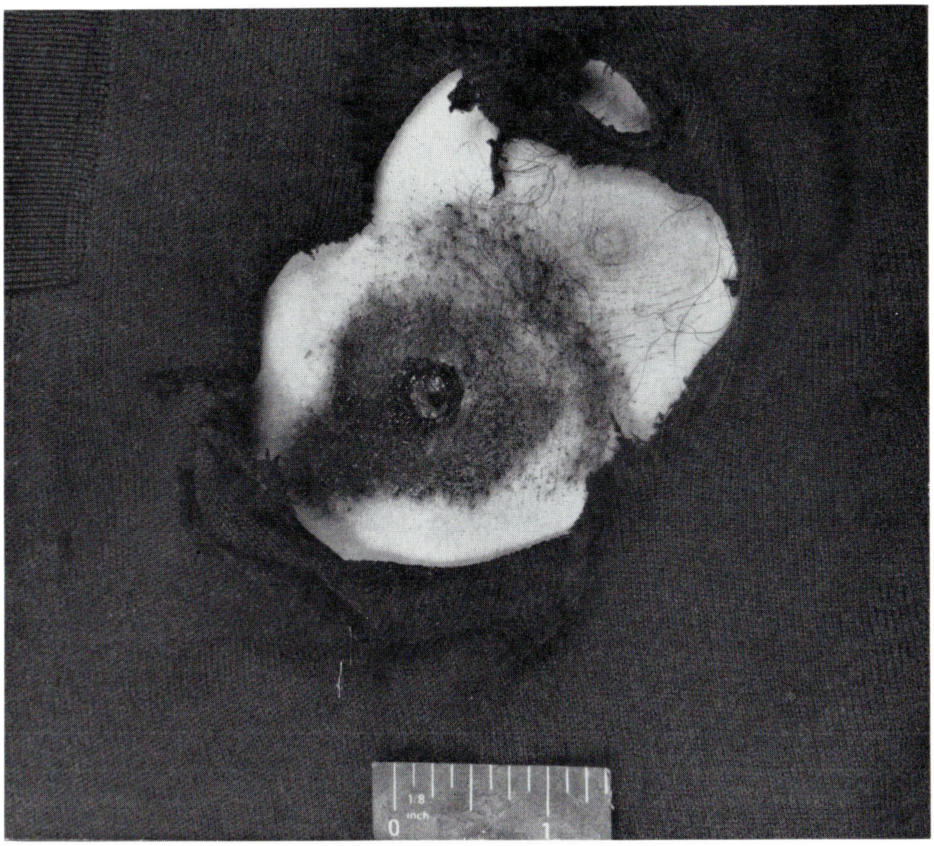

FIGURE X-14. Near-contact suicidal shot of the chest. The synthetic fabric of the shirt is scorched. The skin is superficially burned around the bullet wound, and the hairs in the area are singed. Only a few specks of gunpowder are scattered on the skin surface.

the target, but only a few granules of gunpowder may be scattered on the surface. Most of the gunpowder is propelled into the bullet wound (Fig. X-14).

Evidence of scorching is noted on microscopic examination of near-contact bullet wounds. A comprehensive microscopic study of dermal gunshot wounds was described by Adelson.[4]

The high concentration of carbon monoxide in gunsmoke transforms hemoglobin into carboxyhemoglobin. A characteristic cherry red discoloration of the musculature under a contact bullet wound enables identification of carboxyhemoglobin in the tissue. Chemical confirmation of the presence of carboxyhemoglobin is useful, particularly in cases where the range of fire is unknown. Perforation of the chest wall involving the lung, as by a stab wound or a distant gunshot wound, may also cause a transient bright red discoloration of the musculature around the site of the injury. This, however, results from perfusion of the area by oxygenated blood and must not be mistaken for carboxyhemoglobin.

## Close-range Shot

A close-range shot is one that is fired from a distance at which gunpowder residue, as well as particles of primer and small fragments of metal from the bullet, may be identified around a bullet hole (Figs. X-15 to X-19).

On naked-eye examination these particles are indistinguishable from one another. The diameter and density of the pattern of particles on the target are useful in evaluating the distance between the weapon and the target. These pat-

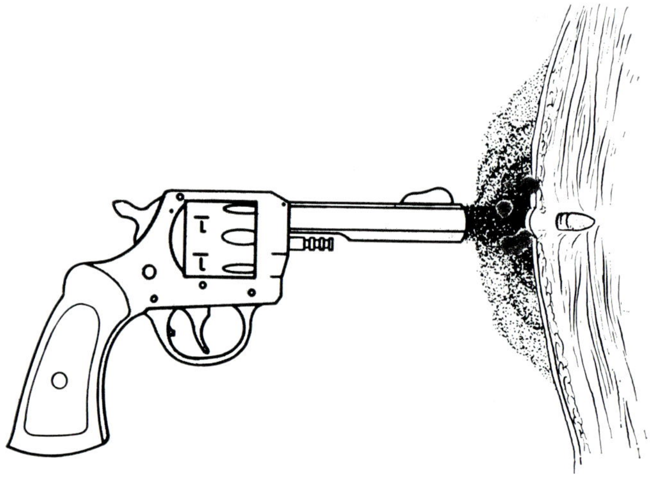

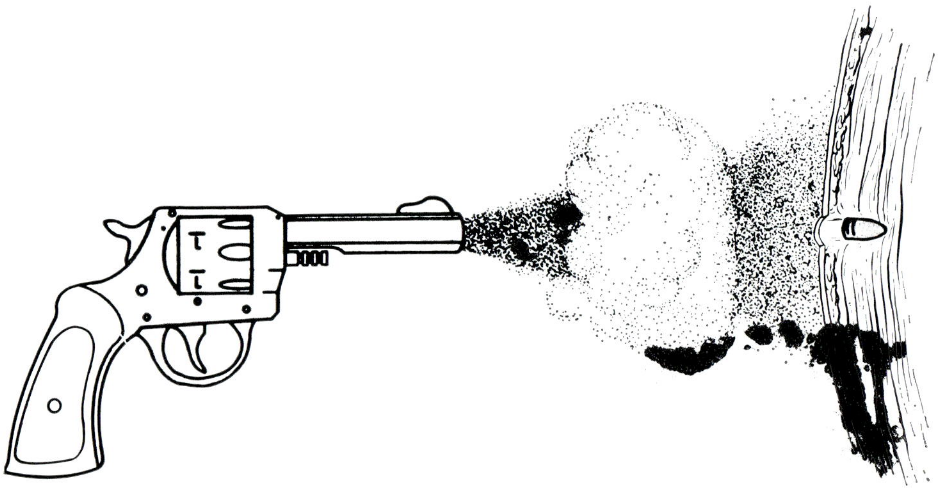

FIGURE X-15. Diagram of close-range shots with a handgun. (a): At a distance of 1 to 2 in. from the target, particles of gunpowder are centered around the bullet hole, while *waves* of soot disperse over a much wider area. (Fig. X-2a illustrates this point.) (b): As the muzzle-to-target-distance increases, the dispersion of particles on the target increases in diameter, while the density of particle scattering decreases. At a distance of 6 or 7 in., abundant gunpowder and little if any soot are deposited on the target (*see also* Fig. X-2b).

terns vary widely with different guns and different types of ammunition. For most handguns, demonstrable residues on skin are found at firing distances of up to 12 to 18 in. For rifles, this may reach several feet. At greater distance, the small particles of gunpowder that are emitted from the barrel at the time of firing lack the inertia required to reach the target. As mentioned earlier, the approximate distance from which a close-range shot was fired can be evaluated only by test firing the particular weapon, using the same type of ammunition as that used in the shooting case under consideration. A frequent source of error with respect to the evaluation of the distance from which a gun was fired is the comparison of a test pattern on a white paper or cloth with the pattern of the wound on the skin. Scattered specks of gunpowder are certainly not as conspicuous on the skin as they are on a smooth white background such as cloth or paper. This discrepancy should be considered when test patterns are evaluated.

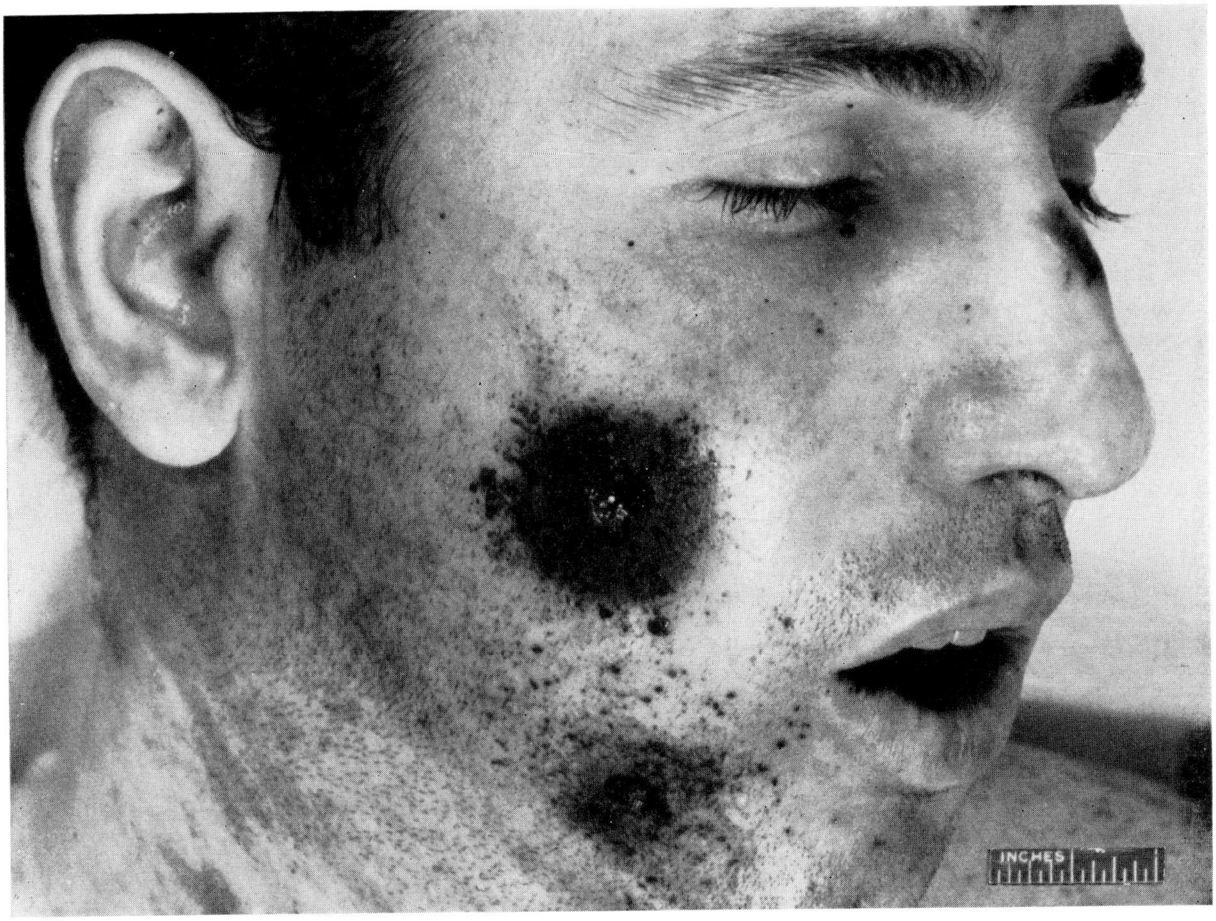


FIGURE X-16. Two homicidal shots of the right side of the face. The upper shot shows abundant soot and very little gunpowder around the wound. This shot was fired at near-contact with the skin. The lower shot is surrounded by a small amount of soot, while particles of gunpowder are scattered over a diameter of about 2 in. This shot was fired from a distance of a few inches.

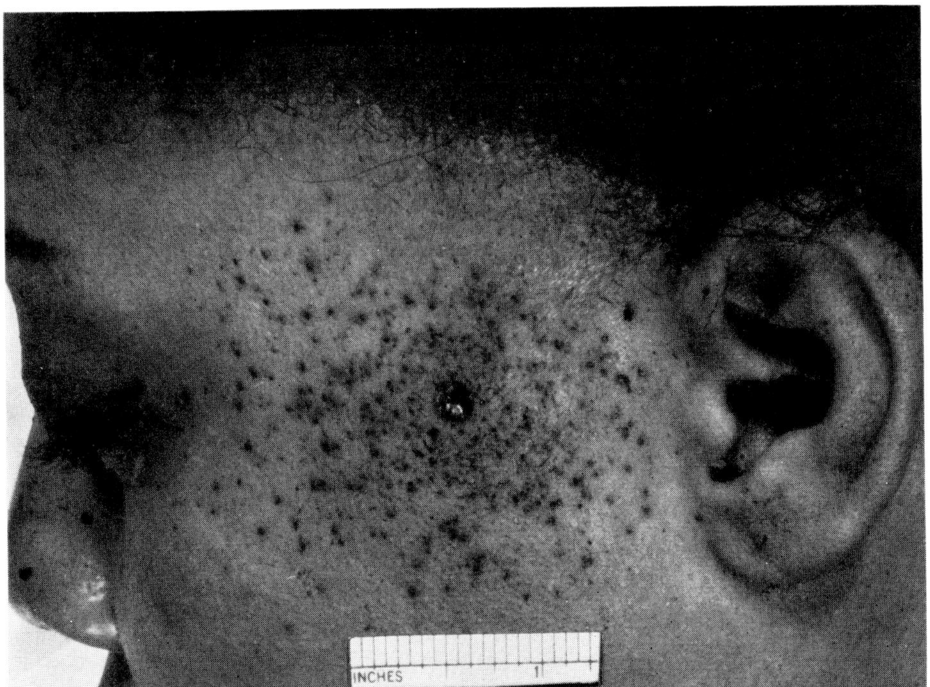


FIGURE X-17. Homicide: Close-range shot of the left temple. Densely scattered powder particles but no soot indicate a shot fired from a distance of several inches.

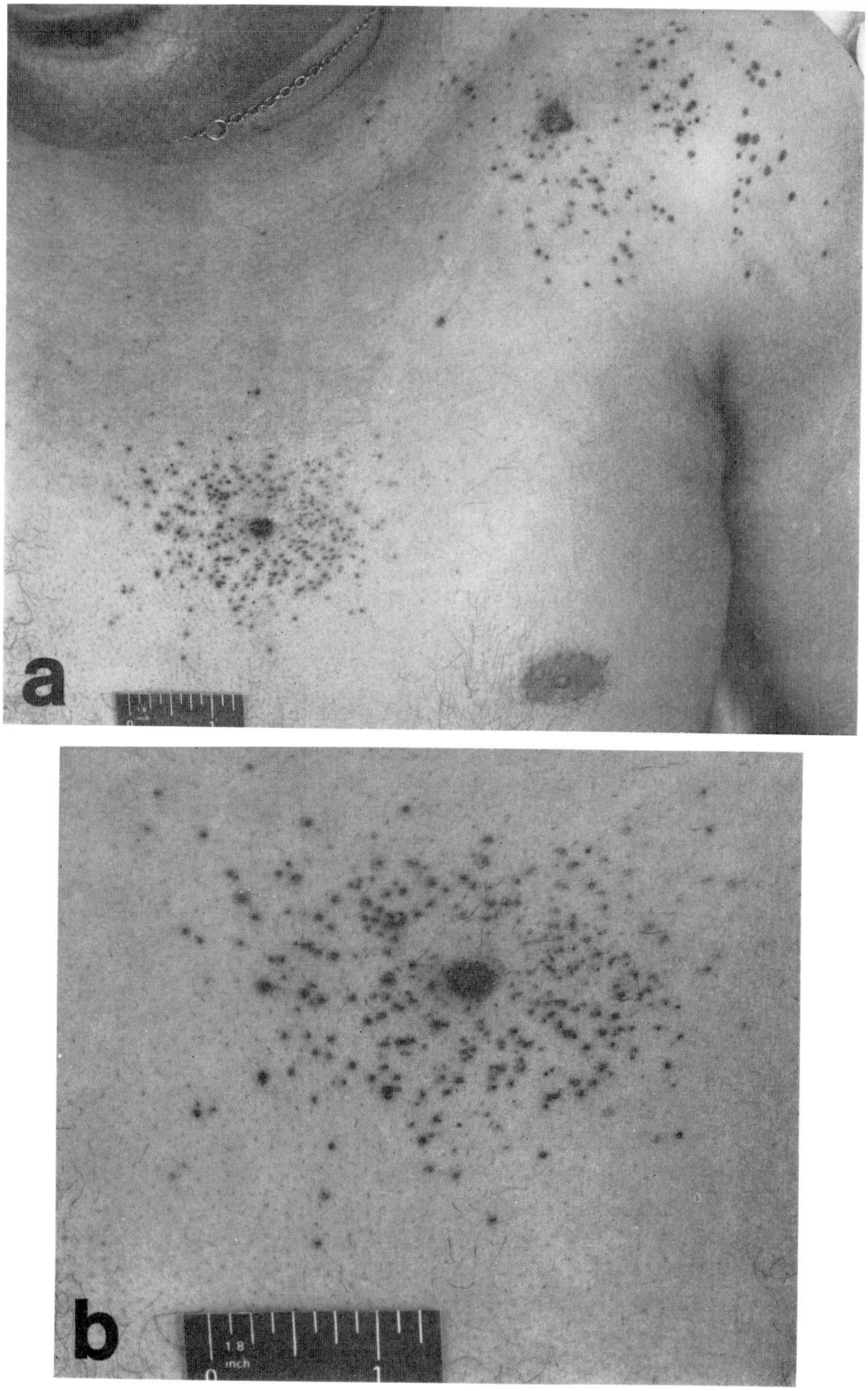


FIGURE X-18. Two close-range gunshot wounds involving a .25 caliber automatic pistol using Western ammunition. (a): The lower wound was obviously inflicted at closer range, as indicated by the greater density and lesser spread of the gunpowder stippling compared to the shoulder wound. (b): In the closeup of the lower wound, the individual gunpowder stipples appear punched out and circular, suggesting that the fired round was loaded with ball powder.

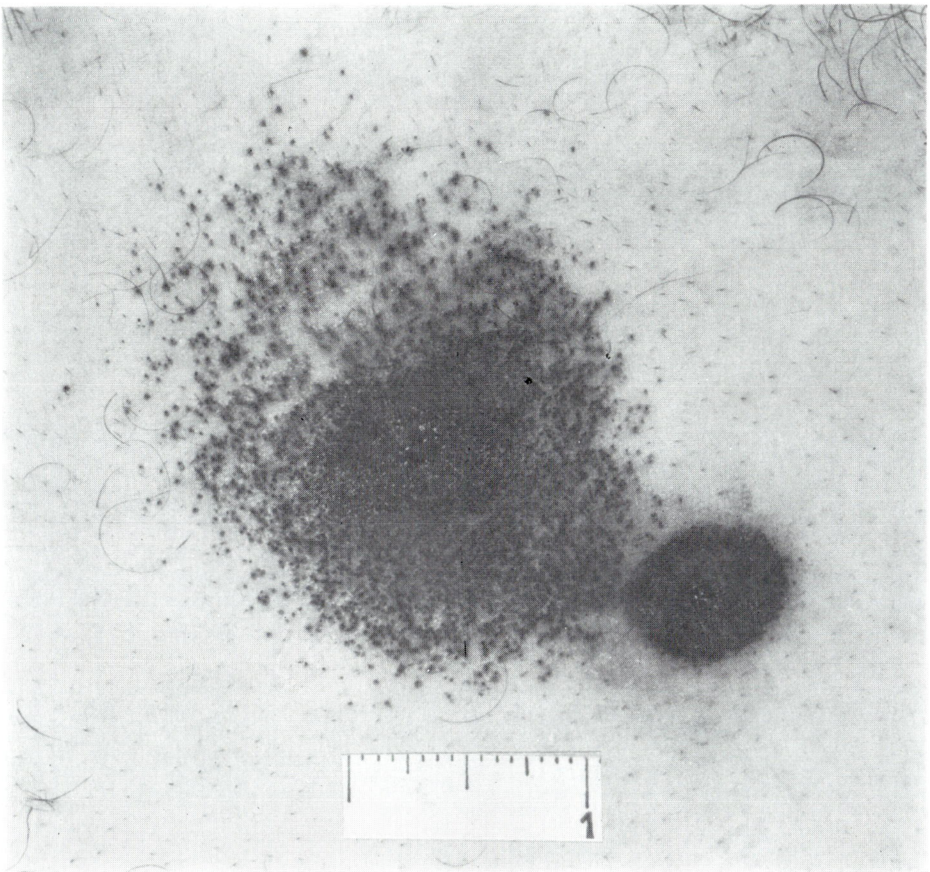

FIGURE X-19. Young man who committed suicide by shooting himself in the chest. The bullet wound on the right is surrounded by a well-demarcated *ring* of soot, and the wound margins are scorched. This injury was inflicted at near-contact with the skin. The adjacent injury (left) is surrounded by densely scattered powder stipples, with a small amount of soot deposited in the immediate vicinity of the wound. This injury was inflicted at close range (2 to 3 in.), as determined by test firing of the weapon (.22 caliber Ruger revolver, using .22 caliber magnum ammunition). The direction of this shot was from left to right and upwards.

The length of the barrel of a firearm has considerable bearing on the diameter of the pattern of gunsmoke deposited on the target. For example, a snub-nosed revolver with a 2 in. barrel spreads gunsmoke over a considerably larger area than a target pistol having a 6 or 8 in. barrel, fired from the same distance and employing the same type of ammunition (Fig. X-20). A useful rule of thumb for handguns is that gunpowder residue may still be identified by naked-eye examination of the target at a distance of double the length of the barrel.[5]

Ammunition manufactured by different companies can produce different patterns of powder residue at a given distance with the same gun. This is due to gunpowder peculiarities, such as the use of *ball* or *flake* gunpowder, as well as other manufacturing characteristics. The powder charge in some *magnum*-labeled handgun ammunition is significantly larger than that in ordinary ammunition of the same caliber. This difference can be observed when such a cartridge has been discharged at close range. The spread of stippling on the skin extends over a larger diameter, and the density of scattering of individual powder flecks is significantly greater than that produced by regular ammunition (Figs. X-21 and X-22).

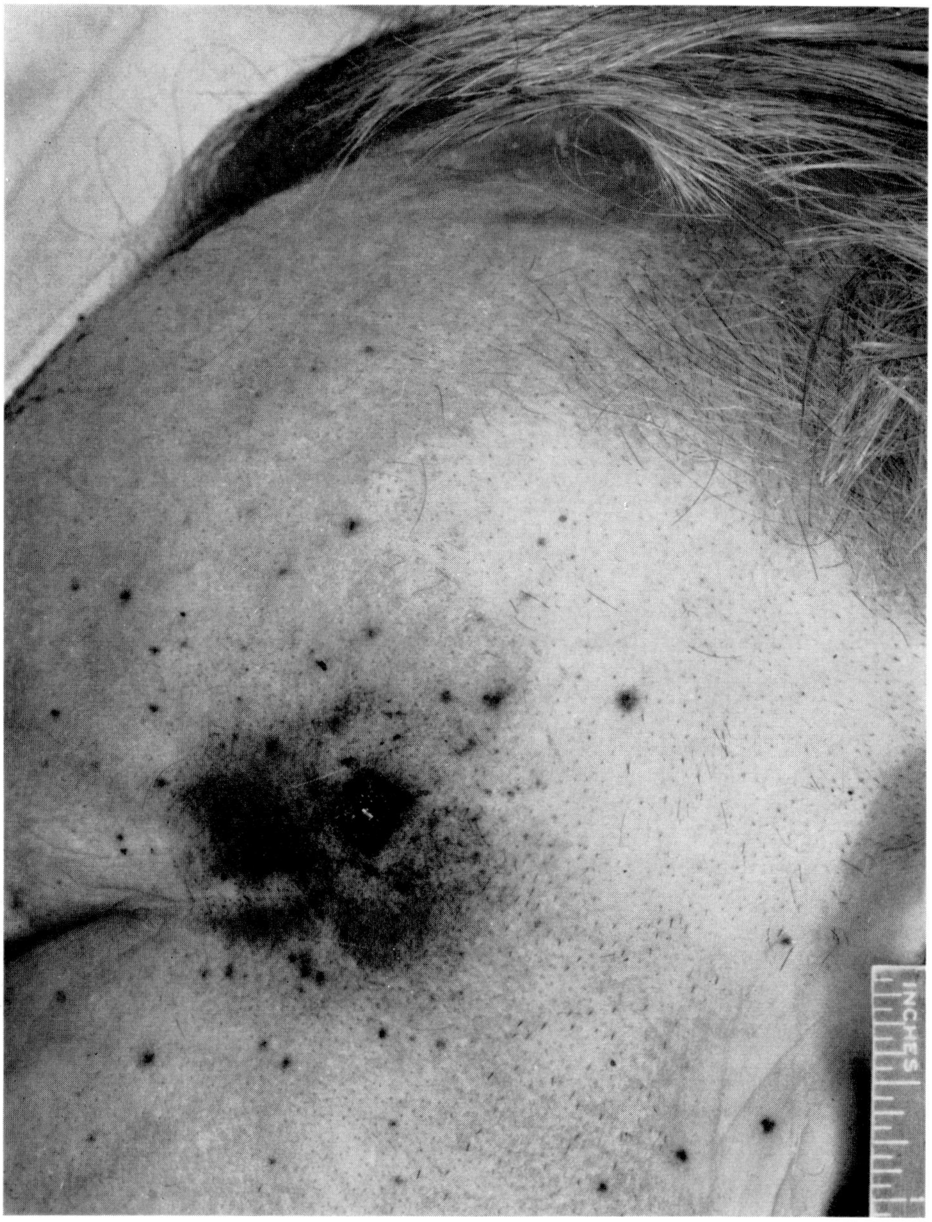

FIGURE X-20. Homicidal gunshot of the left temple during an attempted holdup. The weapon was not recovered, but a .38 caliber nonjacketed bullet was found in the brain. Note the soot centered around the bullet wound, while gunpowder particles are scattered over a diameter of close to 3 in. The relative distribution of soot and gunpowder around this injury suggests that a short-barrelled gun had been used. Test shots confirmed this assumption. A pattern similar to that in this photograph was obtained with a *snub-nosed* (2 in. barrel) .38 caliber Special, firing matching ammunition.

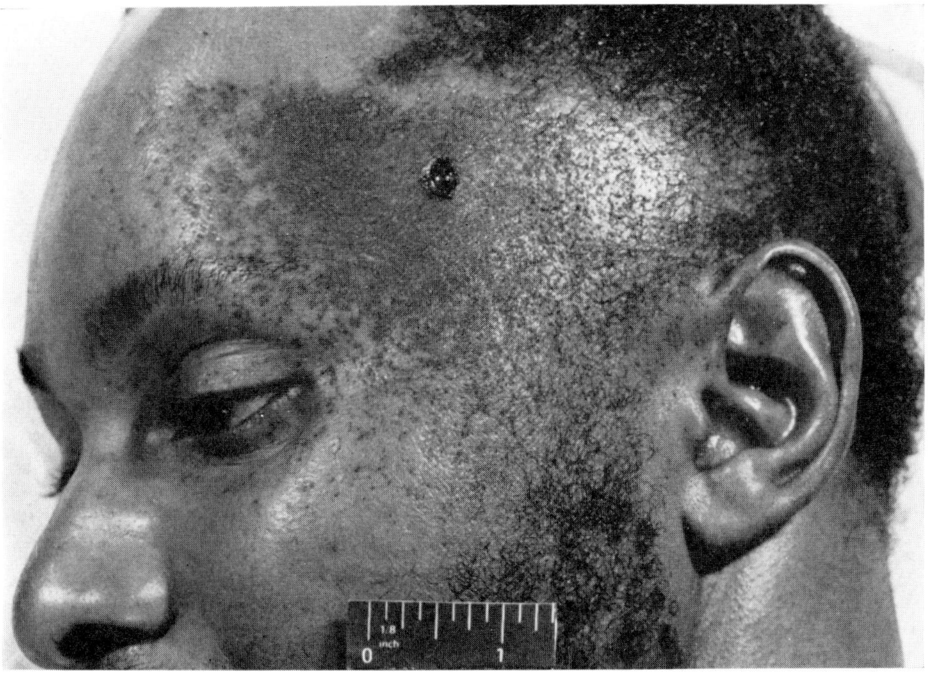

FIGURE X-21. Close-range shot of the left temple with a .357 magnum. The gunpowder particles in the skin in proximity of the bullet wound are so densely scattered that there is no undamaged intervening skin, giving the impression that the area was abraded. The lack of gunpowder stippling along a straight edge above the wound is due to the fact that the deceased was wearing a hat when he was shot.

Generally speaking, as the distance between the muzzle and the target increases, the pattern of particles on the target increases in diameter and the density of particle dispersion decreases. In handguns, at distances up to 6 or 7 in. from the muzzle, abundant gunpowder and diminishing amounts of soot are deposited on the target. On a human body no soot can usually be noted in shots fired from a distance greater than 6 in. In close-range shots of the head, dense hair may prevent powder particles from reaching the scalp at all (Fig. X-23). This obviously hinders any attempt at evaluating the distance from which a shot was fired; it may be possible to identify gunpowder particles in hair using neutron activation analysis or chemical tests as outlined earlier in this chapter.

Clothing will also often filter out soot and gunpowder particles so that none may be seen on the skin (Fig. X-24). The victim's clothing must, therefore, be removed and handled carefully to prevent dislodging of loose particles.

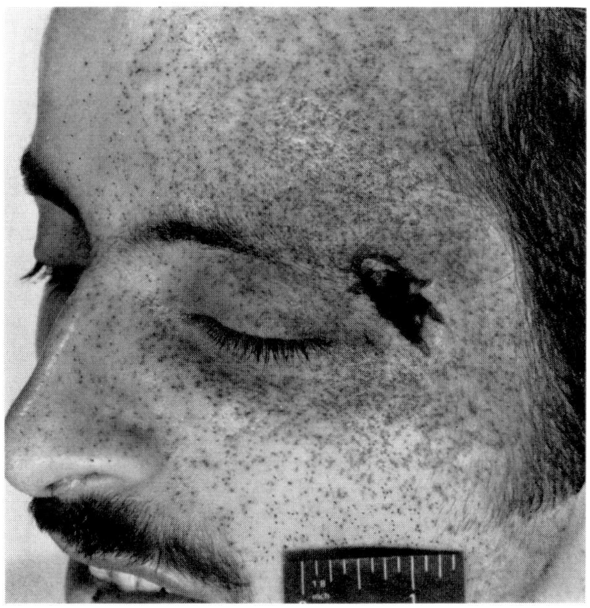

FIGURE X-22. Close-range homicidal gunshot wound of the left temple. The abundance and density of gunpowder in the skin suggests that a round with a magnum load was used. In the case of a through-and through shot, when no missile is recovered, this information may be of considerable significance.

Measurement of the spread of particles on the target is mandatory for subsequent comparison with patterns obtained by test shots to evaluate the range of firing. Photography is recommended if available, and inclusion of an accurate scale of size in the same plane is essential.

The terms *tattooing*, *powder stippling* and *powder burns* are often used to describe the dispersed grains of gunpowder and primer around a bullet wound. The term *fouling* is reserved for small fragments of metal derived from the bullet. Particles that are ejected from the barrel of the gun can usually be identified on the skin without difficulty, as they are embedded in the superficial layers of the skin and cannot be removed by wiping or even shaving of the area. Careful removal of any matter embedded in the skin can permit the identification of the type of gunpowder used in the ammunition or identify it as lead shaving or other material. Each particle produces a small superficial wound. In a case of survival, evidence of powder stippling becomes accentuated due to onset of inflammation associated with the process of healing (Fig. X-25). This is in contrast to soot, which is situated on the skin surface and is easily removed by improper handling.

Silencers mounted on firearms to muffle the sound of discharge significantly reduce the amount of gunsmoke ejected from the muzzle. A silencer extends the length of the barrel and absorbs some of the powder residue. Hence, the use of a silencer may cause misinterpretation of the distance from which a gun was fired. According to FBI reports, powder residue on

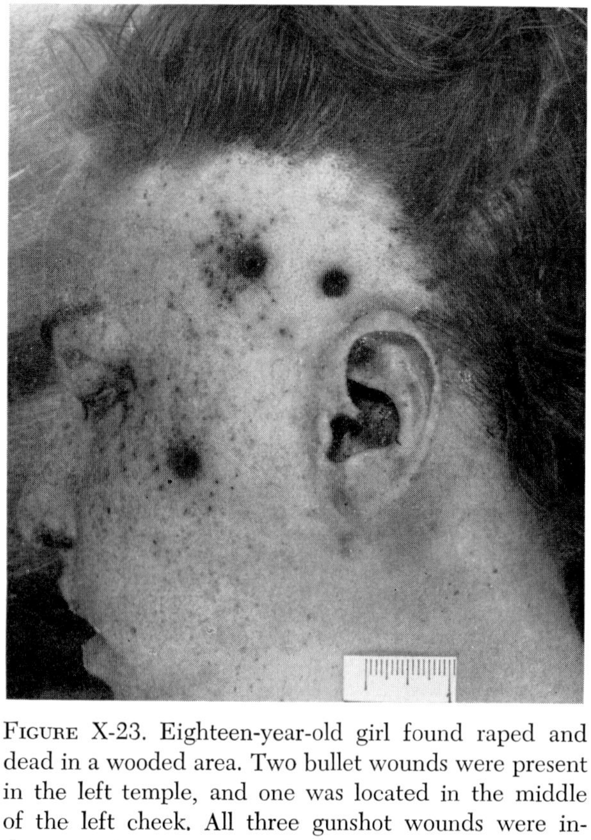

FIGURE X-23. Eighteen-year-old girl found raped and dead in a wooded area. Two bullet wounds were present in the left temple, and one was located in the middle of the left cheek. All three gunshot wounds were inflicted at close range, but the one above the ear showed no evidence of powder stippling because of the filtering effect of the hair in that area. The wound thus resembled one sustained from a great distance.

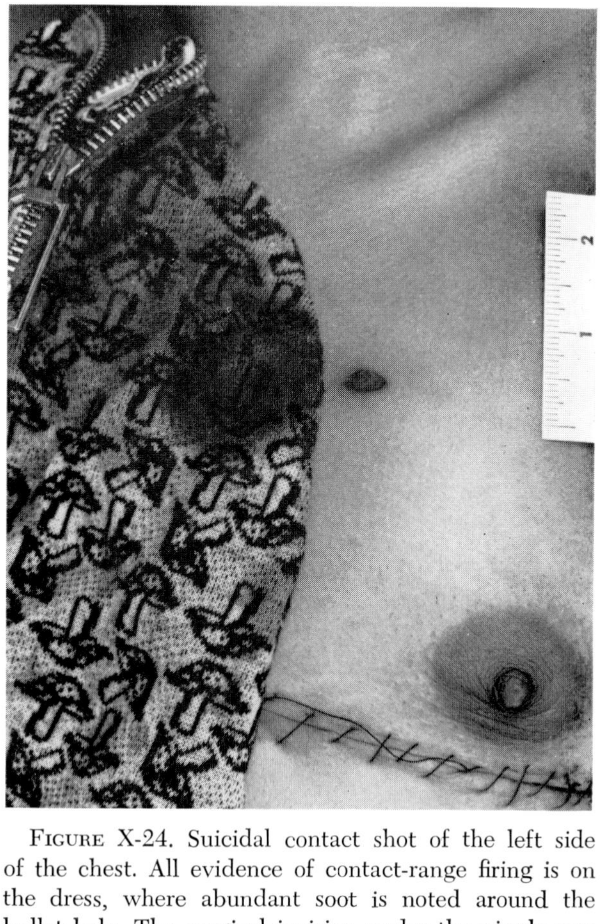

FIGURE X-24. Suicidal contact shot of the left side of the chest. All evidence of contact-range firing is on the dress, where abundant soot is noted around the bullet hole. The surgical incision under the nipple was made in an attempt to resuscitate the deceased. Any soot that may have been present in the bullet wound or on the surrounding skin was probably scrubbed away at the hospital.

clothing or a body may be entirely absent if weapons equipped with certain types of silencers were used. The .22 caliber is the only production-model handgun that can be effectively silenced. This may account for the large number of *execution-style* murders committed with .22 caliber automatic pistols.

### Distant Shot

A distant shot is one that is fired from a distance at which gunsmoke will not reach the target. In the case of most handguns, this distance exceeds 12 to 18 in. depending again on the weapon and the type of ammunition that were used. In the absence of gunsmoke around

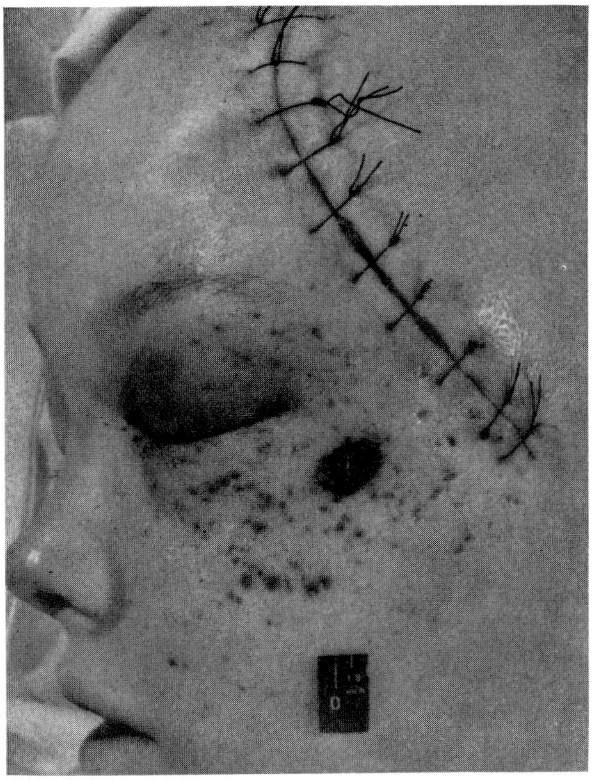

FIGURE X-25. Homicidal through-and-through shot of the head. The victim survived for twenty-four hours. Unlike the soot, which was cleaned away during surgical intervention, gunpowder stippling, evidence of close-range firing, is still present due to onset of the healing process.

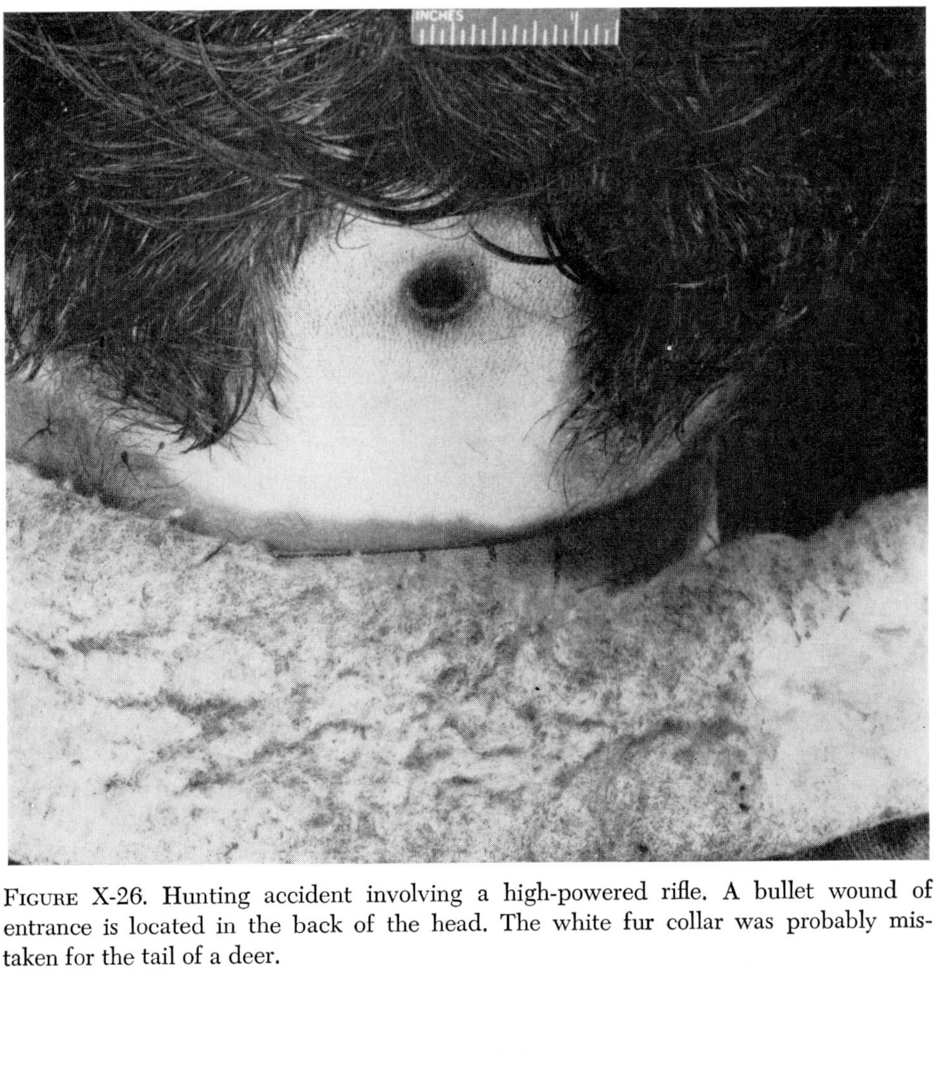


FIGURE X-26. Hunting accident involving a high-powered rifle. A bullet wound of entrance is located in the back of the head. The white fur collar was probably mistaken for the tail of a deer.

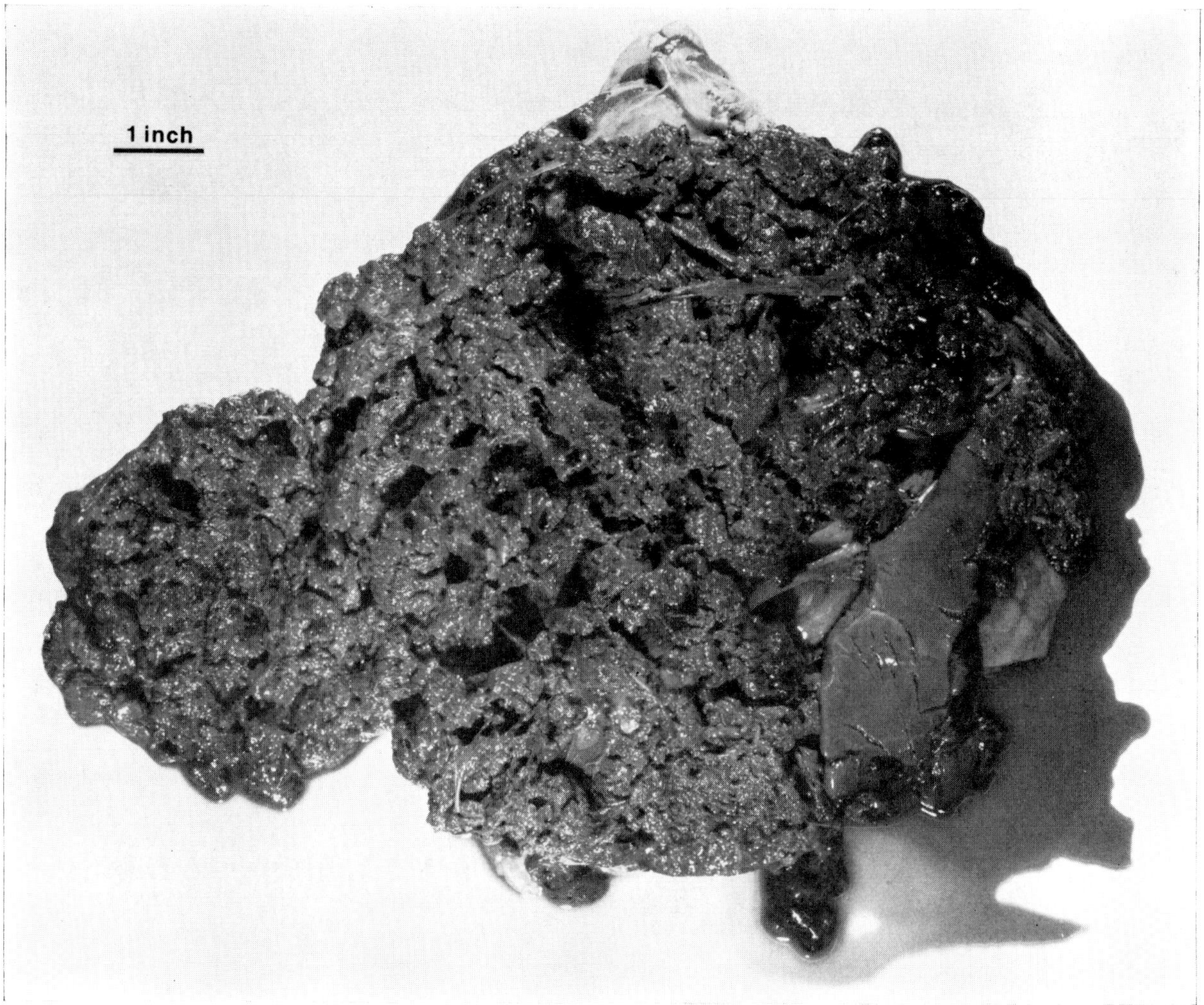


FIGURE X-27. Disintegration of the liver due to a shot from a 30-30 rifle fired from a distance of 20 ft. In a through-and-through shot this injury permits the conclusion that a high-powered weapon was used.

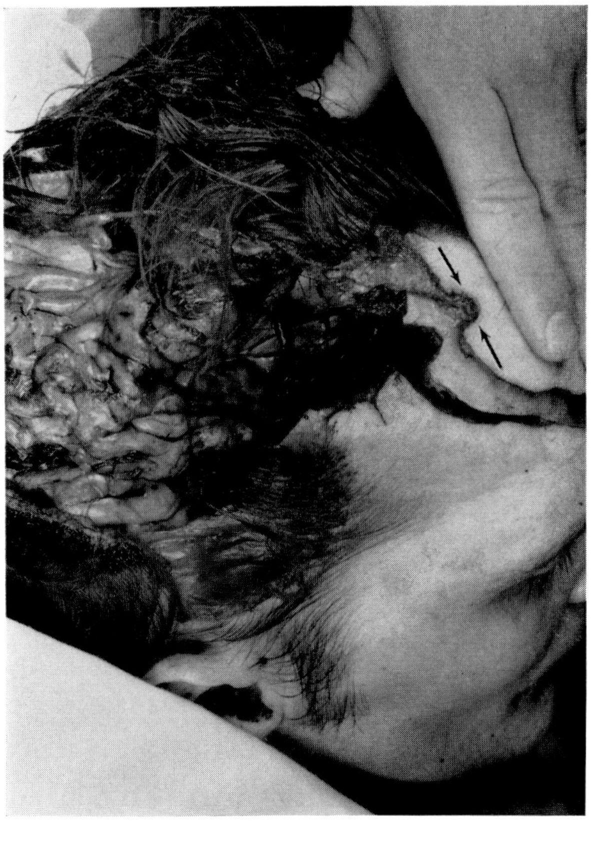

FIGURE X-28. Shot from a 30-30 rifle, fired from a distance of about 60 ft. The wound of entrance is indicated by arrows.

a bullet hole, no distinction with respect to distance can be made between one distant shot and another. Consequently, the appearance of a bullet wound inflicted from a distance of 6 ft. does not differ from one inflicted from 16 or 60 ft. In evaluating a bullet wound, consideration must be given to any intermediary target that may account for the absence of gunpowder residue around the bullet wound. For example, a shot fired through a door from a distance of a few inches, wounding a person on the other side of the door, will produce an injury that lacks all evidence of close-range firing due to retention of powder residue around the site of penetration on the door.

In the case of a high-powered rifle, the ex-

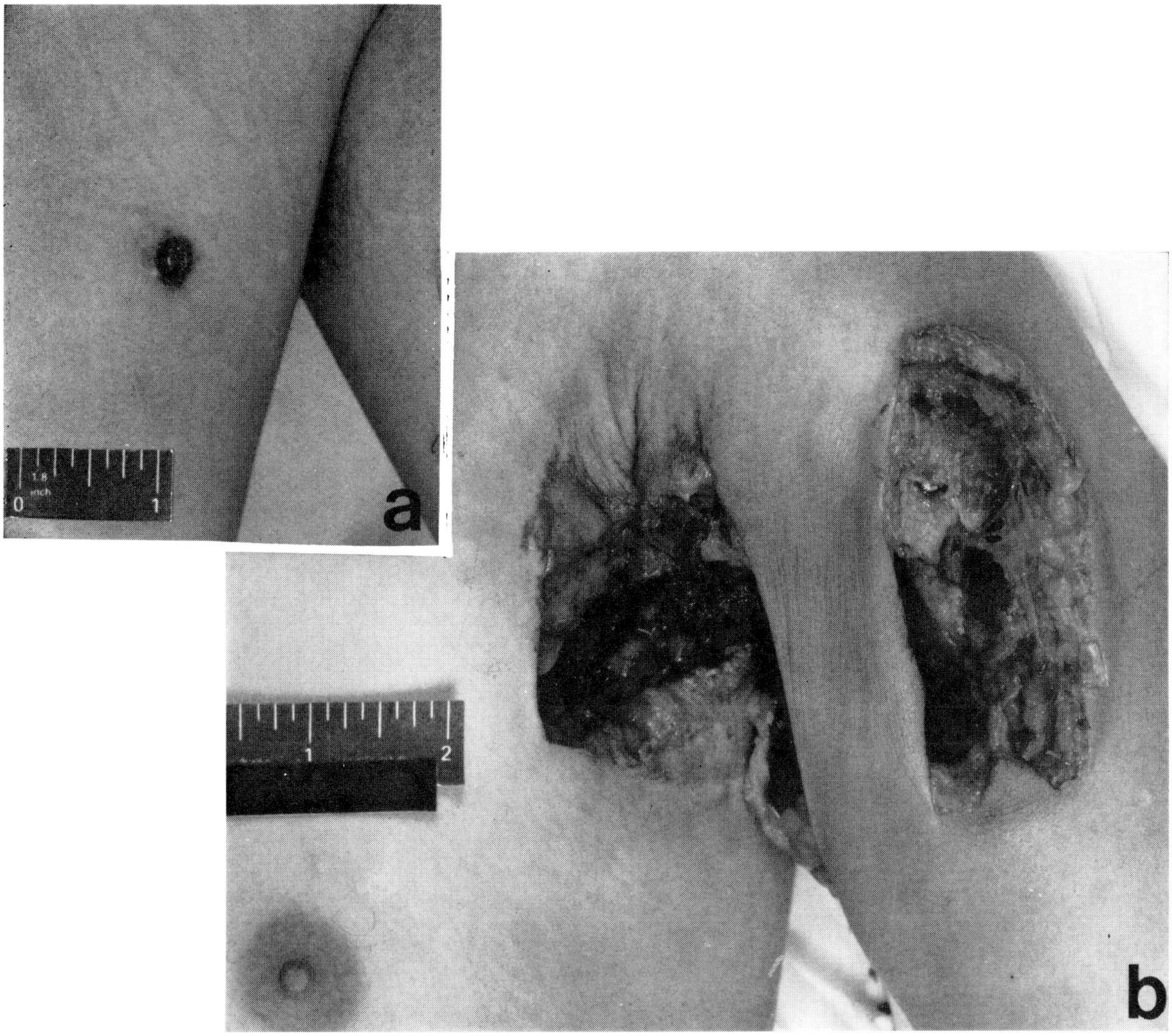


FIGURE X-29. Gunshot wound with a .308 Winchester high-powered rifle. (a): The entrance wound in the right side of the back. (b): The exit wounds through the left chest and arm. The shot was fired from a distance of 25 to 30 ft.

ternal appearance of the entrance wound does not materially differ from that of a gunshot wound inflicted with a handgun or an ordinary rifle (Fig. X-26). However, internal destruction is usually considerably more severe. Soft tissues collapse into a vast temporary cavity produced in the wake of the bullet. The skull, including the base, is often shattered, and in solid organs such as the liver, the wound track may be 3 or 4 in. in diameter (Figs. X-27 and X-28). We have observed large, gaping tears of the heart where the wound track passed through the chest but did not directly involve the heart. The size of the temporary cavity depends in great part on the kinetic energy of the bullet, $E_{kin} = \frac{m}{2} v^2$. It is the location of the temporary cavity with respect to vital organs that produces varying degrees of incapacitation.

The exit wound of a high-powered rifle shot is frequently large and ragged and quite out of proportion to exit wounds produced by other types of firearms as discussed later in this chapter (Fig. X-29). If no bullet is recovered and the weapon is unknown, the extent of external and internal damage often suggests that a high-powered rifle had been used.

The body of a sixteen-year-old boy was found in a wooded area. An entrance bullet wound that measured ¼ in. in diameter was noted in the back of his head (*see* Fig. X-26), and a large, gaping exit wound was located in the center of the forehead. The entire skull was shattered. Subsequent investigation disclosed that the boy had been accidentally shot with a .35 caliber Remington high-powered rifle during a deer-hunting expedition.

High-powered rifle ammunition is known to fragment upon striking a firm target, spraying a large area with shrapnel. The fragments of an exploded bullet may be so small and numerous as to simulate a shotgun wound, gunpowder stippling or both. Small superficial perforations of the skin produced by fragments from the original target may significantly compound the wound pattern (Figs. X-30 and X-31).

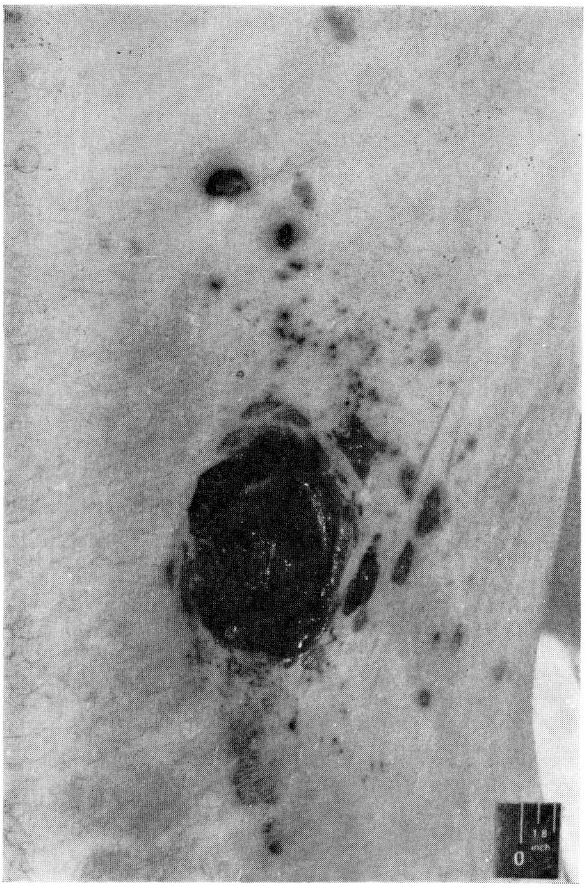

FIGURE X-30. A 30.06 shot through the door of an automobile. The bullet disintegrated, and numerous fragments of different sizes struck the passenger.

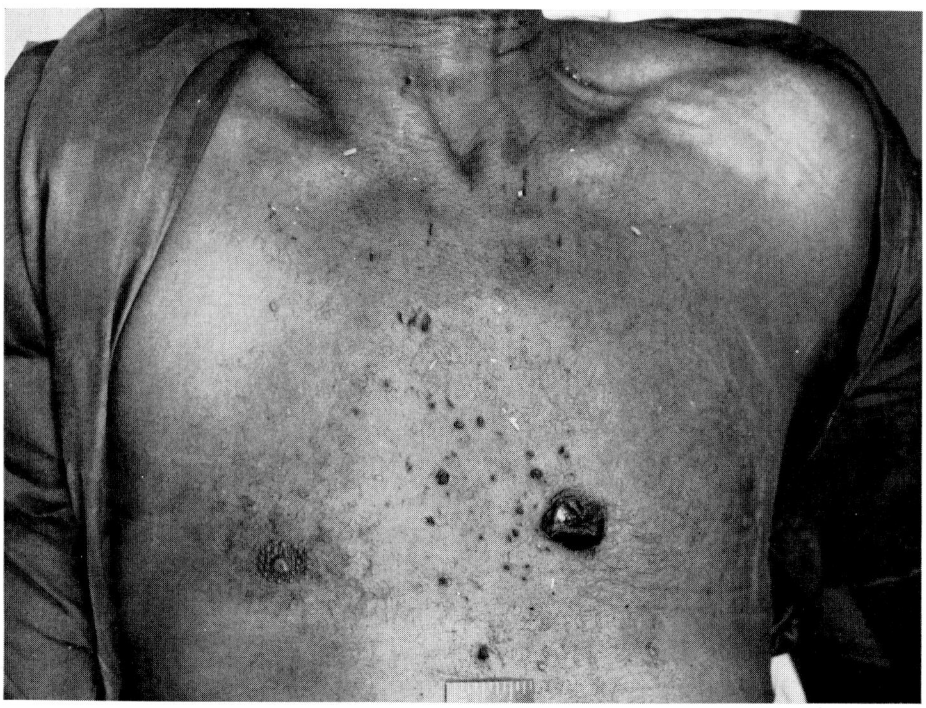

FIGURE X-31. This man was struck by multiple fragments of metal from a .30 caliber slug. The bullet fragmented when it passed through a wooden door. Some of the smaller injuries were caused by wood splinters.

## DIRECTION OF FIRE

The direction of fire may be derived from the relationship of entrance to exit wounds, although internal deviation of the bullet, as by impact on bone, must be considered. For this purpose it is essential that the wound of entry be distinguished from the wound of exit. The presence of gunsmoke around or within a gunshot wound indicates an entrance wound, inflicted with the weapon in contact with the skin or at close range. A larger amount of gunsmoke deposited on the skin on one side of the bullet wound indicates that the bullet struck the body at an angle. The same applies to the outer garment.

In the case of a distant shot, a decision regarding the direction of fire is often difficult; however, regardless of the distance from which a shot was fired, a characteristic feature of a bullet wound of entrance is circumferential marginal abrasion (Fig. X-32). This results from scraping of the wound margins by the passing missile. As in the case of abrasions due to other mechanisms, the abrasion around an entrance bullet wound becomes darker and consequently more conspicuous when drying of the area sets in. The abrasion is circular and of uniform width if the bullet strikes the body perpendicularly. Under such circumstances, the scraping by the bullet is equal on all sides of the wound. However, if the bullet strikes the body at an angle, the wound itself is round but the marginal abrasion is oval, due to increased width on one side resulting from scraping of the skin by the side of the bullet (Figs. X-33 to X-37). The actual width of the abrasion at this point depends on the angle at which the bullet struck the body. A grazing shot thus produces an abrasion from which there is proceeding a furrow-shaped tear of the tissue (Fig. X-37). If the bullet strikes at a very acute angle, a grazing shot may cause only an abrasion of the approximate width of the bullet but no tear of the skin.

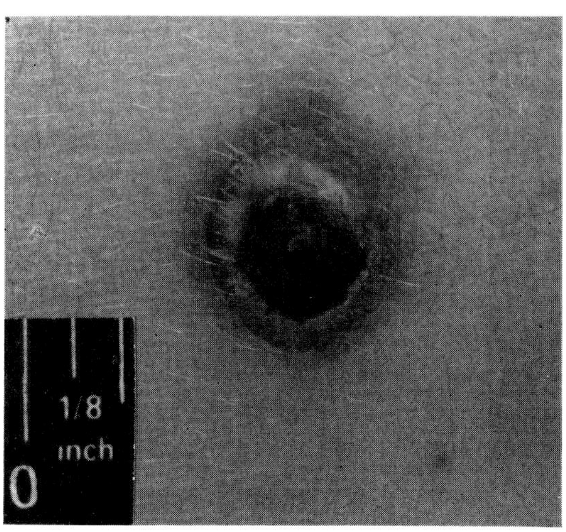


FIGURE X-32. Characteristic circumferential marginal abrasion of an entrance bullet wound. The abrasion is dark as a result of drying.

Irregular and occasionally patterned abrasions adjacent to entrance bullet wounds are sometimes caused by coarse articles of clothing scraping on the skin (Fig. X-38). This phenomenon is probably the result of the percussion wave produced by the missile upon striking the target. When such atypical findings are present, careful examination of the clothing will facilitate the proper interpretation of the wound (Fig. X-39).

Marginal abrasion of an exit wound is rare, and when present it may confuse even the experienced examiner. It occurs exclusively if a firm object such as a belt, necktie or brassiere is pressed against the body at the site of the exiting bullet or if the body is leaning against a hard surface such as a wall, floor or pavement. Under such circumstances, the exiting bullet crushes the skin against the hard surface, thus abrading the area immediately around or adjacent to the exit wound (Figs. X-40, X-41 and X-42).

Dirt and lubricant from the gun barrel and bullet and metal rubbed off from the bullet surface may be deposited on the edges of a bullet hole in clothing (Figs. X-43 and X-44). This phenomenon may be observed with both jacketed and nonjacketed bullets. The black deposit is particularly conspicuous on a light-colored garment, and the inexperienced observer may mistake it for soot. The *ring of dirt,* as it is called, is sharply outlined and appears as if it were

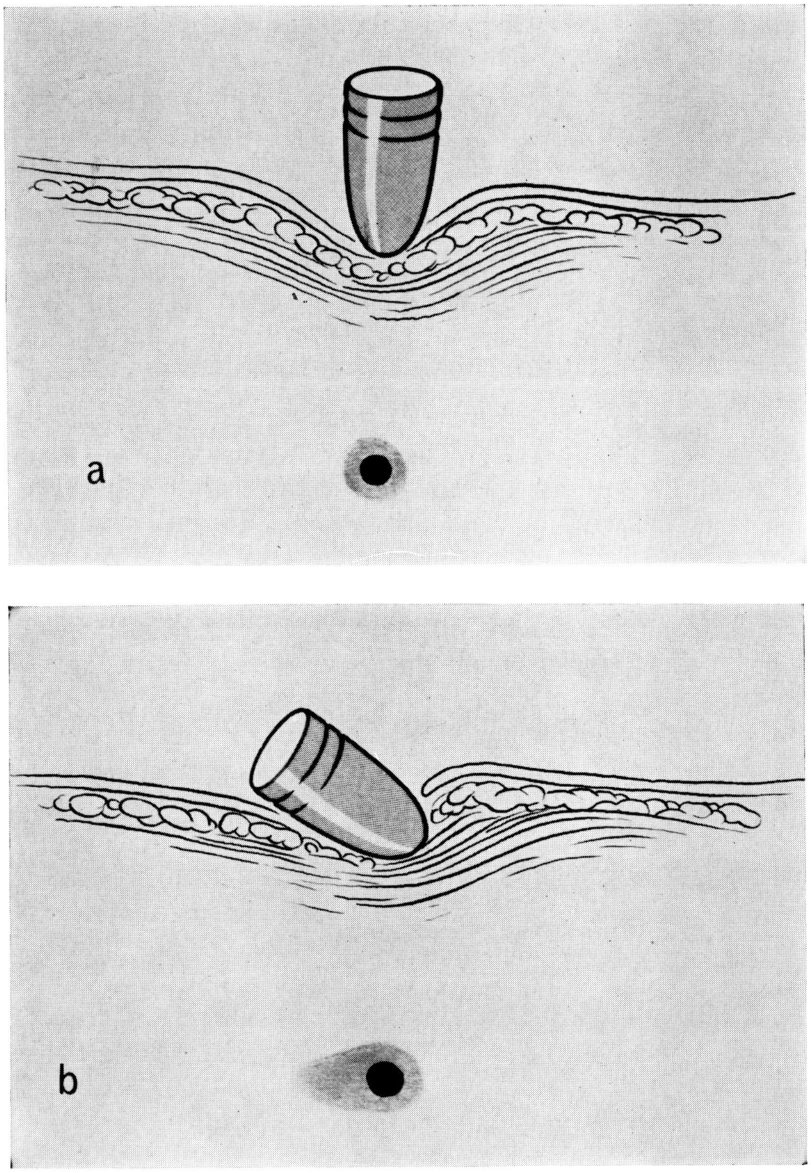


FIGURE X-33. Diagram showing different configurations of the marginal abrasion of an entrance bullet wound, depending on the angle at which the bullet strikes the body. (a): Bullet perpendicular to body. (b): Bullet at an acute angle.

FIGURE X-34. Gunshot wound of chest, between the nipples, inflicted from a distance of several feet. The semilunal abrasion on the right side of the wound (left side in the photograph) indicates the victim was shot from right to left. The bullet was recovered from the left chest wall.

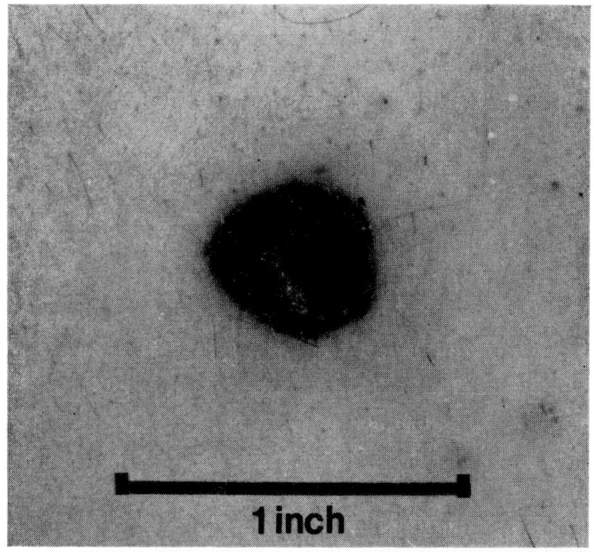


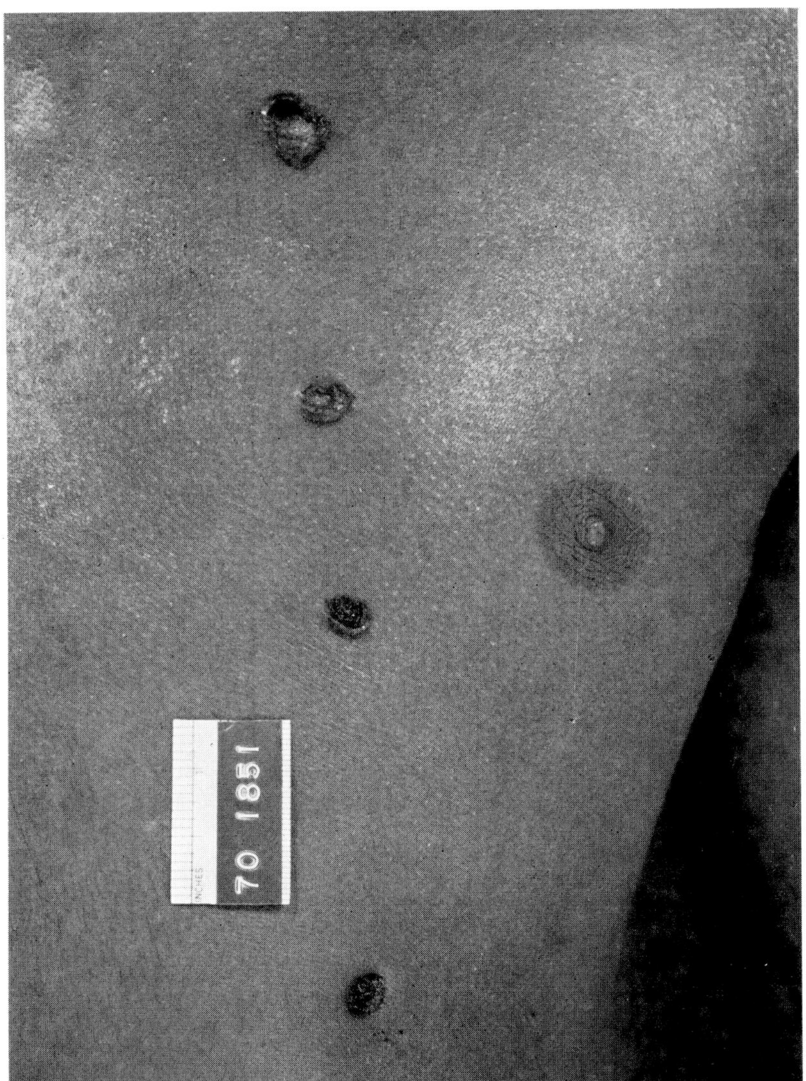


FIGURE X-35. Homicide: The abrasions along the lower margins of these entrance wounds indicate the upward course of the bullets. It is interesting to point out that the close proximity of these bullet wounds and their arrangement in a straight line at first suggested that an automatic weapon had been used. However, the murder weapon was a .38 Special revolver.

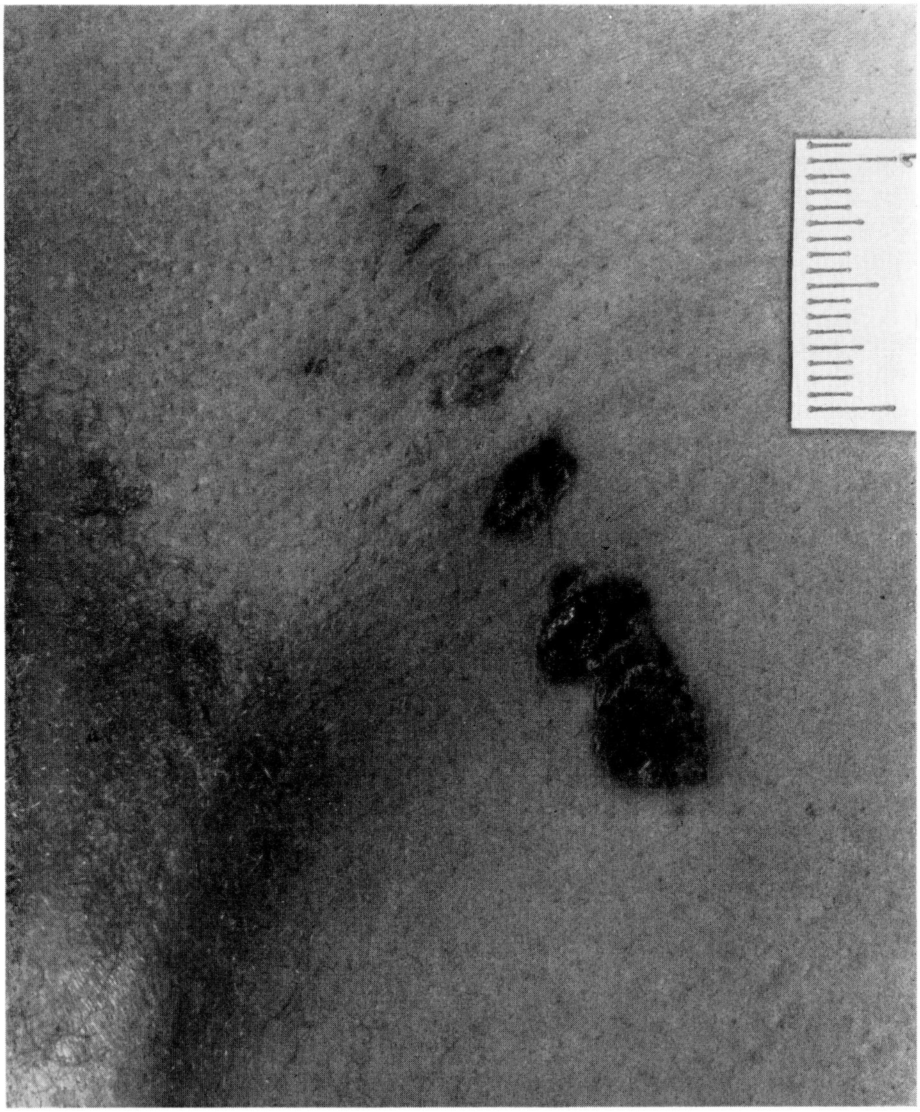

FIGURE X-36. Single shot of the left groin, simulating several bullet wounds due to skin folds. The lowest wound is the primary entrance wound, showing a wide abrasion, which indicates the upward pathway of the bullet. The bullet then exited and reentered several times before proceeding into the abdominal cavity.

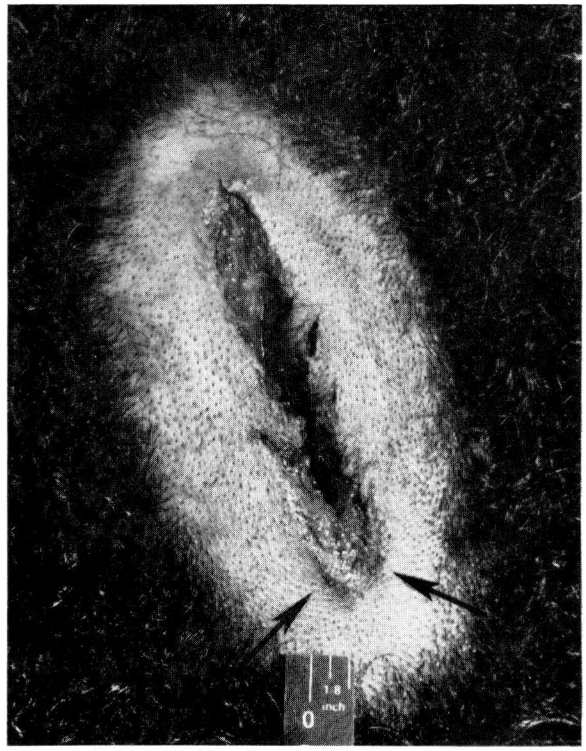

FIGURE X-37. Grazing bullet wound of the head. The actual entrance wound is indicated by arrows.

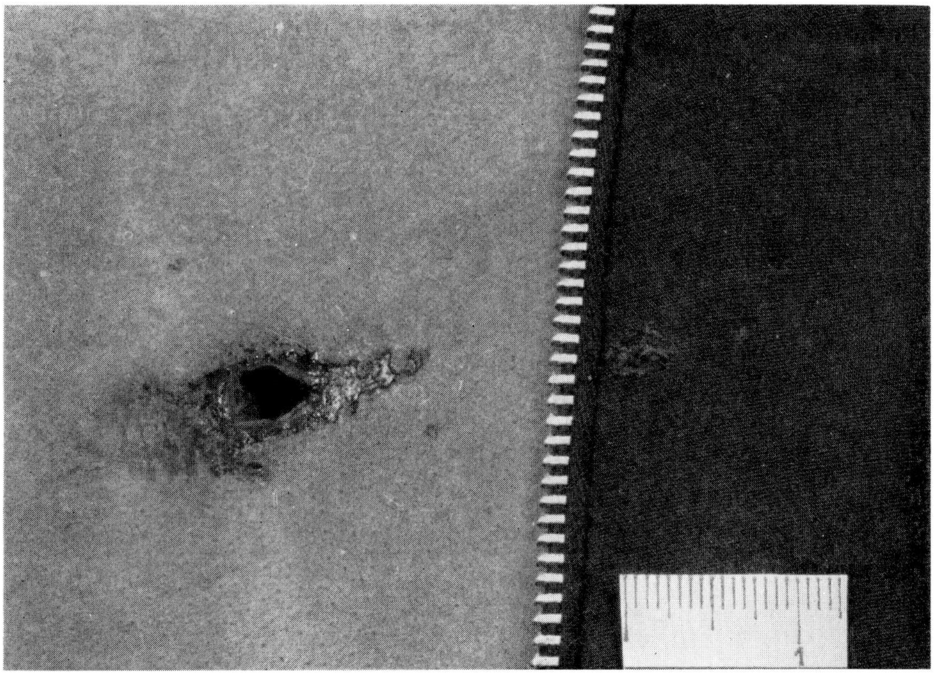

FIGURE X-38. The abrasion adjacent to this entrance bullet wound was caused by the zipper, which was scraped on the skin by the passing bullet.

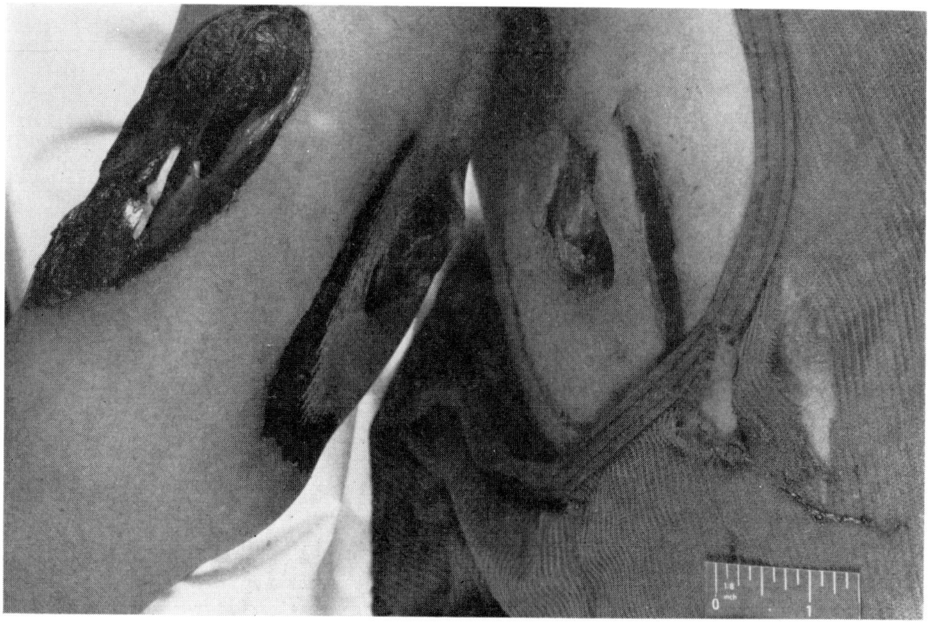

FIGURE X-39. Shot with a Mauser rifle in the left arm. The bullet passed through the chest, exited on the right side, reentered and exited through the right arm. The humerus was shattered. Note that the band of the undershirt with some of its weave pattern abraded the skin around the exit wound of the chest and the reentry wound of the arm. This was caused by the percussive effect of the passing missile. The size of the injury is suggestive of a high-powered weapon.

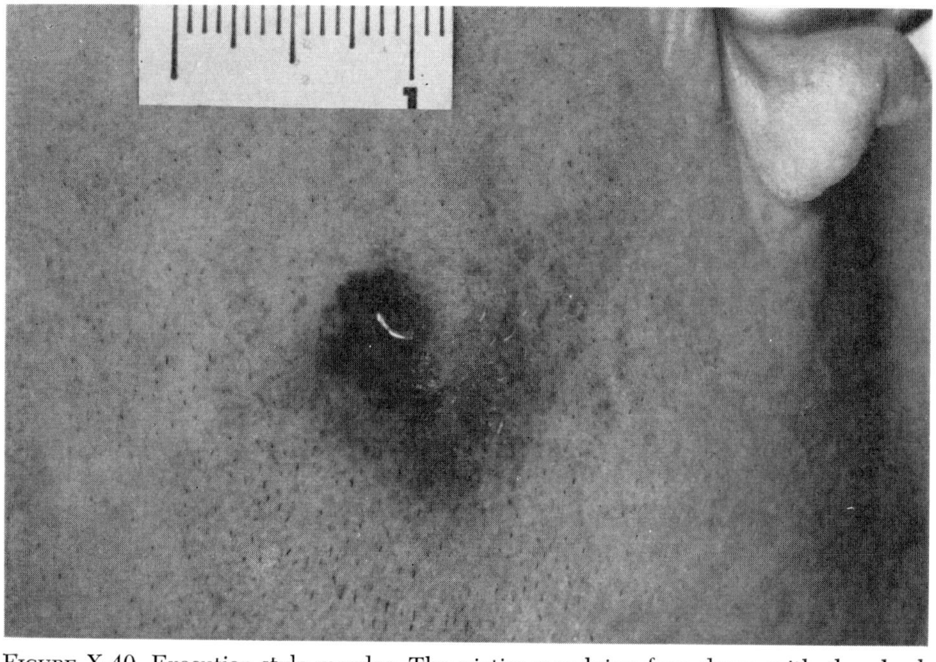

FIGURE X-40. Execution-style murder. The victim was lying face down with the cheek against the cement floor. The entrance wound was a contact shot under the lower jaw on the opposite side. A jacketed .32 caliber slug is seen in the wound. The abrasion around the wound was caused by crushing of the skin against the floor by the exiting bullet. The percussive effect produced by the exiting slug accounts for the large area of abraded skin.

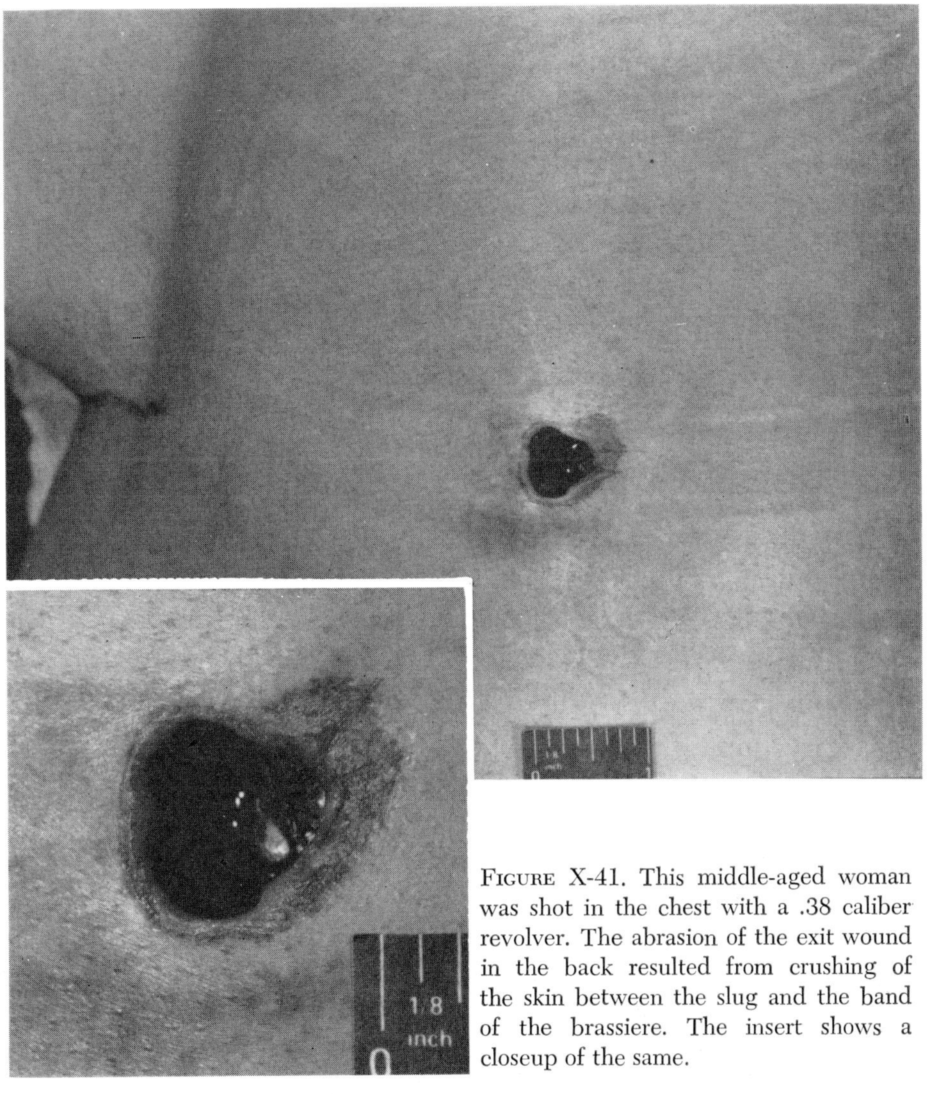


FIGURE X-41. This middle-aged woman was shot in the chest with a .38 caliber revolver. The abrasion of the exit wound in the back resulted from crushing of the skin between the slug and the band of the brassiere. The insert shows a closeup of the same.

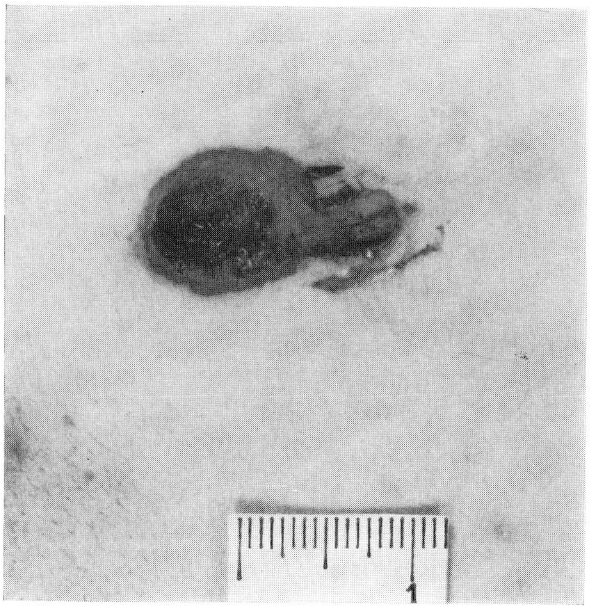


FIGURE X-42. Marginal abrasion of an exit bullet wound on the back. The victim was leaning against a concrete wall.

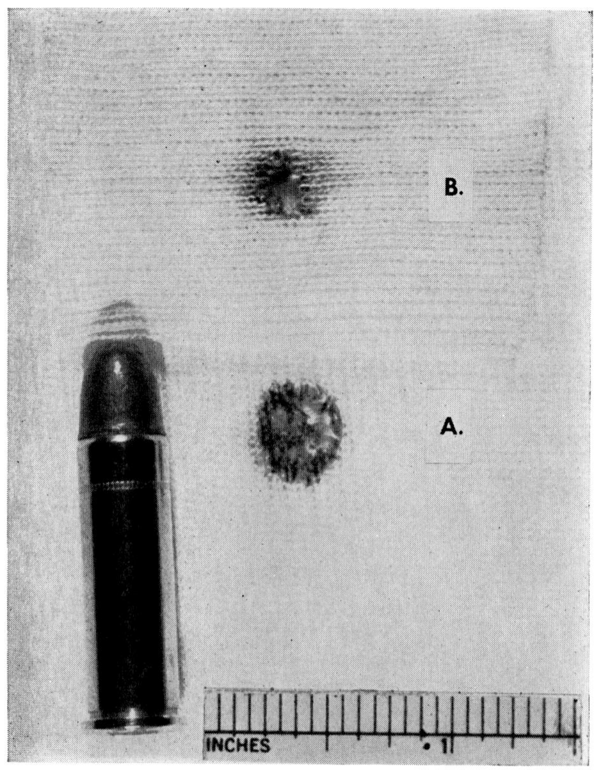


FIGURE X-43. *Ring of dirt* produced by test firing a .38 caliber bullet into a white garment. (A): Outer surface; (B): Inner surface. Care must be taken not to mistake the *ring of dirt* for the deposit of soot associated with close-range firing.

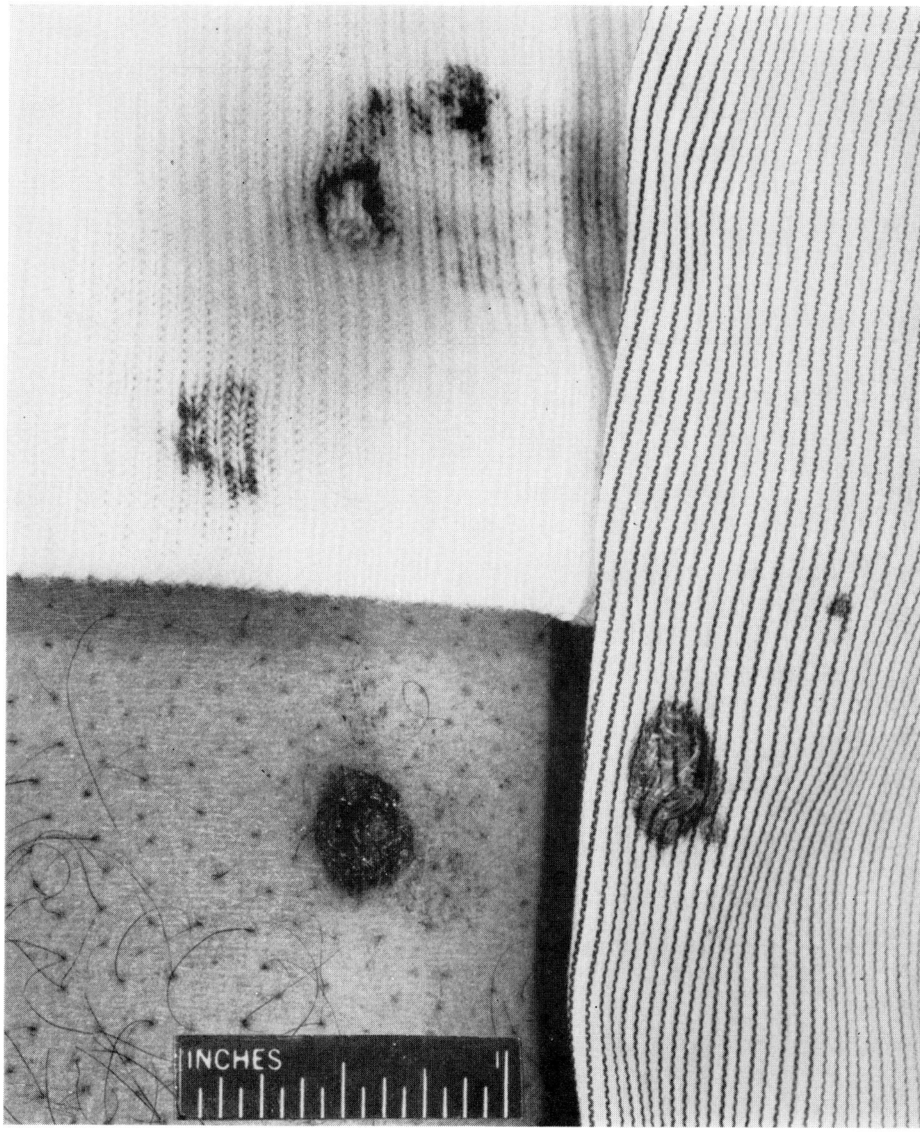


FIGURE X-44. *Ring of dirt* in the shirt of a homicide victim who was shot from a distance of about 15 ft. The adjacent injury is the entrance bullet wound in the left side of the abdomen.

printed on the fabric. Soot, by contrast, is dark in the center and fades toward the periphery. In questionable cases, laboratory examination will resolve the problem. The *ring of dirt* is not recognizable on skin, and any suggestion that the dark edge of a bullet wound may be caused by dirt or lubricant is strictly erroneous.

The frayed edges of a bullet hole in a garment follow the path of the bullet in most cases, depending on the type of fabric (Fig. X-45). This may be helpful in the distinction of an entrance from an exit wound in questionable cases.

As mentioned earlier in this chapter, pieces of fabric may be carried into the wound track and are sometimes found in proximity of the entrance wound. It is extremely rare, however, that such pieces are carried through the wound and deposited at the exit, except if the gunshot involves a thin part of the body, such as a hand, or in a case of a grazing shot.

Whereas bullet wounds of entrance usually conform to a set pattern, exit wounds may vary considerably in size and appearance. A bullet wound of entry is often smaller than the caliber of the bullet, while the exit wound is frequently considerably larger. The skin is overstretched by the penetrating bullet, and it returns to its former position after the bullet has passed, accounting for a small entrance wound. Consequently, a conclusion concerning the caliber of a bullet based on the diameter of the entrance wound is speculative and inadvisable (Fig. X-46).

In the case of an exit wound, tissues, including bone, are often pushed ahead by the bullet, causing a larger defect. Added to this is the tumbling effect of the bullet, which results from the resistance of the tissues as it passes through the body. Obviously, if the bullet exits sideways, a larger wound results. Slitlike exit wounds are

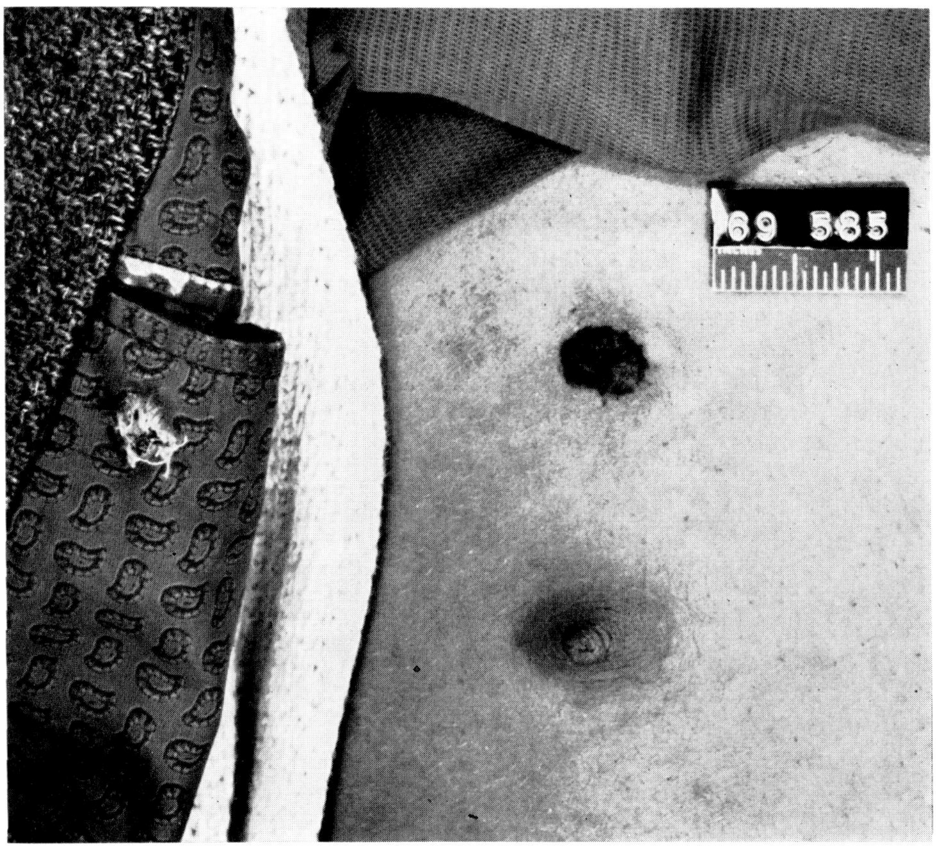


FIGURE X-45. The frayed edges of the bullet hole in the jacket point in the direction of the wound track. In cases of doubt, this finding may be important to distinguish an entrance from an exit wound.

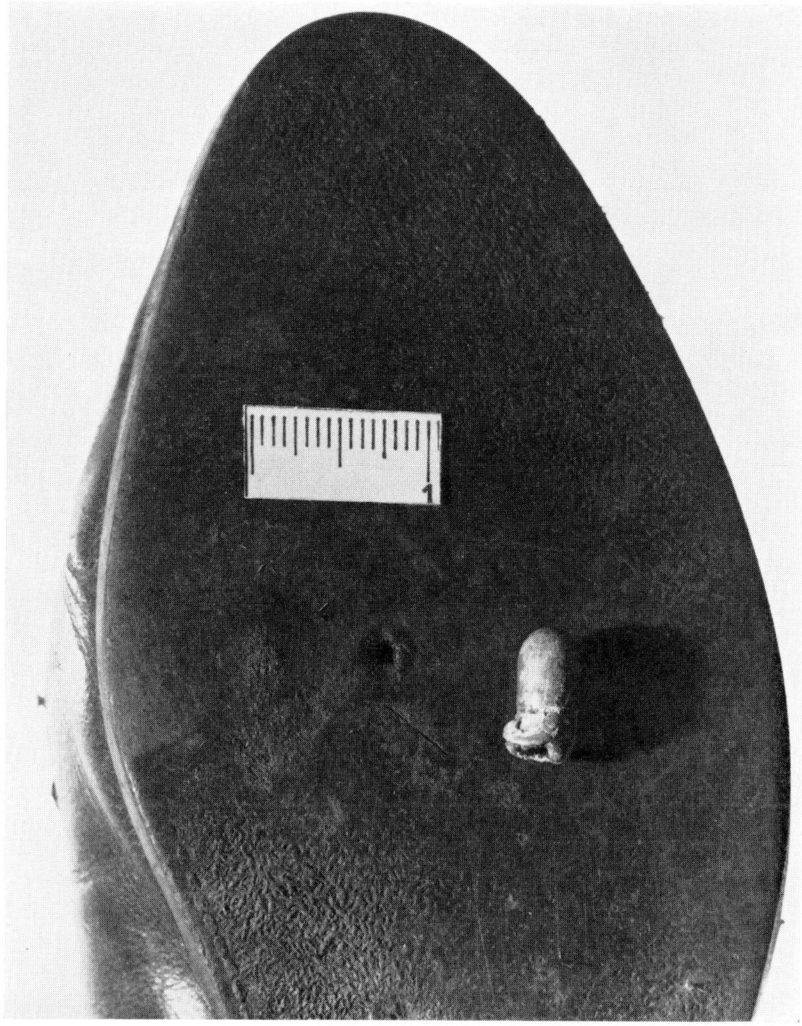

FIGURE X-46a. The caliber of a bullet cannot be determined by the size of the defect in the garment or the skin. This .38 caliber bullet passed through the hole in the rubber sole of this shoe. The elasticity of the rubber provides for the discrepancy in size. Note the *marginal abrasion* surrounding the defect in the sole of the shoe.

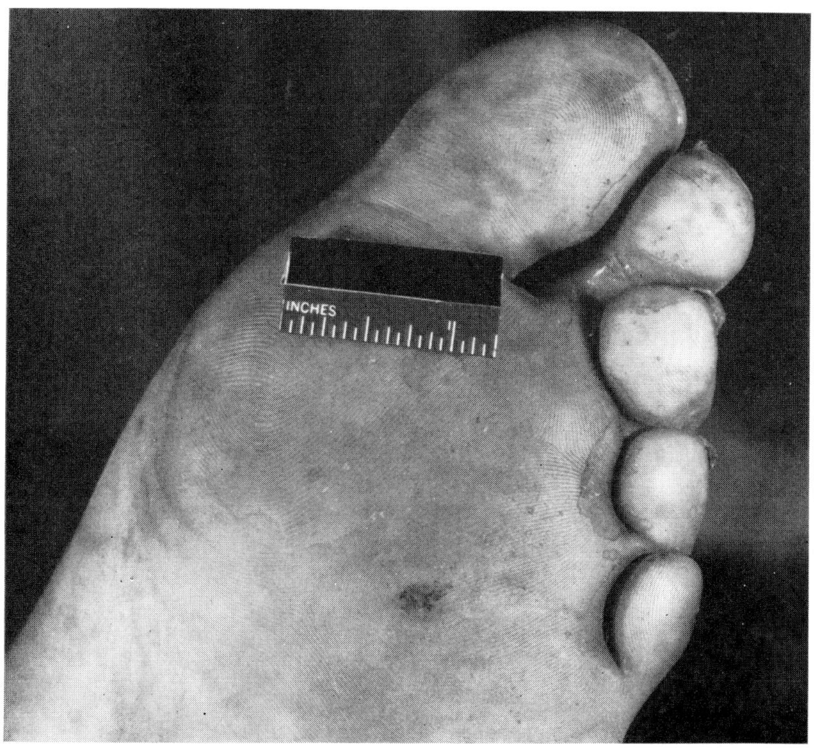


FIGURE X-46b. The small wound in the sole of this foot was caused by the same bullet (.38 caliber). The spots around the bullet wound are dry blood. The slug was found in the exit wound on the dorsum of the foot.

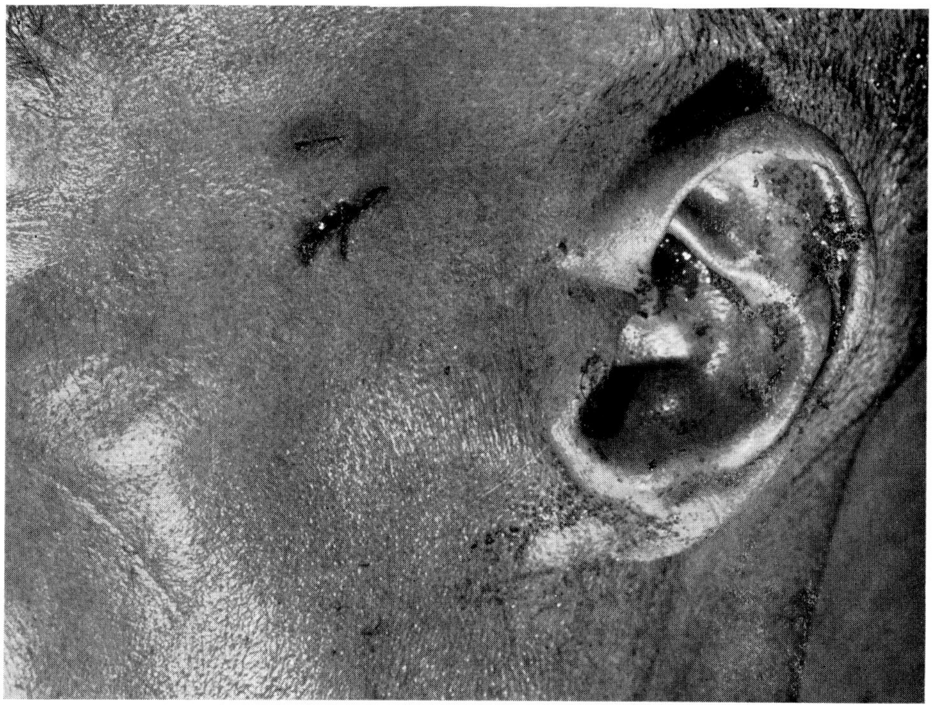

FIGURE X-47. Two exit wounds. Obviously it cannot be determined which one was caused by the bullet and which by a fragment of bone. A complete but deformed .38 caliber slug was recovered from a wall.

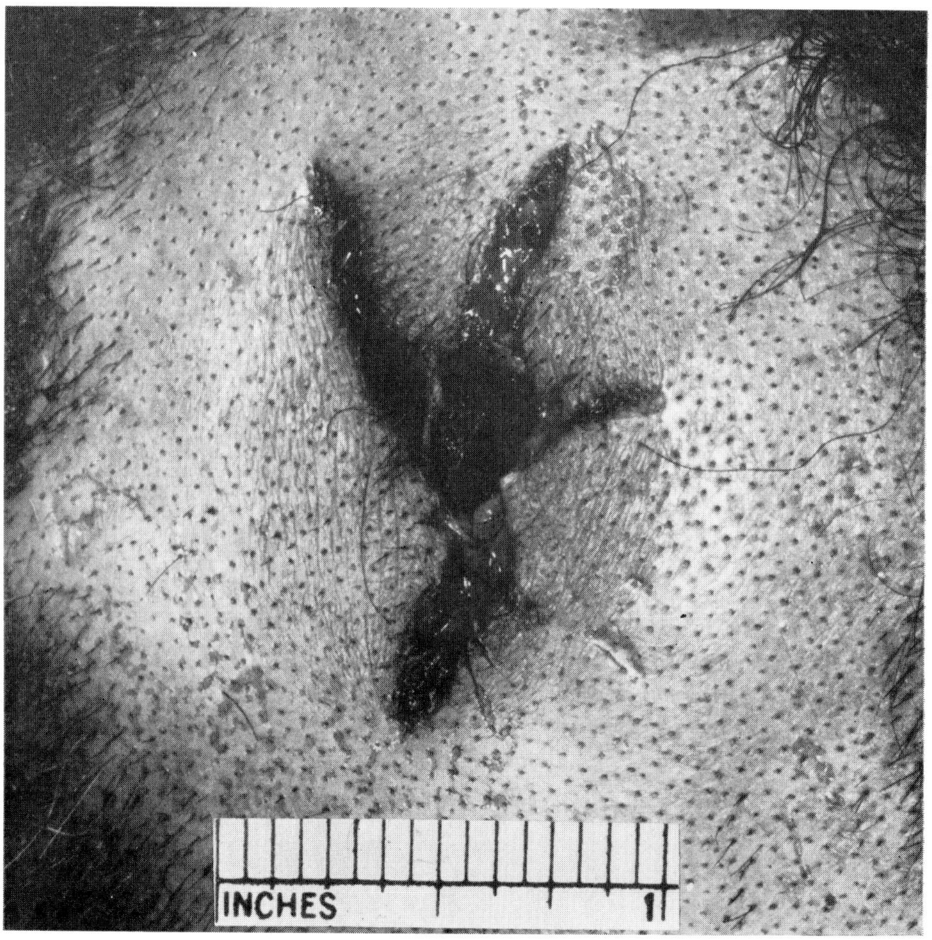


FIGURE X-48. Exit wound on the top of the head. This was a homicide. The bullet entered through the left eye. Note the absence of marginal abrasion.

occasionally encountered. They are attributed to deformity of the bullet, caused by impact on bone. An exit wound of a fragment of bone may also be slitlike, while the bullet remains in the body (Fig. X-47). Such wounds are mostly seen on the head and over the shoulders. Care must be taken not to mistake such wounds for stab wounds, since the similarity is often striking.

Exit wounds of the head are frequently star shaped, resembling contact entrance wounds except for the absence of marginal abrasion and gunsmoke in the depth of the wound (Fig. X-48).

An entrance wound may assume a bizarre shape if the bullet is deformed by striking a firm object before entering the body. A bullet deformed in this manner is referred to as a *ricochet bullet*. A wound caused by ricochet, even though it often is of unusual shape and size, has abraded edges, as has any ordinary entrance bullet wound. Bullet wounds that are more atypical than those caused by ricochet are produced by bullets that have passed through one part of the body before proceeding into another. For example, a bullet that has passed in and out of an upper extremity may cause an unusually large and peculiarly abraded, ragged wound in the chest or abdomen as a result of tumbling and also due to the percussive effect of the limb against the area of reentry (Figs. X-49 and X-50). Recognition of reentry wounds is essential for correct interpretation of the position of the victim and other far-reaching conclusions.

Occasionally, an entrance and an exit wound in the head are located within an inch or two of each other, and at autopsy a subcutaneous

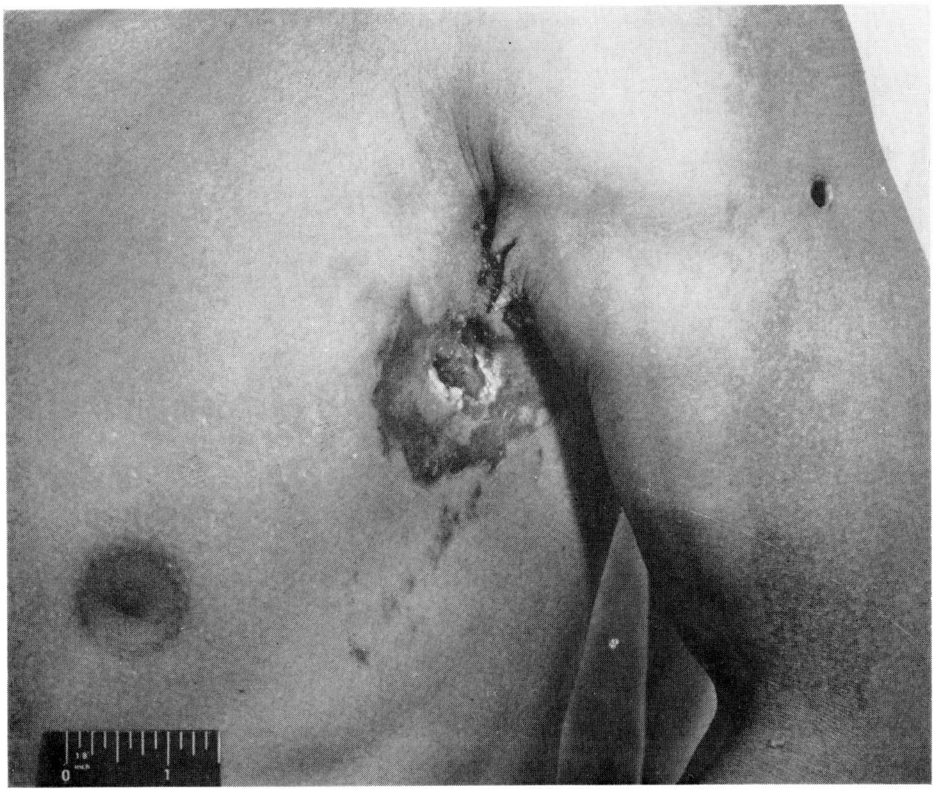

FIGURE X-49. Entrance bullet wound on the outer surface of the left arm. The high-powered .30 caliber rifle slug passed through the arm, fractured the bone and reentered the chest at the armpit. The reentry wound is ragged, unusually shaped and irregularly abraded. The peculiar wound is due to the percussion of the arm against the chest associated with the passage of the missile.

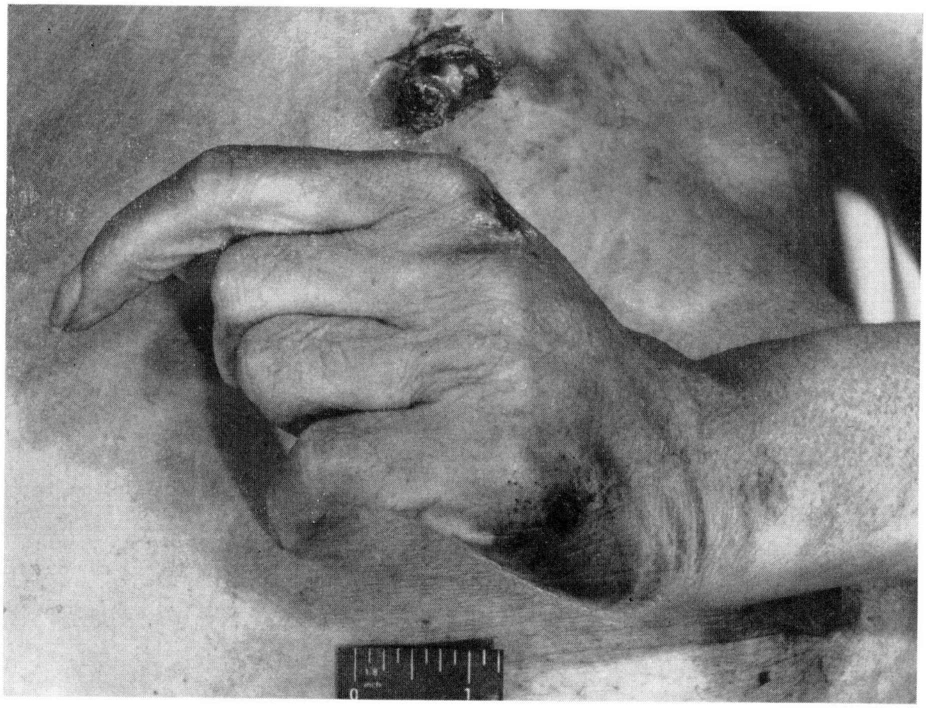

FIGURE X-50. Close-range shot of the left hand, showing soot and gunpowder stippling. The .38 Special slug exited at the knuckle of the index finger and reentered the chest. The reentry is large and unusually abraded.

wound track connects the two injuries. When this occurs, it is usually due to separation of a fragment of metal from the bullet during its passage through the skull (Fig. X-51). The separated fragment proceeds under the skin until it exits or remains lodged between the skull and the skin, while the major part of the bullet enters the skull and may exit in a different location. Under such circumstances, two exit wounds may be caused by the same bullet.

Bullets sometimes disintegrate upon impact on bone. In the head many metal fragments may be found scattered in the brain and, on x ray film, occasionally resemble a shotgun injury. More commonly, the wound track produced by the missile after striking or grazing bone is outlined on an x ray film by a deposit of *metallic snow*. This consists of punctate particles of metal scattered along some distance of the wound track, indicating the direction of the shot, as particle dispersion is wider in the direction of travel. X ray films taken during the autopsy of President John F. Kennedy indicate a fine metallic snow in the lower right neck area, suggesting that a lateral vertebral process was fractured by the jacketed rifle bullet.

Contact shots fired into the back of the head suggests *execution-style* murder. We have observed four such shots in one individual. None of the .22 caliber slugs penetrated the bone but were found flattened against the outer surface of the skull. Death was probably due to brain injury caused by the concussive effect of the impacts. Such a finding suggests defective, possibly old, ammunition. In another case a .22 caliber slug fragmented on striking the occipital bone. The major fragment of lead remained under the scalp, whereas *metallic snow* was found scattered along the wound track in the brain (Fig. X-52). Frangible bullets, used in shooting galleries and cattle stunning, have been described as giving a similar picture.[6]

Sometimes the jacket of a bullet separates from the core upon impact on a firm object, such

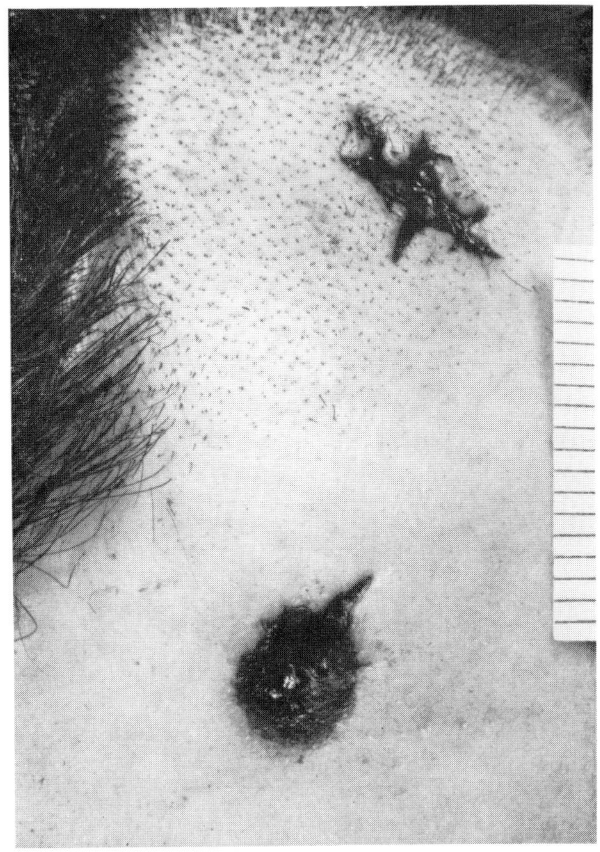

Figure X-51. Entrance wound of the forehead. A fragment of the slug was *shaved off* at the time of penetration of the bone. The fragment continued its course under the skin to exit an inch or two above the entrance wound. The shot was fired from a distance of several feet, and the weapon was a .38 caliber Colt. Each division of the scale in the photograph equals 1/16 in.

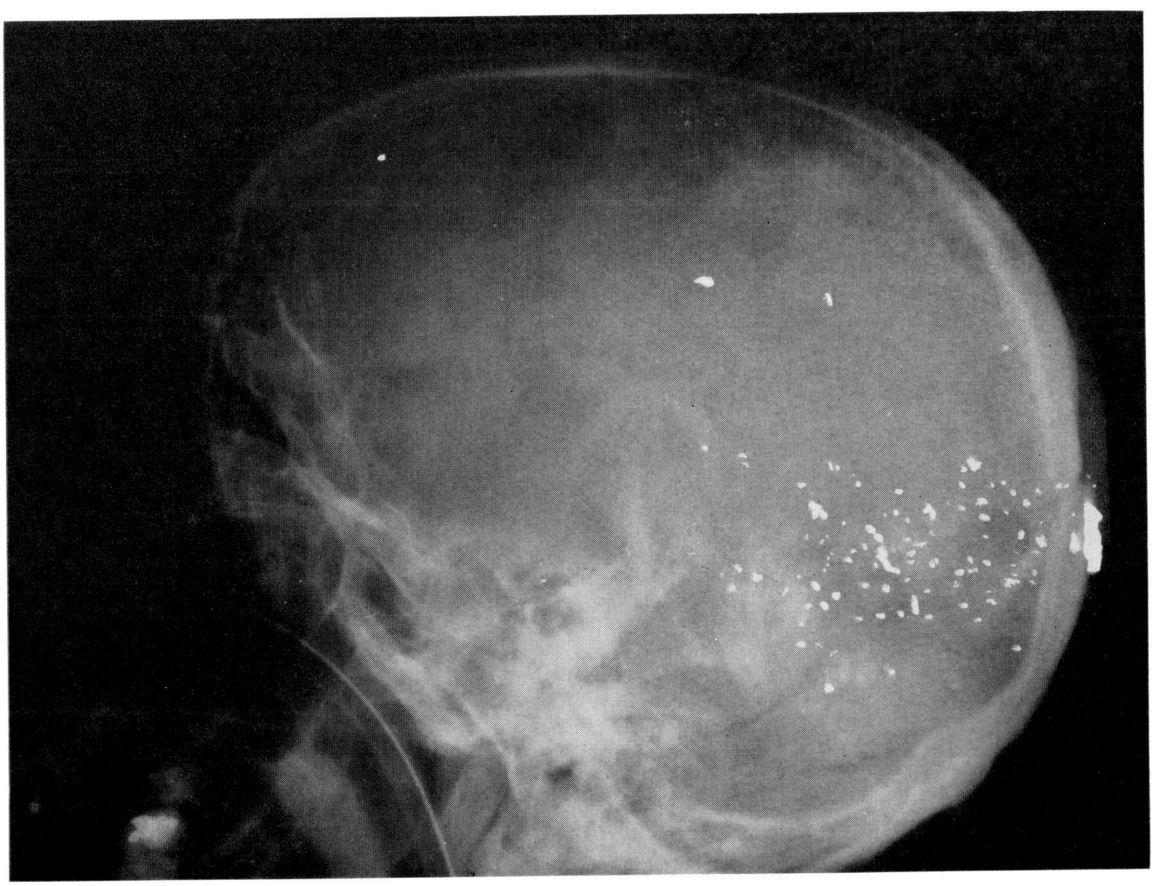

Figure X-52. A .22 caliber shot into the back of the head. The major fragment of the lead slug is situated on the outer surface of the occipital bone. The remainder of the missile fragmented, and *metallic snow* is scattered along the wound track in the brain.

as a button, a coin in the pocket or bone. In such cases the jacket and the core each assume separate tracks. Whereas the core may leave the body, the jacket very seldom does. Although fragments of the jacket may break off, in our experience the major portion of the jacket of a bullet remains intact and should invariably be recovered. Recovery of the jacket is of particular importance for identification of the suspected weapon, as the jacket carries the rifling marks.

In the case of a gunshot wound of the head, the direction of fire may be readily apparent from the appearance of the bullet holes in the skull. An entrance hole is bevelled inward; the defect on the inner surface of the bone is larger than that on the outer surface (Fig. X-53a). An exit hole in the skull is bevelled outward; it is larger on the outer than on the inner surface of the bone and may justly be referred to as crater shaped (Fig. X-53b, c). The same phenomenon is sometimes observed in a plate glass window struck by a BB pellet. Asymmetry of the bevelling may aid in assessing the angle of fire. Symmetrical bevelling usually indicates that the bullet struck the skull at right angles.

A rare observation in gunshot wounds of the head in which the bullet strikes at an angle is deflection of the bullet from its trajectory by impact on the bone to produce a continuous wound track under the skin without penetration of the skull. The subcutaneous pathway sometimes proceeds for a considerable distance, the bullet following the curvature of the skull. In the same manner, a bullet striking a rib at an angle sometimes passes under the skin, partly encircling the chest and possibly exiting the opposite side without having penetrated the pleural cavities. A shot fired at a curved part of the head at an acute angle often causes a typically inward-bevelled entrance hole adjacent to an outward-bevelled exit hole, producing in the skull a *keyhole*-shaped defect (Fig. X-54). A fragment of the slug *shaved off* at the entrance hole may penetrate the brain. Occasionally, in contact shots of the head, the same entrance hole in the skull is bevelled both inward and outward, due to chipping of the outer layer of

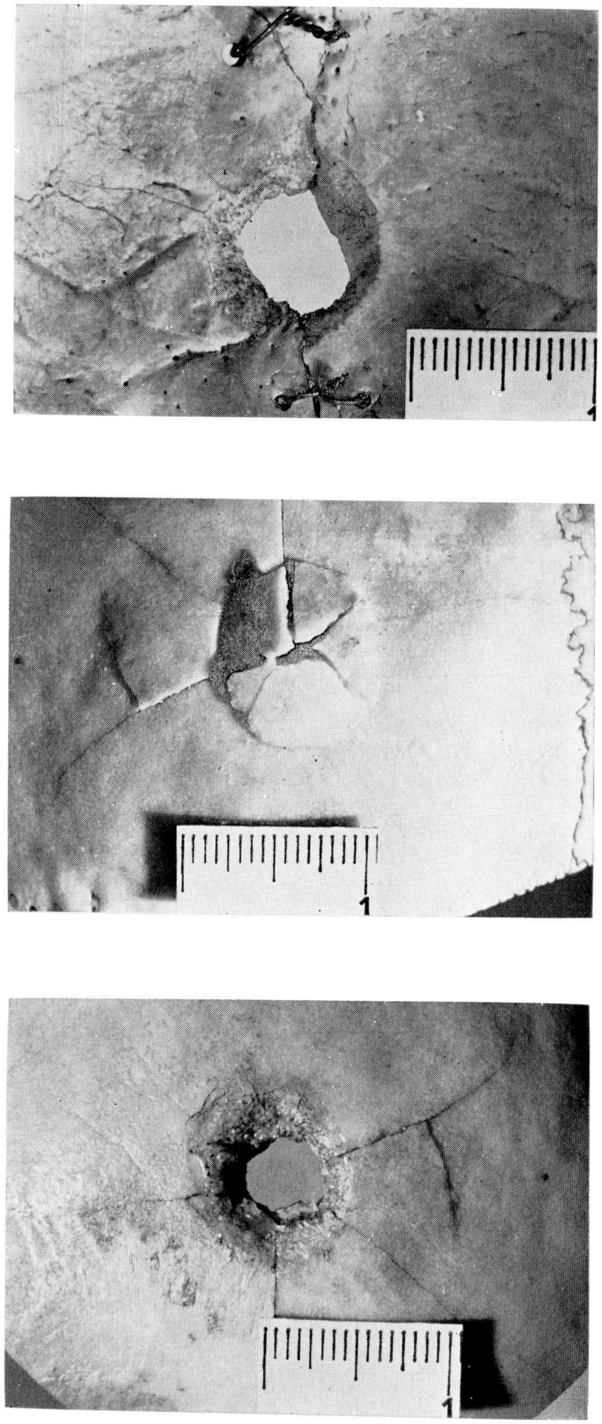

FIGURE X-53. Upper: Internal surface of the skull, showing inward bevelling of the defect in the bone under an entrance wound. Middle: Outer surface of the skull, to show the mechanism of outward bevelling at the exit. Note the raised bone fragments by the exiting bullet. The actual hole is shown in the lower photograph. Lower: Outer surface of the skull, showing outward bevelling of the exit defect.

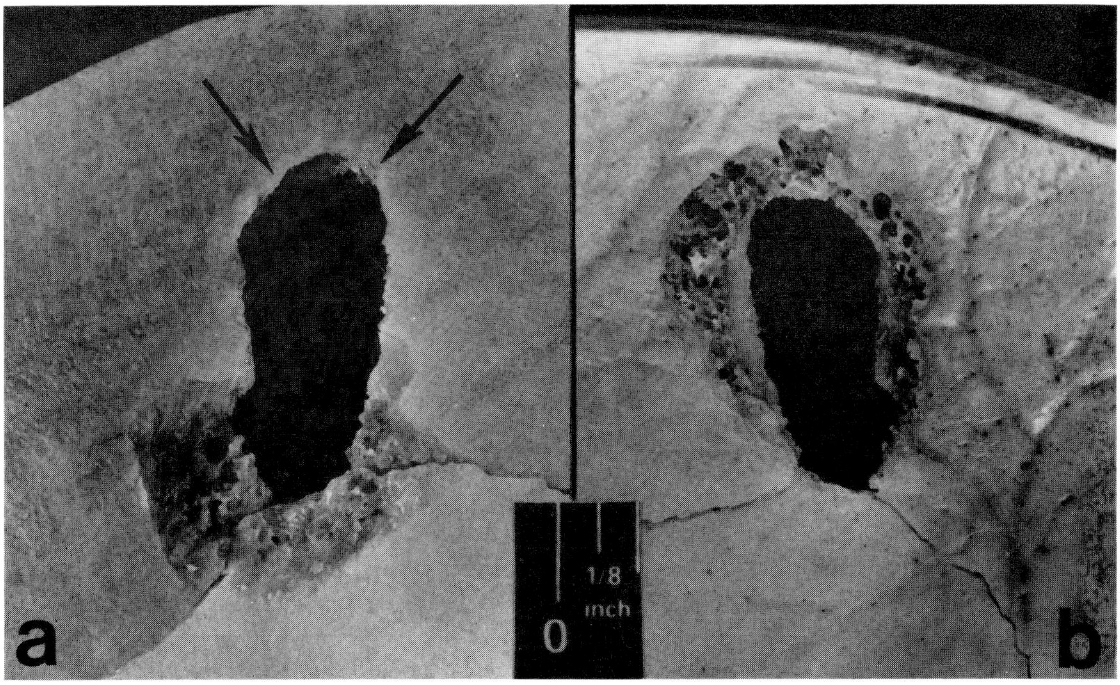


FIGURE X-54. Keyhole-shaped defect in the parietal bone of the skull due to a tangential gunshot. Figures 54a and 54b are the outer and inner surfaces of the bone, respectively. The entrance of the slug is marked by the inward bevelled part of the keyhole (arrows); the exit, at the lower part of the defect, is bevelled outward.

the bone around the defect by the forceful return of gases through the bullet hole or by the twisting force of the rotating bullet. Other parts of the skeleton may also enable recognition of the direction of fire by the inward displacement of bone fragments adjacent to the entrance wound in contrast to outward displacement of the fragments near the exit. The ribs and pelvis are common sites for this to occur.

A task often asked of the pathologist is to place the parties involved in a gunfight by using the pathways of the bullet or bullets in a victim's body. For this purpose, evidence regarding the position of the assailant at the time of the shooting is required to reconstruct the position of the victim, while the position of the victim must be established to ascertain that of the assailant. For example, a horizontal wound track results if the victim is standing upright when confronted by the assailant or if the victim is lying on the ground and the assailant is standing over him.

Other information that can be obtained from the postmortem examination of a shooting victim is given in the following sections.

### Homicide, Suicide or Accident

Distinction between homicide, suicide or accident may be difficult and sometimes impossible, yet it is the first question asked by the crime investigator in every death involving a shooting. Certain criteria are used by pathologists to define the manner of death within reasonable medical certainty. Among these, evaluation of the range of fire is of utmost importance. It is obvious that a distant shot could not have been self-inflicted in the absence of a contraption specifically designed for this purpose. The presence of gunpowder stippling, soot or both around a bullet wound are consequently of great significance. In the absence of grossly recognizable gunpowder residue, sensitive laboratory analyses may turn up findings missed by naked-eye examination. Examination of the clothing over the gunshot wound area should be included in the search for powder residue, particularly as this may be the only site to yield a positive result. It should be emphasized that gunpowder is by no means always found inside of contact bullet wounds. For instance, a contact shot of the heart area may be devoid of identifiable powder residue due to the fact that the powder is spread and partly washed out by extensive bleeding as long as the heart is pumping. Under such circumstances gunsmoke may be still detectable on the inner surface of the garment, as mentioned earlier in this chapter. In the case of close-range shots, where gunpowder is expected to be scattered on the target, it is interesting to note that clothing of a body drenched in decomposition fluids may completely lose any evidence of gunpowder; hence, estimation of the range of fire based on the presence of powder residue may not be feasible.

A gunshot wound in an area of the body not accessible to the victim, or only so with difficulty, e.g. in the back of the head or between the shoulder blades, is suspicious of homicide. The vast majority of suicidal shots is in the temple, the heart, the forehead and the mouth. Among these, the temple area is used most frequently.

Right-handed individuals are more likely to shoot themselves in the right side of the head, but a contact shot of the right temple does not necessarily imply that the victim was right-handed. We have observed many times where a right-handed individual shot himself in the left temple and vice versa.

Gunsmoke deposits on the hand that fired the gun are sometimes seen (Figs. X-55 and X-56). This gunsmoke originates in part from

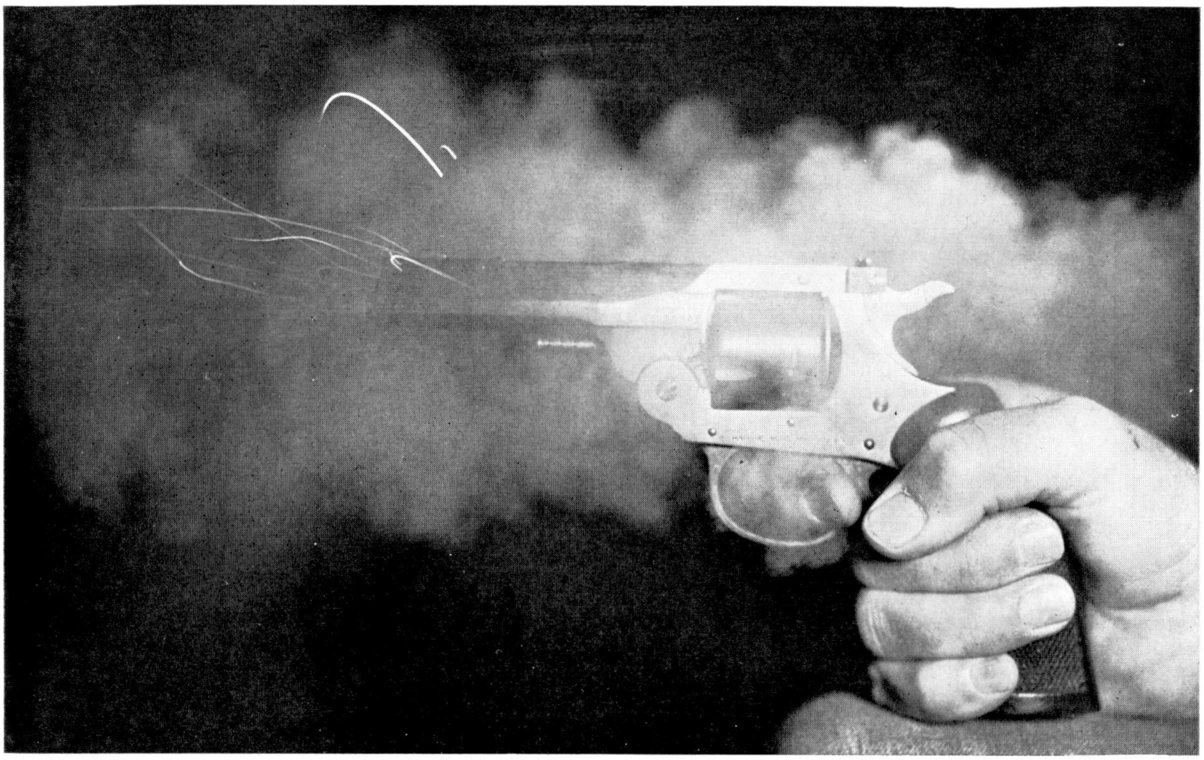

FIGURE X-55. Cloud of gunsmoke engulfing the hand of the individual who fires the weapon. The presence of gunsmoke deposits and their distribution on the hand are important for the determination of whether a bullet wound was self-inflicted. The light streaks emerging from the muzzle of the gun are glowing particles of gunpowder. (The author gratefully acknowledges the cooperation of Donald M. Flohr of the H. P. White Laboratories, Bel Air, Maryland, for the preparation of this photograph.)

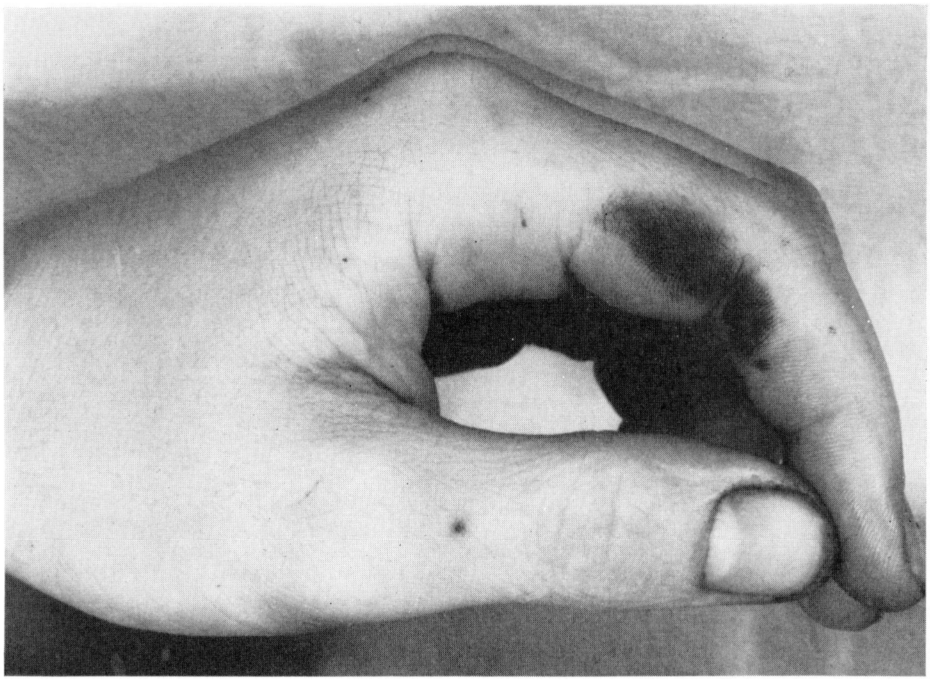

FIGURE X-56. Deposit of soot on the index finger of an individual who shot himself in the head.

the blow back associated with the muzzle blast as well as from loose fittings in the frame of the weapon. Thus, revolvers, especially if poorly constructed, such as the notorious *Saturday night specials,* are more likely to deposit gunsmoke on the firing hand than pistols of good quality. With rifles and shotguns in good condition, it is very unlikely that identifiable gunsmoke will be found on the hand that pulled the trigger. Different firearms tend to deposit gunsmoke in different patterns. This may be useful in the determination of whether a bullet wound was self-inflicted. Laboratory experiments involving handguns have shown that the index finger, thumb and connecting web area of the shooting hand are most likely to be contaminated with gunshot residue. Occasionally, gunsmoke deposits are noted on both hands, especially on the one that was used to steady the weapon while the other pulled the trigger.

A twenty-four-year-old woman was found in her bedroom wedged between bed and dresser. On the bed were male undershorts smeared with blood. Near the body on the floor was a male shoeprint pointing away from the body. A .38 caliber Colt revolver was in her left hand, the index finger in the trigger guard. A near-contact gunshot wound was present on the right cheek (Fig. X-57a, b). On the palmar surface of the hand, just below the index finger, were two parallel ¼ in. long pinch marks surrounded by faint brownish discoloration due to gunsmoke (Fig. X-57c). The fired cartridge in the cylinder of the revolver was at six o'clock. The weapon was clean, apparently freshly oiled.

The boyfriend, a gun collector, free on probation, was seen driving away from the house after a shot was heard, and he was not apprehended until late that night. He stated that they had had an argument following which she shot herself. He took the weapon from the pool of blood on the floor and wiped the blood on a pair of shorts. When it occurred to him that possession of the gun might incriminate him in a murder charge, he cleaned and oiled the weapon, then placed it back into her hand. His statement sounded credible. When the cocked gun was held in the right hand with the thumb pulling the trigger and the muzzle pointing toward one's own cheek and the left hand placed over the cylinder to steady the weapon, the downcoming hammer inflicted a pinch of the same appearance and in the same location as on the left hand of the deceased.

Gunsmoke deposits on hands obscured by

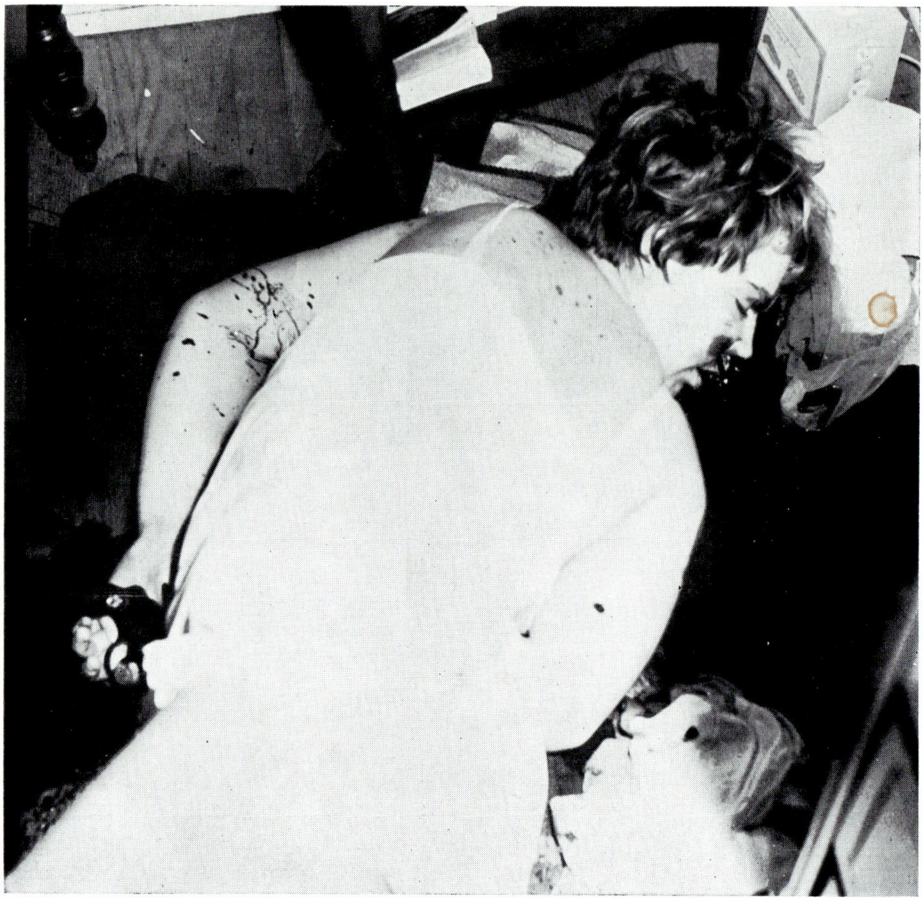

(a)

(b)

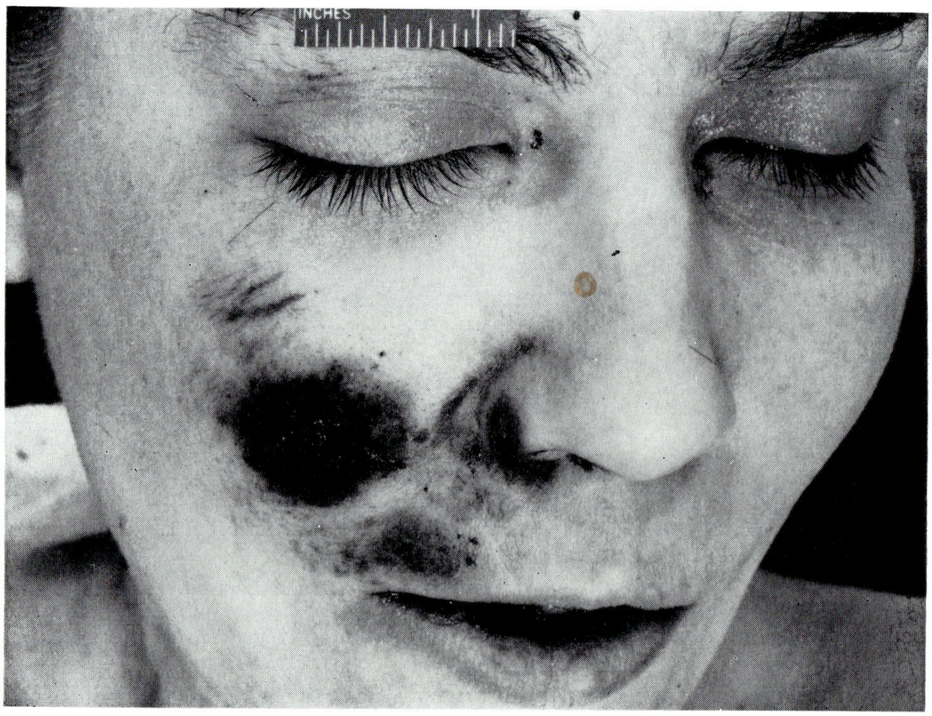

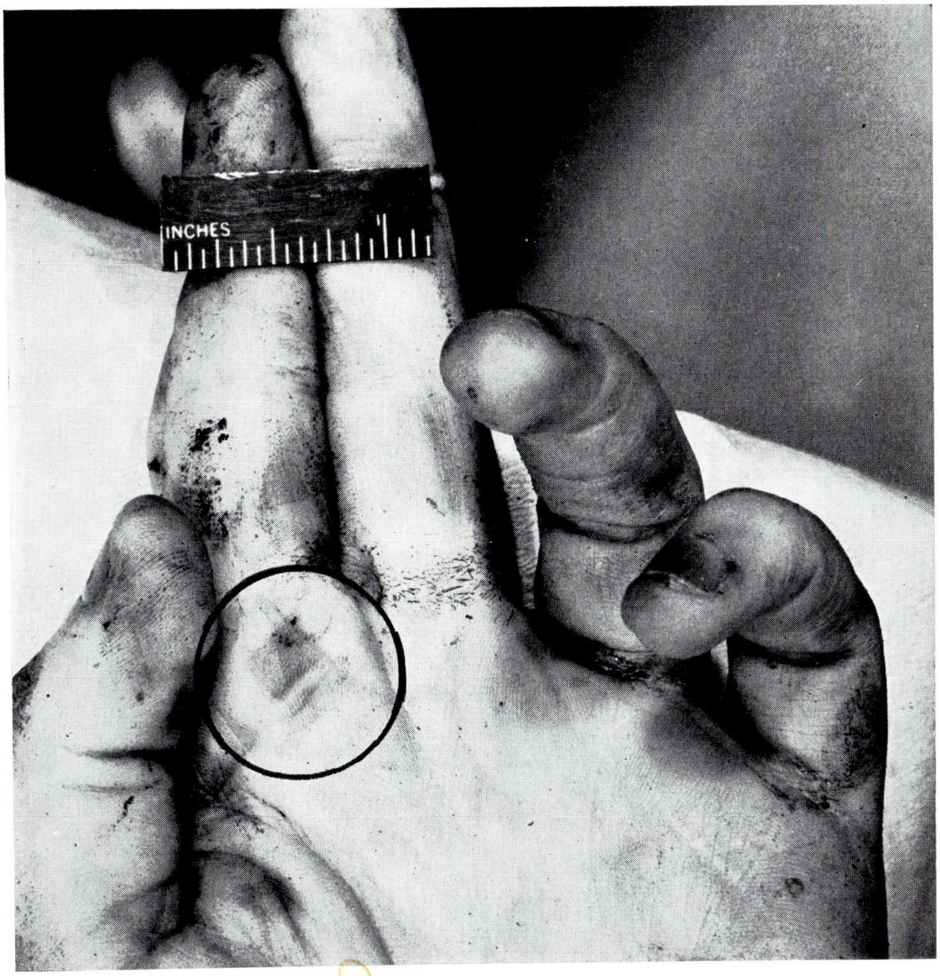


(c)

FIGURE X-57. (a): The body of the victim wedged between bed and dresser. A .38 caliber Colt revolver is noted in her left hand; the index finger is in the trigger guard. The right cheek displays a near-contact wound. (b): Closeup of a near-contact bullet wound of the right cheek. (c): Two parallel ¼ in. long *pinch marks* surrounded by faint brownish discoloration from gunsmoke on the palm of the left hand. This hand was apparently used to steady the weapon when it was fired.

extensive blood soiling can be identified by gentle rinsing of the hand under running cold water, which dissolves even dried blood without scrubbing.

Hands suspected of having fired a gun should never be fingerprinted until after proper examination for powder residue. In some cases the results could mean the difference between homicide and suicide, although the absence of visible gunsmoke deposits on the victim's hand does not imply that the gun was fired by another person. Laboratory procedures ranging from relatively simple chemical tests to complex neutron activation analysis, using a nuclear reactor and complicated electronic equipment, are capable of detecting gunsmoke even when none can be seen on gross examination. One of the earliest and most widely known tests is the so-called paraffin or nitrate test.

Melted paraffin at about 120° F is brushed on the surface to be tested. After hardening, the wax is pulled off. The inner surface of the wax cast is then treated with diphenylamine or diphenylbenzidine reagent; a blue color develops in areas where residue is present. It must be noted that this test is not specific for gunpowder residue. Any substance containing soluble nitrates will give a positive result. Among these are soil, tobacco, certain cosmetics, many types of fertilizer and urine; many other substances will also give a false positive result. For this reason, the FBI laboratory has abandoned using this method for determining whether a person has recently fired a weapon.[7]

A more specific method for the detection of gunshot residue is that developed by Doctor Harrison, Professor of Chemistry at the University of Rhode Island. This procedure is based on the finding of primer elements, barium and antimony, on the hand that fired the weapon. The residue is removed from the suspect's hands with a small piece of cotton cloth. The cloth is then treated with two reagents, triphenylmethyl-arsonium iodide and sodium rhodizonate. Colored spots are produced in those areas of the cloth that are contaminated with the metallic elements of the primer. This method is rapid and specific but of poor sensitivity. Its application is therefore limited.

Neutron activation analysis has a sensitivity that surpasses by far that of any other test. As in the Harrison method, barium and antimony from the primer are the components of residue that are identified and accurately measured. However, some recently developed primers contain neither barium nor antimony. In such cases neutron activation analysis is obviously of no value. Nevertheless, it has been the method generally used in recent years. Deterrents to this method are the substantial investment, high operating costs and limited availability of the equipment. Flameless atomic absorption spectroscopy provides sensitivity that approaches that of neutron activation analysis and is sometimes used as an alternative for the detection of firearms discharge residue.

For either method, the residue from the suspect's hands is removed for testing either by the ordinary paraffin cast or simply by swabbing the backs of the hands with cotton-tipped swabs moistened with dilute nitric acid.

In the case of suicide by rifle fire, the victim

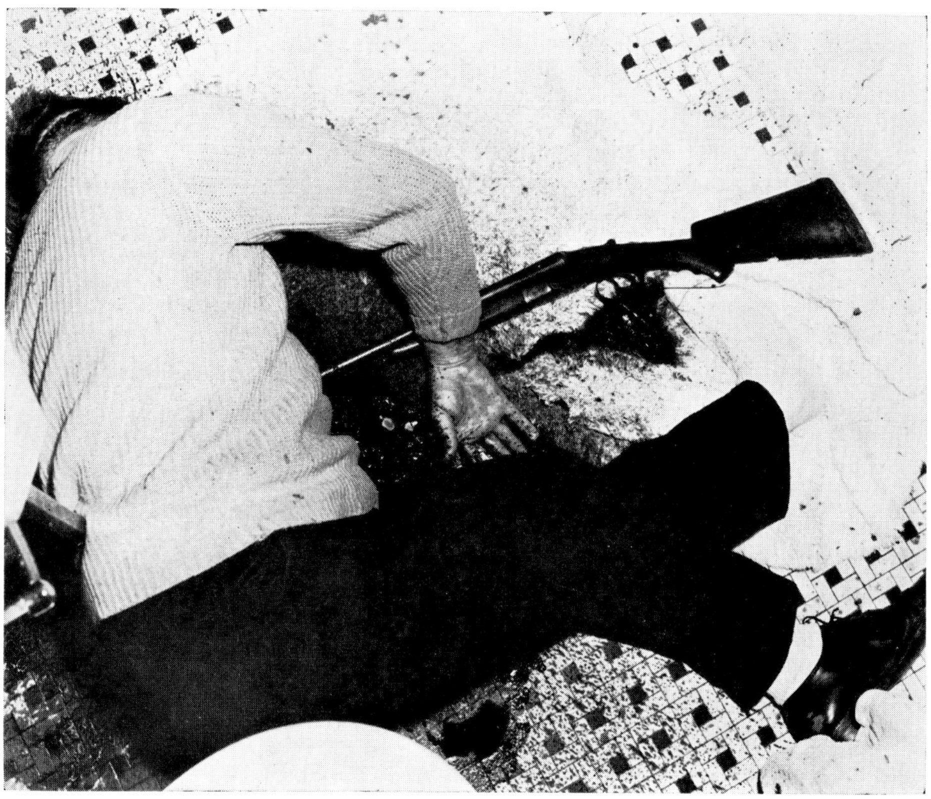

FIGURE X-58. Suicidal shot of the chest. A coat hanger was used to pull the trigger.

may be in practically any position to fire the gun. Nevertheless, depending on the position in which the victim is found, it is sometimes necessary to verify whether he was capable of reaching the trigger. Measurement of the victim's arm length yields the required information. It must be noted that the trigger may be moved as easily by using a toe, stick or coat hanger. These methods are not at all uncommon (Figs. X-58 and X-59).

Multiple bullet wounds invariably arouse a suspicion of homicide. However, in certain cases suicide must also be given consideration. Multiple suicidal shots commonly involve the same general area of the body. It is highly unusual to find the shots scattered. Under such circumstances, homicide should be suspected.

In a case on file at this office, a forty-three-year-old man addressed a suicide note to his wife before shooting himself three times (Fig. X-60). A superficial graze was

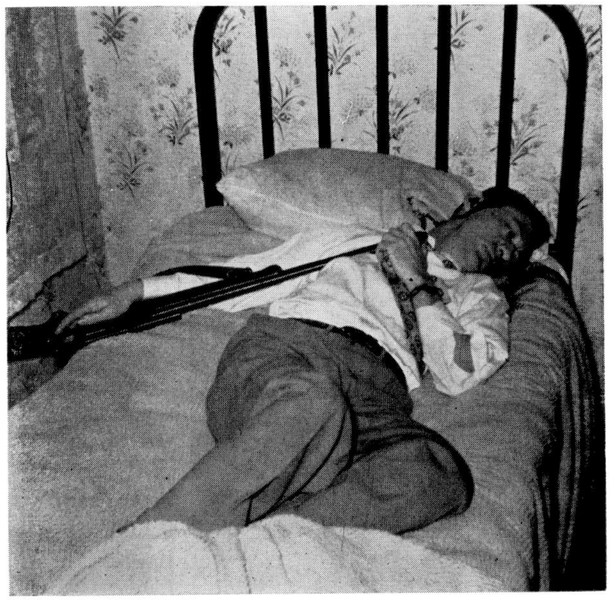

FIGURE X-59. The length of the victim's arm is important in determining whether he could have fired the weapon himself.

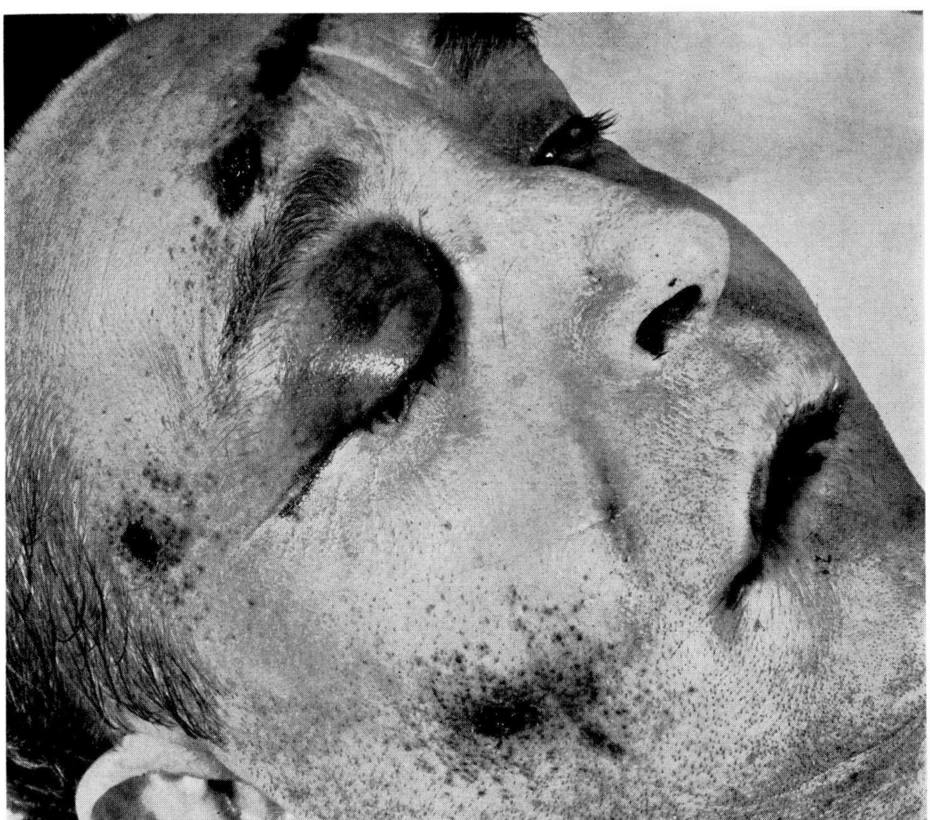

FIGURE X-60. Suicide with three close-range gunshot wounds: graze of the forehead, through-and-through bullet wound of the cheeks not involving vital organs and fatal shot of the right temple.

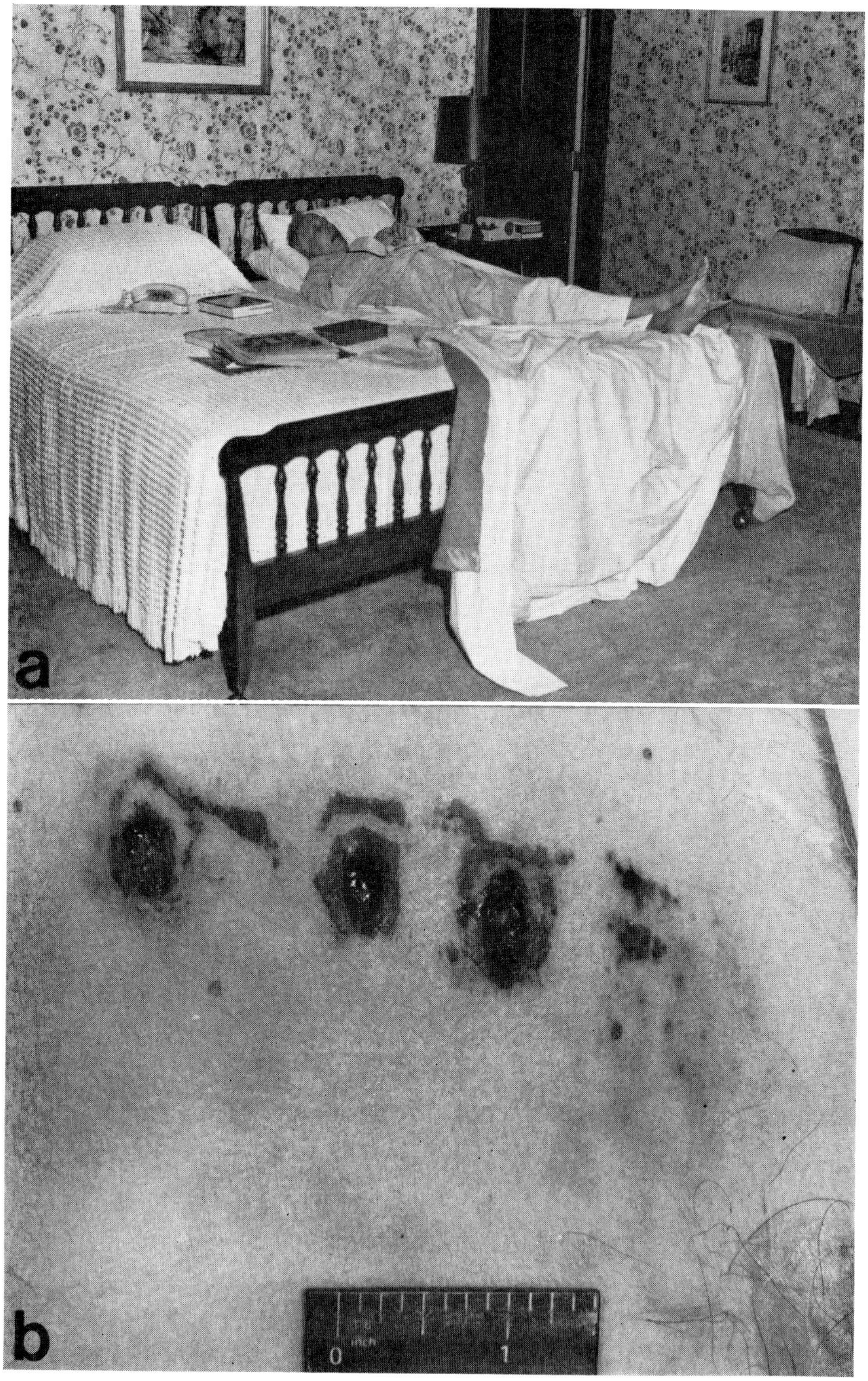


FIGURE X-61. (a): Seventy-two-year-old man found lying peacefully on his bed. The scene appears to be quite uneventful. Practically no bleeding was noted anywhere. The pistol and cartridge cases were in the bathroom, seen with the door open. (b): Three contact shots in the left side of the chest above the nipple. Each injury shows the muzzle imprint of the .25 caliber pistol that was used.

noted in the forehead, another bullet pierced both cheeks and a gunshot of the right temple (no doubt the third by chronological order) proved lethal by penetration of the brain. The sequence of the shots in the forehead and the cheek could not be ascertained.

Any attempt to establish the sequence of shots must take into consideration the degree of incapacity that results from each shot. This will enable the examiner to determine which was the fatal shot and allow conclusions regarding the physical activity of the victim following the other shots. In the case of the man mentioned earlier, one may wonder whether the graze of the forehead and the shot of the cheek were *hesitation shots* similar to hesitation cuts outlined in Chapter VIII.

In another case a seventy-two-year-old man committed suicide by using a .25 caliber pistol and firing three contact shots into his chest (Fig. X-61). The incident occurred in the bathroom. After the shooting, he walked to the bedroom and lay on his bed. The body was found the next day. At autopsy it was found that all three shots perforated the heart.

Occasionally in gunshots of the head, it may be possible to ascertain the sequence of the shots by the pattern of fracture lines that radiate from each defect. The fractures that extend from the second bullet hole are arrested by those that originated from the first (Fig. X-62). This is in keeping with characteristics of fractures of the skull due to blunt trauma as outlined in Chapter VII.

Another point in the distinction of homicide from suicide is the observation that suicides frequently remove the clothing from the area they intend to shoot. Thus an open shirt is not unusual in suicidal shots of the heart area.

An accidental gunshot can be distinguished from a homicidal or suicidal injury only by the circumstances that surround the incident. It is the task of the pathologist, on the basis of his findings at the postmortem examination of the victim, to confirm or dispute the account that was given of the circumstances, i.e. to prove whether the injury is consistent with the manner of injury that was described. The availability of photographs and diagrams of the scene is most helpful in this regard.

Russian roulette is termed *accidental* by many pathologists. This is a betting game in which the players hold a revolver loaded with a single cartridge (the position of which in the cylinder is unknown) to their temple and pull the trigger. It is our contention that these deaths are suicidal due to the significant element of deliberate self-destruction involved.

### Ricochet

A ricochet is a missile that is deviated from its course by striking an intermediary object. Such missiles are commonly deformed. The degree of deformity varies depending on the texture of the bullets, the angle of impact and the consistency of the object which is struck. Jacketed bullets have a greater ricochet potential than nonjacketed ones.

The path of a ricochet is unpredictable, although in the case of a ricochet on a body of water, the angle of incidence equals the angle of reflection. The missile penetrates the water for a short distance. The same may occur with a shot fired at a block of wood. In no other case can injury by ricochet be inflicted intentionally. These missiles are, therefore, of considerable legal significance.

It is important in the case of a suspected ricochet that the missile be examined for possible foreign inclusions originating from the intermediary target. Such inclusions are common in lead bullets because of the softness of the metal. Sensitive analyses are now available to identify these substances.

An entrance wound produced by a ricochet is not necessarily different from that produced by an ordinary bullet, although it may assume a bizarre shape due to the deformity of the missile.

A twenty-two-year-old woman who witnessed an argument between her husband and two men suddenly slumped over dead when the husband fired his gun at his opponents (Fig. X-63a). At postmortem examination she had an injury in midforehead, resembling a typical contact gunshot wound except for the absence of gunsmoke (Fig. X-63b). The weapon used was a 9 mm Luger with corresponding ammunition. The husband was found guilty of murder despite his contention that he had not fired in the direction of his wife.

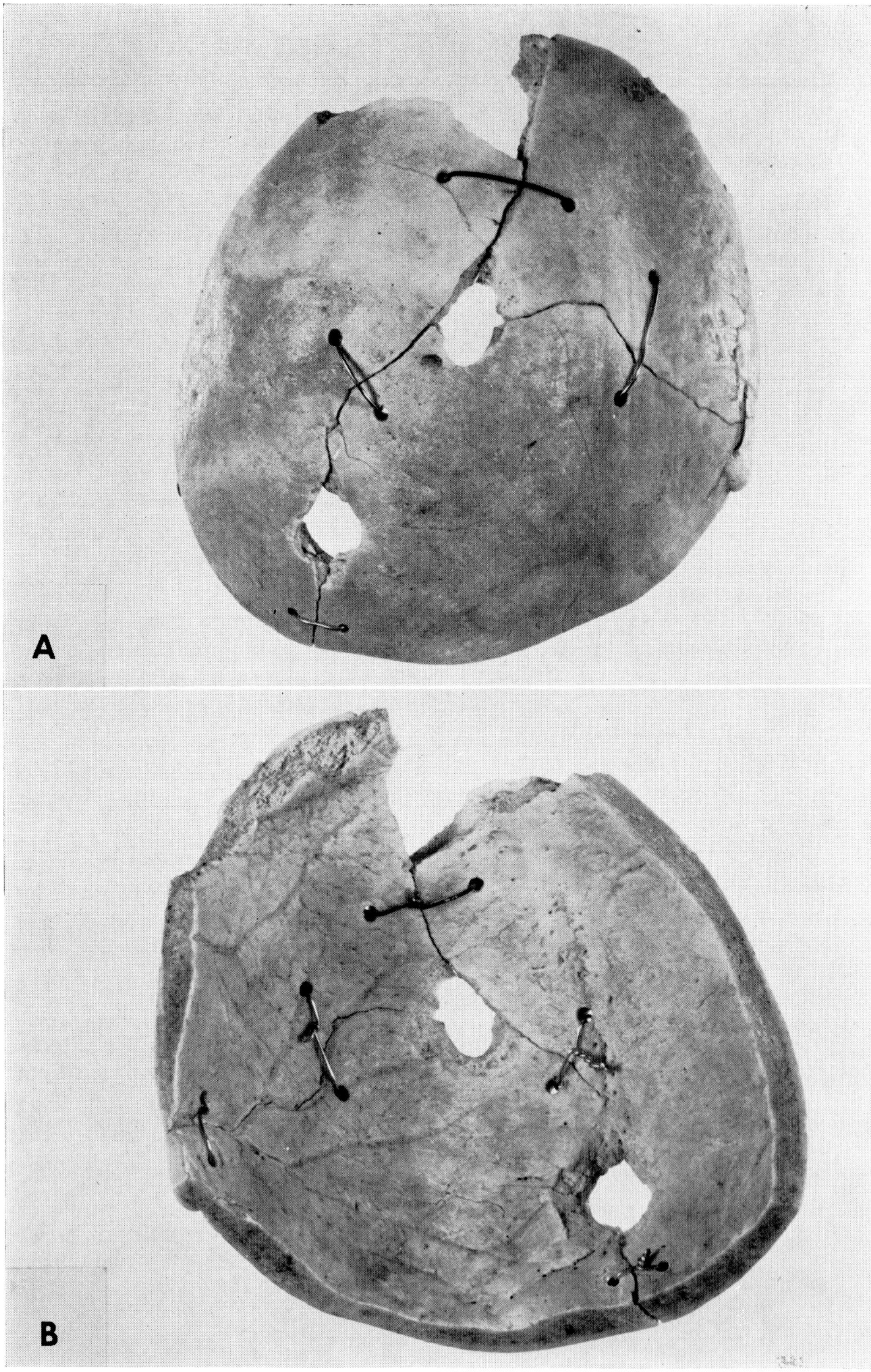


FIGURE X-62. Exterior (A) and interior (B) aspects of a skullcap with two experimental entrance bullet holes. The pattern of the fracture lines which radiate from the holes and the interrupted bevelling of the upper defect indicate that the lower wound must have been inflicted first.

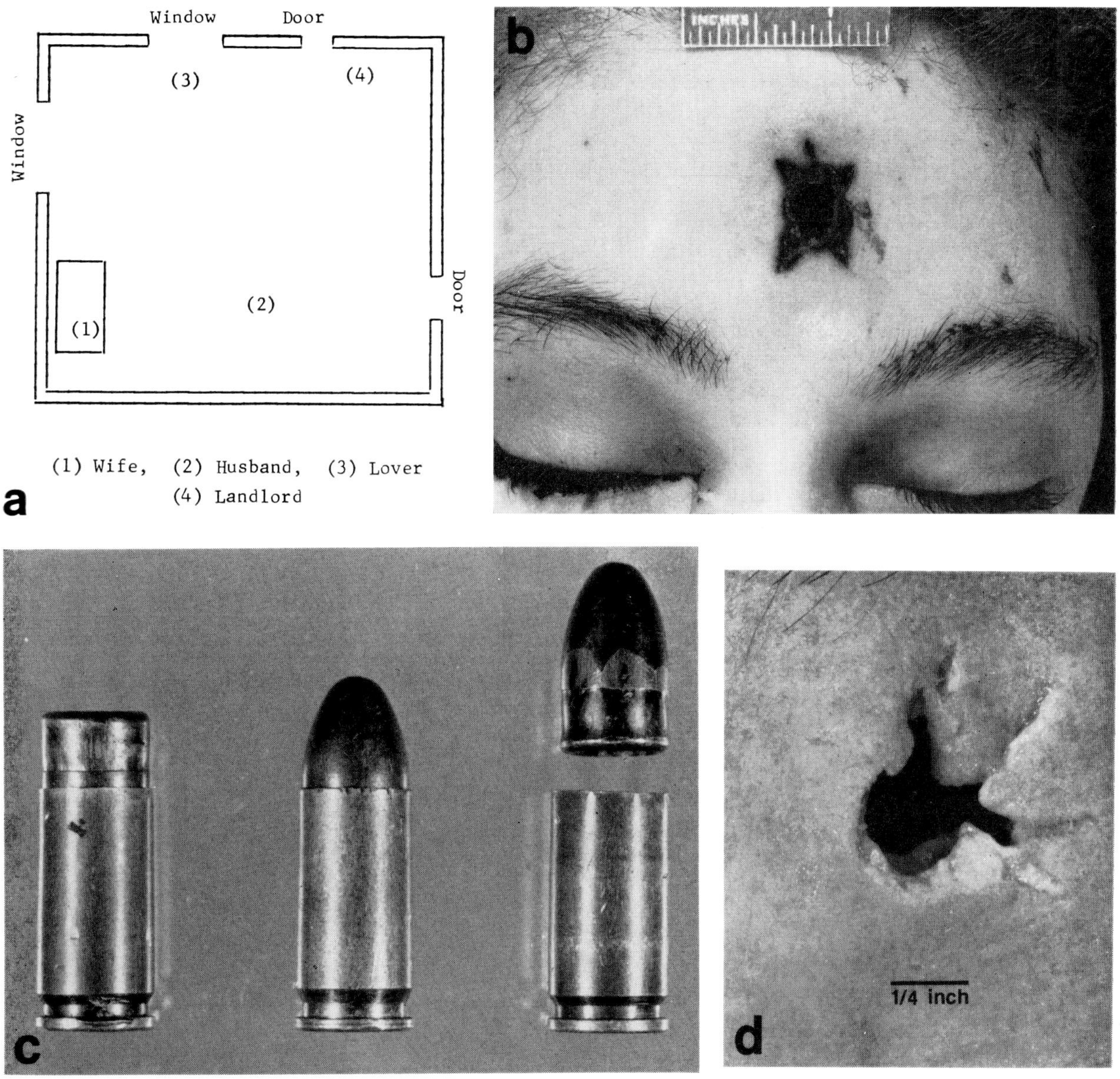


FIGURE X-63. Ricochet. (a): Layout of the room and position of the parties. (b): Entrance bullet wound in the forehead of the victim resembling a contact shot but showing no presence of soot or gunpowder. (c): The bullet in the center is original Luger ammunition. A slug inverted in the cartridge case is displayed on the left. (d) Injury bearing similarity to the bullet wound of the victim is obtained by a test shot from a distance of 9 ft. using Luger ammunition with inverted slug. (Figure X-63 reproduced from Spitz, W. U.: Rikoschett- oder Kontaktschussverletzung. *Dtsch Z Ges Gerichtl Med, 66:*153, 1969. Courtesy of Bergmann Verlag, Heidelberg.)

Puzzled by the absence of soot and gunpowder within and about the bullet wound, close-range firing seemed doubtful, and the possibility of a ricochet was entertained. Test firing of the same gun with matching ammunition was carried out at contact with the skin as well as from a distance of 7 to 9 ft. Injuries bearing similarity to that of the deceased could be obtained only when the slugs that were used were inverted in their cartridge cases, thus striking the target base first (Fig. X-63c, d). These results gave rise to the probability that the woman was struck by a deformed bullet, namely a ricochet. When the Luger bullets were fired as manufactured, the injuries that resulted had the expected appearance.

On the basis of this new experimental evidence, the trial was reopened and the case was dismissed.[8]

In another case an eighteen-year-old boy was found dead beside a narrow path in a forest. He had a bullet wound of the groin, and autopsy showed that death had resulted from blood loss due to laceration of the iliac artery and vein. A lead bullet was recovered from the soft tissues of the pelvis. Meanwhile, the friend of the victim surrendered to the police, claiming that the death of his friend was accidental. They had been playing *chicken*, a game of courage, the object of which is to avoid taking cover while shots are fired by the other player. He had definitely not shot at his friend but admitted shooting in the same general area when suddenly his friend collapsed and was dead a short time later. At this point the bullet that had been removed from the victim was examined. The tip of the bullet was flattened on one side, and the base bore the imprint of the weaving pattern of the victim's trousers. A few threads of the fabric were actually trapped in the lead. It was thus evident that the bullet struck the victim base-first after it had apparently glanced off one of the trees between the two players. The flattened tip of the bullet and numerous grazes in the bark of the trees in that section of the forest gave credence to this version. Criminal charges were thereupon dropped.

## PHYSICAL ACTIVITY FOLLOWING FATAL INJURY BY GUNFIRE

Contrary to popular belief, the physical activity of a person who is fatally shot is not necessarily arrested immediately following the injury. Missile wounds of the brain are common exceptions because unconsciousness develops rapidly. A bullet that severs the neck segment of the spinal cord would cause immediate collapse due to paraplegia, but death may be delayed, depending on the exact location of the injury. Death is instantaneous if the medulla oblongata is involved.

A study of 111 homicidal firearm and stabbing cases with regard to the duration of activity of the victims before they collapsed was published by Spitz et al. in 1961.[9] Gunshot wounds of the heart and lung are often followed by extended activity until blood loss causes shock, followed by death. Many of the fatally injured attempt to reach help. Some crawl, run or call.

One thirty-nine-year-old man, who was shot in the chest with a .32 caliber pistol, ran seven city blocks before he collapsed and died two hours later at the hospital. Autopsy of the victim showed that the bullet had severed intercostal vessels and proceeded through the right lung. There was 1 quart (approx. 900 ml) of blood present in the pleural cavity in addition to a large amount of blood found at the scene.

A thirty-one-year-old man was shot in the chest with a .38 caliber bullet. He was witnessed to have crawled about 55 ft. following the injury and then collapsed. He died a few minutes later.

Autopsy showed that the wound track traversed the left lung and the heart, resulting in massive hemopericardium.

In general, capability to act is shorter in victims of shooting than in victims of stabbing. The dissimilar nature of these wounds accounts for this difference. Whereas gunshot wounds cause an actual hole, a stab wound causes a slitlike opening, which tends to *seal* after the knife is withdrawn.

## DIVERSE CHARACTERISTICS OF LESS COMMON AMMUNITION AND THEIR EFFECTS

Many types of ammunition are available. Most are conventional varieties that produce known patterns of injury. Occasionally, however, gunshot wounds are observed that exhibit unusual characteristics.[10]

### *Super Vel® Ammunition*

This .38 caliber ammunition has replaced some of the .38 Special in use by many police departments in the United States. The Super Vel bullet is lightweight, partially jacketed and is propelled at high velocity. It is available in two designs: a flat-nose soft-point and a hollow-point. Muzzle velocity of Super Vel is 1370 ft./sec., compared to 855 ft./sec. of the .38 Special. The muzzle energy of Super Vel bullets exceeds that of the standard .38 Special by nearly 200 ft./lb. Test firing of Super Vel ammunition shows that entrance wounds in the skin by soft- and hollow-point Super Vel bullets are identical to those inflicted with standard .38 Special. In deeper structures, however, the defects are two to three times the diameter of wounds produced with conventional .38 rounds. A comparison of hollow- and soft-point Super Vel ammunition indicates that hollow-point bullets are more devastating, producing a larger and more irregular wound track than the soft-point variety. The increased destructive effect of the hollow-point bullet seems to result from its greater tendency to mushroom on impact and to expand by opening than is exhibited by the solid-nose soft-point bullet.

### *Plastic Ammunition*

Plastic ammunition is intended for indoor target practice. The cartridge case and the projectile are both made of plastic. The propellant is a pistol primer. Muzzle velocity is advertised at 500 ft./sec.

Test firing of this ammunition in contact with the skin and at distances up to twenty feet supports the manufacturers' claim of relative safety. The wadcutter-shaped projectile does not pierce the skin, except for a circular *cut* of the epidermis less than $\frac{1}{16}$ in. in depth; damage to the eyes may be expected, however.

### *KTW® Ammunition*

This ammunition is available in a variety of calibers, including .30 carbine. The Teflon®-coated tungsten alloy bullet is designed to pierce the body or the engine block of an automobile. The ricochet potential of this bullet is very great. A half-jacket of gilding metal serves to seal the bore and spin the bullet. Muzzle velocity is 700 ft./sec. for the .38 Special.

Test firing to determine impact characteristics and on-target effectiveness shows that injuries sustained by *KTW* do not differ from bullet wounds due to conventional types of ammunition. However, the half-jacket of the *KTW* bullet tends to separate from the core and to pursue an independent course. It usually remains within the body. The core usually exits, even after traversing bone.

As the barrel markings of the gun are engraved on the half-jacket, identification of the gun by bullet comparison in the absence of the jacket cannot be done. This implies that an autopsy in the case of a death involving *KTW* ammunition is imperative, even in the presence of an exit wound, for recovery of the half-jacket.

### *Frangible Bullets*

A type of .22 caliber ammunition, frangible bullets are used in shooting galleries and to stun and kill cattle in a safe and humane manner. The bullet is manufactured of bonded powdered lead or iron. It disintegrates on striking the target; consequently, frangible bullets do not ricochet. Graham et al.[6] reported a death due to a self-inflicted gunshot of the head involving a frangible bullet. These authors conducted experiments with this type of ammunition to determine its disintegrating and penetrating characteristics, as well as the suitability of such bullets for comparison microscope identification. They concluded that penetration of the skull occurs at distances from 0.5 to 36 in.

Location and recovery of the bullet fragments are greatly facilitated by the use of x rays. Due to the extent of fragmentation and mutilation of these bullets, they are generally unfit for matching under the comparison microscope.

### *Birdshot*

Birdshot is available in a variety of calibers and loads. The more commonly used cartridges are .22 and .38 caliber. Birdshot is considered low-powered and is used for pest control. The .22 cartridge is loaded with approximately 150 pellets of No. 12 shot. At 20 yd. the pellets will barely penetrate thin cardboard. At close range, however, birdshot can be extremely dangerous. DiMaio and Spitz[11] observed a victim of homicide with a shot of the head involving this type of ammunition. The distance from which the fatal shot had been fired was unknown, and test shots were carried out in an attempt to establish the penetration power and wounding characteristics of this ammunition at various distances. The victim had been shot through the temple. X ray showed numerous metallic pellets scattered throughout the brain.

The dispersion pattern of the pellets in the body cannot be applied to the estimation of the range of firing, as demonstrated by Breitenecker et al.[12] Considerable dispersion of the shot within the body occurs if the majority of the pellets strike the target en masse. This dispersion is the result of deflection of the pellets by striking each other at the time of passage through the target (so-called *billiard ball* effect). The same phenomenon occurs in the case of shotgun injuries, which will be discussed in a later section.

Test firings indicated that in the homicide in question the gun had been fired from a distance of less than 6 in.; the possibility of a contact shot should be ruled out.

### *Piggyback Bullet*

A *piggyback* or tandem bullet is one that results from the discharge of a second bullet while the first is still in the barrel. It is thus a projectile composed of two independent bullets, where one is pushed into the rear of the other. The projectile weighs double or nearly double the weight of an ordinary bullet of the same caliber. As in the case of any bullet, parts of this projectile may be chipped off as it penetrates the target. The occurrence of a *piggyback* bullet is rare, but when it happens it is associated with faulty ammunition or a defective firearm.

The body of a fifteen-year-old youth was found in the basement of a vacant house. A gunshot wound, which indicated no evidence of close-range firing, was noted in his chest. The bullet had traversed the lungs and the heart, and a relatively well-preserved .38 caliber lead bullet weighing 140.2 grain was recovered from under the skin of the chest wall on the opposite side. A second bullet wound was noted in the inner angle of the right eye. This injury was surrounded by an abundant amount of gunpowder and soot. A large irregular missile weighing 266.5 grain was found in the center of the brain (Fig. X-64). From the appearance of this missile it was evident that two bullets had been joined together at the time of firing. A defective .38 caliber revolver was later recovered and associated with this homicide.

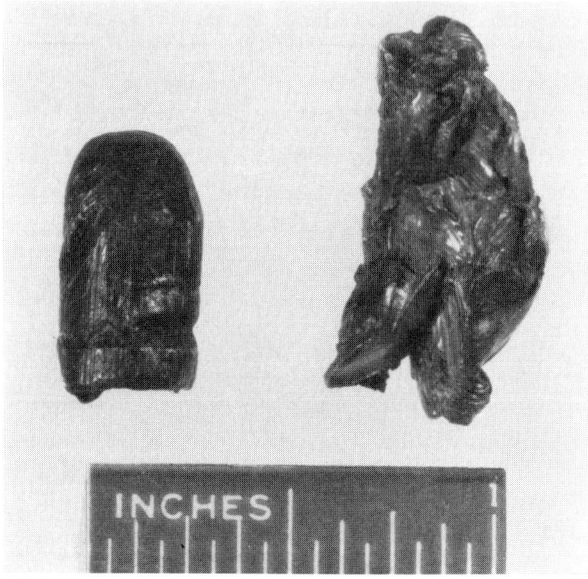


FIGURE X-64. Relatively well-preserved .38 caliber missile recovered from the chest of the victim (left) and piggyback bullet recovered from his brain (right).

### *Blank Cartridges*

A blank cartridge is one with primer, gun powder and wadding but without a bullet. It contains a faster-burning propellant than an ordinary cartridge of the same caliber. Due to the considerable noise produced by this ammunition, it is used for starter pistols, signals, etc. Smokeless powder has largely replaced black powder in blank cartridges. Smokeless powder produces a larger amount of gas than black powder; consequently, blanks loaded with smokeless powder produce larger injuries. Experiments indicate that distant shots with blank cartridges are harmless; however, at a 1 in. distance significant tears of the skin and underlying tissues are noted. At contact with the skin using

.38 and .45 caliber blanks, devastating wounds are produced due to the gas generated by the exploding gunpowder. These wounds measure up to 3 by 2 in. and 2½ in. in depth. A contact shot to the head with a blank cartridge can be fatal as a result of penetration of the skull and the concussive effect on the brain produced by the sudden release of gases under tremendous pressure.

### *Stud Guns (Nail Guns)*

Stud guns are firearmlike tools used in construction work for firing metal studs into steel, wood or concrete. An interchangeable breech plug enables a choice of calibers, depending on the power required for adequate penetration. Calibers usually range from .22 to .38. Due to their marked penetration power, injuries by stud guns are severe. The size and shape of the stud and its tendency to tumble and ricochet are other features that cause atypical and larger wounds than those produced by ordinary bullets.

A series of test shots into human cadavers indicates the destructive capacity of this tool.[13] The shots were fired at close and distant ranges using .22 caliber cartridges. At 27 in., 6 ft. and 9 ft. the studs struck the body sideways. Marginal abrasion of the wound in the skin was absent. The studs traversed the entire body and then penetrated a wooden block. At 3 in. the wound in a thigh was a gaping circular defect measuring 1 in. in diameter. A shot of the forehead from this distance fractured the skull extensively. The stud exited posteriorly and penetrated a wooden block to a depth of several inches.

### *Short-range Ammunition (Short-Stop®)*

Short-range ammunition was designed to be nonricochet for use in congested, enclosed areas, primarily as a hijacking deterrent in commercial airliners. A round of this ammunition consists of a .38 Special/.357 caliber cartridge enclosed in a plastic cap. A collapsed projectile composed of a beanbaglike structure containing fine lead shot is enclosed within the cap. A plastic wad separates the projectile from the gunpowder. When fired, the projectile assumes a pancake shape of 1 in. diameter. Muzzle velocity is greater than 1000 ft./sec., and muzzle energy is 125

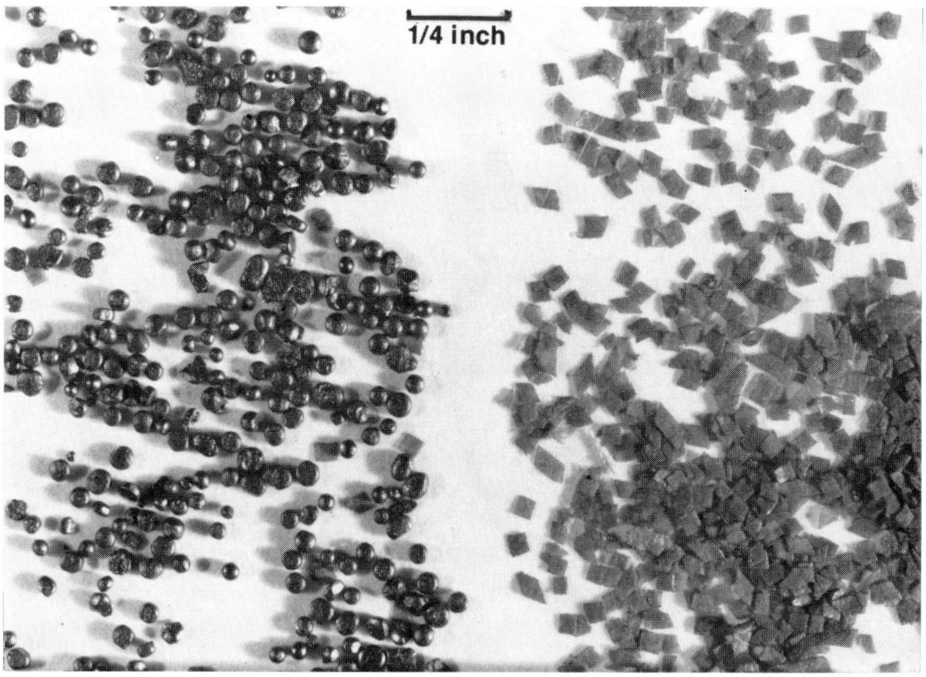


FIGURE X-65. Two kinds of gunpowder. Left: Ball powder. Right: Flake powder (more commonly used).

ft./lb. On striking the body, the *shell* of the projectile ruptures and the pellets are scattered along the wound track.

Testing of this ammunition[14] shows that the projectile never exits the body, regardless of the range of fire. Accuracy is reasonably good, and at ranges of up to 15 ft. with a clothed individual, evidence of substantial injury is noted. At 25 ft., only superficial wounds occur. In an unclothed individual significant damage occurs at distances of 25 ft. but not at 50 ft. At ranges up to 10 ft., wounds that would be fatal are observed. Up to 6 ft., this ammunition perforates the full thickness of a wall of a commercial airliner and produces a ¾ in. hole in the aircraft's Plexiglas® window.

### *Ball Powder*

Ball powder is a variety of smokeless gunpowder in which the grains are spheres rather than flakes or cylinders (Fig. X-65). A bullet fired from a cartridge loaded with ball powder shows typical small indentations resembling *pockmarks* on its base. These are due to the explosion in the cartridge at the time of discharge, which, by increasing the pressure in the cartridge, imprints the spherical grains of gunpowder on the bullet. There is considerable significance to ball powder, as it is mainly used in Winchester-Western ammunition. Since most ammunition is not loaded with ball powder, it is important for exclusion purposes to determine when it is used.

## THE AUTOPSY

In addition to general information that is applicable to every autopsy protocol, the autopsy of a victim of gunfire should include at least the following observations: (a) description of clothing, (b) pertinent findings regarding bullet wounds, (c) cause of death, (d) toxicological and serological analyses.

The autopsy file should also include an adequate police report with a concise description of the scene where the body was found. Appropriate sketches and photographs of the scene are desirable. Further guidelines concerning the medicolegal autopsy and different techniques of the postmortem examination are outlined in Chapters XXIV and XXV.

### Description of Clothing

The body is to be disrobed with care. The clothing should not be torn or cut, and the examiner must be alert to the possibility of finding bullets among the clothing items. List all items and their condition and the extent of bloodstaining. Record the number and location of bullet holes. It usually suffices to describe the number of bullet holes in the outer garment and to add that the bullet holes in the remaining items correspond in location to those already mentioned. The location of bullet holes in clothes is described in relation to the distance from collar, seams, pockets, etc. Several holes may result from a single bullet due to the presence of creases in the garment, thereby simulating more than one shot.

Observe any evidence of close-range firing. Measure the extent of soot and gunpowder distribution, and note the density of powder stippling. This will enable subsequent comparison with test shot patterns for evaluation of the distance from which the weapon was fired. Record the size of the bullet hole in the garment. Mention whether the fibers of the fabric are turned inwards or outwards; this may aid in determining the direction of the shot, particularly if evaluation by other criteria is tenuous. Photography of pertinent findings is often helpful but does not replace a good description.

The clothing should be retained for subsequent examination by the police crime laboratory and a receipt obtained when handing over the items. If soiled with blood or otherwise wet, the clothes should be dried before storage. The pathologist must observe that his part in maintaining the chain of custody is preserved at all times.

### Pertinent Findings Regarding Bullet Wounds

Number entrance and exit wounds and grazes, naming them accordingly. Lengthy descriptions tend to confuse. In the case of multiple gunshot wounds, it is advisable that a number be assigned to each wound, disregarding whether the wound was caused by entry or exit of a bullet.

The location of each wound should be described in relation to its distance from the top of the head (or the sole of the foot) and from the midline of the body, as well as from a recognized and relatively fixed landmarks, e.g. "in the abdomen, 31 in. below the top of the head, 4 in. to the right of the midline and 6 in. below the umbilicus is located an entrance bullet wound. . . ." A diagram or a photograph showing the location of the numbered wounds is helpful. Following a close search for the presence of gunsmoke, hairy areas such as the scalp should be shaved to insure adequate documentation on a photograph.

It is advisable that the wound in the skin and the wound track through the body be recorded in one section entitled *Evidence of Injury.* A description of the injuries in this sequence will facilitate future recall and enable rapid reference. Two separate paragraphs are helpful.

### *External Evidence of Injury*

Include the characteristic features of the bullet wound that distinguish it as an entrance or an exit wound. Describe the shape of the wound, such as stellate, round, slitlike or jagged. Record the width of the marginal abrasion, particularly if it is oval, as in the case of a shot that strikes the body at an angle. Measure the extent of powder residue deposits. If the distance from which a shot was fired is unknown and the presence of gunpowder within the wound suspected, excision of the wound for microscopic examination is advisable. However, a bullet wound must never be excised until its description and measurements have been recorded and the autopsy has been completed. Because the elastic fibers of the skin are severed during excision of the wound, neither dimensions nor the exact appearance of the wound can be preserved for adequate evaluation.

### *Internal Evidence of Injury*

Describe the wound track in anatomical order. The path of the bullet is best documented by following the track of hemorrhage through the organs before their removal from the body. This will usually obviate the need for x rays for finding the bullet.

Finally, a resume of the missile path through the body should be given in relation to the planes of the body, e.g. "the wound track passes from front to back, from left to right, and slightly downward. . . ." Angular estimates with respect to the horizontal, vertical and sagittal planes of the body are also useful in completing the description.

In the absence of an exit wound (more common with small-caliber bullets), it is often rewarding to palpate the body opposite the wound of entrance in an attempt to locate the bullet under the skin. If the bullet is felt in this manner, it may be removed through a small incision and the location described.

Damage to the bullet during its removal from the body must be avoided. Handling the bullet with forceps or hemostats will destroy the features required for matching the missile with a specific firearm. Particular care to avoid scratching of the bullet must be exercised in removal of a bullet from bone. Excision of the segment of bone containing the bullet, followed by manual bending and prying of the specimen, will usually release the missile without actually handling it. All bullets and as many bullet fragments as possible should be recovered for subsequent firearm identification.

Occasionally a bullet penetrates a hollow viscus and the wound track is interrupted. For example, a bullet in the stomach may be moved into the intestines while peristalsis is in progress. A bullet that penetrates the aorta may be transported with the bloodstream anywhere in the body. This is referred to as a bullet embolism. A wound track may also be interrupted by surgical procedure and as a result of healing, in cases of prolonged survival. Obviously, the use of x ray in such situations is an invaluable timesaver. An explanation in the autopsy report as to the reason for discontinuity of the wound track is advantageous.

Whenever a bullet is found, its appearance should be described accurately: intact, deformed or fragmented, lead or jacketed and the caliber if known. The bullet should be marked for subsequent identification. The initials of the prosector are used ordinarily, but the case number or the initials of the victim serve the same purpose. The base of the bullet, which is devoid of identifying characteristics, is usually chosen for marking.

Each bullet should be preserved in a separate envelope stating the name of the victim, date and number of the autopsy and location of the bullet, as well as the name of the prosector.

X rays are sometimes used for assessing the caliber of a bullet, particularly in living patients if surgical removal of the missile is not indicated. It must be remembered, however, that the dimensions of an object on the film depend on its distance from the film. Magnification and vagueness are increased the further the object is removed from the recording plane (Fig. X-66). Anteroposterior and lateral roentgenograms are therefore mandatory. Even with such x ray films the exact caliber of a bullet remains speculative. Peculiar characteristics of a bullet, such as its shape and the presence of cannelures, are identifiable features.

The use of x ray is of value in the case of skeletonized bodies. Bone fractures may be due to blunt injury or postmortem mutilation by animals. A fracture caused by a perforating bullet must also be considered. Roentgenograms of bullet tracks through bones may reveal the presence of minute fragments of metal along fracture sites. The composition of these fragments may be analyzed and compared to that of projectiles found among the remains or in the immediate vicinity of the remains.

The skeletonized remains of a young male were found in a remote area of a public park. The upper half of the skeleton was resting on a wooden board to which was caked a cluster of approximately fifteen shotgun pellets. In the neck area, resting on one of the vertebrae, a .38 caliber lead bullet was found. No fractures were noted in that region. Three ribs overlying the heart area showed fractures, and one rib had a track through it that measured the size of the lead pellets that were found behind the body. X ray of the skeleton showed minute metallic deposits along the rib fractures (Fig. X-67). Analytical comparisons of this metal with the

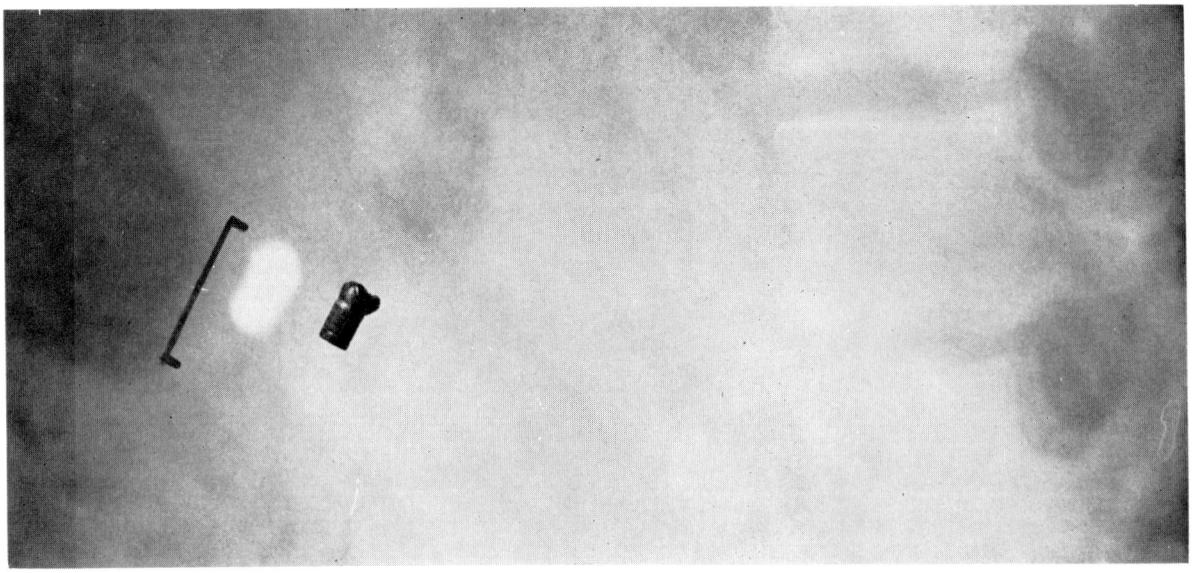

FIGURE X-66. Lateral (left-right) x ray, displaying the shadow (white) of a .22 caliber bullet in a homicide victim. The bullet was located under the skin of the left side of the chest. After the autopsy the bullet was placed on the x ray film adjacent to the shadow and photographed to show the discrepancy in size. The line on the right is a 1 in. scale.

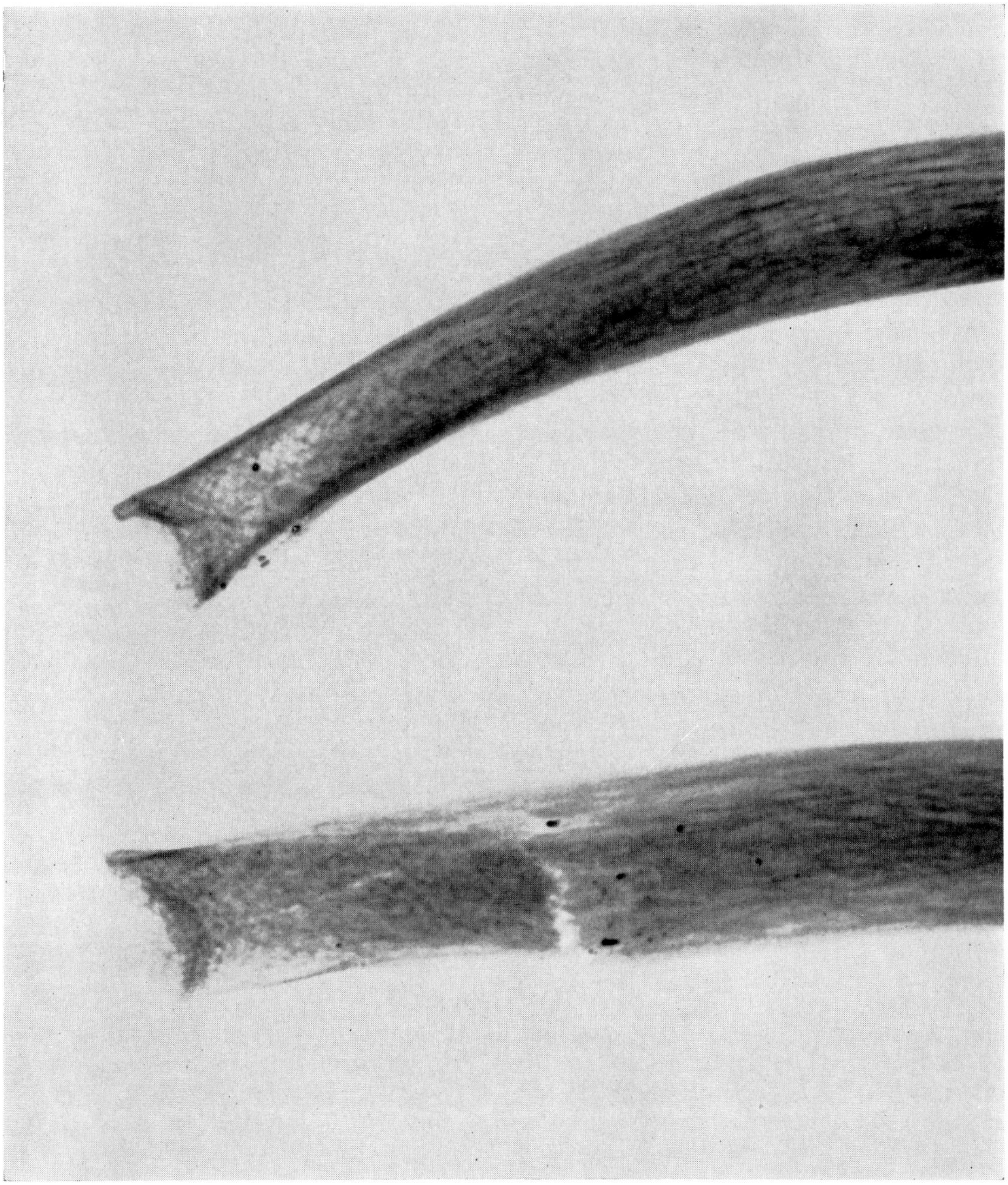

FIGURE X-67. X ray of ribs of an individual who was killed by a shotgun blast of the chest. Minute fragments of lead are deposited in the ribs along the pellets' pathways.

shotgun pellets showed an identical composition, indicating that the fractures were caused by the shotgun pellets and that death was due to a shotgun blast of the left side of the chest.

The .38 caliber bullet could not be associated with a specific injury, considering that no metallic deposits from this bullet were found in any of the bones. It could not be ascertained that this bullet had not been present in the victim following a prior shooting incident.

### Cause of Death

Hemorrhage is by far the most common cause of death in victims of gunfire. Depending on the organ or blood vessels involved, death from bleeding usually occurs within a few minutes to several hours. In gunshots of the abdomen with several days' survival, infection is the prevalent cause of death. Peritonitis develops due to leakage of contents from the perforated intestines into the abdominal cavity. Death from peritonitis may not occur until months after the injury.

Pneumonia develops frequently in cases of prolonged prostration and is especially common in gunshot wounds of the head with extended unconsciousness. Pulmonary embolism is a less frequently encountered complication of injury by gunfire and usually results from migratory clots originating in the calves as a result of prostration or if the extremity is immobilized due to fracture. Other complications of gunshot wounds occur, but because of their relative rarity they will not be listed.

### Toxicological and Serological Analyses

Analysis should include determination of the blood alcohol concentration of the victim and his blood group. The latter may furnish additional circumstantial information relating bloodstains found at a crime scene to the victim. The finding of a different blood group in stains would positively eliminate the victim as a source of this blood. In the case of several hours' survival, a urine determination is often of value (see Chapter XXII).

## REFERENCES


1. Federal Bureau of Investigation (C. M. Kelley, Director): *Uniform Crime Reports of the United States,* 1976. Washington, D.C., U.S. Govt. Print. Office, 1977.
2. Eastman Kodak Company: *Applied Infrared Photography.* Kodak Technical Publication M-28. Rochester, New York, Kodak, 1968.
3. Gilmore, H. R.: Medical aspects of the assassination of Abraham Lincoln. *Proc R Soc Med, 47:*103, 1954.
4. Adelson, L.: A microscopic study of dermal gunshot wounds. *Am J Clin Pathol, 35:*393, 1961.
5. Sellier, K.: *Schusswaffen und Schusswirkungen.* Lübeck, Schmidt-Römhild, 1969, p. 44.
6. Graham, J. W., Petty, C. S., Flohr, D. M., and Peterson, W. E.: Forensic aspects of frangible bullets. *J Forensic Sci, 11:*507, 1966.
7. Federal Bureau of Investigation Laboratory: Gunpowder and shot pattern tests. *FBI Law Enforcement Bulletin,* September, 1970.
8. Spitz, W. U.: Rikoschett- oder Kontaktschussverletzung. *Dtsch Z Ges Gerichtl Med, 66:*153, 1969.
9. Spitz, W. U., Petty, C. S., and Fisher, R. S.: Physical activity until collapse following fatal injury by firearms and sharp weapons. *J Forensic Sci, 6:*290, 1961.
10. DiMaio, V. J. M., and Spitz, W. U.: Variations in wounding due to unusual firearms and recently available ammunition. *J Forensic Sci, 17:*377, 1972.
11. DiMaio, V. J. M., and Spitz, W. U.: Injury by birdshot. *J Forensic Sci, 15:*396, 1970.
12. Breitenecker, R., and Senior, W.: Shotgun patterns. I. An experimental study on the influence of intermediate targets. *J Forensic Sci, 12:*193, 1967.
13. Spitz, W. U., and Wilhelm, R. M.: Stud gun injuries. *J Forensic Med, 17:*5, 1970.
14. Smialek, J. E., and Spitz, W. U.: Short range ammunition: A possible anti-hijacking device. *J Forensic Sci, 21:*856, 1976.

*Part 2*

## SHOTGUN WOUNDS

RUSSELL S. FISHER

SHOTGUNS OR SCATTER GUNS were developed as an alternate to the single-missile rifle or handgun in order to enable the gunner to spray a wide area with shot and thus kill birds and other small animals too difficult to hit with single-missile weapons. The use of shotguns on humans has unfortunately become common, and indeed, special improvisations, such as the *sawed-off* shotgun, testify to their effectiveness. The inherent differences in these weapons and their ammunition are reflected in differences in the typical wounds resulting from shotgun fire as compared to bullet injury, but in general the targets and the pattern of the shot allow reconstruction of range of fire and direction of fire in a fashion similar to the single-missile weapons. The prime difference is in the multiplicity of the missiles which vary from 1, as in the rifled slug or *punkin ball,* through 9 to 12 in 00 buckshot, to as many as 270 in the 12 gauge No. 9 birdshot. The respective diameters of 00 buckshot and No. 9 birdshot are .33 and .08 in.

The gauge of a shotgun indicates the inside diameter of its bore. It is an antiquated measure defined as the number of round lead balls, each of the same diameter as the bore, required to weigh one pound. Thus, for the 12 gauge, a lead ball of the same diameter as the inside of the barrel (bore) would weigh 1/12 lb. or 1⅓ oz. This measure is still used in all except the .410 gauge, where the diameter of the barrel is .410 in. The 12 gauge is by far the most commonly used shotgun and, with a variable choke, is a most versatile weapon.

The smooth bore of the shotgun may be uniform in diameter, in which case it is referred to as *cylinder bore,* or it may be narrowed at the muzzle end to a lesser or greater degree, as in the *medium* and *full choke* guns. The degree of choke obviously modifies the spread of exiting shot from the muzzle and governs the size of the shot pattern at a given distance from the muzzle.[1] The choke of a gun barrel is usually expressed in shot percentages that fall within a 30 in. circle at 40 yd.:

| | |
|---|---|
| 65%-75% | full choke |
| 55%-65% | modified |
| 45%-55% | improved cylinder |
| 35%-45% | cylinder bore |

### Contact Shotgun Wounds

The characteristics already described for small arms fire, particularly those of close-range shots, are also observed in shotgun wounding. Thus, at loose contact or close range there is considerable scorching and soot and powder residue soiling on the target surrounding the entrance wound itself. Marginal abrasion similar to that caused by single-bullet entrance is observed as the shot enter the body in a conglomerate mass. There may also be annular abrasions surrounding the defect but separated from it by up to 1 in.; this is caused by the *blow back,* which stretches the skin around the wound (Figs. X-68, X-69 and X-70).

Occasionally there will be stellate lacerations due to the extreme force of the *blow back* phenomenon as gases expand beneath the skin and lacerate the margins of the wound as they exit through the original entry wound. Contact shotgun wounds of the head, where the gases have restricted space for expansion, are commonly associated with extreme mutilation due to the explosive effect that is thus created. Destruction of the entire contour of the face and head occurs, and the actual point of muzzle impact or entry wound may be difficult to locate, especially when the muzzle is put into the mouth. In this case bone and soft tissues may be scattered over a wide area, and the entire brain may be eviscerated and shredded.

Superficial and deep tears at the inner angles

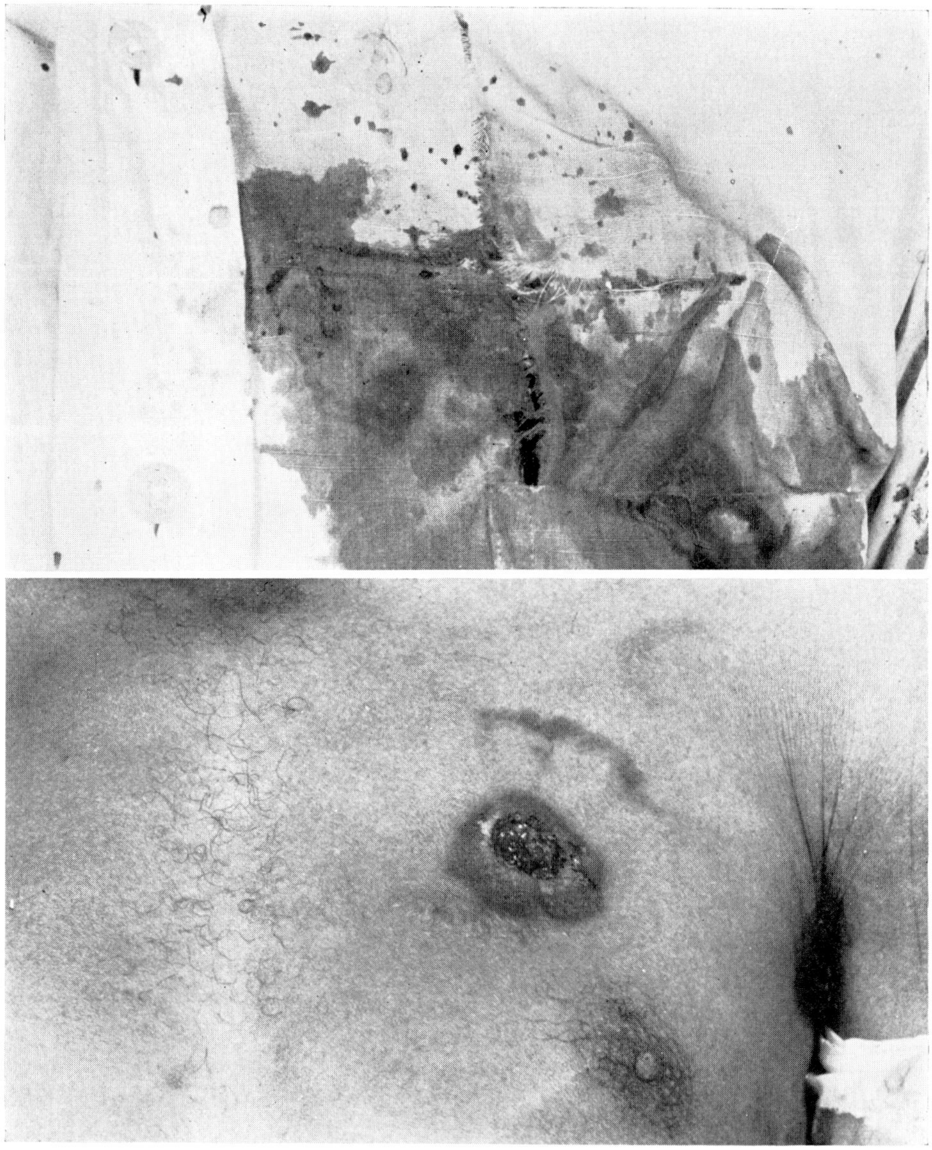

FIGURE X-68. Suicidal wounding at contact range with 12 gauge shotgun. Note that no fabric of the shirt is missing, even though it is torn. This is explained by the fact that the victim inserted the muzzle under the shirt, between the buttons. The blast was therefore outwards as *blow back* occurred. The gun was fired with the toe as the victim sat on a chair and held the muzzle in his hands. The abrasion of the edges of the wound and the abraded area above the wound are due to stretching of the skin by the *blow back* and the gases expanding beneath the skin.

of the eyes, the sides of the nose and mouth and in front of the ears may occur as a result of overstretching of the skin by the large amount of gases *injected* into the head, especially in shots into the mouth and contact shots below the chin (Fig. X-71).

### Close-range Shotgun Wounds

With close-range shots varying up to as much as 4 to 5 ft., the shotgun charge enters the body as a single conglomerate mass, producing a round defect somewhat larger in diameter than the bore of the barrel. The margins of such wounds, in addition to showing abrasion, are apt to display some scalloping, which in gunners' terminology is frequently described as the *cookie cutter* etching (*see* Figs. X-80a, X-81a and X-86).

Beyond this range the diameter of the wound increases as the shot begin to fan out and stray shot make tiny entrance wounds separated from the main defect. The minimal distance for the latter phenomenon to occur is extremely variable. It may be 3 or 4 ft. with some *sawed-off* shotguns but tends to be 6 ft. or more with cylinder bore guns and as great as 18 ft. with full choke guns (Figs. X-72 and X-73). At distances up to 4 or 5 ft. there may be considerable powder and some soot and smoke soiling of the clothing or skin. Another phenomenon sometimes seen in contact or close-range wounding by shotgun is the presence of annular or linear abrasions in the immediate vicinity of the wound. These abrasions are caused by the impact of clothing against the stretched skin during the penetration of the shot en masse. Such abrasions are therefore frequently observed in wounds caused by rifled slug, when the bulk of lead pushes the clothing forward into the wound. Obviously, rough clothing tends to have a more abrading effect (Figs. X-74 and X-75).

### Distant Shotgun Wounds

The pattern made by a shotgun from a distance of over a few feet varies with the choke, the length of the barrel, the load of the powder, the size of shot and the gauge of the gun and is further modified by varying designs of inner liner within the shotgun shell (Fig. X-76). For example, the Remington power piston and post wad, the Winchester AA trap and skeet shot shell and the Winchester winwad are all variants of devices built into the shell itself that will modify the pattern (Fig. X-77). In general these are designed to improve the pattern by cutting down on stray shot or by compressing the pattern into a tighter circle, but some have the opposite effect.

With small shot the individual pellets entering the skin produce round defects with narrow marginal abrasion; in the case of buckshot the individual wounds closely resemble bullet wounds (Fig. X-78). The rifled slug represents the largest bullet fired by any low velocity weapon available outside of military channels. In addition to the holes in the skin made by entering shot, the target frequently shows larger contused and abraded areas, circular or elliptical in shape, which are due to impact of the shotgun wadding. This will carry as much as 30 to 35 ft. and cause a typical injury as illustrated in Figures X-72 and X-78. The wadding may, of course, follow the main bulk of shot into the interior of the body, but, due to dispersion of the pellets at ranges of fire in excess of 10 to 12 ft., the wadding does not usually penetrate the body. It is of importance that the wadding be recovered whenever possible, since it may give useful clues to the gauge of the gun or the manufacturer of the ammunition used. Plastic wads retain their shape and diameter within the body, but felt and cardboard wads soak up blood and fluids and swell, causing the diameter to be altered.

### Patterns of Shotgun Wounding

In suicide cases the shotgun wound is obviously nearly always contact or very close range, since the length of the barrel and of the individual's arm do not allow true distant self-infliction. However, one occasionally finds shotgun wounds that are self-inflicted with the use of a stick to push or a string to pull the trigger. Another common pattern is for the sui-

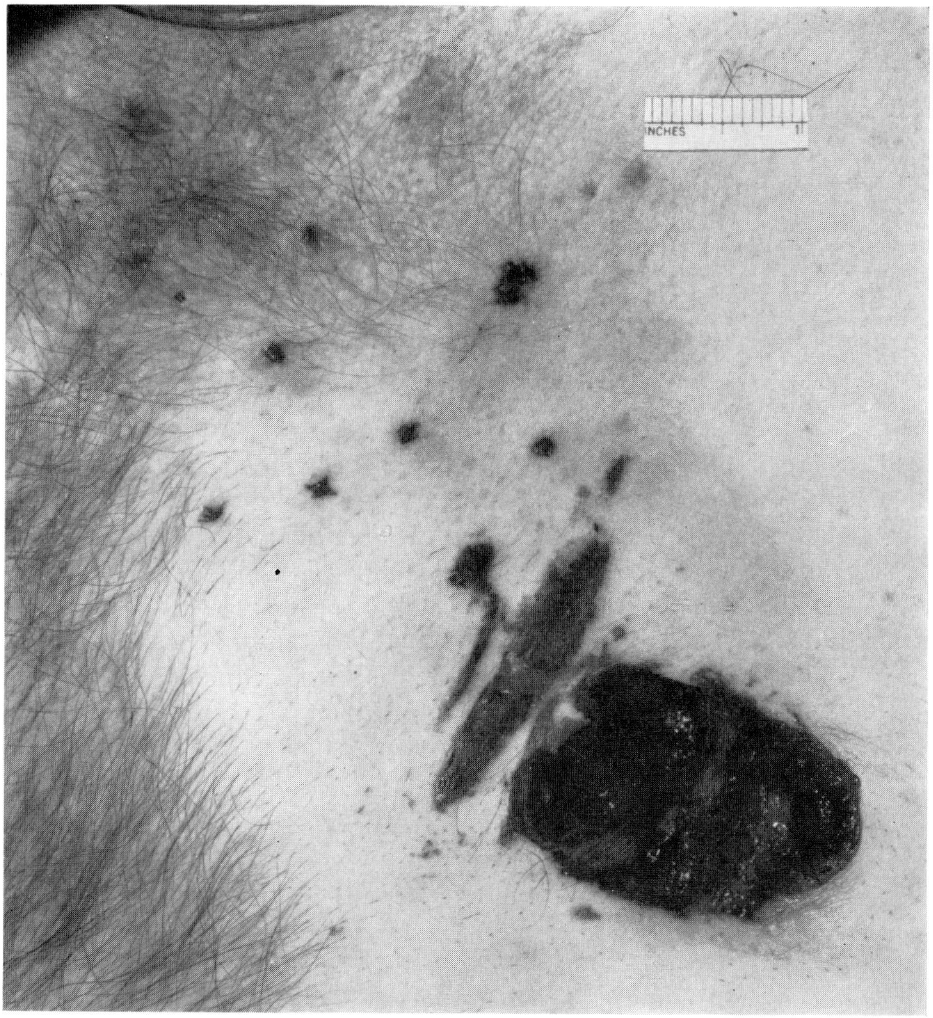


FIGURE X-69a. Elliptical contact shotgun wound of the left chest. The elliptical shape is due to an acute angle from below, upwards and to the right. The linear abrasions are due to stretching and impact of the skin over the muzzle and a ball-point pen in the pocket as *blow back* of gases occurred. The discrete perforations are due to exiting shot ricocheting from the main pattern.

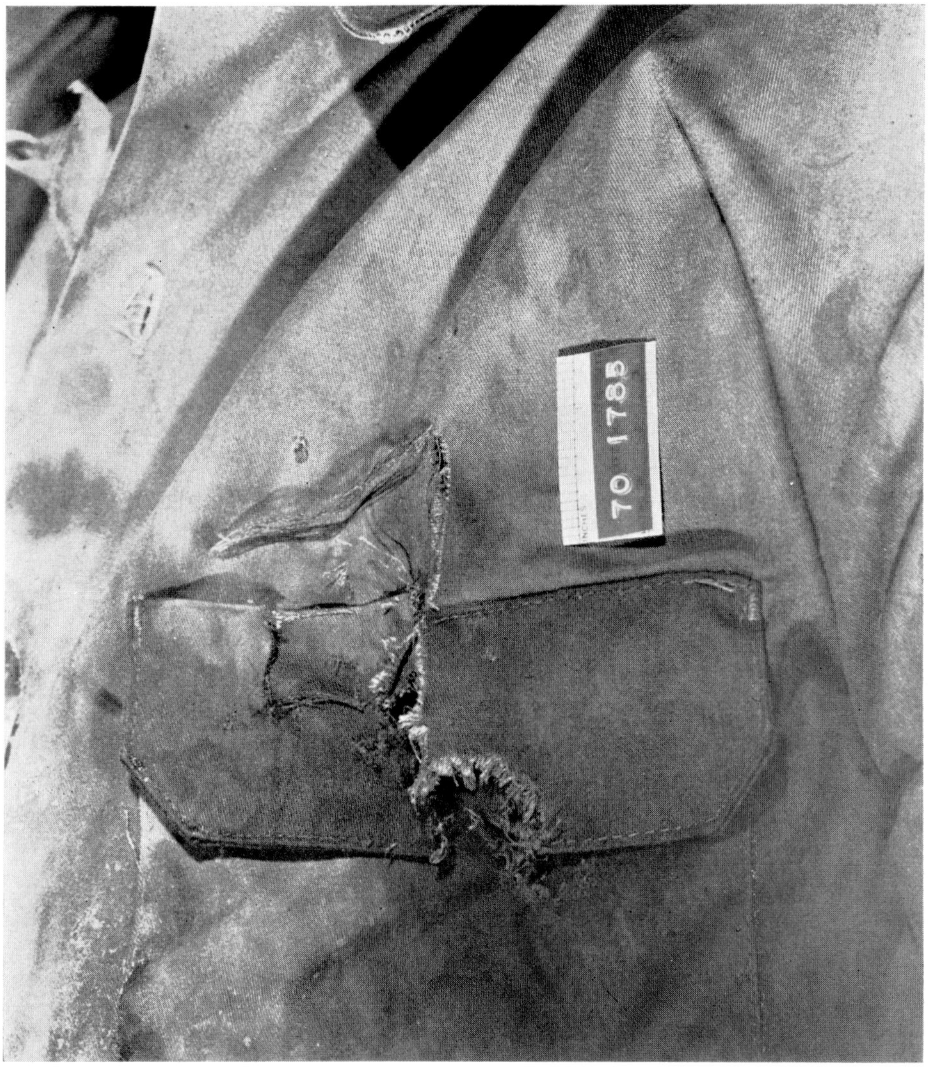


FIGURE X-69b. Clothing from the victim shown in Figure X-69a. Note the elliptical entry hole at the bottom edge of the pocket flap and the tearing above due to *blow back.* These tears are in the same areas as the linear abrasions above the wound in Figure X-69a.

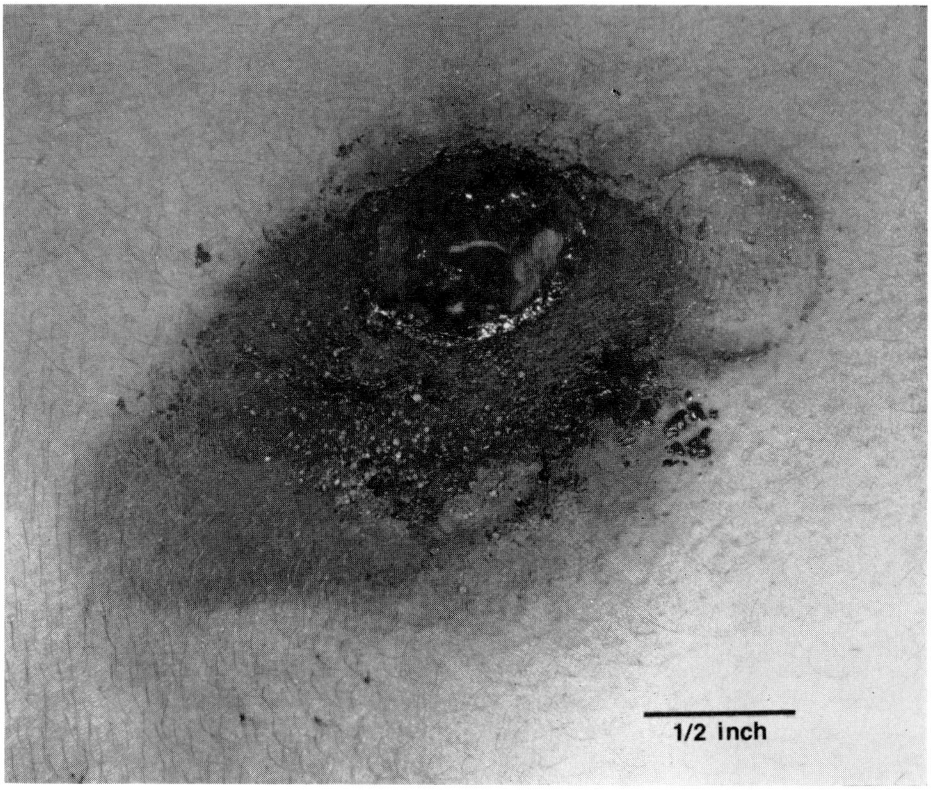


FIGURE X-70. Self-inflicted shotgun wound of the chest. The muzzle imprint of a double barrel 20 gauge shotgun fired at contact with the body is evident. Only the left barrel was discharged. Note the impression of the right barrel due to *blow back* as the gases expanded under the skin.

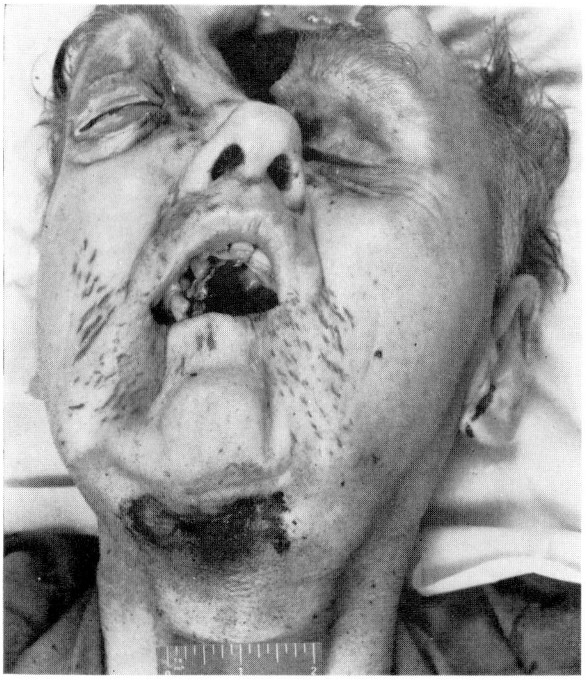

FIGURE X-71. Suicidal shotgun blast of the head, using a 12 gauge shotgun loaded with No. 6 shot. The contact entrance wound is below the chin. The facial skeleton is fragmented, and tears caused by overstretching are noted on both sides of the mouth and the inner angles of the eyes. The shot partly exited from the top of the head.

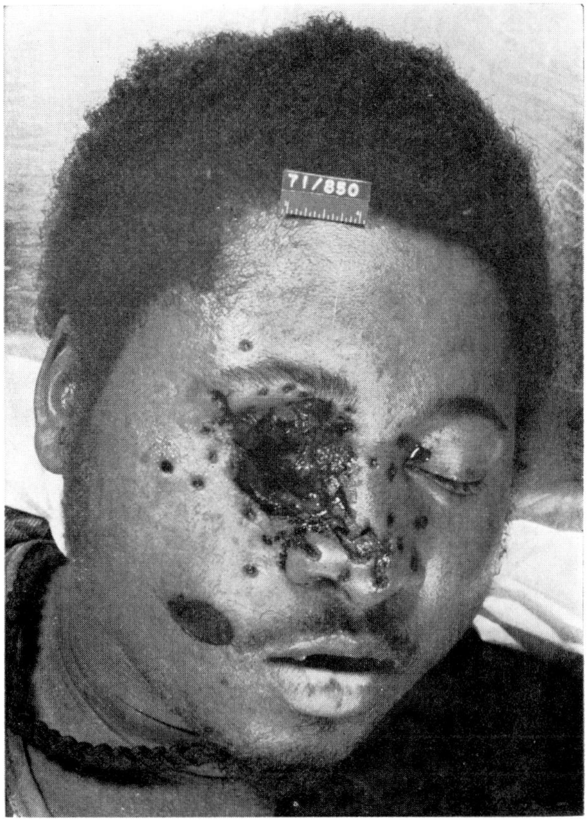


FIGURE X-72. Shotgun wound showing beginning spread as a few shot veer off from the main charge. The weapon was a 12 gauge shotgun, cylinder bore, loaded with No. 6 shot and fired from a distance of 10 ft. The oval abrasion at the right side of the mouth was caused by wad impact.

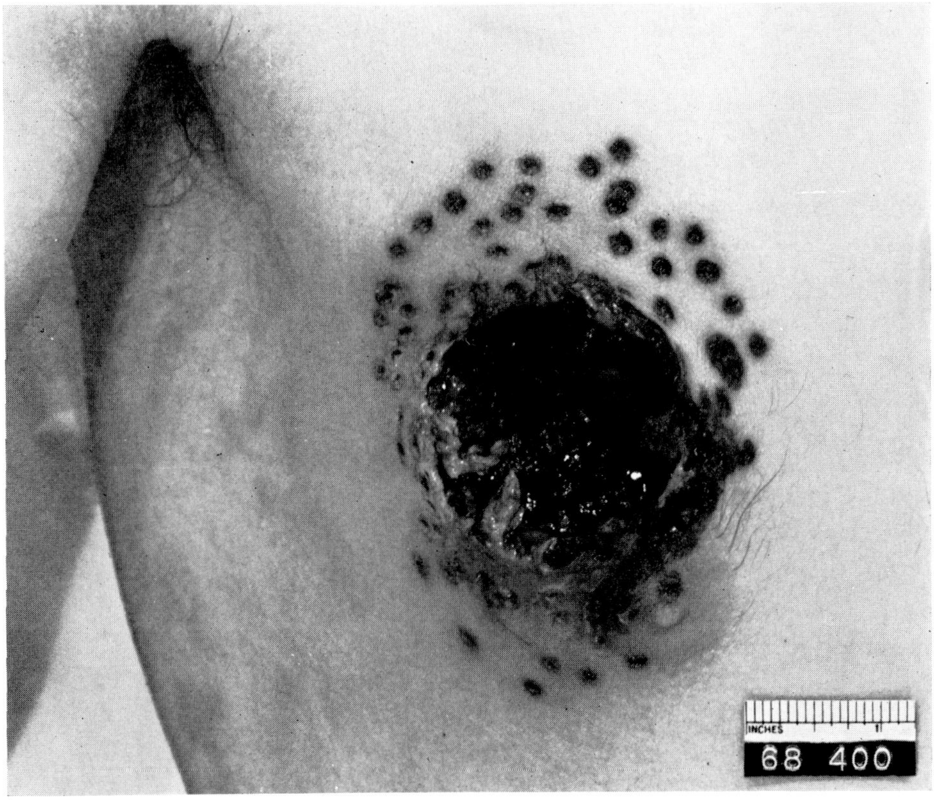


FIGURE X-73. Homicidal assault with a 12 gauge pump action shotgun and No. 5 shot from a distance of 10 to 12 ft.

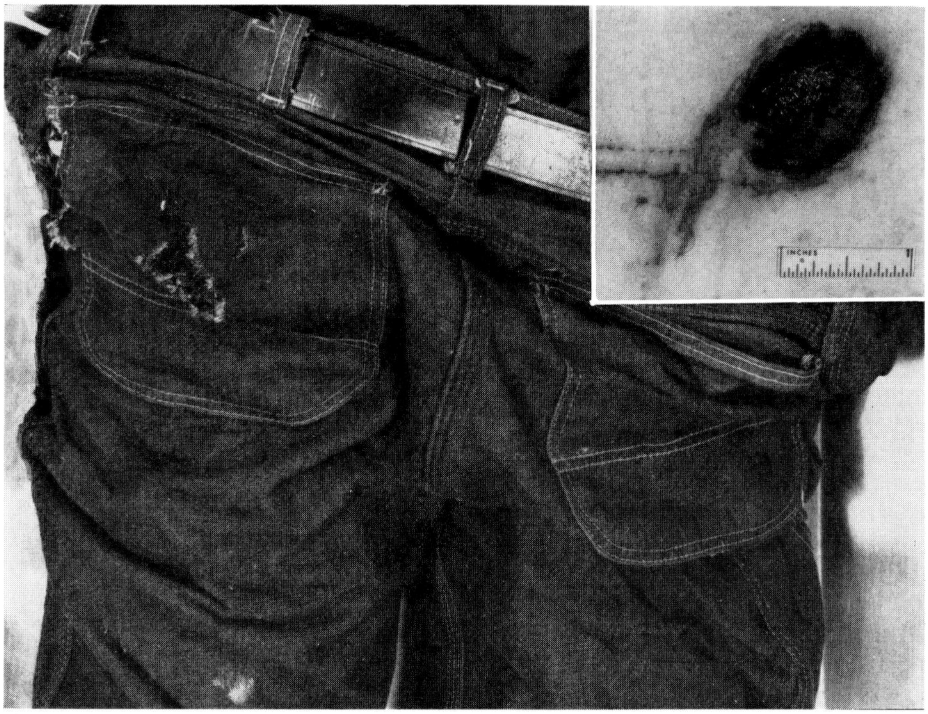


FIGURE X-74a. Rifled slug injury from a distance of 40 ft., caused by a *sawed off* shotgun with an 18 in. long barrel. Note the pocket seam of the denim pants imprinted on the skin (insert). Compare with Figure X-75, which shows a similar phenomenon.

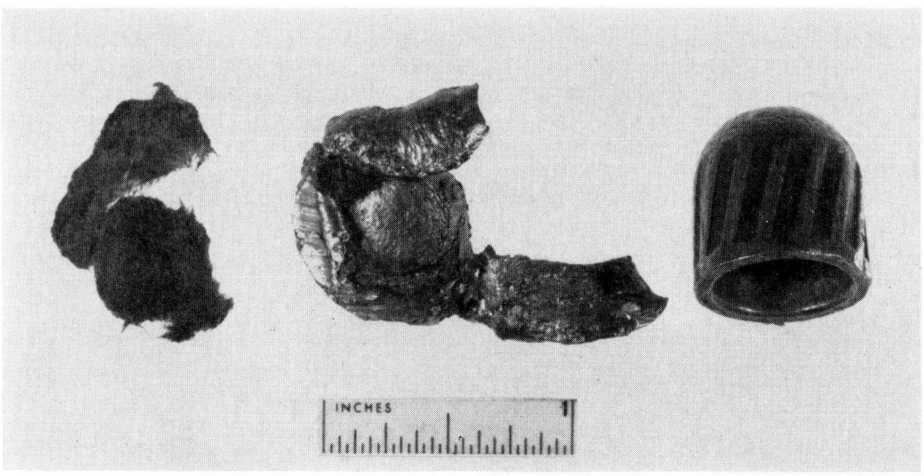


FIGURE X-74b. Same case as shown in Figure X-74a. Deformed slug (center) and wadding (left) removed from the body. An intact rifled slug is shown on the right for comparison.

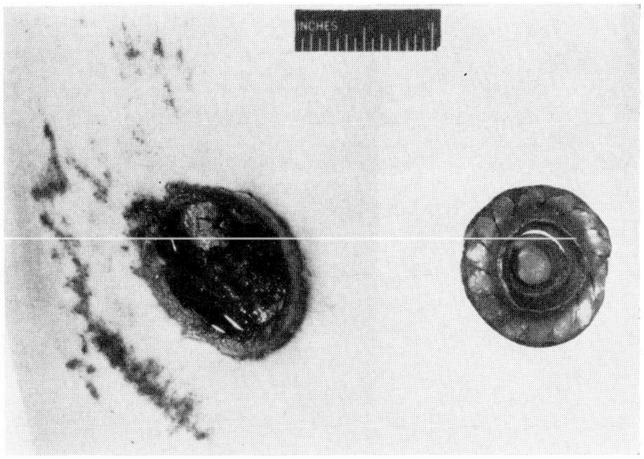


FIGURE X-75. Rifled slug injury by a 12 gauge shotgun, inflicted from a distance of 100 ft. Evident is the characteristic marginal abrasion, but there is also an unusual annular abrasion and contusion of the skin, due to impact of the leather jacket, which was stretched by the entering slug. These injuries are readily misinterpreted as evidence of contact injury. Compare with Figures X-69a and X-74a. The deformed rifled slug was recovered within the body and is shown on the right.

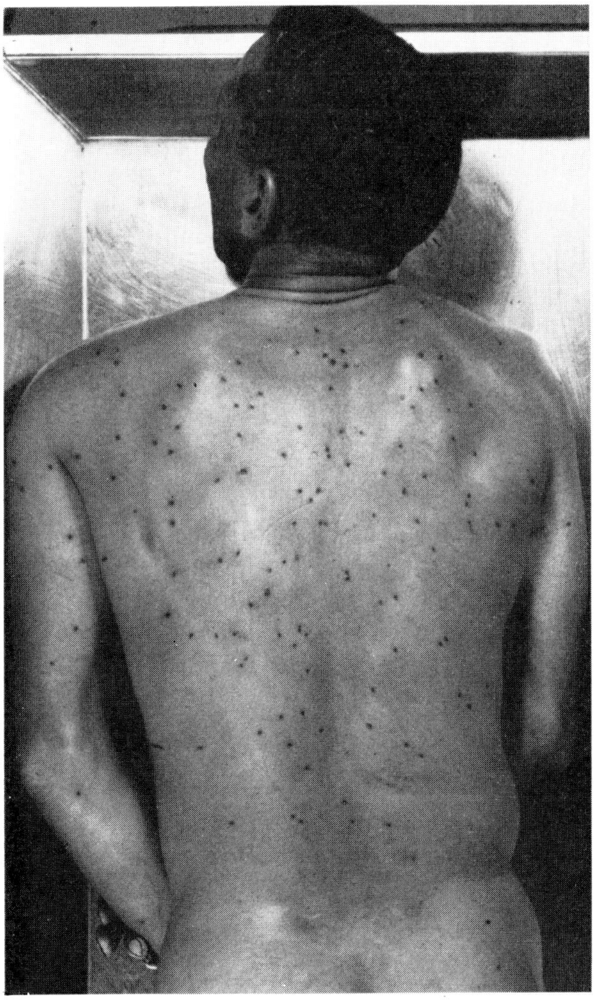

FIGURE X-76. Injury produced by a .410 gauge shotgun and No. 7½ shot from a distance of over 20 ft. The pattern measured 19 × 17 in. and had 114 birdshot.

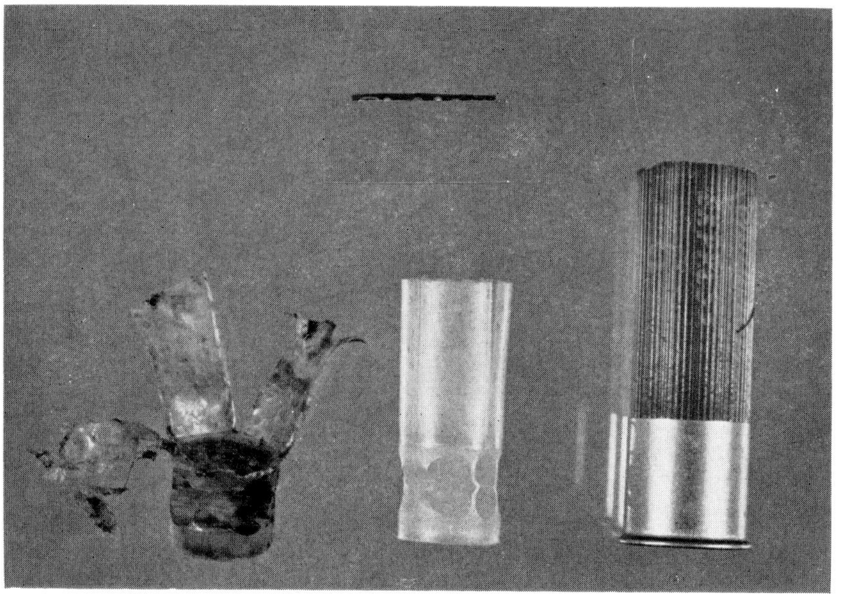

FIGURE X-77. Remington Express, 16 gauge shotgun shell. The plastic post wad (left) was removed from the cranial cavity after a self-inflicted close-range shot. The central structure is an undamaged post wad from another shell. This inner lining of the shotgun shell produces a uniform dispersion of the shot, so that a 16 yd. target is the same diameter as a 25 yd. target made with standard loading.

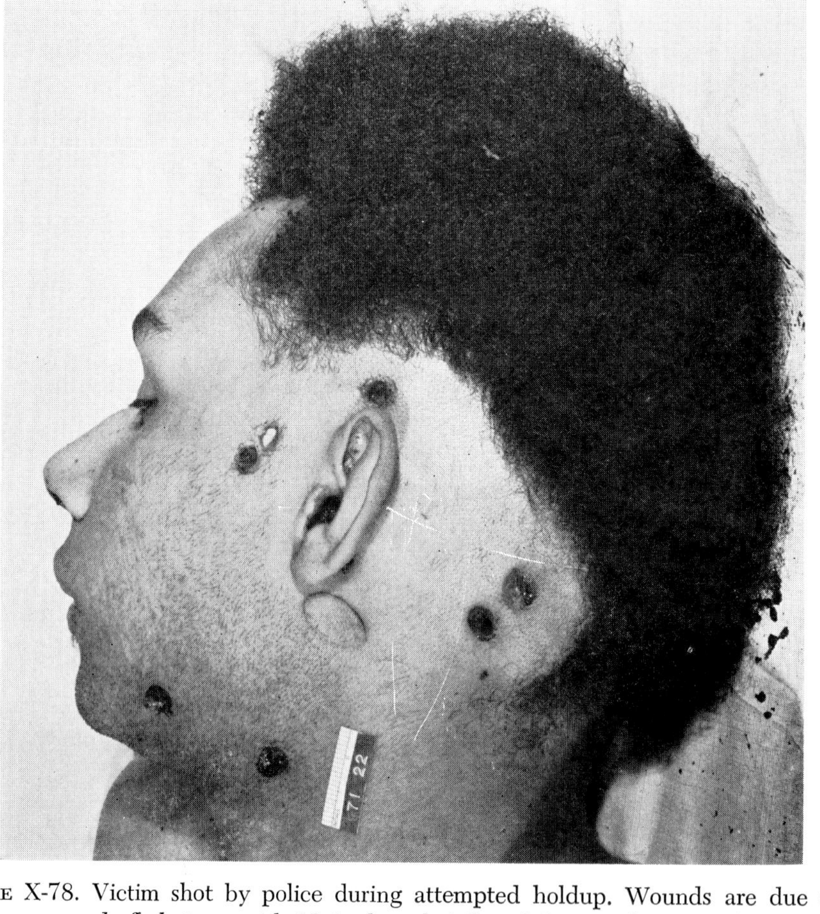


FIGURE X-78. Victim shot by police during attempted holdup. Wounds are due to a 12 gauge *sawed-off* shotgun with 19 in. barrel, inflicted from a distance of 9 ft. using 00 buckshot. The injury below the ears was caused by the plastic inner liner from the shell.

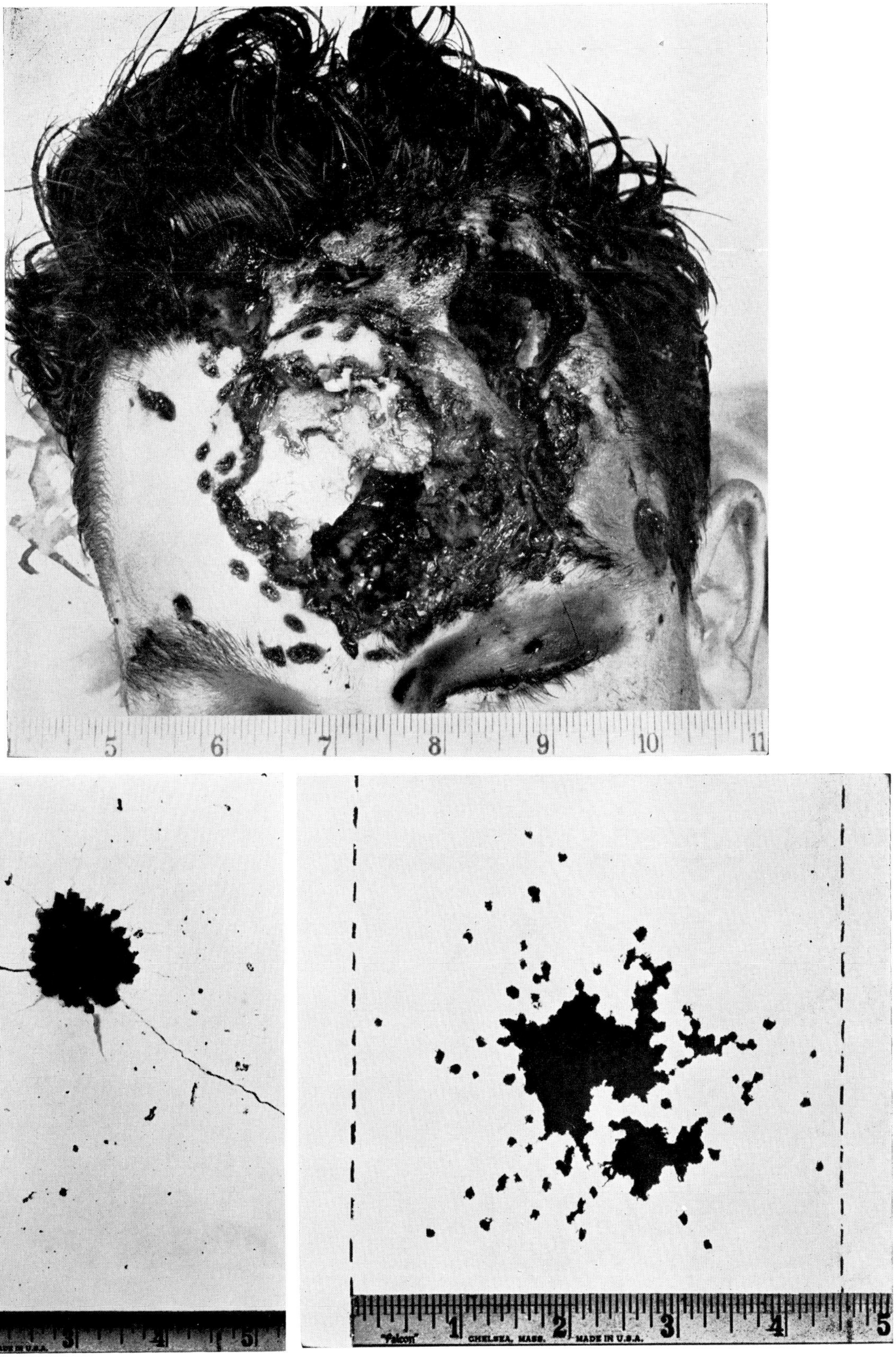


FIGURE X-79. (a): Shotgun wound of the head, at first alleged to be suicide. Diameter of the wound is approximately 4½ in. (b) Pattern at 3 ft. is 1⅜ in. in diameter, obviously ruling out self-infliction. (c): Pattern at 10 ft. is similar to that of the deceased, who was in fact shot from a doorway of a bedroom in which he was asleep in bed in the opposite corner.

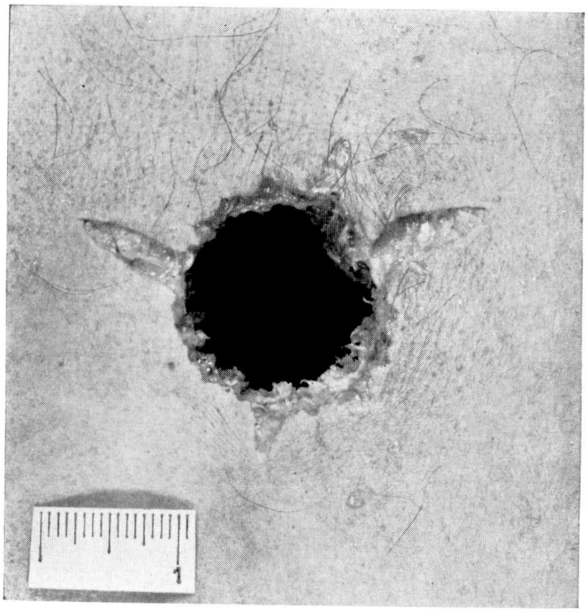

FIGURE X-80. Experimentally produced billiard ball ricochet effect, using a 12 gauge shotgun loaded with No. 6 shot. Note the different skin wounds (a and c) but nearly identical x-ray patterns of disseminated shot in the body (b and d). (a—top left): Wound inflicted from a distance of 4 ft. It shows the scalloped *cookie* but nearly identical x ray patterns of disseminated shot entrance wounds (compare with Figures X-81a and X-86). The stellate shape of the wound is not usually seen in shotgun injuries inflicted from this distance. It is attributed to congealing of the subcutaneous fat tissue in the cadaver used for this experiment. (b—bottom right): X ray of the shot pattern associated with the wound in Figure X-80a.

(a)

(b)

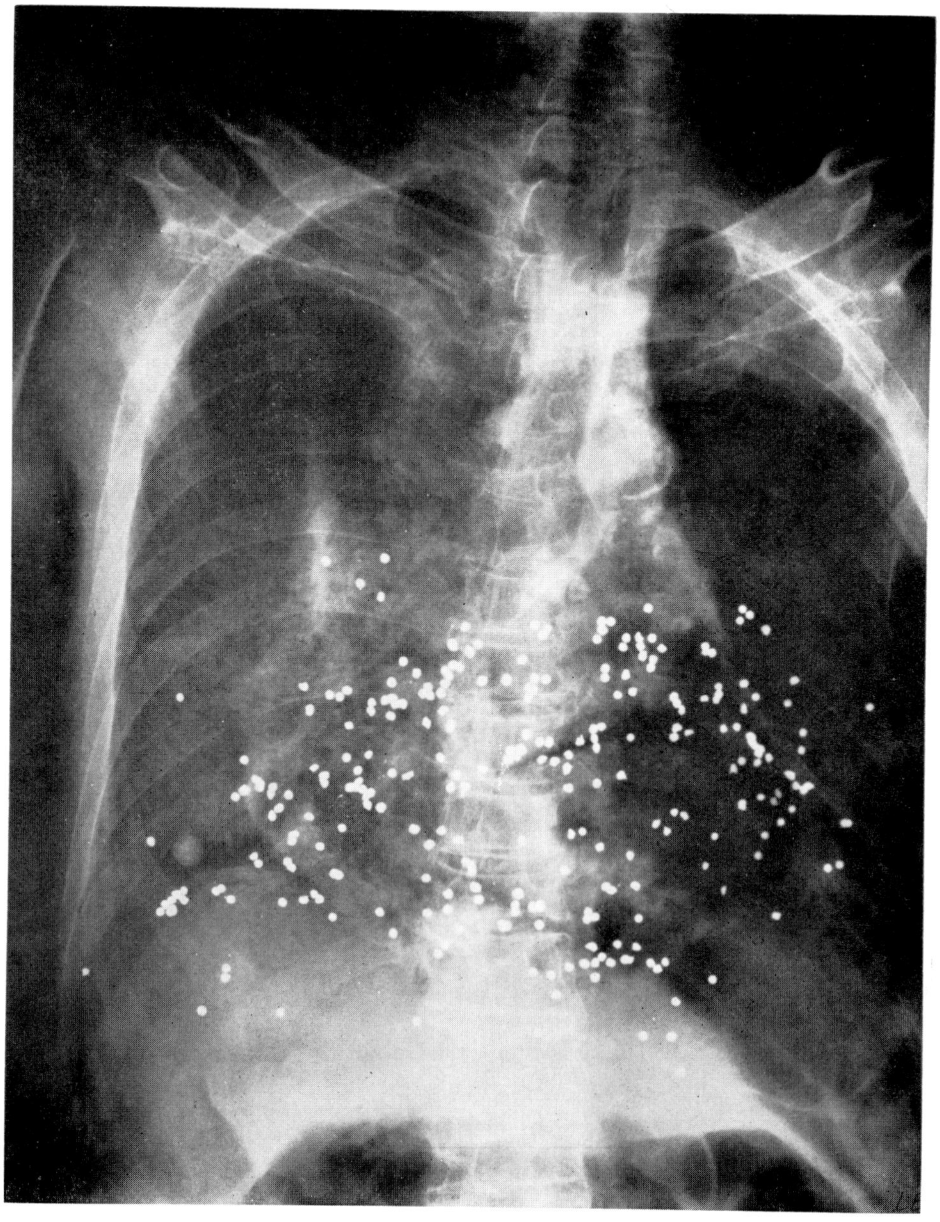

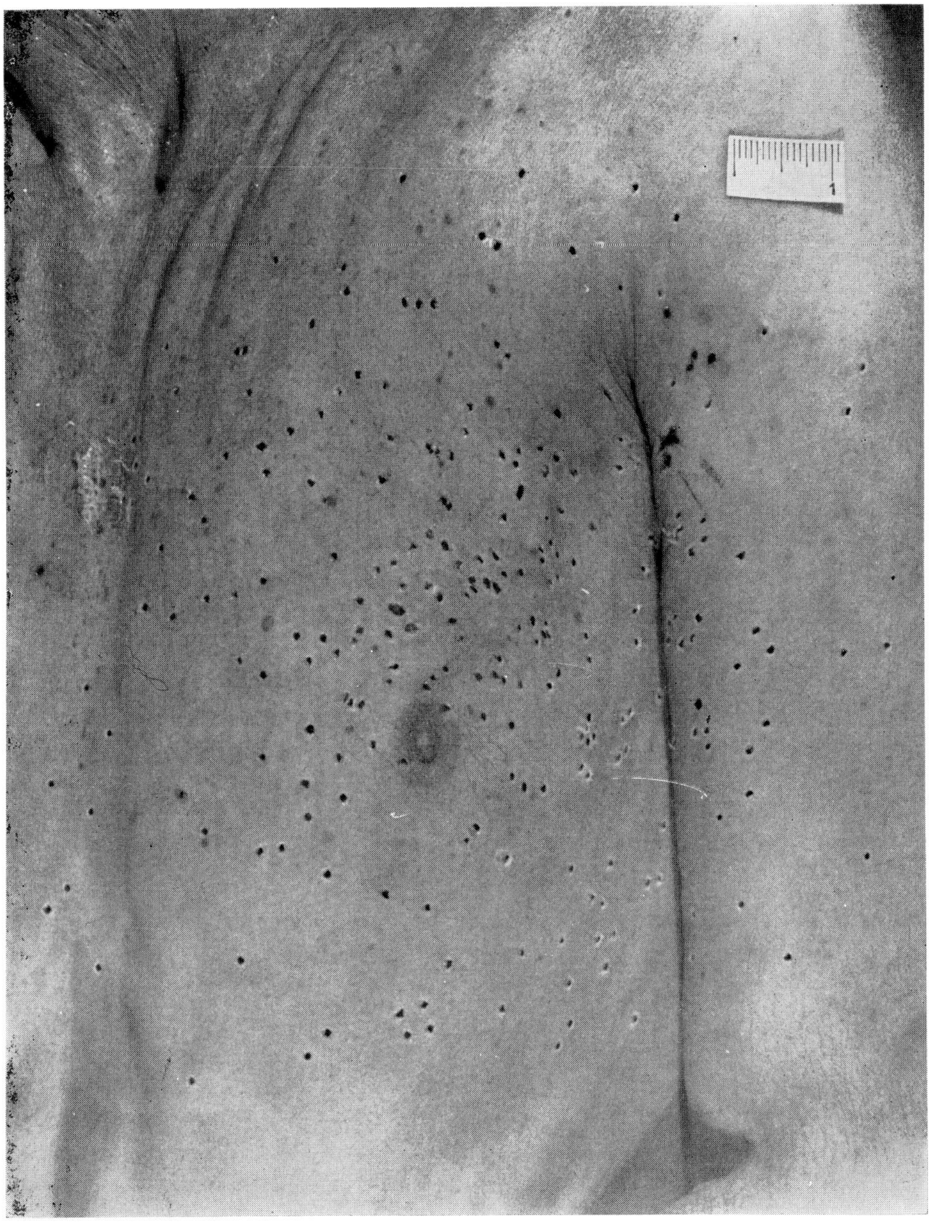

FIGURE X-80c. Wound inflicted from a distance of 16 ft.

cidally bent individual to push the trigger with his toe. Not infrequently, a deceased person will be found with the barrel of the shotgun in his hand or lap, with one shoe and stocking removed and a shotgun wound of the abdomen or chest. Such action as removing a shoe obviously is important in evaluating the case and ruling out an accidental manner of shooting. Suicidal individuals will frequently place the shotgun muzzle in the mouth, with consequent tremendous destruction of the head.

Accidental shotgun wounding shows many variants principally related to carelessness in handling the gun. It is, of course, possible to establish the range of fire with considerable assurance, provided one has the shotgun in question and the ammunition that was used to inflict the wound under investigation.

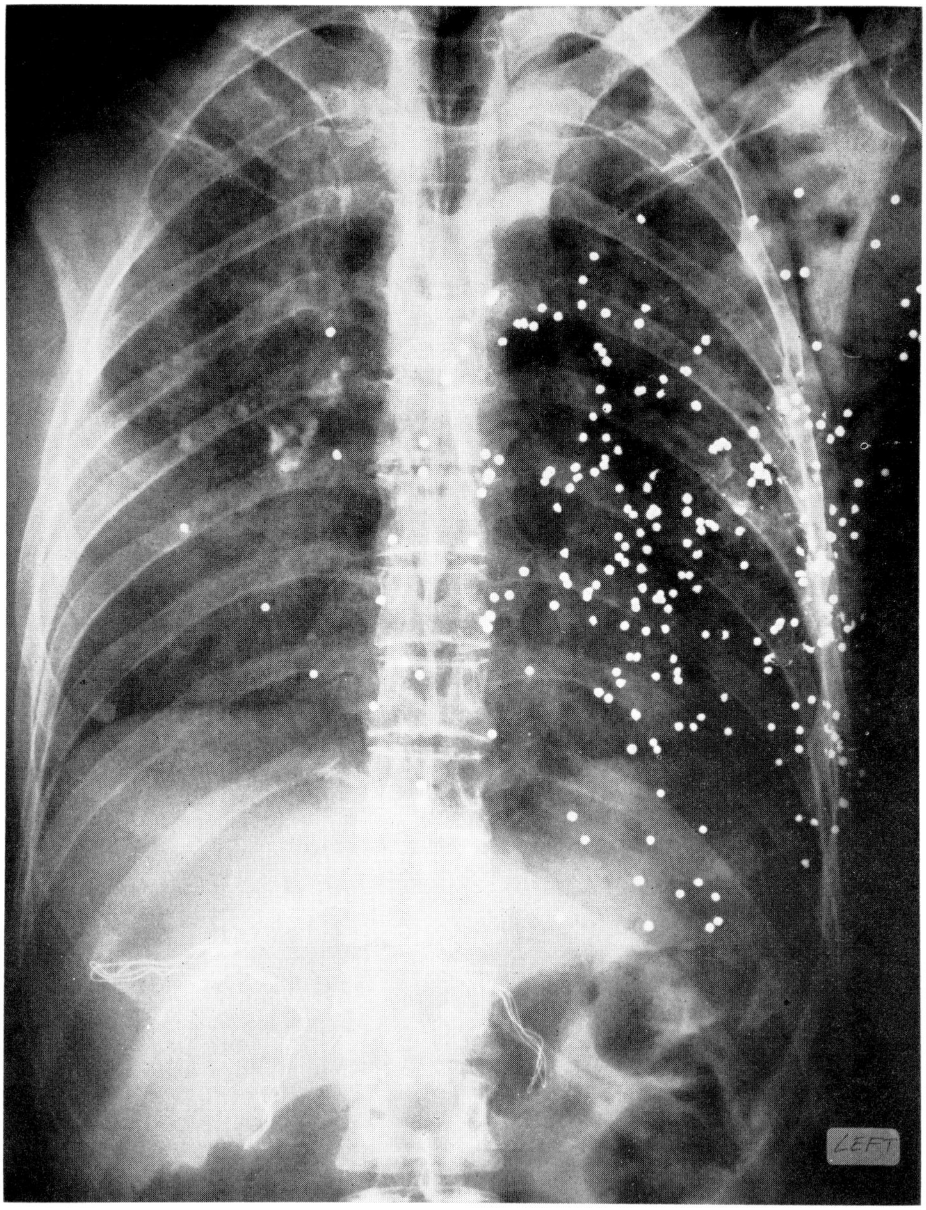


FIGURE X-80d. X ray of the shot pattern associated with the wound in Figure X-80c.

A twenty-four-year-old man had reportedly committed suicide by shooting himself in the head. Investigation revealed that there had been an altercation between the deceased and his landlord. Examination of the wound indicated that it had been inflicted from a distance of several feet, thus excluding the likelihood of suicide. The weapon, an old single-shot 12 gauge shotgun, was test fired using the same ammuniton as in the case under consideration (No. 6 shot). The test shot from a distance of 10 ft. closely resembled the pattern of the wound in the victim, indicating that the deceased was shot from approximately that distance. The landlord was charged with murder and confessed to the crime (Fig. X-79).

Whenever there is allegation of accidental shooting in an attempt to mask a homicide, test firing at different ranges to produce a target pattern similar in size and density of shot to the victim's injury should be done. This enables the investigator to evaluate the circumstances and thereby test the alibi of the individual who claims the shooting was accidental.

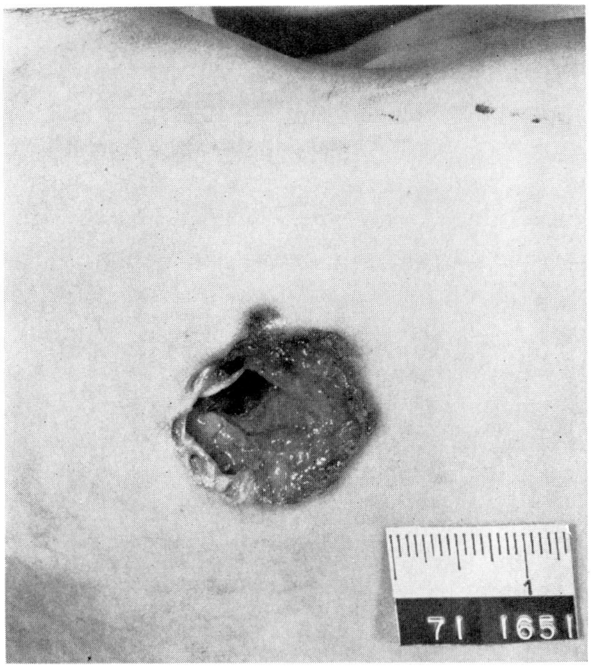


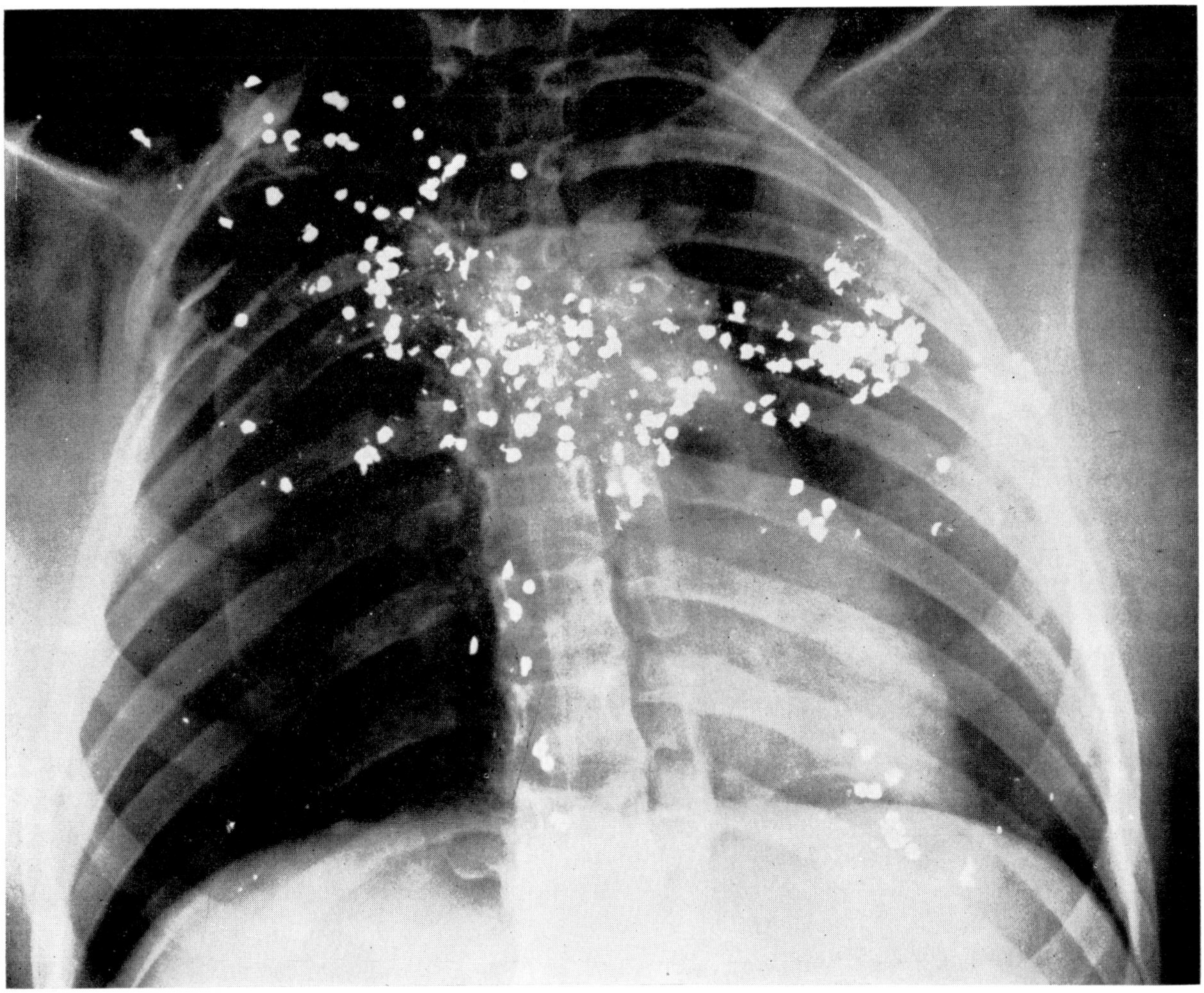

FIGURE X-81. (a): Homicidal shotgun wound of the right shoulder, inflicted from a distance of 4 to 5 ft. with a 12 gauge shotgun and No. 6 shot. The shot struck the body *en masse*, producing a single wound with typical scalloping of the wound margins (*cookie cutter* edges). The x ray (b) shows a wide spread of the shot *(billiard ball ricochet effect)*.

In determining the range of fire in decomposed and burned bodies where the skin pattern cannot be seen, x rays may be of considerable assistance. X rays of bodies revealing shot patterns, however, must be interpreted in the light of the fact that the charge consists of many small shot. At close range, while the shot are bunched, they strike one another upon impact with the primary target, such as the skin or clothing of the victim, and spray out in a wide pattern as they continue on into the body.[2, 3] This produces a wide dispersion of the shot and may lead to the conclusion of a greater range of fire than actually occurred. The same holds true if the shot strike any other intermediary object, such as a door or a window, before reaching the victim. The phenomenon may be compared with billiard balls hit at the break by the cue ball and is appropriately termed the *billiard ball ricochet effect.* Only when the range of fire is great enough that the shot are spread out before striking the target (and thus collisions of the shot do not occur) will the final shot dispersion, as shown by x ray, yield a true picture of the range of fire (Figs. X-80 to X-85).

The billiard ball effect may not occur with old shotgun cartridges. Corroded pellets often adhere to each other and will not separate upon striking an intermediary target. This may change the pattern of injury and lead to considerable error in estimating the range of fire.

### Shotgun Exit Wounds

Shotgun exit wounds are uncommon even in contact or close-range shots, except if the victim is very lean or if the shot strikes the body at an acute angle and no major bony structures are situated in the pathway of the pellets. Large shot sizes tend to pass through the body somewhat more frequently due to their greater mass and energy as compared to bird shot (Figs. X-86 and X-87). More common is the accumulation of large numbers of shot immediately beneath the skin opposite the entry wound (Fig. X-88).

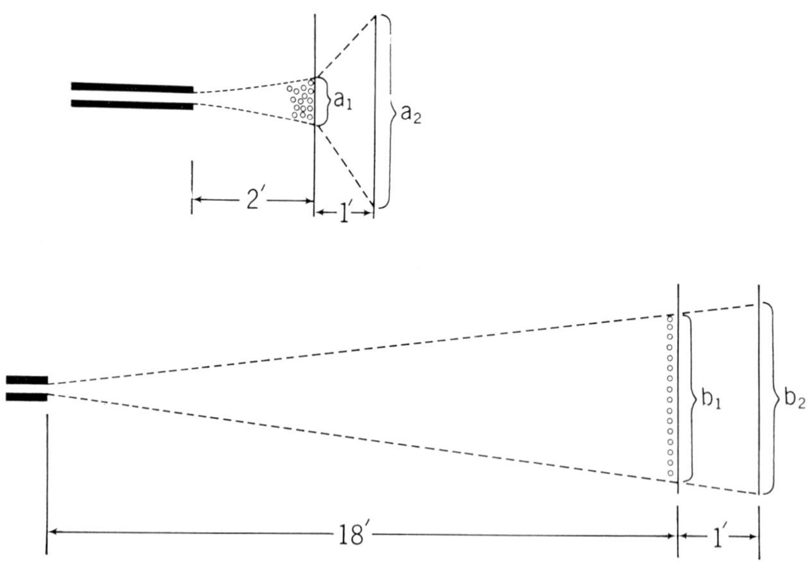


FIGURE X-82. Schematic representation of the *billiard ball ricochet effect.* The heavy black parallel lines on the left represent the shotgun barrel. At close range the shot are bunched, and as they strike the primary target ($a_1$), the leading shot are slowed and are hit by the after-coming shot, causing them to veer off in a wide pattern as billiard balls do when hit at the break by the cue ball. At greater distances, at which the shot are spread out, such collisions of the shot do not occur. Hence, for example, the secondary target ($a_2$) may show the same spread as $b_2$, where the ranges are 2 ft. and 18 ft. to the primary targets.

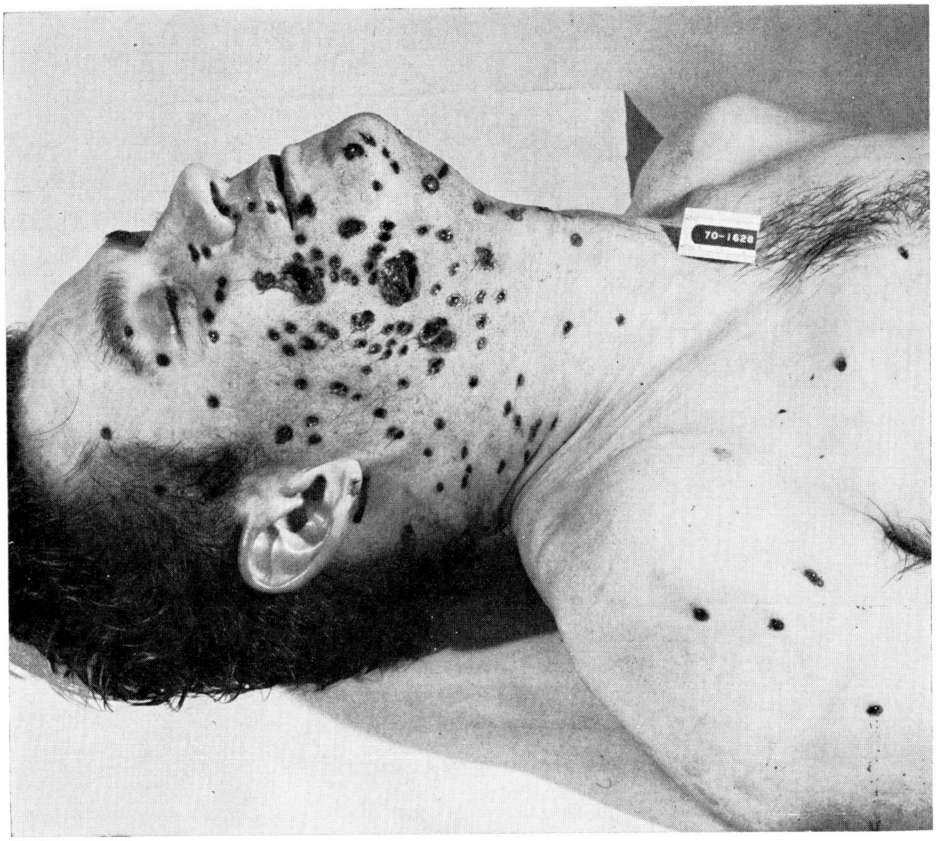


FIGURE X-83. Shotgun injury inflicted with a 12 gauge Browning automatic, loaded with No. 4 shot, fired through a window from a point 9 ft. from the window. The target is larger than expected due to the *billiard ball ricochet effect*. Note the wad injuries.

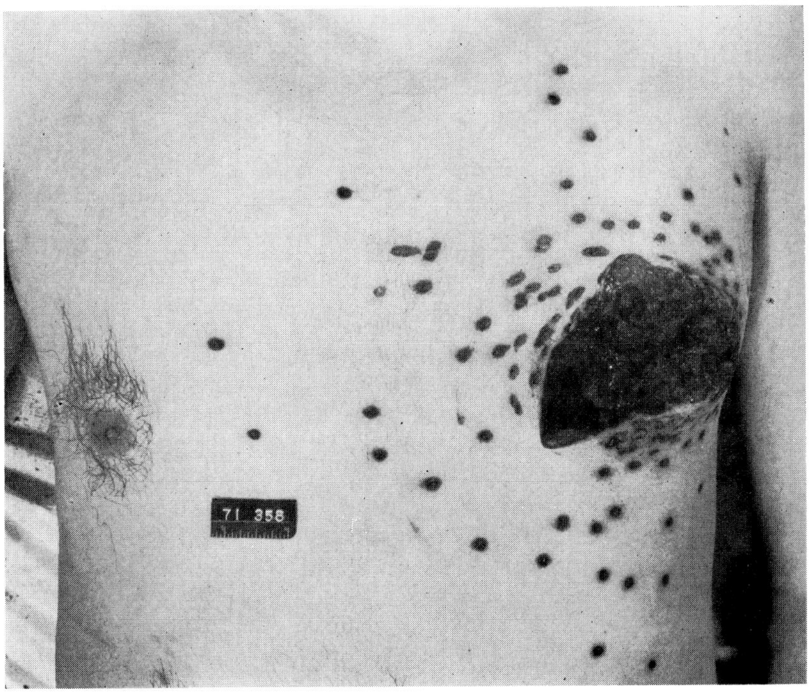


FIGURE X-84. Shotgun wound inflicted with a 12 gauge shotgun, No. 6 shot, through a thin wooden door, at a distance of 4 ft. (2 ft. muzzle to door and 2 ft. door to subject). The wide pattern at this distance is partly due to the scattering produced by ricocheting as the shot struck the primary target, the door.

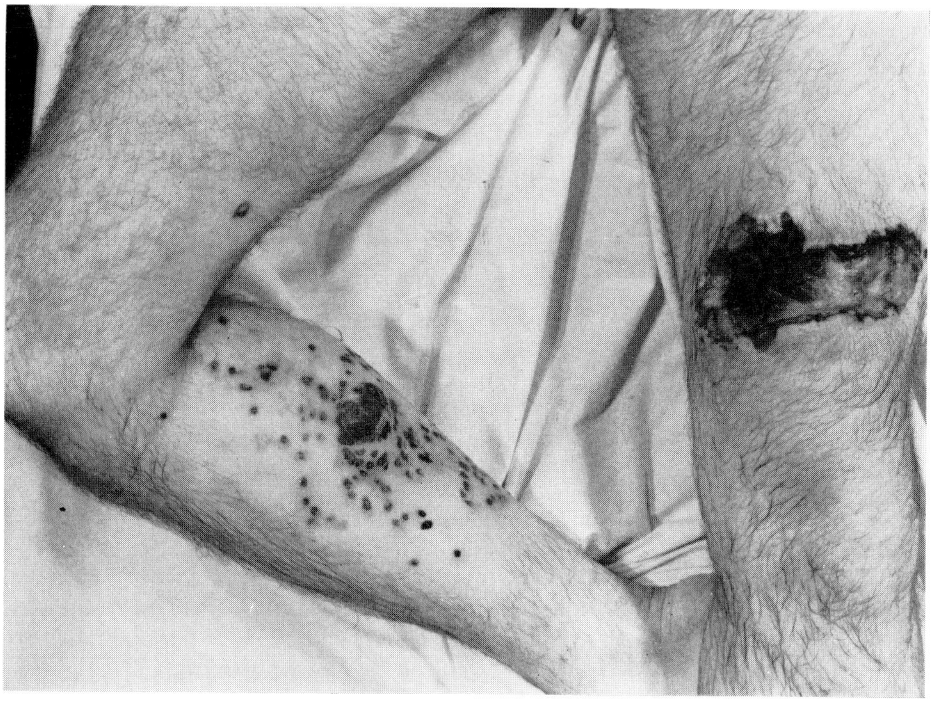

FIGURE X-85. *Billiard ball ricochet effect.* The shot, fired from a distance of about 5 ft., grazed the left thigh, causing the shot to scatter over a wide area, as indicated by the wounding pattern on the right leg.

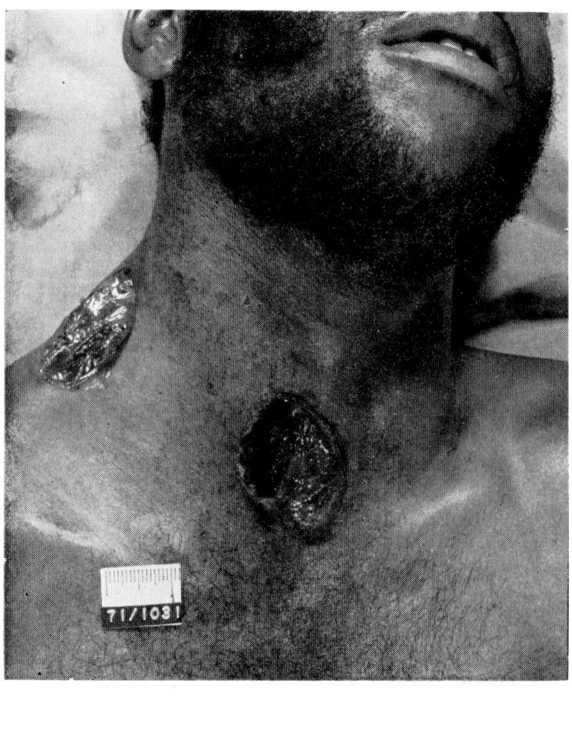



FIGURE X-86. Injury in the front of the neck caused by a 12 gauge shotgun, loaded with No. 6 shot, fired from a distance of about 5 ft. Most of the shot exited through the wound in the side of the neck, but the plastic and cardboard wadding were recovered from the soft tissues near the exit wound.

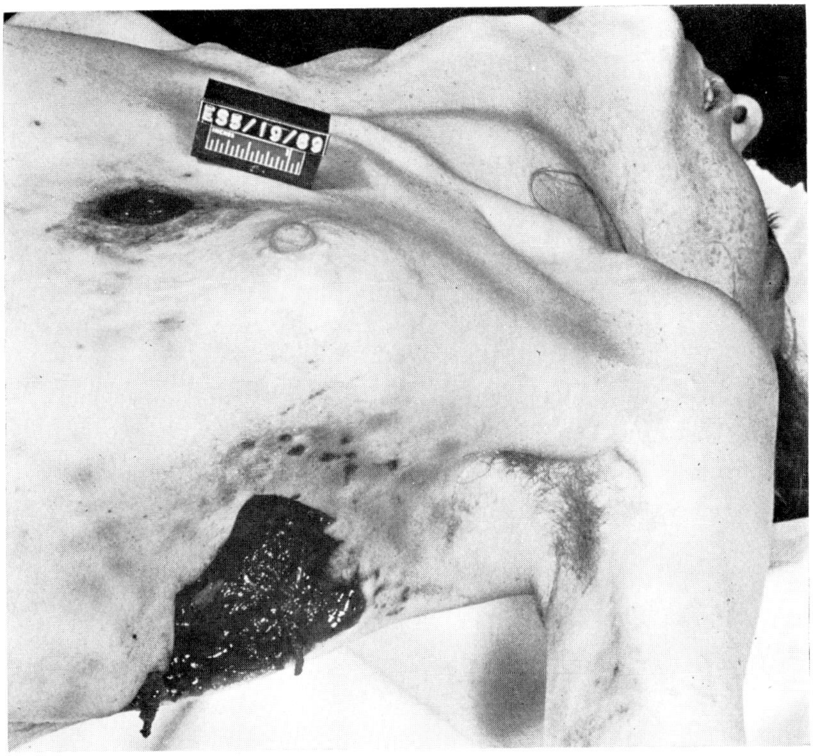

FIGURE X-87. Self-inflicted contact shot of the left chest and a gaping exit wound with individual small perforations made by exiting pellets under the armpit. The deceased was 5′6″ tall and weighed 85 lb. A 20 gauge shotgun, loaded with No. 5 shot, was used.

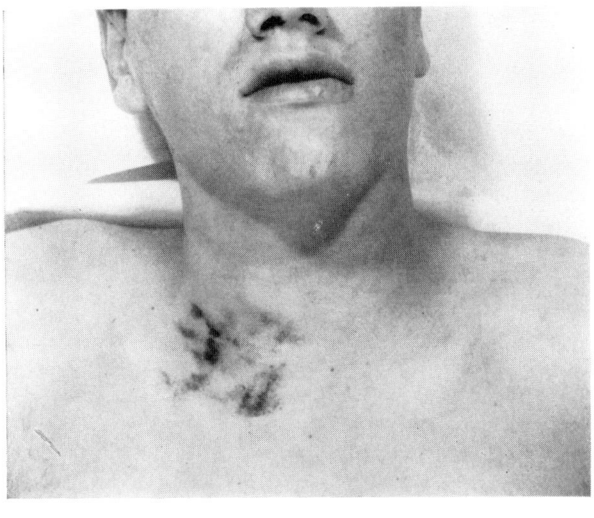

FIGURE X-88. Shotgun wound between the shoulder blades, inflicted with a 12 gauge shotgun, No. 4 shot, from a distance of approximately 2 ft. The injury shown includes points of exit of two pellets and extensive abrasion of the skin by shot that failed to break through the skin.

### The Survivability of Shotgun Wounds

As with small arms fire, shotgun wounds, particularly when relatively small shot are used, are quite variable in their effect upon the victim. At contact or close range the blast effect, as well as shot damage, may cause instantaneous death due to major destruction of the head or body. In fact, death can be caused by the blast effect and wadding injury even with *blank* shells if the range of fire is under 1 or 2 ft. At greater ranges, where only a few shot reach the victim, the injury may be insignificant or there may be considerable delay in the development of blood loss sufficient to cause collapse of the victim.

A fifty-five-year-old man was rabbit hunting with a friend when he was shot from approximately 20 ft. with a 12 gauge shotgun, cylinder bore, loaded with No. 5 shot. Only three of the shot struck the body; one of these produced an insignificant skin wound, but the two others penetrated the back and perforated the aorta in the abdominal area. The individual realized he was injured and started to walk to the nearest road, where his friend meanwhile had gone to pick up their car. He did succeed in walking more than 1000 yd. and was able to get into the car by himself, but upon arrival at the hospital twenty minutes later he was dead. He died as a result of blood loss into the retroperitoneal area caused by the two perforating wounds of the aorta made by the birdshot.

The ability to walk more than 1000 yd. while fatally wounded is remarkable. Furthermore, this case illustrates that a fatal shotgun injury can occur with small shot, even from a relatively great distance.

## REFERENCES

1. Guerin, P. F.: Shotgun wounds. *J Forensic Sci, 5:* 294, 1960.
2. Breitenecker, R., and Senior, W. J.: Shotgun patterns. I. An experimental study on the influence of intermediate targets. *J Forensic Sci, 12:*193, 1967.
3. Breitenecker, R.: Shotgun wound patterns. *Am J Clin Pathol, 52:*258, 1969.

*Chapter XI*

# THERMAL INJURIES

WERNER U. SPITZ

THERMAL BURNS remain a prominent cause of death both in civilian life and in modern warfare. The chances of survival following this kind of injury have changed dramatically since World War II. Until 1941 it was generally expected that a burn involving 50 percent or more of the body surface would prove fatal. Nowadays patients with 80 percent burns of the body need not necessarily succumb to their injuries. Nevertheless, the age of the victim greatly influences the clinical outcome of a burn injury; the very young and the elderly are particularly vulnerable to lethal complications.

Burns are commonly classified according to the depth of tissue destruction:

1. First degree burns are superficial. The damage is limited to the outer layer of the skin. Blisters do not form, but peeling may follow. The burned area is red, swollen and painful.
2. Second degree burns typically show blistering. The upper layers of the skin are destroyed. Healing takes place from the margins and from small epithelial remnants. Nevertheless, scarring sometimes results.
3. In third degree burns the entire thickness of the skin (epidermis and dermis) is destroyed. Pain is commonly absent because the nerve endings themselves are destroyed. Healing is from the edges of the injury, and scarring is the rule. Skin grafting is usually necessary in treatment.
4. More severe thermal injury, such as charring and complete destruction of skin and underlying tissue, is commonly referred to as fourth degree burning.

The extent of the burns should be specified. It is conveniently estimated using the *rule of nines* (Fig. XI-1). The severity of the burns depends directly on both the intensity of the heat and the duration of exposure. Among other factors, temperatures in a fire differ depending on the substances that are burning. Some chemical fires may rapidly reach several thousand degrees, whereas the ordinary house fire seldom exceeds 1200° F; hence, it is unlikely that the body of an adult will burn so completely in a house fire as to leave no trace. Disposal of a homicide victim by setting fire to a building is, therefore, usually unsuccessful (Fig. XI-2).

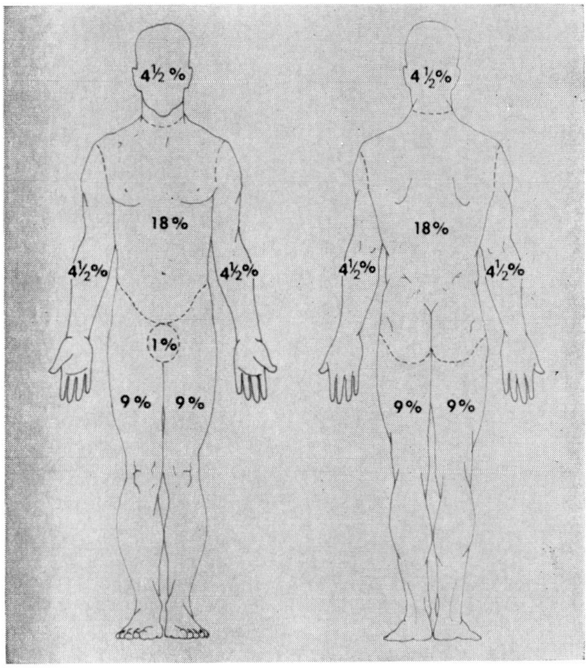


FIGURE XI-1. Body surface expressed as percentages using the *rule of nines.*

The bodies of two badly burned women were recovered following a house fire. The unburned body of a man was found in a part of the house that was not damaged by the flames. Subsequent investigation of the circumstances led to the conclusion that all three had been drinking when an argument developed, during which the man stabbed the women and attempted to dispose of their bodies by setting fire to the premises.

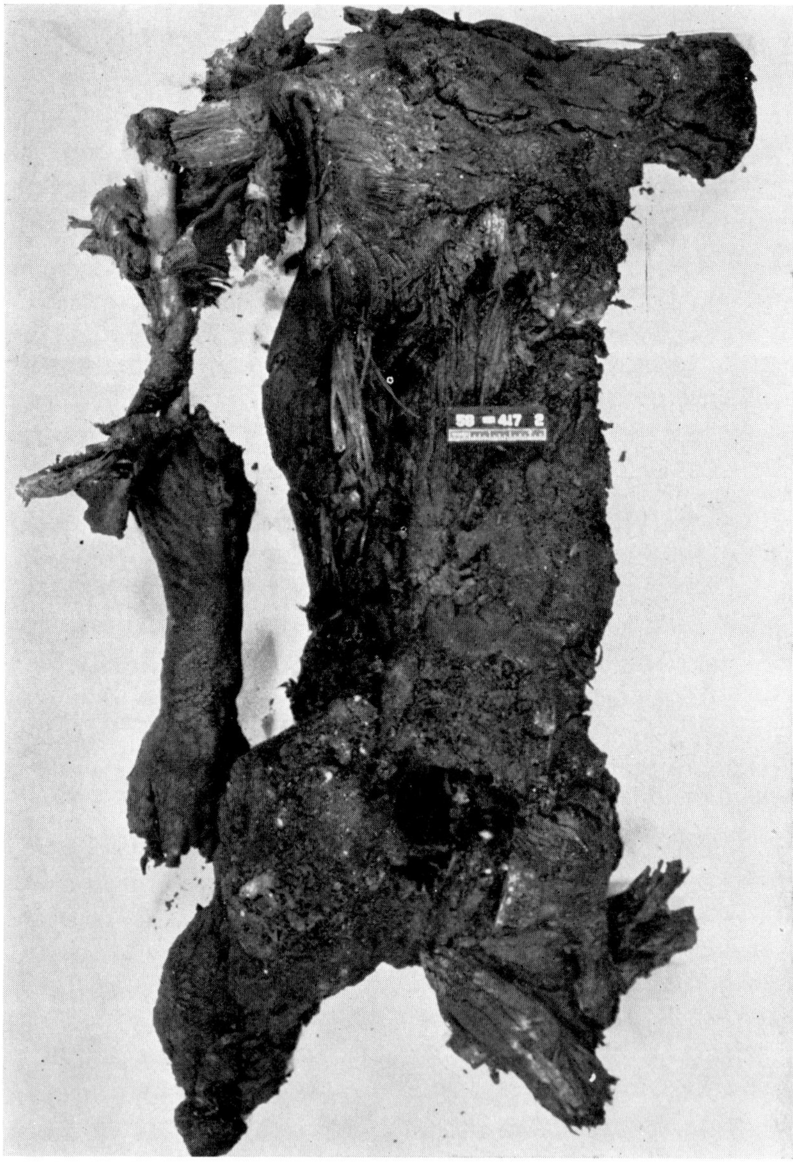

FIGURE XI-2a. Human body profoundly mutilated by fire.

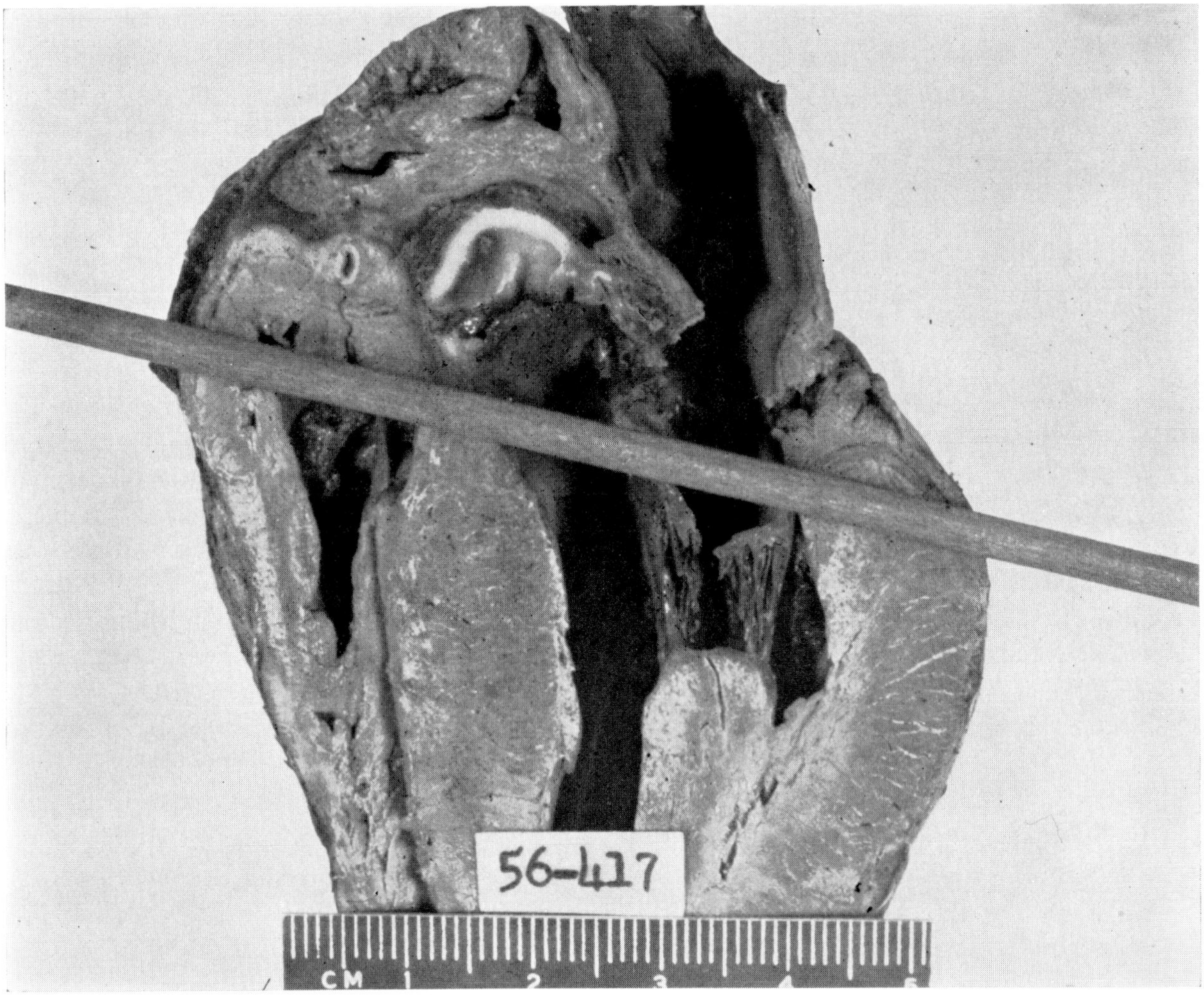


FIGURE XI-2b. Same case as shown in Figure XI-2a. Despite external charring, the internal organs were preserved, and the heart showed a bullet track as indicated by the probe.

To exculpate himself, he went to sleep in another part of the house, but he succumbed to inhalation of carbon monoxide with a blood saturation of 65%. He also had a blood alcohol level of 0.28%. The two women were likewise markedly intoxicated. Autopsy showed that both had died of multiple stab wounds and that both were dead before the fire had started, as evidenced by negative carbon monoxide levels in the blood.

By contrast, the body of a child within the first few years of life may be reduced to a few ounces of ashes in a relatively short time by a fire that would not similarly affect the body of an adult.

The charred body of an adult was found in the rubble of a burned-down log cabin. Anthropologic studies and dental records identified the remains as a certain thirty-two-year-old white woman, who had lived there with her three-year-old daughter. No remains of the child could be recovered after a thorough search. A death certificate was finally issued after a court decided that the child had, indeed, perished in the flames.

It is interesting to note that the body of a newborn child can be burned away in an ordinary stove in less than two hours.[1]

A clothed body is destroyed in a fire more rapidly and more completely than an unclothed one, and the body of an obese individual is consumed more thoroughly than that of a lean person. The heat of the fire exposes the body fat, and the clothes act as a wick, providing for more complete combustion. In a ravaging house fire a body is usually badly charred in less than twenty minutes. As a point of comparison, it has been said that timber is charred to a depth of ½ in. in about the same time.[2]

Peculiar, characteristically curved fractures are often noted in bones exposed to very high temperatures. The bones of the extremities as well as the skull may show this type of fracture. No other means is known that is capable of breaking bone in a similar fashion. Experimentally, these cracks occur after the bone is removed from the fire and cooling has begun (Fig. XI-3).

A fire in the open, as in a field, will not usually permit complete combustion of a human body. An example of this point may be found in the attempted disposal of Hitler's body by one of his aides at the end of World War II. In spite of the use of gasoline to enhance the fire and resultant widespread charring of the body,

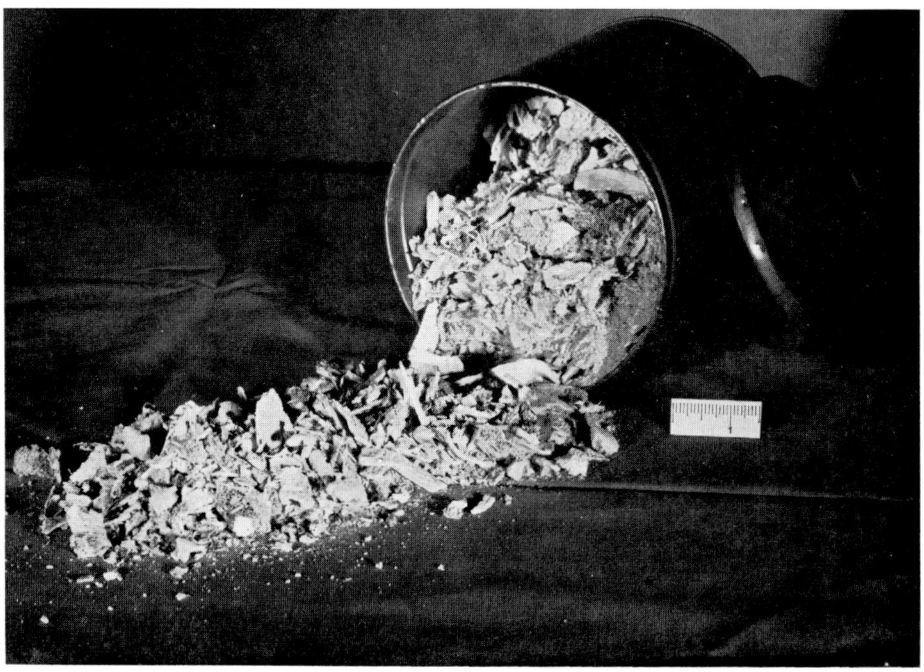

FIGURE XI-3. Half-gallon tin can containing human remains following cremation.

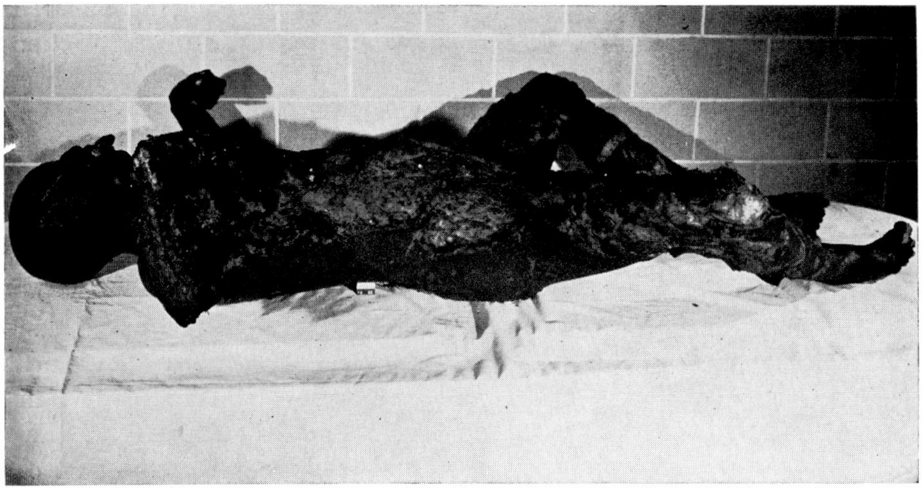

FIGURE XI-4. Extensive disfigurement by fire. Note the position of the extremities due to contraction of the musculature by the heat. This posture of a fire victim resembles that of a boxer and is commonly referred to as *pugilistic attitude*. Note the protruding tongue due to contraction of the tissues of the neck and face.

positive dental identification was made without difficulty.[3] Cremation in an outdoor pyre is the orthodox mode of corpse disposal among the Hindus. The pyre is allowed to burn for three days before the remains are collected for later consignment to the Ganges. Even at this stage, large pieces of bone are still recognizable among the ashes.

Generally, if the teeth of a body recovered from a fire are charred while the internal organs of the chest and abdomen are significantly less affected by the flames, it is conceivable that an attempt may have been made to obliterate the identity of the victim by starting the fire in the head area. In this case, arson should be suspected. The use of accelerants, such as kerosene or gasoline, in an effort to dispose of a body by fire often causes patchy charring. If the adipose tissue of the body is ignited, prolonged local smoldering sometimes results in severe skeletal damage, which may include amputation.

The death of an individual in a fire often occurs a considerable time before the conflagration can

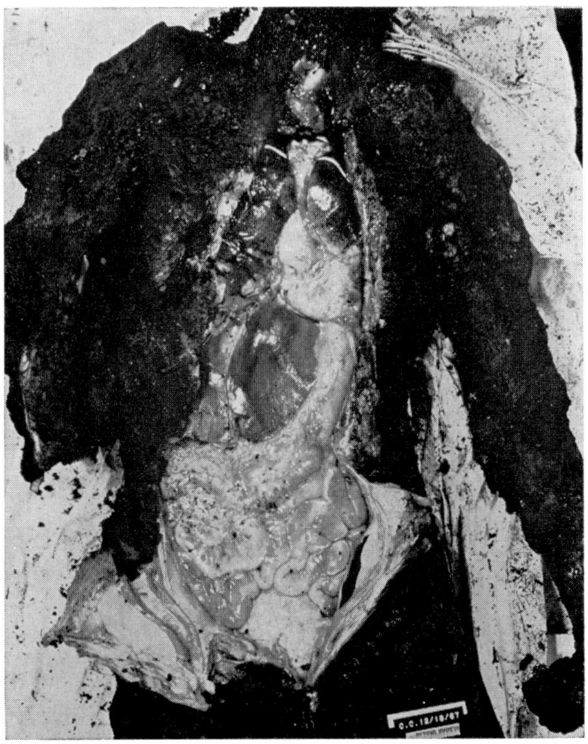

FIGURE XI-5. Preservation of the internal organs in spite of charring: Liquid blood was present in the heart and was removed for chemical analyses.

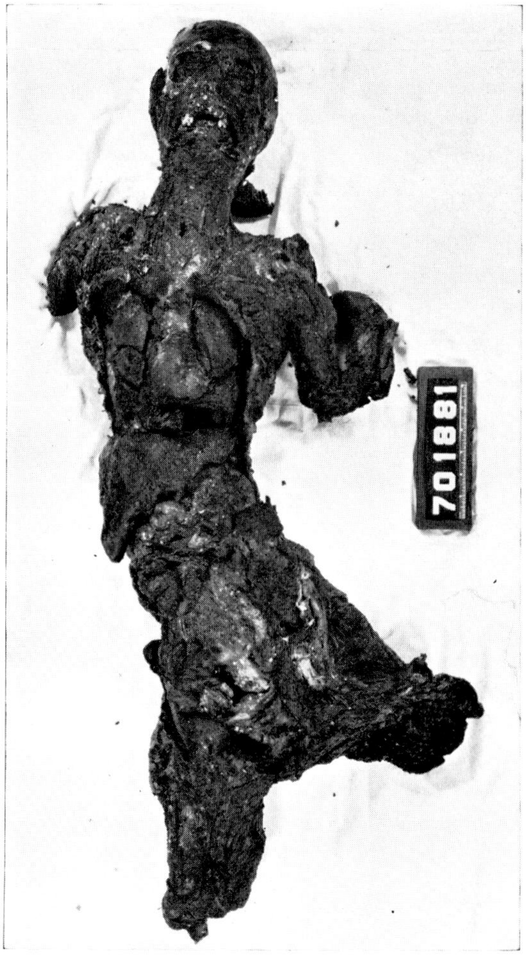


FIGURE XI-6a. Charred remains found among debris of a burned-down house. Note exposure of the chest and abdominal organs as a result of the fire.

be brought under control. It is obvious, therefore, that the extensive mutilation frequently seen in victims of fire has largely occurred after death. Charring of the body under such circumstances is common (Fig. XI-4). Regardless of how severe the surface destruction may be, the organs are usually well enough preserved that a meaningful autopsy may subsequently be carried out, and tissues are usually available for carbon monoxide and alcohol determinations as well as for other chemical analyses (Fig. XI-5).

It should be mentioned in this regard that the autopsy is best done on the body before embalming, since crystalline formalin, sometimes sprinkled on charred bodies (in lieu of the injection of embalming fluids), interferes with the determination of alcohol because of alcohol-soluble perfumes that are part of its composition. These materials diffuse into the interior of the organs and render even deeper tissues unsuitable for such chemical analysis.

The charred remains of a fifty-two-year-old woman were found on the living room floor of her one-story frame house. The house was completely demolished by fire. Even though the chest and abdominal walls were burned extensively, at autopsy the organs were relatively well preserved (Fig. XI-6). A blood carbon monoxide saturation of 25% was found. It was further established that the victim had suffered from advanced arteriosclerosis of the coronary arteries. A blood alcohol determination was not performed because scented salts had been sprinkled on the body. (A negative alcohol level in this body would have indicated that the deceased had a negative blood alcohol content at the time of death.)

The examination of a body found at the site of a conflagration involves primarily the following objectives: (a) identification of the victim, (b) determination of the cause of death.

## IDENTIFICATION OF THE VICTIM

The identification of the victim is generally carried out according to the outline in Chapter III. Certain principles, however, are peculiar to the victim of a fire. The weight and length of a charred body are unreliable, as desiccation of the tissues, skeletal fractures and pulverization of the intervertebral discs resulting from the heat may significantly alter these dimensions. Body length may be shortened by several inches, and weight loss may amount to 60 percent. Also, the skin is tightened and contracted, thus changing the features. An ear, for example, may shrink to two-thirds or less of the size of its undamaged counterpart. Cataract as a result of coagulation of proteins in the lens of the eye has been observed to occur at environmental temperatures as low as 150° F (Fig. XI-7).

Identifiable peculiarities of the body surface,

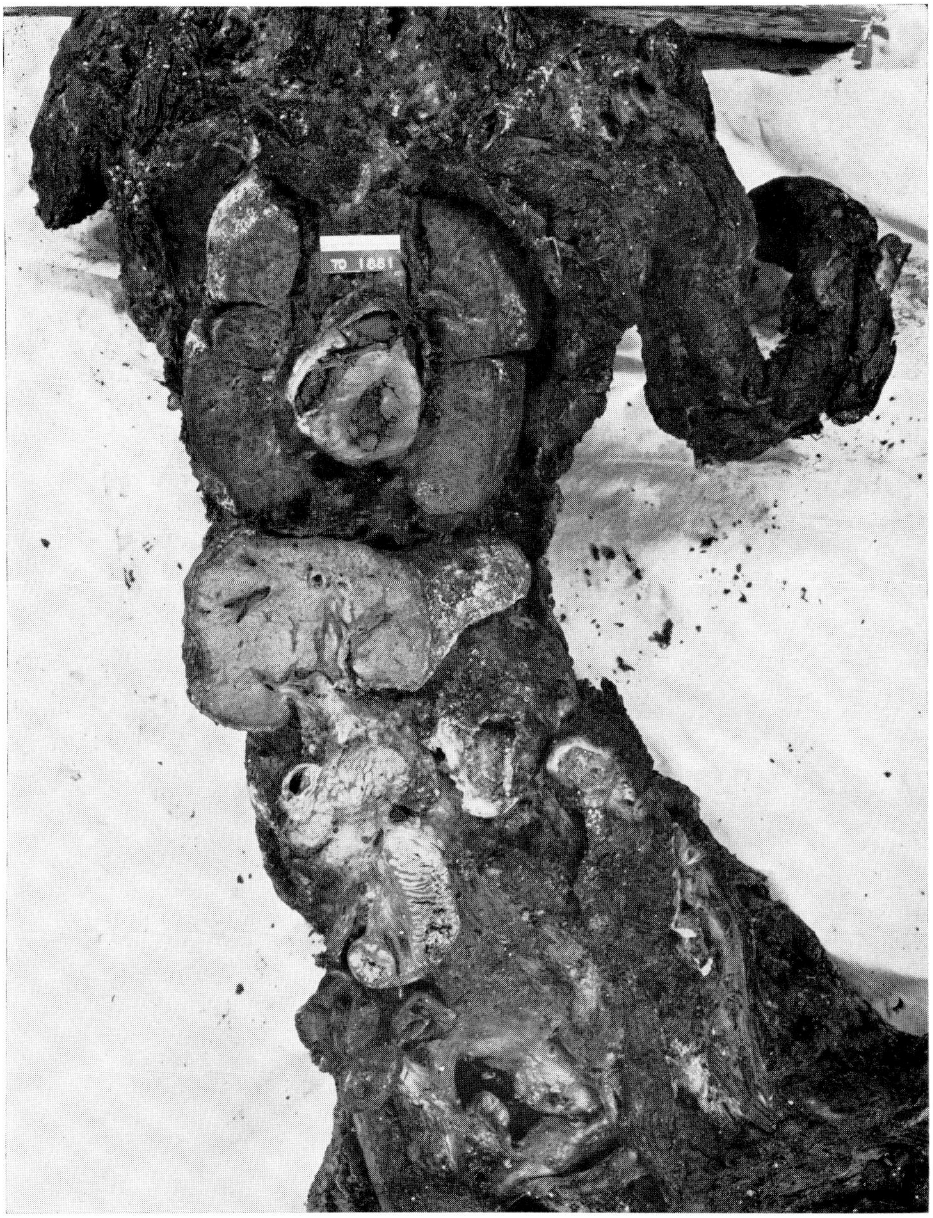

FIGURE XI-6b. The organs were hardened (cooked) by the heat. Nevertheless, clotted blood that could be utilized for toxicologic analyses was found in the heart. The architecture of the organs was relatively well preserved, as the sections demonstrate.

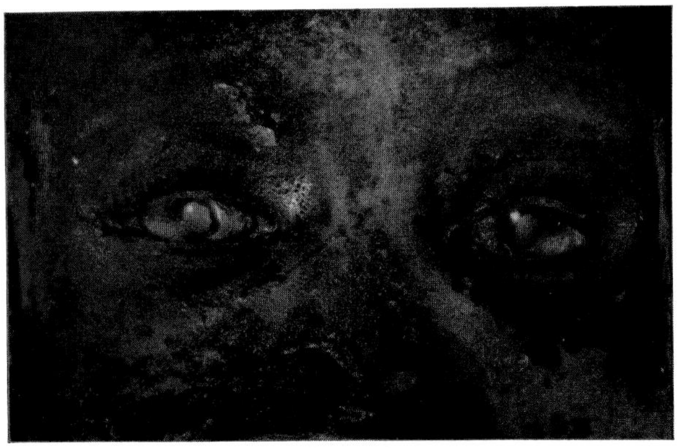

Figure XI-7. Postmortem opacity of the lenses (cataract) of both eyes, caused by heat coagulation of the lens proteins. The deceased was found face up on the kitchen floor, her head in close proximity to the open oven door. The oven was set at 400° F. The room temperature was described as "extremely hot."

Sometimes skin and hair in the armpits are spared. The gums are also often preserved. Since they are brown or mottled in a large number of Negroes, this finding may lead to racial identification. Another frequent observation in Negroes is the dark gray deposit of melanin in the arachnoid membrane around the medulla oblongata and in the area of the olfactory nerves at the base of the frontal lobes.

Light hair changes color on exposure to heat, depending on the temperature. At about 250° F gray hair turns brassy blonde, and ten to fifteen minutes at 400° F imparts a slight reddish hue to brown hair. Black hair does not change color.

Complete body x rays of the victim are advisable to locate possible old fractures, bony ab-

such as scars, tattoos and moles, are frequently destroyed. The presence of a surgical scar may nevertheless be deduced from the autopsy findings, such as a missing appendix or evidence of an old gastrectomy.

Distinction between the sexes can be made by examination of the internal genital organs and breast tissue. The appearance of the female breasts with respect to the estimation of the age of a fire victim is often misleading, since heat causes loss of fluids from the tissues with resultant shrinkage, erection and increased firmness of the breasts, regardless of age.

For racial identification despite extensive charring, the pathologist should look for patches of intact skin. The most likely sites are under tight clothing, such as the belt, shoes, brassiere or buttoned collar. Unburnt skin about the wrists and ankles may indicate the victim was bound before the fire started. A straplike, horizontal undamaged area on the neck suggests ligature strangulation.

The badly burned body of a twenty-four-year-old black female was found in a field (Fig. XI-8). Remnants of clothesline were found on the neck. The underlying skin was not burned. Death was determined to be due to ligature strangulation. The burns were caused by a subsequent attempt to dispose of the body or obliterate its identity.

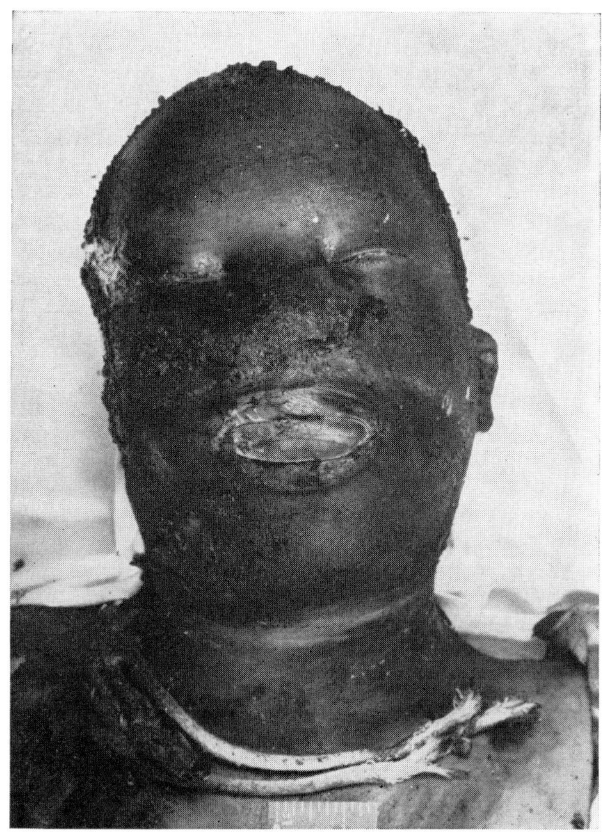

Figure XI-8. Body of a young Negro woman found charred in a field. The undamaged straplike area of skin on the neck was caused by the unburned clothesline that was used as a ligature. A fairly pale horizontal band of skin across the left cheek and the upper lip suggests the deceased was gagged.

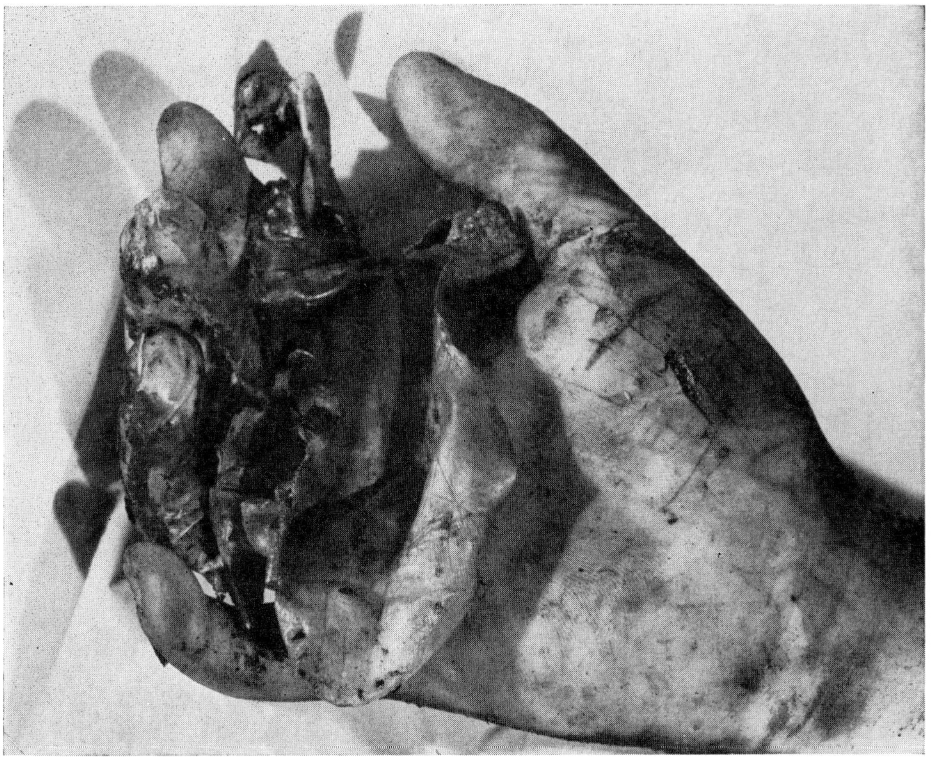

FIGURE XI-9. The skin of the hand detaches as a *glove*, due to the effect of heat. The *glove* includes the fingernails. Both the *glove* and the underlying skin are still suitable for obtaining inked impressions for fingerprint comparisons. Care must therefore be taken to preserve this peeled-off skin when handling such a body.

normalities or foreign bodies that might otherwise escape observation. X rays of the teeth may reveal metal pins used for root canal treatment and fillings that were not detected on direct examination. The dental examination is much more difficult when the heat and flames have fragmented the enamel and when soot and smoke have been deposited on the teeth. Generally, however, teeth and restorations are remarkably resistant to heat, and unless they are struck directly by the flames, adequate preservation is probable in most cases. When heat contractures have tightly locked the jaws and preclude detailed visual examination, especially of the molars, the alternative is to disarticulate the mandible and excise the upper jaw. The technique is described in Chapter XXIV. Since the charred remains of a fire victim are not injected for the purpose of embalming and are not viewed by the relatives, excision of the jaws to facilitate examination by the pathologist does not usually excite objection.

Frequently in severely burned bodies tissue fluid collects between the layers of skin. In the hands the skin detaches as a *glove*, including the fingernails. Either the detached *glove* or the remaining hand, whichever is less damaged, may be used to obtain fingerprints (Fig. XI-9). The skin of the feet may detach in like fashion. A similar process occurs in decomposition and following prolonged immersion.

Removal of the superficial layers of the skin by wiping or rubbing renders a tattoo better recognizable. The pigment of the tattoo is situated deeper than those layers of skin that are removed. Wiping areas thought to be tattooed may reveal a tattoo previously obscured (Fig. XI-10).

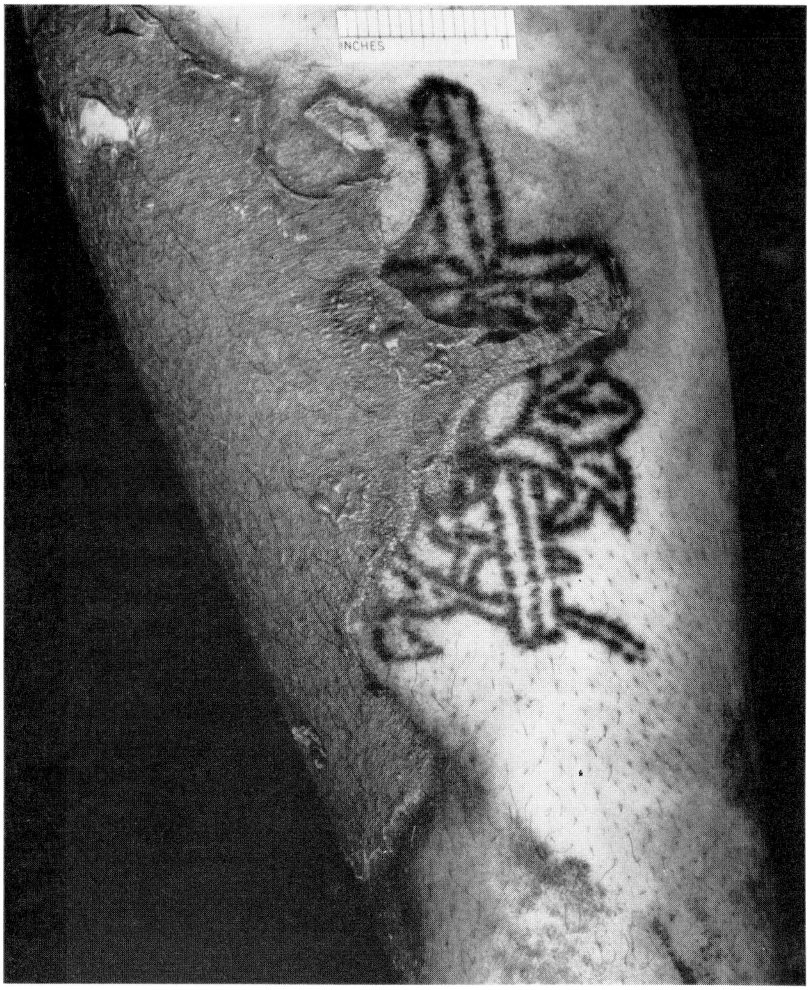


FIGURE XI-10. Tattoo on forearm of a Negro male made apparent by wiping off the burnt superficial layers of the skin. This may be an important finding if identification is a problem.

## DETERMINATION OF THE CAUSE OF DEATH

To determine the cause of death the examiner must first establish whether the victim was alive at the time of the fire. While the presence of carbon monoxide in the blood (carboxyhemoglobin) is proof of life when the fire started, its absence does not necessarily exclude this possibility. Carbon monoxide (CO) is frequently absent in victims of flash fire, as in the conflagration of a chemical plant, in warfare or in an explosion, when death is practically instantaneous. An individual stoking an industrial fire, for instance, may also be the victim of a flash fire. Flame throwers in wartime cause death in a similar fashion. As a rule, flames that hit the face are liable to cause death extremely rapidly due to inability of the victim to breath. Inhalation of superheated air causes edema of the airway and death by suffocation within a few hours.

It may be interesting to speculate regarding the toxic effect of inhalation of combustion products of some synthetic materials, particularly in conjunction with inhalation of carbon monoxide. Plastic furniture, upholstery, etc. are being used with increased frequency in all echelons of life, and it is possible that chlorine, phosgene, cyanide and the oxides of nitrogen, etc., that are released by such burning materials may aggravate the anoxic effect produced by carboxyhemoglobin. This was demonstrated in the Coconut Grove fire in Boston in the early 1940s, where the burning of plastic drapes high in nitrogen gave rise to poisonous nitrogen oxides responsible for lung damage in many of the surviving victims. Generally, however, the amounts of these materials within the fumes are quite small and, in our opinion, are of negligible significance.

Carbon monoxide is generated in all conflagrations, especially if household items such as furniture and clothes are on fire. A smoldering mattress is a particularly generous source of carbon monoxide. Careless smoking in bed, especially following consumption of alcohol, is the most common cause for this type of circumstance (Fig. XI-11). A few inhalations of a CO-rich atmosphere suffice to build up a significant carbon monoxide blood level.

The blood carbon monoxide level in victims of fire who are found dead at the scene may differ, depending on their age and general state of health. In a healthy middle-aged adult who dies in a conflagration, a blood saturation level of 50% to 70% is usually found. Somewhat lower levels are found in children and in the elderly. A high carbon monoxide level in an elderly victim suggests a good state of health. In the presence of emphysema, advanced arteriosclerotic heart disease or anemia, death would occur before carbon monoxide could build up to a high level. Chain smokers may have a CO level of 8% to 10% saturation from the CO in cigarette smoke; therefore, the interpretation of a low CO blood level must be done with care. In a nonsmoker a similar blood level may be considered evidence of smoke inhalation and consequently that the victim was alive after the fire started (Fig. XI-12). (For additional information regarding death associated with carbon monoxide inhalation, the reader is referred to Chapter XII.

Infants and children build up a fatal carbon monoxide level in less time than adults exposed to the same atmosphere. This is because of the increased respiratory exchange (breathing volume in proportion to blood volume) in early life. It is, therefore, not unusual in cases of conflagration to find that an infant sleeping in the same room as his parents is dead of CO poisoning while his parents are but little affected. A dog or a cat in the same room is also likely to die early, supposedly due to the greater metabolic rates in these animals and consequent rapid buildup of a fatal level of carbon monoxide.

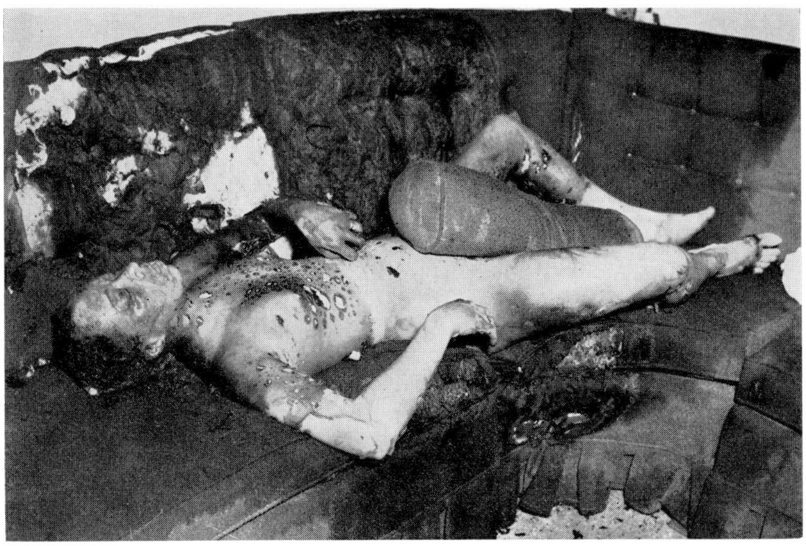

FIGURE XI-11. Thirty-six-year-old woman who fell asleep while smoking a cigarette. The autopsy showed that death resulted from inhalation of smoke, and the blood carbon monoxide level was 65%. The burns are postmortem. The fire was limited to the sofa.

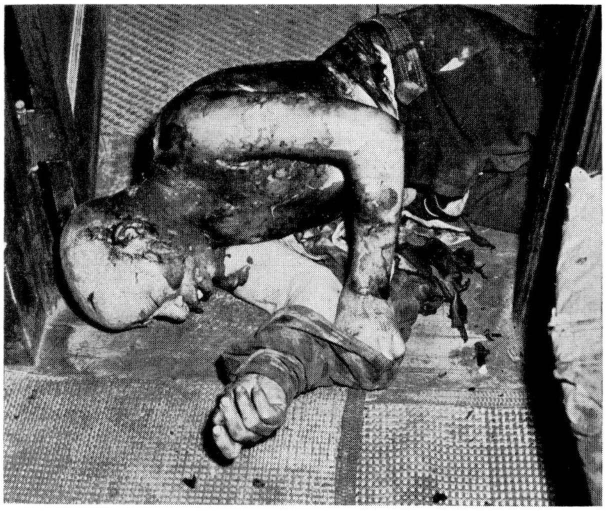

FIGURE XI-12. Seventy-six-year-old man, known heart patient, with marked pitting edema of the legs and ankles. His shirttail caught fire on a hot plate while he was cooking his dinner. He was a nonsmoker; his carbon monoxide level was 10%, indicating that he was alive at the time the fire was in process. It appears probable that he sustained a heart attack as a result of the commotion associated with the fire while trying to remove his burning shirt.

The question of carbon monoxide diffusion across the placental barrier is undecided. According to Gonzales et al.,[4] the gas does not pass into the fetal circulation, while Mueller,[5] quoting Dérobèrt[6] and Franke,[7] maintains that it does, even though the blood level is slightly lower in the fetus. Wiener[8] states that the placenta is no barrier to the CO in the maternal blood. The more rapidly the mother dies of a lethal concentration of CO, the less CO will enter the fetal blood.

Inhaled smoke is readily shown in the nostrils and the mouth as black particles of soot (Fig. XI-13). At autopsy, such particles are mixed with the mucus covering the congested lining membranes of the airways (Fig. XI-14). The soot frequently extends deep into the lungs. Occasionally, soot is swallowed and may be recovered from the esophagus. When soot is present, it is better seen by spreading a thin film of mucus on a clean sheet of white paper.

Contrary to the general belief, blisters in the skin do not necessarily indicate that the victim

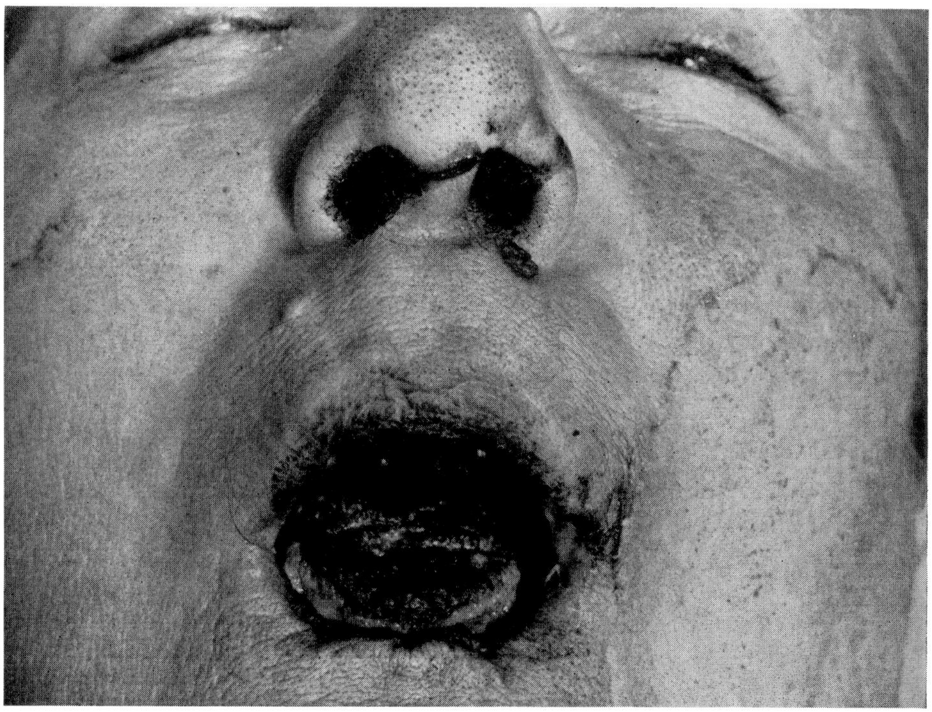

FIGURE XI-13. Soot in the nostrils and mouth of a body recovered from a smoldering fire that started in a mattress.

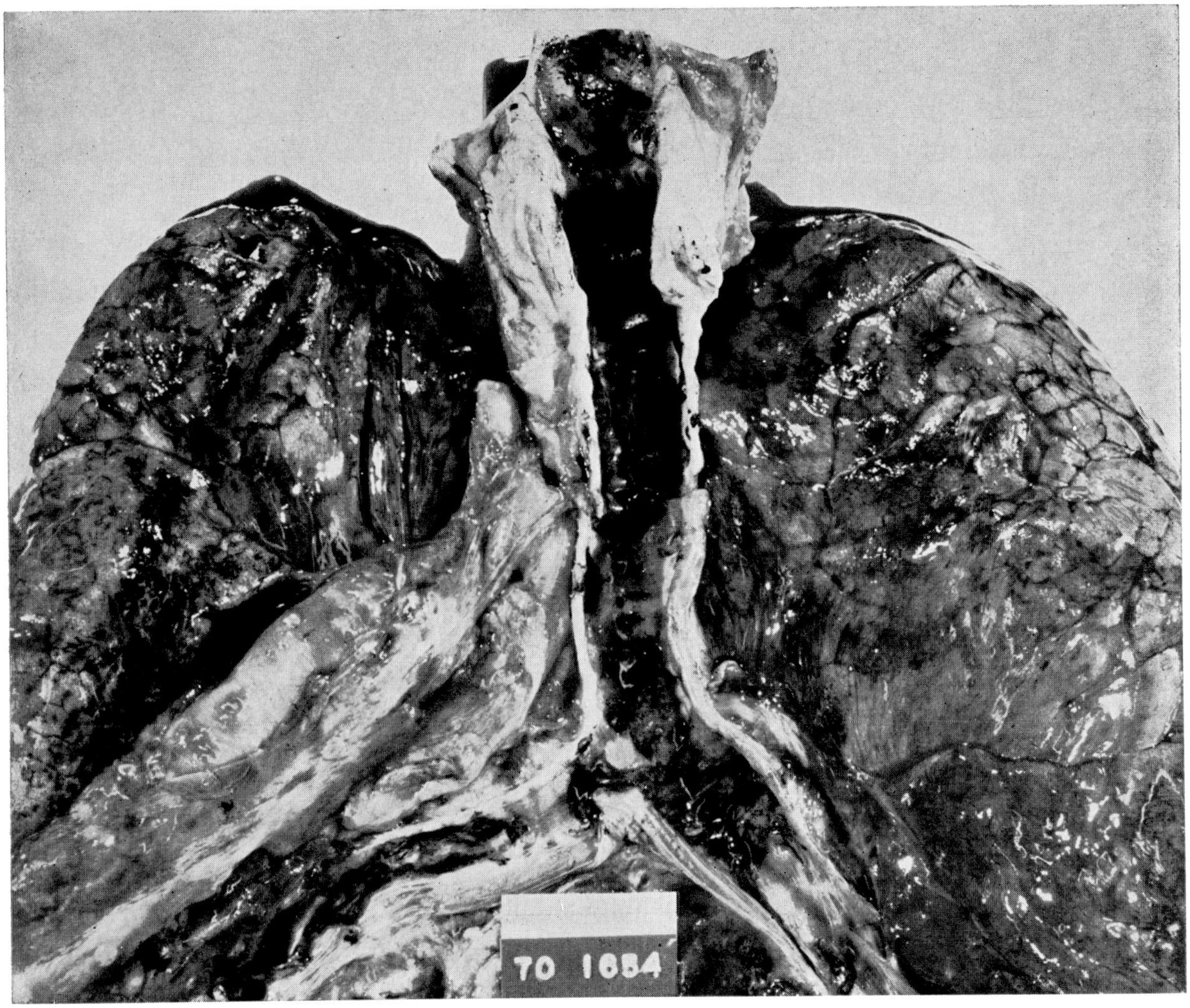


FIGURE XI-14. Soot deposits in the airways of a fire victim. This indicates that the person was alive when the fire was in progress.

was alive at the time of the fire. Similarly, the narrow red border surrounding indurated brown areas of burning results from the accumulation of blood and tissue fluids pressed out of the areas that are affected by the heat and is not indicative of early inflammation (Fig. XI-15). Instantly fatal electrocution burns and experimentally produced postmortem burns often show this red peripheral border zone due to the same mechanism (Fig. XI-16). Thus, it is not possible to determine, either by naked eye or by microscopic examination, whether burns occurred shortly before death or thereafter. Also, distinction cannot usually be made between the blisters of a second degree burn sustained shortly before or after death and slippage of the skin seen in the early phases of decomposition. An adequate investigation of the circumstances surrounding the case is mandatory to provide the answer.

A fifty-eight-year-old woman was found dead on her bathroom floor, leaning against a hot radiator. Initial investigation suggested foul play. Postmortem examination, however, revealed that death was due to massive spontaneous bleeding in the brain associated with hypertension. A patterned injury on the left arm and shoulder was a postmortem second degree burn, sustained by contact with the radiator ribs (Fig. XI-17).

Blisters over joints, such as those that are known to occur in cases of carbon monoxide

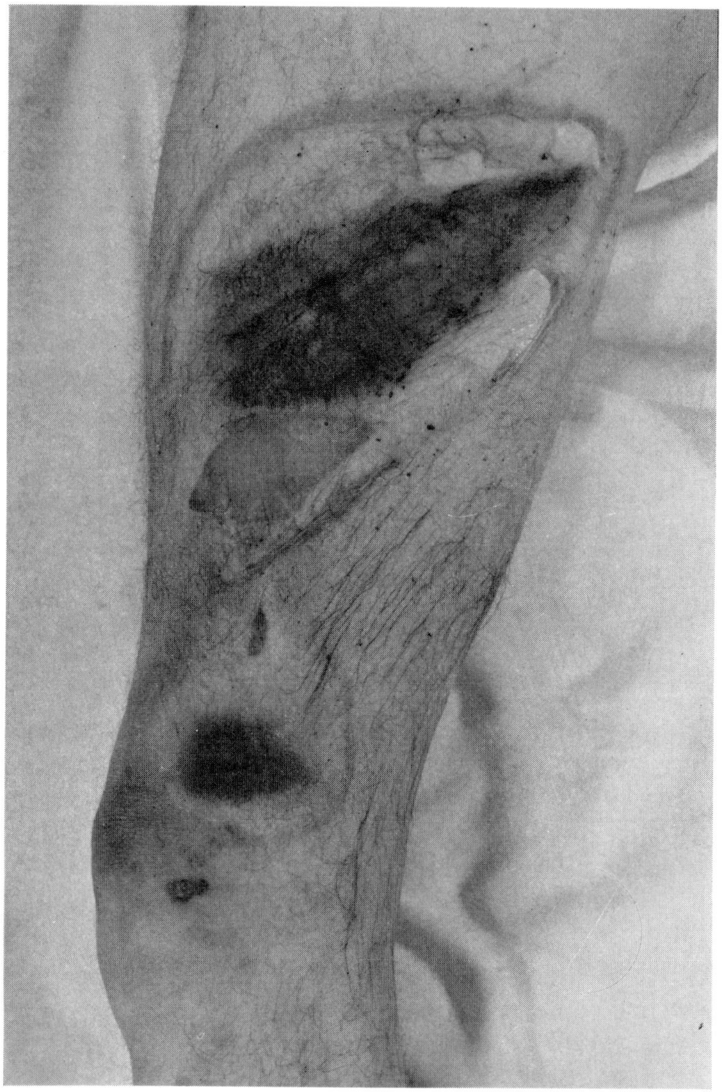

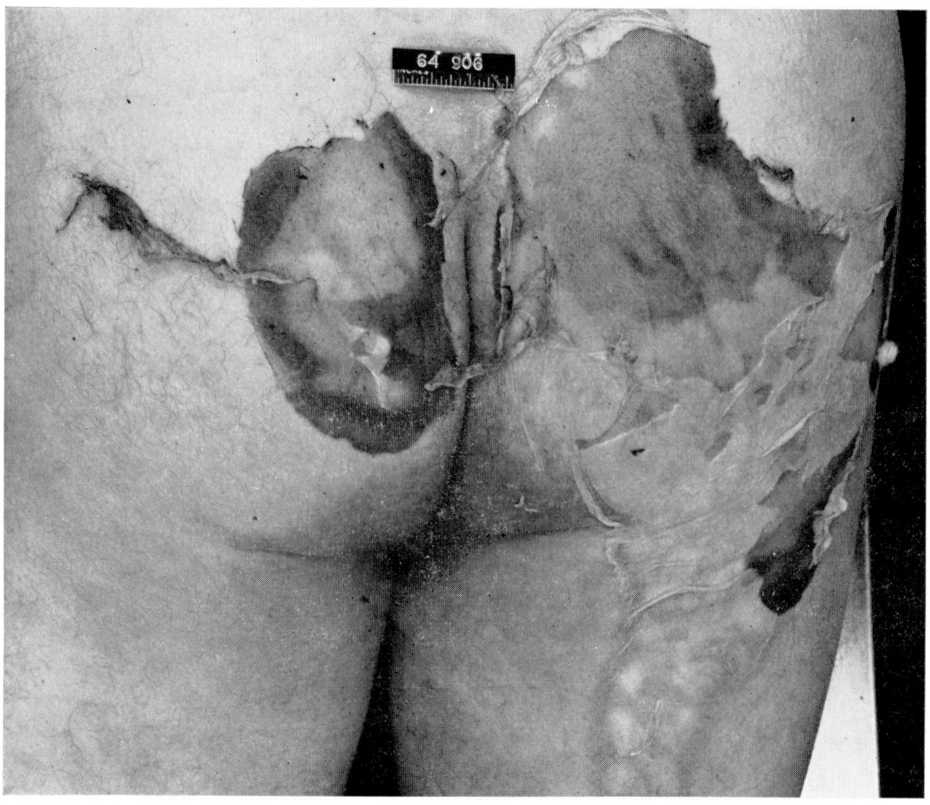
64 906

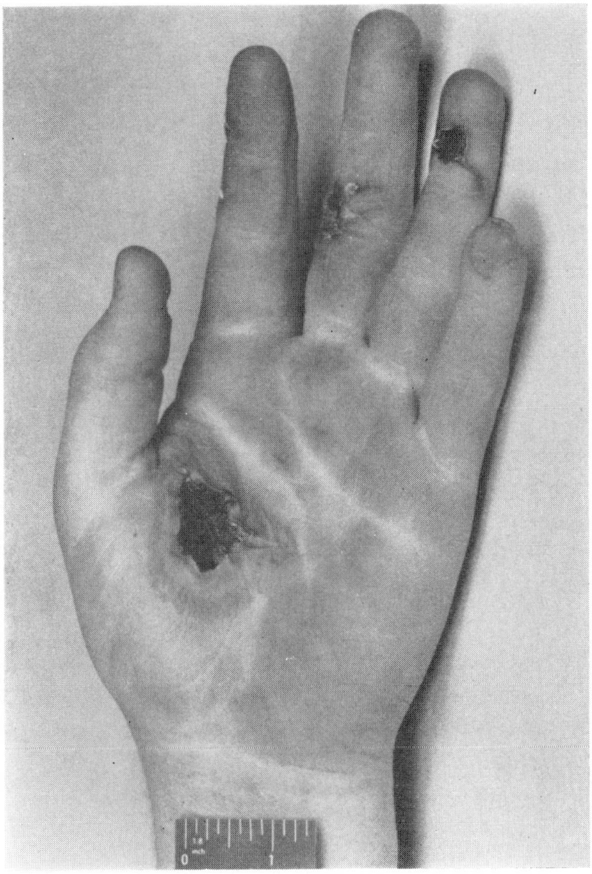

FIGURE XI-16. Electrocution. The burn in the palm consists of a charred, depressed center, elevated edges and a peripheral pale zone surrounded by a narrow red ring. The latter consists of blood and fluids pushed out of the burned area and represents an artifact unrelated to whether the electrocution occurred during life or after death.

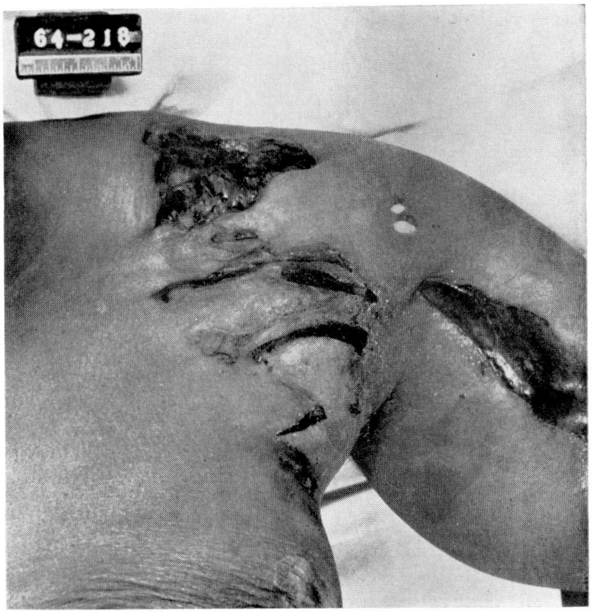


FIGURE XI-17. Second degree postmortem burns sustained as a result of contact with radiator ribs.

poisoning and in other deaths following deep coma, are also indistinguishable from second degree burns and are frequently mistaken for such. After bursting, these various types of blisters leave behind a pale, moist, raw surface, which turns yellow, tan and eventually dark brown and leathery as it dries. Gasoline exposure, either ante- or postmortem, causes skin slippage indistinguishable from some second degree burns when observed in occupants of overturned automobiles with a front gas tank. It requires special care to avoid misinterpretation of the findings.

The presence of fat droplets in blood vessels of the lungs must be interpreted with care, and fat embolism due to blunt injury should be considered. However, a small amount of fat in the vessels of the lungs may result from the effects of heat alone and is occasionally observed in individuals who are known to have died before the fire started. This results from a physicochemical alteration of fats already present in the blood.

Fractures of the extremities in fire victims are caused by excessive shrinkage of the muscles, which exerts unduly great pull on the tendons and bones (Fig. XI-18).

Artifactual fractures of the skull resulting from heat are occasionally seen in bodies re-

←

FIGURE XI-15. Examples of postmortem burns. Note the peripheral dark zone and marginal blistering surrounding the burned areas. These phenomena result from the accumulation of blood and tissue fluids which are pressed out of the areas affected by the heat. This is a frequently observed artifact which must not be confused with the onset of inflammation.

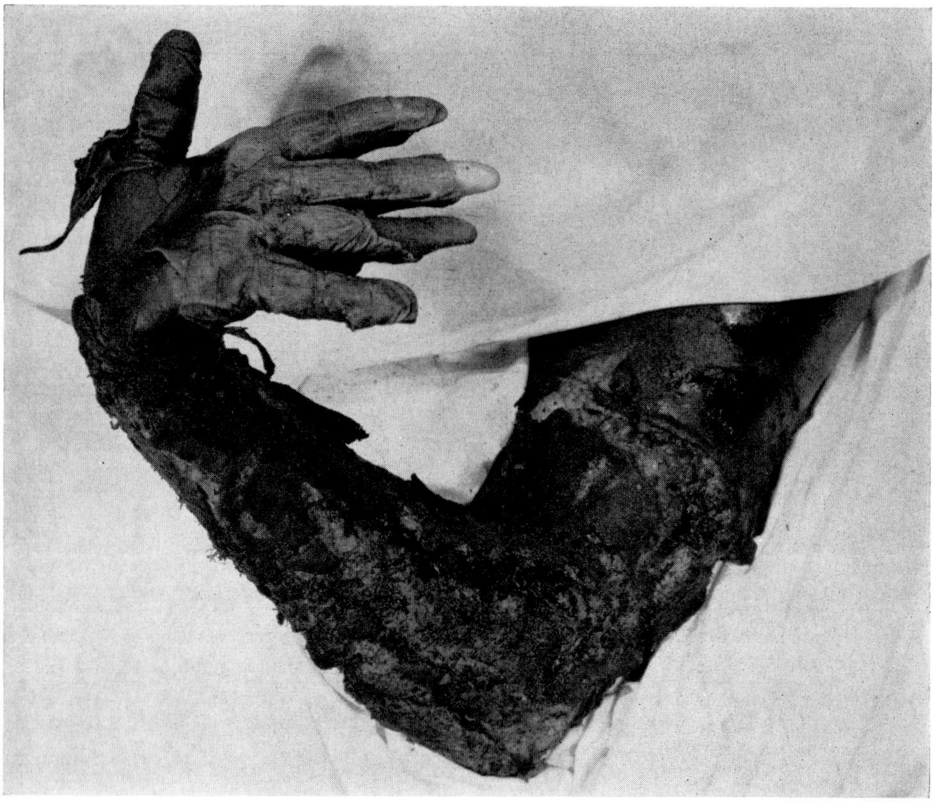

FIGURE XI-18. Heat shrinkage of the forearm muscles caused the backward pull of the hand of this body recovered from a fire.

covered from fire. These *cracks* are commonly located on either side of the skull above the temples. Sometimes they may be bilateral. Characteristically, they consist of several lines radiating from a common center (Fig. XI-19). Commonly, outward bursting of the bone flaps and protrusion of brain tissue through the defect may occur as a result of steam pressure within the skull (Fig. XI-20). Cracks of the skull are rarely limited to the external table. If the appearance of the fracture is not typical, distinction from a fracture sustained during life may occasionally be difficult.

Curiously, heat fractures do not generally involve the sutures of the skull, even in young individuals with open sutures. Heat fractures may cross a suture line, but it is unlikely that a suture will gape by steam pressure alone. Complete burning of the scalp and exposure of the skull is common. The bone becomes brittle, particularly if contacted directly by the flames. Blood and marrow are expressed from the skull bones by the heat and accumulate between the undersurface of the bone and the dura mater, forming a clotlike structure that may be easily mistaken for an epidural hematoma sustained during life (Fig. XI-21). The overlying bone is commonly badly damaged by the flames, but fractures need not necessarily be present. The brain is usually shrunken, firm and yellow to light brown due to cooking (Fig. XI-22). The dura mater is leathery and without evidence of injury. The presence of blood *under* the dura mater (subdural hemorrhage) in a victim of conflagration always indicates an injury sustained while the victim was alive and is not related to the effect of the heat or flames. Such subdural blood should invariably be retained and submitted to the laboratory for chemical analyses. A positive alcohol level in these clots indicates that the deceased had been consuming alcoholic beverages before he sustained his head

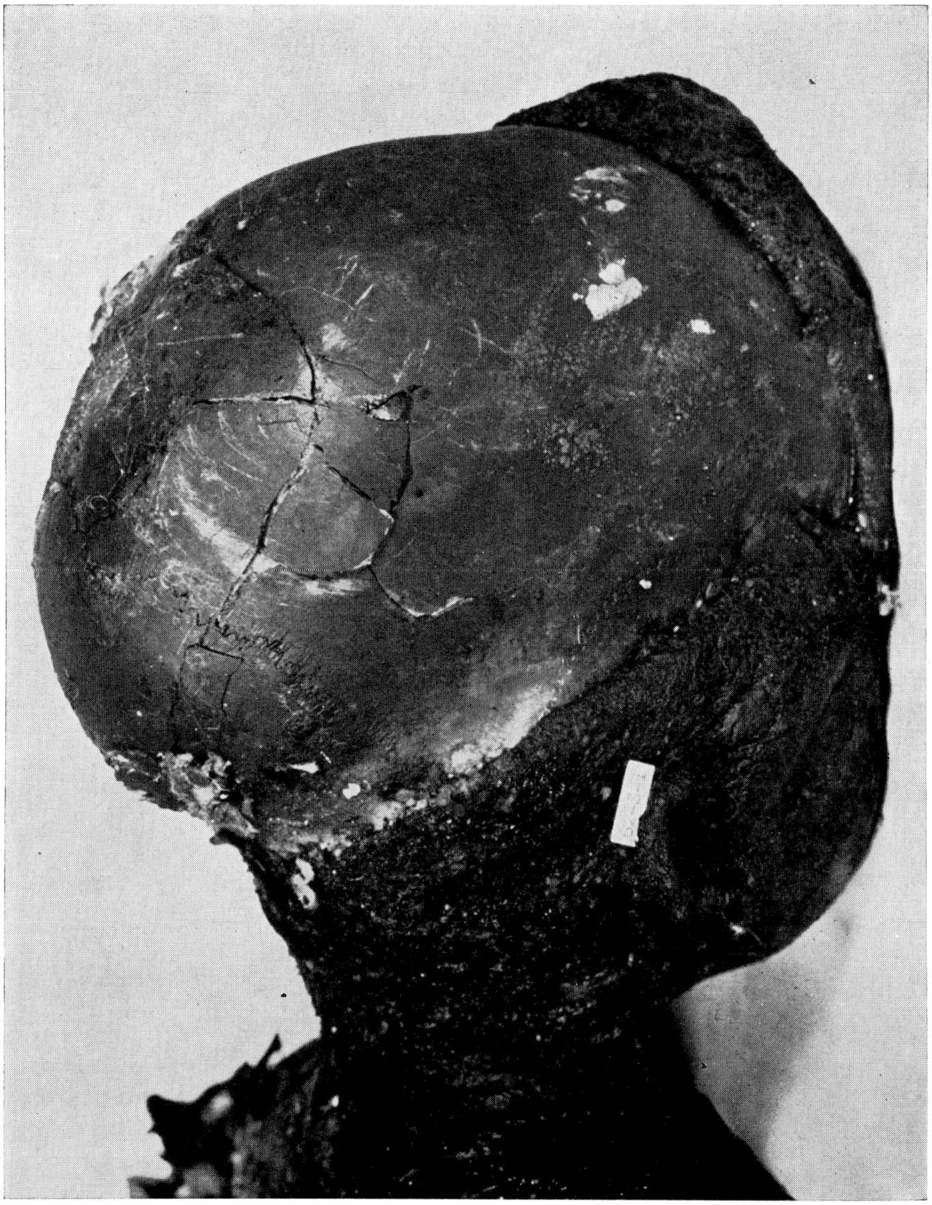

FIGURE XI-19. Heat fracture of the skull; the bone fragments are bent outward due to the steam pressure within the skull.

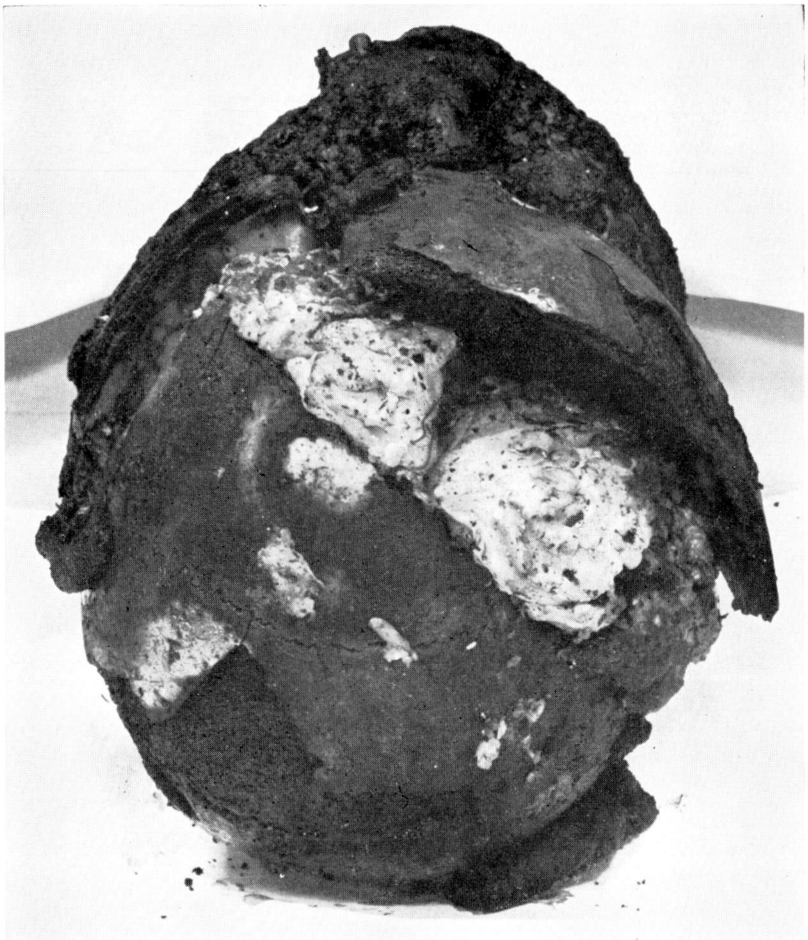

FIGURE XI-20. Outward bursting of bone flaps and protrusion of cooked brain tissue in a victim of fire.

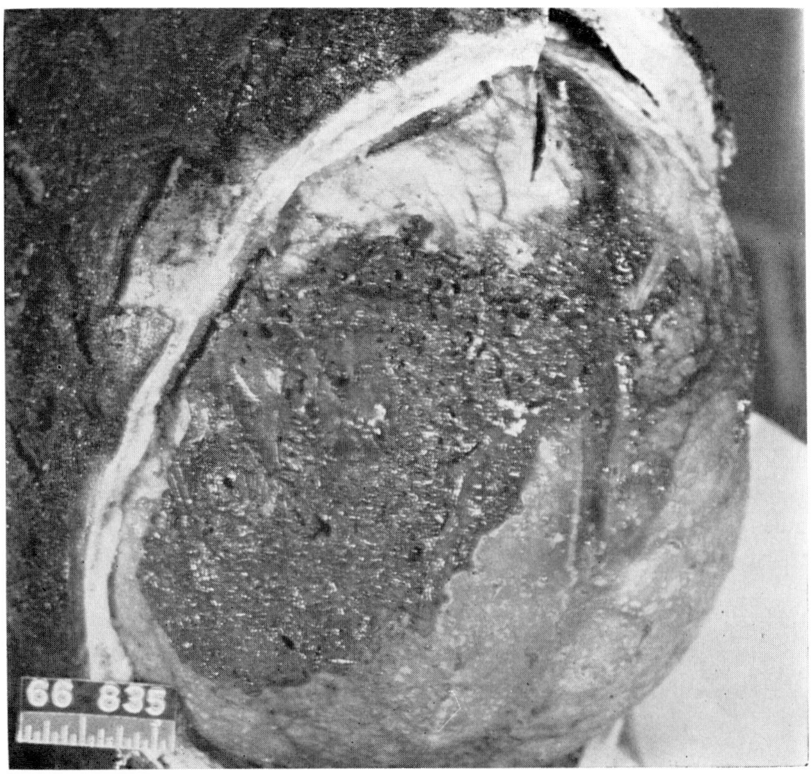


FIGURE XI-21. Epidural hematoma caused by heat. The calvarium has been removed. The dura mater is intact. The clot is due to blood and marrow expressed by the heat from the bones of the skull. Steam pressure moved the released blood and marrow to one place, forming a single clot.

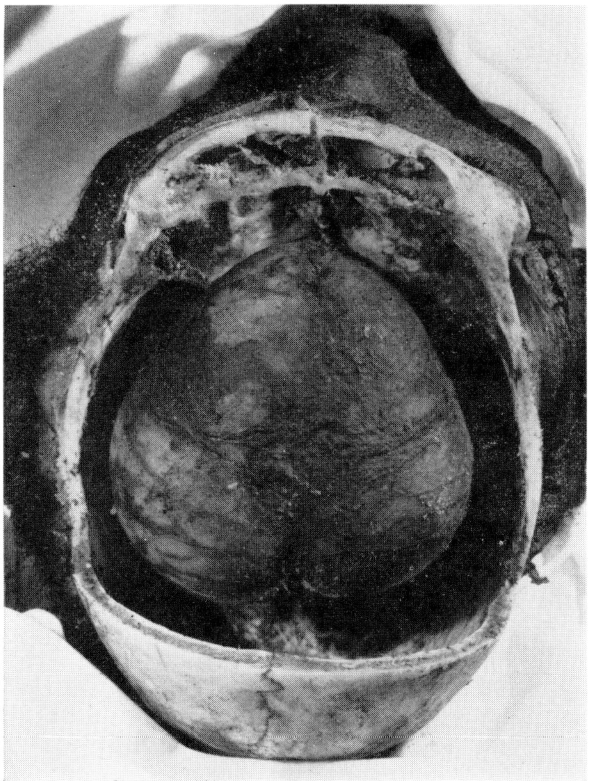

FIGURE XI-22. Shrinking of the brain within the skull of a fire victim. The brain is enclosed in the intact dura mater.

injury. Several days may elapse between the injury and death. In this period the alcohol in the peripheral blood may have been metabolized. It is thus conceivable that a subdural clot may show the presence of alcohol while the peripheral blood of the same individual indicates a negative alcohol level.

Heat that builds up in the chest of a fire victim is sometimes associated with blood pressed out of the lung tissue into the alveoli, airway, mouth and nostrils in much the same fashion as blood and bone marrow are expressed from the skull, forming an epidural clot. The condition may simulate blood that was inhaled during life, suggesting injury.

Splitting of the skin in a fire victim occurs in much the same fashion as the heat fractures of the skull. The abdominal cavity may be exposed. It is important to distinguish these postmortem splits from antemortem cuts and slashes (Fig. XI-23).

In a fire victim the anus is occasionally dilated due to shrinkage of the perianal tissues by the heat. This could be mistaken for sodomy or homosexuality. The same phenomenon sometimes occurs as a result of increased abdominal pressure from gas buildup caused by ordinary putrefaction.

### Injury Due to Scalding

Liquids at temperatures above 130° F will usually cause injury to the skin. The mucous membranes of the mouth and throat are considerably more resistant. We can, therefore, eat and drink foods too hot to touch with our hands. The severity of injury will depend on the temperature, the duration of contact and the sensitivity of the skin. The skin of a child is more sensitive than that of an adult; certain areas of the body are more sensitive than others. For example, the palmar surface of the hands is markedly more resistant to heat than the face, the abdomen or the genitalia. Household hot water is generally 130° to 140° F and may reach 160° F. Second or third degree burns may result if a hot water tap is opened inadvertently while bathing or if a child spills the contents of a hot cooking pot on himself. In industry, steam from a boiler will do the same. It should be emphasized that scalding may occur through clothing. The extent of the damage is in no way comparable to that caused by fire.

Singeing of hair does not occur as a result of scalding. This enables distinction of a second degree scald from a similar burn caused by fire.

It is frequently mandatory to differentiate between accidental scalding due to spilling or splashing and scalding due to deliberate pouring or throwing of hot liquids. Immersion of a child in hot water by an abusive parent or sibling is sometimes the cause of scalding. It is important under such circumstances that the distribution of the scalds be evaluated in light of the manner in which the injury was supposedly sustained. This will indicate the compatibility of a certain scalding pattern with a given history.

Inhalation of hot vapor may cause death with-

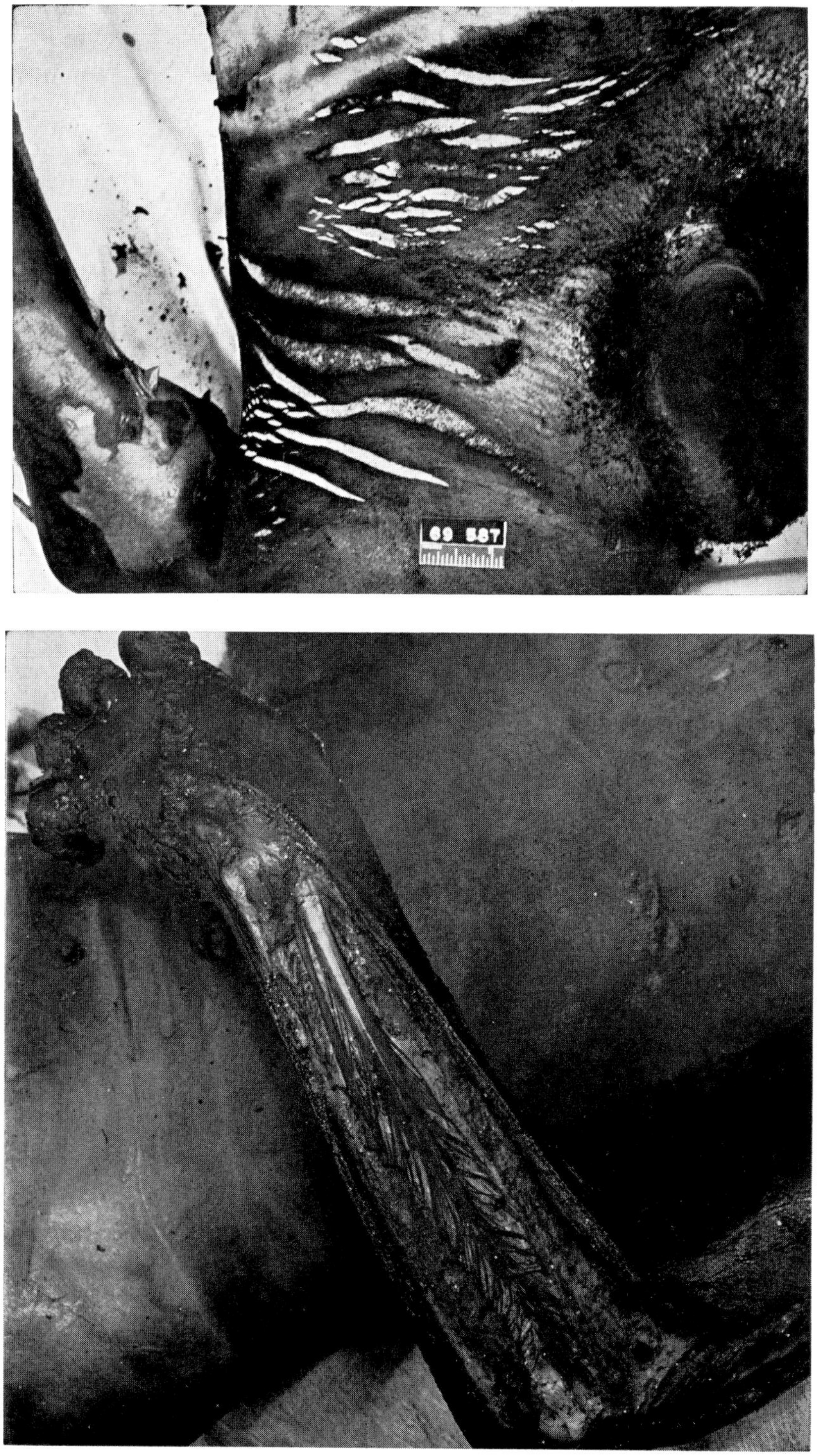


FIGURE XI-23a and b. Splitting of the skin as the result of heat. Only the skin is involved, while the underlying tissues are intact.

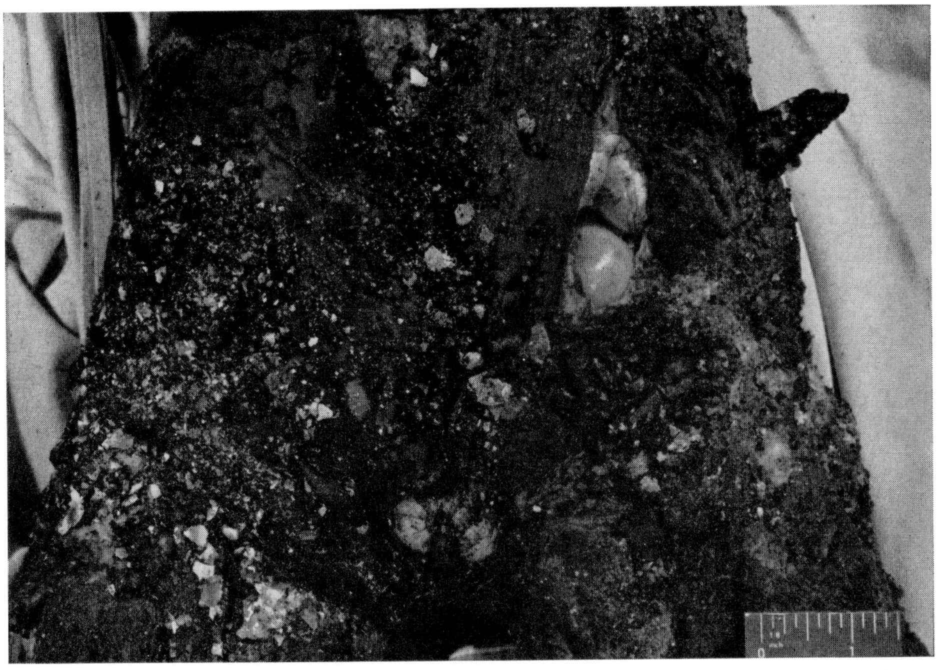

FIGURE XI-23c. Charred body of a young boy with a stab-wound-like split of the abdominal wall. The split is vertical between muscles (rather than *through* muscle substance) and is a result of increased abdominal pressure caused by the heat. Loops of uninjured bowel protruded through the gap and were replaced before this photograph was taken. There was no bleeding into the abdominal cavity.

out external manifestations of injury. It follows a short asymptomatic period, gradually developing into a progressively worsening shortness of breath and asphyxia resulting from obstruction of the airway by edematous swelling of its lining membrane.

## MEDICOLEGAL CONSIDERATIONS OF BOMB EXPLOSIONS

The postmortem examination of an explosion victim involves two main objectives: (a) identification, (b) reconstruction of the events.

With the wave of bombings in the United States and elsewhere, this subject matter has markedly increased in importance. There were close to 8000 separate bombing incidents in the United States alone in 1970, and several fatalities have occurred. There is no reason to believe that this form of violence will abate in the near future.

Procedures for identification of explosion victims are the same as those for identification in general, but certain complications result whenever there is wide dispersion of body parts by the blast. Destruction of the face places particular emphasis on other means of identification. The jaws and fingers may be blown off and must be retrieved for identification by dental comparison or fingerprints.

With respect to reconstruction of the event, location and extent of the injuries are of foremost significance.

In a case involving an explosion in an automobile,[9] examination of the two victims established who was the driver and who the passenger in the right front seat. It was further determined that the bomb was located on the floorboard between the passenger's feet and that he was bending over and most probably holding the bomb when the blast occurred (Fig. XI-24). On-the-scene examination of the automobile by explosion specialists confirmed the conclusions of the medical examiner and added that the explosive charge was definitely not in the glove compartment or affixed to the vehicle under the floorboard, which would have indicated sabotage.

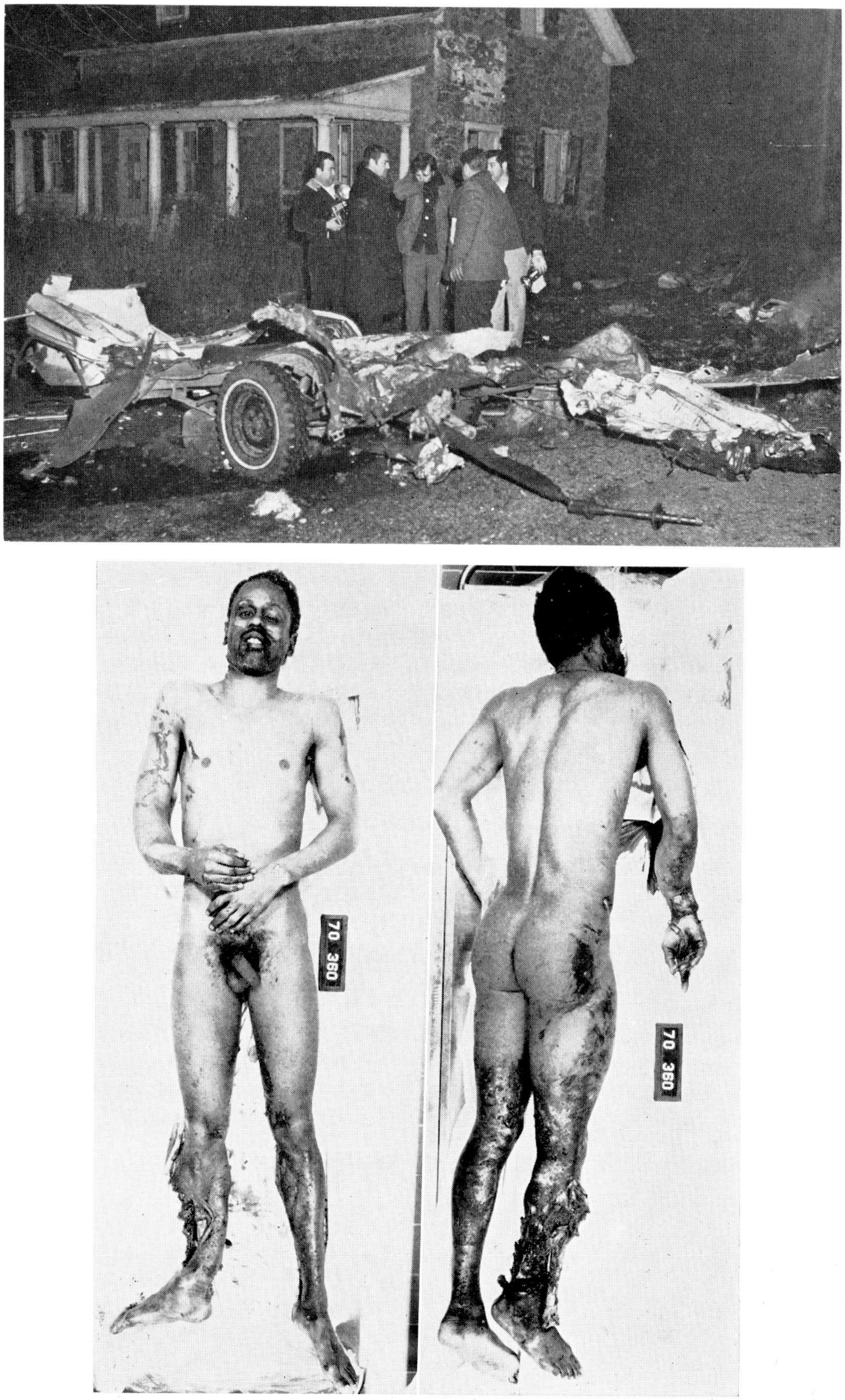


FIGURE XI-24. (a): Explosion scene, showing the extensive destruction of the automobile. Fragments were found 162 ft. away from the center of the explosion. (b): Front and back view of the driver of the automobile, showing that the injuries are confined to the right side. The right forearm and the right leg are fractured. The back and the buttocks are intact.

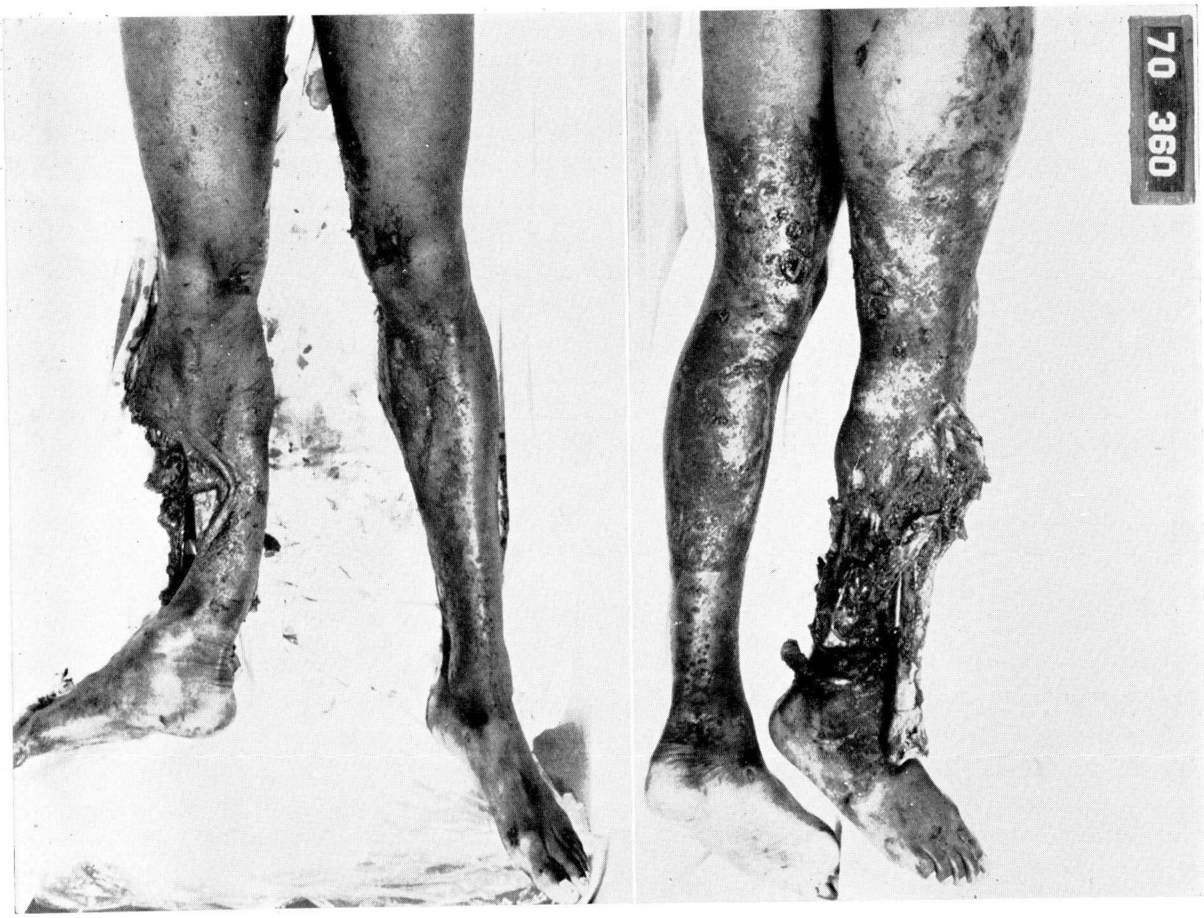


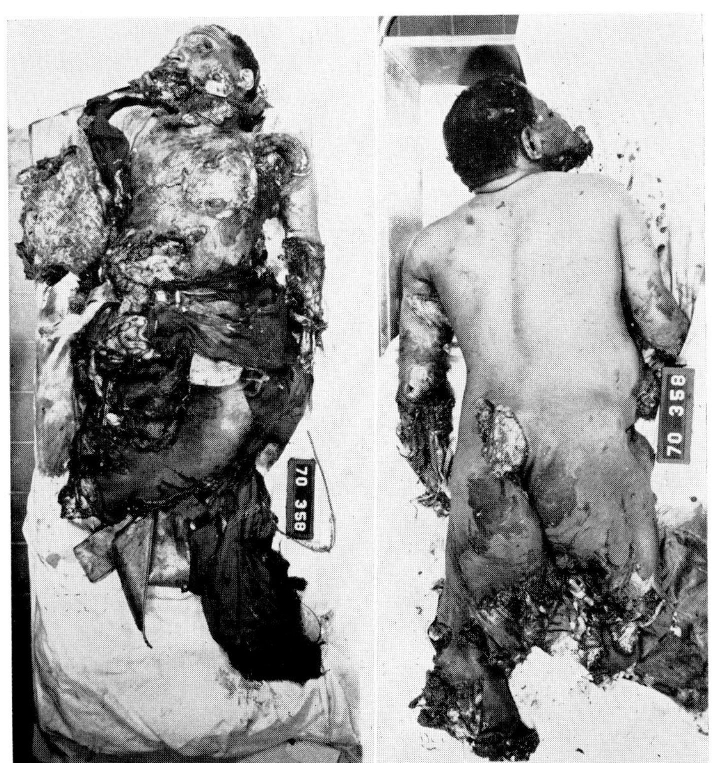


FIGURE XI-24. (c): A closer view of the lower extremities of the driver shows the shredding of the musculature of the right leg with particular involvement of the outer aspect of the leg. The inner aspect of the left leg is singed to the shinline, and in the rear singeing is limited by a vertical plane through the middle of the calf. (d): The body of the passenger of the right front seat shows extensive mutilating injuries with partial amputation of the extremities and partial exposure of the abdomen and lower chest. A narrow strip of intact skin was preserved under the belt. The pattern and the distribution of the injuries permitted the conclusion that the bomb was situated between the feet of the victim and that he was probably slightly bent over, holding the bomb at the time of the explosion. The facial skeleton was fragmented and features unrecognizable. (Figures XI-24b through d courtesy of Callaghan & Co. From Spitz, W. U., Sopher, I. M., and DiMaio, V. J. M.: Medicolegal investigation of a bomb explosion in an automobile. *J Forensic Sci, 15*:537-552, 1970.)

The combined results of the independent investigations by the medical examiner and the police left no doubt that the explosion occurred accidentally when the bomb was being transported by the occupants of the vehicle. Test explosions conducted by the FBI indicate that twelve sticks of 40% dynamite placed on the right floorboard of an automobile are required to produce damage equivalent to that of the automobile in question.

Death due to an explosion may be associated with extensive external injuries, as seen in the passenger mentioned previously. Multiple external injuries may also be caused by falling debris or cave-in and burial under rubble. However, in some instances death may occur without external manifestations of trauma. These deaths result from massive hemorrhages in the lungs due to the shock wave following the blast. This is a concussion-type injury, and death may be practically instantaneous.

Extensive confluent hemorrhages were noted in both lungs of the driver of the vehicle described earlier. The same injury was reported as the prevalent cause of death in individuals who were not injured by shrapnel or fire but who were situated within the blast diameter of exploding bombs in the London blitz of World War II.[10]

A large variety of bombs are used, many of which are homemade. It is important after an explosion that an attempt be made to ascertain the materials that were used in the construction of the bomb, since this may provide leads to the identity of the perpetrator. Complete body x ray of the victims is imperative before the clothing is removed. Fragments of the bomb may be trapped within the body tissues or the clothing. In the case of the automobile explosion mentioned previously, x ray films of the passenger revealed a number of metallic objects in the skull and trunk. Subsequently, at autopsy, a 1.5 v mercury battery was recovered from within the skull, and other remnants, including a small portion of a spring, several rivets and two ½ in. long, thin metallic wires, were removed from the chest and abdomen. Some of the fragments used for the firing system of the bomb were identified as originating from a key-wound clock movement characteristic of a specific manufacturer.

It is of utmost importance that the clothing be retained for chemical analyses, since this too may reveal the presence of trace evidence with respect to the type of explosive that was used. It should be mentioned in this regard that victims who are close to an explosion may be found partly or completely nude. Their clothes are blown off by the blast and may be recovered in shreds at a considerable distance from the victim. Tight articles such as a belt, a buttoned collar, or lace-up boots are commonly retained on the body.

While explosives are notorious for their blasting and fragmentation effects, incendiary bombs primarily cause burns. Napalm belongs to this category. Napalm consists of a combination of oil and gasoline in a jellied form. It generates a temperature of close to 1800° F. Phosphorus and magnesium are frequent additives to incendiary bombs and grenades. Under such circumstances temperatures may exceed 3500° F. Systemic poisoning by the added chemicals is sometimes observed.

The *Molotov cocktail* is another variety of incendiary bomb. It is designed to be hand thrown and has been frequently used by terrorists and in guerilla warfare. It has a considerable psychological and devastating effect. A crude version of this bomb consists of a bottle filled with gasoline and a rag to serve as a wick. The wick is lit, and the cocktail is thrown at the target. Addition of various acids and chemicals enhances the destructive effect of the device.

## REFERENCES

1. Svensson, A., and Wendel, O.: *Crime Detection.* Amsterdam, Elsevier, 1955.
2. Richards, N. F.: Fire investigation—Destruction of corpses. *Med Sci Law, 17*:79, 1977.
3. Bezymenski, L.: *The Death of Adolf Hitler.* New York, HarBraceWorld, 1968.
4. Gonzales, T. A., Vance, M. V., Helpern, M., and Umberger, Ch.J.: Asphyxiating gases. In *Legal*

*Medicine Pathology and Toxicology,* 2nd ed. New York, Appleton, 1954, p. 502.
5. Mueller, B.: Blut-, Atmungs- und Fermentgifte. In *Gerichtliche Medizin.* Berlin, Springer, 1953, p. 693.
6. Dérobèrt et al.: Cited in Mueller, B.: Blut-, Atmungs-, und Fermentgifte. In *Gerichtliche Medizin.* Berlin, Springer, 1953, p. 693.
7. Franke: Cited in Mueller, B.: Blut-, Atmungs- und Fermentgifte. In *Gerichtliche Medizin.* Berlin, Springer, 1953, p. 693.
8. Wiener, M. F. Carbon monoxide poisoning: Basic concepts and current clinical-pathologic implications. In Sunderman, F. W., and Sunderman, F. W., Jr. (Eds.): *Laboratory Diagnosis of Diseases Caused by Toxic Agents.* St. Louis, Green, 1970, pp. 259-277.
9. Spitz, W. U., Sopher, I. M., and DiMaio, V. J. M.: Medicolegal investigation of a bomb explosion in an automobile. *J Forensic Sci, 15:*537, 1970.
10. Zuckerman, S.: Experimental study of blast injuries to the lung. *Lancet, 2:*219, 1940.

*Chapter XII*

# ASPHYXIA

Werner U. Spitz

Asphyxia is a broad term encompassing a variety of conditions that result in interference with the uptake or utilization of oxygen together with failure to eliminate carbon dioxide ($CO_2$). The tissues of the body cannot function without oxygen. Subnormal oxygen in the blood supply to the brain causes rapid unconsciousness. The brain is most sensitive to oxygen deprivation, and for this reason it is the organ most intimately affected in all types of asphyxial death.

In all forms of asphyxia heart action may continue for several minutes after respiratory standstill. This is of critical importance in effecting resuscitation.

For practical purposes, asphyxia falls into one of the following categories:

1. *Compression of the neck,* with or without blockage of the airway, as in
   a. Hanging
   b. Strangulation (throttling)
2. *Obstruction of the airway,* as in
   a. Smothering
   b. Aspiration of foreign material
   c. Swelling of the lining membranes, as in certain allergic and inflammatory reactions or following a blow to the neck
3. *Compression of the chest* sufficient to prevent adequate respiratory movements
4. *Exclusion of oxygen* by depletion and replacement by another gas or by chemical interference with its uptake and utilization by the body.
   a. Carbon dioxide poisoning
   b. Carbon monoxide poisoning
   c. Cyanide poisoning

## COMPRESSION OF THE NECK

### Hanging

Death by hanging usually results from arrest of the arterial blood supply to the brain or obstruction of the venous return from it. In either case the brain tissue is deprived of oxygen, resulting in loss of consciousness in less than two to three minutes. The amount of pressure on the neck that can bring about loss of consciousness is surprisingly low.[1] Loss of consciousness is followed by increased pressure on the neck from the added weight of the suspended limp body. This, in turn, completely occludes the arteries, and death supervenes as the oxygen is depleted. The insidious and inadvertent loss of consciousness accounts for a large number of accidental hangings, particularly in children. An example of this gradual transition into unconsciousness may be found in the following case:

A seventeen-month-old child was playing in his crib with a toy telephone and was heard by his mother, who was in an adjacent room. When the mother heard no sound from the child for a *few minutes,* she checked and found him dead, with the telephone cord around his neck. The receiver was beside the child; the phone had slipped from the mattress and was suspended between the bars. The weight of this phone was sufficient to interfere with the cerebral blood supply. There was no evidence of a struggle; the nonfitted sheet was in order, and the child was not heard to have cried out (Fig. XII-1).

A very similar situation occurs in the so-called autoerotic deaths *(vide infra).* Judging from the circumstances in which these individuals are found, there is certainly no indication that this is an *unpleasant* mode of death. It seems as though the individual has gone to sleep, unfortunately to be found in this predicament.

Actual compression of the airway by the noose in hanging cases is not as common as is

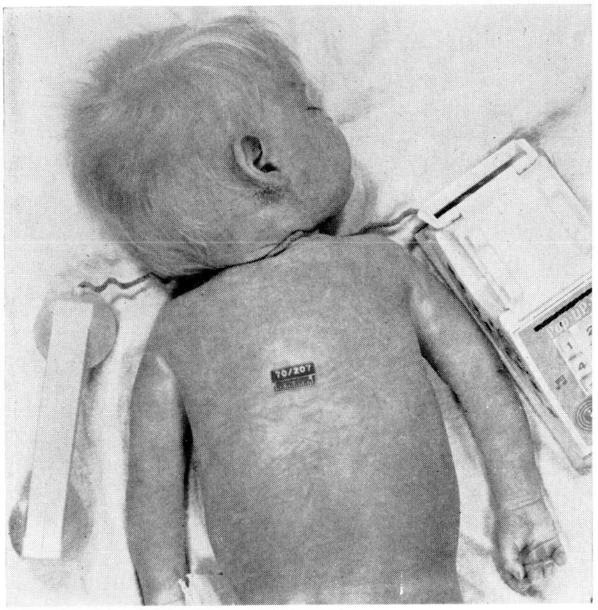

FIGURE XII-1. Seventeen-month-old child, showing toy telephone cord around the neck. The pressure exerted by the weight of the phone hindered the blood flow to and from the brain.

generally believed. Supporting evidence for this includes the finding of vomitus in the bronchi of numerous hanging victims. Suicidal hanging by persons with an artificial opening into their airway (tracheostomy) below the level of the noose[2] may equally serve to illustrate this point (Fig. XII-2). Such individuals continue to breathe while dying of hanging. Occlusion of the airway invariably elicits a struggle, a dramatic condition commonly referred to as *air hunger*.

A mode of death that is now rarely seen in hanging is fracture of the odontoid process of the second cervical vertebra. When hanging was the prevalent form of judicial execution, such fractures caused almost instantaneous death by pressure of the dislodged bony process on vital nerve centers of the brain (medulla) controlling respiration and heartbeat. The weight of the individual to be hanged was directly proportional to the distance he was made to drop.

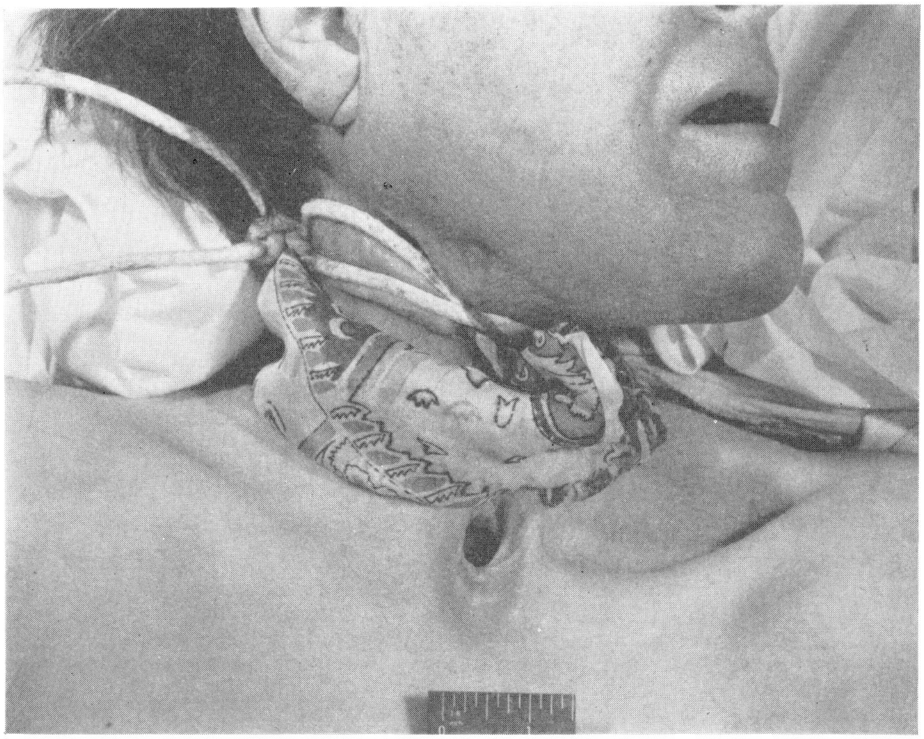

FIGURE XII-2. Sixty-one-year-old woman who committed suicide by hanging. She was despondent because of the removal of a cancerous larynx. A tracheostomy is noted below the noose.

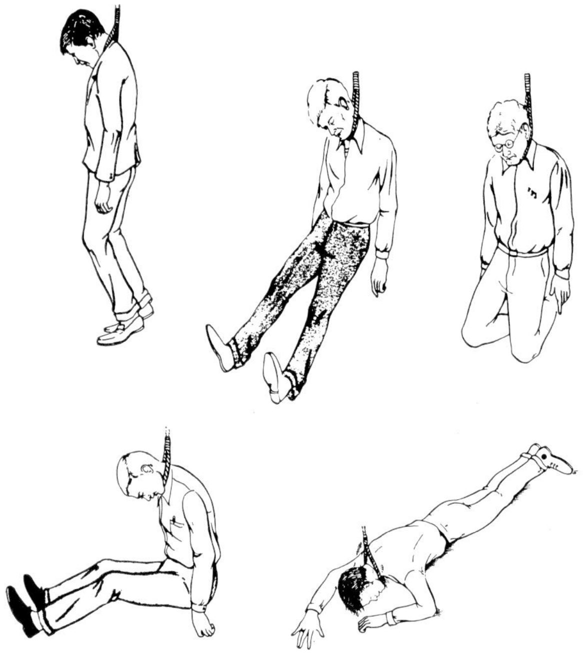

FIGURE XII-3. Hanging can take place in any position.

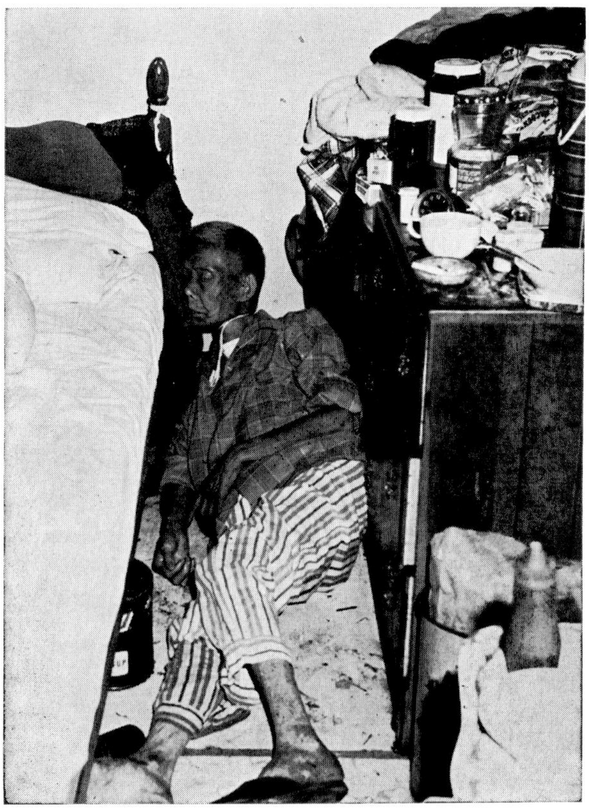

FIGURE XII-4. Fifty-two-year-old man who lived alone and had been despondent. A neighbor found him hanging from the bedpost in the position shown. The neighbor cut the rope and called the police.

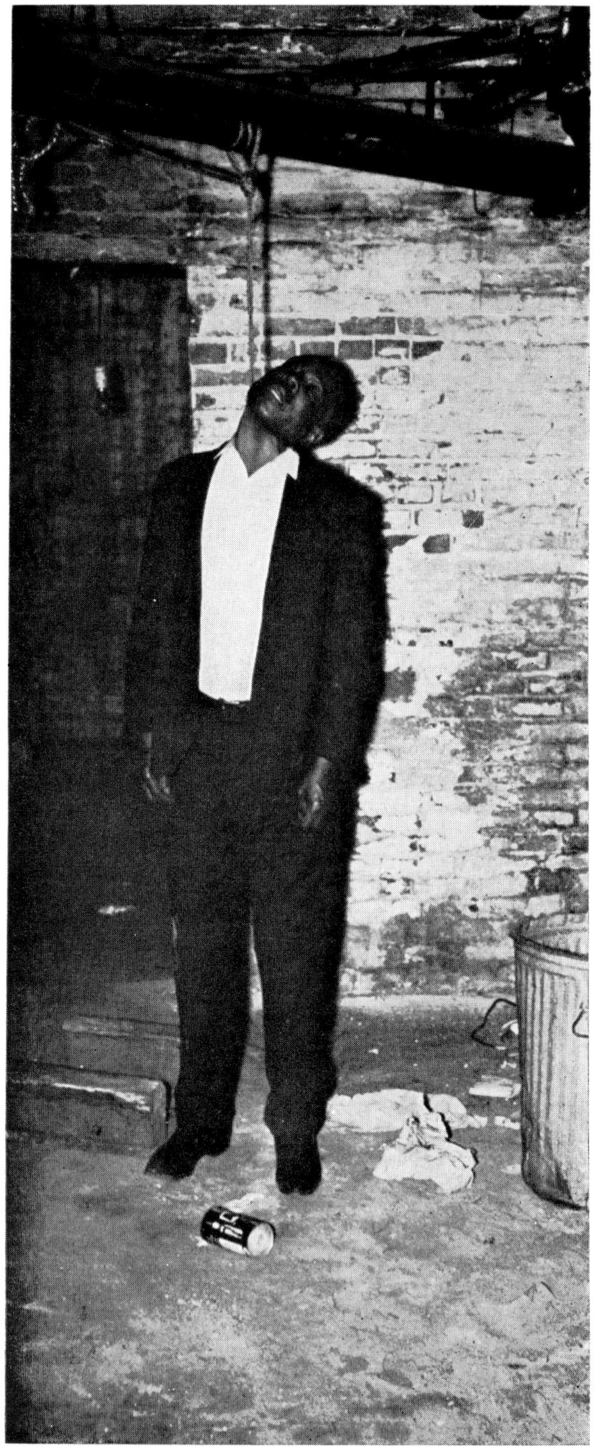

FIGURE XII-5. Forty-five-year-old janitor who hanged himself in the basement of the building in which he worked. Note the erect position of the victim: both feet are on the ground.

The knot was positioned in a manner to effect a sudden backlash of the head at the same time as the body was brought to an abrupt halt at the end of the rope. According to Pierrepoint, the former hangman of London, in his testimony before the Royal Commission on Capital Punishment in 1950, the knot must be situated under the left side of the jaw to throw the head back and snap the neck at the moment of the drop. If the knot were on the right side, the head would be thrown forward and cause strangulation.[3]

Hanging can take place with the victim in any position (Fig. XII-3), provided the pressure on the neck is maintained above that necessary for vascular occlusion. Hanging in a semireclining or standing position is thus not at all unusual (Figs. XII-4 to XII-7). Due to the relative ease with which hanging can be effected, almost any type of noose around the neck will suffice. Children occasionally hang themselves in the crib by various means. As an example, the case of a fifteen-month-old child who slipped between the mattress and the side of his crib, remaining semisuspended by the neck while his feet dangled on the floor, may be cited.

Such accidents result from the use of defective, usually old, cribs in which the lower side rail has come loose, permitting it to be pushed outward (Fig. XII-8).[4]

Hanging usually leaves definite, readily recognizable evidence, even if the individual has been cut down and the scene altered to suggest a different mode of death. A groove (or furrow) in the neck may suggest the type of loop used (Fig. XII-9). The weave of the rope may be imprinted on the skin, permitting a match of patterns. In a typical suicidal hanging the arms of the loop pass around the neck and climb toward the knot. An abraded area of skin often marks the site of the knot. Hanging grooves should be thoroughly examined. When fresh they may be considerably less conspicuous than after drying for several hours. Hanging may occur, however, without visible marks on the victim's neck. A loop made of soft material, as a towel or a scarf, will probably leave no noticeable injury, although the knot, if there was one, may well produce a patterned abrasion due to its firmness (Fig. XII-10). Clothing is often used in suicidal jail hangings.

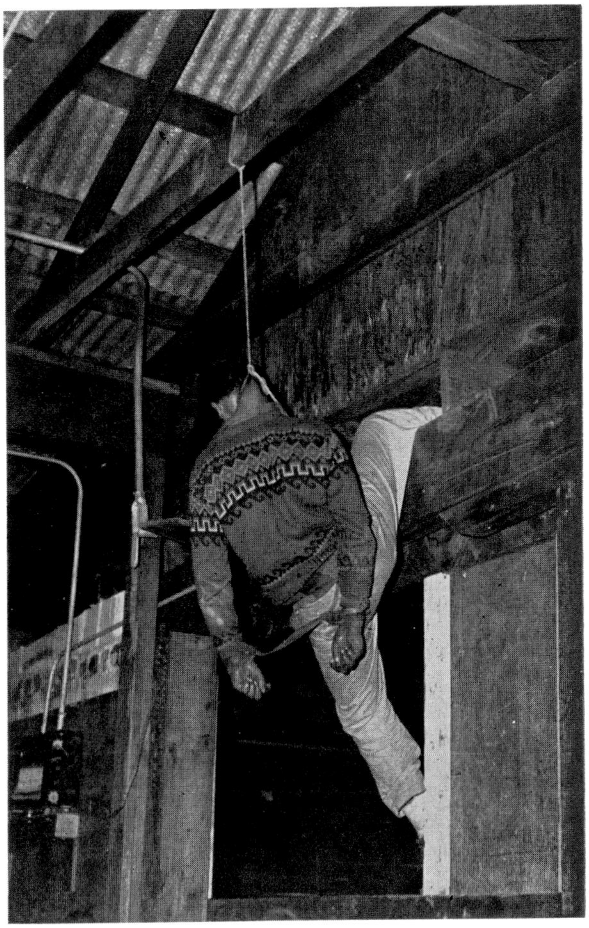

FIGURE XII-6. The body of this man was found in an abandoned warehouse, suspended from a rafter above the floor. The scene suggested foul play; however, there was no evidence of a struggle. A suicide note in a stamped and sealed envelope, addressed to the police, was found in the pocket of the victim. It read as follows: "This is Albert, I am sorry if i put yours a lot off mess. But i thout that God was going to forgive me for what i have done. I did not want to run from God or no one. i am Sorry."

Skin folds on the neck in obese persons or in infants may resemble a noose mark, particularly after refrigeration of the body has caused congealing of the subcutaneous fat. Conversely, the hanging groove is soon obliterated with decomposition of the body.

Scattered pinpoint hemorrhages are often present in the face of the hanging victim, par-

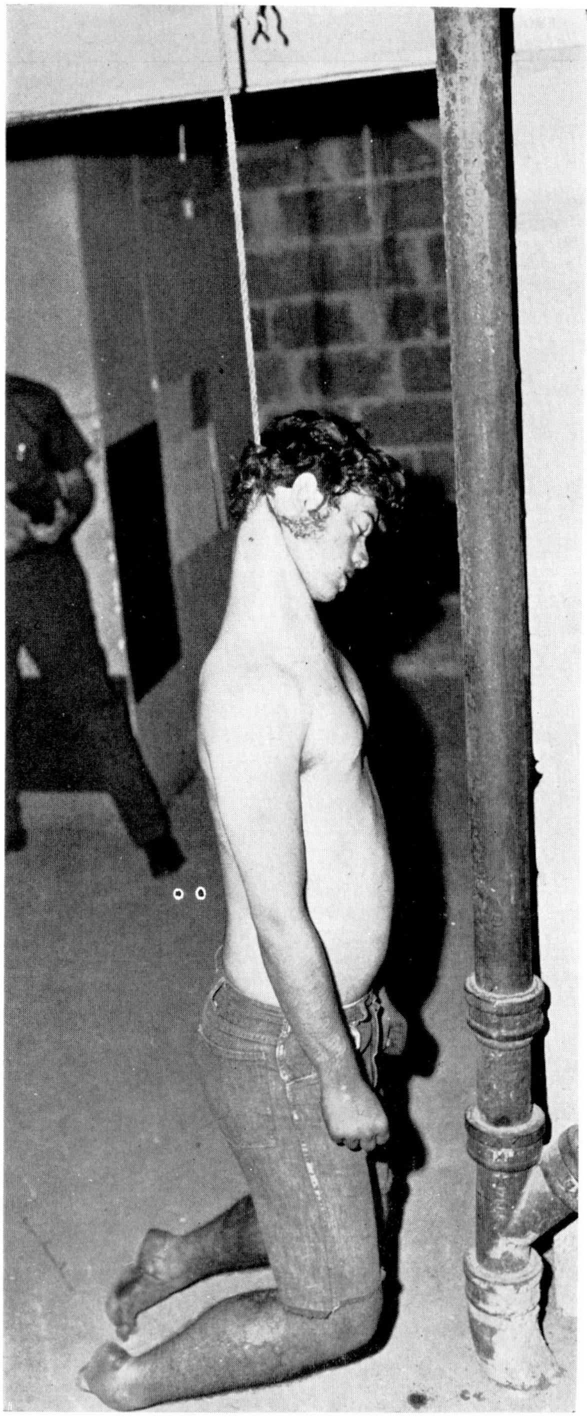

FIGURE XII-7. Twenty-year-old college student found in the basement of his residence. He was in semikneeling position, suspended from a beam in the ceiling.

ticularly in the conjunctivae and eyelids. Occasionally they may be observed in the mucosa of the mouth and throat, as well as in the muscles of the temples and under the serosal surfaces of the pleura and the epicardium. They were first described by Tardieu and are commonly referred to as *Tardieu's spots.* He considered them indicative of asphyxial death. It has been shown, however, that petechial hemorrhages are by no means always indicative of death by suffocation. Identical hemorrhages, especially in the conjunctivae and the skin, are often found in cases of natural death with marked facial lividity, particularly in plethoric and obese individuals and in those who died of acute right heart failure with markedly elevated venous pressure.

In cases where the hanging victim is found with his body *partially* supported, the face is dusky purple, congested and often slightly swollen. Pressure on the neck is insufficient to occlude both arteries and veins, and only the veins, which are nearer the surface as compared to the arteries, are closed. This causes blood carried into the head by the arteries to be trapped. The eyes are frequently protruberant and firmer than usual, apparently as a result of this congestion. The pinpoint hemorrhages of the face may extend to the level of the noose, but none are found below it.

When the body is found *completely* suspended, with feet off the ground, pressure on the neck is such that all blood supply to and from the head is interrupted. This causes the face to be pale, and the changes described earlier, including pinpoint hemorrhages, are not observed. Superficial incision along the groove produced by the noose may show small hemorrhages in the underlying layers of the skin. These hemorrhages, however, are not the result of congestion but are caused by direct trauma inflicted by the noose.

Injuries to the neck musculature are rare in hanging, and fracture of the thyroid cartilage or the hyoid bone are the exception rather than the rule. The latter in particular is fractured quite rarely. Such fractures are more likely to occur in elderly individuals who *jump to their death* and remain suspended after a *long drop,* due to calcification of the cartilage and fragility of the bony structures. A small horizontal tear of the inner lining of the

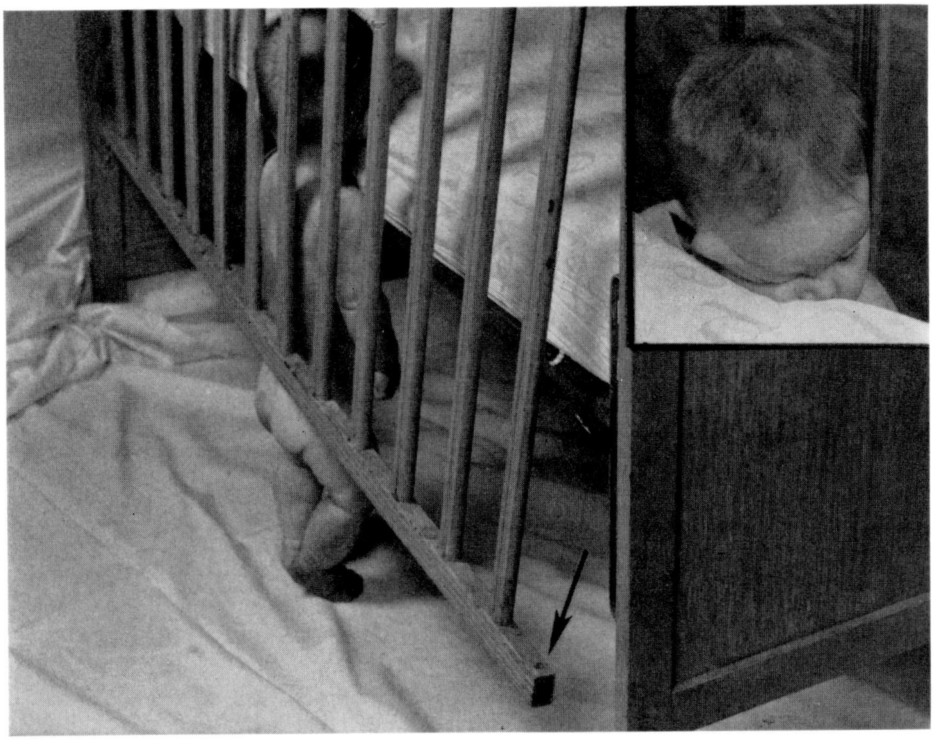

FIGURE XII-8. Infant trapped between the mattress and the side of the crib. The latter had been repaired but came loose (arrow), allowing the child to slip into the gap, causing compression of the head and neck.

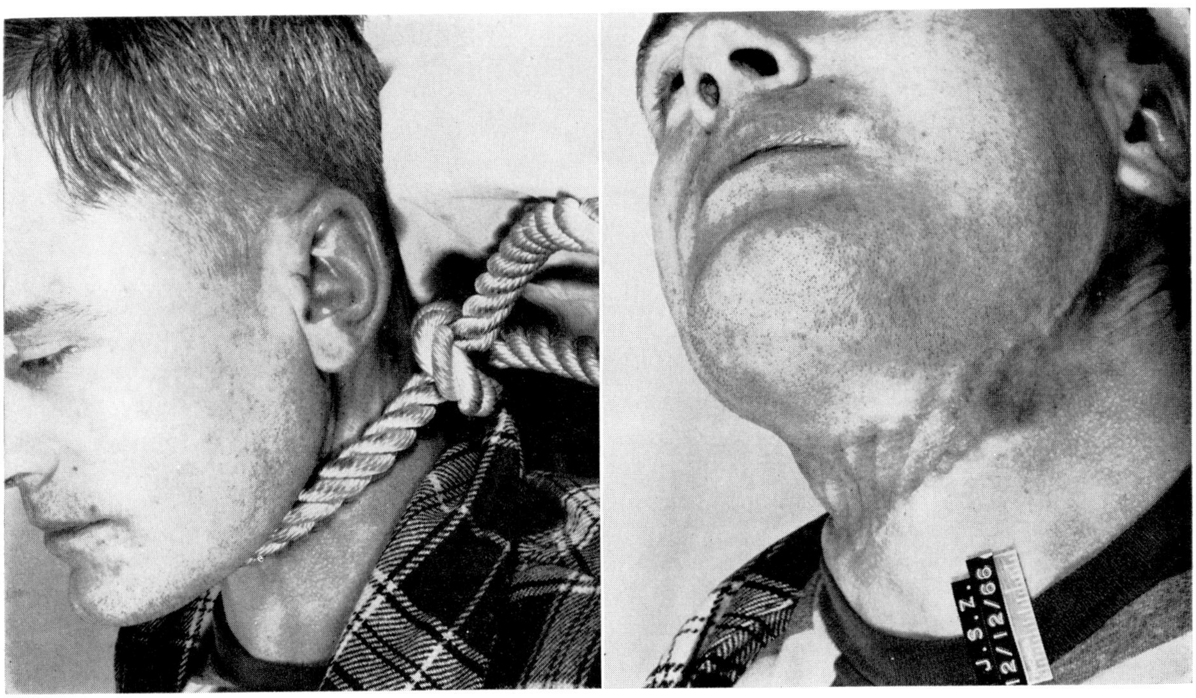

FIGURE XII-9. Suicidal hanging. Note the pattern of the rope imprinted on the neck. The dark discoloration of the imprint is due to drying.

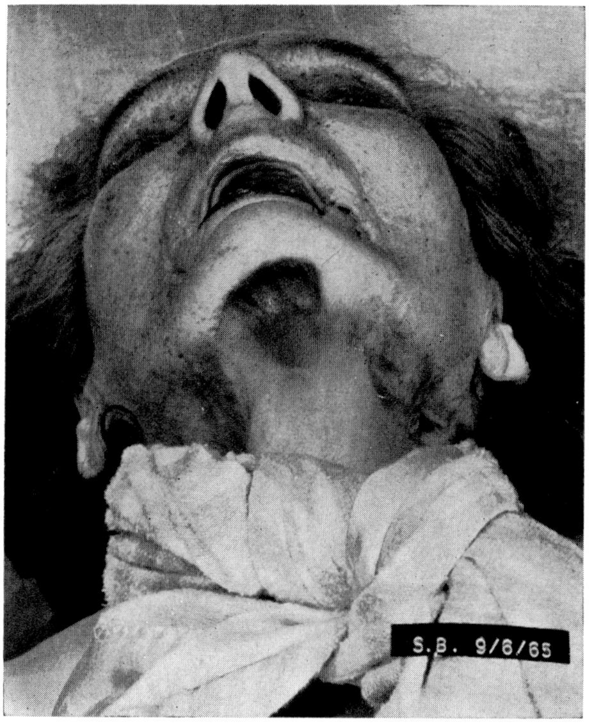


FIGURE XII-10. Elderly woman who hanged herself using a soft blanket attached to a door hinge. The imprint of the knot is well demonstrated on the chin, while the neck shows a faint mark made by the noose, visible as a result of drying. When the body was first viewed, the mark on the neck was not noticed.

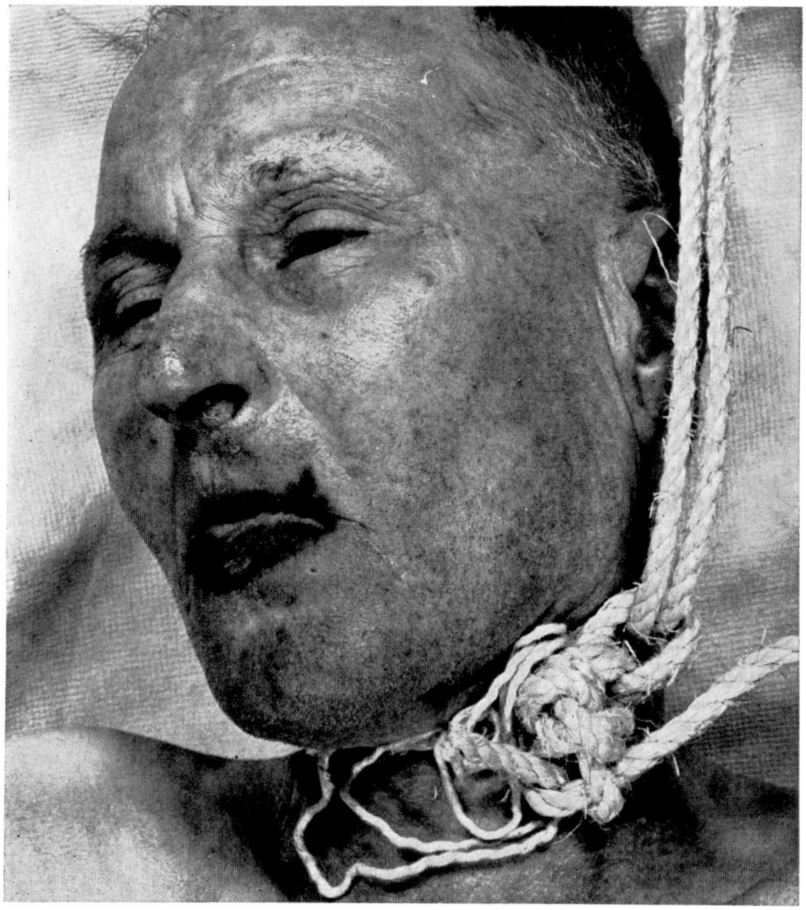

FIGURE XII-11. Upward pressure on the neck organs by the noose causes elevation and protrusion of the tongue. The exposed part becomes dark brown, even black, as a result of drying.

carotid artery with adjacent hemorrhage in the vessel wall is seen under the groove in a considerable number of hangings. These injuries result from friction of opposite sides of the vessel due to the pressure exerted by the ligature. Polson[2] attributes them to the *traction* associated with hanging. If *traction* were the case, one would expect to find a larger number of tears, not necessarily limited to the level of the ligature. Several horizontal intimal tears scattered along the carotid arteries at different levels are sometimes found in hanging associated with a *long drop* and in falls from height. In the latter they are often associated with a transverse tear of the first segment of the aorta.

Demonstration in the carotid arteries of frictional intimal tears surrounded by hemorrhage is important supplementary evidence that the victim was alive at the time of the hanging. This is in sharp contrast to a homicide followed by suspension of the body to suggest suicide. Opening the carotid arteries to the level of the mandible may be necessary to demonstrate these intimal tears. This procedure will interfere with subsequent injection of embalming fluids by the undertaker unless the arteries have been cannulated with tubing that is tightly secured in place at the time of autopsy. In this case the preparation of the body will not be affected.

The tongue frequently protrudes from the mouth of the hanging victim. The mechanism for this phenomenon is upward pressure on the neck organs by the noose, causing elevation of the tongue. The protruding part of the tongue is commonly dark brown or even black as a result of drying (Fig. XII-11). Protrusion of the tongue may also be seen in other modes of death.

Slight hemorrhage or bloody mucus may exude from the nose of the hanging victim, and some blood may be found under the body. This results from rupture of engorged blood vessels and should not be mistaken for evidence of foul play. Fluidity of the blood (absence of usual postmortem clotting), which is a constant feature in all types of asphyxial death, may well contribute to such bleeding. Where putrefaction has set in, dark red-brown and foul-smelling fluids that resemble blood may accumulate

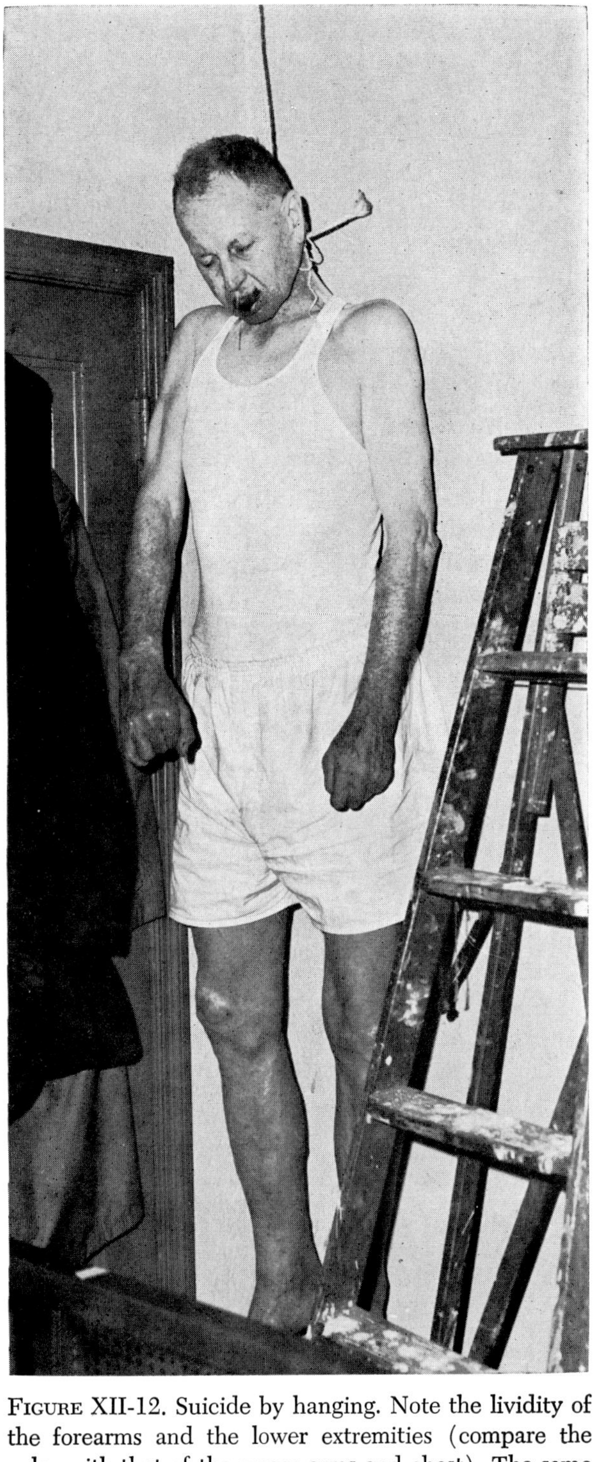

FIGURE XII-12. Suicide by hanging. Note the lividity of the forearms and the lower extremities (compare the color with that of the upper arms and chest). The same phenomenon is noted in Figure XII-7. Bloody mucus exudes from the nose.

under the body. Such fluids originate from the decomposing tissues and do not constitute evidence of injury. Hemorrhage into the middle ears is also seen occasionally in victims of hanging. This is due to excessive congestion and is not specifically associated with hanging or other modes of asphyxial death.

Postmortem lividity in the hanging victim suspended in the upright position is limited to the lower half of the body, including the hands and forearms (Fig. XII-12). If the body is cut down within four or five hours after death and is placed in the supine position, postmortem lividity in the extremities will fade and new areas of lividity will appear along the back and buttocks. This may be of importance if for publicity or insurance reasons a hanging suicide was placed in bed to suggest death from natural causes.

Scattered pinpoint and larger hemorrhages are often noted in areas of lividity in the hanging victim. These petechiae result from excessive engorgement, i.e. they represent an accentuation of the postmortem lividity. Their mechanism is identical to that of the petechiae in the face (Tardieu's spots), as mentioned earlier in this chapter.

A sixty-eight-year-old woman used a piece of a soft thin blanket to hang herself on a door hinge. She was found by her daughter, who cut her down, removed the blanket and placed her in bed. She then called the police and insisted she found her mother in that position. The daughter stated further that her mother had suffered from a heart condition and had been under the care of a physician. The latter, however, refused to sign the death certificate, as he had not seen the patient recently. Postmortem examination immediately suggested hanging due to pronounced lividity in the lower half of the body, while the back was quite pale. Pinpoint hemorrhages were noted abundantly in the conjunctivae, the face and on the legs. There was no impression of the loop on the skin of the neck, as the blanket was too soft and too wide, but the knot caused a typical abrasion under the chin. Upon questioning, the daughter admitted to changing the scene because she had been concerned about losing insurance benefits.

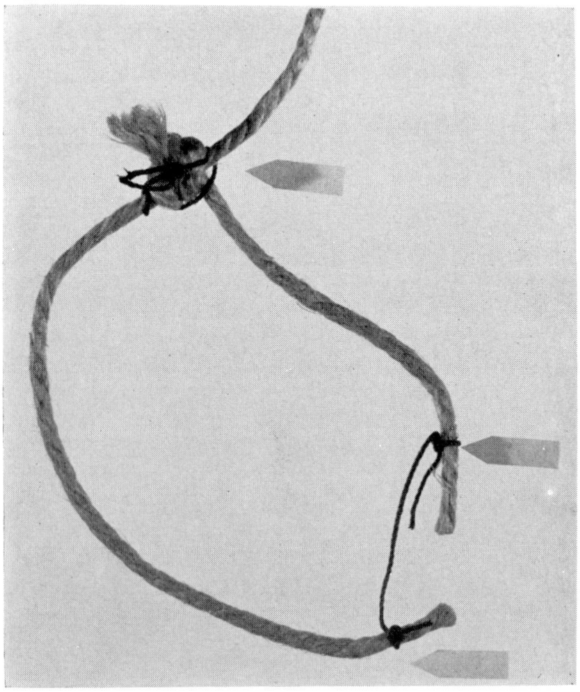

FIGURE XII-13. The noose of a hanging victim should be preserved. This is best done by cutting the noose away from the knot and securing the ends with string or wire. To assure preservation of the knot, it may be necessary to secure it independently.

Certain types of knots and nooses may suggest involvement of another party in what initially is an apparent suicide. In order to enable subsequent examination of a given noose, the knot should not be undone. Removal of the noose from the deceased is done by cutting the noose away from the knot and tying the cut ends with string or wire. This will enable adequate preservation (Fig. XII-13).

### Strangulation (Throttling)

Strangulation may be homicidal, suicidal or accidental. Homicidal strangulation may be manual or by ligature. Manual self-strangulation is impossible, as pressure on the neck depends on voluntary action, which is discontinued when the power of decision is obliterated with loss of consciousness. Manual strangulation, therefore, is always homicidal. A sexual motive to the crime must be considered. Detailed examination of the external and internal genital organs, including acid phosphatase determination on vaginal washings and microscopic search

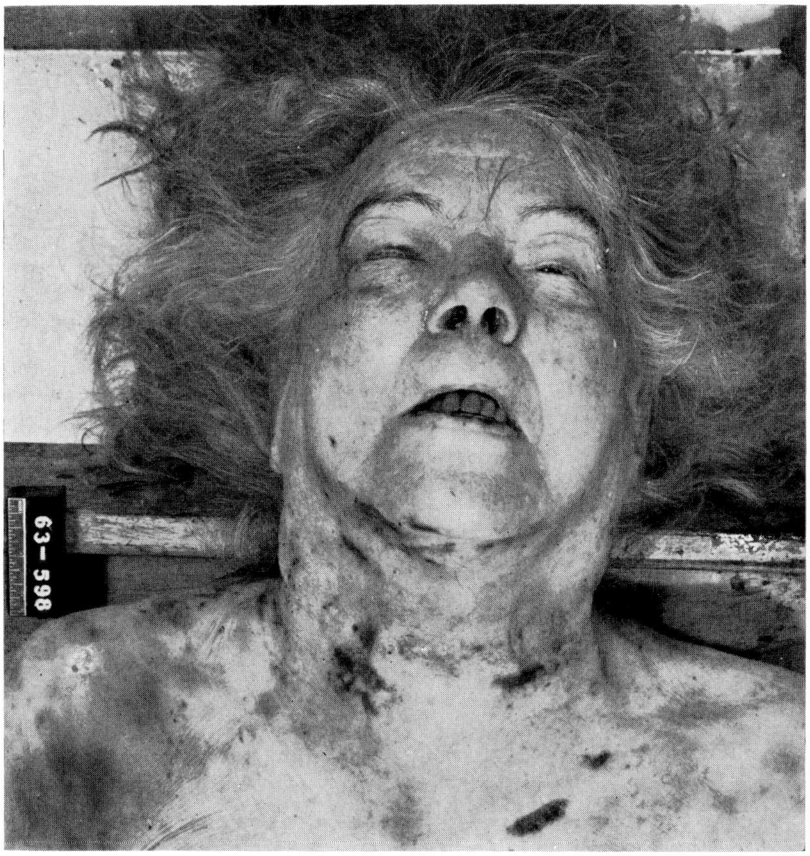


FIGURE XII-14a. Sixty-seven-year-old woman found dead in the bedroom of her apartment. She was raped and strangled. Note the extensive bruising on the neck. The upper chest and shoulder bruises indicate a struggle.

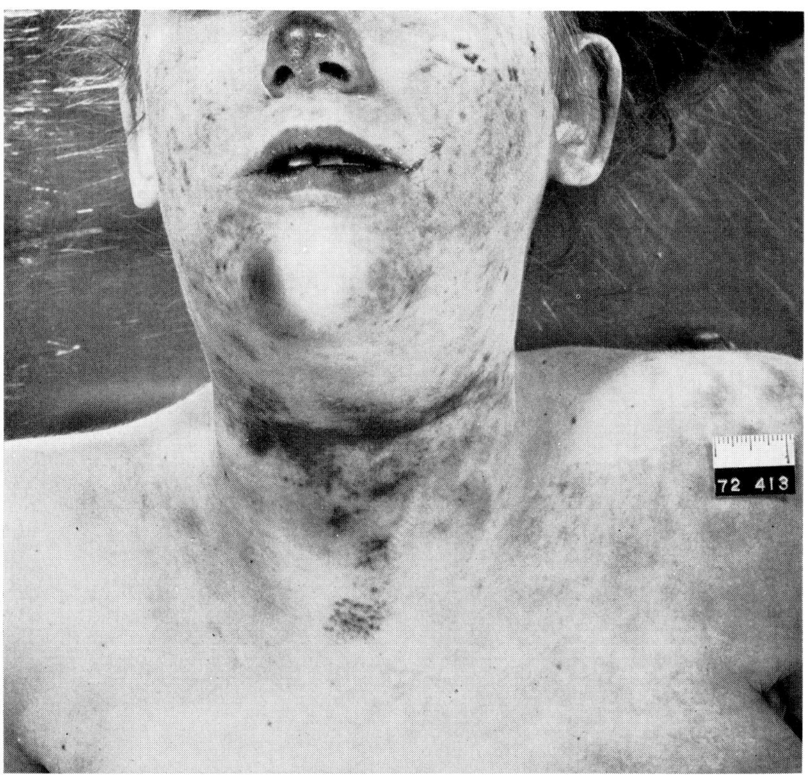


FIGURE XII-14b. Body of an unidentified young girl found beside a highway. The injuries on the neck indicate throttling by twisting the zippered front of the sweater she was wearing. The imprint of the zipper is noted on the left side of the neck.

for spermatozoa, should be performed. Fingernail scrapings and pubic and head hair from the deceased should also be retained for possible later examination by the police crime laboratory. Accidental strangulation will be discussed under *sexual asphyxia* at the end of this chapter.

The hallmark of manual strangulation is fingernail marks on the neck of the victim, though their absence does not preclude throttling. In many cases of manual strangulation there is extensive external injury to the neck, while in many others there are few or no external manifestations of trauma (Fig. XII-14). The characteristic fingernail mark is a thin linear or crescentic abrasion of the skin. Inferences regarding the way in which the hand of the assailant may have been applied to the victim's neck based on the direction of the curved abrasions should not be attempted. Too many variants, such as the shape of the nails[5] and their length, as well as inherent qualities of the skin, render such conclusions extremely tenuous. In rare instances, if the fingernails of the assailant are long and firm, injuries resembling small *cuts* may be produced (Fig. XII-15). A wet body may not show fingernail marks until drying of the skin has occurred.

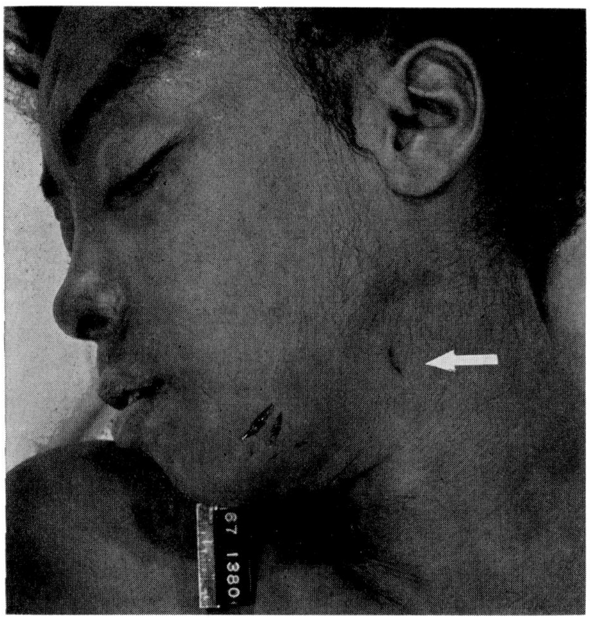


FIGURE XII-15. Middle-aged woman found in a dufflebag in a public park. Note the typical nail mark under the left angle of the jaw (arrow). The two superficial *cuts* on the left side of the chin are believed to also have been inflicted by the long fingernails of the assailant.

A young black female was found dead, submerged in a bathtub. Initial examination on the scene showed *only two small whitish areas resembling scars*. At autopsy five hours later unequivocal nail marks were noted on all sides of the neck. The drying of the body after removal from the water and the subsequent color change of the *whitish areas* during the five hours permitted proper interpretation (Fig. XII-16).

Hemorrhage in the subcutaneous tissues and the musculature underlying nail marks is usually scant when compared with the external injuries. Conversely, the absence of nail marks on the skin does not imply absence of bruising in deeper structures. A single small area of bruising in any muscle of the neck, but commonly on either side of the midline and usually over the thyroid cartilage or the hyoid bone, may be all that is found in a given case of manual strangulation.

To best visualize these bruises and eliminate the possibility of artifacts, the pathologist should first elevate the shoulders on a wooden block, then eviscerate the body, leaving the neck organs in place, and remove the brain. When the blood has stopped draining, layerwise dissection of the neck can begin. This technique assures a dry dissection field and obviates the subsequent difficult task of distinguishing true from artifactual soft tissue hemorrhages.

Fractures of the larynx, including the hyoid bone and the thyroid and cricoid cartilages, are frequently associated with manual strangulation. The hyoid bone is a horseshoe-shaped structure situated at the base of the tongue. Just below it is the thyroid cartilage. The signet ring-like cricoid cartilage is smaller but thicker and stronger than the thyroid cartilage and is located between the latter and the trachea. The ends of the hyoid bone, also known as horns, and similar projections of the thyroid cartilage are the weak areas of these structures and consequently are more likely to fracture in cases of trauma. Strangulation is mostly responsible

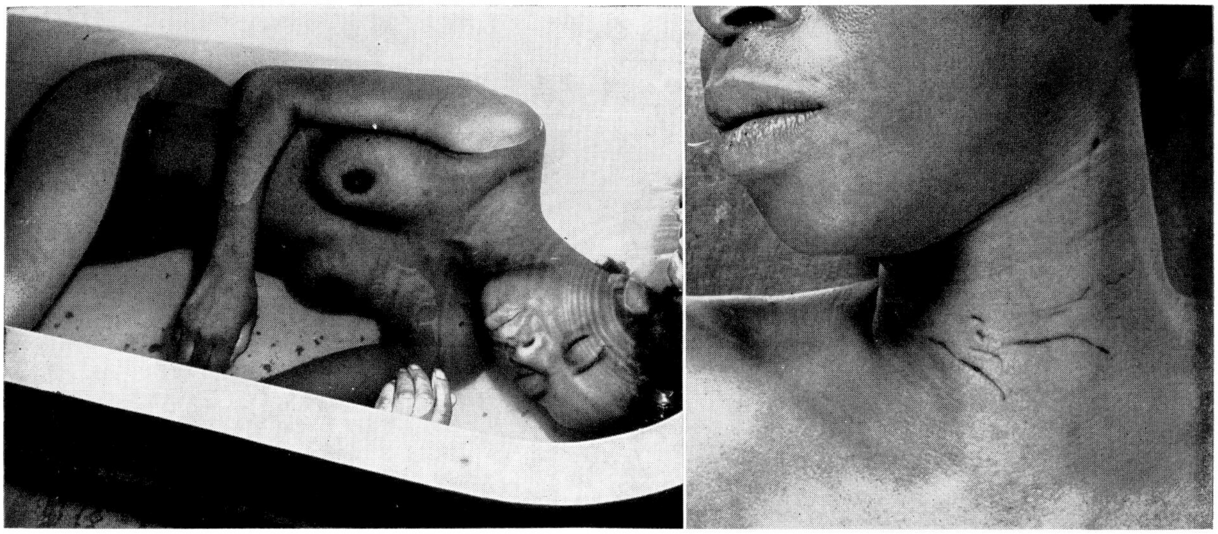

FIGURE XII-16. (a): Body of a young woman submerged in a bathtub. No injuries were seen on the neck until the skin dried. (b): Same individual as in Figure XII-16a, five hours after removal from the water. Extensive fingernail marks are visible over the entire neck.

for these fractures, although fractures of the upper horns of the thyroid cartilage, particularly in an elderly individual with calcification of this cartilage, may sometimes occur as a result of a fall or forceful direct impact on the neck. I have never seen a hyoid bone fractured by a blow to the neck. The hyoid bone is well protected behind the mandible unless the head is extended. However, fracture of this bone as a result of a fall is sometimes seen.

A young soldier was charged with the murder by strangulation of his middle-aged female companion. During the trial it became evident that the woman's fractured hyoid bone was incurred by a fall on the steering wheel of her parked automobile while she was markedly intoxicated by alcohol.

Fractures of the larynx may sometimes occur during removal of the neck organs at autopsy. Focal hemorrhage, however, always surrounds a fracture sustained during life and distinguishes it from a postmortem artifact. The hemorrhage surrounding such a fracture may be minute, and only a careful search when the specimen is first examined may reveal this fundamental piece of evidence. The importance of documenting focal hemorrhage at the site of a laryngeal fracture became a controversial issue in the trial of Doctor Carl Coppolino at the Monmouth County courthouse in Freehold, New Jersey, in 1966. At this trial, diametrically opposed medical testimony was given by three renowned forensic pathologists regarding the presence of hemorrhage at the site of a fractured cricoid cartilage in an embalmed body three years after burial.[6] Doctor Coppolino, a physician, was being tried for the murder by strangulation of the husband of his mistress.

In a decomposed body, where public viewing can no longer take place but where strangulation is suspected, the neck organs may be best removed at autopsy by beginning the incision of the skin below the chin rather than by the customary Y-shaped incision. This technique permits a direct and easy approach to the neck organs and eliminates the likelihood of artifactual fracture of the larynx during autopsy. Furthermore, in a decomposed body, putrefaction of soft tissues in the neck may produce areas that closely resemble hemorrhage. In such cases, the presence of laryngeal fractures

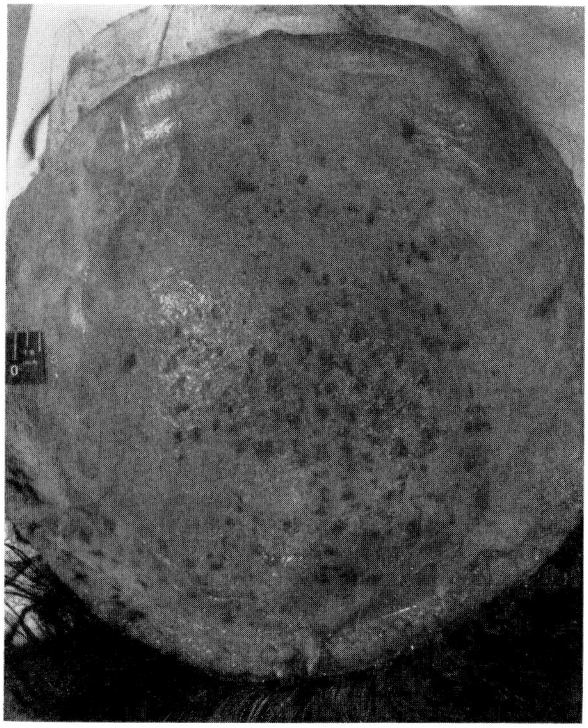

FIGURE XII-17. Reflected scalp at autopsy showing multiple small hemorrhages produced by tearing the tiny blood vessels that pass between the scalp and the vault of the skull. These hemorrhages bear no relationship to the cause of death.

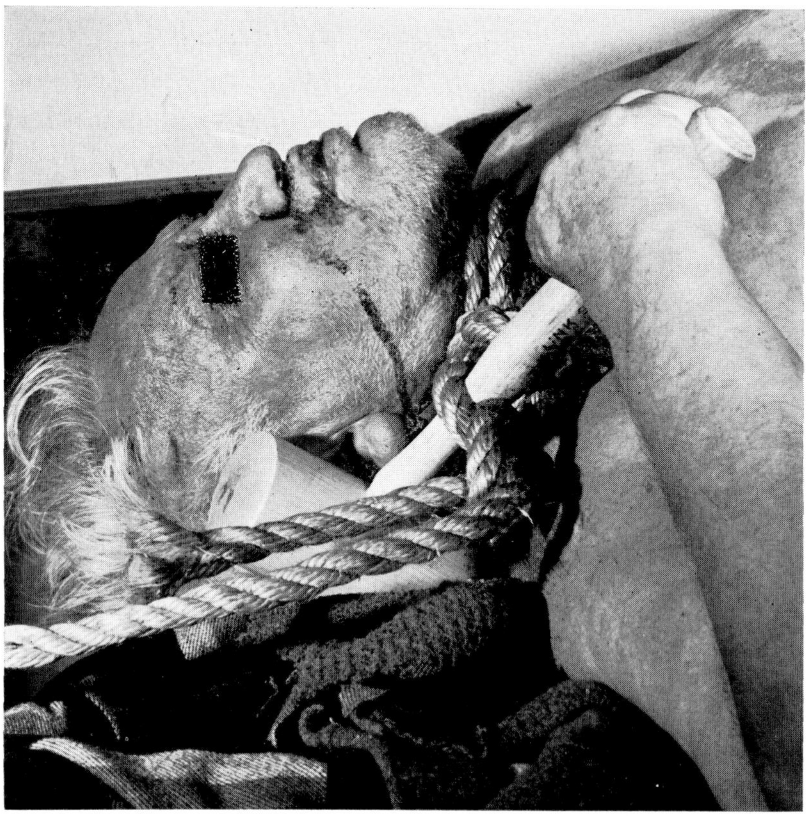

FIGURE XII-18. Suicidal strangulation: An elderly carpenter found dead in his shop. The noose was tightened by the handle of the mallet.

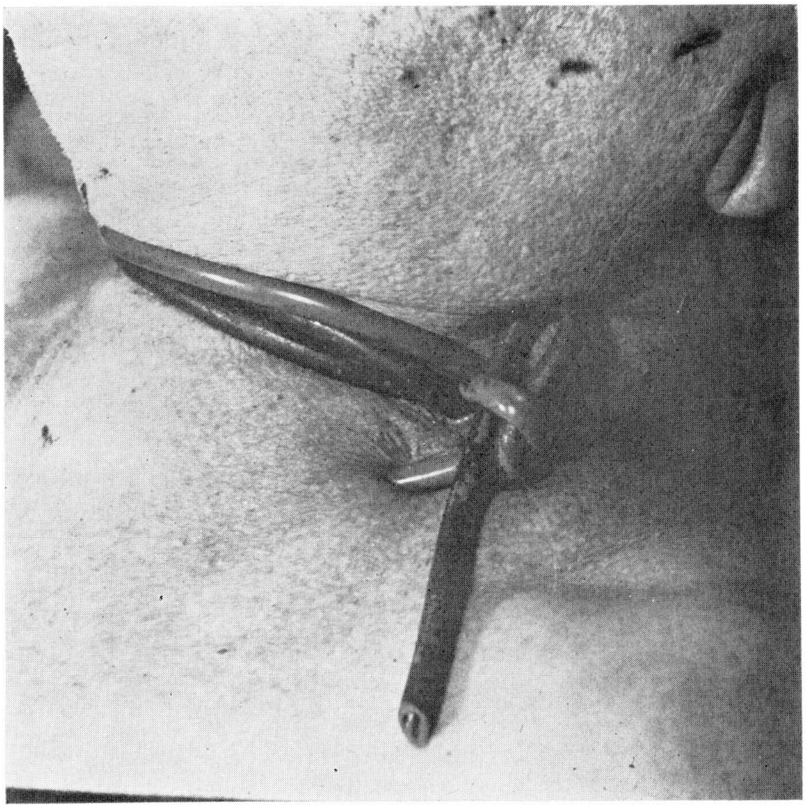

FIGURE XII-19. Elderly man who strangled himself with a telephone cord after prolonged depression. Note the tourniquetlike knot, which could have been released by pull on one end. (Courtesy of Dr. Dominick DiMaio, New York City.)

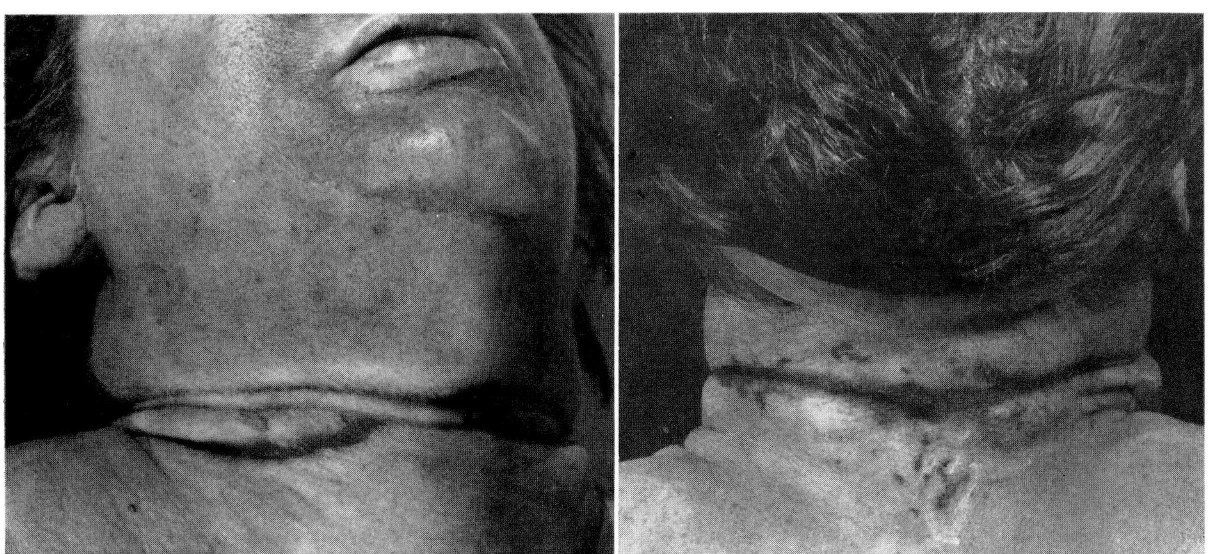

FIGURE XII-20a and b. Middle-aged woman who was strangled with a nonspiral telephone cord. The photographs of the front and back of the neck show the horizontal imprint of the ligature. Figure 20b shows superficial scratches of the nape of the neck and upper back. These corresponded with the zipper of the woman's dress. The assailant apparently subdued the victim from the rear.

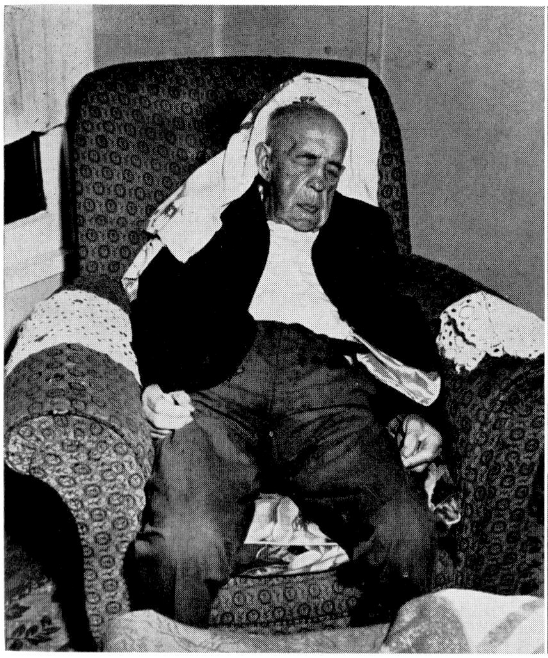

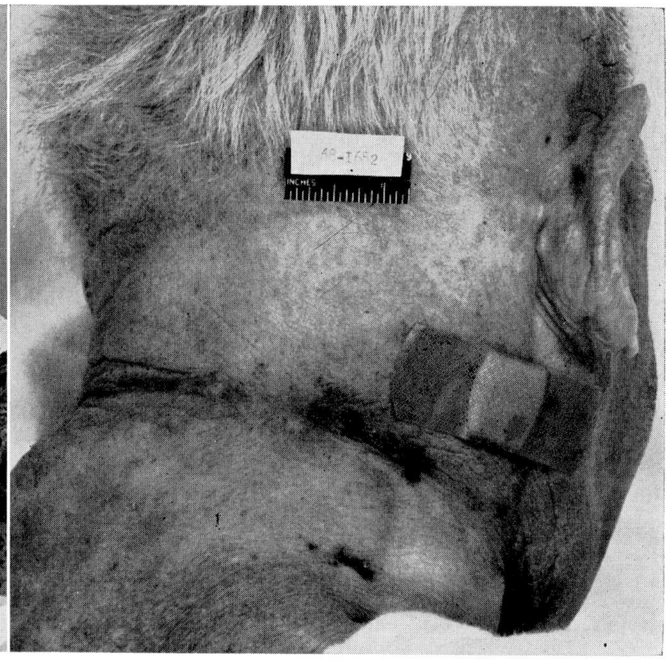


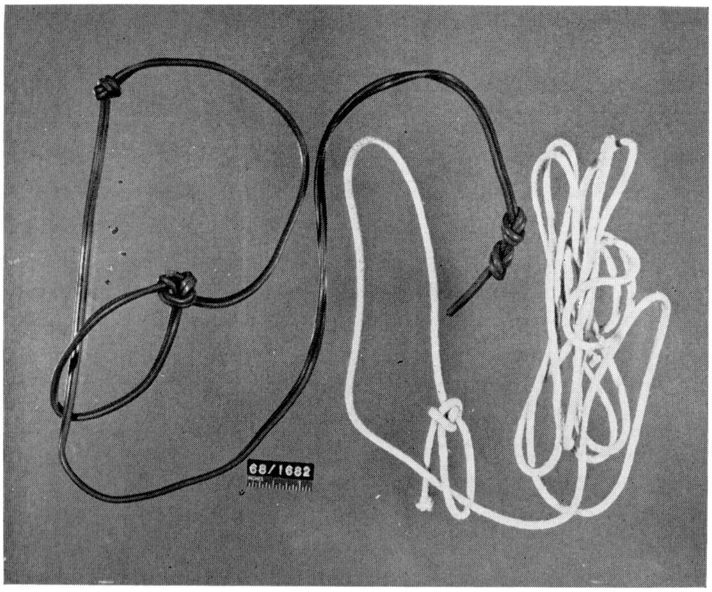


FIGURE XII-21 a, b, c. This sixty-five-year-old man was found sitting in an armchair in a beach house. He did not live at this address. He was initially believed to have died of natural causes. Postmortem examination showed a faint horizontal furrow around the neck, some fresh areas of bleeding and abrasions covered with an adhesive bandage. The findings prompted the conclusion of homicidal strangulation by ligature, and the premises were searched. The rope and electric cord in Figure 21c were found in a trash can outside the house. The owner of the beach house was suspected but denied the charge until confronted with the results of the postmortem examination.

assumes vital importance, and any possibility of artifactual fractures must be eliminated.

If putrefaction is advanced, the entire body and, of course, the neck may be considerably swollen by decomposition gases. A scarf or other piece of clothing around the neck may become very tight as a result of such swelling and may be mistaken for a ligature. To avoid misinterpretation, the length of the ligature may be compared with the collar size of the shirt of the deceased.

As a point of interest, the degree of calcification of the neck skeleton varies with age to the extent that in older individuals the hyoid bone and thyroid and cricoid cartilages become firm and unyielding. When pressure is applied to the neck of an elderly person, these structures break easily, much more easily than in a young individual. Consequently, the degree of calcification and fragility of the neck skeleton is of great significance and should be noted in autopsy reports of cases of suspected strangulation.

As in some cases of hanging, pinpoint and slightly larger hemorrhages are often noted in the face of the strangled victim, especially in the conjunctivae and the eyelids. The presence of these so-called *Tardieu's spots* is supportive evidence of death by asphyxiation but as a sole finding must not be considered specific. Occasionally these pinpoint red spots are so densely spread on the eyelids and upper part of the cheeks that they impart a brownish hue to the skin, resembling makeup. Slight downward pull of the upper eyelid will straighten wrinkles and cause separation of the spots, thus distinguishing pinpoint hemorrhages from artifact.

Hemorrhages resembling *Tardieu's spots* are sometimes seen at autopsy in the reflected scalp, especially if it is congested. These hemorrhages are caused by the tearing of small blood vessels when separating the scalp from the vault of the skull and have no bearing on the cause of death (Fig. XII-17).

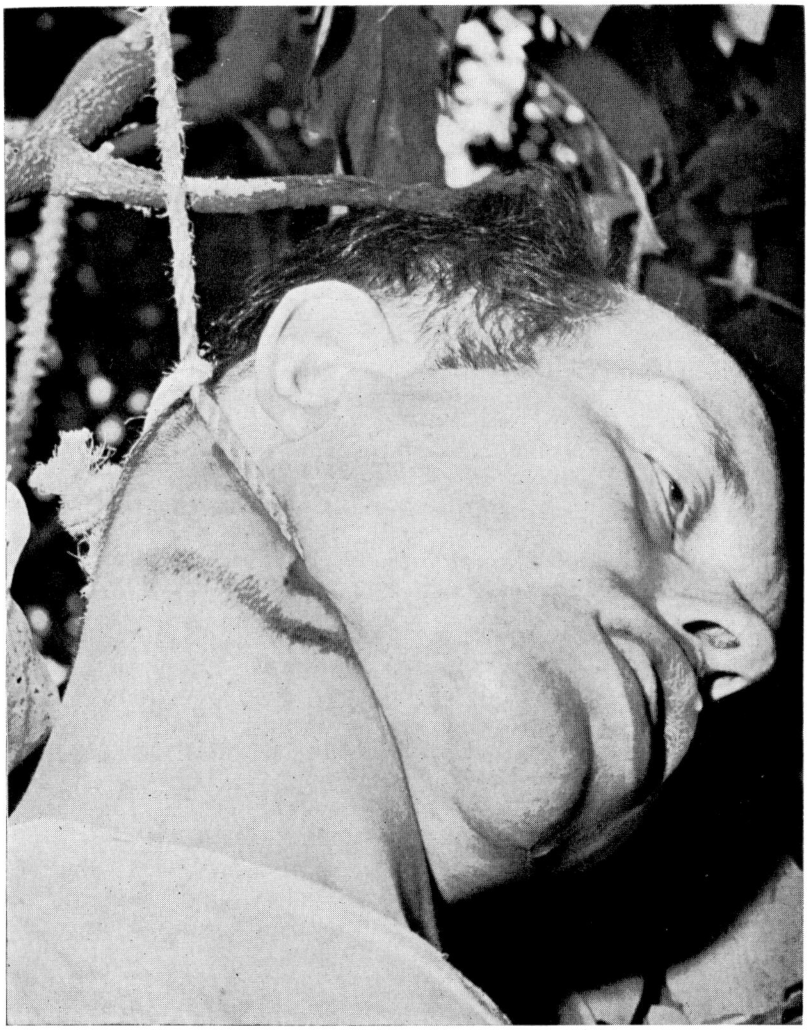

FIGURE XII-22. Thirty-two-year-old man found hanging from a tree 12 ft. above the ground in the backyard of his home. He had climbed up the tree with a ladder. Note the horizontal abrasion made by the rope before it slipped to the upward position seen on the picture.

Cases of suicidal ligature strangulation are distinctly uncommon. The possibility of second party involvement must always be carefully scrutinized. Distinction between homicidal and suicidal strangulation by ligature is often impossible on the basis of the anatomical findings alone, although fractures of the larynx in suicidal strangulations are unknown. The construction of the noose and the knot in particular, as well as the number of *turns* of the ligature around the neck and the general circumstances under which the body is found, may suggest the manner of death. A history of mental depression, allusions to suicide or past suicide attempts provide presumptive evidence in a given case (Figs. XII-18 and XII-19).

Cases of homicidal strangulation by ligature and subsequent hanging of the victim to simulate suicide are rare. Yet, because some cases have been described in the literature, crime investigators everywhere are alert to this type of homicide. Certain features permit the distinction between hanging and strangulation (Figs. XII-20, XII-21 and XII-22).

Defense wounds on the body of the strangulation victim are a frequent finding, although it should be noted that an occasional nail mark, even on the neck, may be self-inflicted, as when the victim tries to free himself from the strangling grip. During an episode of terminal air hunger, as in an asthmatic attack or following an overdose of heroin, an individual may also clutch his own neck in an effort to *open* the airway.

Also, in suicidal hanging the victim is sometimes found with nail marks and bruises on the neck and with fingers wedged under the noose, as if attempting to remove the constriction. This is a reflex action to preserve life and is not in any way related to deliberation.

| *Strangulation by Ligature* | *Hanging* |
|---|---|
| Mark on neck is commonly horizontal. | Mark on neck passes upward toward the knot; may be horizontal, as in strangulation, if hanging is carried out while lying down. |
| Mark on neck is commonly below the level of the thyroid cartilage. | Mark on neck is commonly in the level of the thyroid cartilage or above it. |
| Hyoid bone and/or thyroid cartilage are sometimes fractured. | Hyoid bone and thyroid cartilage are usually intact, except in hanging with a *long drop* or in elderly individuals. |

## OBSTRUCTION OF THE AIRWAY

### Smothering

Blockage of the nose and mouth causes death by asphyxia due to inability to breathe. This may be effected in a variety of ways, such as by gagging, holding a pillow over the face of the victim or shutting his airway with one's hands.

Smothering is homicidal in the majority of cases. Accidental smothering is comparatively rare, as in the case of an infant who gets entangled in his bed linen. Death in an avalanche is another form of asphyxia. Obstruction of the airway by a plastic bag exemplifies suicidal or accidental smothering (Figs. XII-23 and XII-24). Until the late 1960s, the latter increased proportionally with the popularity of *glue sniffing*. Water vapor accumulating in the plastic bag that contains the glue contributes to the adherence of the plastic to the skin, sealing off outside air. The lungs, liver and blood should be retained at autopsy for chemical analyses to demonstrate the solvent. The presence of the solvent in the lungs indicates that the material has been inhaled, while a positive finding in the liver or the blood indicates systemic absorption. Pathologic changes in the liver, kidneys, brain and bone marrow have been described following repeated glue sniffing, although they are nonspecific in nature.[7]

Deaths associated with the sniffing of aerosols without the use of plastic bags are also known. These individuals use paper bags or make a tent of their clothing, into which they spray the aerosol. The deaths are attributed to an overwhelming allergic reaction and possibly an arrhythmia of the heartbeat, as shown experi-

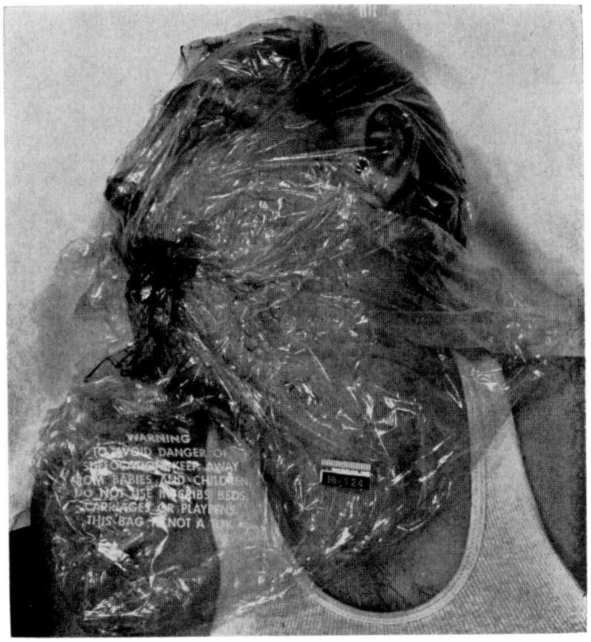


FIGURE XII-23. Fifty-five-year-old alcoholic who committed suicide with a plastic laundry bag. He had repeatedly spoken of his intention to commit suicide. Such cases are rare in this age group compared to the accidental asphyxia in glue-sniffing teenagers.

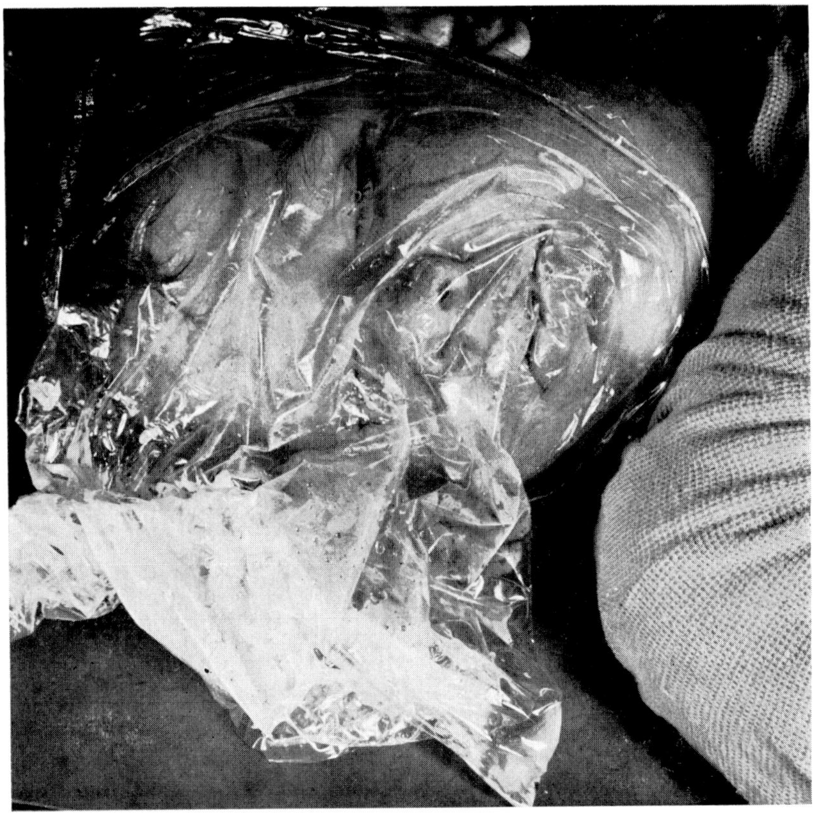

FIGURE XII-24. Eleven-year-old boy found in a wooded area with a plastic bag over his face following a glue-sniffing *orgy*. Plastic bags and emptied tubes of airplane glue were scattered in the area. Note the water vapor in the plastic bag. A small amount of glue is also still present in the tip of the bag. Subsequent police investigation disclosed that the area had been frequented on different occasions by a group of boys who met there for the express purpose of glue sniffing.

mentally by Taylor and Harris.[8] In the last few years glue and aerosol sniffing has diminished to the point that deaths resulting from this fad have become a distinct rarity.

The findings at autopsy in cases of smothering are nonspecific. Slight, acute emphysema and edema of the lungs with scattered areas of atelectasis, petechiae and congestion constitute the major findings. An important area to examine in a suspected homicidal smothering is the inside of the cheeks. Hemorrhages and tears of the mucosa by forceful closure and pressure against the dentition may be the only findings suggesting trauma to the face area.

Until a few years ago, cases of sudden death in infancy, or so-called *crib death,* were attributed to smothering. This was primarily due to the failure to find an obvious cause of death while at the same time observing at postmortem examination some of the usual changes of asphyxia. In recent years, however, smothering has been abandoned as the cause of sudden death in infancy, although the true explanation of these deaths is still far from understood.

### Aspiration of Foreign Material

Aspiration of foreign material may be fatal by occluding or severely narrowing the airway. Aspiration of vomitus occurs mostly in unconscious or semiconscious individuals, with or without contributory factors such as drugs or alcohol. A healthy but grossly intoxicated individual who begins a meal, suddenly turns blue, coughs violently, then collapses and dies should be suspected of having asphyxiated by aspirating food. At autopsy a large piece of poorly chewed food (bolus) may be found obstructing the larynx. The condition is referred to as *cafe coronary* because it mimicks a heart attack. Dislocation of one's denture into the airway is not necessarily associated with alcoholic intoxication. It may occasionally occur in traumatic cases, particularly with sub- or unconsciousness.

A forty-year-old woman inhaled her partial denture during a coughing spell. She lapsed into unconsciousness in front of her husband, who thought she had fallen asleep. At autopsy her blood alcohol level was negative, and she was not under the influence of medication.

Food aspiration following suppression of the gag reflex by tranquilizing drugs is a common phenomenon in mental institutions.

Infants and children occasionally aspirate a variety of objects, such as nuts, marbles, coins and rattles. Less frequently occurring hazards are certain imported pacifiers with a small diameter plastic guard and a rigid handle.[9] Children may sometimes inhale into the airway a pea or grain of corn. If small enough, such a grain will not obstruct the air passage completely; however, its presence will produce a progressively worsening cough as the adjacent lining membrane of the airway swells from irritation and the grain begins to germinate in this moist and warm environment.

### Swelling of the Lining Membranes of the Larynx

Insect bites, notably those of bees, wasps and hornets, and drug reactions, such as those that may follow the administration of penicillin, can cause swelling of the lining membranes of the larynx and death within a few minutes due to an allergic reaction. In one case I had examined, a hornetlike insect stung the neck of a five-year-old-girl. In several minutes the child developed extreme difficulty breathing and was dead on arrival at the hospital. The autopsy showed near-occlusion of the larynx due to edema. In another case a forty-two-year-old man attempted to remove a wasp nest by sawing it off a tree limb. He was stung many times on the face, arms and legs. Within a very short time he developed severe respiratory distress. He reached the hospital in time for an artificial airway (tracheotomy) to save his life.

Inflammation of the throat as sometimes seen in diphtheria and infectious mononucleosis may cause swelling of the airway to the point of obstruction. A blow to the front of the neck may cause severe swelling of the lining membrane of the airway due to edema and hemorrhage. Fracture of the cartilages of the larynx or the trachea is not an essential finding.[10] Rupture of the trachea has occurred without a blow to the neck in straining during labor, during a bout of coughing to dislodge a foreign body or even as a result of a sudden backward extension of the head.[2]

Severe swelling of the lining membrane of the airway is frequently observed following intubation for the purpose of artificial respiration.

## COMPRESSION OF THE CHEST

Compression of the chest to the extent of preventing respiratory movements may occur in a wide variety of ways. Examples include persons buried under the rubble of a collapsed building, those crushed to death when panic in a crowd leads to stampeding, or the individual crushed by the automobile under which he was working when the jack under the car slipped. Homicide by compression of the chest, as by kneeling on the victim, is rare. The autopsy shows the usual changes of asphyxia. In addition, the face is frequently markedly congested, appearing purple-blue and with numerous pinpoint hemorrhages scattered in the skin and mucous membranes. Discoloration of the face is due to the fact that a heavy load on the chest will primarily compress the thinner and less potent right side of the heart, which receives the blood from the head, while the more powerful left side of the heart continues to pump. This causes a tremendous overfilling (congestion) of blood in the head area, resulting in the purple-blue discoloration (Fig. XII-25). Another frequent observation is small hemorrhages in the neck and chest muscles, particularly near bony attachments. They probably result from rupture of individual muscle fibers during forceful breathing attempts against the restraint. For best demonstration of these hemorrhages, the pathologist should follow the dissection guidelines outlined under *strangulation.*

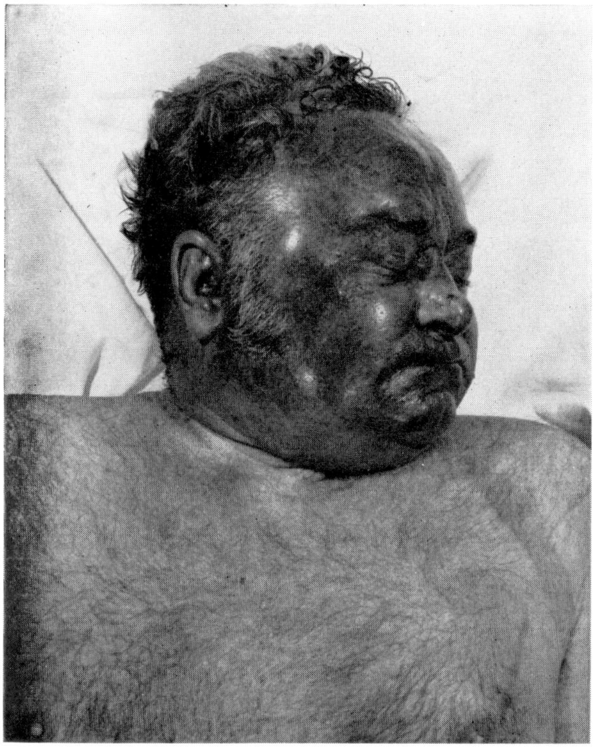

FIGURE XII-25. Marked congestion of the face in a driver of a tractor trailer that was carrying several tons of rolled steel. Following a sudden stop, the metal rolled forward, crushing the driver.

## EXCLUSION OF OXYGEN

Exclusion of oxygen may take place by depletion and replacement by another gas or by chemical interference with its uptake and utilization by the body.

### Carbon Dioxide Poisoning

Carbon dioxide ($CO_2$) may cause asphyxia by excluding oxygen. $CO_2$ is heavier than air, and therefore it settles when it accumulates in the absence of turbulence. Common places that may contain $CO_2$ in excess include manholes, wells, silos and occasionally cellars. Carbon dioxide may also cause asphyxia when it accumulates within a small closed space as a result of oxygen depletion from consumption due to rebreathing. The glue sniffer found dead with a plastic bag over his head pulled snugly around his neck with a tube of airplane glue in the bag is a classic example. With the onset of unconsciousness from inhalation of the volatile hydrocarbon in the glue, he cannot respond to the rising $CO_2$ or to the decreasing $O_2$ levels, and

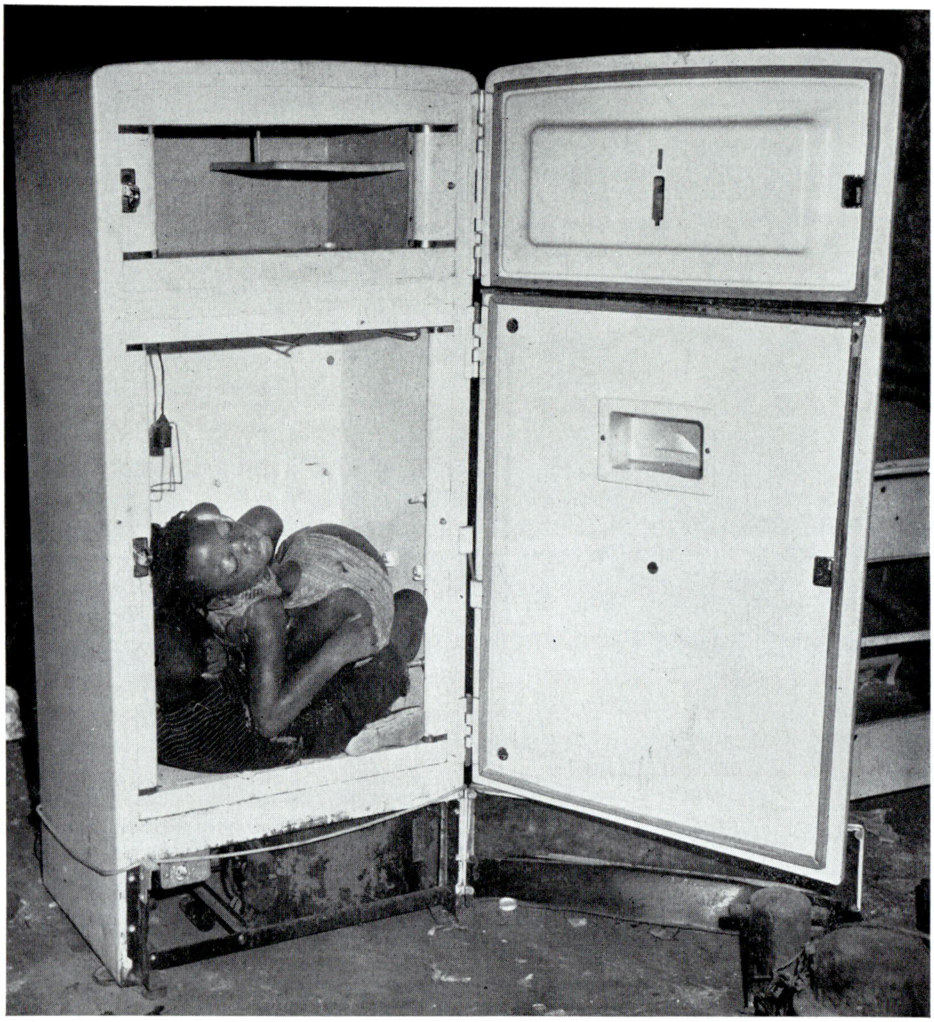

FIGURE XII-26. Three children discovered in a discarded refrigerator in an unused garage two days after having been reported missing by their parents. They had been playing *hide-and-seek*.

death ensues. Other examples are the tragic asphyxial deaths in the 1950s of children who hid in discarded refrigerators or washers while playing. Those appliances could only be opened from the outside. Since then, laws in most states require that the door be removed or secured before such appliances are discarded (Fig. XII-26). Doctor Dominick DiMaio, formerly Chief Medical Examiner of New York City, reports a case of suicide in an elderly woman who placed herself in her kitchen refrigerator (Fig. XII-27).

The autopsy in carbon dioxide poisoning shows the usual changes of asphyxia. Blood $CO_2$ content determinations have no diagnostic significance, since $CO_2$ rapidly accumulates postmortem. Of critical importance, however, is the collection of an air sample from the scene and analysis of the sample for its $CO_2$ content.

### Carbon Monoxide Poisoning

Carbon monoxide (CO) causes asphyxia by blocking the respiratory pigment of the red blood corpuscles (hemoglobin) from carrying oxygen to the tissues and from returning carbon dioxide to the lungs. Hemoglobin has an affinity for carbon monoxide 250 times greater than for oxygen. Carbon monoxide is an odor-

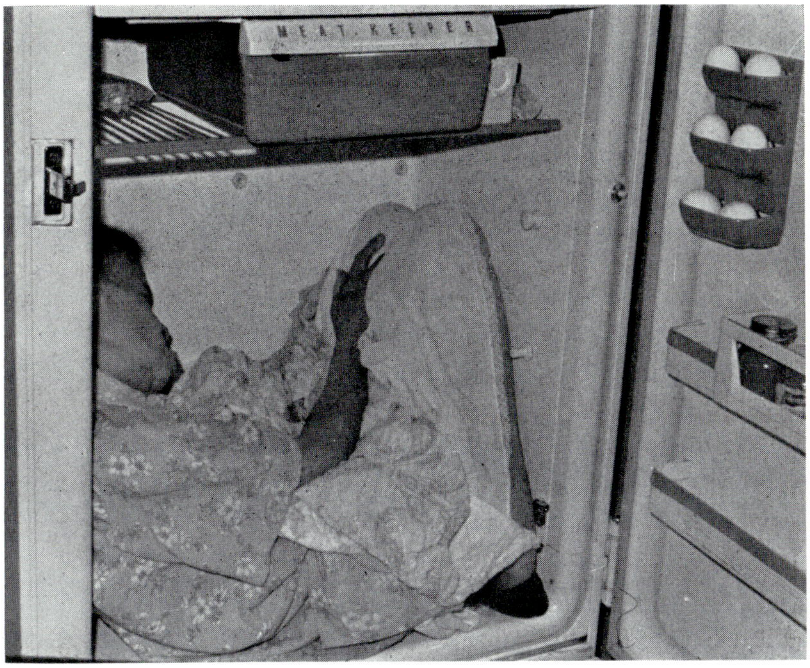


FIGURE XII-27. Suicide in kitchen refrigerator. (Courtesy of Dr. Dominick DiMaio, New York City.)

less, colorless, nonirritating gas, slightly lighter than air. It results from incomplete combustion of carbon-containing material; consequently, it is abundant where soot is produced. Its presence in the fumes of fire, in exhaust gas, in illuminating gas and in tobacco smoke makes it a constant hazard. The amounts of carbon monoxide in tobacco smoke vary considerably. For example, cigarette smoke yields approximately 1% by volume, pipe smoke 2% and cigar smoke 6%.[11] Some heavy cigarette smokers may have a carbon monoxide blood level up to 8% or 10%. Automobile exhaust fumes supposedly contain 3 lb. of CO for every gallon of fuel that is burned.[12] With over 100 million motor vehicles in the United States, the internal combustion engine is considered the greatest single source of carbon monoxide.

While the postmortem diagnosis of carbon monoxide poisoning is not difficult, the blood levels and their significance may vary considerably. In a healthy middle-aged individual a CO blood saturation greater than 50% to 60% is considered fatal. In some conditions far lower concentrations may be found. Among these are all illnesses in which the oxygenation of the tissues is in some way impeded. Anemia, chronic lung diseases (particularly emphysema) and arteriosclerotic heart disease are some of the more common diseases in which carbon monoxide blood levels may be appreciably lower than in healthy persons who were similarly exposed. The carbon monoxide level in these people depends on the severity of the disease. A blood carbon monoxide level of 15% resulting from exposure to a fire in an individual with far-advanced coronary heart disease may unquestionably represent "the straw that broke the camel's back." Another factor that must be considered in the interpretation of CO levels in the blood is the rapid loss of CO observed when the still-living person is removed to fresh air. Generally, in an acute exposure, 40 to 50 percent of the carbon monoxide is eliminated in the first hour if oxygen is administered rapidly. The remaining CO is eliminated at the rate of 8 to 10 percent per hour. Nevertheless, the poisoned victim may die despite the clearance of

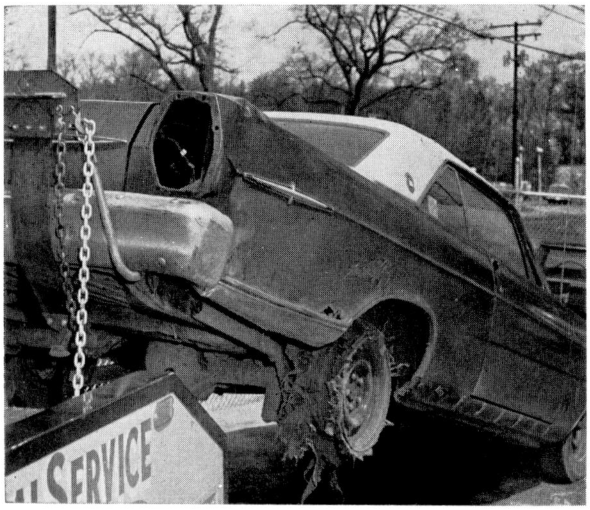

FIGURE XII-28. The driver of this automobile was found dead in his parked car. The windows were rolled up. The blood CO saturation level was 40%, and the blood alcohol level was 0.11%. Investigation revealed that this driver had been stopped by police several hours earlier at the same location for driving on a flat rear tire. He was told to change the tire before driving on. The carbon monoxide seeped into the trunk, then the passenger compartment through the opening of the missing taillight. Directly beneath the opening was the broken and shortened tail pipe.

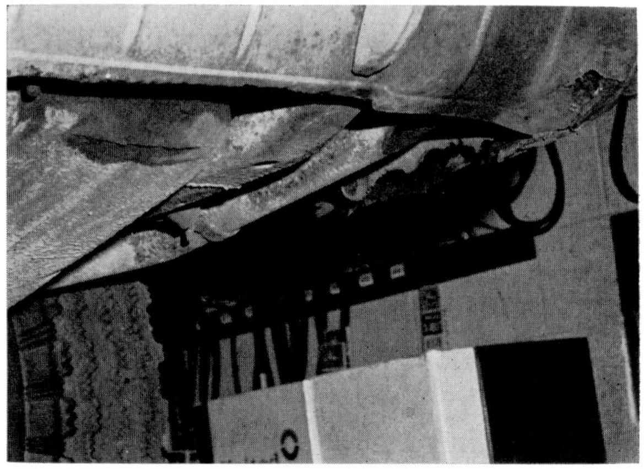

FIGURE XII-29. The forty-four-year-old driver of this automobile was found dead in his car, which was parked in front of his rural home. The engine was running, since it was a cold winter night. The cause of death was a 60% carbon monoxide blood saturation. The blood alcohol level was 0.12%. The source of the CO was a defective exhaust system. The tail pipe outlet was suspended too close to the undercarriage of the vehicle, and fumes could not escape adequately due to deflection by the bumper and the rear trunk area. The adjacent rear fender panel showed rust perforations, which allowed fumes to seep into the passenger compartment.

CO because of irreversible brain damage sustained while the high CO concentration persisted. Some survive weeks or months in coma before succumbing to infection. In investigating self-limited house fires or defective burners that produce CO, the possibility that the CO concentration will have fallen to a low level in the

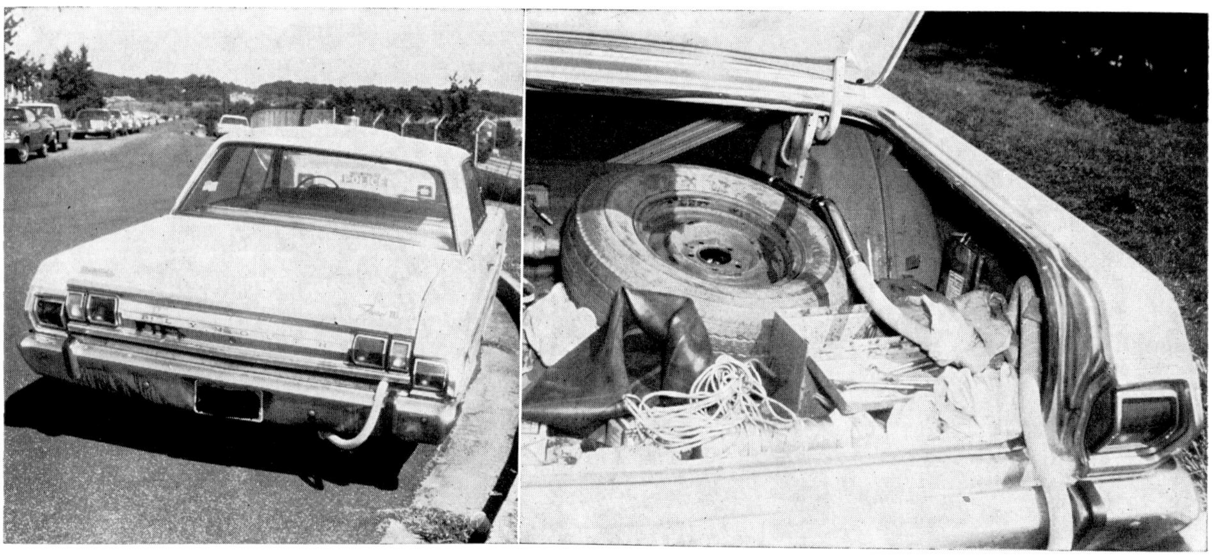

FIGURES XII-30a and b. A vacuum cleaner hose connecting the exhaust pipe with the interior of the automobile by way of the trunk. A suicide note was found at home on the kitchen table. (Courtesy of Maryland State Police.)

victim as the source abated is occasionally important in interpreting the evidence.

Alcohol, barbiturates, sedatives and many other drugs are other common factors that potentiate the toxic action of carbon monoxide. For instance, a CO saturation of 35% or 40%, from which a healthy individual would probably recover after temporary disability, may be fatal in the presence of a blood alcohol concentration of 0.2%. Numerous automobile accidents are due to the combined action of alcohol and CO on the driver. The CO is usually traced to faulty exhaust pipes, with leakage of fumes into the interior of the car (Figs. XII-28 and XII-29).[13] Suicidal CO inhalation of automobile fumes is relatively frequent. A garden or vacuum cleaner hose is commonly used to connect the tailpipe with the vehicle's interior, but other methods have been used (Figs. XII-30 and XII-31). A level of carbon monoxide sufficient to cause death accumulates in five to ten minutes in a single-car garage if the door is closed and the engine of the automobile is running.

Investigation of the scene in cases of carbon monoxide poisoning is imperative for determination of the manner of death. A closed garage door is usually quite suggestive of intent, while scattered tools or an open hood would be presumptive evidence of accident (Fig. XII-32). We have observed a number of deaths where people backed their cars into the garage to warm up the engines and opened the garage door to release the exhaust fumes. The fumes engulfed the rear of the car and seeped into the passenger compartment of the vehicle.

Pathologic changes attributable to CO poisoning include bright cherry red discoloration of the blood, musculature and the livor mortis. The fingernails are involved in lividity in most deaths and are consequently purple; in CO poisoning, however, they appear red or pink—one might say *alive*. It is a good policy to use one's own fingernails for comparison. The fingernails are a particularly good place to look for this bright redness, especially in Negroes, in whom the discoloration of the skin is usually not noticeable. Cyanide poisoning and exposure of the dead body to cold may cause redness indistinguishable from that due to CO. If the cherry redness is visible, the concentration of CO in the blood usually exceeds 30%. With concentrations less than 20% to 25% the color might

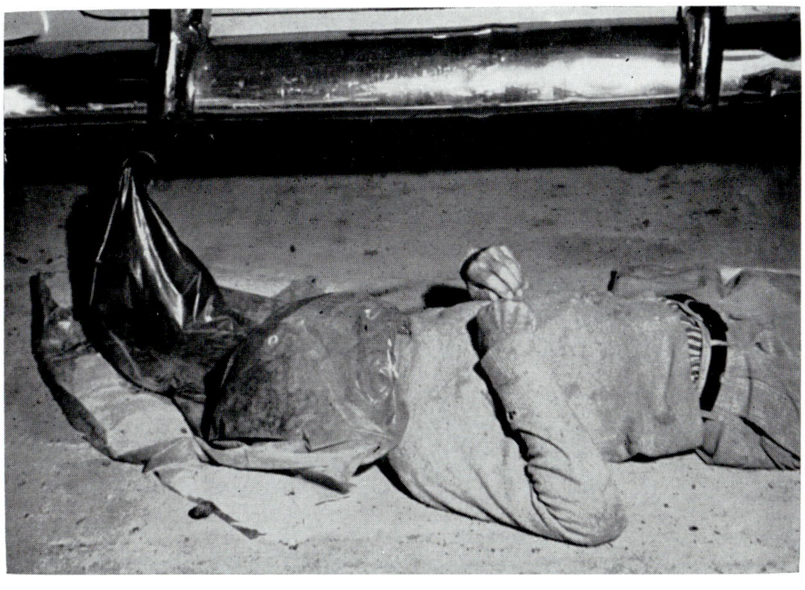

FIGURE XII-31. Suicide by inhalation of automobile exhaust fumes from a plastic laundry bag connected to the tail pipe.

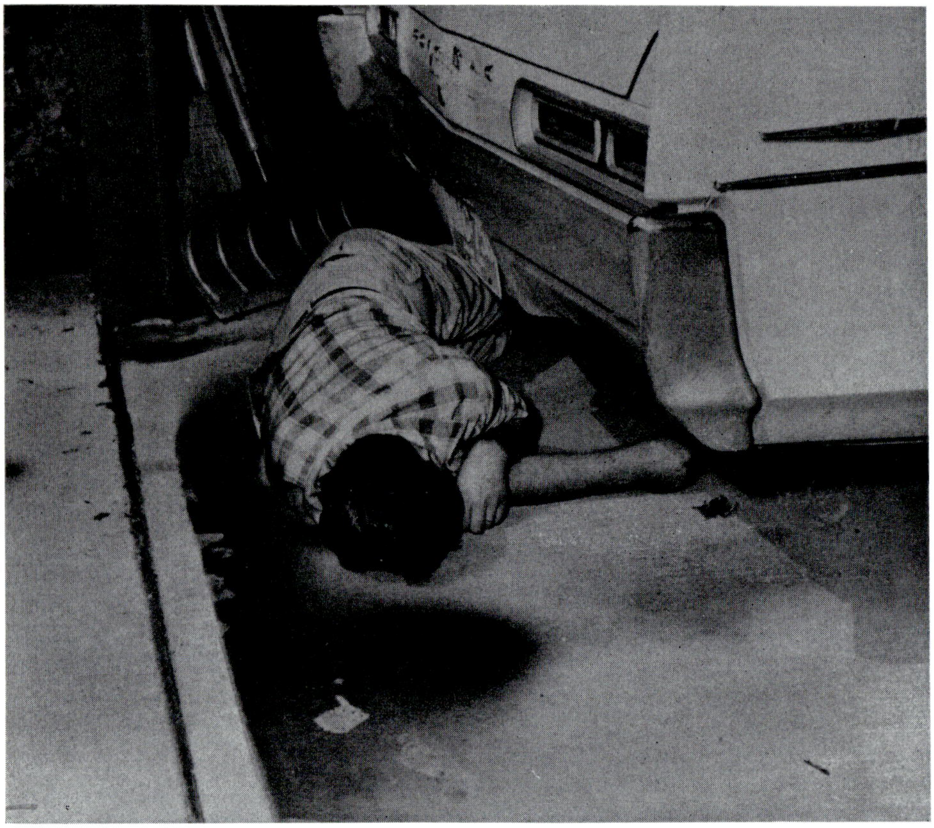

FIGURE XII-32. Forty-three-year-old man found dead, partly under the rear of his automobile in the family garage. The car's ignition was still on, but the engine was not running due to an empty gas tank. The garage door was closed, as shown by the soot pattern on the floor. The blood carbon monoxide level was 80%. No autopsy was performed. The family sued for accidental death benefits, maintaining that he had had a heart attack and collapsed. The high carbon monoxide level suggested that his heart was healthy or he would have succumbed with a significantly lower level. Furthermore, the position of the deceased, partly under the vehicle, corroborated the hypothesis of suicide. The court denied award of double indemnity payments.

go unnoticed. It is essential, therefore, that the blood be analyzed for CO in all automobile occupants killed in a crash.

Fluidity of the blood is a feature shared by carbon monoxide poisoning with other types of asphyxia. Blisters or bullae of the skin containing a clear serous fluid are frequently seen in cases of carbon monoxide or barbiturate poisoning where death follows deep coma. These blisters are often mistaken for burns because their rupture leaves a red, raw surface that later dries to a brown parchmentlike area. They are most common over the joints of the extremities; the knees and wrists are most commonly involved. Occasionally an entire side of a forearm or a thigh is blistered (Fig. XII-33).

Changes associated with anoxia and coma and seen in individuals who survive an acute episode of carbon monoxide poisoning but die later of other causes are symmetrical necroses in the globus pallidus. These structures are particularly vulnerable to anoxemia due to their unique blood supply. The necrotic areas later change to form pea- or lentil-sized brown cysts. Identical lesions have been observed in barbiturate poisoning and in cases of marked arteriosclerosis of the vessels of the corpus striatum.[14] Multiple punctate hemorrhages in the white matter of

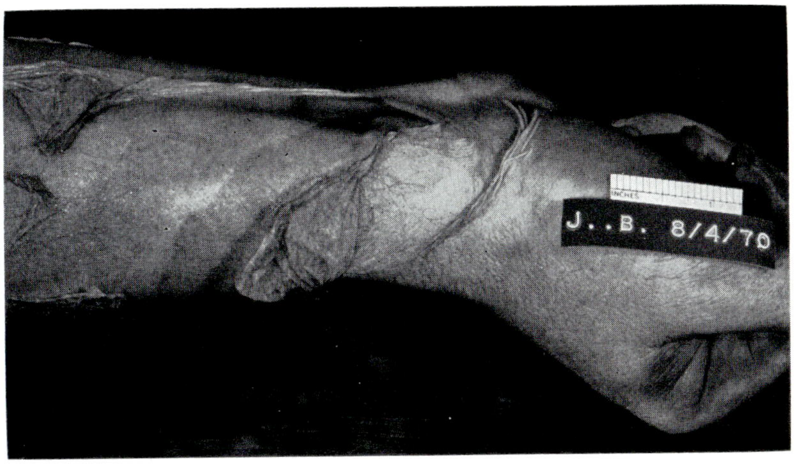


FIGURE XII-33. Blister formation in suicidal carbon monoxide poisoning. The CO level was 60%.

the brain and in the heart muscle, as well as focal myocardial nccroses, are other occasional findings.

The cherry red discoloration seen in CO poisoning changes to dark green, then to brown with the onset of decomposition. Carboxyhemoglobin, however, persists for many weeks and may be detected even after embalming and prolonged burial. Decomposition of the body does not produce carbon monoxide, nor is a significant amount of the compound absorbed by the tissues as a result of exposure to a CO-contaminated atmosphere.

### Cyanide Poisoning

Cyanide (hydrogen cyanide–HCN; potassium cyanide–KCN) asphyxiates by blocking the utilization of oxygen by the tissues through poisoning of respiratory enzymes. (Cyanide inhibits the action of cytochrome oxidase, carbonic anhydrase and probably other enzyme systems.) Cyanide paralyzes vital functions, and death occurs within seconds. In about half the cases the body is bright cherry red, because oxygen remains in the red cells as oxyhemoglobin. Since cyanide is lethal in very low quantities, the total amount of poison in the body may be insufficient for a generalized cherry red discoloration. In such cases the lividity closely resembles that seen in deaths due to other causes. Hydrogen cyanide smells like bitter almonds, and this odor exudes from the body. It is particularly noticeable when the body is opened in a warm autopsy room. Chemical proof clinches the diagnosis. Not all persons are able to detect the odor of bitter almonds; this ability is inherited as a sex-linked recessive trait.[15]

Potassium or sodium cyanide taken orally causes extensive corrosion of the stomach. Vomiting or postmortem reflux of stomach contents may corrode the esophagus and the mouth as well as the cheeks and neck. The stomach mucosa reacts intensely alkaline after ingestion of these cyanides.

## SEX-ASSOCIATED ASPHYXIAS

Various means of accidental asphyxia associated with sexual perversion are encountered. A large proportion of these deaths are discovered under bizarre circumstances, which sometimes defy the imagination by their complexity and hence arouse suspicion of foul play. The scene is often the victim's own home: his bedroom, bathroom or the basement are the usual locations. The door is commonly locked from the inside. Sometimes a motel or a secluded wooded area is chosen. In our experience, sex-associated asphyxias involve males exclusively,

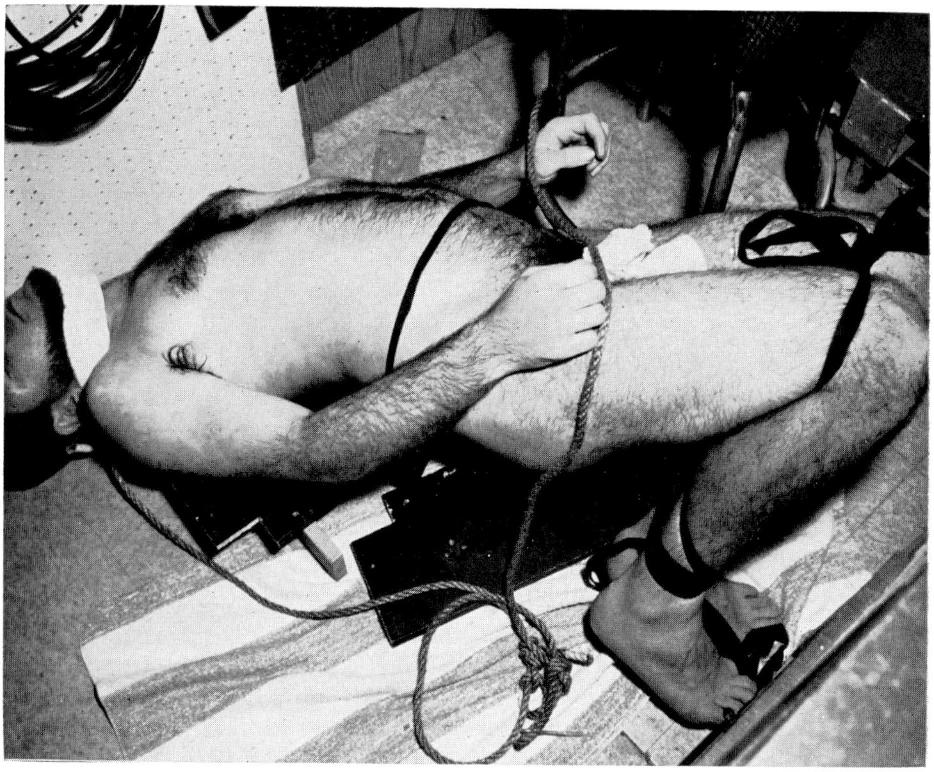

FIGURE XII-34a. Thirty-two-year-old mailman, married, with two children, found in the basement of his home. The ankles and knees were tied together. A cloth was wrapped around his genitals and secured by a rubber band. The padded rope around the neck passed over a water pipe in the ceiling and back down, ending in an eye-hook fastened in a vise.

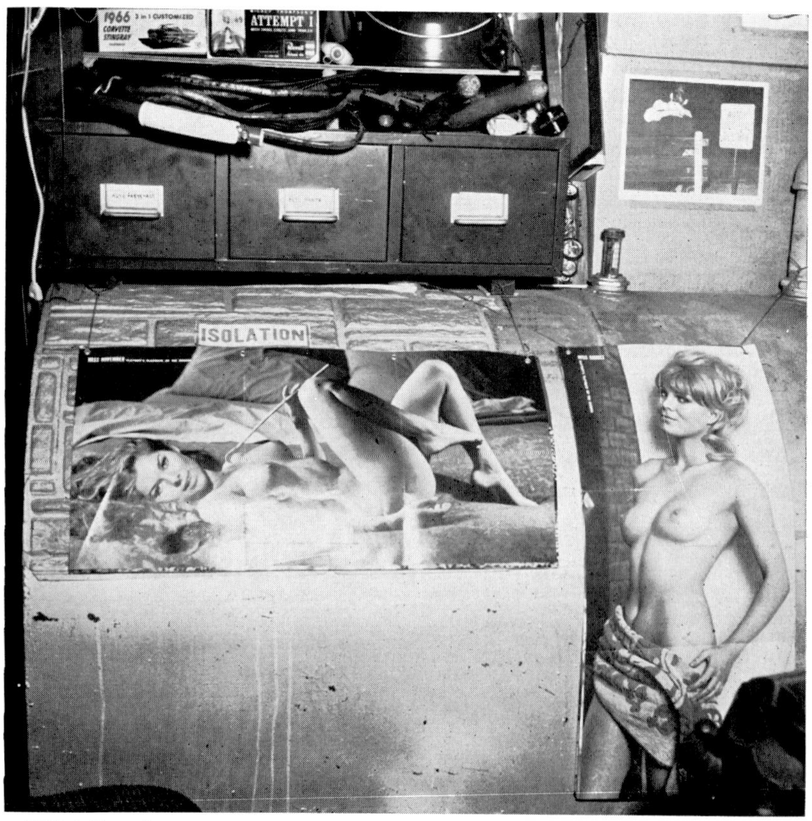


FIGURE XII-34b. These photos were in full view of the deceased shown in Figure XII-34a.

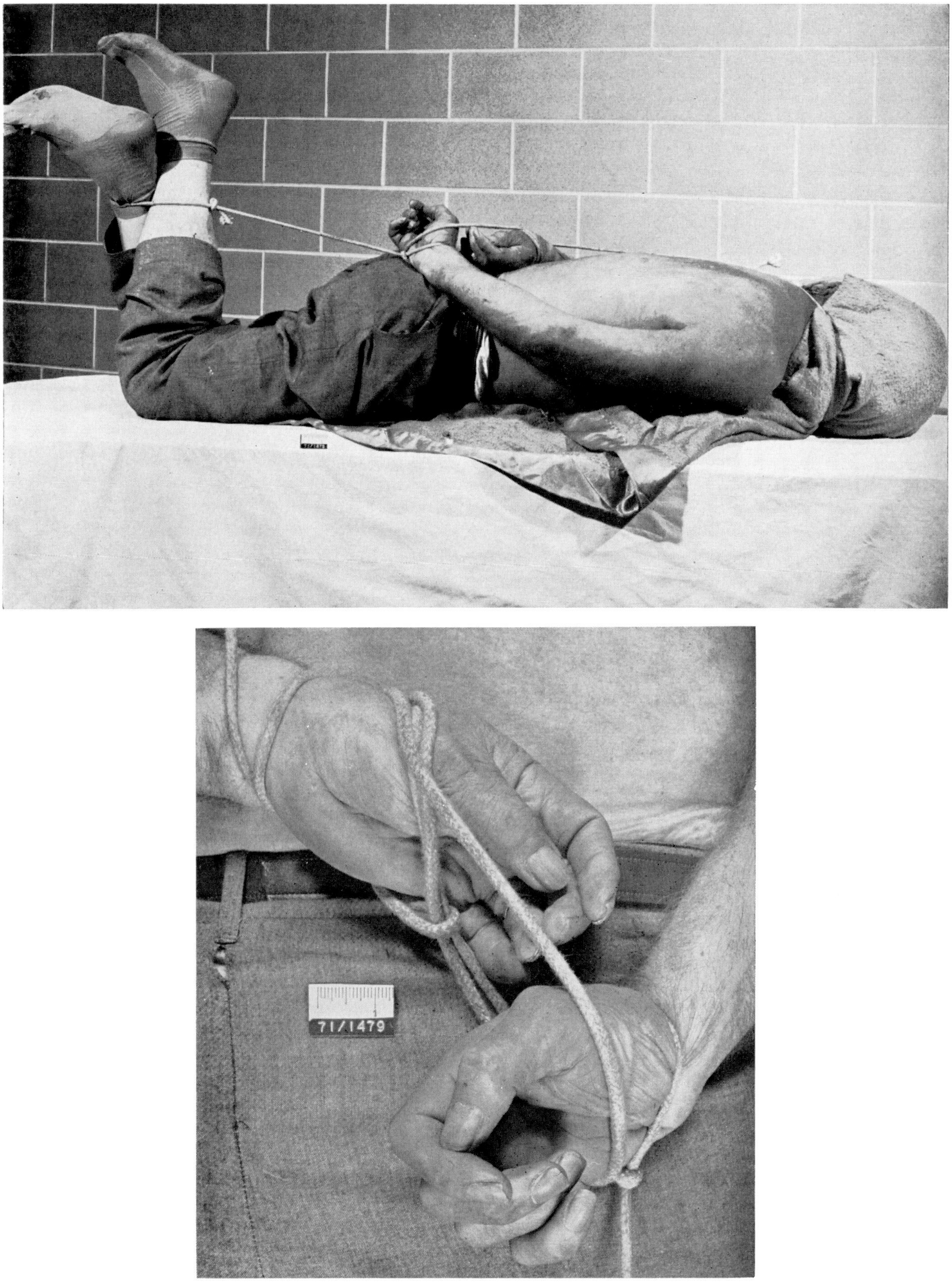


FIGURE XII-35a and b. Seventy-seven-year-old man who lived alone was found dead on his kitchen floor. The blanket over the head and neck served as padding. Straightening of the legs tightened the noose. The hands of the victim were tied behind his back, a finding that led the police to suspect homicide. However, the manner in which the hands were secured led to the conclusion that the victim had done this himself as part of the sexual ritual.

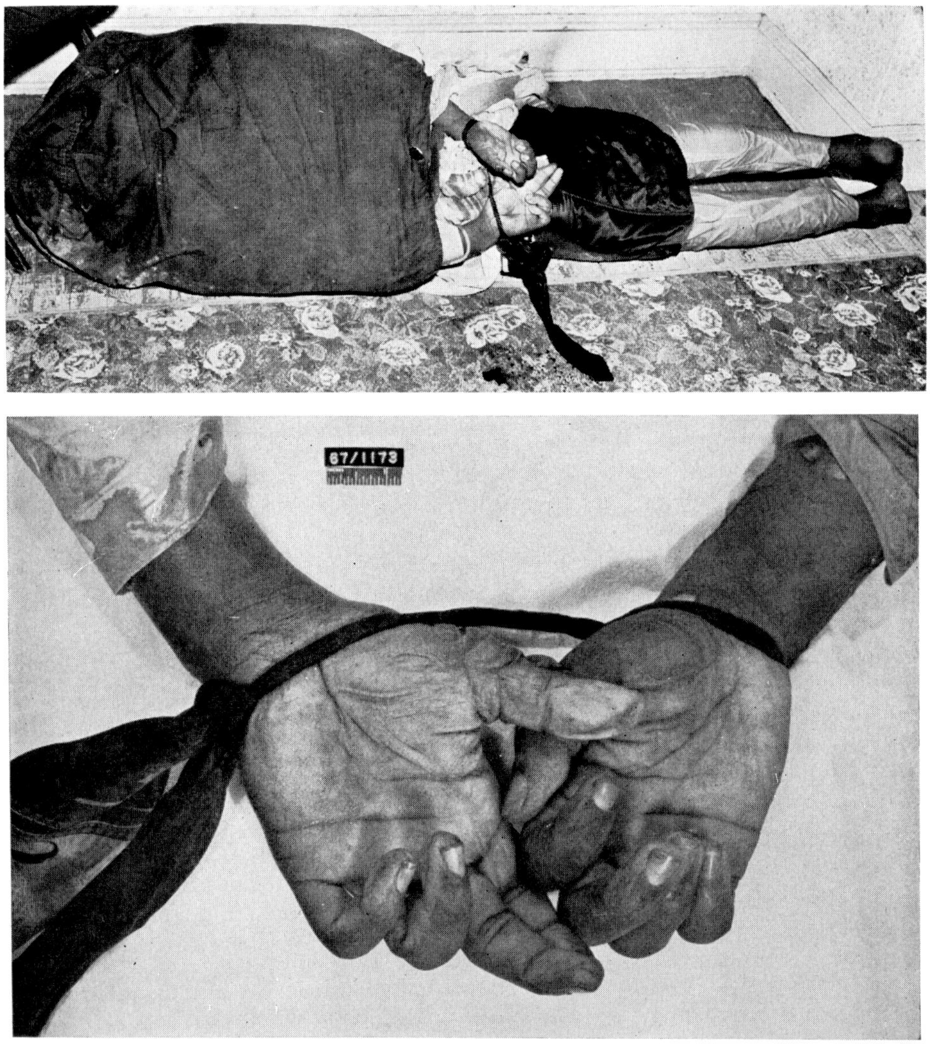


FIGURE XII-36a and b. Nineteen-year-old male college student, found dead wearing a brassiere, girdle, shirt and plastic raincoat, wrapped in a blanket, covered by a plastic laundry bag, with a duffle bag pulled over the upper half of the body. A book was wedged between the girdle and the genitals. The hands were secured in the back by a necktie, which was first knotted into a loop, then the wrists twisted in order to tighten as shown in Figure 36b. This case was first believed to be a homicide until it was ascertained that it was indeed possible for the victim to have tied his own wrists after placing the multiple layers of clothing on himself.

from boys to old age, although Henry in 1971 described the first such case in a nineteen-year-old female.[16]

The victim may be found hanged, strangled or with a plastic bag over his head. Binding the extremities, tying the wrists or handcuffing are quite frequent. Contrary to expectation, the genitalia are not necessarily exposed. Frequently the body is clothed in female attire, particularly underwear. Within the victim's view may be found pornographic pictures, mail order catalogues opened to women's wear, etc. Occasionally the victim is apparently happily married and has a number of children. The psychiatric background for these undertakings is complex and not totally understood. It is believed that reduction of the blood supply to the brain stimulates and heightens the sexual response (Figs. XII-34 to XII-37).

The presence of sperm on or near the body of a male victim of asphyxia is believed to be associated with stimulation of certain nerve centers in the brain by the asphyxial process, as well as with contraction of the musculature of the seminal vesicles by rigor mortis, causing the extrusion of seminal fluid. The latter may occur in any mode of death. Some swelling of the penis in a hanging victim is also artifactual, resulting from postmortem accumulation of blood and fluids in the lower half of the body.

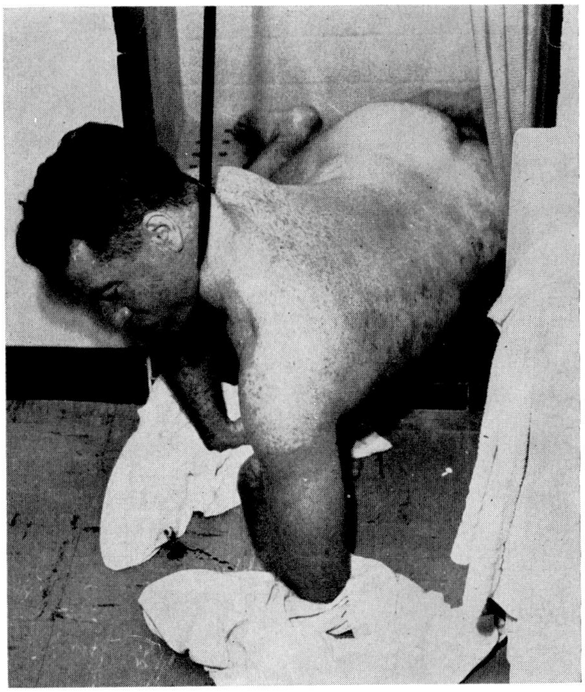

FIGURE XII-37. Thirty-nine-year-old salesman who accidentally hung himself with a belt tied to the shower curtain rod. Note the towels used to pad the elbows. The blood on the floor under the mouth and nose is due to extreme congestion in the head associated with the hanging.

## REFERENCES


1. Brouardel, P.: La pendaison, la strangulation, la suffocation, la submersion. Paris, Baillière, 1897.
2. Polson, C. J.: *The Essentials of Forensic Medicine.* Springfield, Thomas, 1965, pp. 278-374.
3. Teeters, N. K.: *Hang by the Neck.* Springfield, Thomas, 1967, p. 156.
4. Smialek, J. E., Smialek, P. Z., and Spitz, W. U.: Accidental bed deaths in infants due to unsafe sleeping situations. *Clin Pediatr, 17:*10, 1977.
5. Shapiro, H. A., Gluckman, J., and Gordon, I.: The significance of fingernail abrasions of the skin. *J Forensic Med, 9:*17, 1962.
6. Holmes, P.: *The Trials of Dr. Coppolino.* New York, NAL, 1968.
7. Glaser, H. H., and Massengale, O. N.: Glue sniffing in children. *JAMA, 181:*90, 1962.
8. Taylor, G. J., and Harris, W. S.: Cardiac toxicity of aerosol propellants. *JAMA, 214:*81, 1970.
9. Mihalakis, I.: Asphyxia from pacifier. *Md State Med J, 20:*53, 1971.
10. Zeuch, L. H.: *Ill Med J, 41:*451, 1922. Cited in Polson, C. J.: *The Essentials of Forensic Medicine.* Springfield, Thomas, 1965, p. 355.
11. Volle, R. L., and Koelle, G. B.: Ganglionic stimulating and blocking agents. In Goodman, L. S., and Gilman, A. (Eds.): *The Pharmacological Basis of Therapeutics,* 4th ed. New York, Macmillan, 1970, p. 591.
12. Wiener, M. F.: Carbon monoxide poisoning: Basic concept and current clinical-pathologic implications. In Sunderman, F. W., and Sunderman, F. W., Jr. (Eds.): *Laboratory Diagnosis of Diseases Caused by Toxic Agents.* St. Louis, Green, 1970, p. 260.
13. Sopher, I. M., and Masemore, W. C.: The investigation of vehicular carbon monoxide fatalities. *Traffic Dig Rev, 18*(11):1-11, 1970.
14. Gonzales, T. A., Vance, M., Helpern, M., and Umberger, Ch. J.: Asphyxiating gases: Carbon monoxide. In *Legal Medicine Pathology and*

*Toxicology,* 2nd ed. New York, Appleton, 1954, p. 505.
15. Camps, F. E. (Ed.): *Gradwohl's Legal Medicine,* 2nd ed. Bristol, Wright & Sons Ltd., 1968, p. 616.
16. Henry, R. C.: "Sex" hangings in the female. *Medico-Legal Bulletin,* No. 214. Richmond, Virginia, Office of the Chief Medical Examiner, February, 1971.

*Chapter XIII*

# DROWNING

WERNER U. SPITZ

BETWEEN 7000 and 8000 deaths by drowning occur in the United States each year; this represents the fourth leading cause of accidental deaths.[1] Our knowledge of the events that take place in the drowning victim is by no means complete. It is primarily derived from animal experiments and to some extent from observations on humans where the drowning was witnessed and reported.

Submersion is usually followed by a panicky struggle to reach the surface. When energy reserves are exhausted, the struggle subsides and actual drowning begins. Several phases are recognized in the drowning process:

1. Breath holding lasts for a variable length of time until carbon dioxide accumulation in blood and tissues reaches a level at which stimulation of the respiratory center in the brain leads to inevitable inhalation of large volumes of water.
2. Swallowing of water, coughing, vomiting and progressive loss of consciousness follow in rapid succession. Escape of air remaining in the lungs and replacement by water lead to the next phase.
3. Profound unconsciousness and convulsions associated with gasping precede respiratory standstill, which is followed by failure of the heart. Irreversible changes in the brain and death supervene within a very short time.

It is remarkable that when drowning is interrupted before terminal gasping has set in, spontaneous recovery sometimes occurs.[2] Drowning is commonly thought of as a form of asphyxia; however, the mechanism is very much more involved than mere deprivation of air. True asphyxia is *said* to occur in only 10 or 12 percent of all drowning deaths. This supposedly results from closure of the larynx by a protective reflex mechanism that seals the airway and prevents inhalation of liquid into the deeper air passages. It is unexplained why precisely 10 to 12 percent of *drowning deaths* are believed to be associated with this mechanism. Spastic closure of the airway is not detectable at autopsy because of relaxation of the tissues in the early postmortem period. The finding at autopsy of *dry lungs* indicates neither that water was inhaled nor that it was not *(vide infra)*.

In any case, in the vast majority of instances death by drowning is associated with inhalation of large volumes of liquid. This causes some degree of anoxia as well as acute disturbances in the composition of the blood.

The mechanism of death by drowning differs, depending on the chemical composition of the drowning liquid; consequently, freshwater and seawater drowning must be considered separately.

## DROWNING IN FRESH WATER OR BRACKISH WATER

Because of the low salt (sodium chloride) content of these waters (brackish water has approximately 0.5% salinity), precipitous absorption into the circulation takes place. This results in hemolysis and dilution of the blood constituents associated with an abrupt violent increase in blood volume (Fig. XIII-1a). The heart is rapidly overburdened by this increased load, and pulmonary edema becomes manifest. Arrhythmias of the heartbeat, which culminate in ventricular tachycardia and fibrillation, lead to death within three to five minutes from the

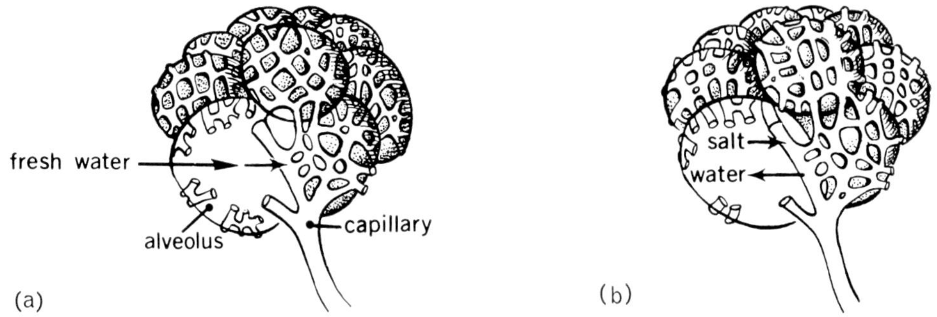


FIGURE XIII-1. Diagram of events in fresh- and saltwater drowning. (a): Drowning in fresh or brackish water is characterized by rapid absorption of the water into the bloodstream because of absent or low salt content in these waters. (b): Submersion in seawater is followed by rapid diffusion of salts into the bloodstream, while water is drawn from the circulation into the lungs to establish osmotic balance.

start of submersion. Exhaustion due to a prolonged struggle in the first phase of drowning tends to shorten this interval.

If results of animal experiments are extrapolated to humans, the amount of water that is inhaled and absorbed by an adult may approach six pints or more.

## DROWNING IN SEAWATER

In contrast to fresh water, seawater is strongly salty (usually over 3.0% sodium chloride concentration). Due to this high salinity, fluids are drawn from the blood into the lung tissue, causing severe pulmonary edema. However, the amount of fluid that is thus shifted is relatively small and in no way compares to that which penetrates the bloodstream in freshwater drowning. Some concentration of the blood occurs. Simultaneously, salts from the water in the lungs move into the bloodstream in an attempt to reestablish osmotic balance (Fig. XIII-1b). In general terms, drowning in saltwater more closely resembles an asphyxial type of death compared with freshwater drowning. Severe arrhythmias of the heartbeat are practically never observed in laboratory experiments. As may be expected, therefore, saltwater drowning usually lasts longer and hence is likely to be more amenable to resuscitation than drowning in fresh water.

The different mechanism in freshwater versus saltwater drowning has significant implications with respect to the blood alcohol concentration of the victim. In freshwater drowning dilution of the blood may be expected to cause a decrease in the alcohol level, whereas in saltwater drowning a slight increase should occur. However, preliminary experiments on rabbits indicate a decrease in both modes of drowning. In the freshwater series, a decrease of up to 33% was observed, i.e. an animal that had a blood alcohol concentration of .21% before submersion has a .14% thereafter.

## DIAGNOSIS OF DROWNING

Drowning is mostly accidental. In a relatively small number of cases it is suicidal. In some cases death in the water is due to natural causes, such as a heart attack or cerebral hemorrhage during bathing or swimming. Disposal of a victim of homicide to simulate drowning is rare, yet because of such possibility, distinction between changes due to drowning and those resulting from postmortem immersion of the body is of prime importance. In recent years we have seen a significant number of adults in their early twenties, all known heroin users, who were found dead and partly or completely submerged in a bathtub. As recounted by witnesses in some of the cases, these individuals collapsed because of an adverse reaction to the injected drug and were placed in a water-filled tub as a means of resuscitation (Fig. XIII-2).

What aggravates these situations is the fact that no reliable tests permitting an unequivocal diagnosis of drowning are available. Thus, the central question in the case of a body recovered from water is whether the individual was alive at the time he entered the water. The scene, the circumstances surrounding the incident with all available background information, the deceased's clothing, all play a significant role in this determination. For example, the finding of an alcoholic floating in the water 20 ft. below a cliff with his zipper open suggests that he had been urinating before he fell. The rare instance of a hand clutching weeds also belongs in this category and permits the conclusion that the deceased may have struggled to stay on the surface. Parenthetically, we do not believe in cadaveric spasm or instantaneous rigor as some prefer to call it; rather, it is our opinion that the weeds remain entangled between the fingers.

From a practical standpoint, the presence of water in the lungs and the stomach of a drowning victim is of no real significance. Water may well reach these organs after death.

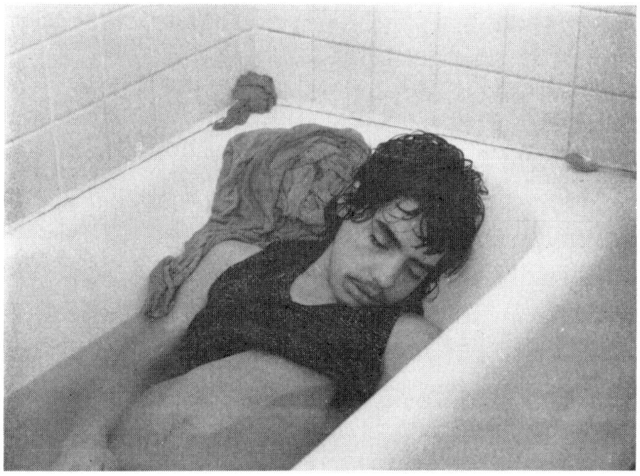

FIGURE XIII-2. Narcotic addict placed in a water-filled tub in a resuscitation attempt following an adverse reaction to heroin. A stocking tourniquet and a spoon *cooker* are noted on the sides of the tub.

The fully clothed fresh body of a young woman was found on a deserted beach just below the waterline. The waves were washing over the body and had swept abundant sand over the clothing. A large amount of sand was present in the creases and in the pockets. At autopsy a contact gunshot wound was noted in the center of the forehead. The airway, including all its major tributaries, was filled with sand and seaweed to the extent of forming a solid cast. A small quantity of sand was present in the stomach and the first part of the small intestine. As death was believed to have occurred practically instantaneously, the sand and seaweed must have been washed into the body after death.

At autopsy, the lungs of a drowning victim commonly resemble those seen in deaths associated with severe pulmonary edema, as in cases of arteriosclerotic heart disease.

A fifty-six-year-old worker was standing on a concrete platform painting a bridge support. Suddenly, he was observed to fall and slide into the water which was very shallow at that point. He was picked up *within a few seconds.* He was unconscious at this time, but breathed heavily until arrival at a hospital ten minutes later. The attendant in the ambulance said that the decedent was foaming from the mouth as they were approaching their destination. He was pronounced dead fifteen minutes later. At autopsy no injuries were noted. The lungs were heavy, and on incision large amounts of fluid and foam exuded from the cut surfaces. The appearance of the lungs suggested that death was due to drowning. The coronary arteries showed far-advanced arteriosclerosis.

At a later hearing before the Workmen's Compensation Commission, a fellow worker, who had been painting next to the deceased, testified that his friend had complained of severe chest pain and that he particularly emphasized that he felt *as if a rope were being tied around* his chest a few minutes prior to his fall. The coworker further stated that the deceased's head and shoulders had not been submerged at any time, as he held the victim to prevent this. On the basis of this testimony it was decided that death was due to an acute heart attack. Death benefits were consequently denied by the Commission.

The body of a known epileptic or alcoholic recovered from the shallow end of a pool or found face down in a roadside puddle may equally pose a considerable diagnostic problem (Fig. XIII-3). Edema of the lungs is a common finding in deaths that occur during an epileptic seizure or due to alcoholic intoxication.

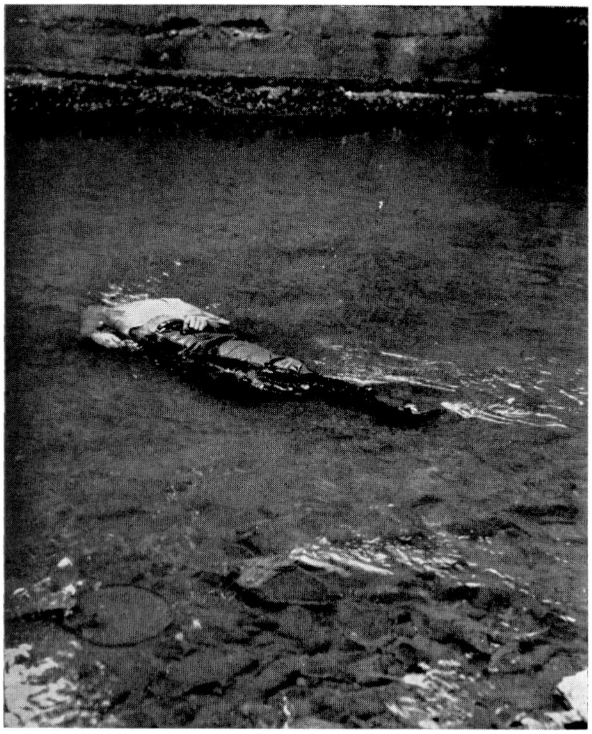

FIGURE XIII-3. Young man found in a shallow stream (water depth about 18 in.). Autopsy showed no injuries but a fatty liver and early cirrhosis, consistent with chronic alcoholism. His blood alcohol level was 0.32%.

A young woman, known epileptic with evidence of gingival hypertrophy (Fig. XIII-4), was found in a ditch beside the road, her face submerged in about eight inches of water. The rest of the body was dry. No one saw this woman collapse. The autopsy showed no recent injuries and no other changes, except for an old injury of the left parietal region of the brain and severe edema of the lungs. Some sand and muddy water identical to that in the ditch were found deep in the trachea and in some of the major bronchi. Chemical analysis of the blood showed an alcohol level of 0.12%. No phenobarbital or diphenylhydantoin used for the control of epileptic seizures were found. It seemed logical to conclude that the deceased had suffered an epileptic seizure, fallen into the ditch and died as a result of drowning.

Drowning in the bathtub poses a considerable medicolegal problem. In our experience such drownings occur only if unconsciousness is brought about by disease (epilepsy, heart disease, etc.) or after consumption of alcohol and/or drugs (Fig. XIII-5). An excellent review of this subject is given by Geertinger and Voigt.[3] These authors reviewed fifty-one bathtub deaths, which accrued over an eight-year period.

The diagnosis of strangulation in a body recovered from water, particularly in the absence of characteristic injuries to the neck, is another example in which conclusions regarding the cause of death would be tenuous.

Accidental drowning in the swimming pool sometimes results from jumping off the diving board. Impact of the forehead on the floor of the pool may cause hyperextension of the head and loss of consciousness, with subsequent inhalation of water. Common anatomical findings under such circumstances consist of hemorrhages in the deep neck muscles in the region of C-1 and C-2, with or without vertebral fractures. The autopsy technique to document these injuries in the upper cervical area is described in Chapter XXIV. Evidence of injury to the forehead is usually minimal and may be absent, especially if the impact is alleviated due to a slippery pool bottom. It is often necessary that the galea be incised after reflection of the scalp to show minimal bruising of the subcutaneous tissue.

A riddle to pathologists are the sudden

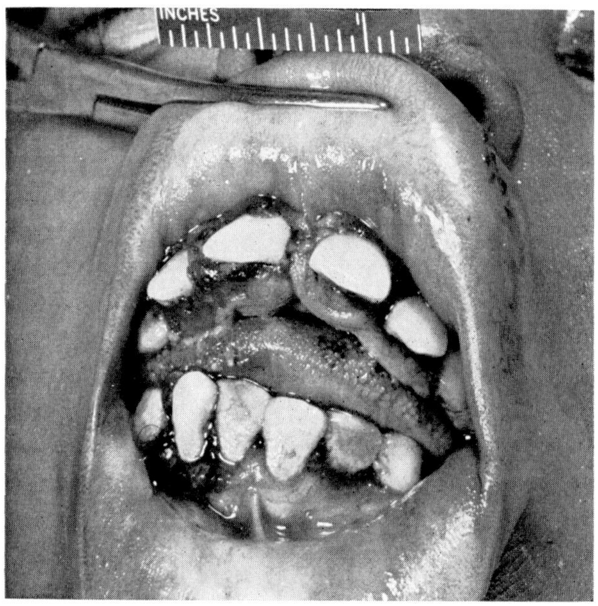


FIGURE XIII-4. Gingival hypertrophy following treatment with diphenylhydantoin used for the control of epileptic seizures.

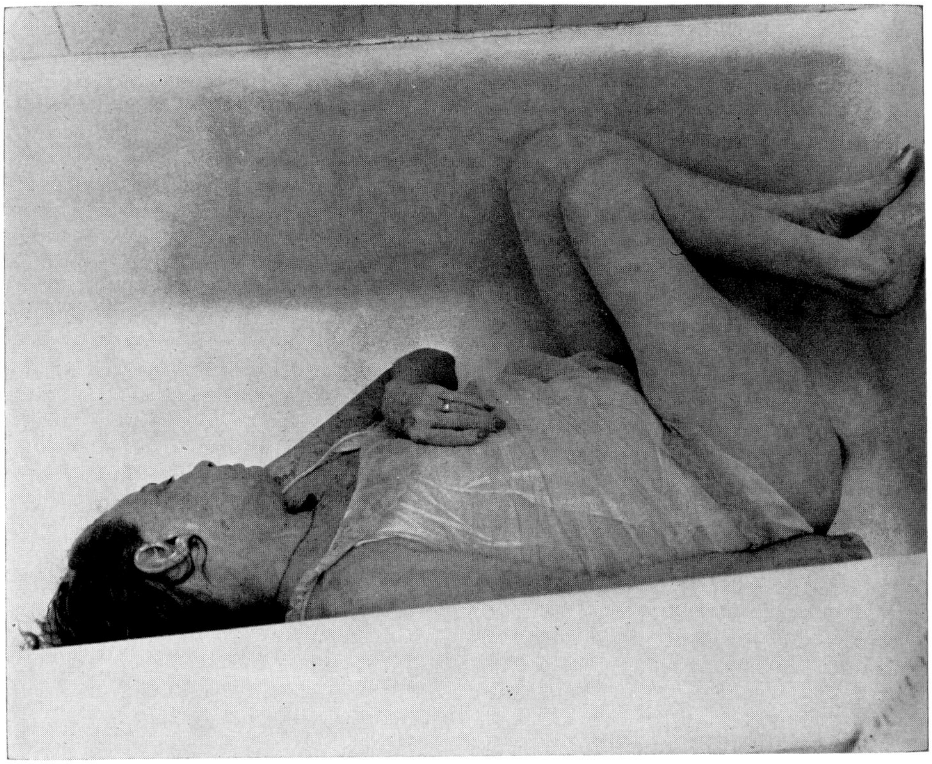

FIGURE XIII-5. This fifty-four-year-old woman was found submerged in the bathtub in her apartment. A suicide note was appended to the bathroom door. She had a blood alcohol level of .20% as well as 1.2 mg% of a short-acting barbiturate.

drowning deaths of young healthy individuals while engaged in underwater swimming. Mostly these are underwater endurance tests where people hyperventilate before entering the water. A plausible explanation is that overbreathing followed by exercise under water causes the arterial oxygen tension to fall to a level at which consciousness is lost and water is inhaled.

Abundant foam is usually noted exuding from the mouth and nostrils of a drowning victim (Fig. XIII-6). This foam may not be apparent when the body is first recovered from the water, but it appears when pressure is applied to the chest, as by attempted resuscitation or during removal of the victim's clothing. The foam is produced by the mixture of air, mucus and water in the presence of respiratory movements. Hence, the presence of foam in the airway indicates beyond doubt that the victim was alive at the time of submersion. Frequently the foam is bloodstained, not as a result of injury to the chest but due to tears of the lung tissue by the increased pressure within the lungs, which is part of the drowning process. When decomposition sets in, the foam is rapidly changed to a foul smelling, brown, somewhat bubbly fluid.

The significance of bloodstained foam in the respiratory passages of a body recovered from water was an important issue at a 1969 court hearing in Wilkes-Barre, Pennsylvania, regarding the death of Mary Jo Kopechne. At this hearing, arguments were heard regarding whether or not Miss Kopechne's body should be exhumed for autopsy to determine the cause of death.

The judge refused to order an exhumation based on the testimony that a large amount of pinkish foam exuded from her nose and mouth after she was recovered from the water. This finding led to the conclusion that Miss Kopechne had to be alive, and therefore drowned, when the car in which she was a passenger drove off a bridge at Chappaquiddick Island, near the Massachusetts coast.

Drowning cases with relatively dry lungs are occasionally observed. Heart action in

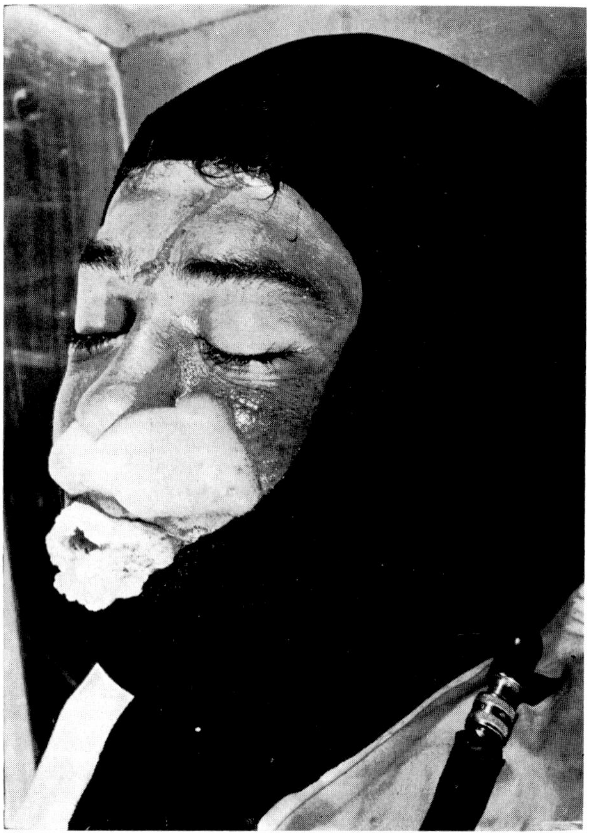

FIGURE XIII-6. *Mushroom of foam* emerging from mouth and nostrils of a drowned victim.

drowning continues after cessation of respiration, and, whereas meaningful heartbeats are maintained for only a brief period of time, this suffices to absorb the water from the lungs into the bloodstream. No significant amount of water reaches the alveoli after inhalations have stopped. The same is believed to occur if circulation of the blood remains functional for a short time after recovery of the victim from the water or if resuscitative measures were instituted.

Spotlike hemorrhages in the lungs, especially under the pleura, are often noted in drowning cases. These hemorrhages result from overdistension of the lungs by the drowning liquid; hemolysis and dilution account for their pink or red washed-out appearance. An occasional small hemorrhage may be seen in a conjunctiva of a person who drowned. However, multiple pinpoint hemorrhages in the eyelids and the conjunctivae, as in strangulation or hanging, do not occur in drowning.

Hemorrhages in the middle ears and mastoid air cells are occasionally encountered in persons recovered from water. Some have associated these hemorrhages with death by drowning.[4] It appears logical, however, to consider middle ear hemorrhages the result of pressure changes, not unlike those that are sometimes associated with underwater swimming or diving. Lanphier[5] has observed hemorrhage in the sinuses and in the middle ears and rupture of the eardrums in cases of unequalized descent to a depth of 10 ft., and Behnke[6] reports striking changes in the ear resulting from slight differences in pressure such as 1 to 2 psi, which is equivalent to 2.3 to 4.6 ft. of water.

The inhalation of water alone does not seem to adequately explain middle ear hemorrhage, except as a result of extreme congestion. Congestion of similar severity occurs in all types of asphyxial death, as well as in a large number of other conditions. Severe congestion may be seen in cases of heart failure. Possibly the added pressure developing in a part of the body as a result of lividity may contribute to the occurrence of spotlike hemorrhages.

An elderly, obese and hypertensive man who died of an acute myocardial infarction was found on his bed, his head hanging down over the side. His face was deep purple with lividity. At autopsy bleeding was noted into both middle ears.

Wrinkling of the skin of the hands and feet seen in individuals recovered from water is frequently referred to as *washerwoman's skin* (Fig. XIII-7). It is not associated with the process of drowning but is strictly due to prolonged immersion. Wrinkling of the skin cannot be used to determine the length of time a body was in the water, although at a water temperature of 50° to 60° F, wrinkling is manifest as early as thirty minutes to one hour. After a certain time, depending on the temperature of the water and length of immersion, the superficial layers of the skin peel like a *glove,* including the nails. In cold water, several days may elapse before the glove separates, while in warm

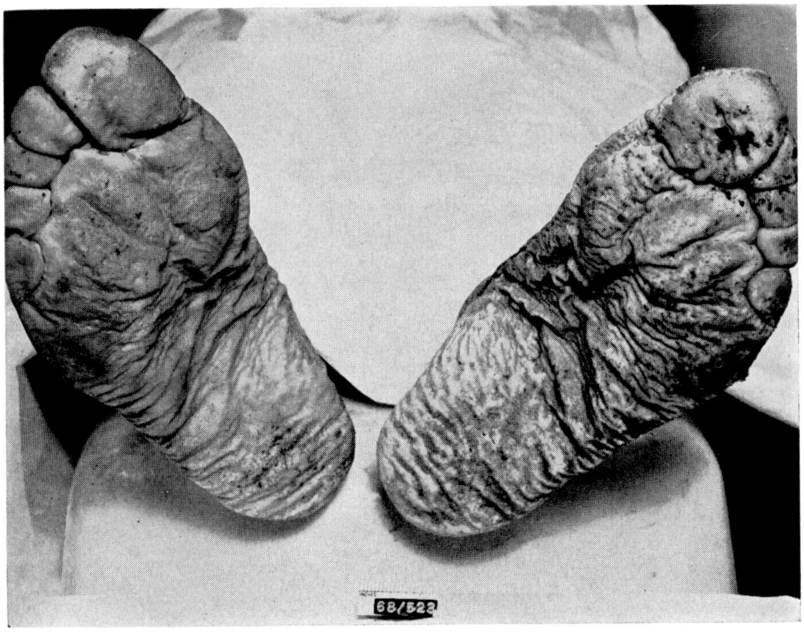

FIGURE XIII-7. *Washerwoman* skin due to prolonged immersion.

water several hours suffice. The glove may be used to obtain fingerprints for the purpose of identification.

An elderly woman had a heart attack while taking a bath. She was found eight hours later sitting in lukewarm water while hot water was trickling from the tap. The skin of her hands and feet was peeling and could easily be removed (Fig. XIII-8).

In second degree burns and in decomposition, peeling of the skin from the hands and feet occurs in a similar fashion.

The microscopic findings in the lungs in drowning are not characteristic, yet they differ to some extent, depending on whether drowning occurred in fresh water or in seawater. In freshwater drowning the lungs are overdistended, alveolar walls are torn and structures in the way of the inundating fluid are disrupted. This picture is sometimes referred to as *aqueous emphysema*. In seawater drowning the architecture of the lungs is often better preserved and aqueous emphysema is less pronounced. Perivascular infiltrates of leukocytes may be noted, ranging from a few leukocytes to marked focal perivasculitis. Occasional small intra-alveolar hemorrhages are common in both types of drowning. This causes the pink or red staining of the foam in the airway. It appears likely that the different appearance of the lungs in the two conditions is related to the differences in salt content (osmolality) of the two drowning media.

Numerous laboratory criteria for diagnosing drowning, some believed to be more dependable than others, have been reported since the turn of the century. Each of these was accepted by forensic pathologists for some time until experience showed their questionable value.

Carrara[7] in 1902 established disproportionate dilution of left heart blood in freshwater versus saltwater drowning on the basis of specific gravity, freezing point and electrical conductivity determinations. In 1903 Placzek[8] emphasized the diagnostic value of the specific gravity method. In 1921 Gettler[9] published a test for drowning involving the determination of chlorides in blood from the right and left heart chambers: a difference of 25 mg/100 ml between the chloride concentrations of the two sides of the heart indicated that death was due to drowning. In freshwater drowning the chloride level in the blood in the left side of the

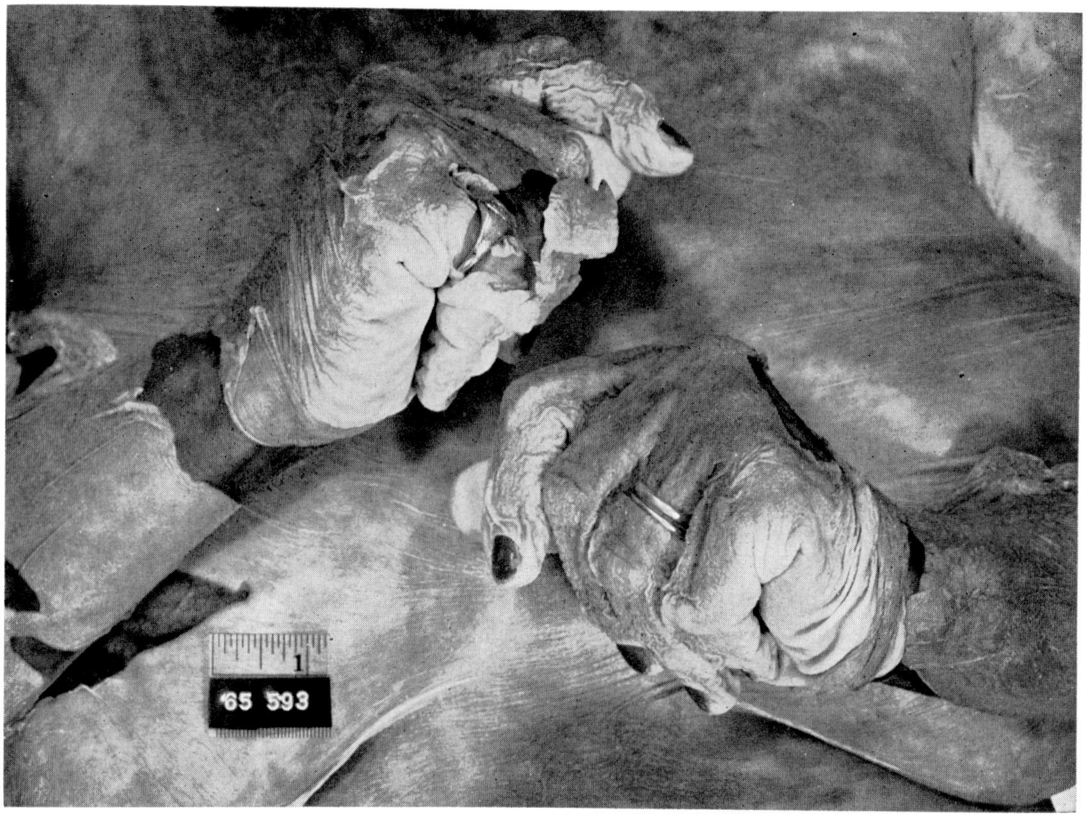


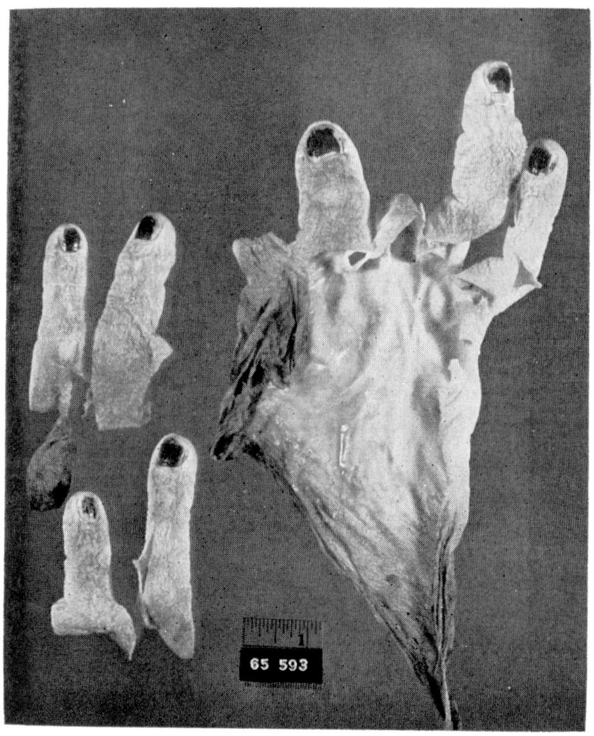


FIGURE XIII-8. (a): Peeling of skin from the hands after eight hours immersion in warm water. (b): The *glove* of skin includes the fingernails. Excellent fingerprints can be obtained from such specimens.

heart was lower than that in the right side; the reverse situation was noted in saltwater drowning.

Gettler's observations have since been challenged repeatedly. It has been shown that changes in the chloride levels after death occur in blood in both sides of the heart simultaneously and not in any constant fashion. In 1944 Moritz[10] suggested magnesium as being more reliable than chlorides, particularly for the determination of seawater drowning, and in 1955 Freimuth et al.,[11] using specific gravity values of heart plasma, concluded that negative differences between the left and the right side may be obtained in either drowning or nondrowning cases, while positive values usually indicate that death was caused by means other than drowning. Since then others have investigated the changes that occur in serum electrolyte concentrations as a result of drowning, and their

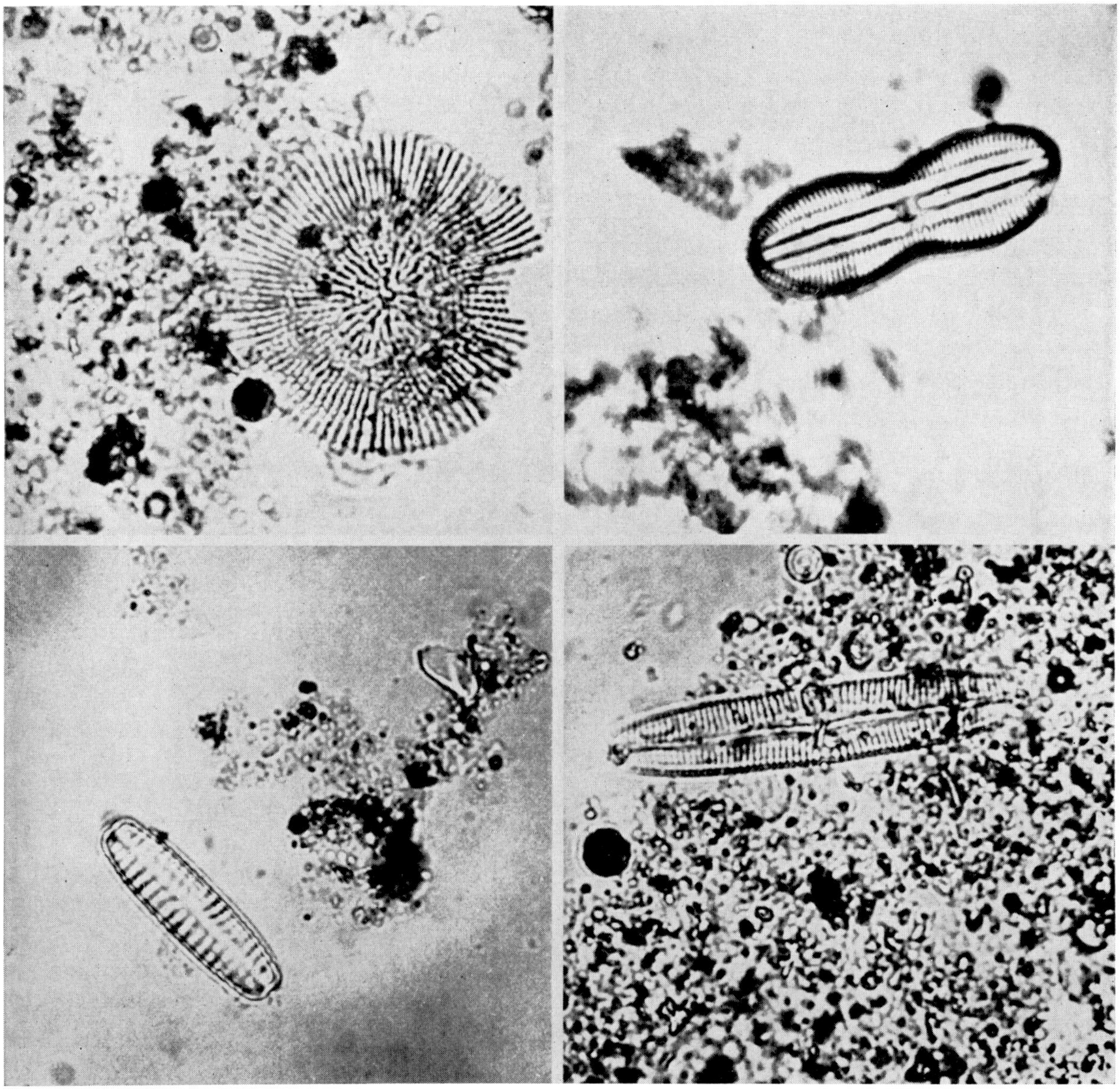

FIGURE XIII-9. Various forms of diatom shells recovered from the ashes of incinerated air filters. The material in the background is mostly carbon. The diatom in the upper left corner measures 42 $\mu$ in diameter.

results shed considerable doubt on the reliability of diagnostic tests based on electrolyte changes.[12]

Now, as before, there persists discrepancy and uncertainty with respect to all chemical tests used for the diagnosis of drowning. There are a number of factors that hinder the reliability of chemical drowning tests. A major obstacle is, no doubt, the rapidity of onset of postmortem changes in the blood and in the tissues. The publication, therefore, by Incze[13] in 1941 of the finding of diatoms in the lungs and the systemic circulation of individuals recovered from water as a diagnostic test for drowning, even after advanced decomposition, was a widely acclaimed event, particularly in Europe. The finding of diatoms in the lungs was considered indicative of the inhalation of water in which these silica-coated algae find their natural habitat.

The portal of entry of diatoms into the bloodstream was believed to be via the lungs, through microscopic tears of alveolar walls that occur in the process of forceful water inhalation.[14] It was after the diatom method for the diagnosis of drowning was established in Europe that it began to spread to several North American medicolegal departments, but in 1963 we questioned the validity of this method by the recovery of diatoms in the liver and in other organs of individuals who had died of causes other than drowning.[15] We also showed diatoms in significant numbers in the air.[16] The ubiquity of diatoms has been known to meteorologists for many years but was never considered by forensic pathologists (Fig. XIII-9).

How diatoms enter the circulation in the nondrowning victim is not clear. Could it be that they are absorbed from the gastrointestinal tract? The relationhip between diatoms and the diagnosis of death by drowning has since given rise to a large volume of literature of pros and cons, and there is hardly a medicolegal journal that has not taken part in the "war of diatoms" in one way or another.

Quantitative assays of peroxidase in animal lungs (rats) yielded values close to 800 units in freshwater drowning and 6400 units in saltwater drowning. Experimental asphyxia and pulmonary edema showed levels of intermediate order (but close to the saltwater series) between these two drowning groups.[17, 18]

Refinement of these experiments or other enzyme studies may someday find applicability in the determination of drowning deaths. At this time there has not yet been developed a test that might be referred to as a *drowning test*, as some like to believe. Only an evaluation of all possible criteria, especially the findings at autopsy and the circumstances in a particular case, together corroborate the diagnosis.

Determination of tissue catecholamines has been proposed as a means to distinguish sudden natural death followed by a fall into the water from the drawn-out death associated with a fight for survival, as is known to occur in victims of actual drowning. The levels of adrenalin and noradrenalin are known to rise under conditions of stress and shock.

## POSTMORTEM CHANGES

A body in water will sink unless air trapped among the clothes keeps it afloat. The body will resurface when gas is formed as a result of putrefaction. Putrefaction in the water proceeds at a considerably slower rate than in the air, but once the body is removed from the water, postmortem changes progress far more rapidly than is usual under the same prevailing environmental conditions. Putrefaction is slower in seawater compared to fresh water because high salinity retards bacterial growth. In stagnant waters where bacteria abound, putrefaction occurs rapidly.

The time until reappearance of the body depends on the temperature of the water. It may take two or three days in the summer and weeks or months in the winter. In deep and very cold waters, as in some of the Great Lakes, gas formation does not occur, and the body may never resurface. The same is true if the body is trapped

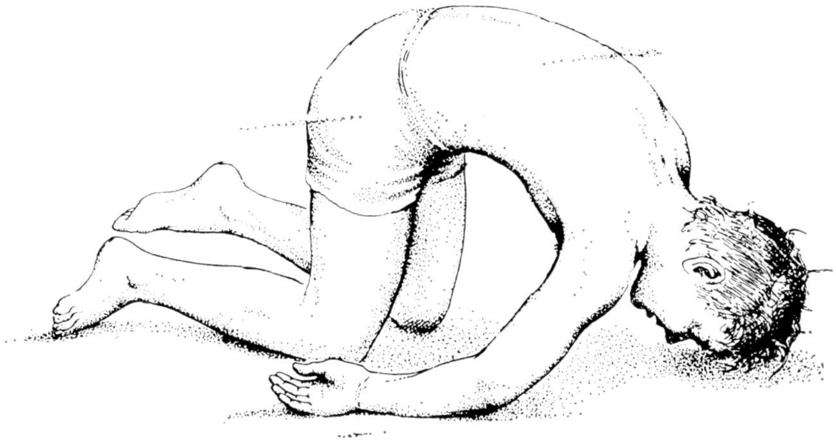

FIGURE XIII-10. Areas of the submerged body that are exposed to injury by drifting below the water surface. The back of the hands, the forehead and the toes are especially vulnerable. (Courtesy of Hospital Publ. Inc. From Spitz, W. U.: Drowning. *Hosp Med*, 5:11, 1969.)

among rocks or caught in underwater shrubbery. While the body is under water it is subject to injuries by wildlife, by drifting along the ground (Fig. XIII-10),[19] by propeller blades of boats and ships (Fig. XIII-11), rocks, etc. Injuries by spear guns are occasionally seen. It is important that these injuries be recognized and that they be distinguished from injuries sustained during life. A victim of drowning tends to bleed more readily, and more blood usually oozes from a wound of such an individual compared to a person who died from another cause. The lack of postmortem blood clotting in drowning and the draining and leaching of blood from

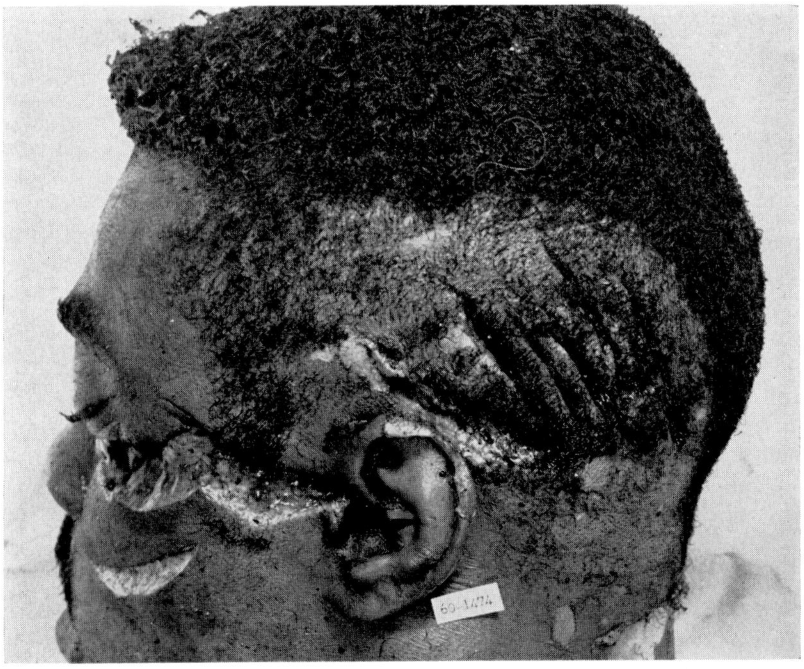

FIGURE XIII-11. Parallel cuts of the scalp and face in a victim of drowning. The body was found floating in the harbor area. These postmortem injuries were inflicted by the propeller blades of a boat's outboard motor.

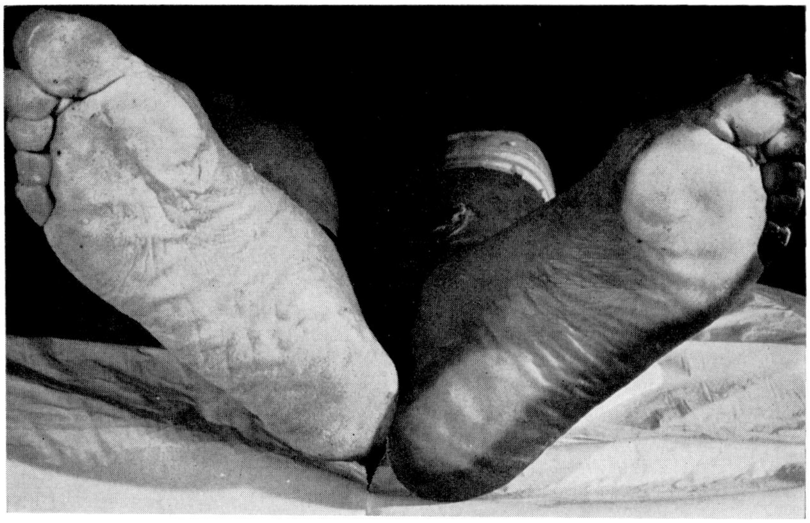

FIGURE XIII-12. The deceased was found collapsed over his kitchen sink while hot water from the faucet was trickling down his right leg. The sock on his right foot was thoroughly wet, while the left was dry. Note the absence of postmortem lividity from the right foot due to swelling and loss of transparency of the upper layers of the skin as a result of prolonged immersion.

an open wound may alter the appearance of a wound and make the determination of ante- versus postmortem occurrence difficult or impossible.

Postmortem lividity is often difficult to recognize in a body recovered from water due to swelling and loss of translucency of the upper layers of the skin; the skin becomes water-

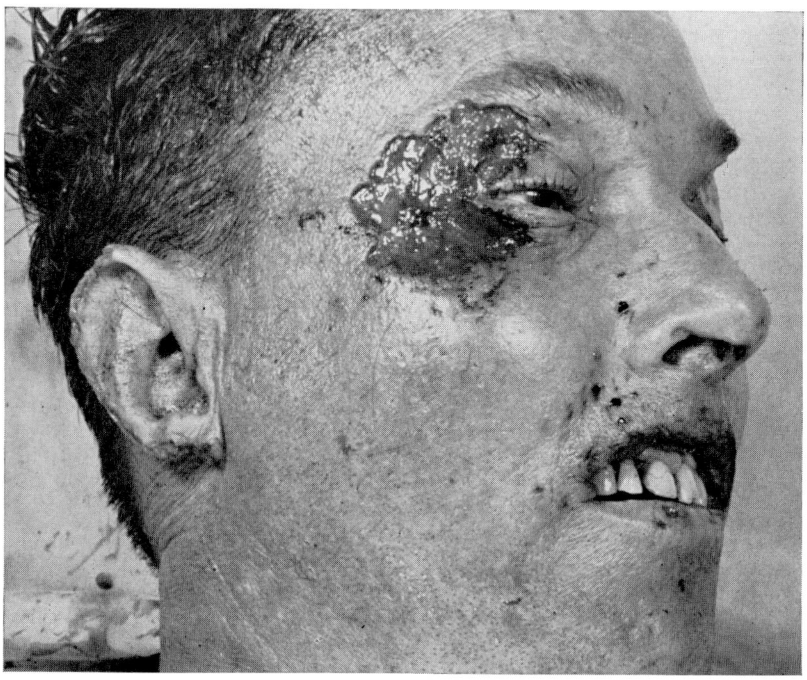

FIGURE XIII-13. Injuries of the eyelids, the ear, the nose and the lips by crabs and crayfish. In their early stages these postmortem injuries resemble abrasions.

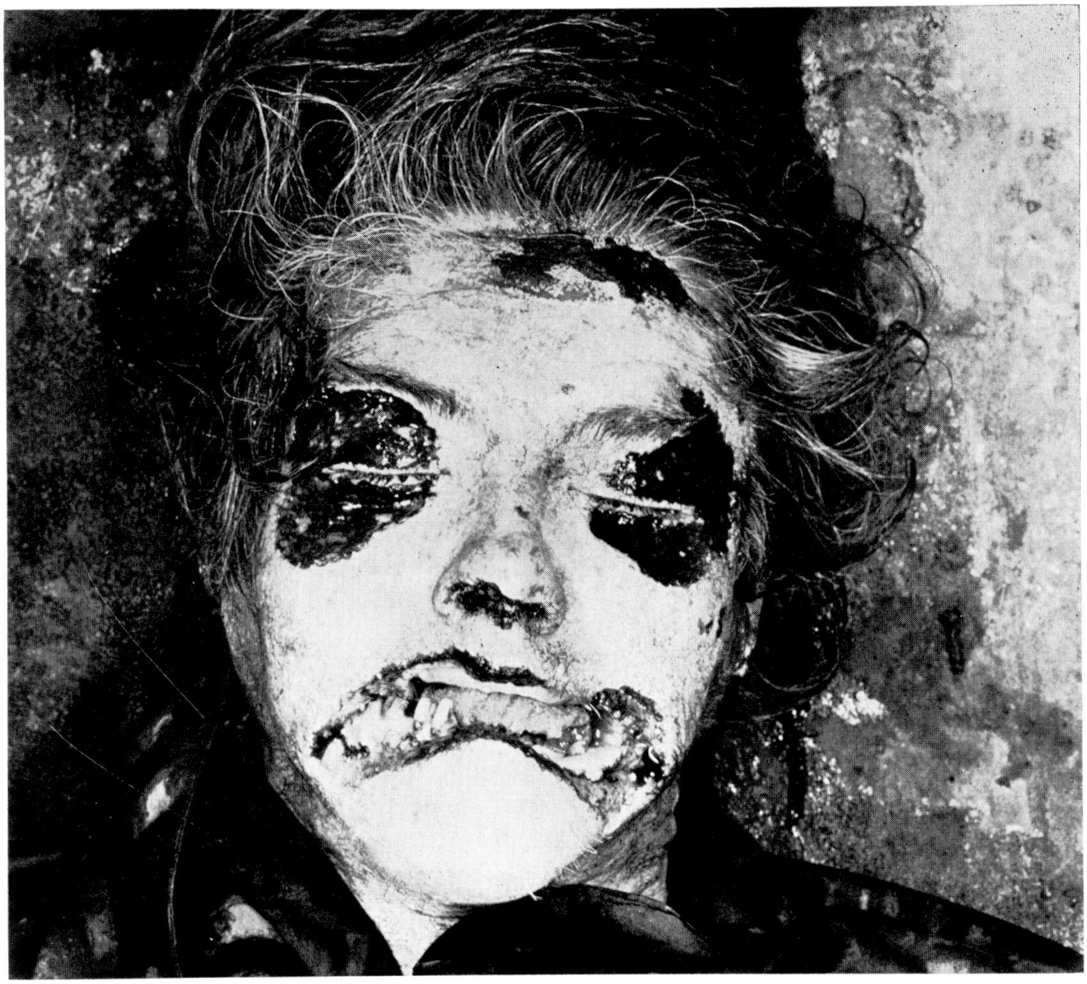

FIGURE XIII-14: Growth of algae on areas of the face exposed by marine life.

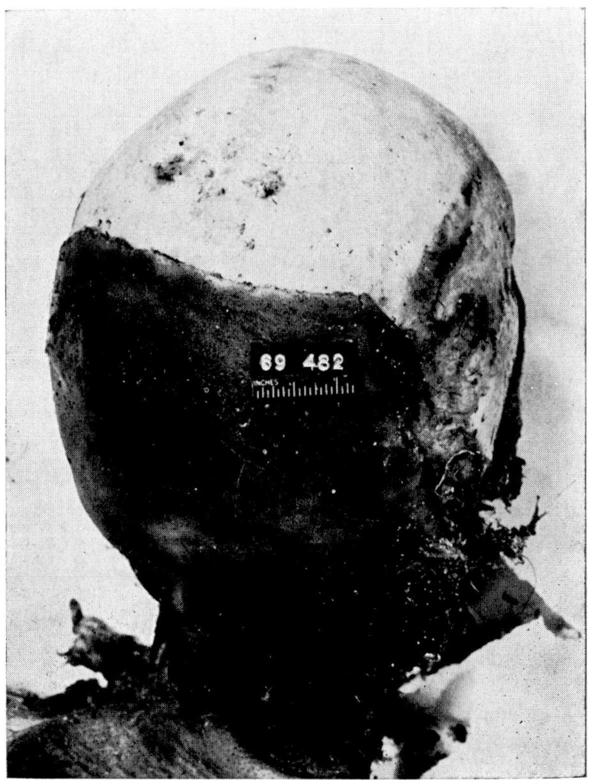


FIGURE XIII-15. This body was found in July drifting in the waters of the Chesapeake Bay a short distance offshore. The entire back of the body, which was exposed to the air, was mummified, while the submerged front was skeletonized. The victim had been reported missing eight months earlier. The head shows the horizontal water line above which the skull was exposed. Skeletonization in this case is believed to be due to the combined effects of postmortem marine life feeding and putrefaction.

logged, particularly if immersion was prolonged (Fig. XIII-12). The internal organs, however, display lividity in the usual fashion.

Crabs and fish feed particularly on the soft parts of the face (Fig. XIII-13), i.e. the eyelids, the lips and, to a lesser extent, the ears. Algae subsequently grow on these exposed parts, imparting a profound green or black color to these areas (Fig. XIII-14). A body recovered from the waters around the lower two-thirds of Michigan in the summer will be covered with algae so extensively as to make the identification of the individual appreciably more difficult. The entire body appears as if covered with mud. The layer of algae cannot be removed except by scrubbing, causing concurrent removal of the skin.

Mummification does not occur in water, but drifting in shallow waters may expose the back of the victim while keeping the front submerged. Under these circumstances mummification of the back is sometimes observed (Fig. XIII-15).

Adipocere, a condition in which tissues become soaplike (*see* Chapter II), is common in victims of submersion. Since the putrefactive process stops when adipocere is fully developed, the soft tissues of the body may be preserved for a long period of time. This renders futile any attempt to evaluate the time of death in a body altered in this fashion. Bodies found in the water in winter months, when marine animal activity is absent, develop adipocere in areas of the face that may be mutilated by aquatic life in the summer. This may provide a crude estimate of the length of time the body has been in the water.

## DIVING

Deaths associated with diving have become more numerous in recent years due to the increase in popularity of this sport. The two common types of diving are skin diving and scuba diving.

Skin diving is practiced mostly by amateurs for the purpose of spear fishing, photography, underwater exploration, etc. Only a simple mask and fins are used. The time under water depends on the ability of the diver to hold his breath and is consequently limited by his activity during this period. In general, since great depths are not usually attained in this type of diving, skin diving may be considered an extension of swimming, and the hazards are similar.

Scuba diving implies the use of a self-contained underwater breathing apparatus (SCUBA), which enables prolonged independent stay under water. Hence, depths are reached that are not usually attained by skin divers. Hazards of scuba diving, other than drowning, are those due to pressure changes associated with descent and ascent (baro-trauma). The bends (caisson disease), acute pulmonary emphysema, pneumothorax, air embolism and related conditions are some of the more common examples. Carbon monoxide intoxication occurs rarely *(vide infra)*.

*The bends* (caisson disease, decompression sickness) occurs if the diver remains for a prolonged period of time at depths at which changes of ambient pressure cause the formation of bubbles in his blood and tissues. The bubbles consist predominantly of nitrogen, but variable amounts of $CO_2$, $O_2$ and water vapor may also be found. In addition to significant individual variability, a large number of extrinsic and intrinsic factors predispose the body to the formation of bubbles. Among the latter, uptake of gas by the blood and tissues, gas solubility, diffusion, tissue vascularity and the biophysics of bubble formation and growth are relevant. Except in extreme cases, death from decompression sickness is rare, as even delayed therapy is often successful. At autopsy the findings consist of foci of ischemic necrosis, especially in the brain. The lungs show hemorrhages, edema, atelectasis and areas of emphysema.

*Acute pulmonary emphysema, pneumothorax and air embolism* may be considered together, as they are all different stages of the same phenomenon. The mechanism responsible for the development of these conditions, singly or in combination, is excessive pressure in the lungs. This may occur in less than fifteen feet of water due to inadequate breathing.

In acute emphysema small tears of alveolar walls cause hemorrhages in the lungs. In pneumothorax air leaks into one or both pleural cavities. Mediastinal and subcutaneous emphysema may complicate the pulmonary overpressure by dissection of air along the interstitial tissue in the lungs. Air embolism results from escape of air into the lung capillaries. It is imperative that the autopsy on a diver begin with a check for pneumothorax and air embolism. The techniques for these procedures are described in Chapter XXIV.

*Carbon monoxide inhalation* is an infrequent complication of scuba diving. The cause of carbon monoxide inhalation may be contamination of the inhaled air by exhaust fumes of the scuba, or it may result from a faulty air tank containing carbon monoxide. This may occur if an oil-contaminated air compressor is used to fill the scuba tanks. Sudden onset of unconsciousness and drowning may follow, or death may be due to carbon monoxide poisoning.

A comprehensive study of the various aspects of diving may be found in the U.S. Navy Diving Manual.[20]

## DEATH IN COLD WATER

Prolonged immersion in cold water is a far greater hazard than is commonly realized. Except in tropical waters warmer than 68° F, the main threat to life during prolonged immersion is cold or cold and drowning combined.[21] The length of immersion and the temperature of the water are the two factors that determine survival time. A chart issued by the U.S. Coast Guard[22] illustrates this relationship.

| *Water Temperature* | *Expected Time of Survival of Men Immersed in Seawater* |
|---|---|
| Less than 35° F | Less than ¾ hour |
| 35°-40° F | Less than 1½ hours |
| 40°-50° F | Less than 3 hours |
| 50°-60° F | Less than 6 hours |
| 60°-70° F | Less than 12 hours |
| Over 70° F | Indefinite (depending on fatigue) |

It should be emphasized that the above figures are based on the assumption that the individual is clothed in ordinary clothes, is in good physical health and, when immersed, wears a life preserver.

Thick clothing increases the times quoted in the chart appreciably. Also, unusual body builds tend to cause considerable deviations from the times mentioned. According to observations by Keatinge,[21] thin men become helpless more rapidly than obese men; very obese men may survive almost indefinitely in near-freezing water if they are warmly clothed, although they cannot do so without clothing. Consumption of alcohol generates hyperthermia and consequently helps maintain body temperature. Contrary to expectation, exercise in cold water reduces chances of survival.

With regard to the general problem of death by undercooling of individuals immersed in cold water, it may be interesting to cite the sinking of the *Titanic* with 2207 people on board after this ship struck an iceberg in the North Atlantic Ocean. At the time of the sinking the water temperature was approximately 32° F. Within one hour and fifty minutes, another ship appeared and picked up the survivors. Seven hundred and five people in lifeboats were rescued, while all others who were in the water were dead.

It should be noted that submersion in cold water may reduce the metabolic rate of a person so drastically that a state of suspended animation sets in. The chilly environment markedly reduces oxygen requirements of vital centers, enabling successful resuscitation after periods of submersion that would have proved fatal much sooner under ordinary circumstances. Several such cases presumably occurred in individuals who fell into icy waters.

## REFERENCES


1. National Safety Council: *Accident Facts.* Chicago, National Safety Council, 1969.
2. Kvittingen, T. D., and Naess, A.: Recovery from drowning in fresh water. *Br Med J, 1:*1315, 1963.
3. Geertinger, P., and Voigt, J.: Death in the bath. *J Forensic Med, 17:*135, 1970.
4. Niles, N. R.: Hemorrhage in the middle-ear and mastoid in drowning. *Am J Clin Pathol, 40:*281, 1963.
5. Lanphier, H.: Diving medicine. *N Engl J Med, 256:*120, 1957.
6. Behnke, A. R.: Physiologic effect of pressure changes with reference to otolaryngology. *Trans Am Acad Ophthalmol Otolaryngol, 49:*63, 1944.
7. Carrara, M.: Untersuchungen über den osmotischen Druck und die specifische elektrische Leitfähigkeit des Blutes bei der Fäulnis. *Vierteljahrsschr Gerichtl Med, 24:*236, 1902.
8. Placzek, M.: Die Blutdichte als Zeichen des Ertrinkungsvorganges. *Vierteljahrsschr Gerichtl Med, 25:*3, 1903.
9. Gettler, A. O.: A method for the determination of death by drowning. *JAMA, 77:*1650, 1921.
10. Moritz, A. R.: Chemical methods for the determination of death by drowning. *Physiol Rev, 24:* 70, 1944.
11. Freimuth, H. C., and Swann, H. E.: Plasma specific gravity changes in sudden deaths. *Arch Pathol, 59:*214, 1955.
12. Modell, J. H., and Davis, J. H.: Electrolyte changes in human drowning victims. *Anesthesiology, 30:*414, 1969.
13. Incze, Gy.: Fremdkörper im Blutkreislauf Ertrunkener. (*Verh Dtsch Ges Ungarisch Pathol,* 1940/41), cited in *Zentralbl Allg Pathol, 79:* 176, 1942.
14. Mueller, B., and Gorgs, D.: Studien über das Eindringen von corpusculären Wasserbestandteilen aus den Lungenalveolen in den Kreislauf während des Ertrinkungsvorgangs. *Dtsch Z Ges Gerichtl Med, 39:*715, 1949.
15. Spitz, W. U.: Diagnose des Ertrinkungsvorganges durch den Diatomeen-Nachweis in Organen. *Dtsch Z Ges Gerichtl Med, 54:*42, 1963.
16. Spitz, W. U., Schmidt, H., and Fett, W.: Untersuchungen von Luftfiltrationsstreifen aus verschiedenen Gebieten der Bundesrepublik auf ihren Diatomeengehalt. *Dtsch Z Ges Gerichtl Med, 56:*116, 1965.
17. Spitz, W. U., Burfitt, H. P., Freimuth, H. C., and Michaelis, M.: Enzymologic approach to the diagnosis of death by drowning. *Am J Clin Pathol, 47:*704, 1967.
18. Spitz, W. U., Hebel, J. R., and Michaelis, M.: Enzymatic changes in asphyxia, experimental pulmonary edema and drowning. *Am J Clin Pathol, 51:*102, 1969.
19. Spitz, W. U.: Drowning. *Hosp Med, 5:*8, 1969.
20. United States Navy Department: *U.S. Navy Diving Manual. Navyships 0994-001-9010.* Washington, D.C., U.S. Gov. Print. Office, March, 1970.
21. Keatinge, W. R.: *Survival in Cold Water.* Oxford, Blackwell, 1969.
22. United States Coast Guard: *National Search and Rescue Manual.* (FM 20-150; NWP 37(A); AFM 64-2; CG 308) Amendment No. 6, April, 1970.

*Chapter XIV*

# ELECTRICAL AND LIGHTNING INJURIES

RUSSELL S. FISHER

## ELECTRICAL INJURY

THE PASSAGE of electric current through the human body is capable of producing a wide variety of effects, ranging from insignificant localized muscle spasm and little or no contact burns to instantaneous death with little or no burns or extremely severe burning without death.[1–4]

Not all current flow is dangerous. Diathermy, where the frequency of oscillation of current is 1,000,000 cycles/sec. and the voltage as high as 40,000, is incapable of producing shock but does induce heat at flow rates of 1 to 2 ma. Another variant of this high frequency current is the surgical diathermy knife, which actually cuts by inducing high but very localized current flow. Electroshock therapy used in the treatment of certain mental disturbances utilizes as much as 200 ma of current through a bifrontal circuit of the head. This is excited by 60 cycle AC, and this amount of flow is capable of inducing cardiac arrest were the patient to be inadvertently grounded.

In cardiac defibrillation the current flow is enormous, but of such short duration that it stops the fibrillating heart rather than inducing fibrillation. It is given by a capacitator discharge at up to 3,000 v potential through an inductive system that may produce as much as 30 amp. but only for 50 msec. This polarizes the myocardium and obliterates the chaotic electrical activity of fibrillation, allowing the physiologic pace maker to regain control of the heart's rhythm. The discharge must be delivered at an appropriate time during the cardiac cycle to prevent induction of fibrillation or standstill. This is accomplished by an additional circuit, which monitors the heart and triggers the capacitor at an appropriate time.

The physiological effects of electrical current that may result in a fatality impinge either upon (a) the brain stem and the cervical spinal cord or (b) the heart, depending upon the location of the contacts between the *live* conductor and the body and between the body and the *ground.*

Circuits from any of the extremities to the head clearly involve the brain stem and the upper spinal cord, while arm-to-arm circuits may also involve the upper portions of the spinal cord. Death, when it occurs in association with circuits involving the brain stem, apparently is the result of respiratory paralysis, since the electrical current passing through the brain stem cells so disturbs their function that they are no longer able to generate impulses necessary for the stimulation of the respiratory muscles of the chest and abdomen. Furthermore, persistent or tetanic muscle contraction may be so prolonged that asphyxia ensues before the shocked fibers can relax.

Arm-to-arm, or left-arm-to-either-leg circuits obviously involve the heart, particularly since it appears that most of the current flow follows the large blood vessels. In such circuits either ventricular fibrillation or cardiac arrest without fibrillation may occur. It appears that ventricular fibrillation occurs most frequently with 60 cycle AC and that instantaneous cardiac arrest is apt to be seen only with the rare DC exposures incident to old-style home-generated electricity or certain industrial applications. The amount of current flow necessary to cause fatal cardiac fibrillation is a subject of considerable variation of opinion among experts, but it would appear that as little as 70 ma can cause fatal fibrillation in exposures involving the cardiac axis. There are reports of cardiac fibrillation where as little as .1 ma passed through the tissues, caused by inadvertent shorting of

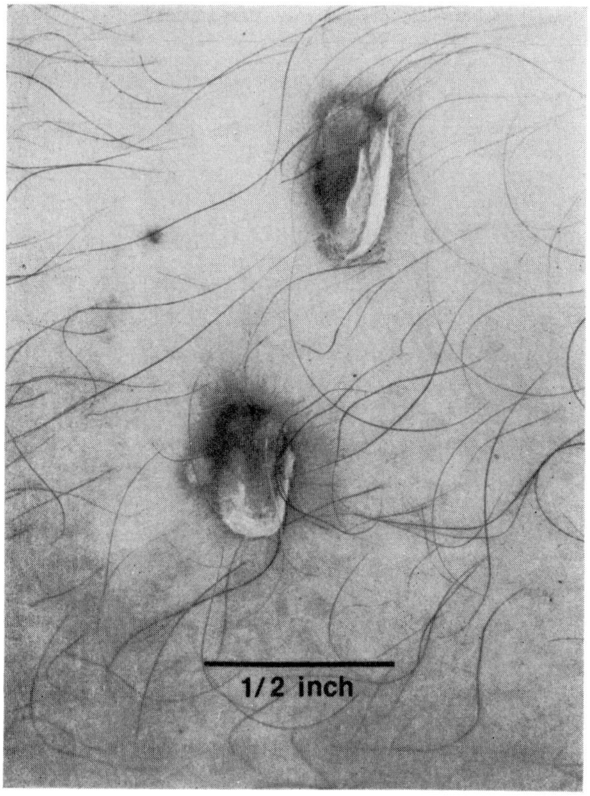


FIGURE XIV-1. *Punched-out* electrical contact burns, 220 v alternating current. The victim was electrocuted while attempting to repair a motor.

internal electrodes (such as pacemakers) applied directly to the heart.

The amount of current flow through the body is determined by two major factors: first, the available voltage and second, the nature of the contact. Since the resistance of intact skin is high, the passage of current through skin produces heat locally. This is the explanation of electrical burns that may be as tiny as pinpoints or deeply seared and contracted if contact is allowed to continue for a long period of time or if extremely high voltage is applied (Figs. XIV-1 to XIV-6). It must be borne in mind, however, that fatal electrocution can occur with no visible skin burning where the area of contact is relatively large, as may occur when one grasps a *hot wire* with a wet hand. When the body is damp with perspiration, the entire skin surface, being bathed in *salt water*, becomes a conductor. With such a large *electrode*, not enough current passes through any minute portion of it to generate sufficient heat to directly burn the epidermis or the underlying collagenous tissue where the major part of the resistance is concentrated.

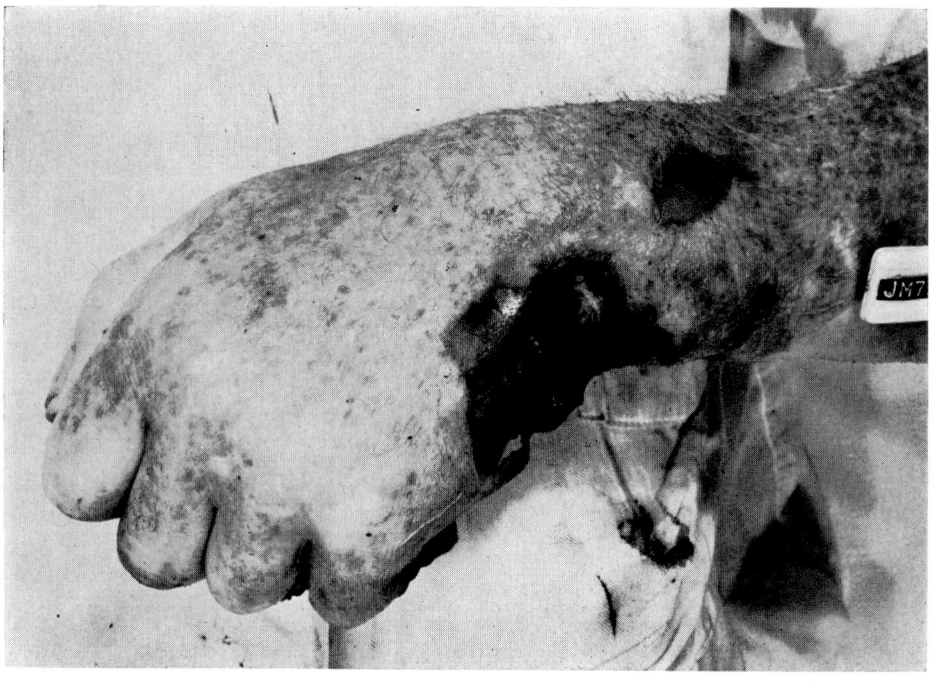

FIGURE XIV-2. Severe burning due to electrocution. The subject attempted to move a live power line with a wet stick after a severe storm had blown it down.

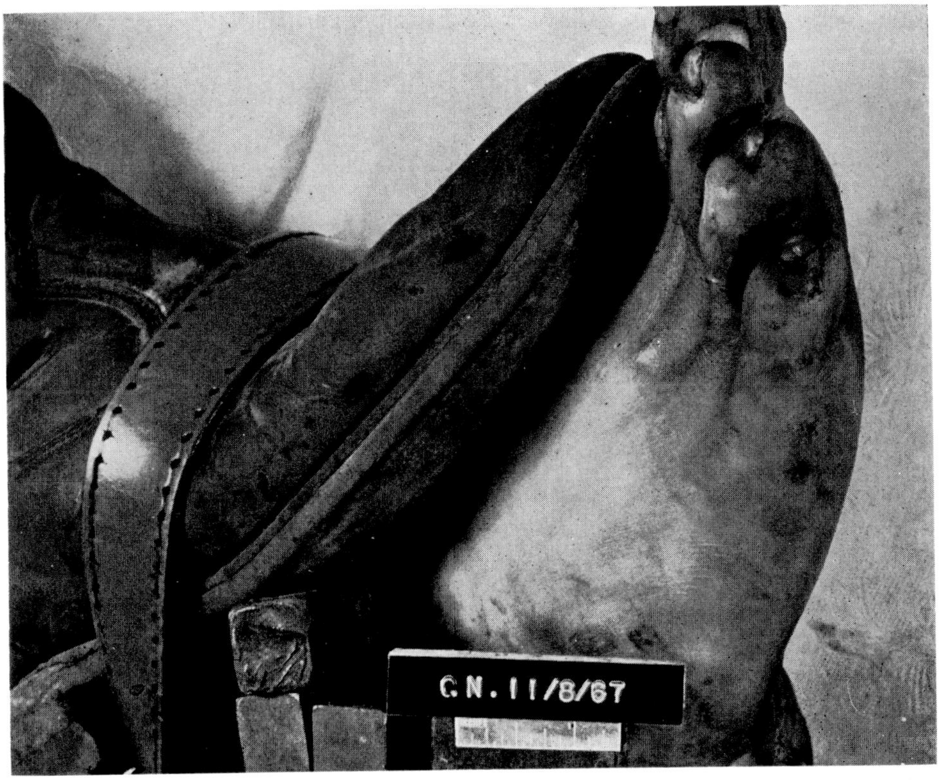


FIGURE XIV-3. Burns on the foot with associated punched and burned holes in the shoe. The subject was in contact with a swinging boom when the upright member hit a high tension line.

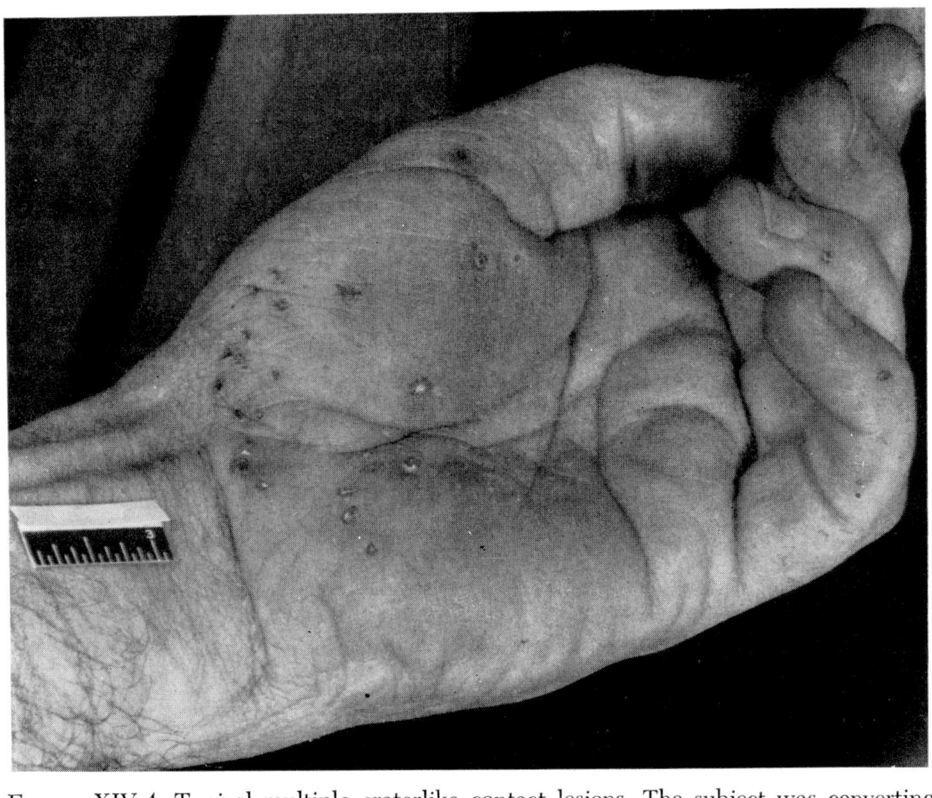

FIGURE XIV-4. Typical multiple craterlike contact lesions. The subject was converting a transformer from 4,000 to 13,000 v.

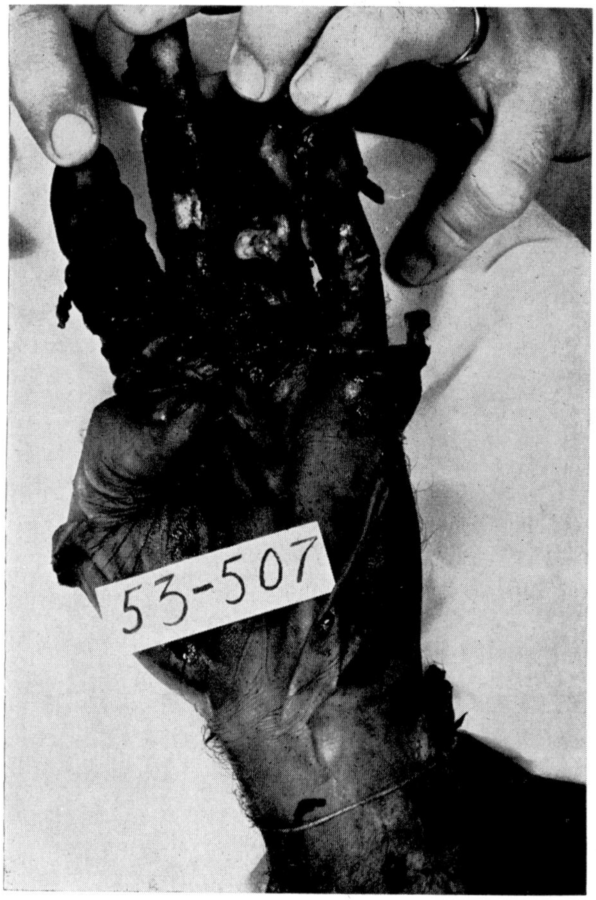


FIGURE XIV-5. Extensive retracted and dessicated electrical burn where contact with high tension line continued after the individual was dead.

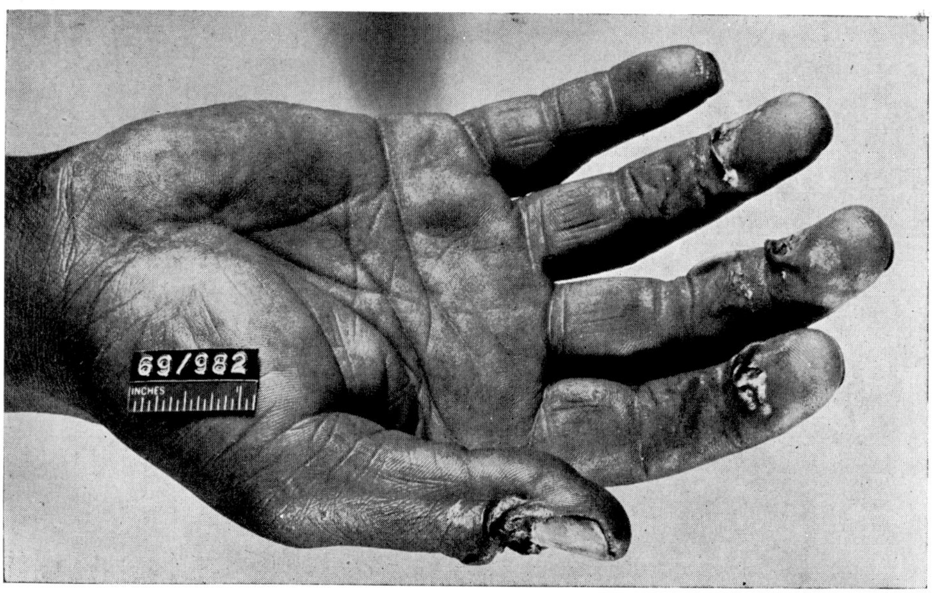


FIGURE XIV-6. Typical grasp pattern where an individual reached up and grabbed a hot wire—550 v overhead train power line. More severe burning would have occurred, but he fell free of the line to the ground below.

Secondary burning due to the ignition of clothing is common and indeed may produce more severe injuries than the electrical current itself. High tension electrical injury may cause multiple discrete lesions due to arcing from the conductor to the body of the victim, though no direct contact is made. In such cases the arc seems to *dance* over the body surface, producing multiple seared or punched-out lesions.

Electrical burns usually represent very high temperature burns, and this produces characteristic findings of severe thermal denaturation of the collagen, causing it to stain blue in the ordinary hematoxylin and eosin stain. The epidermis is elevated with microblisters developing within the squamous epithelium as well as in the external horny layer. These blisters result from the *cooking effect* on the tissue and represent defects through which the steam exited (Fig. XIV-7). Large vacuoles produced by the heat also appear within the epidermal cells. In addition, the nuclei of the epidermal cells at the site of an electrical burn show a peculiar distortion, with stretching and narrowing of the contour to produce a palisade-type appearance. This change, called *streaming of the nuclei,* is shown in Figure XIV-8.

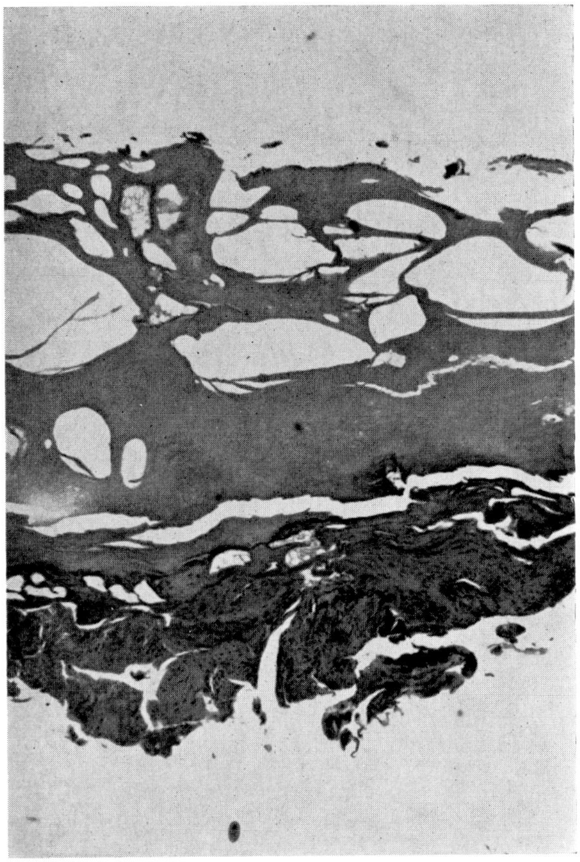

FIGURE XIV-7. Microblisters in the epidermis characteristic of electrical burns.

Other microscopic changes associated with the passage of electric current through the body have been described by Jellinek.[1] These include alterations in the nuclei of endothelial lining cells and of the fibroblasts in the media of blood vessels. According to Jellinek, the nuclei of the vascular media tend to be twisted to resemble spirals, and this may occur at points quite distant from the site of contact with the electrode. It is suggested that they are localized in the arterial walls because blood is a good conductor of electricity, and indeed most current passage within the body is via the blood vessels. In addition to the nuclear alteration in blood vessels, there is a tendency to localized degeneration of the intima. Blood vessels having a strong elastic lamella are especially prone to this type of change. Tearing of elastic fibers and the overlying intima occurs commonly and is apt to cause secondary thrombosis. Should this involve one of the major arteries to an extremity, gangrene of the extremity may follow. It should be noted that all of these changes characteristic of electrical burning can be produced after the death of the individual as well as during life. Nevertheless, their recognition as evidence of the passage of current supports the assumption that the same current was fatal.

The occurrence of hemoglobin in the urine and degenerative kidney changes associated with breakdown of muscle myoglobin have also been described. This would be expected if there were extensive muscle damage due to the passage of a high current in a nonfatal circuit, when the muscles degenerate and release their myoglobin content. In such cases, renal shutdown as a result of lower nephron nephrosis may occur, as it does following extensive crushing injury.

One of the most remarkable features of elec-

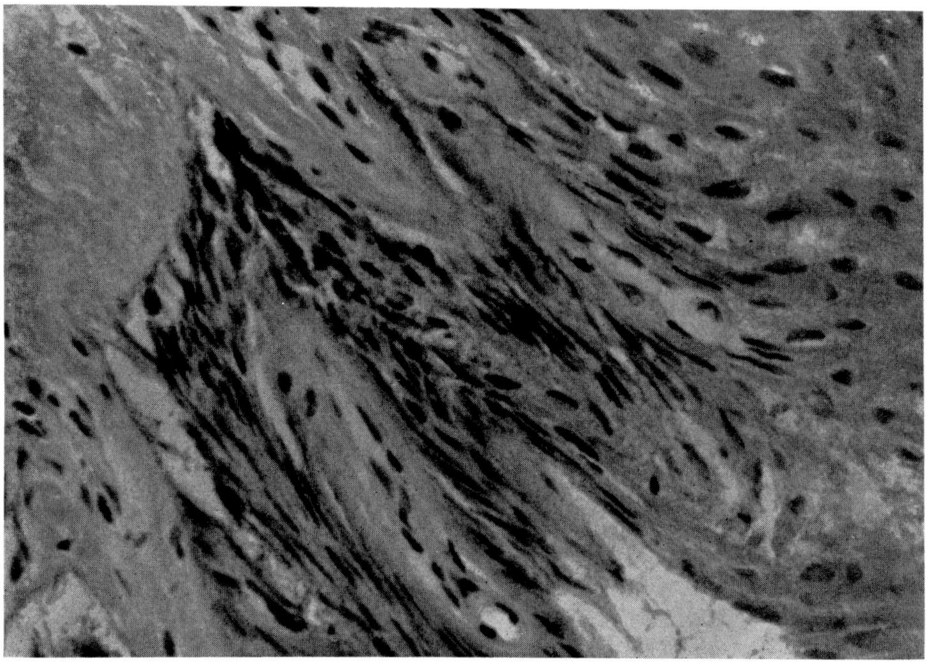

FIGURE XIV-8. *Streaming* of epidermal nuclei characteristic of electrical burns.

trocution is the fact that death need not be instantaneous.[5] The Medical Examiner's Office in Maryland has several documented cases where individuals came in contact with strong electrical current and were able to walk some distance and talk before the onset of collapse and death.

Two men were working on a 600 v transformer at the top of a utility pole when one leaned forward and his chest touched a live wire. He was able to push himself back from the electrode, and his coworker asked him, "Are you alright?" He answered, "Yes, I think I will be alright, except I've got a burn." Thereupon he collapsed, and by the time he was carried to the ground and resuscitation commenced, it was too late.

In another instance, an individual was working behind a large electrical panel. Another man elsewhere in the room heard him curse and state, "I've electrocuted myself." He came walking out from behind the panel and reached the middle of the room some ten or fifteen feet away before he collapsed. Even though immediate resuscitative efforts were started, it was apparent that he had sustained a cardiac fibrillation, and in the absence of a defibrillator, his heart rhythm could not be restored.

These two instances do not prove that the onset of fibrillation was not instantaneous but only that a number of seconds may follow before coma occurs, even though cardiac function is interrupted. This same phenomenon may occur with ventricular fibrillation from any cause. Thus, it is no longer uncommon for occasions to arise in which a cardiac patient on a television monitor exhibits the onset of ventricular fibrillation in the electrocardiogram, and the defibrillator, which is already attached, is activated to return the patient's heart to a normal rhythm without the patient losing consciousness or even realizing the event until it has passed. Patients have related that the shock of the defibrillator comes as a great surprise in these circumstances.

In judicial electrocution the head is shaved and moistened with a conducting paste and a caplike electrode applied. The legs are similarly fitted with electrodes, so that large areas of contact are insured. An alternating current of several amperes is then passed through the body by impressing 1,700 v. After a minute or two the voltage is reduced, and the current is allowed to flow for several additional minutes. Skin burns are usually insignificant, if present at all, but the temperature within the brain at autopsy, immediately after execution, may reach 114° F.

## INJURY BY LIGHTNING

The effects of lightning resemble those of other very high voltage electrical discharges. They are, of course, to be regarded as direct current rather than alternating and surprisingly are by no means always fatal. It has been estimated that less than half of the individuals struck by lightning are killed. Apparently when death does occur it is a result of passage of the current through *fatal* circuits involving either the heart or the brain stem. This can occur without evidence of injury to the surface of the body or with only minor singeing of the hair if the head is one contact. It is extremely rare to see truly severe burning from lightning strike per se, although tremendous local heat develops where arcing occurs as the *bolt* strikes a metallic ob-

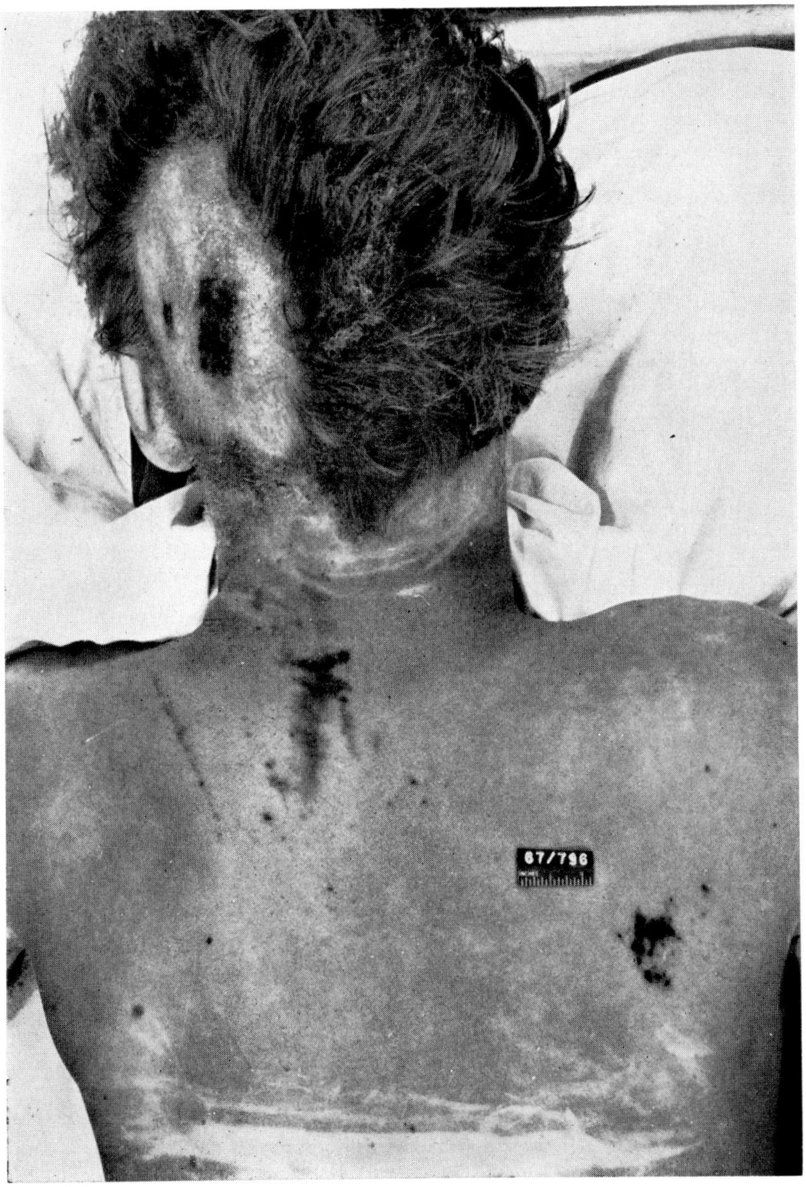

FIGURE XIV-9. Lightning injuries. The hair, some of it singed, has been clipped to show the scalp lesions. The lightning *impact* caused local subarachnoid hemorrhage under these injuries. The burns on the back are also due to the lightning.

ject. We have seen belt buckles, earrings or car keys and similar items melted, even though there was little if any burning of the body. One finding that is invariably evidence of lightning strike is the occurrence of a peculiar fernlike pattern of erythema in the skin, usually located over the shoulders or the flanks. Whether this develops in a few minutes postmortem or whether it is instantaneous has never been determined. It is not associated with burning and appears more probably to be the effect of breakdown of the red cells within the skin capillaries with escape of hemoglobin in the loose perivascular tissues. This mark may be the only evidence that lightning strike occurred and should be carefully searched for in any instance where death occurred under circumstances suggesting that lightning may have been the cause (Figs. XIV-9, XIV-10 and XIV-11).

Another effect associated with lightning strike, especially in those who survive, is the development of intense edema of the skin at points of current entry. This is probably to be explained by paralysis of local capillary and lymphatic vessels as a result of electrical injury to the nerve supply of the vessels or to the cells of the vessels themselves. The resulting dilatation of the blood vessels allows fluid to escape and local edema to form.

Despite the characteristically insignificant-appearing bodily injuries associated with lightning strike, the explosive force associated with the extreme air pressure changes adjacent to a bolt of lightning quiet commonly rips the seams of the shirt, pants and even shoes worn by the victim.

Late sequelae of lightning strike, also seen with high tension electrical contact, include trophic changes in the skin, apparently due to

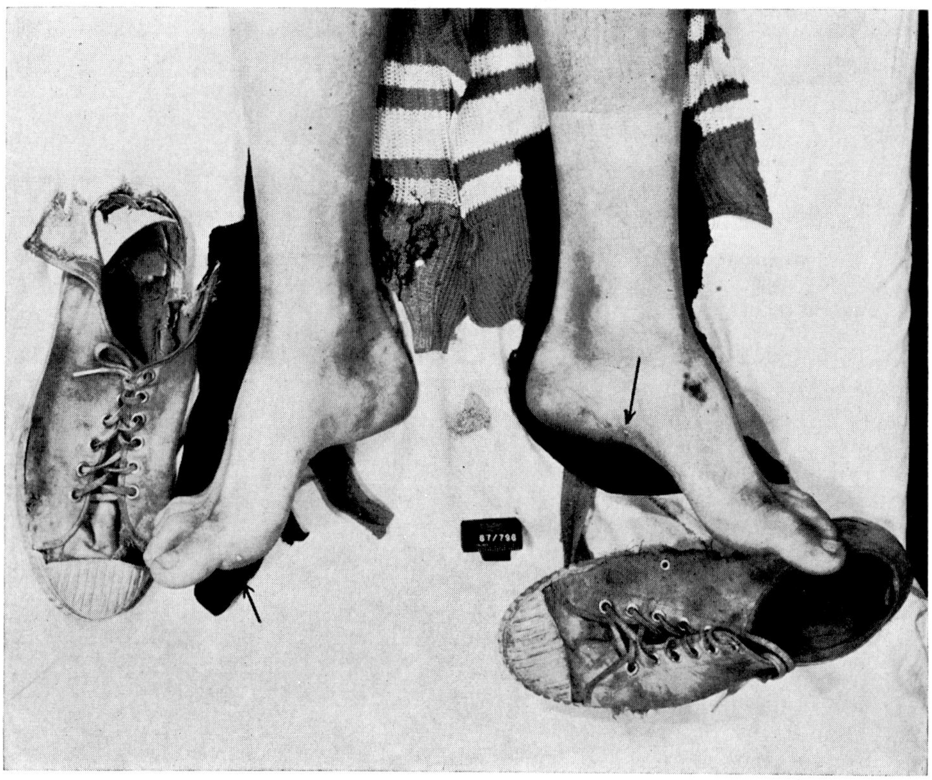

FIGURE XIV-10. Feet and shoes of the same victim as in Figure XIV-9. Note the destruction of the right shoe and a typical small electrical burn at the base of the right great toe and the sole of the left foot (arrows). The right nylon sock is melted at the ankle.

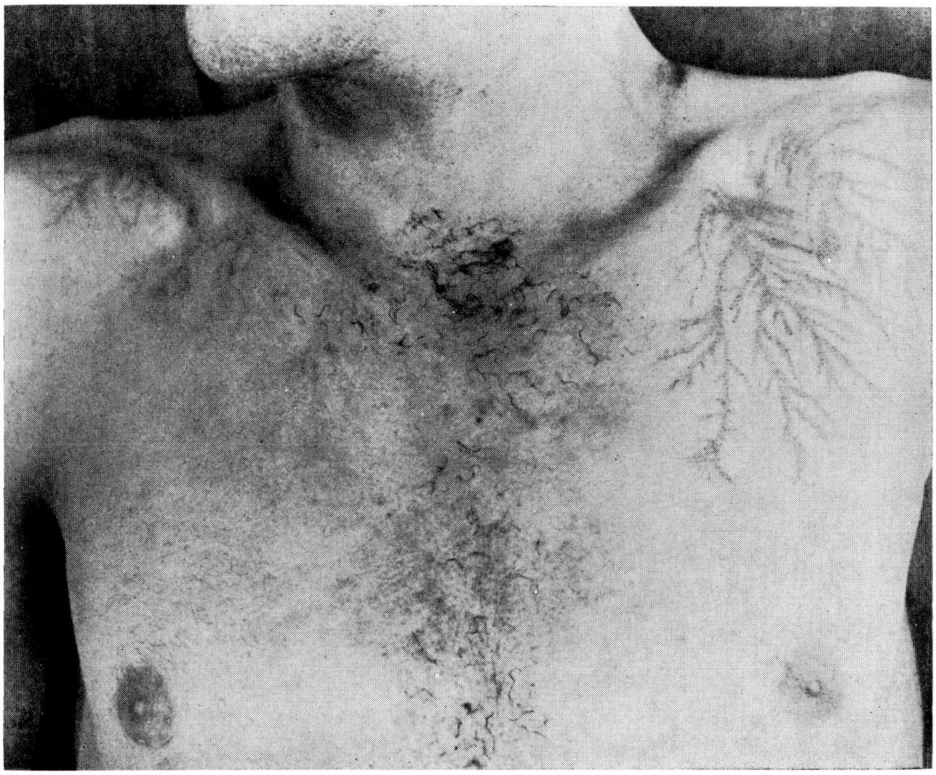

FIGURE XIV-11. Lightning effect. Dendritic pattern of erythema on the left shoulder in a victim who was standing under a tree that was struck by a lightning bolt. Note also singeing of chest hair.

nerve damage to peripheral nerve branches or to the cutaneous blood supply. Neuritic pain, tingling and other sensory disturbances, especially in the extremities, persisting for months or years have also been described after both types of high tension *strikes.*

## THE AUTOPSY IN ELECTRICAL INJURY CASES

As in many other medicolegal investigations, the examination of the scene may be far more important than the examination of the body at the autopsy table. This is especially true where no characteristic burns or other injuries are noted on the body and the only clue is the finding of electrical short circuits or defective wiring in such apparatus as home laundry machines, electrical drills, saws and other hand tools.

The medicolegal investigator, unless he has had considerable experience, is well advised to call upon an expert electrician and have him test the apparatus with devices available to him under circumstances as similar to the death situation as can be devised. It is not sufficient to simply impound the suspect apparatus and place it in a dry situation for hours or days before the examination takes place. The drying out of wet insulation may indeed restore the electrical apparatus to its original effectiveness, and testing of the apparatus at that late stage may not reveal the defect that allowed the victim to become part of the circuit between the power source and the ground when he attempted to use the defective instrument.

The gross autopsy findings characteristic of fatal electrical injury are not specific and consist of severe congestion of internal organs, edema of the lungs and fluidity of the blood. These are merely evidence of an asphyxial type of death. Occasionally there will be encountered local hemorrhages or tears in the muscles, especially in the extremities. These are due to forcible contraction and spasm induced by the passage of current, usually described inaccurately as *tetanic convulsion*.

The microscopic examination of small lesions on the extremities or wherever electrical contact may have occurred is frequently a helpful step, and adequate specimens should be taken at the time of the autopsy.

Another examination that may be useful is low power microscopic inspection of hairs from the margin of any suspected electrical burn. Arcing of the current may produce pitlike defects on the surface of the hair that are characteristic of electrical effect. Too much emphasis cannot be placed on the examination of the clothing of the individual in electrical cases, particularly where high voltage or a lightning strike is concerned, since the destructive changes in the clothes may be far more revealing than the injuries to the body. Finally, if particulate material is found in the margin of a suspected electrical burn, spectrographic and/or histochemical tests may be helpful in identification of the material as tiny fragments of metallic conductor, melted and fused to the wound margins.

Color tests depending on reagents that react with copper to produce a purplish color and with iron to produce a blue color may be used in studying electrical burns. Traces of the metal conductor left at the site of the contact burn, either as oxidized iron (rust) or as electrolytically deposited or molten particles of copper, are detected by these tests. Identification of these metallic substances may serve as evidence that the burn came from electrical contact.

The test is performed by gently wiping the burned area with filter paper or dye transfer paper moistened with a drop of dilute ammonia, then adding a drop of the specific reagent. This is a 1% solution of rubeanic acid in acetone for the copper test and a 1% aqueous potassium ferrocyanide solution for the iron test. If nickel is present instead of copper in the rubeanic acid test, the color will be blue-green. For more details and variants of these spot tests, reference to Feigl[6] is advised, since different conditions of acidity and the presence of other metallic substances may alter the color of the spot. It would seem that neutron activation techniques might be more useful to identify metallic elements in such burns.

## REFERENCES

1. Jellinek, S.: *Elektrische Verletzungen*. Leipzig, Barth, 1932.
2. Jaffe, R. H.: Electropathology. *Arch Pathol, 5:*837, 1928.
3. Fisher, R. S.: Toxicity from electrical and chemical burns. In Sunderman, F. W., and Sunderman, F. W., Jr. (Eds.): *Laboratory Diagnosis of Diseases Caused by Toxic Agents*. St. Louis, Green, 1970, p. 554.
4. International Labour Organizations: Meeting of Experts on Electrical Accidents and Related Matters. Record of Proceedings, October 1961. Geneva, Occupational Safety and Health Branch, International Labour Office, 1962.
5. Spitz, W. U.: Befunde bei vorübergehender Wiederbelegung nach Elektrounfall. *Münch Med Wochenschr, 106:*495, 1964.
6. Feigl, F.: *Spot Tests. Inorganic Applications,* 5th ed., vol. I. Amsterdam, Elsevier, 1958.

*Chapter XV*

# THE ROAD TRAFFIC VICTIM

WERNER U. SPITZ

## CORRELATION OF POSTMORTEM FINDINGS WITH ROADSIDE EVIDENCE

THIS CHAPTER may not furnish detailed definitions of traffic accident injuries, but it will facilitate recognition of certain injuries occurring with some regularity and enable those concerned with the investigation of traffic deaths to corroborate autopsy findings with available roadside evidence.

Traffic police are instructed to furnish thorough accident reports, which frequently include photographs and detailed diagrams. This information is invaluable to the pathologist who handles the postmortem examination. All too often the autopsy of the traffic victim is conducted in great detail, yet only a listing of the injuries and the determination of the cause of death are recorded in the official autopsy protocol. Any attempt by the pathologist to draw conclusions from the injuries with respect to the reconstruction of the accident is generally avoided. The important point to be made is that the assessment of a traffic casualty must include not only the victim but also the vehicle and the circumstances of the accident. Only by the incorporation of all available data can a better understanding of the mechanism of the crash and causation of injuries be established for later use as evidence. In due course such handling of the cases will counteract the general apathy by law enforcement agencies, attorneys and judges that has developed regarding expert medical testimony in courts of law dealing with traffic deaths.

The recognition and careful evaluation of wounds characteristic of known crash patterns frequently permit reconstruction of the accident with a degree of accuracy not commonly appreciated and, therefore, mostly neglected. On the other hand, overinterpretation of the postmortem findings is equally undesirable, since it must be remembered that it is usually impossible to attribute a specific causative mechanism to each and every injury on the victim's body. In contrast, patterned injuries, which by virtue of their location are known by experience to be caused in a specific way, are vital to accident reconstruction. Examples of such injuries are the circular abrasion on a driver's chest or face from impact on the steering column or the steering wheel or the imprint of the headlight on the thigh of a pedestrian struck by an automobile (Fig. XV-1).

For complete injury documentation, incisions should be made in certain areas of the body that show no external evidence of injury but by experience are known to be frequently traumatized. Such incisions will *map out* hidden injuries, not only according to their distribution but also in regard to their appearance, thereby permitting the documentation of all points of significant impact.

### The Pedestrian

The postmortem examination begins with a thorough investigation of the clothing of the deceased. In a case concerning a hit-and-run vehicle the clothing of the pedestrian requires particular attention. Small fragments of paint and glass from the vehicle involved in the crash may be inadvertently discarded unless undressing the body is carried out on a clean white sheet on which such deposits may be easily seen. Carelessness in handling this part of the postmortem examination may result in the loss of a most valuable link in the investigation. The presence of grease or tire marks on the

Published in part under the title "Essential postmortem findings in the traffic accident victim," in *AMA Arch Pathol*, *90*:451, 1970.

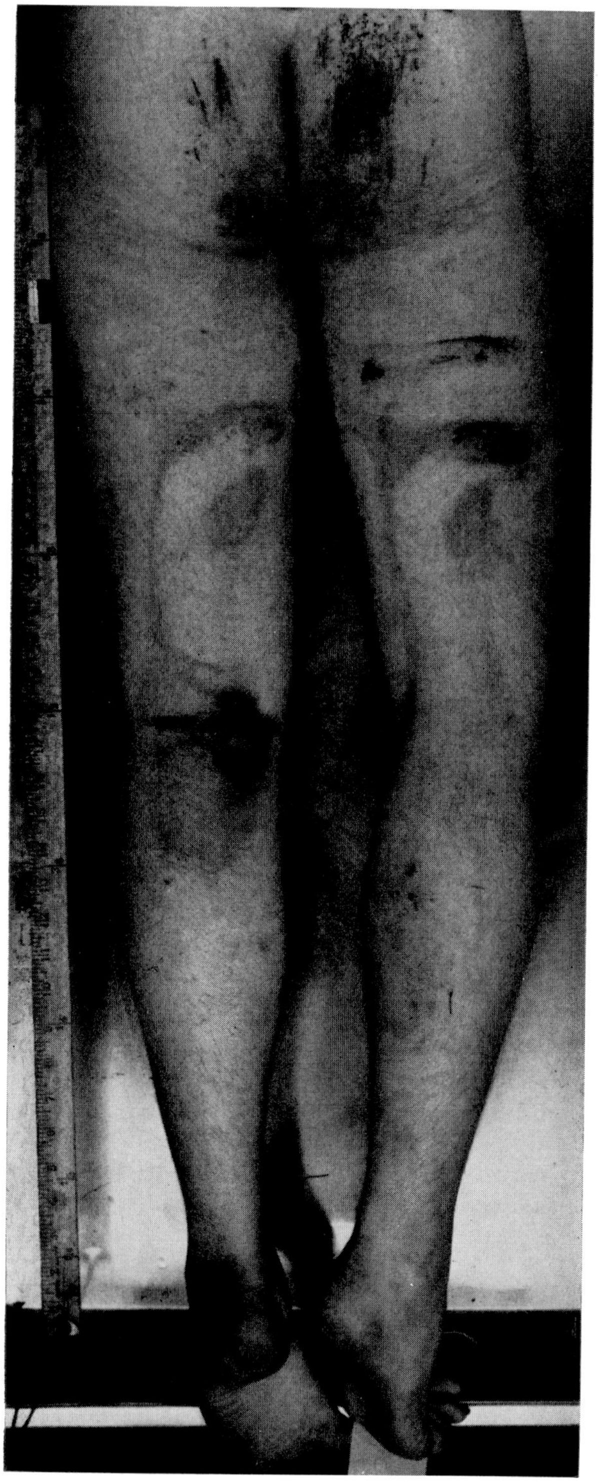

FIGURE XV-1. Pedestrian who was struck from behind by a 1970 Pontiac, receiving a bumper injury on the left leg. Above this injury is noted an imprint by the double headlights of the left side of the automobile. The distribution of the injuries suggests that the victim was standing when struck and that the brakes of the automobile were not applied at the time of impact.

clothing of the victim may further help to determine the circumstances surrounding the accident.

Examination of the vehicle, when possible, adds still another dimension to the investigation and often provides understanding of mechanisms of injury and of phenomena that are otherwise obscure or totally incomprehensible.

The following case exemplifies how an accurate reconstruction of the accident can be accomplished by correlation of autopsy data and examination of the vehicle.

A forty-two-year-old black male pedestrian was struck by a jeep and was dead at the scene. The driver contended that he had not seen the victim before the accident.

The pattern and distribution of the injuries supported the driver's contention by indicating that the pedestrian had not been in front of the vehicle but rather was struck by the side of the car. The victim was struck on his left side; the patterned injuries of the left side of the face resulted from striking the right corner of the vehicle's roof (Fig. XV-2a, b). A dent of the roof corner disclosed several pinhead-size tissue fragments, which were microscopically identified as fat tissue and Negro skin. This finding indicated beyond doubt that this was the impact point on the vehicle. Since there were no brush marks on the front of the vehicle, it was assumed that this had been the site of the primary impact, i.e. where the victim first came in contact with the automobile. A tire mark on the left thigh of the victim, initially believed to have been sustained as the result of having been run over, was in fact due to a sideswipe effect by the spare tire affixed to the right rear of the vehicle (Fig. XV-2c). The spare wheel had indeed been bent outwards by the impact. Interestingly, there was very little hemorrhage underlying these patterned abrasions, and instead of having the edges of the grooves between the treads imprinted on the body as happens in genuine tire marks, the actual tread pattern was depicted on the skin (as if made by a rubber stamp). This indicated the glancing nature of the impact. A circular laceration of the left forearm explained the broken-off right door handle of the jeep.

The deceased had a blood alcohol level of 0.17%. No barbiturates were detected. The autopsy also disclosed evidence of old brain surgery, which corroborated the subsequently available history of posttraumatic epilepsy. Several capsules of an anticonvulsive drug were found in the pockets of the deceased.

The autopsy of an individual struck by an automobile may be most rewarding. In the typical case the adult victim is struck by the front of the automobile, sustaining so-called *bumper injuries* on the legs (Fig. XV-3). These may be severe, with fractures and extensive soft tissue destruction; however, they may also be minimal or even absent on external examination of the body. The extent of these injuries depends upon the speed of the car, the shape of the bumper and the amount of clothing covering the area that was struck. In the winter, when heavy garments are worn, injuries inflicted by the bumpers are frequently overlooked due to the fact that much of the force of the impact is absorbed by the clothing. Incision of the calves and reflection of the skin should be performed in every pedestrian fatality, since this procedure will usually indicate the site of impact. To afford maximum exposure it is recommended that the incision be vertical and extend the entire length of the calves. A vertical incision can easily be sewn together and sealed, causing little interference with subsequent embalming.

Absence of bumper injuries suggests that the *pedestrian struck* the side of the automobile, as could happen if he inadvertently emerged from between two parked vehicles into the path of a passing car. This would result in *sideswiping* of the pedestrian, who would probably sustain head injuries from falling backwards to the ground.

The tibia is frequently fractured as a result of a bumper injury. The bone fragments are displaced, and the skin is often torn opposite the site of impact, i.e. an open fracture. A common observation is a wedge-shaped fracture of the tibia; often, but not invariably, the base of the triangular fragment of bone represents the location of the blow, while the apex points in the direction in which the automobile was travelling (Fig. XV-4).[1]

A preliminary study by Patrick et al.,[2] using a modified automobile on a sled with a total weight of 1,500 lb., indicates that leg fractures (presumably in healthy young adults) first occur at a speed of 14.5 mph and multiple severe fractures at a speed of 25.6 mph. Preliminary experiments conducted by the author appear to substantiate the observations made by Patrick et al. It is conceivable that similar fractures may occur at considerably lower speeds in elderly individuals with skeletal fragility.

The height of these injuries above the soles of the feet should be measured. The height of the heels and the thickness of the soles of the victim's shoes must also be considered.

The level of the injuries obviously varies with the height of the bumper. Photography of the injuries, including a yardstick placed alongside the legs, is advantageous for measurement documentation and for possible later use in court. The average bumper is 20 in. above ground level. However, the front end of the automobile will often *dip* when the brakes are applied, sometimes inflicting such injuries as low as the ankles. Not infrequently, bumper injuries are at different levels on the two legs or absent on one leg, suggesting that the victim was walking or running when struck. In such a case the leg with the higher-placed injury usually represents the one in contact with the ground, supporting the body weight at the moment of impact. This leg acts as an axis upon which the body turns, resulting in an additional but glancing blow by the radiator grill, headlight or front fender. This injury by grill, headlight or front fender is usually located over either hip, thigh, buttock or on the back, depending on the direction in which the vehicle was travelling in relation to the victim. The presence of this secondary glancing injury may be masked by the lack of external evidence of injury or the presence of an insignificant abrasion or a superficial bruise. Palpation of the area may suggest subcutaneous fluctuation, and incision often reveals a large *pocket,* containing blood and lacerated adipose tissue, located between the skin and the muscle fascia (Fig. XV-5). This fascia is usually intact, although the underlying muscles may be torn and extensively bruised. In an obese victim the *pocket* may assume enormous proportions and present a source of major bleeding and fat embolism should the person survive the initial few minutes. In some instances the *pocket* is torn open, with extensive undermining of its margins,

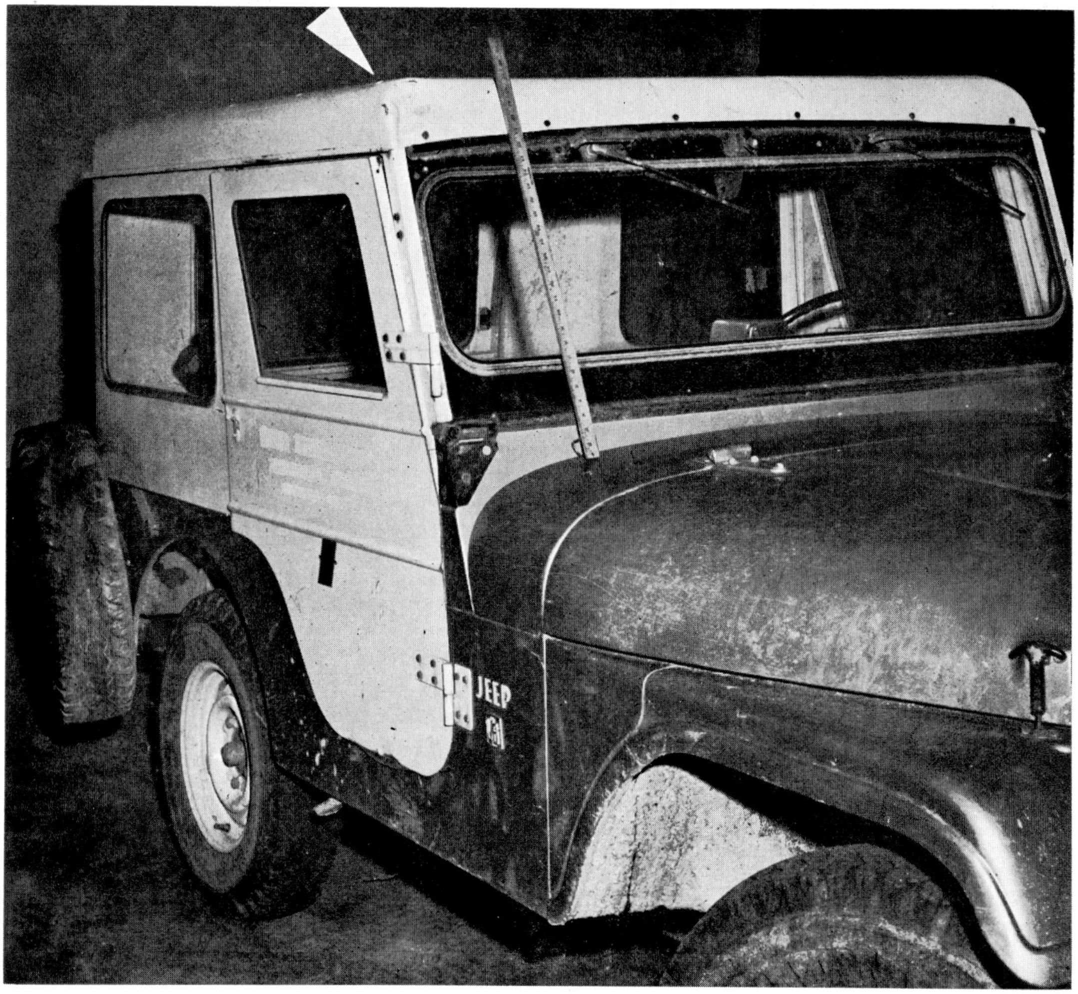


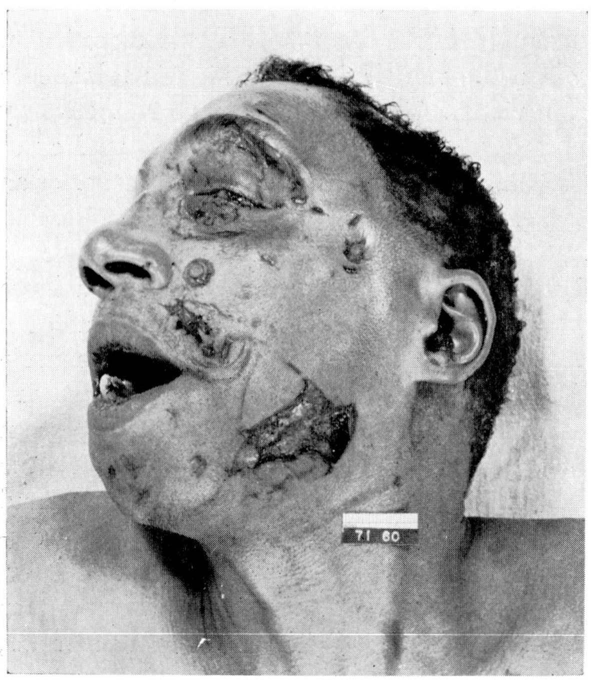

FIGURE XV-2. (a and b): Jeep involved in a collision with a pedestrian. The right upper corner of the jeep (indicated by the arrow) was the point of primary impact and contained minute fragments of skin from the face of the victim. A circular abrasion on the cheek represents a screw, and the angulated abrasion at the corner of the mouth was probably inflicted by the frame of the windshield. Note that the spare tire of the jeep is displaced outward. (c): The tread pattern of the spare tire of the jeep imprinted on the left thigh of the victim is matched with the actual tire, showing a *rubber stamp* effect. Had the victim been run over by the tire, the edges of the grooves between the tread would have been imprinted on the body.

FIGURE XV-2c

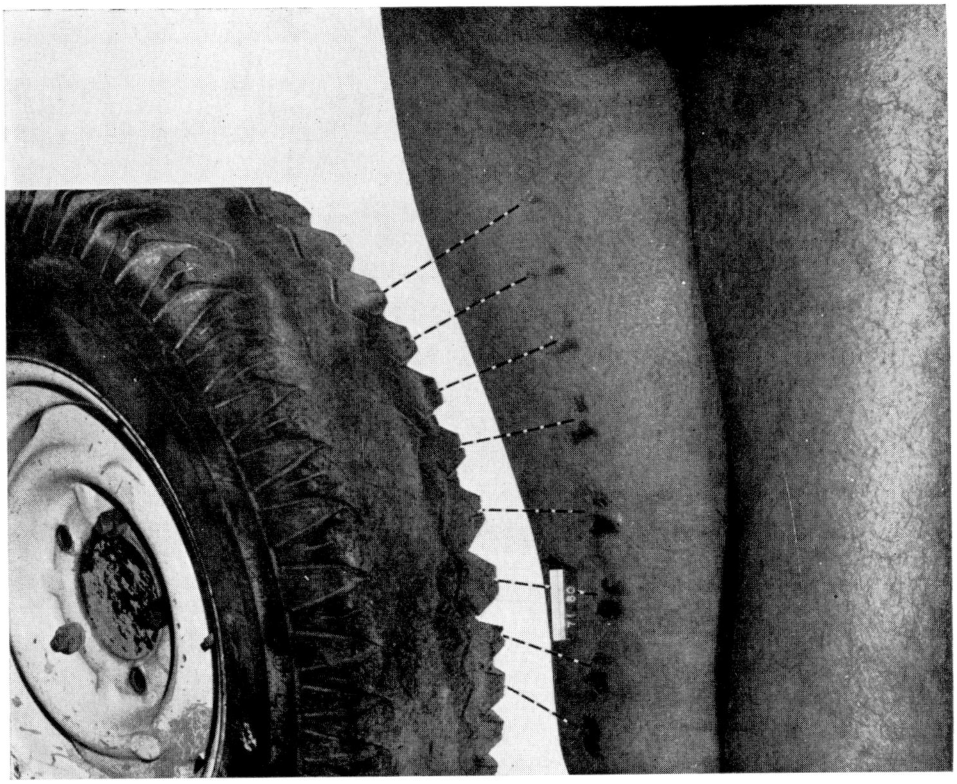

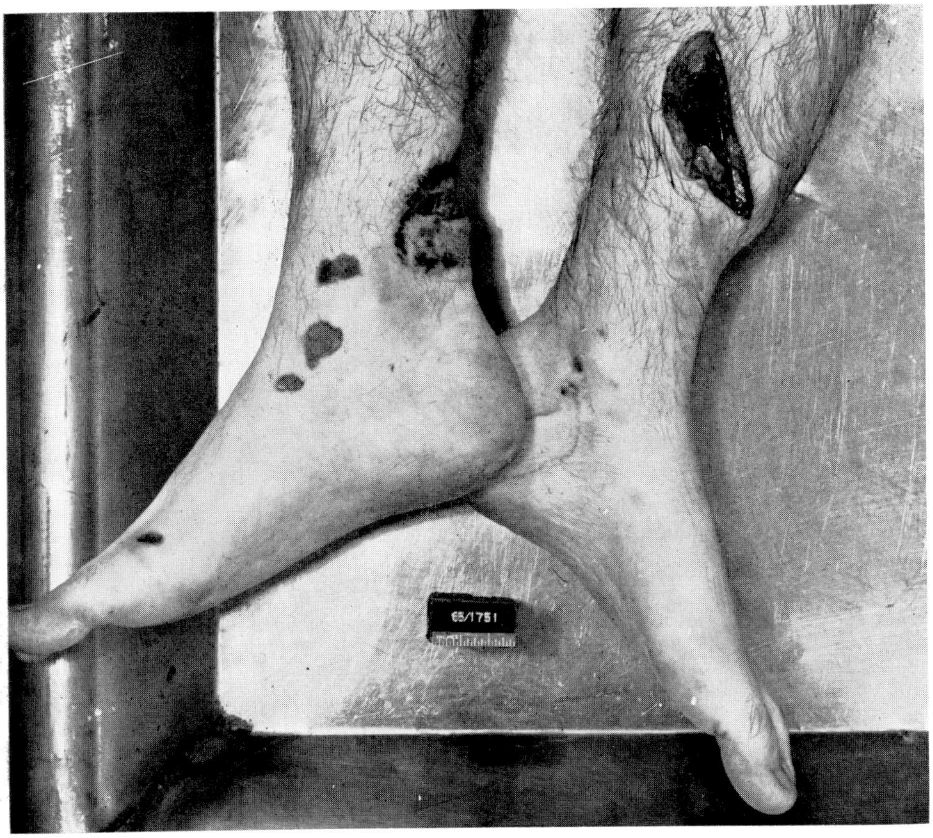


FIGURE XV-3. Bumper injuries. A pedestrian was struck from behind by an automobile, the driver of which was probably applying the brakes. This is indicated by the low level of the injuries, considering that the average bumper is 20 in. above the ground. The laceration on the left leg is due to an open fracture. The different heights of the injuries suggest that the victim was walking when struck. The abrasions on the medial aspect of the right foot and left internal malleolus are probably due to the forward thrust of the feet within the shoes (boots).

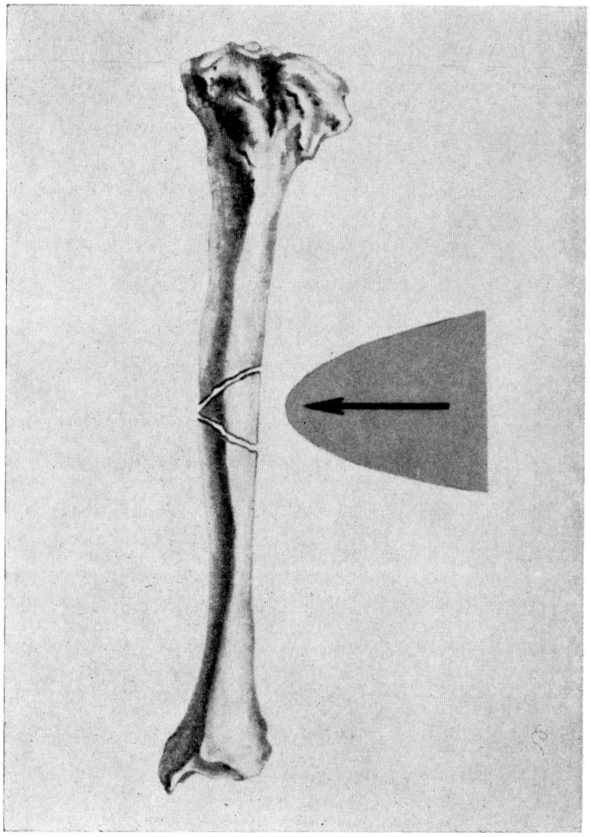

FIGURE XV-4a. Wedge-shaped fracture of the tibia in a pedestrian with bumper injuries. The apex of the triangular fragment of bone often, but not invariably, points in the direction of the movement of the vehicle.

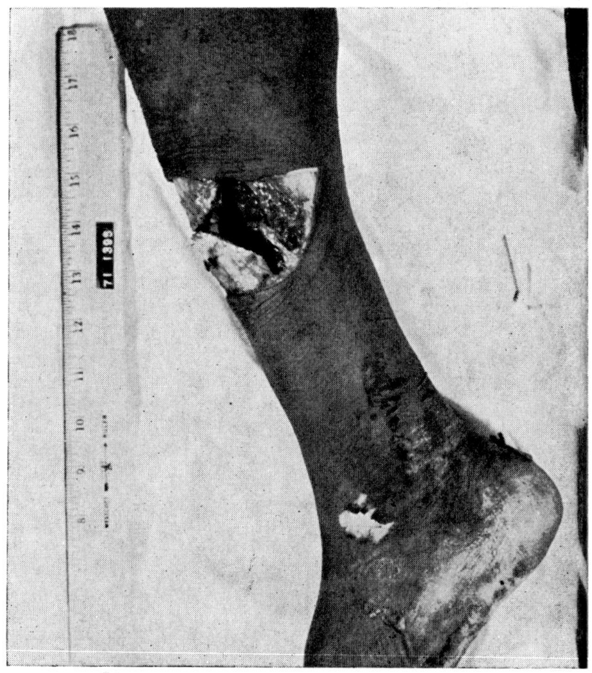

FIGURE XV-4b. Open fracture of the tibia shaft in a pedestrian who was struck from behind by an automobile. Note the triangular shape of the fracture, which points in the direction in which the car was travelling.

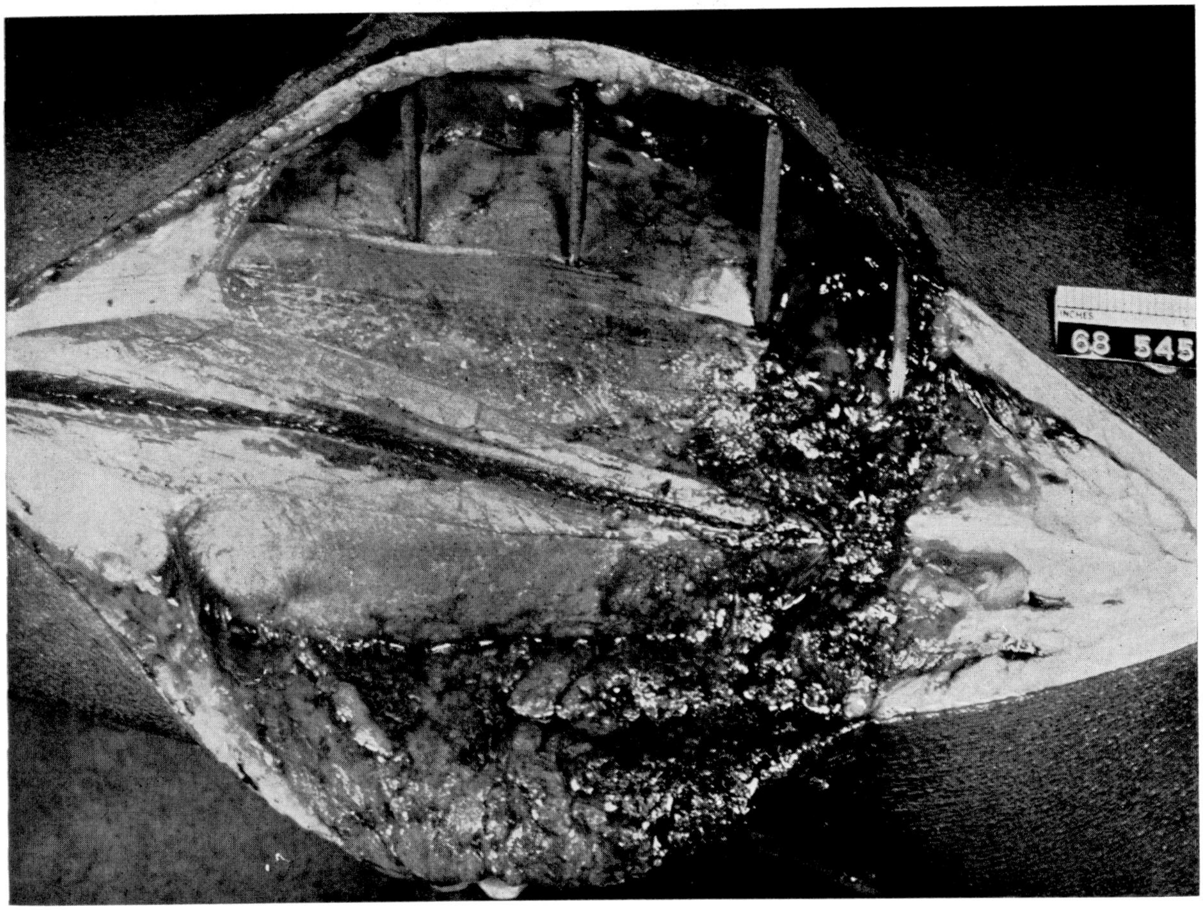


FIGURE XV-5. Pedestrian struck by an automobile. An insignificant abrasion 32 in. above the sole of the foot was noted on the right hip. This was due to a glancing blow by the radiator grill following a primary impact on the legs. Incision of this area reveals a large *pocket* containing blood and lacerated adipose tissue. The *pocket* is limited by intact muscle fascia. The edges of the injury were elevated to show the extent of undermining.

providing an effective *hideout* for fragments of paint and glass from the vehicle involved. Either of these may be of utmost importance for the identification of the vehicle involved in a hit-and-run case. Microscopic examination of a fragment of paint may reveal the number and colors of previous coats, and spectrographic and chemical analyses of the paint may provide conclusive evidence regarding the involvement of a specific automobile in a given crash.

The secondary impact by the radiator guard or the fender also may result in extensive fractures of the pelvis. Commonly, fractures are noted of the pubic rami opposite to the buttock or hip involved. The ilium, particularly the sacroiliac joint, on the same side as the impact is rarely spared. The pelvic fracture pattern resembles the bursting of a wooden hoop when opposite sides of the ring are compressed.

Striaelike superficial tears of the lower abdomen or the inguinal regions due to overstretching of the skin in these areas are not uncommon, particularly if the victim is struck from behind (Fig. XV-6). Deep lacerations due to the same mechanism may occur if the vehicle travels at high speed (Fig. XV-7). The same type of injuries may result if the victim is run over by the automobile, when excessive stretching of

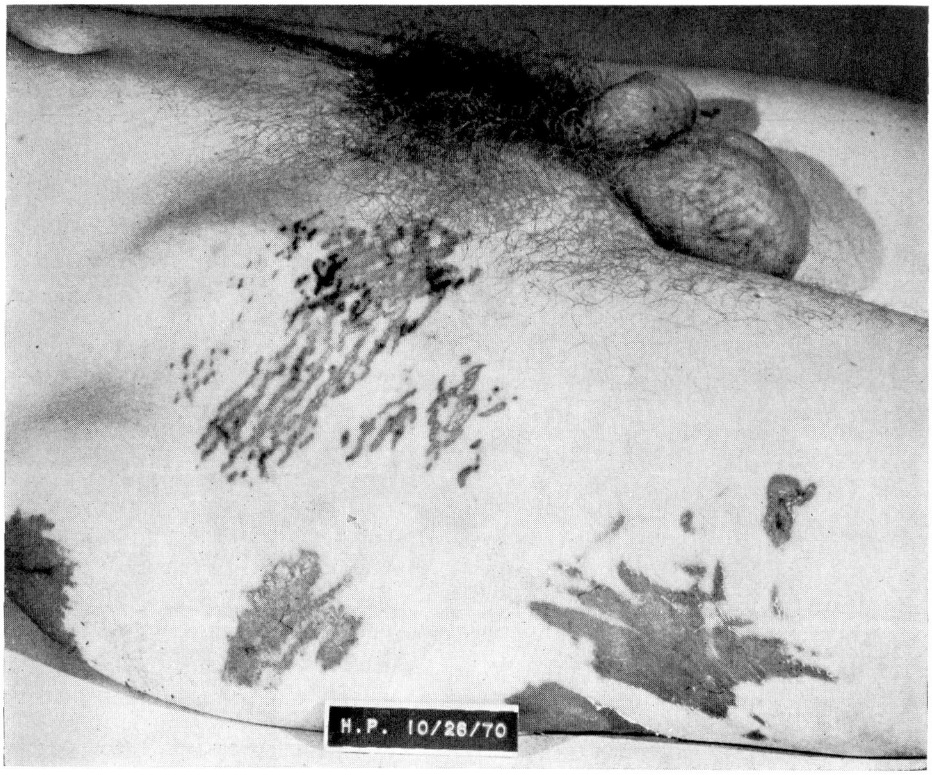


FIGURE XV-6. Striaelike superficial tears of the groin resulting from overstretching of the skin in a pedestrian who was struck from behind. The automobile was travelling at city speed. The injuries are so superficial that bleeding does not occur. The abrasion of the flank and thigh may have been sustained by the fall to the ground.

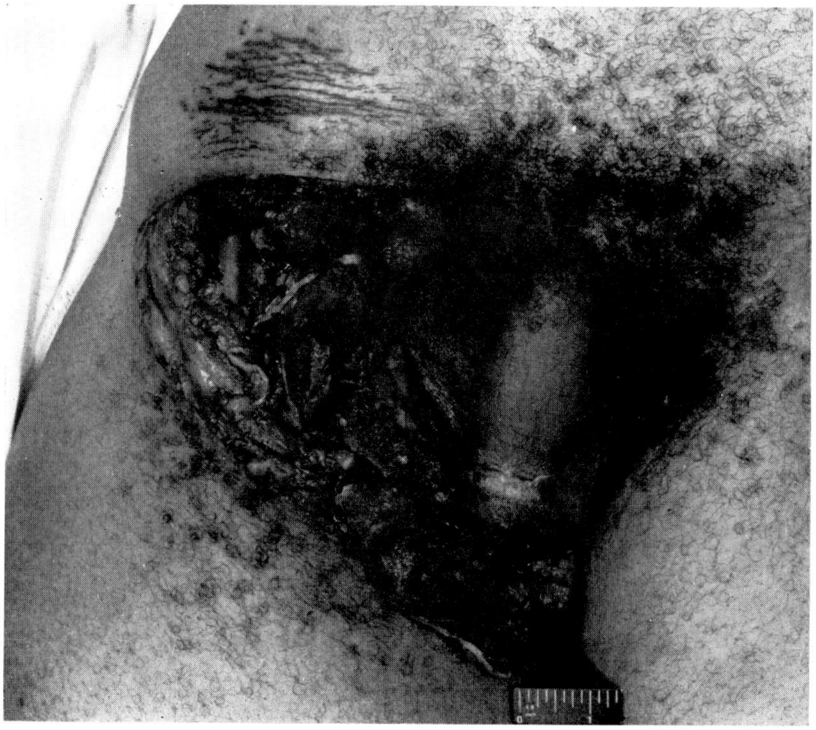

FIGURE XV-7. Deep laceration of the groin by the same mechanism as that described under Figure XV-6: the pedestrian was struck from behind. The automobile in this case, however, was travelling at high speed.

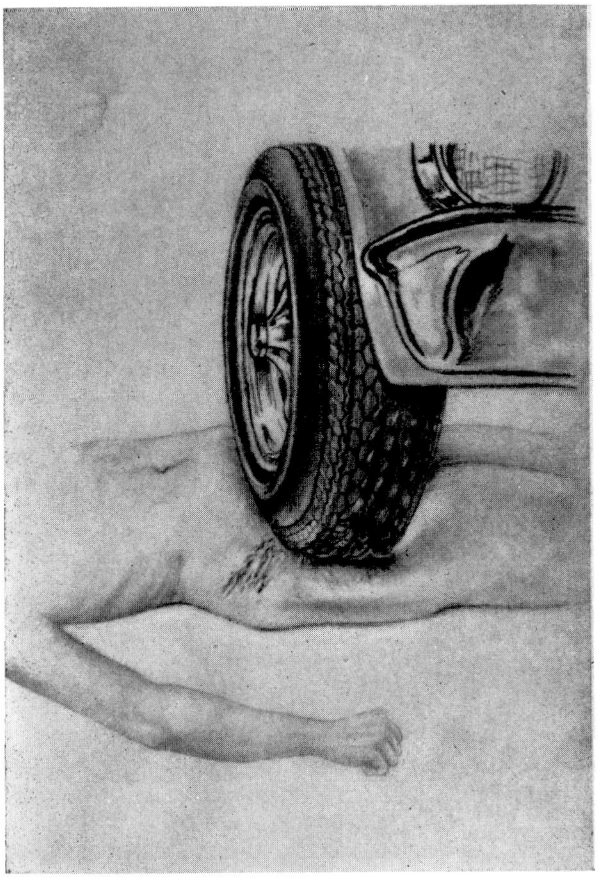

FIGURE XV-8. Diagram showing formation of striaelike tears in the groin of a pedestrian struck and run over by an automobile. The injuries are due to overstretching of the skin by the weight of the automobile.

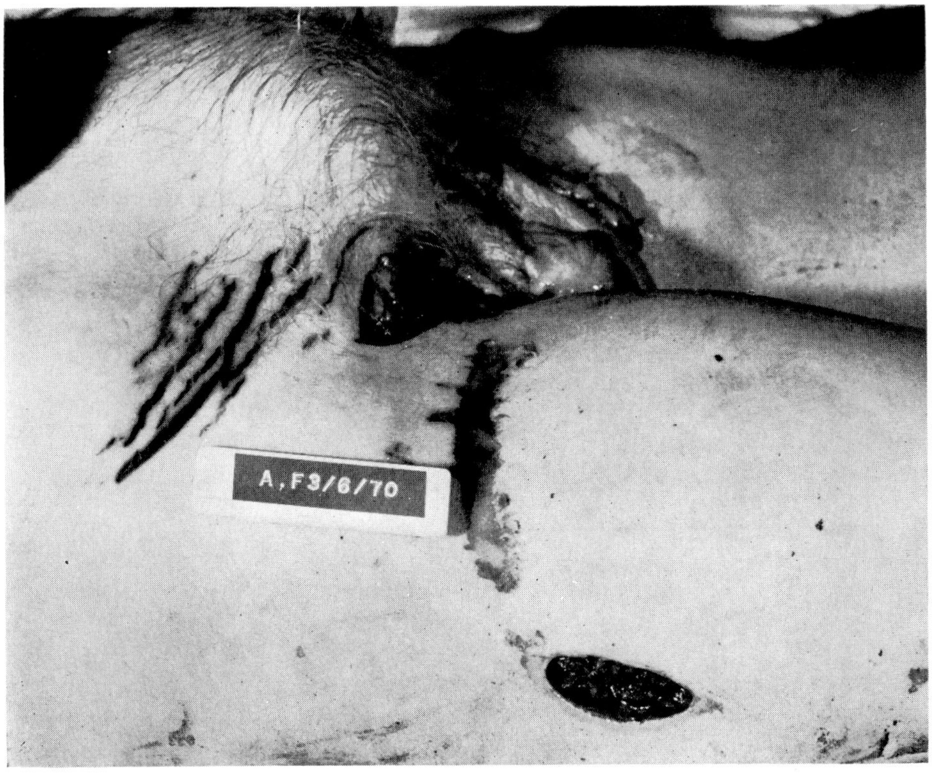


FIGURE XV-9. Pedestrian who was struck by an automobile and thrown into the path of another car, which ran over him. A tire mark is noted over the thigh adjacent to the number plate. Note the striaelike tears in the groin due to overstretching of the skin by the weight of the car.

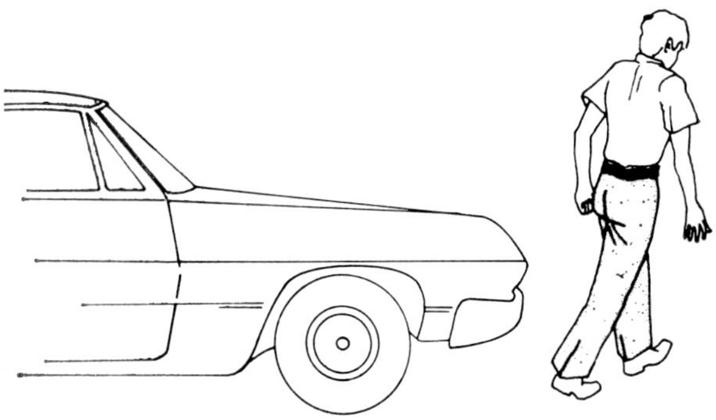

FIGURE XV-10a. Mechanism of injury. An adult victim struck below the center of gravity sustains bumper injuries on his legs and an impact on the hip by the radiator grill.

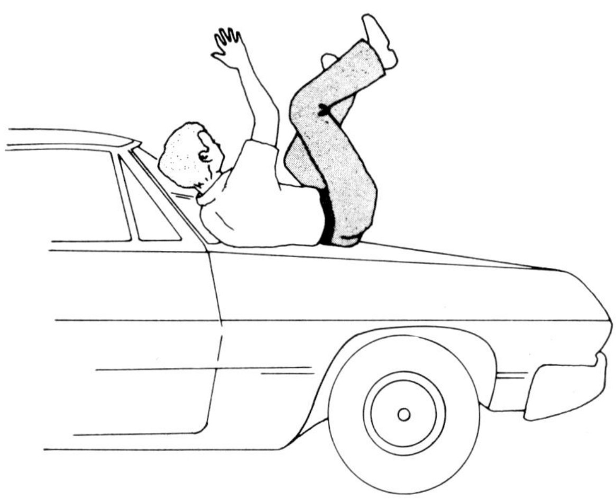

FIGURE XV-10b. At normal city speed, the adult victim is propelled upward after impact by the front end of the vehicle; he slides onto the hood and sustains injuries of the head and shoulders as they come in contact with the windshield. When the vehicle slows or comes to a halt, the victim rolls from the hood to the ground.

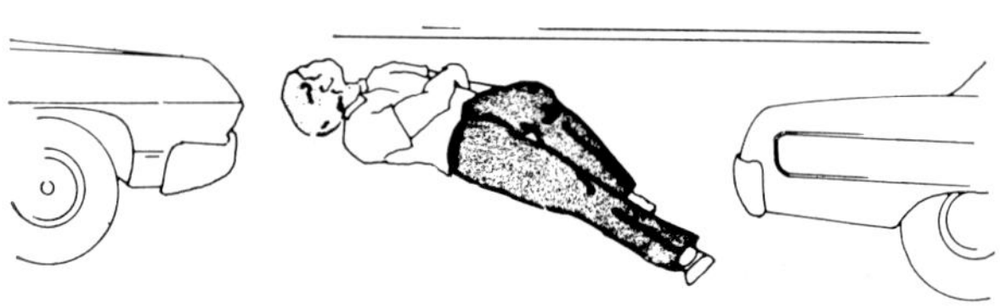

FIGURE XV-10c. At greater speed, the victim may be thrown higher and come to land on the roof of the automobile or on its trunk, or possibly on the road behind the automobile, risking being run over by oncoming automobiles.

the skin is caused by the passing wheel and the crushing weight of the automobile on the body. In this case the presence of tire marks on the clothing or the body will indicate the mechanism of injury (Figs. XV-8 and XV-9).

A certain relationship may be expected between the speed of the vehicle and the nature of the injuries (Fig. XV-10). At normal city speed of 25 to 30 mph, the adult victim, having been struck below the center of gravity of his body, is propelled upward, sliding onto the hood of the automobile and frequently sustaining injuries of his elbows, shoulders and head. These injuries commonly consist of superficial abrasions with little damage to the deeper structures (Figs. XV-11 and XV-12). The victim subsequently slides sideways off the hood, receiving a final impact with the road surface. This impact is usually sustained by the head, resulting in cranial fractures and cerebral injuries. The head injuries are frequently the cause of death in such cases.

On occasion the victim may strike the road surface with the buttocks. Fractures of the sacroiliac joints occur with some frequency, especially in elderly people, as a result of such a fall (forceful sitting). With age the space between the articular surfaces of the sacroiliac joint increases. Manipulation permits significant movement in the joint and at autopsy may lead to an erroneous impression of fracture unless the soft tissues are removed and the joint observed directly.

Fractures and dislocations of the cervical spine resulting from sudden unexpected hyperextension of the neck following initial impact by the vehicle are also common and are occasionally the only injuries capable of explaining the victim's death.

When the automobile is travelling at a greater speed, the pedestrian may be thrown considerably higher and land on the vehicle's roof or trunk, or possibly on the road behind the automobile, with subsequent risk of being run over by oncoming traffic.[3]

In contrast to an auto impact, the circumstances are different in the case of an adult who

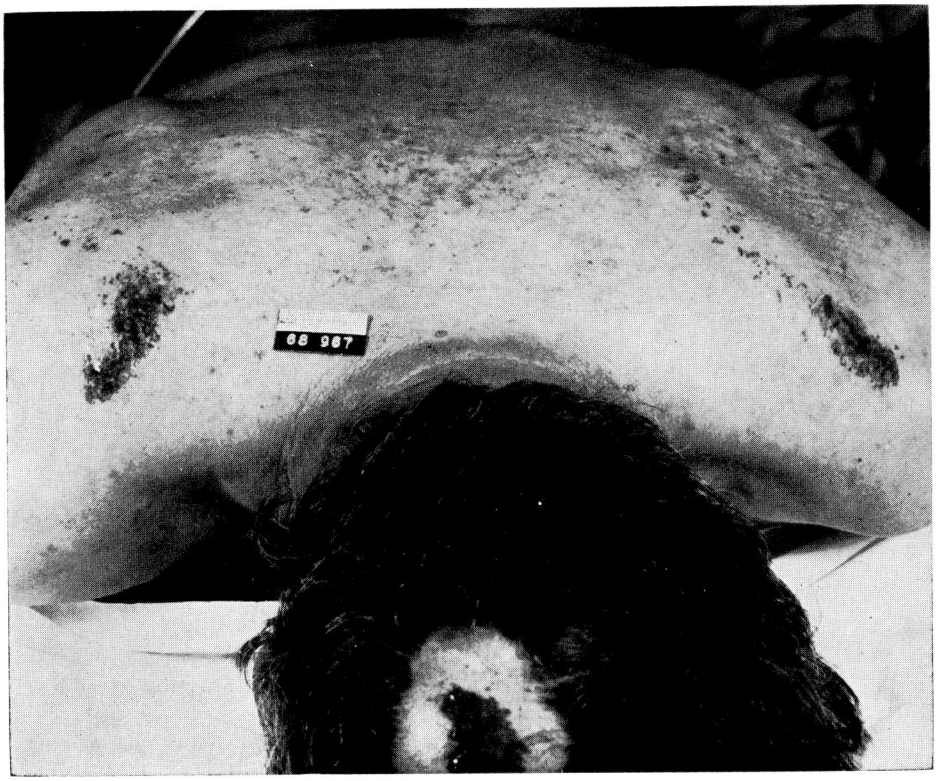


FIGURE XV-11. Pedestrian who was struck by an automobile. The abrasions on the shoulders were sustained by sliding onto the hood. The abrasion of the scalp resulted from impact on the windshield.

is struck by a fast-moving van, truck or bus, all of which have a straight and high front end. The victim when struck is propelled forward or sideways rather than upward, or he may actually be carried or *pinned* on the radiator grill for some distance before falling in front of the vehicle as it slows down or comes to a halt. Running over the victim is common at this time.

With respect to small children struck by automobiles, the mechanism of injury is comparable to that of an adult who is struck by a van, truck or bus. This is due to the fact that in children the primary impact is usually located above the center of gravity of their bodies, frequently involving the head area.

Both adults and children are often run over when struck by a reversing bus or truck. This

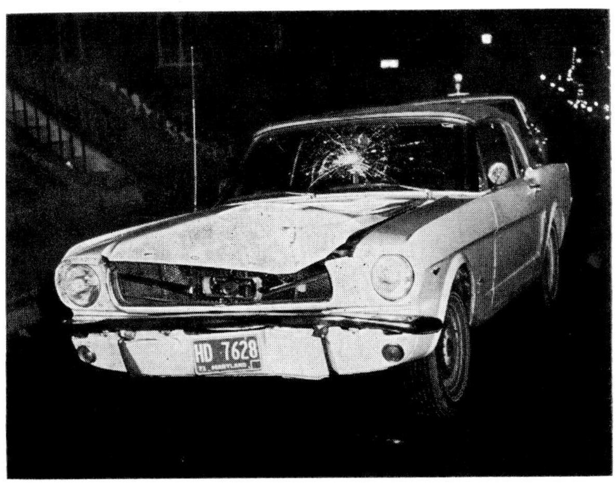


FIGURE XV-12. Fatal pedestrian accident with automobile travelling at city speed. The hood is dented at the point of impact. Fragmentation of the windshield was by the victim's body. The driver of the car sustained no injuries; his head did not strike the windshield.

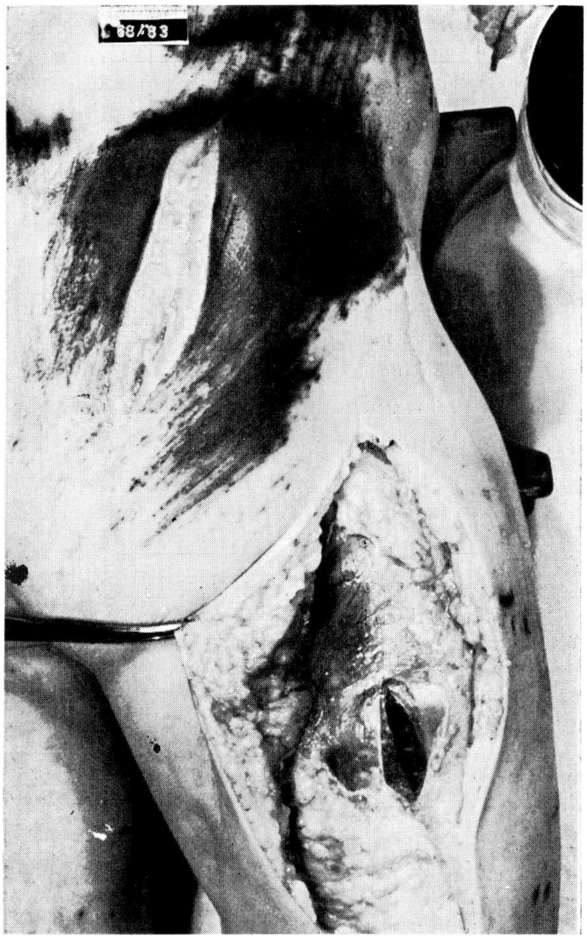

is due to the fact that in both tall and short individuals the point of impact is high and above their respective center of gravity.

For an effective reconstruction of a motor vehicle accident, injuries sustained by dragging or scraping on the ground must be recognized and distinguished from those sustained as a result of a direct impact by or on the vehicle. A helpful criterion for such distinction is that injuries sustained by dragging or scraping are usually superficial, even if spread over large areas, and show typical *brush burning* without significant hemorrhage in the skin and subcutaneous tissue (Fig. XV-13). Depending on the force of impact with the ground, deeper structures may be extensively involved. Due to the friction-type force responsible for brush burns, protuberant parts of the body, such as areas over joints, ribs, and, to a lesser extent, over tendons, are predominantly involved (Fig. XV-

FIGURE XV-13. Pedestrian who was struck by an automobile. Typical brush burn injury of the flank and buttock due to scraping on the road surface was sustained. No hemorrhage is noted in the underlying tissues, except under the site of impact on the thigh.

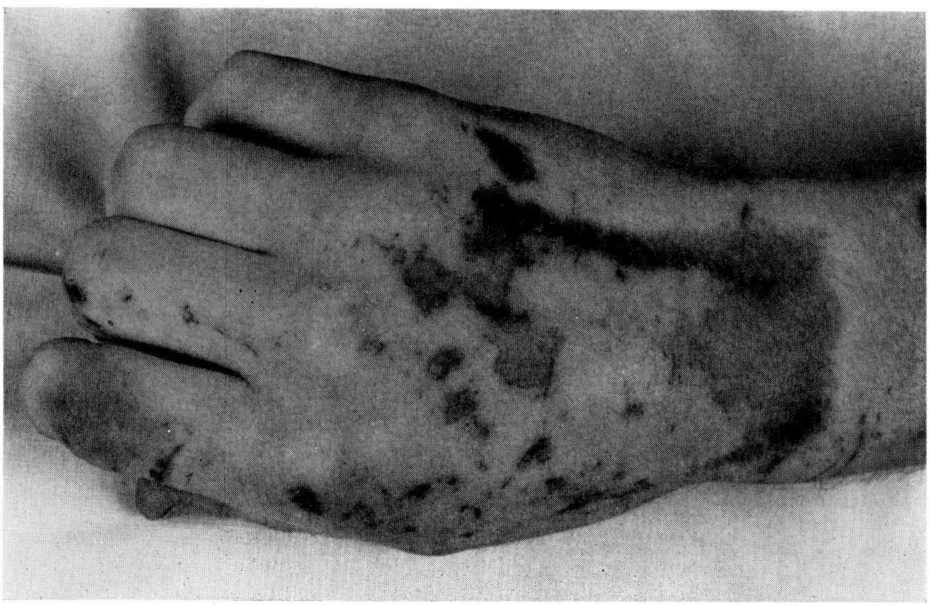

FIGURE XV-14. Brush burns on the back of the right hand and wrist. The protuberant areas are predominantly involved.

14), while depressed surfaces are spared.

Very severe but not necessarily characteristic injuries result when an automobile actually runs over the body of the victim. The grinding action of the wheel commonly causes separation of the skin from the subcutaneous tissue and musculature (décollement). Injury of the skin itself, however, may be slight or altogether absent. If the brakes of the vehicle are applied, the wheels will lock and vast lacerations will be formed due to the shearing action of this tangential type of force. Under such circumstances, complete amputation of an extremity[4] or decapitation may occur (Fig. XV-15). On the other hand, in children run over by vehicles, fractures may be absent due to the considerable elasticity of their partly cartilaginous skeleton. In the case of a three-year-old child, who was run over by a pickup van, there were no fractured ribs or vertebrae, but all thoracic organs and the liver were crushed into a semiliquid pulp.

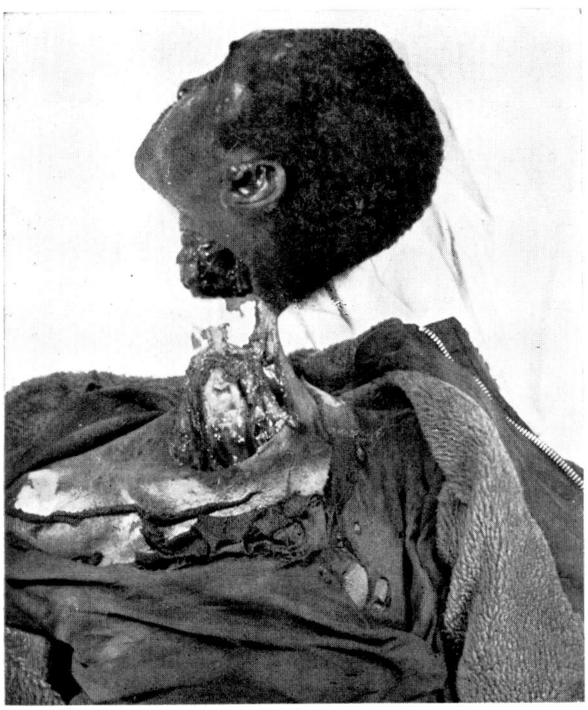

FIGURE XV-15. Pedestrian struck by an automobile and thrown into the path of another automobile, which ran over the victim. The decapitation is due to the shearing action of the tire resulting from application of the brakes.

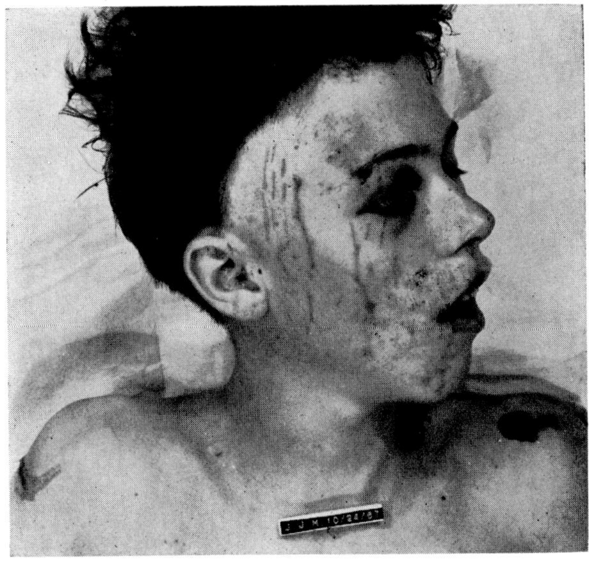

FIGURE XV-16. Pedestrian run over by a car, showing tire marks on his face.

Avulsion of an ear almost always occurs if a tire passes over the head of the victim. The ear is literally *pulled off* by the moving wheel; consequently, the tear is behind the ear if the vehicle rolls from back to front in relation to the victim, and it is located in front of the ear if the vehicle travels in the opposite direction.

Tire marks often remain as trace evidence on the body of the victim or his clothes (Fig. XV-16). Tire marks may be especially helpful in establishing the identity of the vehicle involved in the accident. No two tires are alike, due to small imperfections in the pattern of the tread that are specific for each tire. A useful procedure for comparing the pattern on the body with that of a suspected tire is to copy the imprint from the skin or clothing onto a sheet of transparent parchment paper. Such a tracing permits easy side-by-side comparison with the tire print and can be filed for possible later use as evidence. The importance of photography should likewise by emphasized. Some spreading of the impression on the skin due to flattening of the body by the weight of the vehicle may have to be considered. The side of the body in contact with

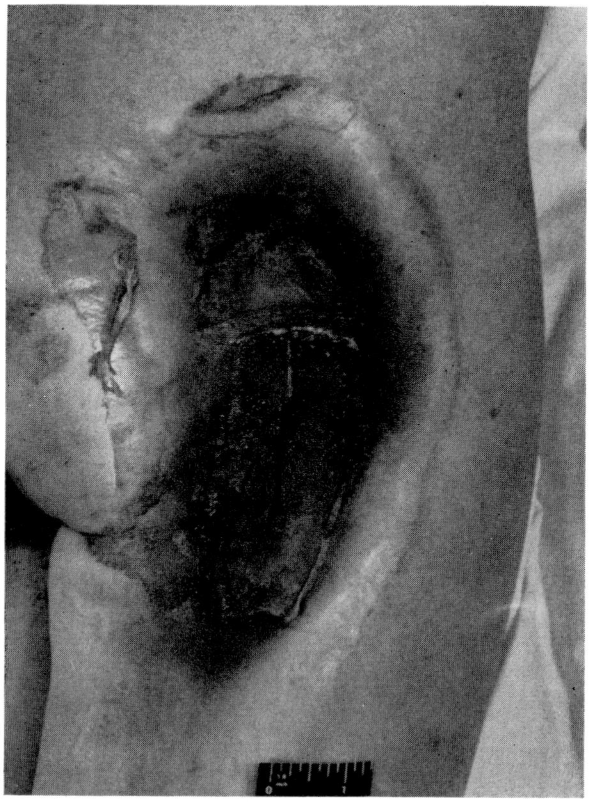

FIGURE XV-17. Charring of the skin by an automobile exhaust pipe. The car struck the deceased and came to rest on his body.

the road surface in the course of being run over commonly shows typical abrasions of the brush-burn nature.

A treadless tire obviously leaves no tire marks. There are other situations where a victim had been run over but no tire marks could be identified on the body or clothing (Fig. XV-17). An opinion as to whether running over occurred must be based on all findings, including the scene and the autopsy.

### The Driver and the Passenger

While injuries sustained by pedestrians usually conform to a certain pattern, those found in drivers and passengers seem to be considerably less uniform. The automobile is a spacious environment in which the unrestrained occupants may be thrown in all directions following a forceful and unexpected impact. Such impacts cause injuries of different severity with an infinite variety of possibilities in respect to their mechanism of occurrence. Frequently, ejection from the automobile further tends to complicate the picture. Nevertheless, while it is important to be aware of the limitations, certain important possibilities with respect to the reconstruction of an automobile accident do exist.

A relatively new Chrysler sedan with automatic transmission was travelling downhill on a major thoroughfare, which intersects and dead-ends with another major highway. On its way, the vehicle ran off the right side of the road, reentered the road, crossed the midline, went up an embankment and hit a tree. The automobile then turned on its right side and came to rest near a telephone pole 75 ft. from the intersection. The latter part of the event was observed by two policemen in a patrol car travelling in the opposite direction. Immediate investigation by these officers showed the victim, a young white woman, to have been thrown onto the door of the vehicle in front of the right front seat. Her face was covered with blood. Swelling and contusion of the right hand were noticed. She was pronounced dead at the scene.

Postmortem examination of the deceased showed multiple fresh typical blunt force injuries of the forehead, the left ear, the scalp, the right hand and the left forearm. The base of the skull was extensively fractured. No other pertinent findings were noted except extensive aspiration of blood and evidence of blood swallowing.

Considering the lack of an adequate anatomical and chronological explanation of the injuries of the deceased on the basis of this apparent accident, it appeared mandatory that the automobile be reexamined. The vehicle showed comparatively little damage, consisting of dents of the left and right sides and fenders. No glass was broken. Clotted blood was noted on and behind the driver's seat, and blood splatters indicating both forward and backward directions in reference to the upright position of the car were found on the ceiling. It was concluded that the woman had been beaten to death in the car and the car dispatched down the hill in an effort to conceal the murder. Additionally, a stone had been found wedged under the rear end of the gas petal, thus applying acceleration to the motor. The husband was convicted of striking his wife with a blunt weapon, probably a piece of metal pipe, then attempting to simulate an accidental death (Fig. XV-18).

Patterned injuries from the steering wheel or the steering column (Fig. XV-19), from knobs on the dashboard or the doors or other protruding objects of definite shapes within the vehicle may be of assistance in establishing the direction of thrust and may possibly give an idea

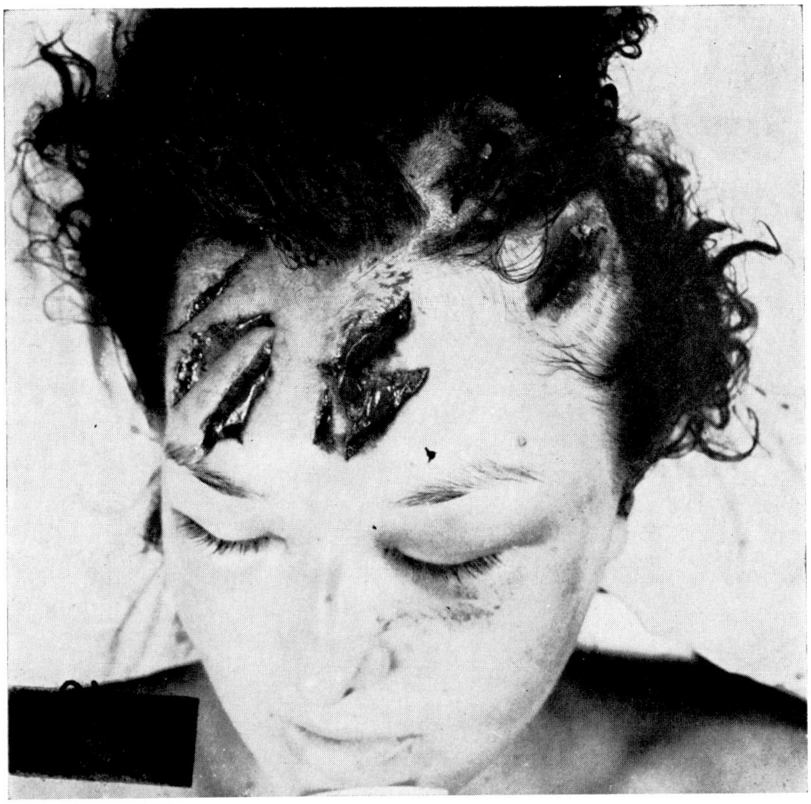

FIGURE XV-18. Multiple injuries of the forehead and scalp inflicted with a blunt instrument (metal pipe).

of how the occupants were seated. Identification of the driver is frequently of prime imporance. One useful criterion in this regard is the pattern of the gas or brake pedal, which is sometimes imprinted on the sole of the driver's right shoe at the time of the collision.

Trauma associated with an impact on the chest by the steering wheel or column is often severe, yet external evidence of injury may be minimal or absent (Fig. XV-20). Multiple fractures of the rib cage as well as tears and contusions of the lungs are frequently observed. Among the less common injuries, central tears of the lung, i.e. without communication with the pleural surface, deserve special mention. Sevitt[5] describes several cases following compression of the chest without apparent injury to the chest wall. With the introduction of the energy-absorbing steering column the frequency and severity of such injuries in drivers has declined appreciably. Nevertheless, cardiovascular injuries still occur far more frequently than current medical statistics indicate.[6] Contusions of the heart are relatively common, and laceration of the aorta at the level of the aortic ligament is by no means rare (Fig. XV-21). In some instances, horizontal and V-shaped superficial tears of the aortic intima in this location are noted due to the same mechanism (Fig. XV-22). One may speculate regarding the occurrence of aneurysms of this segment of the aorta in later life and their association with a previous traumatic episode of this nature.

Facial lacerations and fractures of the facial skeleton in drivers involved in front-end collisions are relatively frequent in automobiles equipped with the energy-absorbing steering column.[7] Compression of the column seems to

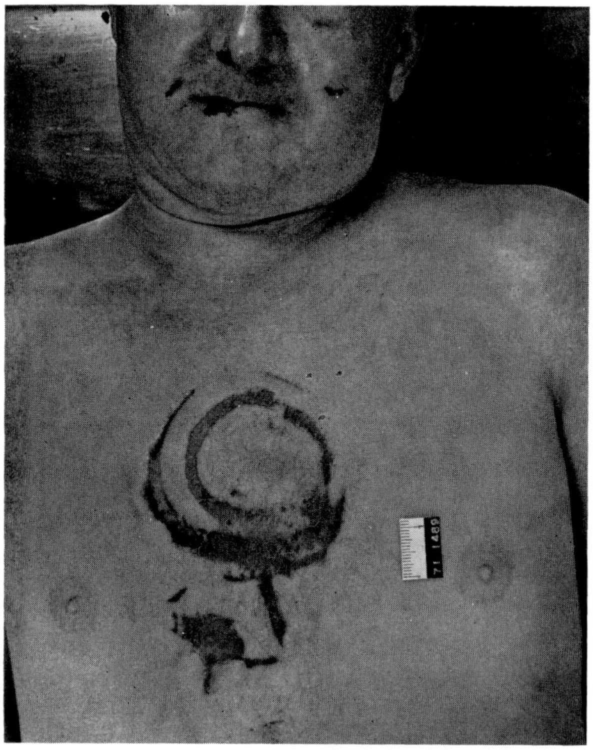

FIGURE XV-19. Fifty-year-old driver of a 1962 half-ton Chevrolet pickup truck, who lost control of his automobile and struck a tree. A typical steering column injury is noted on the chest.

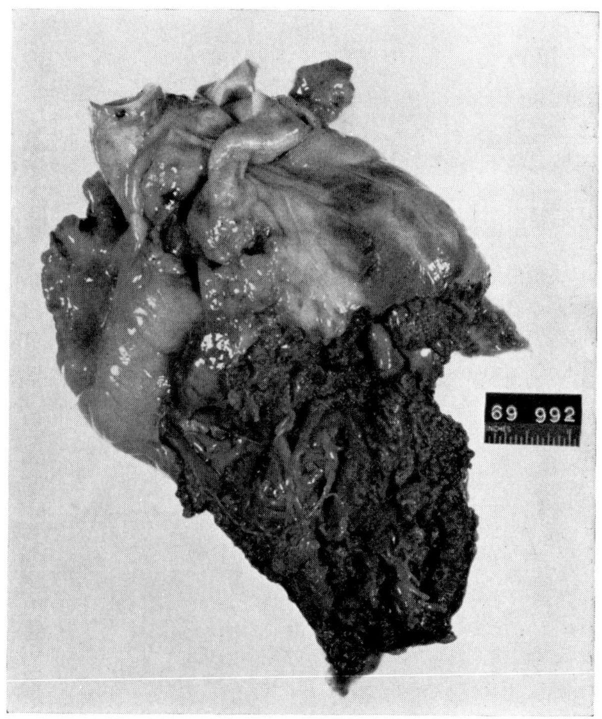


FIGURE XV-20. Driver of a 1966 Ford, who lost control of his automobile, ran off the road and struck a tree. The heart was shredded in spite of minor external injuries of the chest resulting from steering wheel impact.

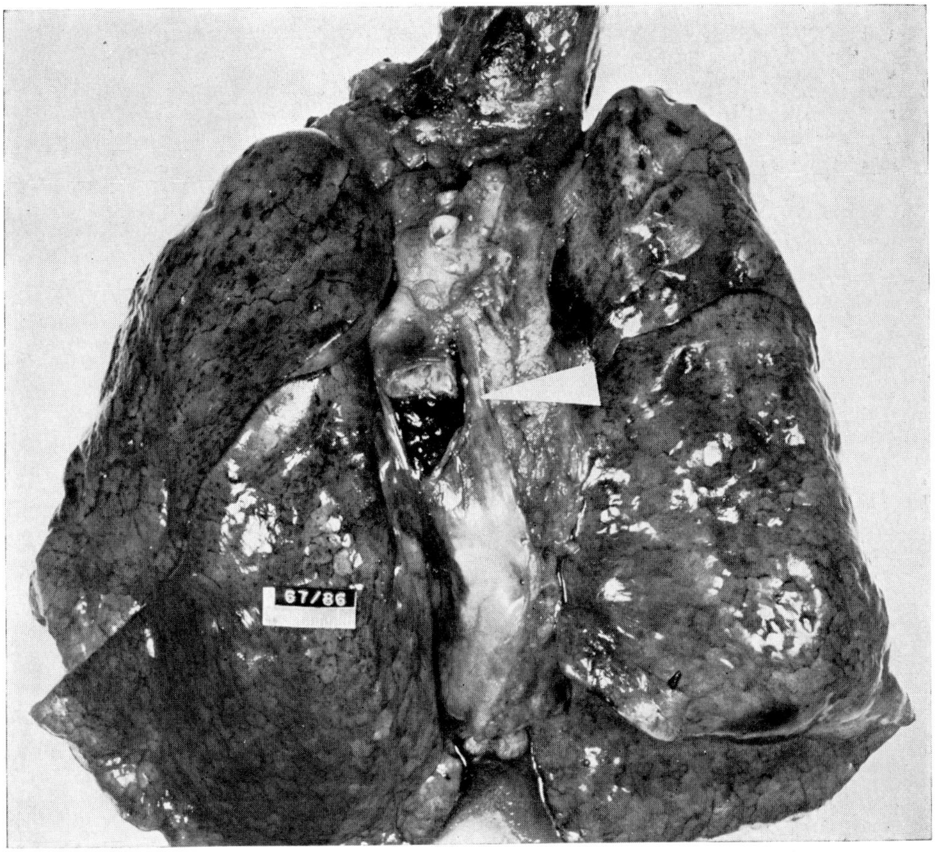

FIGURE XV-21. Aorta viewed from behind. The illustrated aorta is severed in the level commonly seen in steering wheel injuries. This results from compression of the chest between the steering wheel and the vertebral column.

predispose the face to impacts on the steering wheel rim and on the padded dashboard, especially if no seat restraint is worn (Fig. XV-23).

It may be of interest to note that energy-absorbing steering columns have been incorporated in all automobiles manufactured by General Motors, American Motors and the Chrysler Corporation beginning with the model year 1967. The Ford Motor Company introduced the energy-absorbing steering column in the following model year.

Injuries to the neck—so-called whiplash injuries—have been stressed recurrently, particularly in recent years, and prophylactic headrests have become mandatory on new models of automobiles. While fractures and dislocations have been described as occurring particularly in the levels of the fifth and sixth cervical vertebrae, there appears to prevail some controversy regarding the severity of other neck injuries associated with the whiplash mechanism.[8, 9] We have found a significant number of injuries in the atlanto-occipital joints, often with laceration of tendons and joint capsules, intra-articular hemorrhages and separation of the cartilaginous lining of the articular surfaces. Such injuries, while in themselves perhaps of minor importance, are certainly indicative of trauma to this vital area. Visible injury of the medulla is relatively rare. In fatal cases in which no other evidence of injury is found, it may be interesting to speculate whether concussion of the medulla may be the cause of death.

Removal of the atlas through a posterior midline incision permits demonstration of skeletal and soft tissue injuries to this part of the body as well as inspection of the underside of the base of the skull. This incision does not impede

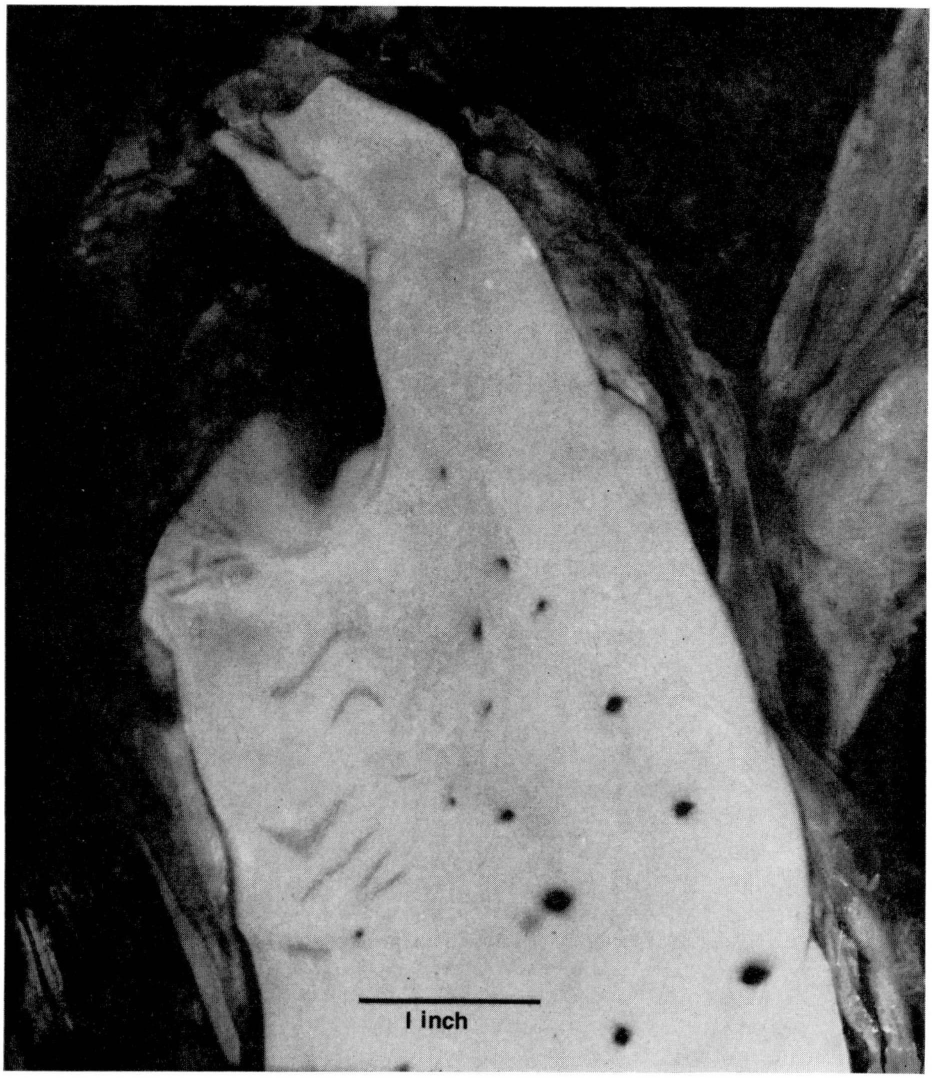


FIGURE XV-22. Superficial tears of the aortic intima in a driver who suffered a steering wheel injury of the chest.

subsequent laminectomy for examination of the spinal cord and does not induce significant mutilation of the body (*see* Chapter XXV). Leakage of embalming fluids through this incision has not, in our experience, been the subject of complaint by relatives and/or funeral directors.

The importance of seat belts in the prevention of injuries resulting from automobile collisions, particularly those due to ejection from the automobile, cannot be overemphasized. Ejection of the occupants from the vehicle is the single most common cause of injury and death in automobile collisions.[10] Nevertheless, isolated cases in which injury is caused by the belt are sometimes seen. Snyder et al.[11] report on the pathomechanics of automotive restraint system injuries and provide a detailed list of pertinent references. The type of seat belt used is believed to have some bearing on the type of injury produced. The diagonal over-the-shoulder strap may be associated with bruising of the chest, fracture of ribs and laceration of the liver. The lap belt may produce injuries to the pelvis, the abdomen and the lumbar spine; since the belt offers no support to the upper half

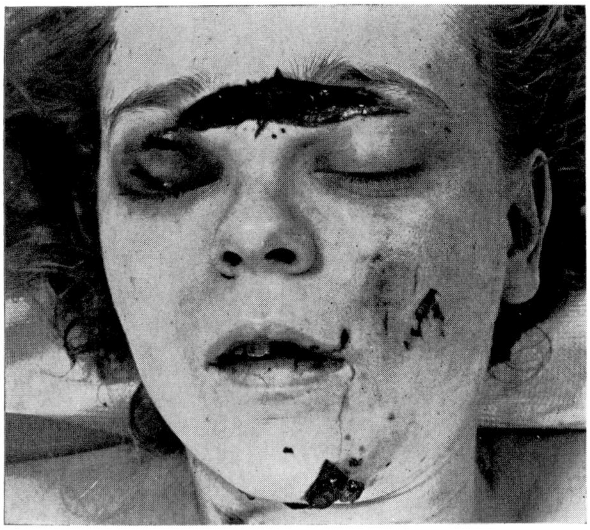

FIGURE XV-23. Laceration of the forehead due to impact on the upper segment of the steering wheel in a driver who struck a bridge abutment. No seat belt was worn. The tissue bridges indicate the blunt nature of the impact and exclude cutting by glass from the broken windshield. Other significant injuries of this victim consisted of extensive crushing of the chest.

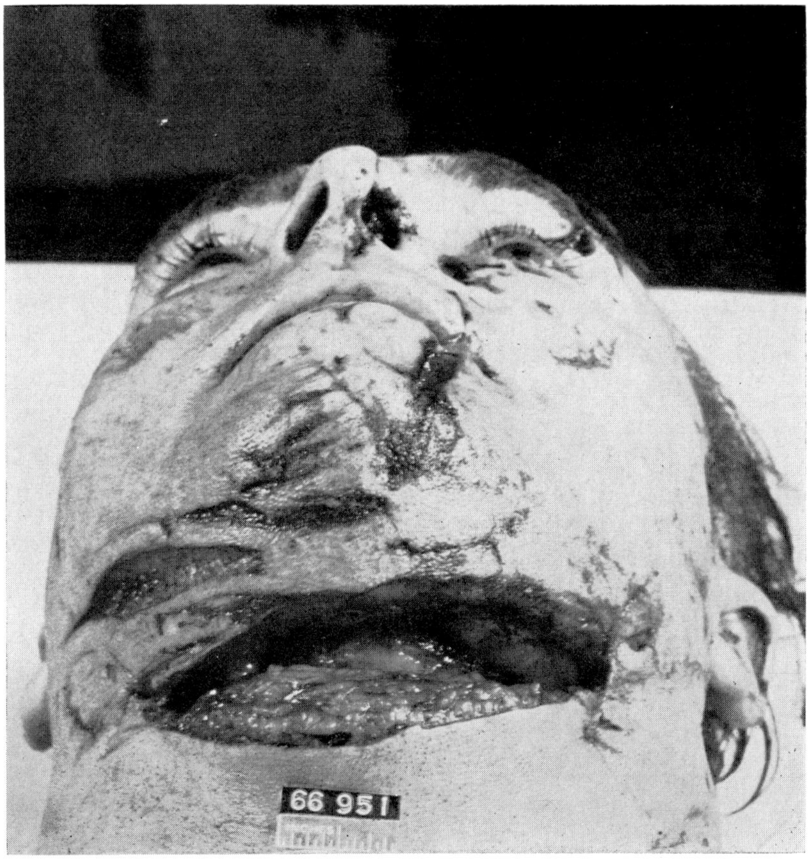


FIGURE XV-24. Driver of 1965 automobile, whose head was thrust through the windshield. The bobbing action of the head after penetration of the windshield caused this gaping cut of the throat.

of the body, the head and chest are free to jackknife over the restraint. Consequently, injuries to the neck were found to occur more frequently if only a lap belt and no shoulder strap were used. Adequate headrests are expected to reduce the frequency of neck injuries.

Present legislation requires that air bags or passive restraint belts must be installed in full-size cars beginning with the 1982 model year and in *all* cars beginning with the 1984 models. It is anticipated that air bags, particularly if used in conjunction with the lap belt, will prevent serious injury of the occupants of the automobile in all seating positions in frontal, angular, lateral and rollover crashes.[12] Preliminary studies show that taking the General Motors Severity Index of 1000 points as fatal, bags reduce this to about 510.

Disfiguring and sometimes fatal injuries of the face and neck by the windshield are common in these deceleration-type accidents. Studies have shown that in head-on collisions the unrestrained front seat occupant moves forward, striking his knees on the dashboard. This halts the forward motion of the lower half of his body, causing the upper half to jackknife about the waist. The head then strikes the windshield. Penetration of the windshield by the head and the severity of the injuries depend on the type of glass. Automobiles and trucks currently in circulation in the United States are equipped with one of two varieties of laminated windshield:

1. The pre-1966 windshield was made by bonding a 0.015 in. thick plastic interlayer between two sheets of plate glass. Severe cuts were sustained by the rigid and jagged edges of this type of windshield, particularly in case of penetration of the windshield by the head. This occurs at head-to-glass speed of about 13 mph (Fig. XV-24).
2. Beginning with the 1966 models, automobiles manufactured in the United States have been equipped with a new type of laminated windshield. This windshield also consists of two sheets of glass, but the plastic interlayer has a thickness of 0.030 in. Furthermore, a lower bond strength between the plastic interlayer and the glass provides for greater energy absorption on impact and for considerable bulging of the windshield before tearing of the plastic allows penetration (Fig. XV-25). The penetration velocity of this windshield is given

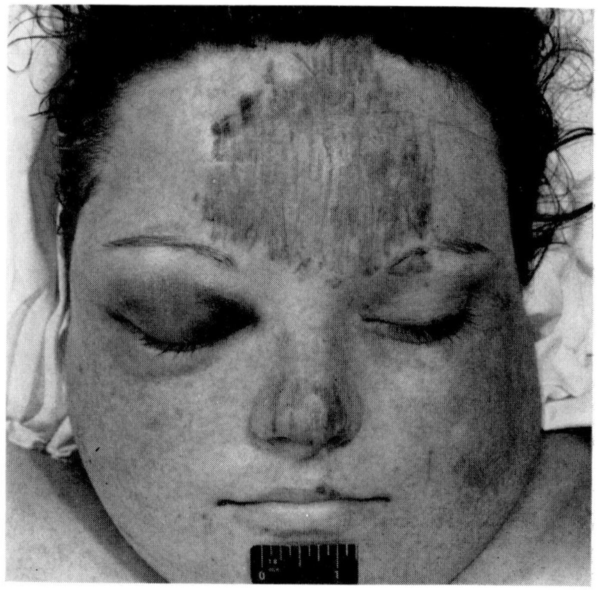

FIGURE XV-26. Unrestrained driver of a 1975 automobile that struck a parked car at low speed. The vertical scratches on the forehead and nose are caused by sliding up or down on the flat surface of the shattered windshield, which was held in place by the plastic interlayer.

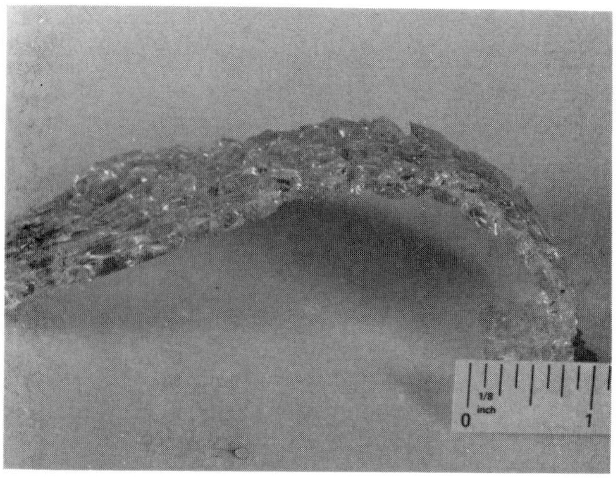

FIGURE XV-25. Section of broken windshield illustrates the *amount of give* upon impact, prior to rupture. A layer of plastic is sandwiched between two sheets of glass.

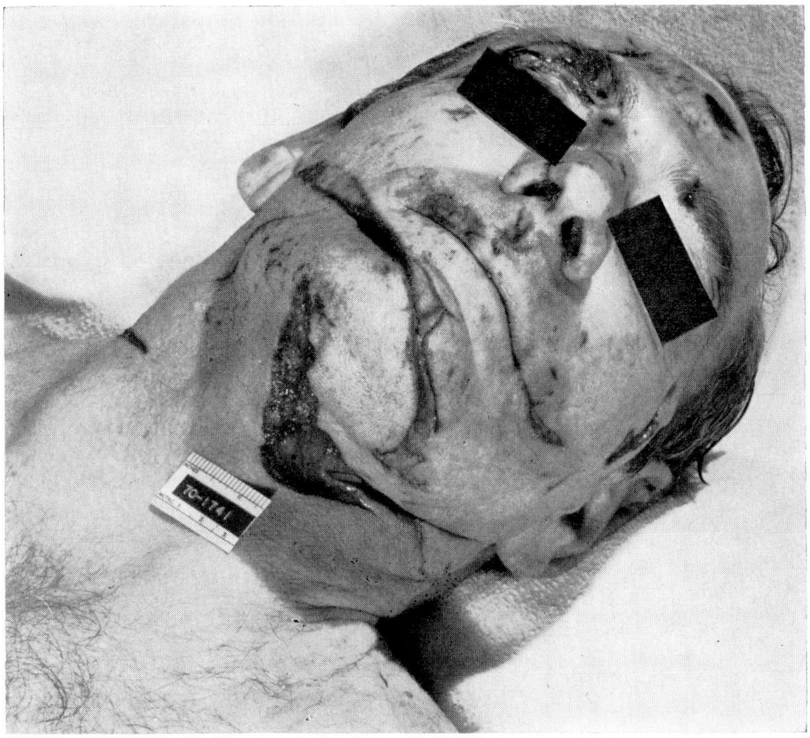

FIGURE XV-27. Driver of a 1970 Cadillac, who travelled at an excessive rate of speed and ran into a bridge abutment. The cuts of the face and neck by the windshield are not materially different from those produced by older types of windshields.

at 25 to 30 mph, or roughly double that of the pre-1966 windshield.

Injuries by this improved type of windshield are consequently reduced both in severity and in frequency (Fig. XV-26). Nevertheless, at high-speed impacts, injuries from this windshield are not materially different from those caused by the pre-1966 variety (Fig. XV-27). Both pre- and post-1966 laminated windshields tend to break in a *spider web* pattern. The central area of the pattern presents the actual point of impact (Figs. XV-28 and XV-29).

The Corning Glass Works has developed a safety windshield that is believed to surpass conventional windshields in being less prone to cause injury.[13, 14] It is equally laminated, but the inner layer is chemically treated and slightly more than half as thick as the inner layer of conventional windshields. According to the manufacturer, this windshield can withstand a short-time bending stress to a 10 in. radius, and when it does break, the fragments are blunt edged and appear to be incapable of causing severe cuts (Fig. XV-30). Some of the 1970 domestic passenger cars are equipped with this feature. Sufficient evidence is as yet lacking regarding the performance of this windshield under actual crash conditions. A windshield manufactured by Libbey Owens Ford and made with two layers of glass, each half of the standard thickness, is presently used almost universally in the United States. This windshield has significantly reduced facial lacerations.

Further improvement may be expected from the Securiflex® windshield used in some European automobiles. This windshield resembles standard United States windshields but has an additional, very thin plastic inner surface, which prevents the occupant from coming into contact with the sharp glass edges when the windshild is struck and broken.

The old-type *safety glass* is now being used

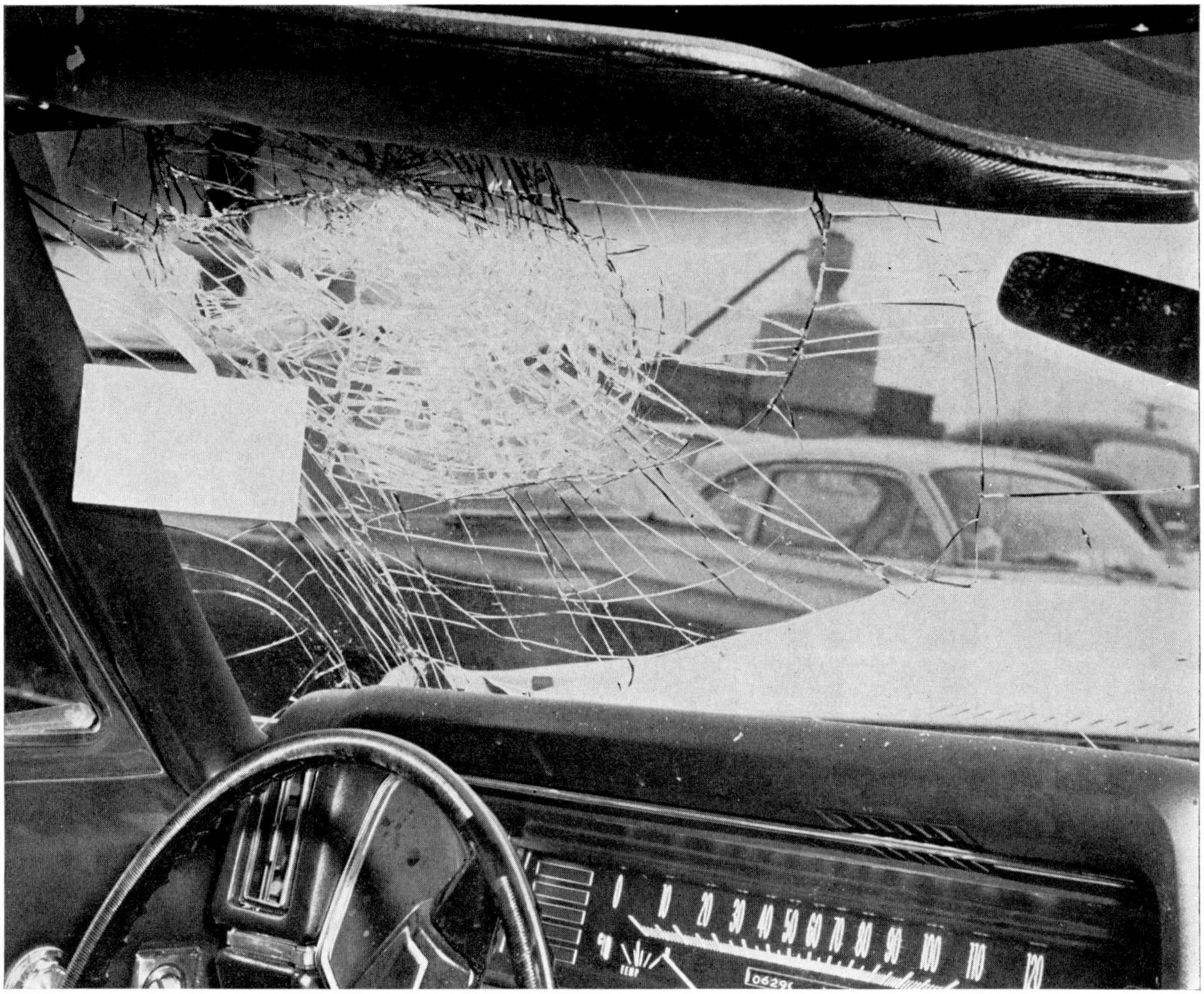

FIGURE XV-28. 1968 Cadillac that struck a tree. Typical *spider web* fracture of the windshield caused by the impact of the driver's head.

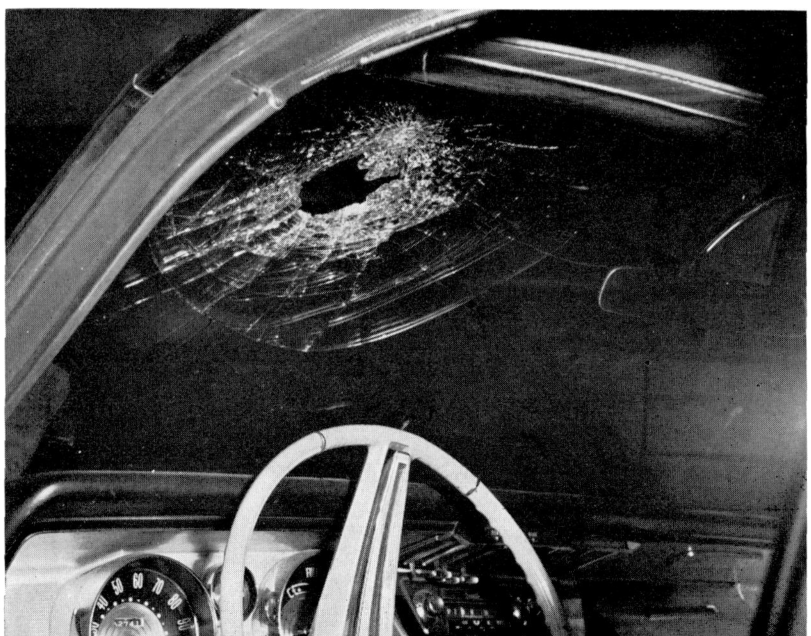

FIGURE XV-29. Head-on collision of a 1966 Buick. The driver's head penetrated the windshield. He sustained severe cuts of the face and neck. Note the punched-out *spider web* fracture of the windshield.

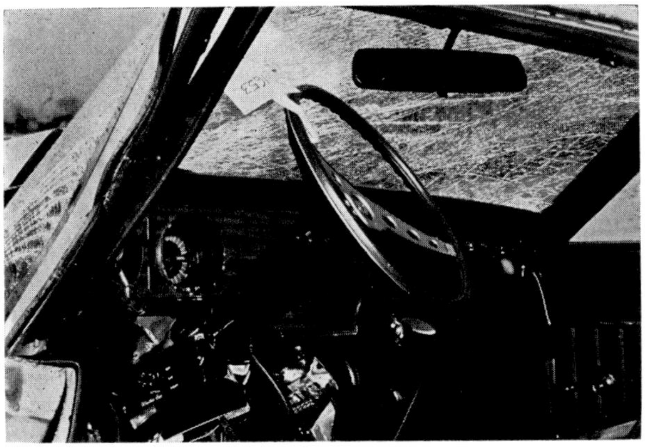

FIGURE XV-30. 1970 AMC Javelin equipped with a new type of safety windshield, which upon impact breaks into multiple blunt-edged fragments, supposedly incapable of causing deep cuts.

for the side and rear windows exclusively. This is a tempered glass that is made from heat-treated plate glass. As a result of this prestressing, the glass retains a high resistance to bending. If this glass is broken in an accident, it disintegrates into small angular fragments (Fig. XV-31). These are commonly ejected from the frame, inflicting superficial cuts, many of which are right-angled. The presence and location of this *dicing pattern* may be invaluable

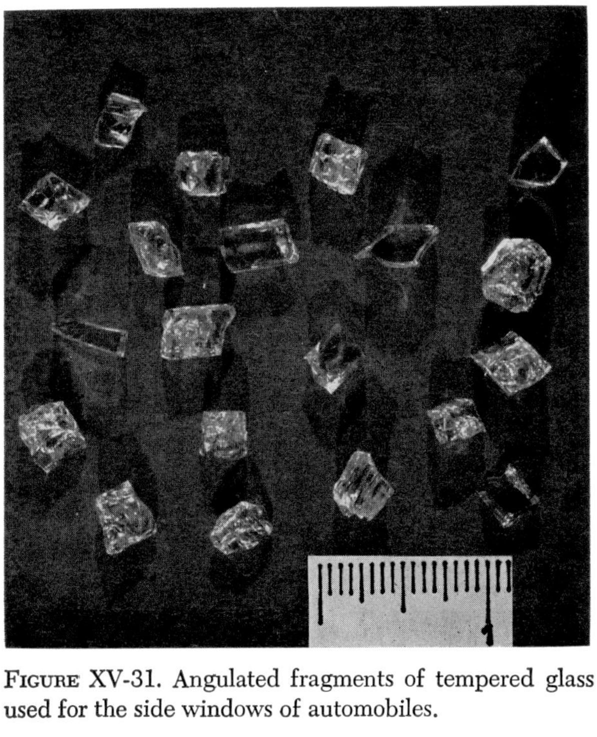

FIGURE XV-31. Angulated fragments of tempered glass used for the side windows of automobiles.

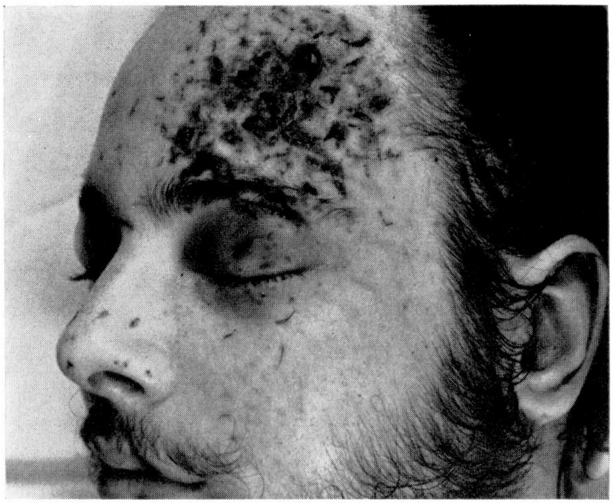

FIGURE XV-32. Driver of a 1969 Chevrolet that skidded into a pole. The driver's side of the automobile sustained the impact. The injuries of the left side of the forehead were caused by chunks and small fragments of tempered glass.

in the reconstrution of a given vehicular accident (Figs. XV-32, XV-33 and XV-34).

Dashboard injuries of the nonrestrained front seat occupants' knees are important insofar as their presence suggests a head-on collision, especially if the injuries are of similar severity on both sides. Contusions, abrasions and lacerations are frequently seen under such circumstances. Fractures of the lower ends of the femurs with separation of the condyles are less commonly observed. Such fractures are due to the fact that in the sitting position, the wedge-shaped patella is forced between the condyles upon frontal impact (Figs. XV-35 and XV-36).

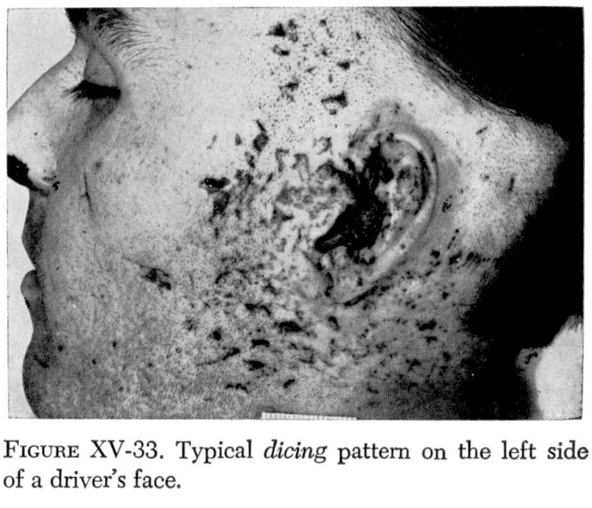

FIGURE XV-33. Typical *dicing* pattern on the left side of a driver's face.

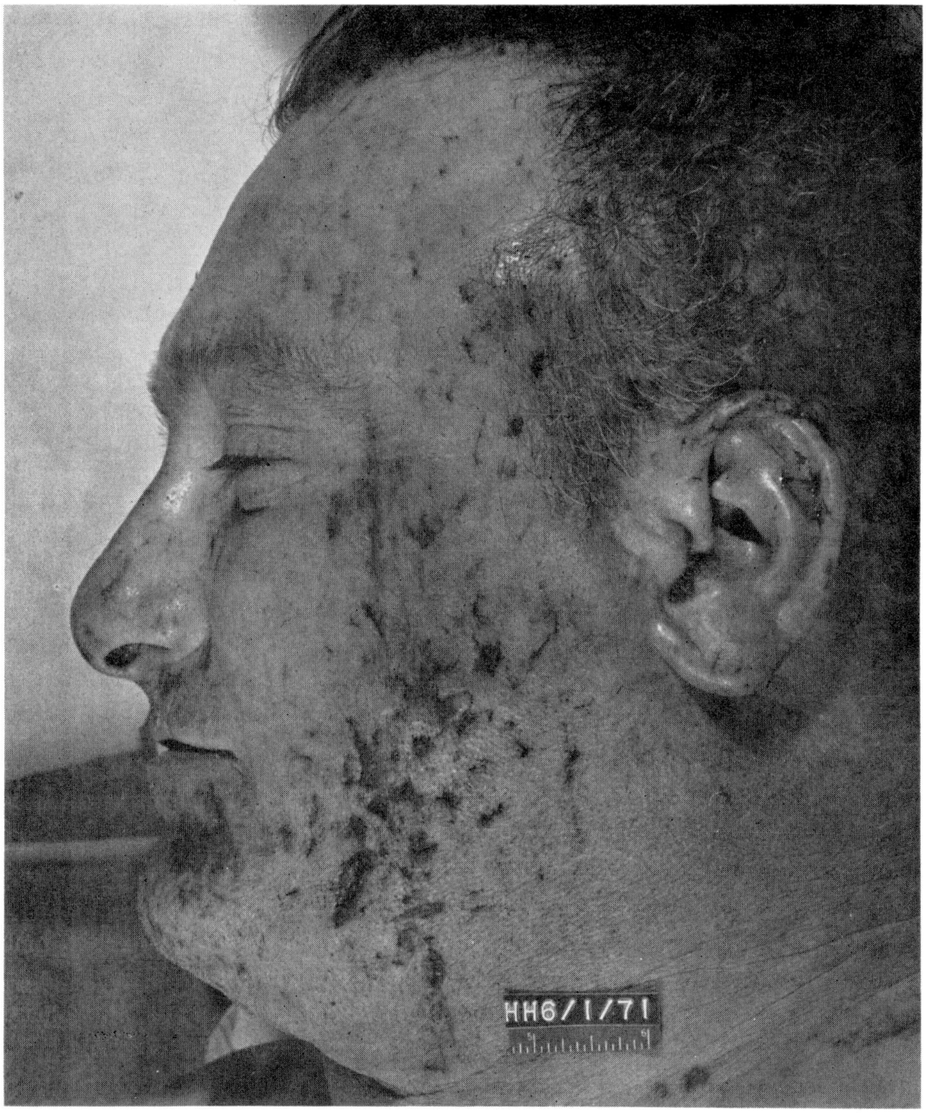


FIGURE XV-34. The victim shown in Figure 34a was the driver, thrown from his automobile after an intersection-type collision in which his car was struck broadside on the right. The victim in Figure 34b was the right front seat passenger. Compare the patterned injuries on both faces. Those in the driver resulted from impact on roadside gravel; these are irregular superficial abrasions with a brush burn noted from cheek to temple. The injury on the passenger's face represents a typical dicing pattern, with numerous superficial angulated cuts inflicted by fragments of tempered glass from the side window.

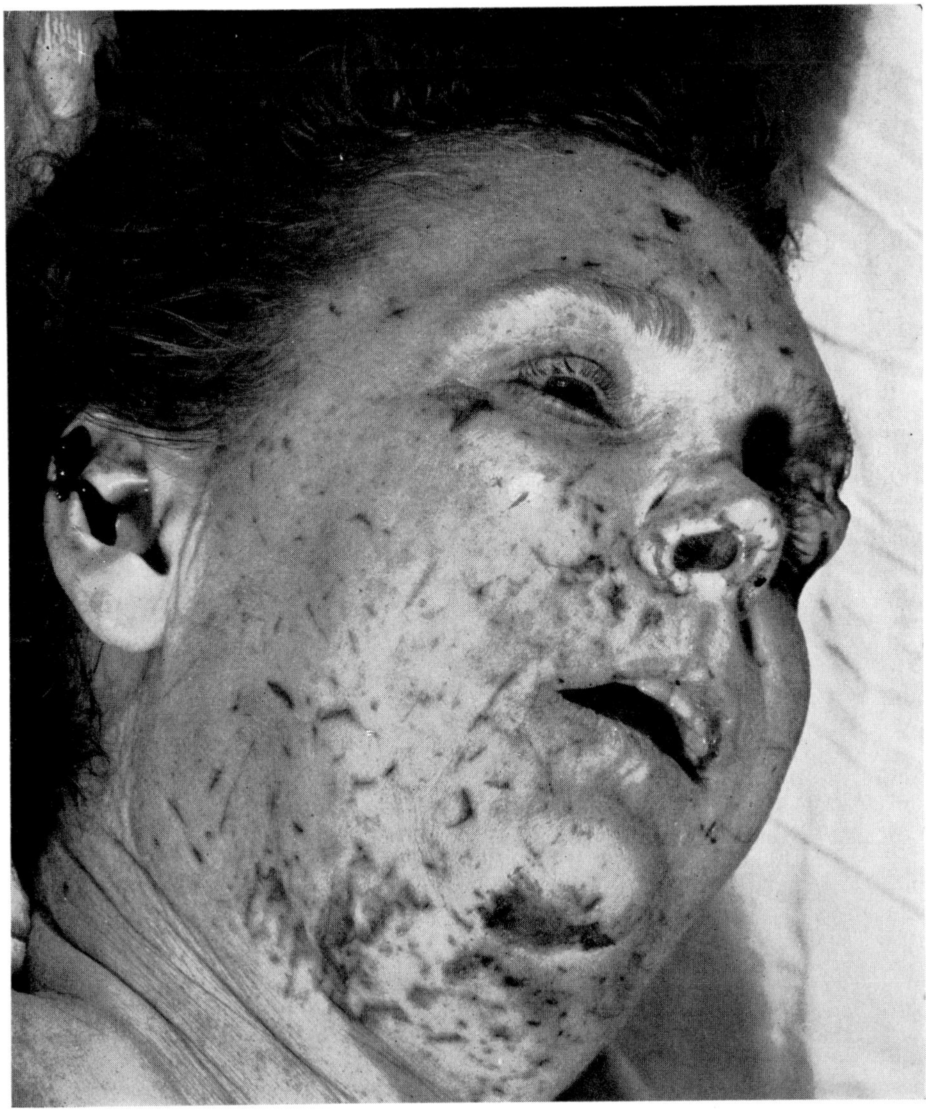

Figure XV-34b

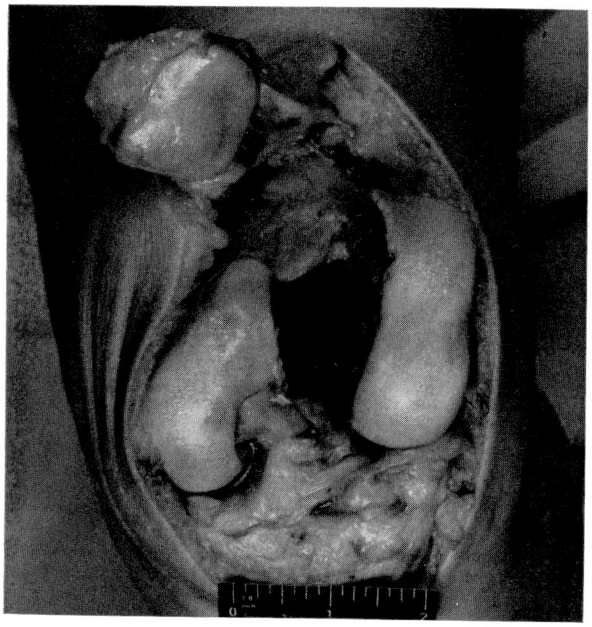

FIGURE XV-35. Incised knee of a driver with a dashboard injury. The condyles of the femur are split as a result of impact on the patella (reflected in the photograph).

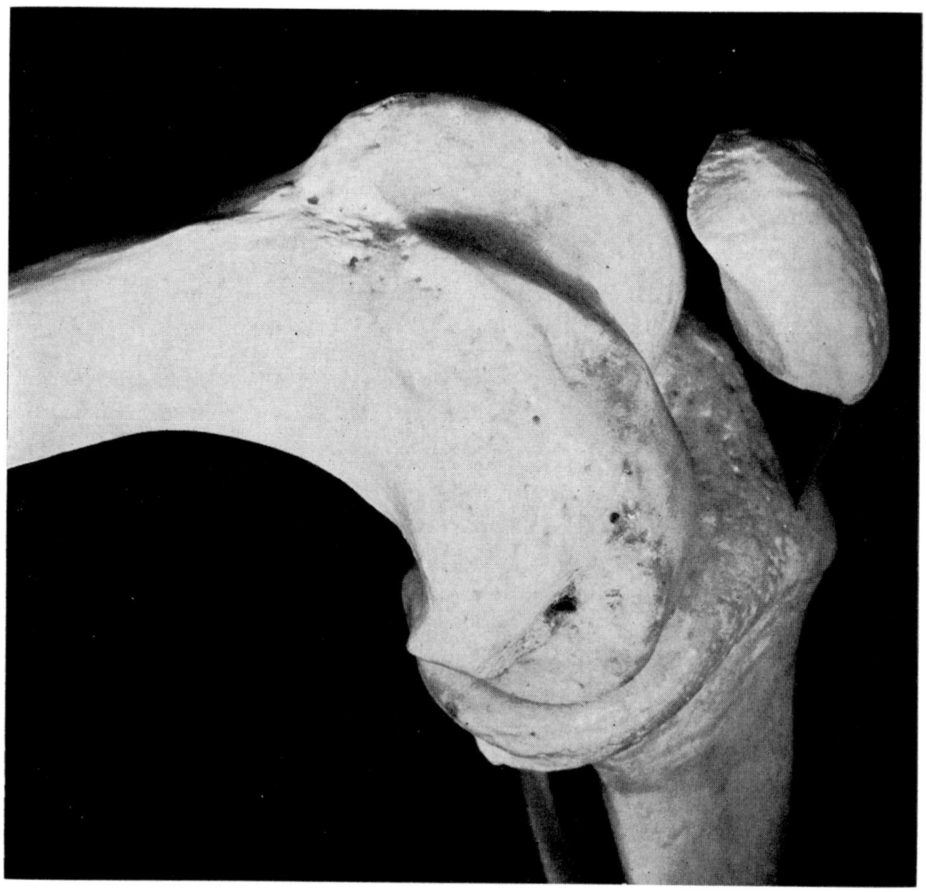

FIGURE XV-36. Knee joint, showing the mechanism of fracture in dashboard impact. The wedge-shaped patella separates the condyles of the femur. Bilateral injuries of similar severity suggest a frontal collision.

The impact velocity, as well as the shape and rigidity of the area that was struck, are factors to be considered in the interpretation of these injuries. External injury to the knees is often minimal or absent.

Another frequent dashboard injury is the dislocation, with or without fracture, of the head of the femur, which is literally pushed out of its socket into the pelvis by the impact of the knee. Again, external evidence of injury may be lacking or minimal.

Head-on collisions may also cause injuries to the feet and ankles of the front seat occupants, often in conjunction with fractures. In the case of the driver these injuries may be due to twisting of the brake or clutch pedal around the foot. More frequently, however, such injury is the result of wedging of the feet under the seat by the backward push of the engine while the seat is thrust forward, trapping the feet under it (Fig. XV-37). The driver's shoes sometimes remain under the seat after his removal. The sole of the right shoe may show the imprint of the gas or brake pedal, indicating which of the two pedals was being applied at the time of the collision.

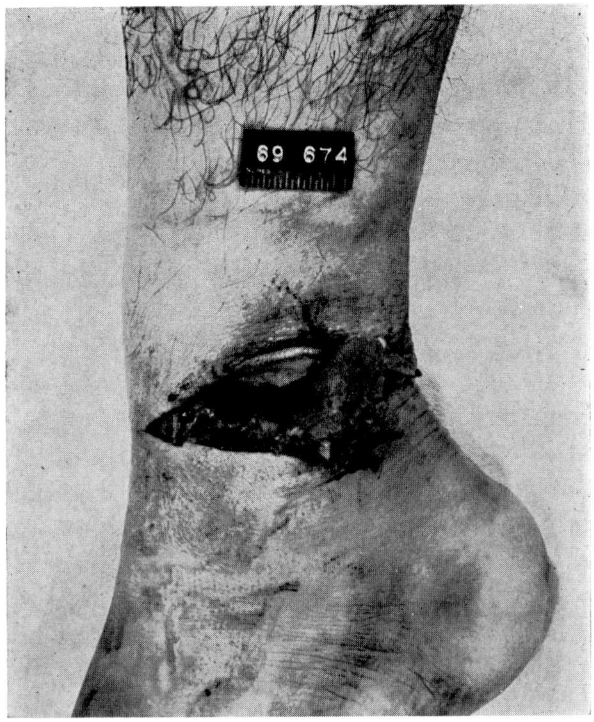


FIGURE XV-37. Fracture of the ankle in a driver. The foot was wedged under the seat, which was thrust forward as a result of the collision while the engine was pushed to the rear.

### Accident or Suicide?

The use of the automobile as an instrument of self-destruction has been postulated repeatedly in recent years. In 1968 Morton[15] reported that life insurance companies had noted a disproportionately high number of fatal automobile collisions occurring in the first year of double indemnity policies. Sociologist David Phillips[16] of the University of California, San Diego, has offered the most convincing evidence to date that a number of suicides deliberately drive to their deaths in the family car. Obviously, there is no way to determine exact figures of the number of suicides by automobile. The main issue is that of deciding whether a decedent consciously and willfully caused his own death. The imprint of the gas pedal pattern on the driver's shoe sole and the absence of skid marks leading to the site of collision are believed by some to be suggestive of suicide, because they indicate that the driver was accelerating his vehicle at the time of impact.

On the other hand, how can it be excluded that the driver fell asleep at the wheel or ignored existing road conditions as a result of alcoholic intoxication? The latter is known to be associated with at least half of all traffic deaths. Also the possibility of carbon monoxide intoxication due to a faulty muffler should not be overlooked. Carbon monoxide causes drowsiness at extremely low concentrations. Drugs, in our experience, contribute to automobile crashes only rarely.

Only unequivocal cases of intentional self-destruction can be certified as suicides. Necessary in this regard is a detailed investigation of all circumstances surrounding the case. The driving record of the victim may indicate previous violations and suggest a problem driver rather than a suicidal intent. More attention should be paid to the psychiatric makeup of the victim, as indicated by Edland.[17] He points out that thirteen of the eighty-six traffic fatalities in the Kansas City area in 1967 resulted from eleven purposely caused collisions. The driver-victims as a group appeared to be immature, unstable persons with recent records of failure in interpersonal relationships.

### Sudden Natural Death at the Wheel

Automobile accidents occur occasionally as a result of sudden death of the driver. Peterson and Petty,[18] in a classical review of this subject, determined that death in 19 percent of all drivers involved in collisions was due to natural causes and that in the vast majority of cases this was due to an acute heart attack. West et al.[19] concur with these observations and ascribe sudden natural death to 15 percent of road accidents in which drivers die. Interestingly, accidents in which these drivers are involved usually are of relatively minor severity, an observation also made by Baker and Spitz.[20] According to their investigation, which involved 591 collisions, natural death of a sober driver does not entail a measurable risk of death or severe injury to his passengers or other persons. Apparently, despite impending death the sober driver is usually capable of reducing the speed of his vehicle and avoiding collision. It is quite different if the driver operates his vehicle while under the influence of alcohol.

### Alcohol and Fatal Crashes

The extent to which alcohol contributes to traffic accidents is best illustrated by the fact that at least 60 percent of fatally injured drivers have positive blood alcohol concentrations. Of these, in over half the cases the blood alcohol level exceeds 0.10% (100 mg/100 ml blood). A large volume of scientific data conclusively show that the driving ability of *all* persons is sufficiently impaired at this blood alcohol concentration to pose a serious threat to public safety. Currently, thirty-six American states have adopted statutes establishing a blood alcohol content of 0.10% as presumptive or *prima facie* evidence of *intoxicated* driving or driving while *under the influence*. Utah and Idaho have adopted 0.08%, and the remaining twelve states have set higher limits, up to 0.15%.[21]

Even blood alcohol concentrations of 0.05% have been shown to cause impairment of driving ability in a large number of people. A blood alcohol concentration of 0.05% would result from the consumption of two or three regular drinks by a person of average weight. To reach a blood alcohol concentration of 0.10%, a 150 lb. individual who drinks following an average meal would have to consume between four and five ounces of 86 proof whiskey or four to five twelve-ounce cans of beer within one hour. This amount of alcohol exceeds that which may be regarded as *social drinking*. In fact, judging by the blood alcohol level of those killed in traffic collisions, the chronic alcoholic or problem drinker plays a far greater role in causing death and injury than is usually recognized.[21] Such observations emphasize the need for alcohol determinations not only in those who die in traffic crashes but especially in all surviving drivers of crashes fatal to others. It appears that most states are reluctant to implement this requirement. Only nineteen states to date have passed laws requiring that a chemical test to determine the alcoholic content be carried out on the bodies of all drivers and adult pedestrians who die in automobile crashes.[22]

In 1926 Norway made it a statutory offense for anyone to drive a motor vehicle if the blood alcohol level was in excess of 0.05%. Sweden soon followed suit and adopted similar legislation, 0.08% was used for some twenty years, but in 1959 this level was reduced to 0.05%. In 1967 Britain reduced the blood alcohol level that constitutes *prima facie* evidence of drunken driving from 0.15% to 0.08%. This was followed by a substantial decrease in the number of road accidents and highway deaths.

## REFERENCES


1. Patscheider, H.: Über Anprallverletzungen der unteren Gliedmassen bei Strassenverkehrsunfällen. *Dtsch Z Ges Gerichtl Med, 54:*336, 1964.
2. Patrick, L. M., and Van Kirk, D. J.: Vehicle accelerator crash simulator. In *Proceedings of the 12th Stapp Car Crash Conference.* New York, Society of Automotive Engineers, Inc., 1968, pp. 402-423.
3. Spitz, W. U.: Reconstruction of accidents: Integration of pathologic and roadside evidence. In Brinkhouse, K. M. (Ed.): *Accident Pathology.* Washington, D.C., U.S. Govt. Print. Office, 1971, pp. 26-35.
4. Nussbaumer, B.: *Die Überfahrung im Rahmen des Strassenverkehrsunfalles.* Basel, Schwabe & Co., 1960.
5. Sevitt, S.: Fatal road accidents: Injuries, complications, and causes of death in 250 subjects. *Br J Surg, 55:*481, 1968.
6. Lasky, I. I., Nahum, A. M., and Siegel, A. W.: Cardiac injuries incurred by drivers in automobile accidents. *J Forensic Sci, 14:*13, 1969.
7. Huelke, D. F., and Chewnin, W. A.: *The Energy-Absorbing Steering Column.* Ann Arbor, Michigan, Highway Safety Research Institute, 1968.
8. Frankel, C. J.: Medical-legal aspects of injuries to the neck. *JAMA, 169:*216, 1959.
9. Gotten, N.: Survey of 100 cases of whiplash injury after settlement of litigation. *JAMA, 162:*865, 1956.
10. Huelke, D. F., and Gikas, P. W.: Ejection, the leading cause of death in automobile accidents. In *Proceedings, 10th Stapp Car Crash Conference.* Alamagordo, N. Mexico, Holloman Air Force Base, 1966, pp. 156-181.
11. Snyder, R. G., Young, J. W., and Townley Price, G.: Pathomechanics of automotive restraint-system injuries. In Brinkhous, K. M. (Ed.): *Accident Pathology.* Washington, D.C., U.S. Govt. Print. Office, 1971, pp. 68-88.
12. Press Release: *Department of Transportation News.* Washington, D.C. National Highway Traffic Safety Administration, March 5, 1971.
13. Patrick, L. M., Trosien, K. R., and DuPont, F. T.: Safety performance of a chemically strengthened windshield. In *Proceedings of the Mid-Year Meeting of the Society of Automotive Engineers, Chicago, May 19-23.* New York, Society of Automotive Engineers, Inc., 1969.
14. Blizard, J. R., and Howitt, J. S.: Development of a safer nonlacerating automobile windshield. In *Proceedings of the Mid-Year Meeting of the Society of Automotive Engineers, Chicago, May 19-23.* New York, Society of Automotive Engineers, Inc., 1969.
15. Morton, J.: The suicide driver. *Traffic Safety, 68:*37, 1968.
16. Phillips, D.: Motor vehicle fatalities increase just after publicized suicide stories. *Science, 196:* 4297, June 24, 1977.
17. Edland, J. F.: Vehicular suicide. In Brinkhous, K. M. (Ed.): *Accident Pathology.* Washington, D.C., U.S. Govt. Print. Office, 1971, pp. 42-45.
18. Peterson, B. J., and Petty, C. S.: Sudden natural death among automobile drivers. *J Forensic Sci, 7:*274, 1962.
19. West, I., Nielsen, G. L., Gilmore, A. E., and Ryan, J. R.: Natural death at the wheel. *JAMA, 205:* 266, 1968.
20. Baker, S. P., and Spitz, W. U.: An evaluation of the hazard created by natural death at the wheel. *N Engl J Med, 283:*405, 1970.
21. U.S. Department of Transportation: *Alcohol and Highway Safety.* Report to the Congress from the Secretary of Transportation, August, 1968.
22. Wagner, M. H.: Where we stand on drinking-driving legislation. *Traffic Safety, 72:*16, 1972.

*Chapter XVI*

# AIRCRAFT CRASH INVESTIGATION

Russell S. Fisher

## INVESTIGATING TEAMS

Federal laws enacted originally in 1939 and amended repeatedly since require an official investigation of all civil aircraft crashes. The responsibility is assigned to the National Transportation Safety Board (NTSB) of the Department of Transportation, with the charge that they determine the probable cause of all civil aircraft crashes in the United States. The NTSB is further charged with the responsibility of making recommendations concerning safety measures or procedures that might have prevented a particular aircraft crash, had they been enforced. The authority of the NTSB to investigate and make recommendations in all civil aircraft accidents is preemptive, and they can mandate the performance of any scientific tests or studies deemed necessary for the successful completion of an investigation. The NTSB is, however, a small agency and must assign the investigative function in certain categories of light plane accidents to other agencies, primarily the Federal Aviation Administration (FAA). In all catastrophic air carrier crashes the investigation is carried out by the Bureau of Aviation Safety within the NTSB.

The investigation will be conducted by a team of individuals representing the following groups: the Bureau of Aviation Safety, the Federal Aviation Agency, the carrier involved, the manufacturers of the power plant, air frame and equipment systems, the airline pilots, flight engineers and air traffic controllers. In addition, representatives of the Federal Bureau of Investigation, the Armed Forces Institute of Pathology and the National Aeronautics and Space Agency are contracted to assist in the investigation by the NTSB or FAA. The NTSB assumed these responsibilities in 1963 when it succeeded to the role formerly delegated to the Civil Aeronautics Board.[1]

Immediately, when a serious plane accident occurs, the Washington headquarters of the Bureau of Aviation Safety is notified and the team to be assigned to the investigation is assembled. While they are proceeding to the scene, representatives of one of the local field offices of the Bureau will ordinarily take charge and arrange with local police authorities to provide security necessary until the investigating team arrives. The investigator in charge establishes headquarters near the scene and promptly convenes a meeting of all concerned personnel, dividing them into groups with specific investigative responsibilities. Usually the groups are designated by such functional names as *Operations, Weather, Air Traffic Control, Witnesses, Human Factors, Structures, Power Plants, Systems* (electrical hydraulic, air conditioning, etc.), *Flight Recorder* and *Maintenance Records.*

The forensic pathologist is ordinarily a member of the *Human Factors* team, and any other physicians or medical personnel will be assigned to that group. The responsibilities of the *Human Factors* team are directed in two general areas: (a) the investigation of the medical histories and autopsy findings of the crew members responsible for operation of the plane; (b) the general identification of the victims. The local coroner or medical examiner is invariably associated with both efforts, since he will ultimately be responsible for certification of the cause of death. Regardless of the limitations of the legal authority vested in the state official, there is a federal law that authorizes the Bureau of Aviation Safety to perform autopsies on all crew members killed in an airplane crash. It is, of course, obvious that a complete autopsy must be performed on those crew members responsible for flying the aircraft, with retention of adequate specimens for microscopic and toxicologic studies.

Toxicologic studies are performed in the laboratories of the Civil Aeromedical Institute (CAMI), a division of the FAA located in Oklahoma City. CAMI provides sturdy self-contained kits containing a list of the specimens to be collected and appropriate containers in which the specimens are to be placed for shipment. Alcohol and carbon monoxide determinations and a general toxicologic screen for drugs and medications are routinely performed. In addition, determinations of the levels of trace elements and unusual toxic substances, such as cyanide, are made if the situation warrants them. In crashes of aircraft used for crop dusting, cholinesterase levels are determined.

## IDENTIFICATION

Perhaps the first and most important step to be taken following an aircraft crash is to establish security of the scene. There is almost always a group of civil defense workers, firemen or other nonmedical personnel who will attempt to remove bodies or body parts or valuable personal items from the scene with the aim of maintaining the security of the valuables. Incalculable harm can be done by these well-meaning individuals. NO ONE SHOULD BE ALLOWED TO APPROACH THE BODIES OR ANY PROPERTY RELATED THERETO, EXCEPT THE SPECIALIZED IDENTIFICATION TEAMS UNDER THE COMMAND OF THE CORONER OR MEDICAL EXAMINER CONCERNED WITH THE IDENTIFICATION PROCEDURES.

In one crash, which resulted from midair disintegration of an airplane, bodies were dropped out of the structure over a pathway encompassing several miles. The local fire teams gathered all the bodies and placed them into a neat pile near the roadway, where the medical examiner's vehicles would haul them away. In so doing they removed wallets and other valuables from each body and collected them in bushel baskets, where they felt security could be obtained. They failed to recognize the cardinal principle that the valuables carried on the body may be the most important item in establishing the identity of that body.

In another instance, where badly fragmented bodies were spread over several acres as a result of a high-velocity crash, a similar impediment to the identification occurred where rings were removed from the dismembered hands of some of the victims. Since rings frequently contain initials leading to identification, the undesirability of this procedure is obvious.

### The Necessity of Identification

With a given airplane crash in which one may assume that all the individuals on board have been killed, one might, theoretically, simply issue death certificates to coincide with the listing of the passengers and crew. The legal status of such procedure, however, is open to serious scrutiny, since the medical examiner's or coroner's authority to issue a death certificate is based upon his actual identification of some part of the body coupled with evidence that such person is dead. Whenever a coroner or a medical examiner cannot issue a death certificate, the *Uniform Absent Persons Act* applies. This generally entails preparation of a petition to a court of record, which may appoint a receiver at any time a person's absence is established *after diligent inquiry* (usually by testimony before the court). Then at a time (generally five to seven years or more) after the date of the original hearing, the court may take further evidence and make a ruling that death has occurred. Meanwhile, at any time upon application to the court and the presentation of satisfactory evidence of the absentee's death, the court may make a final ruling and issue an order that a death certificate be prepared. There is, of course, no presumption of death on a person's merely being missing for any given number of years, and exposure to the specific peril must be considered in each case.

It is fair to presume that within a few weeks

after a plane crash such a court order could be issued and the death certificate and other necessary documents be available. Even this delay is cause of much grief and difficulty for the survivors and should be avoided if possible. Furthermore, this is but one of the many problems in connection with the failure to identify an individual believed to be dead. The orderly settlement of an individual's estate requires copies of the death certificate in support of life insurance claims and in documentation of the responsibility of executors or other persons concerned with the legal matters surrounding the death. Occasionally the marital partner of the deceased may need a death certificate before his or her remarriage.

In addition to the specific legal problems, there is a strong humanitarian reason for establishing the identification of the deceased as quickly and as certainly as possible. Our social system calls for funeral ceremonies and interment or cremation, and these cannot be accomplished without a death certificate. Finally, there is a strong personal desire on the part of the vast majority of people that their loved ones be identified and buried in their chosen burial ground, rather than to be interred in a mass grave as is necessary if identification cannot be effected. Gratitude displayed by bereaved families has in our experience more than merited the extended effort required in identification of victims of a mass disaster.

A temporary morgue facility should be established conveniently near the scene of the crash, and a supply of stretchers, sawhorses, plyboard and other materials for makeshift tables should be procured. If the number of bodies exceeds twenty, one or more refrigerated trucks or trailers should be rented so that the bodies can be maintained with a minimum of deterioration for the several days required for the investigation. We believe it most satisfactory to establish two storage areas: one for identified bodies and parts and the other for bodies and parts awaiting further examination and identification. At this time steps should be taken to provide an office area equipped with as many telephones as possible. Our experience suggests that at least one telephone for each ten victims is the minimum number necessary to allow the information acquisition personnel to operate effectively. Floodlighting of the scene in evening and night hours is helpful for security reasons, as well as in the interest of efficiency and speed.

The identification procedures can be subdivided into three phases: (a) collection of the victims, fragments and valuables from the scene; (b) acquisition of information concerning the victims; (c) autopsy procedures, including fingerprinting, directed at producing information that will ultimately lead to identification.

### Collection of the Victims, Fragments and Valuables from the Scene

In crashes where there is extensive demolition of the plane and spreading of bodies and body fragments over the surrounding areas, it is critical that the location of each recovered item be established. This is best carried out by having a team, including a pathologist and a *property man*, collect the individual pieces, using stakes to mark the site and prenumbered paired tags for each item. One of the tags is affixed to the plastic bag in which the item is to be transferred to the morgue facility, while the other is affixed to a stake at the scene. Individual teams then proceed from item to item until all recognizable parts and property related thereto have been gathered and transmitted to the morgue facility. After all items have been collected, a composite diagram showing the location of each numbered stake is prepared for ready reference in the later stages of the investigation and reassembling of the fragments.

### Acquisition of Information Concerning the Victims

The airline will furnish a list of personnel and passengers aboard the plane, and very early in the investigation the Federal Bureau of Investigation disaster team will join the group concerned with the identification. They will bring with them, or have available within a matter of hours, the fingerprints of all the passengers and crew whose prints are on file in the FBI central fingerprint repository. Additionally, just as early as telephone service is available, clerks assigned either by the airline or by the medical examiner's or coroner's office should begin to contact the relatives of individuals known to have been on the plane to acquire additional information. In some instances the FBI will participate in this activity, using their local offices throughout the country. Regardless, the following information should be established for each victim: (a) name; (b) age; (c) sex; (d) race; (e) weight; (f) height; (g) hair color and style; (h) eye color; (i) skin blemishes, such as moles and scars, including the exact size, location on the body and any other descriptive information available; (j) medical history of the victim. This should include the names of all physicians who may have treated the patient at any time; any known diseases, particularly such conditions as valvular heart disease, gallstones, etc.; the surgical history, including where and when any operation was performed, the name of the surgeon and any other information that will allow contact to be established with the hospital where the procedure was done in order to acquire the medical record. Inquiries should establish, if possible, the blood group and any subgrouping information available. The history of any fractured bones or other abnormalities that may have been disclosed on x rays should be included and details acquired as to where the x rays were taken in order that they may be obtained for comparison with x rays of the victims; (k) dental history, which should include the name, address and phone number of any dentist who may have attended the individual, including dental laboratories where prostheses may have been made. Contact should be established early with the dentist and a request made not only for dental charting but any x rays or other material; (l) jewelry worn by the victim, including detailed description of any kind of costume jewelry with special emphasis on rings that may have identifiable settings or may have engraved initials, dates, etc. It is advisable to get the name of the jeweler who furnished any such personal items as engagement rings or other valuable pieces of jewelry, since the jeweler may be able to make absolute identification of such items; (m) the clothes worn by the victim when the plane trip started. These should be described in detail as to fabric, color, tailoring, etc., including, if available, where purchased, particularly if they were obtained from specialty shops that furnish limited numbers of the style of clothing worn by the victim; (n) shoes. Here again the size and style as well as the manufacturer should be obtained; (o) pictures of the deceased, especially if profile pictures are available, since these may show the ears and other identifiable features; (p) laundry marks. In addition to the manufacturer of the clothing, the names of the launderers or dry cleaners who may have served the deceased should be obtained so that the specific cleaners or laundry marks can be established as a means of identification; (q) fingerprints. In addition to the classification and copies of the prints, information should include where and when the fingerprints were made. If the FBI have the fingerprints on file, their disaster team will undoubtedly have this information available very early in the course of the investigation. Additionally a variety of identification cards made in connection with employment may show one or more fingerprints of an individual. Another occasionally useful source is the baby footprints made of children. These commonly bear on the same card prints of one or more fingers of the mother. A further possibility of obtaining fingerprints, if none are available elsewhere, is the home of the victim, where fingerprints may be found on items that were handled by the victim in the recent past. Suggested are such items as cosmetic bottles in the case of a woman or the spray cans that contain shaving soap or cream and similar items in the case of a man. Hairbrushes with plastic backs are also occasional sources of recognizable fingerprints that can be related to a given individual; (r) samples of hair sufficient to characterize the individual are not infrequently obtainable from hairbrushes.

Steps should be taken to obtain these before they are disposed of by relatives.

In every instance efforts to obtain the information from multiple sources in order to produce a complete record of each victim are essential. Once this information is obtained, a chart listing all information for each of the victims is prepared. The chart should be constructed on a large enough scale that it can be mounted on the wall and readily read at a distance by the various individuals concerned with the identification work.

**Autopsy Procedures, Including Fingerprinting**

The actual examination of the bodies will then be conducted by pathologists, assisted by the secretarial personnel, who can develop a record as the pathologist examines the bodies and related items. Individual items recognizable on the body can be matched rapidly with the wall chart bearing the description of the various victims. In addition to the pathologist concerned, it will be necessary to have fingerprint experts available to make impressions of any printable fingers. These prints can then be related to the original number assigned to the body part when moved from the site and transmitted to the Federal Bureau of Investigation fingerprint experts who will attempt the identification.

The study of the teeth requires the services of one or more dentists who have had some experience in forensic odontology. With intact bodies they can readily establish complete charts, but even with fragmented bodies their skill and ability to recognize specific types of restorations, prostheses or disease processes are essential to the success of the identification task force. Other consultants who may be able to contribute include experts in jewelry, tailors or fashion experts who can help in identifying clothing, radiologists who assist in interpreting x rays and physical anthropologists who may be able to establish age, sex and race on the basis of skeletal parts.

***Intact Bodies***

In cases where relatively intact bodies remain after a low altitude plane crash, the importance of locating the body in the wreckage cannot be overstressed. This is of special importance because, while seating lists are no longer maintained by most carriers, there is a tendency for family groups to be seated together, and useful leads to identification are thus gained if one of the family group can be identified. In our experience the determination of the exact location in the wreckage will be possible only if efforts have been made in advance to acquaint all personnel with the necessity of this item.

Even if identification is made by external means and the cause of death is obvious, a careful listing of the fatal injuries is important. This will enable subsequent assessment as to the rapidity of death. Statutory provisions in most states provide that the estate of an individual passes at the moment of his death to the next of kin or individual designated in the will, and questions frequently arise where both members of a marital team are killed as to which person died first. In a great many cases this cannot be answered, but the pathologist should be alert to the possible importance of his observations at the time of the original examination of the body in regard to determining the rapidity of death after the accident. In addition to a general description of the body with specific emphasis on identifying characteristics, it is recommended that front and side photographs of the face be preserved as a matter of confirmation of identification.

In the case of bodies not immediately identified, a complete autopsy will be necessary not only to document the items already listed but also to list specifically those that have bearing on the age, sex, race and other specific identifying characteristics that might be matched with material obtained through the questionnaires completed by relatives, acquaintances, etc. as described earlier. The pathologist must take special note of the effects of surgery on the body, including location and size of scars and absence of organs such as the appendix, gall bladder, spleen, ovaries or other portions of the genital organs. Other items of importance are evidence of uterine suspension, stomach and intestinal resection, hernia repair, vertebral fusion and abnormalities of the bony structures, whether congenital in nature or the stigmata of diseases such as arthritis or malignancy.

The usefulness of skeletal x rays must be considered, since this may provide information about the age of the victim and reveal specific identifying characteristics such as old fractures and fragments of foreign bodies within the tissue. Of greatest single importance is the dental pattern, since the occurrence of as few as two or three fillings may be sufficient to separate one individual from all others in a given airplane crash.

***Burned Bodies***

Where there has been fire incident to the wreck, there is apt to be extensive destruction of bodies, making fingerprinting impossible. Indeed, the extremities are usually the first portions of the body to be destroyed by fire. Thus, it may be necessary to dissect out the long bones for use of the anthropological formulae to determine height and to examine extensively the pelvic bones and any remaining facial bones for characteristics revealing age, sex and race of the individual. It should also be pointed out that even though a body may be tentatively identified at an early stage of the investigation, other data may be discovered later enabling a positive identification to be made. The absence of the appendix for instance, or the presence of an old fracture of a bone are common examples. Thus, it is advisable to take complete skeletal x rays of burned bodies and to establish items of negative information not ordinarily important in the autopsy of an individual whose identity is well established.

***Fragmented Bodies***

With the crash of modern jet planes, even in the absence of extensive fire, the high speeds of impact lead to disintegration of the aircraft and the passengers therein. In these cases the largest fragment of body found may be only one-third or one-fourth of the original body weight. The extremities in particular are apt to be torn off and thrown long distances. Careful documentation of the site where the given fragment is found continues to be of utmost importance. The examination at the scene, while taking care not to remove rings or disturb items that can be identified with a given portion of the body, is frequently the key to successful identification. In dealing with fragmented bodies the pathologist proceeds from bag to bag of material removed from the field, examines the portions and describes them completely, noting specifically characteristics referable to age, sex, race or specific identifying features. Wherever there are dental fragments, complete description must be made, again emphasizing negative findings such as the absence of fillings or specific teeth, the lack of eruption of third molars, the absence of smoothing off of the occlusal surfaces indicating the relative youth of the victim, etc. It is emphasized that an expert dentist will be able to do a much more satisfactory job in this area than the pathologist. Wherever sizable portions of the dental arches are present, these should be removed and x rayed, since items concealed to naked-eye examination, such as unerupted teeth, root canal fillings and other identifying characteristics, will be revealed by x ray techniques.

The description of the various specimens removed from the scene of the crash should be completed as promptly as possible, and any shorthand notes should be transcribed at the earliest possible opportunity in order that matching with the charted data for each person on board the aircraft can be effected.

## Matching the Collected Information

The identification team begins the analysis of the material described for each of the bodies or body parts when the major portion of the data for the victims is available and charted. Where several specimens can be shown to have been derived from the same body, they should obviously be assembled under one name and probable identity. Despite the fact that indi-

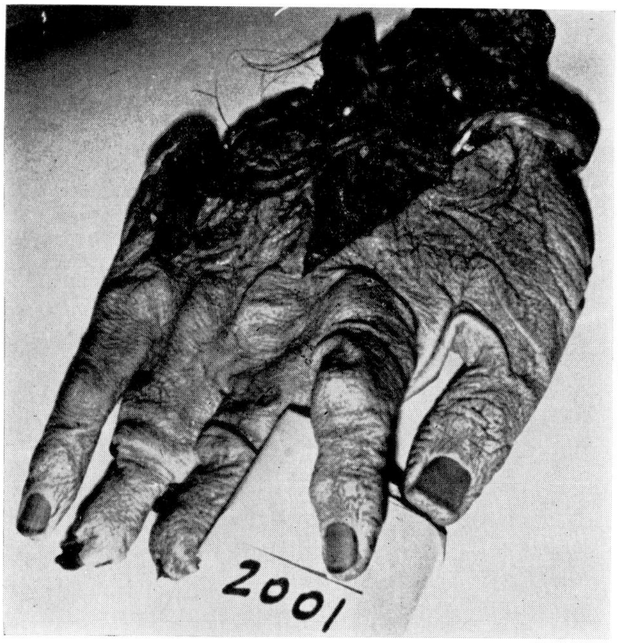


FIGURE XVI-1. Amputated hand identified by *exclusion* as that of an eighty-one-year-old man. X ray was useful in estimating the age and confirming the hypertrophic arthritis.

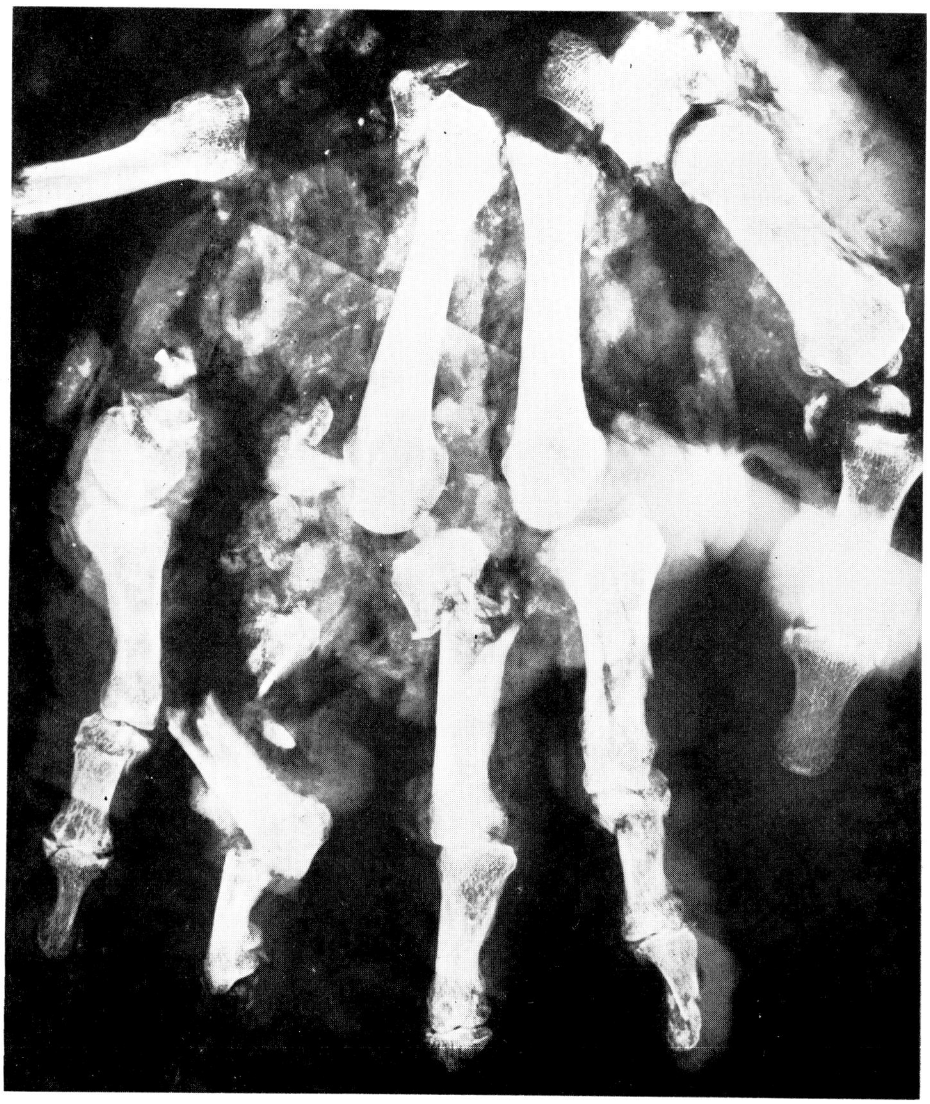

vidual identifications may be made early in the investigation, it is generally inadvisable to release the remains to the funeral directors or next of kin who wish to claim them until the entire investigation is well advanced. The prime reason for this is that even at relatively late stages of the investigation, further portions identifiable as a given body may be recovered, and every effort should be made to assemble as much of the body of a given victim as possible before release to the funeral director. Another reason for delay in releasing the remains is that an occasional *exclusion diagnosis* may require rechecking features of bodies that have already been identified by other means.

In one crash investigation there were among the passengers sixteen men, all over sixty years of age. They were identified by fingerprints, although in several cases only one hand or less was recovered. One man remained unidentified. His age was eighty-one years, and he was known to have advanced hypertrophic arthritis with spur formation in the finger bones. There was also one hand, the prints of which did not correspond to any of the fifteen sets of hands that had been recovered and which related to the fifteen identifications. The anthropologist determined by x ray that this unidentified hand was derived from an elderly and arthritic man. Comparison of this hand with all fifteen identified bodies showed different texture of skin and a type of arthritis not seen in the other fifteen. On this basis it was identified as the hand of the eighty-one-year-old man by exclusion of all others (Figs. XVI-1 and XVI-2). The availability of the hands or parts thereof or fingers of the other fifteen bodies for checking with regard to arthritis was obviously the key to the exclusion process.

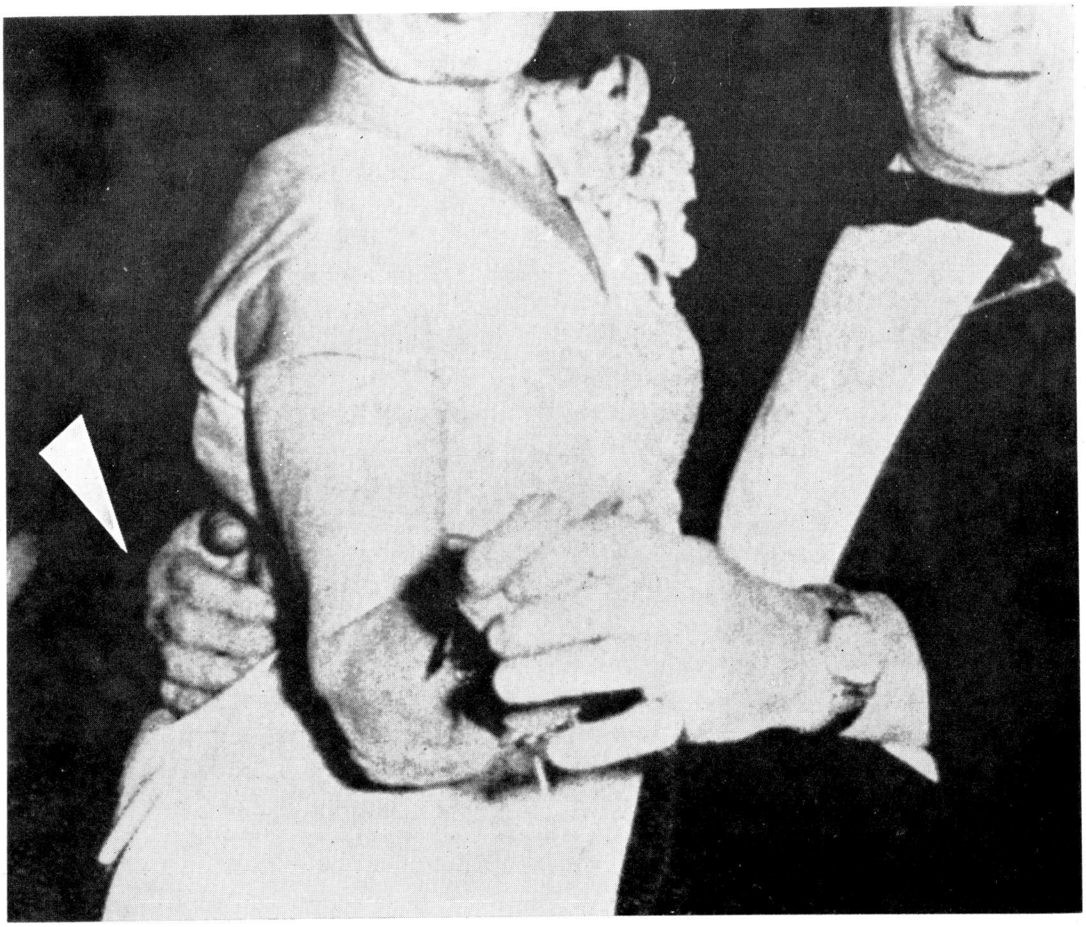

FIGURE XVI-2. Photograph of the eighty-one-year-old man obtained from his family. The picture shows him dancing at a party a few weeks before the plane crash. Compare his right hand with the *knobby* knuckles with the hand in Figure XVI-1a.

Similar exclusion procedures based on combinations of other body characteristics may be necessary, and in such cases it is highly desirable to reexamine the bodies of certain identified individuals to be certain that the part under consideration would not have been derived from one of them. In our experience identifications will be established as *certain* or as *presumptive*. The latter is reserved for those cases where the quality of the information does not justify absolute identification, but where a reasonable presumption can be reached, as in the case of the eighty-one-year-old man cited previously.

## LIGHT AIRCRAFT CRASH INVESTIGATION

Aircraft weighing less than 12,500 lb. at takeoff are defined by Federal Aviation Regulations as being *general aviation* or *light aircraft*. These aircraft are powered by reciprocating single or multi-engines and are used for both personal and commercial purposes. Commercial purposes include crop dusting, passenger carrying such as air charter operations, racing and air taxi operations. These aircraft generally operate at speeds of less than 180 mph and have much lower terminal airspeeds than commercial jet airliners. The injuries sustained in crashes of light aircraft therefore differ qualitatively and quantitatively from those seen in large aircraft crashes, and many of them are survivable.

Several authors have called attention to the distribution of injuries in general aviation accidents and report that lethal injuries of the head, lower extremities, abdomen and chest predominate. Injuries to the liver, heart and thoracic aorta are the most important in the latter two categories. The majority of head injuries result from impact to the face, particularly the point of the chin and below the level of the eyes. Death may result from inhalation of blood following trauma to the soft facial tissues and the facial bones. The second most common lethal injury in light aircraft accidents is rupture of the heart or thoracic aorta. These injuries are caused by compression of the structures between the vertebral column and the sternum, much the same as deceleration steering wheel injuries in automobiles.

Identification of the occupants in light aircraft crashes generally is not a problem. However, the determination of who was actually trying to control the aircraft at the time of the crash, where two or more occupants are involved, may be difficult. This problem is compounded if several of the occupants are thrown clear of the fuselage, and it is further complicated if two or more of the occupants were certified pilots for that particular type of plane. The cardinal rule of flying is the *pilot in command* concept, which is that only one pilot at a time may have charge of the control. This obviously applies to those aircraft equipped with dual controls.

The following procedures should be followed in the investigation of light aircraft crashes:

1. Familiarization with the design of the aircraft controls: this is often best accomplished by examination of an intact aircraft of the same make and model as the one involved in the crash.
2. Complete x ray of the remains, with particular emphasis on the extremities: characteristic fractures and soft tissue injuries suggest which occupant had his hands and feet in contact with the aircraft controls at the time of the impact. Distinct abrasions, bruises and tears are often seen between the thumb and index finger of the hand controlling the stick or wheel, and fractures of the carpal and phalangeal bones, and even avulsion of the thumb, may occur. When the feet are in contact with the rudder pedal, excessive strain is imparted to the heels. This may cause comminuted fractures of the tarsal bones or the ankle. The disintegration of the rudder pedals and linkages may cause penetration of metallic fragments into the soft tissues of the lower extremities. Such fragments are readily demonstrated by x ray.
3. The clothing should be minutely inspected

for marks or impressions made by control surfaces or individual structures on the instrument panel. Conversely, the instrument and control surfaces should be inspected for clothing fragments.

4. As with large aircraft crashes, complete toxicologic evaluation is important. Complete histologic examination is required to rule out the presence of natural disease.

## PUBLIC RELATIONS

It is advisable early in the investigation of an aircraft crash to establish one or more individuals who can handle public relations for the pathologist's identification team. There will be the usual onslaught of newspaper reporters, curiosity seekers and various attorneys and representatives of the relatives who will harass the investigating team to the point of distraction. The appointment of an individual to handle the telephone calls and inquiries, explain why delay is necessary in releasing bodies and identifications and otherwise deal with the public will keep this type of interruption to a minimum and at the same time will assure the public that the work of the identification team is progressing in an orderly fashion.

The following is a summary of the investigation of a crash of a 707 Boeing airliner in 1963, which involved seventy-three passengers and eight crew members (Fig. XVI-3 and XVI-4).[2]

Identification teams, each consisting of a state police officer and a physician from the medical examiner's office, began the removal of the bodies. In each instance where a recognizable portion of a body capable of indicating an identification was found, a number was affixed to the part and a tag bearing the same number affixed to a stake at the site where the part was found

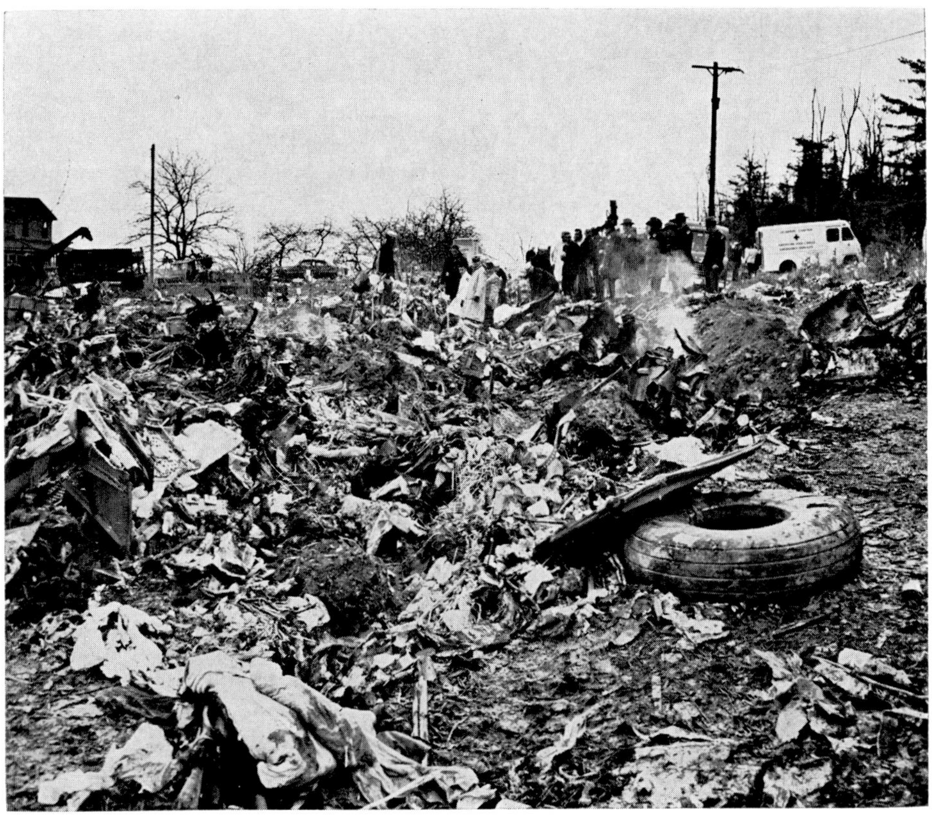

FIGURE XVI-3. Scene at which a Boeing 707 crashed after it was struck by lightning. There were eighty-one people killed. Parts of the aircraft were spread over a circle one-half mile in diameter.

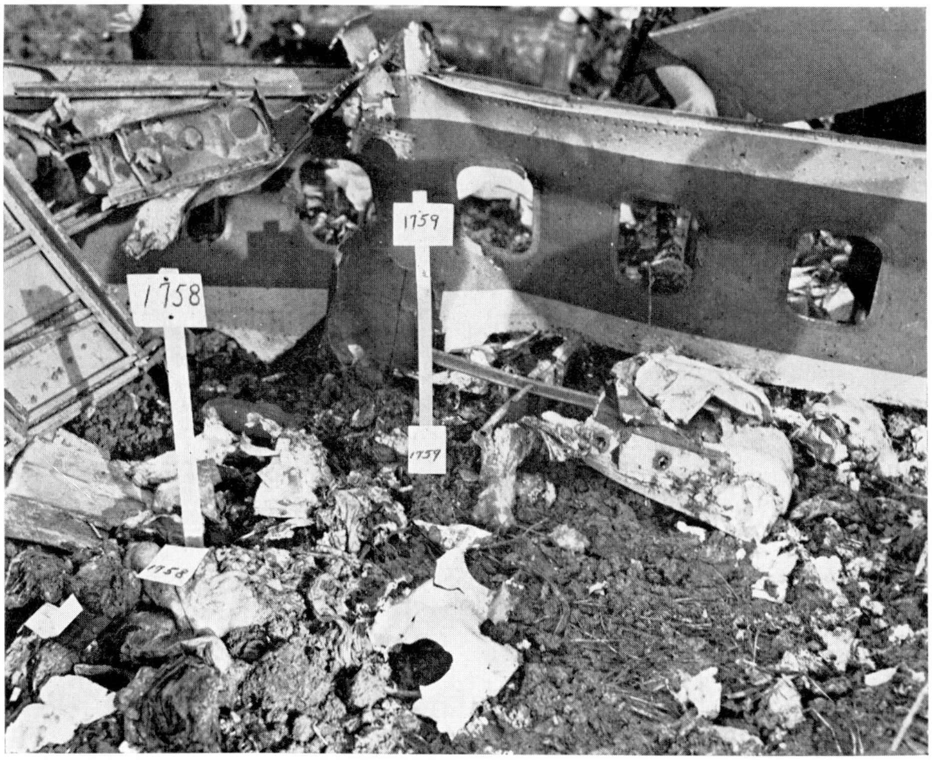


FIGURE XVI-4. Largest single portion of the plane: window section of the fuselage.

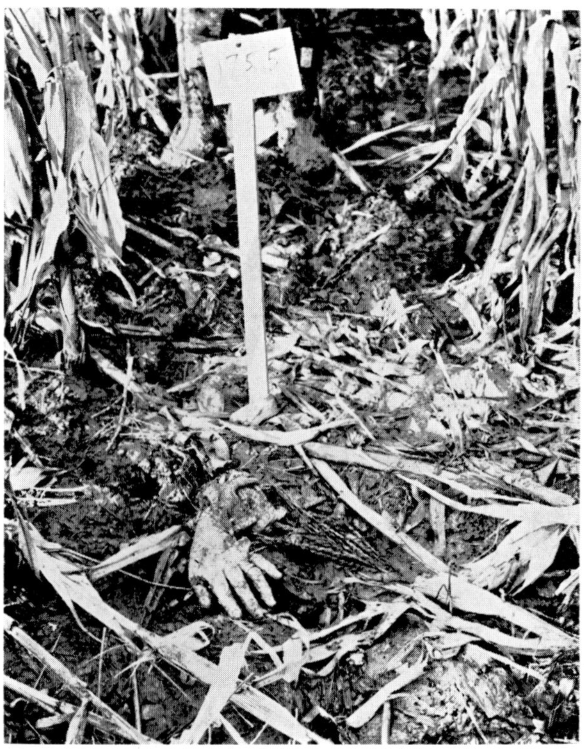

FIGURE XVI-5. Stake erected at the site where a body fragment (left hand) was found.

(Figs. XVI-5, XVI-6 and XVI-7). Individual photographs of each body part and stake were taken by the state police photographers before the part was removed. A chart showing the location of these stakes was subsequently prepared. The body parts were then transferred to the emergency mortuary, where they were examined by pathologists, and in each case where printable material was present, fingerprints were made by the state police. These prints were submitted to the FBI disaster squad who worked with the medical examiner's team for a five-day period.

After all superficially distributed parts had been removed from the field, the site of the actual crash was searched by use of a backhoe to remove the upper layers of dirt and debris, and the process of numbering and staking the site of remains was continued. By the third day all small parts of bodies had been removed from the field, and the total tissue recovered weighed 4,250 lb. Since it was obvious that this accounted for only about one-third of the total weight of the victims, it was decided to excavate the crash site. Accordingly an area paralleling the torso of the plane was bulldozed clean. Thereafter using a front-end loader, the entire area occupied by the torso of the plane was lifted scoop by scoop and sorted by a crew of about forty naval personnel assigned to assist the medical examiner with the task. This procedure took three

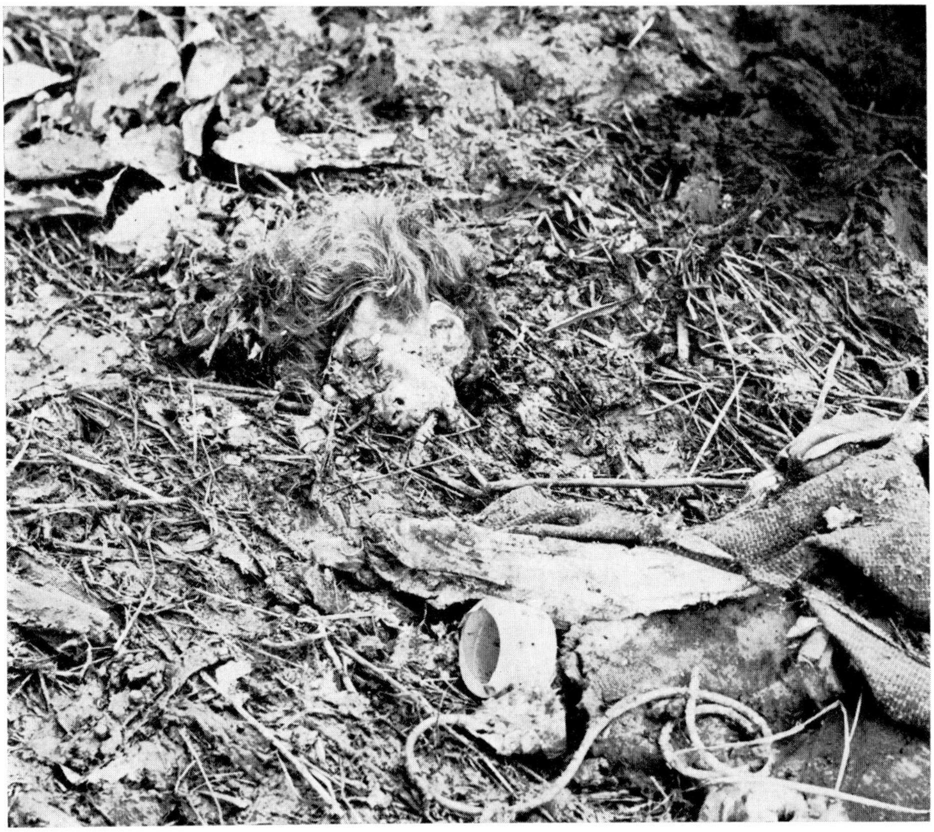

FIGURE XVI-6. Scalp and portion of a face found in the wreckage.

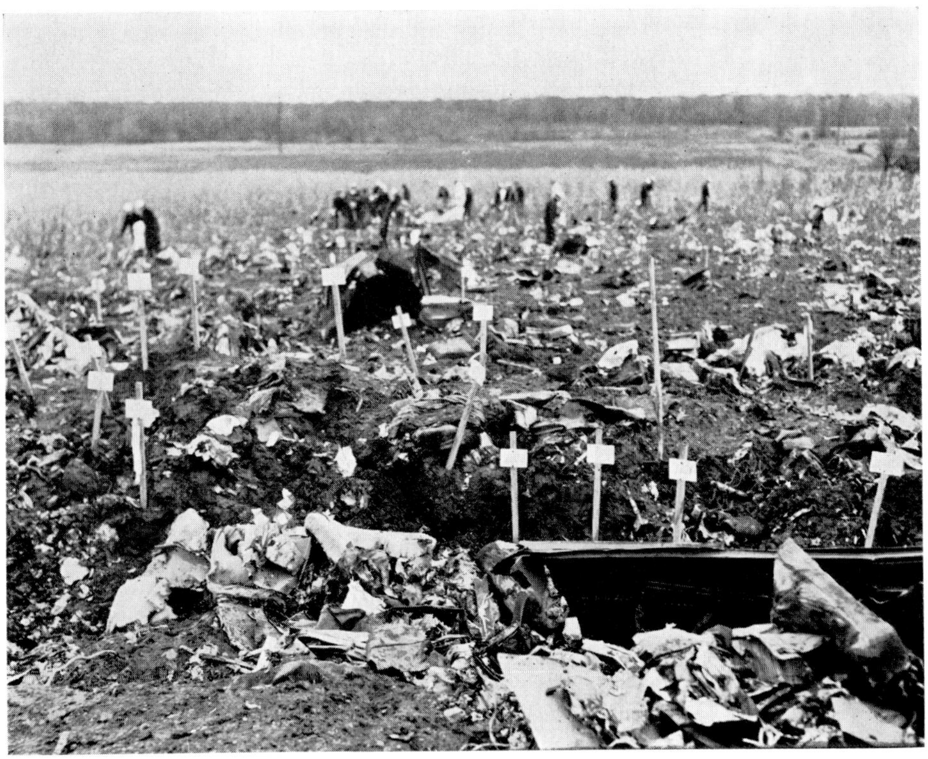

FIGURE XVI-7. After a search of twelve hours, over 100 stakes were set in the field, and the tissue was removed to the mortuary.

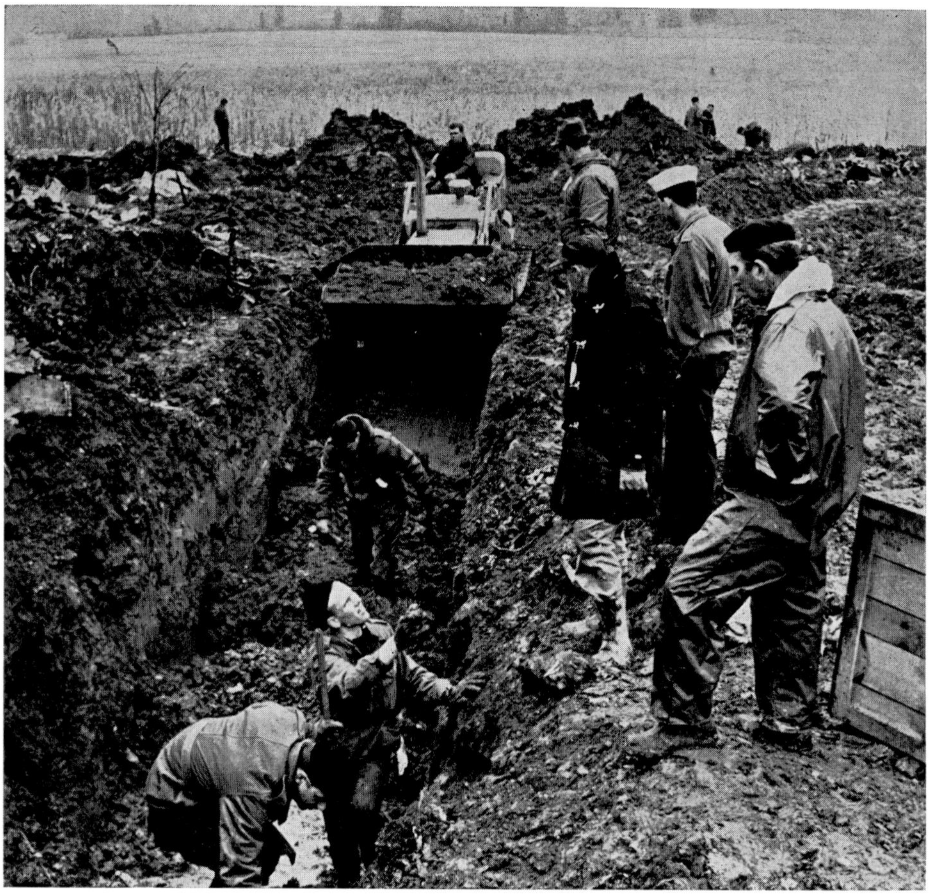

FIGURE XVI-8. After two days of searching the surface, the total weight of remains recovered was only 4,250 lb. (Estimated one-third of the total weight of the eighty-one people.) It was necessary, therefore, to excavate. The entire crash site was removed by a front-end loader to a clear area, and the dirt was sifted as the loader dumped each scoopful. The total excavation was up to 15 ft. wide, 16 ft. deep and over 120 ft. long. The material was resifted as it was replaced. The first sorting yielded 5,450 lb., the second barely 100 more.

days, by which time it was estimated that the entire site occupied by the body of the plane had been excavated to a depth varying from ten to sixteen feet, and the material had been sorted for human remains (Figs. XVI-8 and XVI-9). This procedure raised the total yield of tissue to 9,800 lb., representing approximately 80 percent of the estimated total weight of persons on board the aircraft. Since there was complete disintegration of brain and liver and loss of all blood, it was concluded that substantially all remaining solid tissue had been accounted for.

Meanwhile a team of eight airline employees operating a bank of six telephones and assisted by the local FBI offices in several major cities had accumulated full details of personal information about the passengers and crew.

Identification on the basis of fingerprints and dental studies as well as the autopsy procedures, with matching of personal effects associated with body portions, had continued during the five days. The final analysis of all the material required eleven days, at which time death certificates were issued for all eighty-one persons. Seventy-seven identifications were established with certainty, while four others were presumptive. None of these identifications has been challenged in court since the crash occurred.

Identifications effected by the FBI disaster squad accounted for fifty-three individuals. There was a total of fifty-four complete and four partial sets of fingerprints available. The partial sets were obtained in the case of one stewardess by an identification card in her purse, and in the case of two passengers, from the birth records of a child of each of two mothers who had been killed in the crash. These baby footprint

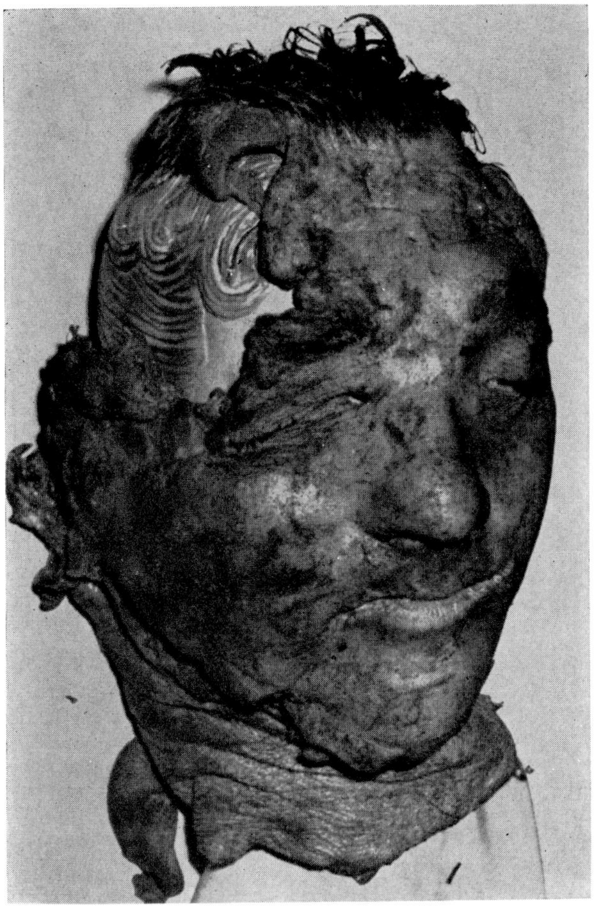

FIGURE XVI-9. Stretching out the scalp and face over a mannikin aided in identification and photography.

records included one or more fingerprints of the mother along with the infant's footprint. Another identification card bearing the prints of one of the crew members was found at the scene.

Among the fifty-three identifications made, many were based on only partial sets of prints, since many of the fingers were unprintable and indeed not all were found. The number of fingers suitable for printing in each case is shown in Table XVI-I. Among the fifty-three bodies identified by fingerprints, thirty-two positive identifications could also be made by other means, such as rings, dentition, physical characteristics or clothing. Among these thirty-two were included ten instances where dentition would have effected identification; seventeen cases where identification could be based on rings; fifteen cases in which identification could be based on clothing; and three cases in which identification could be based on physical characteristics.

TABLE XVI-I
IDENTIFICATION BY FINGERPRINTS

| *Fingers Identified* | | *Number of Cases* |
|---|---|---|
| 1 | | 2 |
| 2 | | 5 |
| 3 | | 6 |
| 4 | | 3 |
| 5 | | 7 |
| 6 | | 7 |
| 7 | | 7 |
| 8 | | 3 |
| 9 | | 4 |
| 10 | | 9 |
| | *Total* | 53 |

Among the twenty-eight bodies for which no fingerprint identification was possible, twenty-four were identified with certainty. Among these were five identifications based on physical characteristics, three by dentition, eight by rings, two by rings and clothing, two by combinations of clothing and physical characteristics, two by combinations of dentition and clothing, one by combination of rings and physical characteristics and one by combination of dentition and rings. The remaining four identifications were classified as *presumptive*. In each case only one specimen was represented; in three of the four the identification was based on physical characteristics and in the fourth on the combination of physical characteristics and clothing.

## REFERENCES

1. Reals, W. J. (Ed.): *Medical Investigation of Aviation Accidents*. Chicago, College of American Pathologists, 1968.
2. Fisher, R. S., Spitz, W. U., Breitenecker, R., and Adams, J. E.: Techniques of identification applied to 81 extremely fragmented aircraft fatalities. *J Forensic Sci, 10:*121, 1965.

*Chapter XVII*

# MECHANICAL INJURIES OF BRAIN AND MENINGES

RICHARD LINDENBERG

THE BRAIN, although well protected against everyday mechanical stress by being encased in the bony skull, is not immune to injury. In fact, in certain types of accidents brain injuries are rather common. In traffic accidents it is estimated that the head and brain are involved in approximately 80 percent of the cases. Since the anatomy of the skull and brain and of its covering meningeal sheaths is more complex than that of other organs, the lesions encountered in head injuries show greater variation in distribution and mechanism than seen elsewhere in the body. Those that are directly related to the injuring force, the so-called primary traumatic lesions, are often associated with additional, mostly circulatory alterations. These may be indirectly related to the primary injury; however, they are most often secondary in nature and caused by the space-occupying effect of primary alterations such as hematomas, by swelling of the brain due to posttraumatic shock, or by posttraumatic respiratory failure and transient cardiac arrest.

For the proper solution of medicolegal problems it is necessary to identify and separate these various types of lesions and to correlate their specific location as much as possible with the functions of the brain areas involved. It is well known that the brain regulates vital functions, initiates and coordinates motor actions, receives sensory impulses and is the seat of emotions and intellectual activities. Each of these functions has its specific location within this large organ, which in weight is second only to the liver. These clinical pathologic correlations are particularly significant for an understanding of the kaleidoscopic range of posttraumatic signs and symptoms. For this reason the description of the pathologic alterations will be supplemented by comments regarding clinical deficits with which they may have been associated.

Since the scope of this presentation is limited, it is not possible to consider all aspects of the lesions, such as histologic aging. The interested reader will find more detailed information and pertinent literature references in the chapters "Trauma of Meninges and Brain," "Oxygen Deficiencies" and "Forensic Neuropathology" in Minckler's *Pathology of the Nervous System.*[1]

## PRIMARY TRAUMATIC LESIONS

The alterations that are directly related to the injuring force, called *primary lesions,* occur at the moment of impact. As is shown in Table XVII-I they are subdivided into two major groups: those that occur outside the brain (extracerebral) and those that are found within the brain (intracerebral).

The extracerebral lesions essentially consist of bleeding due to laceration of blood vessels. If the bleeding is small and thin layered, it is called a *hemorrhage*. If it is space occupying because of its large mass, the term *hematoma* is used. According to the relationship of these alterations to the meningeal coverings of the brain, the dura and arachnoid, they are subdivided into extradural, subdural and subarachnoid bleeding. Since the ventricles are inner chambers of the brain, filled with cerebrospinal fluid flowing into the subarachnoid space, intraventricular bleedings are also listed as extracerebral ones.

The intracerebral lesions are subdivided according to the state of the dura because this membrane constitutes the best barrier against

TABLE XVII-I

PRIMARY TRAUMATIC LESIONS

| *CAUSE:* Impact Force | *OCCURRENCE:* At the Moment of Impact |
|---|---|
| EXTRACEREBRAL | |
| Laceration of Vessels | |
| BLEEDINGS | |
| Extradural – Subdural – Subarachnoid – Intraventricular | |
| INTRACEREBRAL | |
| LACERATIONS or WOUNDS | CONTUSIONS |
| | Hemorrhages – Necroses – Tears |
| Dura Lacerated – Open Injury | Dura Intact – Closed Injury |
| Due to | Due to |
| PENETRATING FORCE | BLUNT FORCE |
| Bullet, Knife, Bone Fragments, etc. | Blow to Head – Fall on Head |

spreading of infection. If the dura is lacerated by the penetrating force of a bullet or any other object, including fragments of fractured bone, or if it is torn due to fracture of the wall of one of the cranial sinuses, one speaks of an *open* injury because it is open to infection. The damage inflicted to the brain by such object is called *laceration* or *wound.* If the dura remains intact, it is called a *closed* injury, irrespective of whether the skull is fractured. In general, closed injuries are caused by blunt force from a blow to the head with a nonpenetrating object or from a fall, the head striking a more or less flat surface or a firm object. The resulting lesions in the brain are in fact bruises called *contusions.* They are subdivided into (a) contusion hemorrhages, (b) contusion necroses, (c) contusion tears. Each one has its special morphologic characteristics.

In describing the various lesions we shall commence with the extradural, subdural and subarachnoid bleedings. Their location and cause are intimately related to normal anatomical facts, which will be briefly reviewed (Fig. XVII-1).

The dura, a strong gray-blue connective tissue membrane, is firmly attached to the skull. It acts as nourishing periosteum for the inner table of the skull and carries along its outer surface the meningeal or dural arteries, the largest one being the middle meningeal artery. These arteries supply the dura and, to a greater part, the bone of the skull with arterial blood. In the adult they often produce an impression in the inner table of the bone by which their course can be identified on x ray. The dura forms the sinuses, which represent rather sturdy, nonelastic and practically noncompressible drainage channels for the venous blood of brain, dura and bone. Extracranial veins also interconnect with the sinuses via *emissary veins.* The most persistent ones are in the mastoid regions. Bacteria from an infected skull wound may follow their course and produce a subdural empyema and/or leptomeningitis.

The space between dura and arachnoid proper is genuine. Although it is very narrow, it contains a small amount of fluid permitting the thin but rather tough arachnoid membrane to move relative to the dura. The cerebral veins must cross this space in order to reach the sinuses. The segments of their stems within the subdural space are referred to as *bridging veins.* The largest bridging vein is the great vein of Galen, which drains into the straight sinus. In normal but forceful movement of the head producing an oscillating motion of the cerebral hemispheres within the skull, the bridging veins

TOPOGRAPHY OF MENINGES

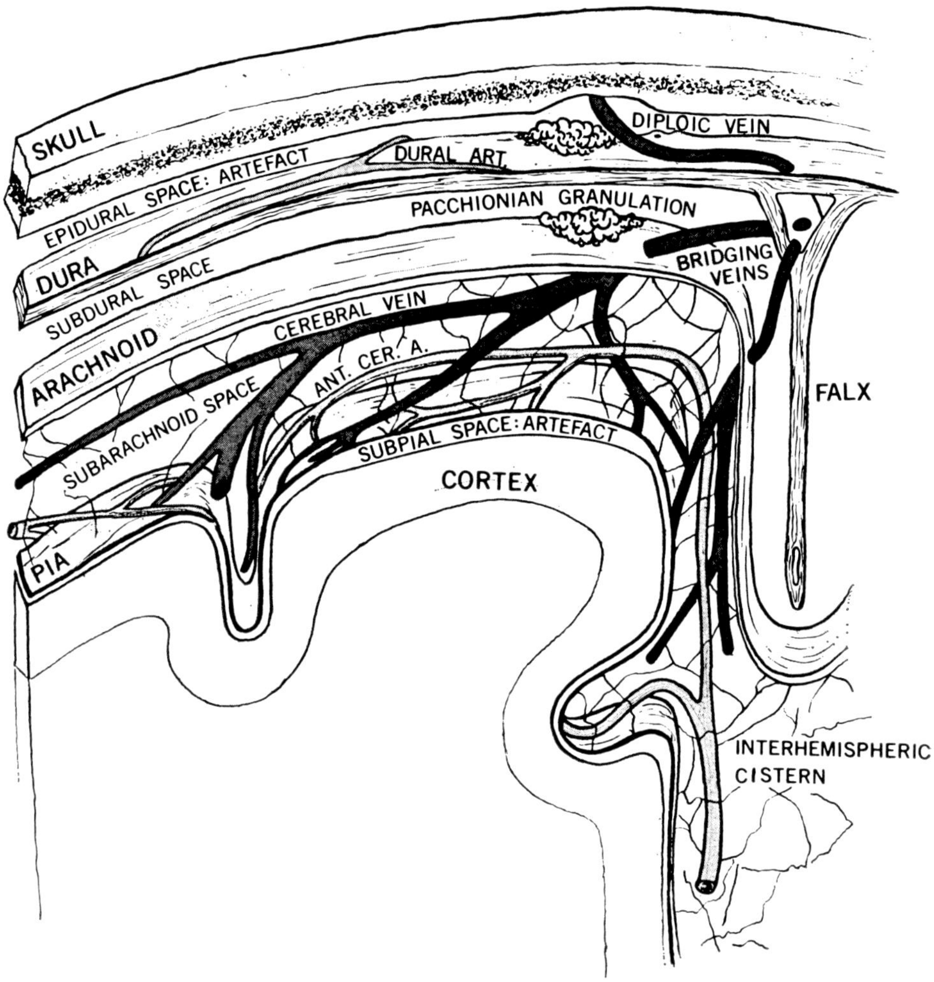


FIGURE XVII-1. Diagram showing the topography of skull, meninges and extracerebral blood vessels.

are protected against damaging stress by arachnoidal, so-called pacchionian granulations, which along most sinuses and particularly along the superior longitudinal sinus fasten the arachnoid to the dura. They are also protected by the dural partitions of falx and tentorium, which act as dampening devices. Otherwise they would easily tear and bleed into the subdural space.

Between the arachnoid membrane and the very thin pia is a second genuine space, the subarachnoid space. It contains the blood vessels of the brain, portions of its cranial nerves and a spider-web-like network of connective tissue fibers. Furthermore, it is filled with cerebrospinal fluid produced by the choroid plexuses of the lateral, third and fourth ventricles. The fluid leaves the ventricles through a small opening in the roof of the fourth ventricle called the *foramen of Magendi*, behind the medulla oblongata and lateral foramens of Luschka, and circulates through the subarachnoid space towards the pacchionian granulations, from where it joins the venous blood in the dural sinuses. The pia follows the surface of the convolutions along the sulci. If the sulci are widened because of a shrinkage of the convolutions or gyri, the increase in the amount of cerebrospinal fluid is called *external hydrocephalus.* Arachnoid and pia together are referred to as *leptomeninges*, meaning thin and delicate coverings of the brain. In leptomeningitis from infection, the cerebrospinal fluid is filled with white blood cells and may appear as thick pus. In trauma, bleeding into the subarachnoid space is very common. Since the subarachnoid space extends continuously all along the spinal cord and along the nerve trunks below the end of the cord, white cells from inflammation and red cells from hemorrhage may reach the lowest portion of this space and be found in a sample of the cerebrospinal fluid removed by lumbar puncture.

## PRIMARY EXTRACEREBRAL LESIONS

### Extradural Bleeding

In the absence of a bone-eroding process and evidence of surgery, extradural bleeding is always traumatic. In the majority of cases an extradural bleeding occurs only in the presence of a skull fracture that causes the dura to separate from the bone, thus producing tears in arteries or their branches or occasionally in veins, predominantly diploic veins. Only in persons with rather elastic skulls, particularly in children, may a skull deformation separate dura and skull and cause an extradural bleeding without a skull

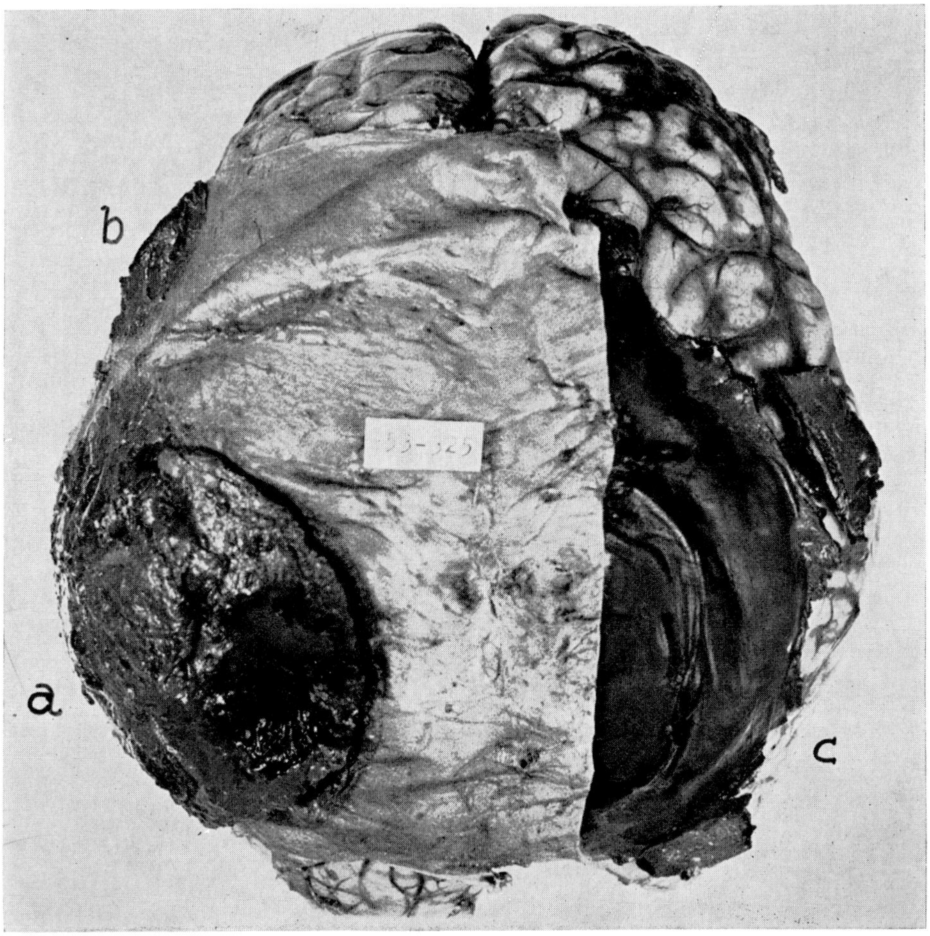


FIGURE XVII-2. Convexity of brain, showing a large (a) and a small (b) extradural hematoma over the left cerebral hemisphere and a subdural hematoma over the right side (c). The injury was received in a fall on the left side of the head. Survival fifteen hours.

fracture being present. In the small number of such cases personally observed, the bleeding was minor in volume. If the bleeding derives from injured veins, its amount is usually also insignificant. The area of predilection for an extradural hematoma is the convexity or the lateral aspect of the cerebral hemispheres. Figure XVII-2 shows an example of a relatively large extradural hematoma over the left cerebral hemisphere (a). In addition there is another smaller hematoma over the lateral aspect of the left frontal lobe (b). There is also a large subdural hematoma on the right (c). Occasionally the smaller of two hematomas may remain undetected at surgery. In a few cases the hematoma develops over the back of the brain and over the cerebellum. At the base of the skull extradural bleedings are rare and usually not space occupying. The hematomas occur in falls on the head as well as in impacts to the stationary head, as for example by a falling brick or by a blow. Although a skull fracture is a prerequisite, the hematoma occurs only in approximately 20 percent of all cases with skull fractures. It may be the sole traumatic lesion and develop rapidly over a period of a few hours. In one of our cases it was fatal by compression of the midbrain thirty minutes after the fall. Few persons survive longer than two days. The patient need not be concussed and rendered unconscious by the impact. There is often a so-called free interval of one or more hours during which the injured may have a headache. This free interval is probably related to a delay in the onset of bleeding due to spasm of the injured dural artery.

As bleeding commences, it first takes place into the preformed space caused by the initial separation of the dura and soon forms a hematoma. As the pressure on the brain increases, the patient first becomes confused and may appear to be drunk. This phase of confusion may not be recognized in a patient who has been drinking and who is not known to have been injured. The confusion indicates that the cerebral hemisphere under pressure is shifting towards the opposite side, thus producing stress on certain structures around the third ventricle and on the uppermost portion of the brain stem, the midbrain. The hematoma may further enlarge by actively separating more dura from the bone around its margin. The added pressure on the deeper brain structures causes sleep, which soon passes into coma. The person cannot be awakened, and it becomes clear to relatives or the guard of the jail that the person is not just sleeping off alcohol intoxication. In this condition the patient may die at any moment from central failure of respiration due to compression of the midbrain region. The examining physician usually finds the pupil on the side of the hematoma dilated and not reactive to the light of his flashlight. This indicates that the medial structure of the temporal lobe, the uncus, exerts pressure on the third cranial nerve, the oculomotor, paralyzing parasympathetic fibers within the nerve that are responsible for contraction of the pupil. Additional procedures such as cerebral angiography may be desirable for making a more precise diagnosis. Usually, however, the state of the patient and the pupillary sign are sufficient reason to explore the situation over the respective hemisphere by making burr holes.

The abnormal pupillary action is not specific for extradural hematoma. It only indicates that the respective hemisphere is shifting and that a space-occupying lesion, such as an acute extra- or intracerebral hematoma, is present. If the extradural hematoma is located in the back over the occipital poles and the cerebellum, the structures around the third ventricle and the midbrain are shifted forward and are less stretched and pressed upon. In such case the injured may remain conscious, develop no signs of confusion and sleep and show no pupillary signs, since the oculomotor nerve is not under pressure. He may die suddenly and unexpectedly because of pressure by the herniated cerebellar tonsils on the medulla oblongata.

Occasionally the hematoma spontaneously becomes smaller by escape of the blood, perhaps through a cleft of the fracture into the subcutaneous tissues, forming a hematoma of the scalp. If the hematoma is of small size and not detected at operation, it often undergoes a slow process of resorption by phagocytes derived from the perivascular cell elements of the dura. Since the dura acts as a periosteum for the bone of the skull, the interposition of the hematoma and the interruption of the blood supply to the skull may result in nutritional changes starting in the inner table of the skull. These changes contribute to the development of a slowly enlarging defect in the skull called *growing fracture*. It is seen most often in infants and children.

### Subdural Hematoma

In contrast to extradural hematomas, not all subdural bleedings are traumatic. They may result from the rupture of an aneurysm or a superficial blood vessel malformation in the brain through the arachnoid into the subdural space. In persons with high blood pressure a superficially located bleeding within the brain may do the same. The great majority of subdural hemorrhages and hematomas, however, are traumatic. Tearing of one or several bridging veins has been cited as one of their causes. Sometimes the arachnoid and dura do not completely separate during the early development of the brain, and a bridging vein, often accompanied by a small artery, may be found in an unusual position at a distance from the dural sinuses. These abnormally located blood vessels are particularly vulnerable to injury. The impact may be so mild that it appears to be insignificant, but if it produces an acceleration of the skull to which the brain does not immediately respond because of its own inertia, these blood vessels may tear. It is possible that an abrupt, forceful movement of the head has the same effect.

Some of the hematomas are arterial in nature, caused by small rents in arachnoid and adjacent cerebral arteries, particularly in branches of the middle cerebral artery in the vicinity of the sylvian (lateral) fissure. Apparently they occur most frequently opposite the side of impact to the head. They may occur without additional contusions of the brain or a significant subarachnoid hemorrhage. In cases of severe cortical contusions associated with bleeding into the adjacent subarachnoid space, the arachnoid may tear and a subdural hematoma may be formed by the escaping blood. In such cases the subdural lesion often extends over the base of frontal and temporal lobes. In contrast to the extradural hematoma, which is always located at the site of a skull fracture, the subdural hematoma shows no such preference. In our large material it was found as often in cases without skull fractures as in those with a fracture.[2]

Most of the subdural hematomas are located over the convexity and lateral aspects of the brain. Occasionally they may develop between the cerebral hemispheres along one or both aspects of the falx, the dural duplication that separates the hemispheres. In the posterior cranial fossa, i.e. around the brain stem and cerebellum, subdural hematomas are very rare. They may develop as fast as an extradural hematoma and become fatal by the same mechanism of brain displacement within hours. Quite often they accumulate gradually and produce mental and emotional disorders, which in younger persons may be mistaken for schizophrenia and in older persons for presenile or senile dementia. With the cessation of bleeding, these psychiatric disorders may become chronic and lead to hospitalization in a mental hospital. If a subdural hematoma is diagnosed in these cases and removed, the patient may remember the injury, which was not known to relatives and friends and which he denied during his state of mental disorder.

Occasionally, subdural hematomas are found over both hemispheres. They may be of equal size. Figure XVII-2 shows the combination of a right-sided subdural hematoma with left-sided extradural hematomas. In these cases there is no or only minimal shifting of one of the hemispheres over the midline. Therefore, the arteriogram may show no displacement of the anterior cerebral artery to one or the other side. As both unci herniate, both oculomotor nerves are pressed upon, and both pupils may show abnormality in size and in reaction to light.

With survival the subdural blood becomes

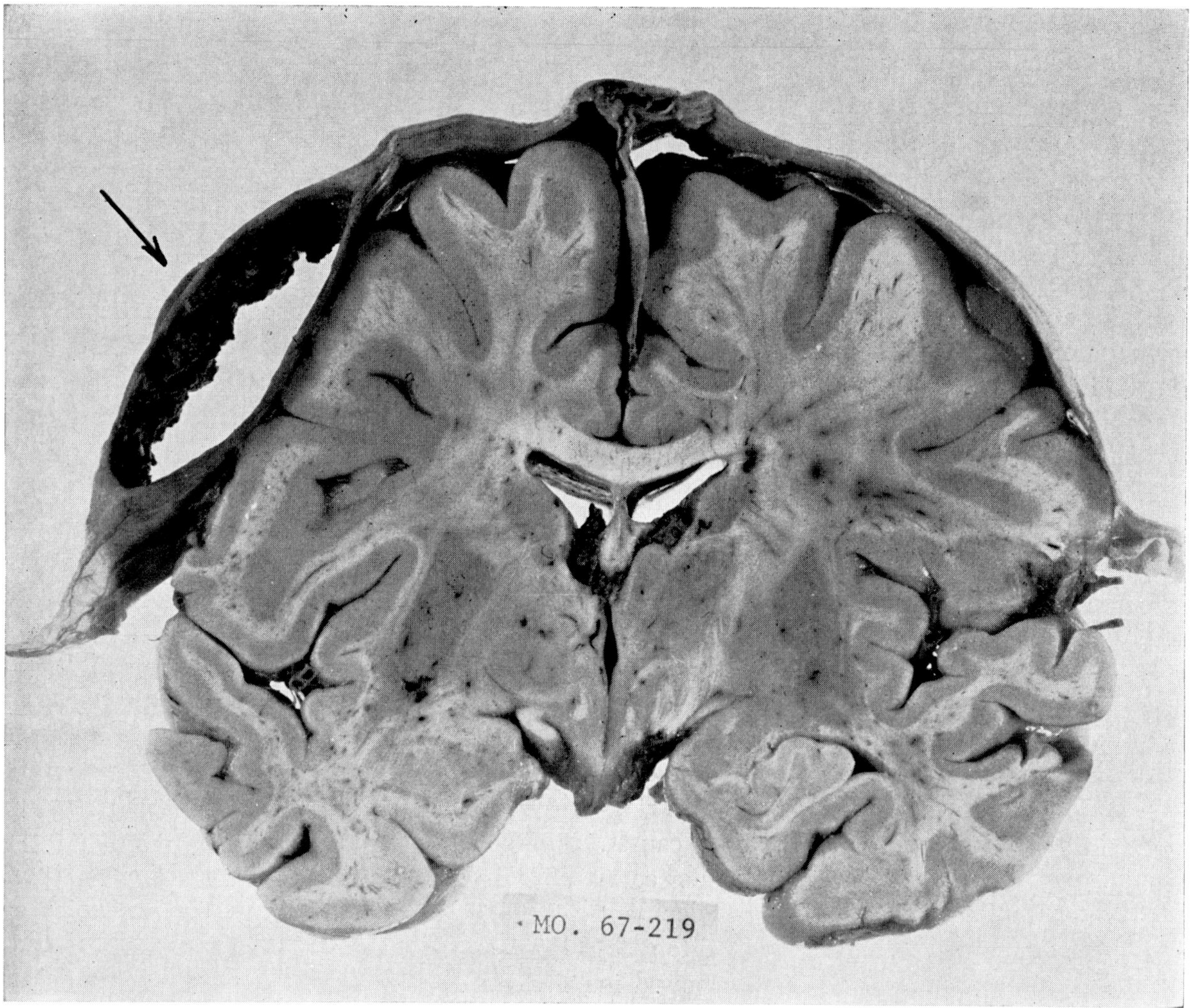


FIGURE XVII-3. Old encapsulated subdural hematoma (arrow) over the left cerebral hemisphere. No swelling of the brain, no noticeable shifting of the left hemisphere to the right, no deformation of the ventricles.

invaded by cells deriving from the dura and its blood vessels. If the layer of blood was relatively thin, these cells form a membrane that consists of strands of connective tissue, harboring phagocytes that contain iron pigment from the digestion of hemoglobin, and newly formed blood vessels. These may turn into small arteries or veins normal in appearance, but in the majority they consist of channels with very delicate, thin walls. These sinusoidal blood vessels may give rise to new localized or diffuse bleeding, which may be spontaneous or provoked by new trauma. The same changes take place along the dural aspect of larger hematomas. In addition, the cells derived from the dura also sprout over the surface of the hematoma facing the arachnoid and gradually encapsulate the mass of old blood.

Such an encapsulated hematoma is shown in Figure XVII-3. The intact arachnoid does not participate in the organization of the membrane; therefore, the capsule is not attached to it and the hematoma can be lifted off the surface of the brain without difficulty. The breakdown

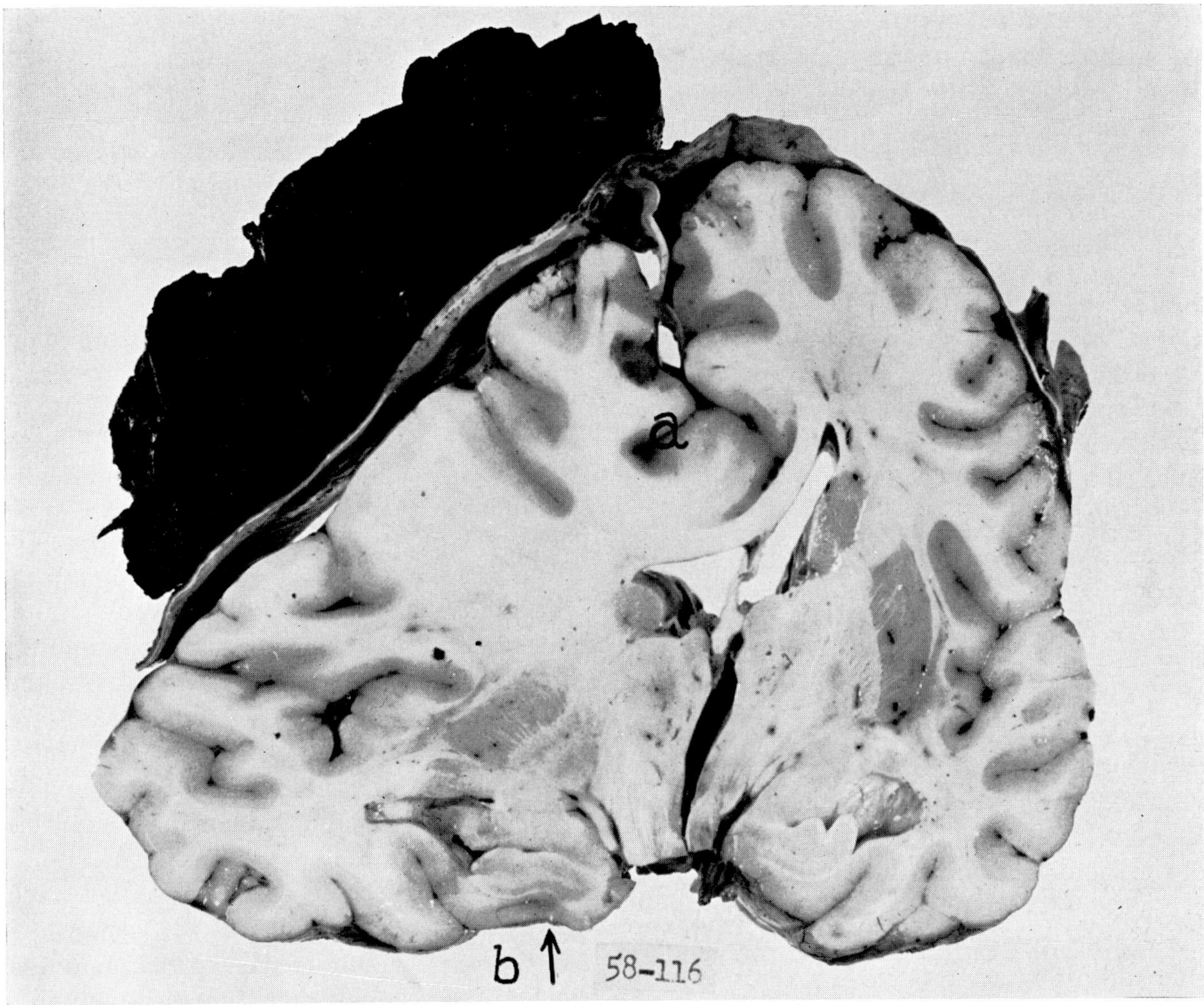


FIGURE XVII-4. Extradural hematoma over the left cerebral hemisphere, causing shifting of the hemisphere towards the right with herniation of the left cingulate (a) and hippocampal gyri (b). Swelling of the white matter of the left hemisphere, severe deformation of the ventricles, no contusions. The injury was sustained in a fall. Survival two days.

of the old blood is very slow. If new hemorrhage occurs within the hematoma, the sac again expands and produces new signs and symptoms. The same is true if the sac is thin and ruptures, filling the subdural space again with fresh blood, thus simulating a bleeding from a new source. Because of the return of clinical signs, clinicians speak of *chronic subdural hematoma*. Some authors attribute the increase in the size of the original hematoma to an osmotic uptake of fluid. Most investigators, however, believe that repeated bleeding causes the enlargement. As can be noticed in Figure XVII-3, a moderately large old hematoma may deform the surface of the brain but cause no shifting of the involved hemisphere towards the other side. This is in contrast to the marked shifting caused by a large recent hematoma, be it extradural, as seen in Figure XVII-4, or subdural. The shifting takes place horizontally through the large opening of the falx and downward into the opening of the tentorium. In many cases such displacement of brain tissues interferes with local circulation, especially in arteries. Tissue changes resulting from such circulatory deficits will be discussed under Secondary Lesions.

### Subarachnoid Bleeding

Bleeding into the subarachnoid space occurs in many nontraumatic conditions. It may develop after death when at the time of removal of the brain from the skull one or the other cerebral vein is torn and empties into the surrounding subarachnoid space. Therefore, it is important that the pathologist inspect the surface of the brain prior to commencing its removal. In trauma, thin-layered subarachnoid hemorrhage, particularly along the sulci, is the most common alteration. Absence of such hemorrhage, however, does not preclude involvement of deeper structures by contusions.

Mild or moderately severe subarachnoid hemorrhage seldom causes significant consequences. Rarely it leads to scarring within the subarachnoid space, particularly over the brain stem and in the basal cistern. The circulation of the cerebrospinal fluid may be retarded or blocked, and a communicating internal hydrocephalus characterized by enlargement of the ventricles may ensue. The enlargement of the lateral ventricles may interfere with the function of the motor fibers responsible for the legs because these fibers encircle the lateral portion of the ventricles on their way to the internal capsule and are rather close to the ventricle wall. Therefore, the patient may complain about an insecure, poorly controlled gait. Distension of the third ventricle and of the anterior aqueduct may produce forgetfulness and confusion or a true psychotic picture, which may persist or present alternate improvement and worsening, depending on changes in the intraventricular pressure or in the circulation in the centrally located structures.

Of particular interest is the subarachnoid hematoma over the base of the brain shown in Figure XVII-5. It is known to occur as the sole traumatic alteration and often is immediately fatal. In these cases it is important that the brain be removed as carefully as possible in order to find the source of the bleeding. The arachnoid, which is seen here as a glistening membrane, should be kept intact during the removal of the brain from the skull. The large feeding arteries—the carotid and vertebral arteries—should be carefully cut. After removal of the arachnoid, the blood is gently removed by running water in order to facilitate inspection of the arteries at the base of the brain, because the hematoma is almost invariably arterial in nature. Perfusion of the arteries with water may help find the leak if no aneurysm or vascular malformation (angioma) can be spotted as source of the bleeding. Sometimes the traumatic tear or tears can be identified by this procedure. However, it should be pointed out that in spite of all care taken, a leak may not be found. The rent in the artery may be obstructed by coagulated blood, or the source of the bleeding may be hidden deep in the sylvian fissure or in cisterns of the subarachnoid space around midbrain, upper pons and rostral cerebellum. It is also possible that the bleeding starts from one of the four feeding arteries at the point where they enter the subarachnoid space. A tear or a miniature aneurysm of the carotid artery, for example, may be found just beneath the stump of the optic nerve.

In most of the cases of traumatic subarachnoid hematomas one will find that the arteries have somewhat thin, delicate walls and that the impact was moderately severe, usually from a blow to the face or forehead. It may have been a fist blow, a blow by a blunt object or even a blow from gases of a firearm discharged near the face. It also occurs in sudden hyperextension of the head, as it did, for example, in a person who, after stepping into a freestanding bathtub, slipped and fell backwards with his shoulders striking the rim of the tub, causing his head to snap momentarily backwards.

Even prolonged backward bending of the head during visual examination of the airways (bronchoscopy) induced in one of our cases a fatal subarachnoid hematoma over the base of the brain. In these cases of hyperextension the bleeding may originate from rents in basal or vertebral arteries. In the cases with impacts to the facial region, particularly to the chin, the arterial injury is more often found in one carotid

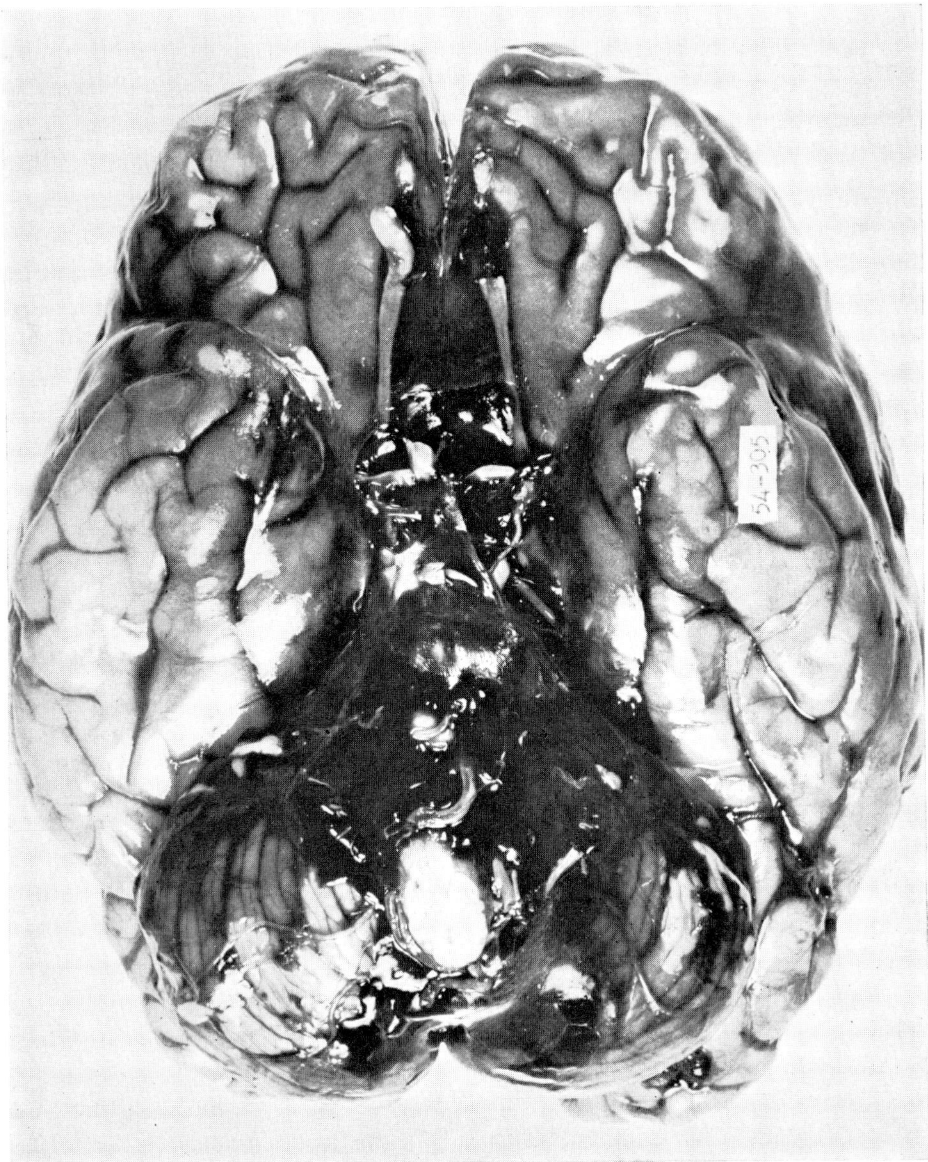


FIGURE XVII-5. Subarachnoid hematoma over the base of the brain as the sole traumatic lesion from a fist blow to the face. Death was instantaneous.

artery or in an artery of the circle of Willis. Here the lesions are most likely the result of a short-lasting oscillation of the brain within the skull following rotational acceleration of the head. Such brain movements were first observed through the plastic skull of monkeys.[3] No subarachnoid hemorrhage occurred in these animals at the base of the brain, but subdural bleeding from torn bridging veins was observed. If the bleeding develops slowly, a subarachnoid hematoma over the base of the brain may be survived.

As subarachnoid bleedings become older, they may be identified for some time by a slightly yellow discoloration of the leptomeninges.

In some cases the blood over brain stem and other basal structures may be an extension of an intraventricular bleeding through the foramens of Magendi and Luschka.

## Bleeding into Ventricles

It is not unusual to find minor intraventricular accumulation of blood in all kinds of craniocerebral injuries. Occasionally subarachnoid hemorrhage enters the ventricles through the foramens of Magendi and Luschka. Sometimes the blood is more condensed around one of the choroid plexuses and apparently originated there. Similarly, the collection of blood next to the septum pellucidum suggests bleeding from one of its veins. There are cases in which the amount of blood is so large that one speaks of an *intraventricular hematoma.* It may be the only traumatic alteration throughout the brain and may lead to a distension of the ventricles, most often of the lateral ventricles. This usually indicates that the bleeding derived from a ruptured artery. Some of these bleedings are caused by tears in the vulnerable septum pellucidum; others, including arterial bleedings, may derive from the choroid plexus, which is highly vascularized. In contrast to the three foregoing kinds of extracerebral bleedings, the true traumatic ventricular bleeding as a sole finding is always the result of the head striking a firm object, i.e. a fall or a fall-like injury. If it is associated with larger contusions, it may have resulted from a contusion hematoma breaking through the wall of the ventricle. Adhesions may ultimately develop between the ventricle wall and the choroid plexus. More often, a traumatic porencephaly remains, similar to that described as a result of injury from a penetrating object.

There is always the possibility that the bleeding is caused by the rupture of an abnormality, known as an arteriovenous fistula, in the wall of the ventricle. Such malformations are not unusual. After careful removal of the mass of blood, one can often see the small defect in the ependymal lining from which the bleeding occurred. It is sometimes associated with local bleeding in the adjacent brain tissues. However, if the hematoma is large, the ependymal lining often undergoes secondary or postmortem changes, making finding of the site of bleeding difficult. Larger angiomas of arteriovenous nature cannot usually be overlooked. They often drain into a vein of the ventricle wall and therefore may bleed only into the ventricles. Also, aneurysms may bleed predominantly into the ventricle system.

An aneurysm of the posterior communicating artery may rupture through the relatively thin layer of cortex and white matter of the anterior hippocampus and bleed into the anterior portion of the inferior or temporal horn of the lateral ventricle. An aneurysm at the end of the basilar artery may break through the floor of the third ventricle. In both instances, little or no local subarachnoid hemorrhage may be present. In cases with hypertensive vascular disease, the first apoplectic bleeding may be so close to the ventricle wall that it does little damage to the surrounding structures, i.e. the caudate nucleus, but fills the ventricles with blood. If the bleeding commences in the areas of the anterior horns or the cella media (the midportion of the lateral ventricles), the septum pellucidum is often disrupted and partially destroyed, giving the impression that the bleeding had originated from the septum.

We mention the nontraumatic together with the traumatic intraventricular bleedings because the question of trauma arises if the person was found lying on the ground and his head showed signs of injury. In the absence of reliable information on the events preceding the fall, it is difficult and often impossible to decide whether the fall was the result of the incipient bleeding or the bleeding resulted from the fall. The presence of contusions is merely evidence that the brain was exposed to a major impact. Their pattern in relation to the external injuries may suggest that the impact was from a blow or a fall. Histologic aging of the contusions and of the area of the source of the bleeding may provide further information of value.

Not all persons with intraventricular bleeding die rapidly. They may linger on for days or survive without major difficulties unless an internal hypertensive hydrocephalus develops from obstruction of the aqueduct or of the foramens of Magendi and Luschka or from obstruction within the leptomeninges over the brain stem and the base of the brain. As evidence of former hemorrhage there may be for a few weeks slight yellow discoloration of the ventricle wall. Storage of iron in the choroid plexus may be more impressive. It persists for a long time.

## PRIMARY INTRACEREBRAL LESIONS

### Brain Wounds

Lesions due to brain wounds, as was stated before, are caused by penetrating objects. The objects either are foreign and have to perforate skin, bone, dura and leptomeninges before reaching the brain, or they are pieces of fractured bone, which have to perforate only dura and leptomeninges in order to damage the brain. The foreign object may be a missile fired or thrown against the head, such as a bullet, a rock or a piece of an exploding body. It may be a falling object, such as a branch of a tree or a brick. It may be a weapon used in a blow to the head, i.e. a hammer, axe, knife, ice pick or a nail attached to a piece of lumber. Finally, it may be a protruding portion of a stationary object that was struck by the head, such as a part of a fence, the handlebar of a bicycle or the blade of a running saw. It is obvious from this list that the shape of the wounds varies to a great extent, as outlined in Chapter VII. In the following pages various types of brain wounds encountered in accidents, homicides and suicides, including stab wounds and wounds from firearms, will be discussed. This will be followed by some remarks on wounds caused by bone fragments.

#### *Stab Wounds*

Stab wounds, caused by an assortment of instruments with a very small impacting surface, such as ice picks, screwdrivers, knives or chisels, often extend deeply into the brain and are considerably more devastating than was expected from the appearance of the small *innocuous* wound in the skin. If the latter is covered by hair and produces little or no external hemorrhage, it may be overlooked by clinician and pathologist alike. The hole in the skull may be missed on x ray. Only a careful examination of the brain will provide the evidence that the patient was stabbed in the head and information on the cross-sectional shape and minimal length of the weapon used.

A man found unconscious in a park was carefully examined at a hospital. He died several hours after admission without the physician being able to arrive at a diagnosis. At autopsy only swelling of the brain was noticed. Upon sectioning, several cutlike wounds with little hemorrhage were found in deeper structures of the brain. They converged towards a small point at the surface of the left lower parietal lobe. The diagnosis of stab wound with an ice pick or ice-pick-like instrument was made. The site of entrance now known, it was possible to identify the small hole in the skull on x ray films, which had escaped attention by the radiologist. The cutlike wounds were obviously caused by wiggling the instrument upon retraction.

Figure XVII-6 shows the intracerebral enlargement of a knife wound by such movement. The entrance wound was above the right eye, and the knife had entered the right orbital lobe after causing a contoured fracture of the orbital roof. Since the knife was held in an oblique position by the fracture, the wound track in the brain enlarged posteriorly in the plane of the blade of the knife. The distance from the entrance wound to the end of the wound track provided information on the minimal length of the knife.

When first seen in the emergency room, the patient was conscious and showed no evidence of cerebral involvement. While the external wound was treated, he went into shock and coma and died a few hours later from swelling of the brain. This swelling was not directly caused by the wound and the bleeding into the wound and the ventricle but was the result of shock, which was probably initiated by the onset of more severe bleeding.

If no shock occurs, a stab wound may be survived; neither the victim of an assault nor the physician in the emergency room may be aware that the brain was injured. In one of our

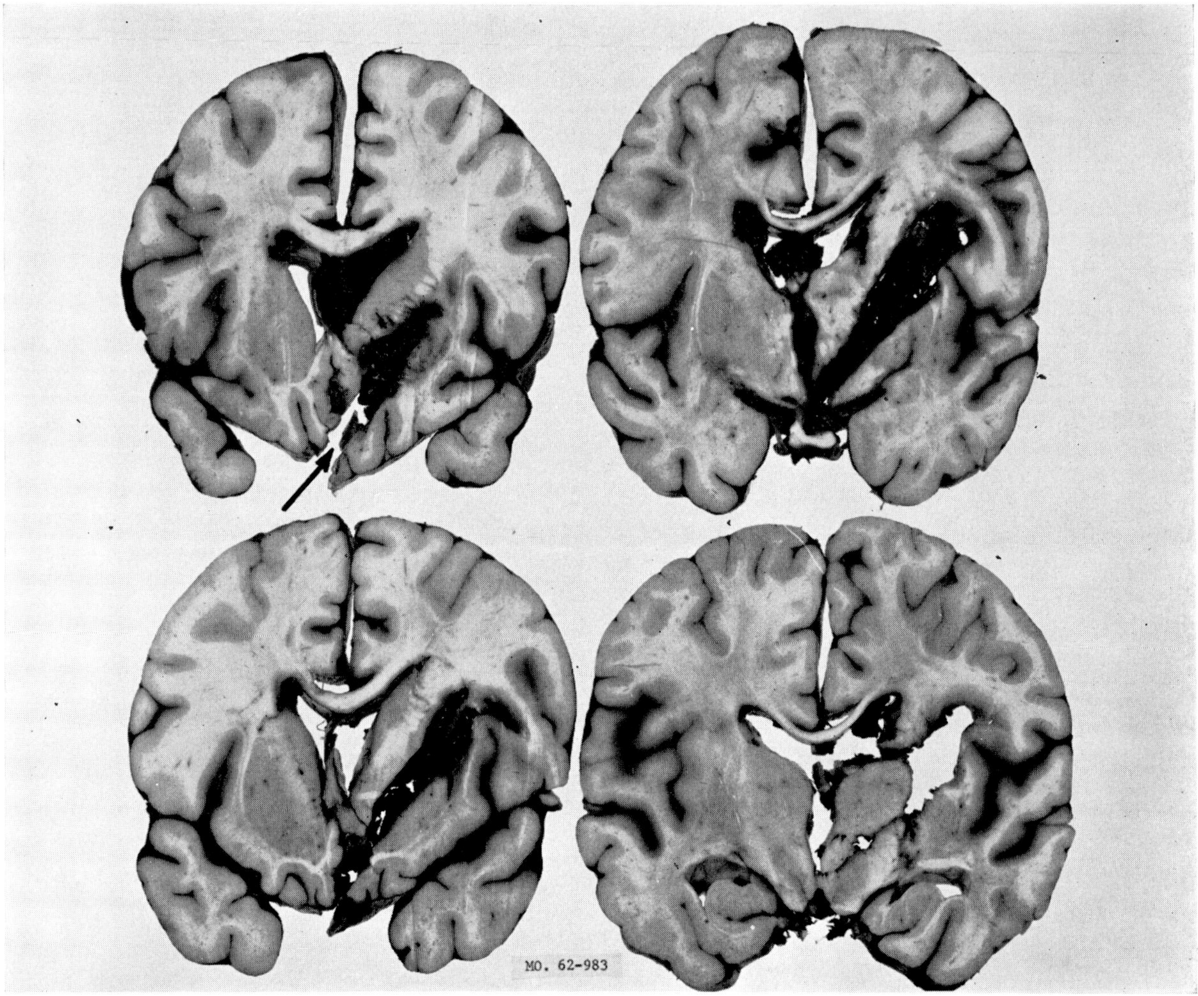


FIGURE XVII-6. Stab wound with a pocket knife above right eye, extending slitlike from the right anterior orbital lobe (arrow) to the level of the midbrain. Posterior enlargement of the wound is due to wiggling of the knife. Survival two and one-half hours.

cases the patient went home after the external wound over the left temple was sutured. Several days later he developed severe headaches and died shortly after admission to the same hospital from meningitis and incipient abscess formation along the wound track. There was almost no bleeding.

In another case, neither the patient nor the physician were aware of a stab wound in the left anterior temporal lobe. A mild weakness of the right side was interpreted as a cerebrovascular accident. When the patient started to complain of acoustic hallucinations, he was admitted to a mental institution. Here he spent the rest of his life as a schizophrenic. At autopsy years later the rusty tip of a penknife, surrounded by scar tissue, was found in his temporal lobe.

If multiple wounds were inflicted by the same instrument over various parts of the body, it may be difficult for the pathologist to determine which of them was the fatal one. In fact, none of the many knife wounds over chest and abdomen exhibited by one of our cases proved responsible for the immediate death. Upon repeated inspection of the body, a small wound in the nape of the neck was detected and found to have extended through the medulla oblongata. Similarly, in cases of survival, the clinical symptomatology may remain unexplained because one of the multiple wounds responsible for these symptoms was overlooked.

The victim of an assault was admitted to a hospital in an unconscious condition with multiple stab wounds, one of them located over the left temporal region without penetration of the skull. A search for extra- or intracerebral bleeding proved negative. During his three months of survival he remained unconscious and continued to show paralysis of the left leg.

The puzzle was solved at autopsy. There was a healed *puncture fracture* over the lower surface of the right cerebellar hemisphere that could not be seen on routine x ray films. From here an old smooth-walled wound track extended upwards through the adjacent brain structure into the upper portion of the midbrain. Because of involvement of the midbrain the patient had remained unconscious. Damage to the motor fibers in the base of the upper pons by twisting and turning the ice pick upon retraction accounted for the persistent paralysis of the left leg.

The depth to which a pointed object may penetrate into the brain is exemplified by the findings in a young boy who accidentally fell with his chin on the unprotected radio antenna of a motor vehicle. From the tiny wound beneath the chin the metal rod had pierced the wall of the nasopharynx, the floor of the skull and the entire brain up to the inner table of the parietal bone at the vertex of the skull.

### *Wounds from Firearms*

The most frequent wounds caused by firearms are bullet wounds. The characteristics of external wounds and fractures produced by bullets are discussed in Chapter X. Here, a few comments are appropriate regarding the wound track within the brain and additional findings at some distance from the wound track.

In general, the destructive effect of a bullet depends on its caliber or mass and to a much greater degree on the velocity with which it passes through the tissues. This is due to the fact that the kinetic energy of a moving body amounts to one-half of its mass times the square of its velocity. This means that doubling the mass but leaving the velocity unchanged merely doubles the amount of energy. However, if the mass remains unchanged and the velocity is doubled, the energy increases fourfold. The energy of the bullet is spent in piercing skin, bone, brain and, in perforating shots, again bone and skin on the opposite side. Part of the energy is expended by the tip of the bullet to break the resistance of the tissues and another part to push the tissues aside. It is this radial displacement producing transient cavitation that is important in regard to the severity of tissue damage.

If the bullet loses almost all its energy during penetration of the skin and bone, including dura, it passes through the soft brain tissues without causing cavitation until it comes to rest. In such a case the effect on the brain is not much more than that of a surgical probe of the same caliber pushed into the brain by the neurosurgeon. However, if the bullet is capable of passing through the brain with great velocity, the wound track expands immediately after the bullet has passed through. This expansion takes only microseconds to develop, and the entire process of cavitation lasts only a few milliseconds. During this short time the brain is suddenly pressed against the inner table of the skull and other firm structures, momentarily bulging out of exit and entrance wounds and collapsing just as fast. The skull fractures, however, occur just prior to cavitation. If they extend beyond the areas of entrance and exit and the cavitation is particularly severe, the skull may burst by the pressure of the brain. Under such high pressure the brain is a firm mass, and large portions of it may be thrown out of the bursting skull and found relatively intact at a short distance from the body. This is referred to as *Krönlein shot* because Krönlein was the first to describe this explosive effect of high energy bullets. If the energy of the bullet is such that this explosion does not take place but cavitation is severe, the sudden pressure on the tissues surrounding the wound track causes it to become immediately necrotic, due to shearing forces acting on submicroscopic structures of cells and their processes. The width of the cylinder of necrosis surrounding the wound track may be taken as an indirect indicator of the severity of cavita-

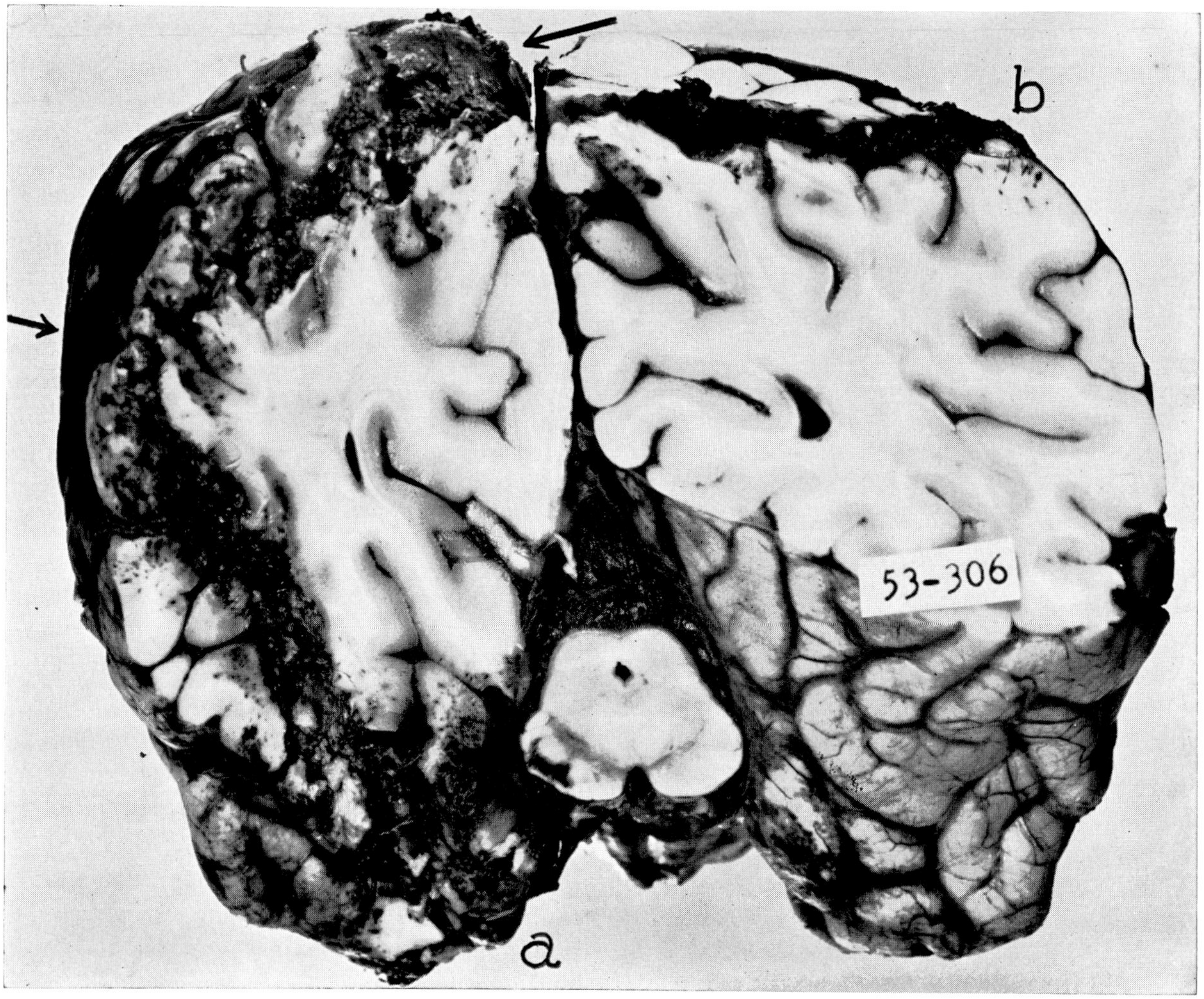


FIGURE XVII-7. Double ricochet of a gunshot. Entrance was in the left anterior temporal lobe (a). The bullet was found in the right parietal area (b). The bullet was deflected on two separate impacts with the inner table of the skull at the points indicated by the arrows.

tion. Outside the necrotic tissue there is often a ring or cylinder of tissue hemorrhages. With survival, it is in this zone in which phagocytic activity starts. Breakdown of the necrotic tissue by phagocytes is a very slow process.

Most of the bullets used in homicides and suicides are small in caliber and of low velocity. They may produce some cavitation but often lack sufficient energy to perforate the head on the opposite side. Sometimes the wound track is relatively small, barely larger than the diameter of the missile, but it is not unusual to find the entire track or one segment of it several times larger. This is not the result of cavitation. It indicates that the bullet either passed sideways through the tissues or tumbled.

Sometimes the bullet does not have enough energy after passing through the brain to penetrate the skull but bounces off the inner table of the skull and performs a ricochet like a billiard ball. It may do this a second time and thereby produce a third wound track, as is seen in Figure XVII-7. If the bullet enters the skull at an acute angle towards the inner table, it may glide along the dura, tearing the leptomeninges and blood vessels, and cause a shallow wound track along the surface of the brain. Since it attempts to follow the course of an inner tangent, one speaks of an *inner tangential course* of the bullet. This may be combined with internal ricochet. The various courses observed by Freytag[4] in forty-four cases of gunshot wound with internal ricochet are shown diagrammatically in Figure XVII-8. They are of particular interest to the clinician because he can never be certain in cases in which the bullet remained in the brain that the bullet took a direct course from the entrance to its final location seen on x ray.

Aside from hemorrhages in the vicinity of the wound track, there are often hemorrhages at a distance from it. These are contusions caused by displacement of portions of the brain due to the sudden space-occupying entrance of the bullet into the brain and by the associated cavitation. They are found wherever shearing forces within the tissues are stronger than the elasticity or cohesive force of the involved blood vessels. Areas of predilection for such distant contusions are the cerebellar tonsils and the cerebellar cortex facing the rim of the foramen magnum. These tonsillar contusions may be the only other lesions aside from the wound caused by the bullet. They occur independently of the location and course of the wound track. In Figure XVII-9 the wound track extends through the orbital roofs and in part through the lower frontal, or, as we call them, orbital convolutions (a). There are practically no hemorrhages in the lacerated tissues. The cerebellar tonsils (arrows), however, show numerous hemorrhages, as does the tegmentum, i.e. the upper portion of the adjacent medulla oblongata (b). Obviously the entering bullet and whatever cavitation it produces give an impulse to the cerebral hemispheres, and they, in turn, momentarily force the tonsils into the only emergency exit of the skull: the occipital foramen. The displaced tonsils again suddenly press on the tegmentum of the medulla oblongata, producing additional hemorrhages there. These tonsillar lesions are called *herniation contusions*, with the understanding that the herniation takes place within a fraction of a second. They also occur in blows to the head with blunt objects, as will be shown later. The contusion hemorrhages in the medulla oblongata are of interest because they are gross evidence that the primary centers for respiration and heartbeat located in this area were under sudden stress, which may have been the true cause of death. On the other hand, the stress on the medulla may be such that concussive fatal paralysis of respiration and/or heartbeat may occur without blood vessels being damaged, because basically death is due to persistent dysfunction of these vital centers.

Figure XVII-10 shows a large wound track through the frontal lobes (a). Cavitation was more severe than in the preceding case, because

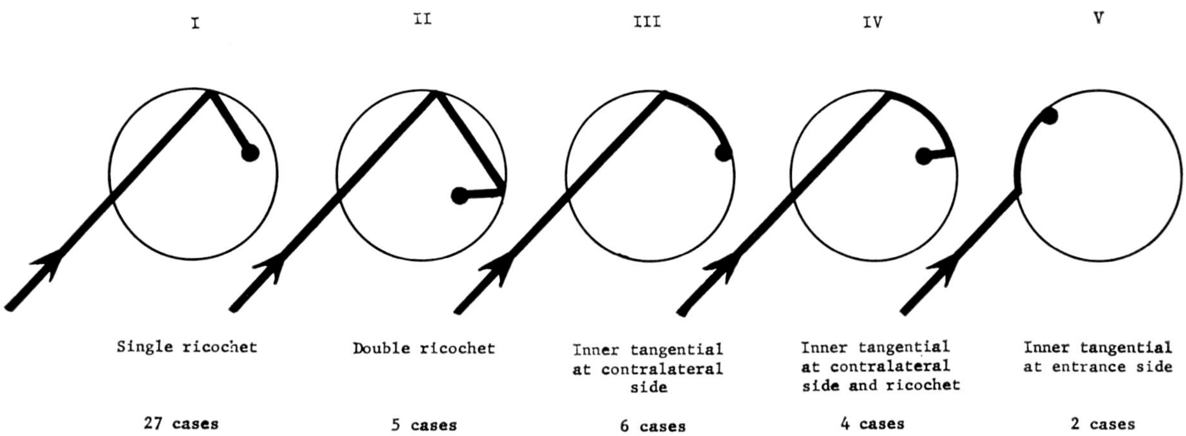


FIGURE XVII-8. Variations of bullet tracks found among forty-four cases of gunshot with internal ricochet. (From Freytag, E.: Autopsy finding in head injuries from firearms. *Arch Pathol, 76*:215, 1963.)

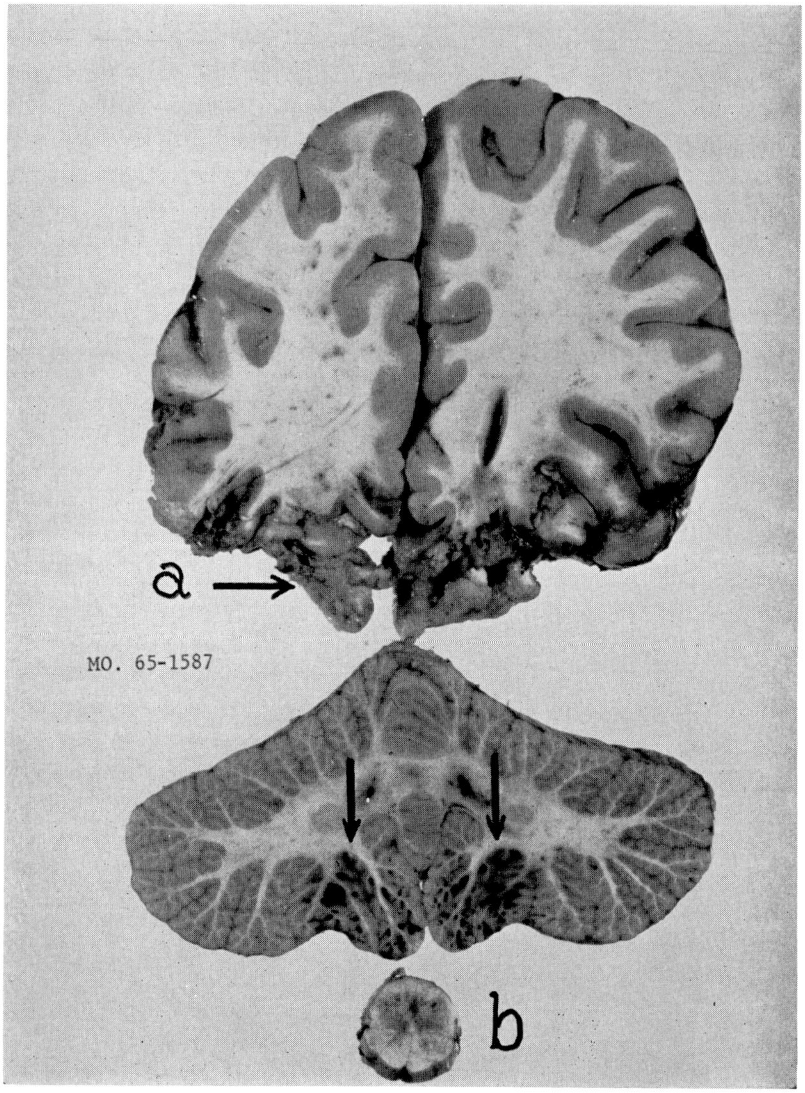


FIGURE XVII-9. Gunshot through orbital lobes (a) causing herniation contusions in cerebellar tonsils (arrows) and medulla oblongata (b). Death was instantaneous.

in addition to tonsillar herniation contusions (arrows), there are many other contusions. The large lesion in the area of the left lower central and adjacent temporal area resulted from craniotomy (b), but the contusions in both orbital lobes (c) and those in the unci (d), right pallidum (e) and near the mammillary bodies (f) are attributable to cavitation. The orbital convolutions were contused by being pressed against the irregular surface of the orbital roof. The pressure was so great that the bony roofs caved in. Such indirect fractures of the orbital roofs are not rare in gunshot wounds and are not dependent on the location of the latter. The contusions in unci and adjacent deep structures were obviously caused by the brain suddenly pressing against the tentorium when the structures around the mammillary bodies attempted to shift into the tentorial opening. This is of interest because the same pattern of contusions will be described again later as a result of a fall on the forehead or the vertex.

Multiple wound tracks caused by internal ricochet are different from multiple wound tracks resulting from a shotgun blast. Here, each individual pellet produces its own track. A

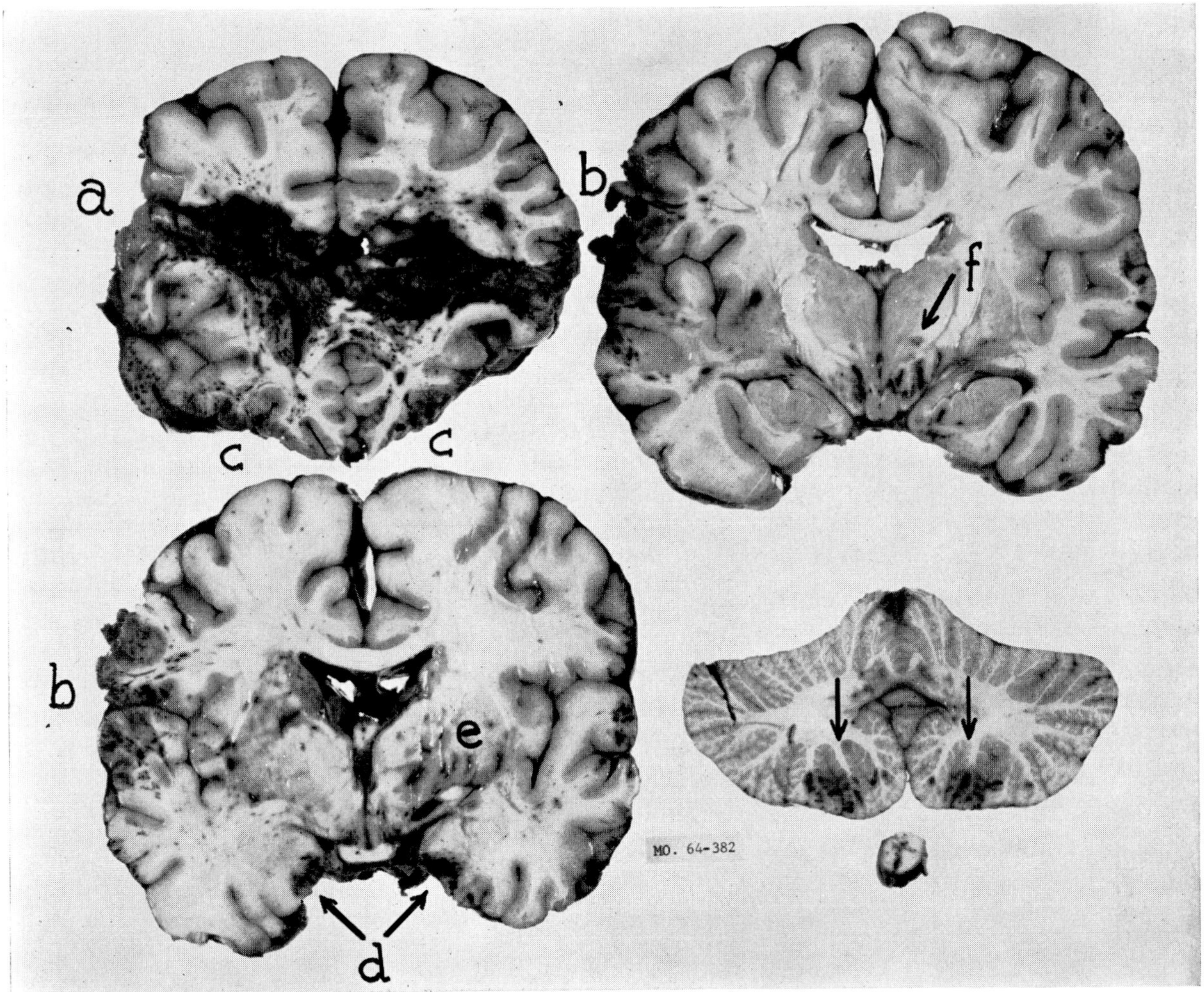


FIGURE XVII-10. Gunshot through the frontal lobes (a) associated with distant contusions in the cortex (c, d) and the deeper structures of the cerebrum (e, f). Craniotomy in the left lower central and temporal area (b). Herniation contusions in the cerebellar cortex facing the rim of the foramen magnum and in the medulla oblongata (arrows). Survival three and one-half hours.

relatively dense pattern of such wounds is shown in Figure XVII-11. The cross section of the wound tracks is seen near the interhemispheric fissure. At the end of one track, near the right lateral ventricle, a pellet can be seen. In spite of the multiplicity of the missiles, their energy is often so severely reduced by perforating the skin and bone that they are unable to cross the entire brain substance. Therefore, cavitation is usually minimal or nonexistent, and distant contusions are rare. One may find, however, *indirect infarcts* from laceration of blood vessels by pellets or bone fragments. Such infarcts may also be seen in other gunshot wounds.

### Lacerations by Bone Fragments

In all kinds of injuries associated with fractures of the skull it is not uncommon that a piece of bone lacerates the brain. In gunshot wounds such pieces may produce short accessory wound tracks. Since these pieces always originate from the fractured skull near the entrance of the bullet into the skull, their presence may be of help in determining which of two

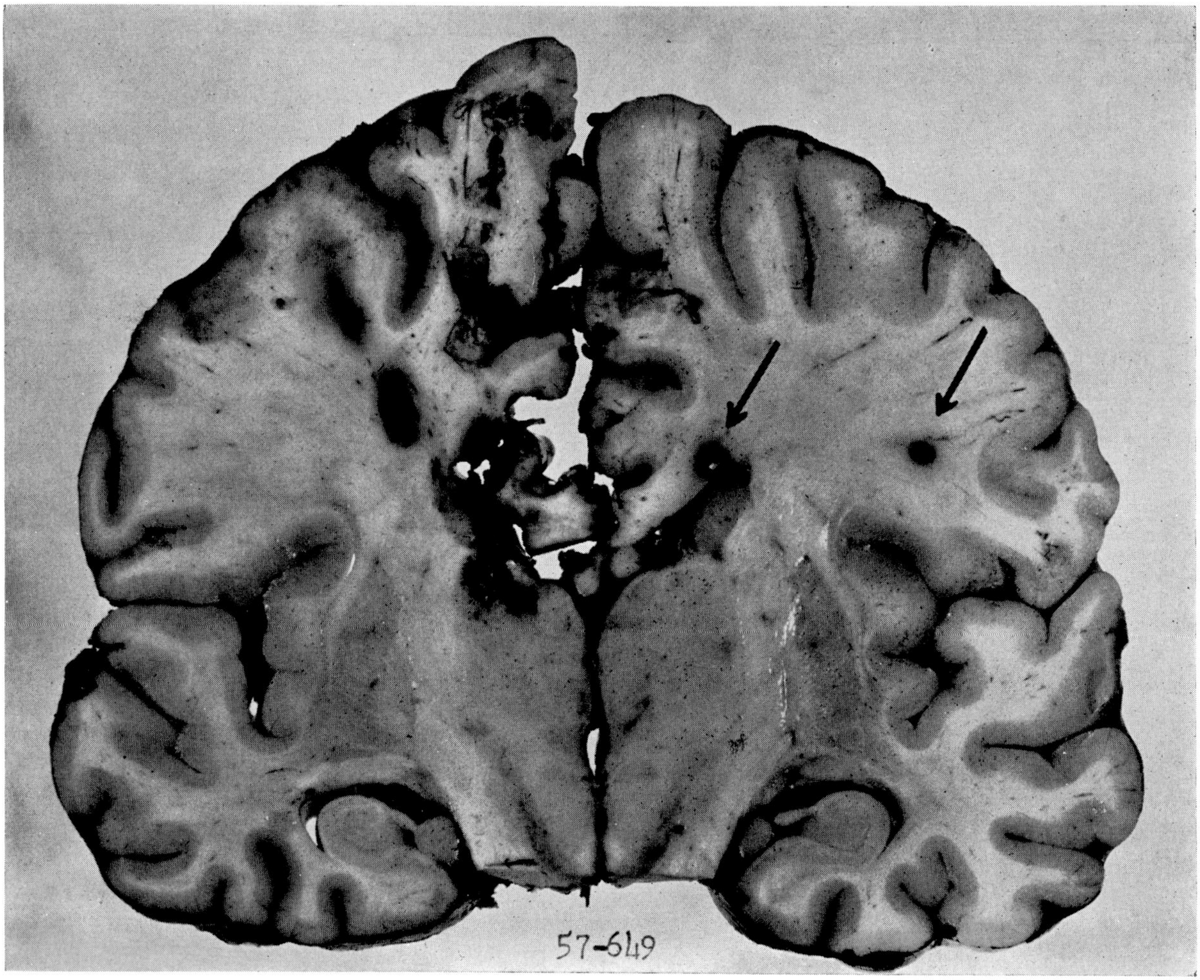


FIGURE XVII-11. Shotgun wound of the brain. A cross section of multiple wound tracks caused by individual pellets in the center of the photograph and two individual wound tracks (arrows). Dead on arrival at the hospital.

ends of the wound track constitutes the wound of entrance if external changes are not conclusive.

In other types of injury lacerations are usually more superficial, because the bone fragment traverses the dura prior to injuring the brain and severe displacement of bone fragments occurs only in the most destructive, immediately fatal injuries. Most frequently the cortex of the orbital lobes is involved, because the bones of the orbital roofs and the roofs of the ethmoidal paranasal sinuses are the thinnest of all bones that form the skull. The lacerations are usually irregular and involve the leptomeninges and the blood vessels in between. It is of interest that these lacerations show no initial hemorrhage and may remain so for one or two hours as result of vasospasm. In contrast to peripheral arteries, cerebral arteries seldom react with spastic contraction unless lacerated. In the case of aneurysms, the reactivity of the respective artery may be so great that touching it during surgery may provoke spasm of such duration that the depending brain tissue becomes infarcted. For this reason, the lack of bleeding in lacerations cannot be used as evidence of instantaneous death. For the same reason, other wounds, and in particular gunshot wounds, may contain little or no blood, although the victim was not instantaneously killed.

## Contusions

As is shown in Table XVII-I, contusions are those primary lesions that occur while the overlying dura is intact. They are the result of shearing forces occurring within the tissues at the moment of impact. They are divided into (a) contusion hemorrhages, (b) contusion necroses, (c) contusion tears.

### *Contusion Hemorrhages*

Some contusion hemorrhages as they occur at a distance from a gunshot wound were shown in Figures XVII-9 and XVII-10. These contusions were related to shearing forces occurring within the tissues due to shifting of the brain away from the path of the bullet because of cavitation. They are the dominant primary lesions in injuries from blunt forces and are found in gray and white matter wherever blood vessels are injured by mechanical stress. Contusions involving the cerebral cortex are the most frequent ones, and their identification is important for proper medicolegal interpretation.

Most hemorrhages occur at the crest of convolutions facing the dura or the dural duplications of falx and tentorium. Both act as stabilizing membranes—the falx between the cerebral hemispheres and the tentorium between the lower temporal lobes and the cerebellar hemispheres. In their early phase the hemorrhages

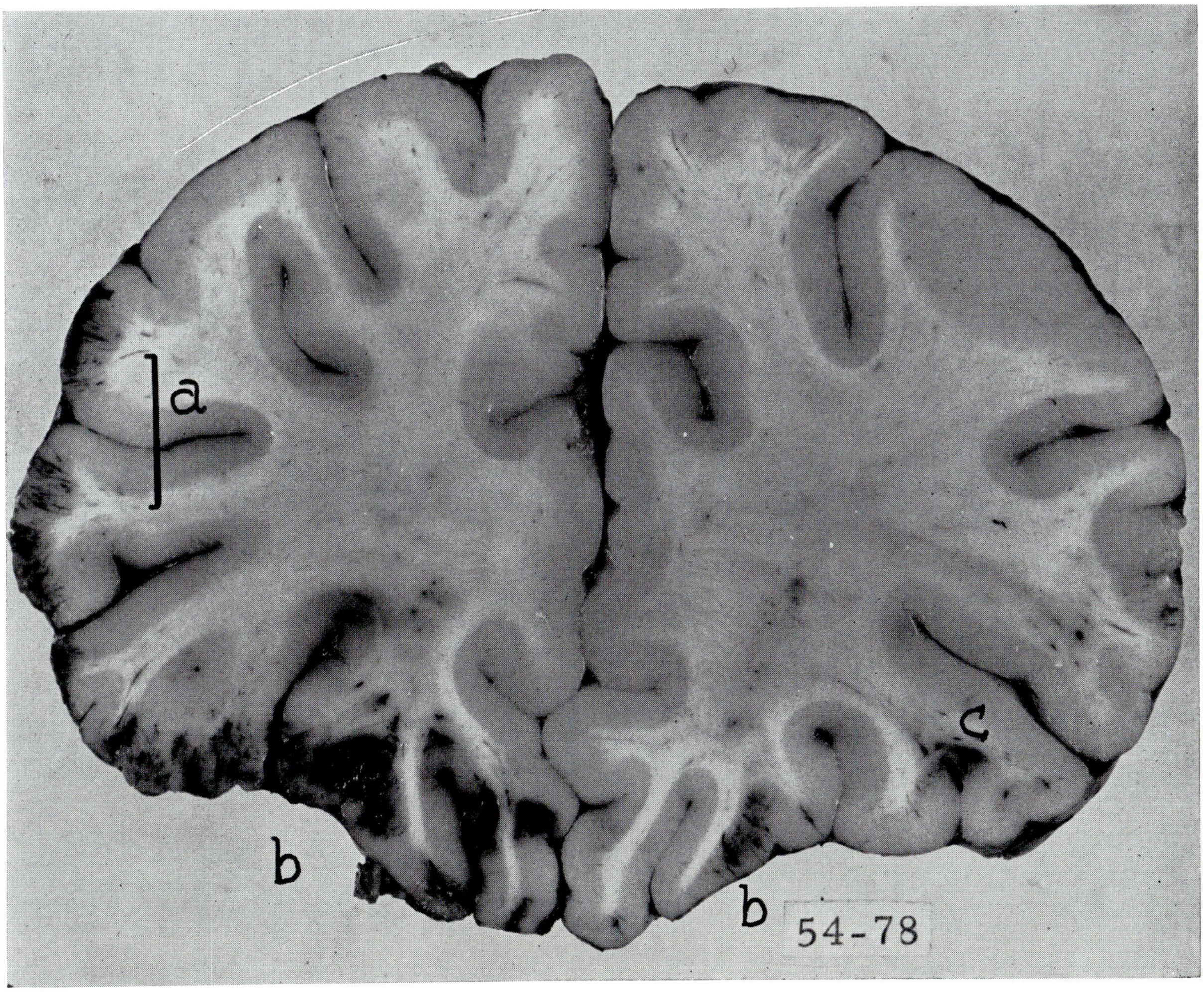


FIGURE XVII-12. Characteristic streaklike, densely arranged contusion hemorrhages in the cortex of the left frontal (a) and both orbital lobes (b). One contusion hemorrhage in the depth of the sulcus (c).

are more or less densely arranged and often elongated, radially pointing towards the white matter. This is illustrated in Figure XVII-12 on a coronal section through the posterior frontal lobes. The tiny, often streaklike hemorrhages characteristically occupy the crest of the second and third frontal convolution on the left (a) and the cortex of both orbital lobes (b) where they face the orbital roof. These hemorrhages should not be mistaken for those occurring in hemorrhagic cortical necrosis, a frequent secondary circulatory lesion in head injuries (*See* Fig. XVII-32). The hemorrhages in such necroses are due to the escape of red blood cells through the damaged walls of congested vessels. Contusion hemorrhages, however, originate from tears in small blood vessels and first accumulate in the perivascular spaces along the shrivelled and collapsed blood vessels. Furthermore, the hemorrhagic necrosis is seldom limited to the crest of a convolution. Instead, it follows the cortex around the sulcus and often involves several convolutions in this way. Occasionally, contusion hemorrhages occur in the cortex facing a sulcus, particularly where it circles around the depth of a sulcus. The hemor-

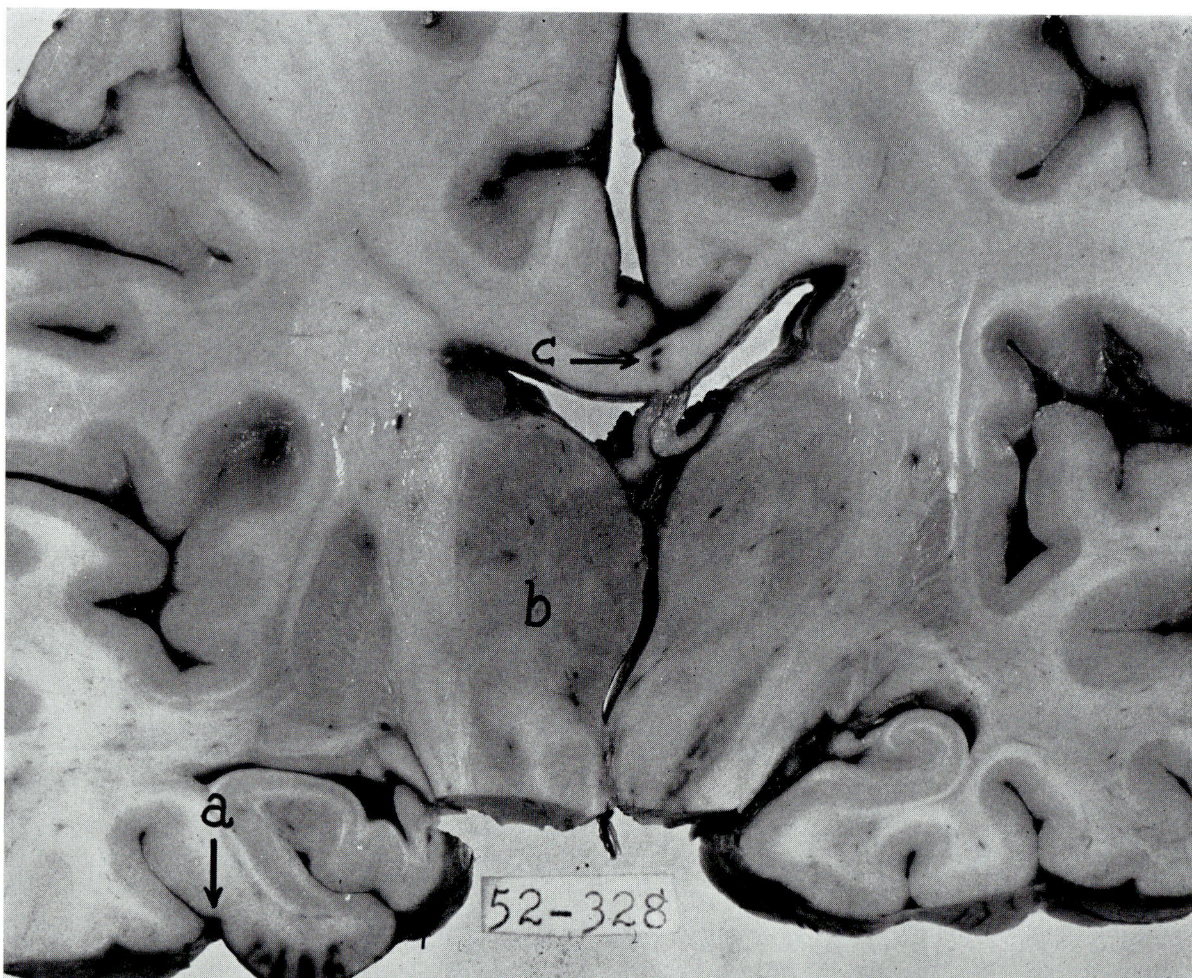


FIGURE XVII-13. Streaklike contusion hemorrhages in the cortex of the left hippocampal gyrus caused at the moment of impact by striking against the tentorial margin, now located medially from tentorial notching (a) due to herniation of the hippocampal gyrus. Shifting of the left thalamus (b) to the right and two punctate contusion hemorrhages in the corpus callosum (c).

rhage seen in the lateral right orbital lobe is an example (c). It is usually associated with some subarachnoid hemorrhage collecting in the depth of the sulcus.

Even if there are only a few contusion hemorrhages at the crest, it is not difficult to recognize them as traumatic lesions by their columnar arrangement perpendicular to the surface of the convolution. This is exemplified by Figure XVII-13, in which such streaklike contusions involve the cortex of the hippocampal gyrus. They occurred when the left hemisphere suddenly shifted downwards and this portion of the cortex was pressed against the margin of the tentorium at a time when this margin was still in normal anatomic relationship to the cortex. In the present case, a subdural hematoma developed over the same hemisphere. It caused shifting of the left thalamus (b) to the right and herniation of the hippocampal gyrus over the margin of the tentorium, which ultimately caused the notching (a) to the left of the contusion hemorrhages. This illustrates that the contusion hemorrhages were present prior to herniation, participated in the shifting of the brain tissues and are now located medially from the tentorial margin. If local pressure necrosis had developed, it would have been located laterally from the area of the contusions where the tentorial notching is seen. The two small sharply outlined hemorrhages in the center of the corpus callosum (c) are also contusion hemorrhages. They occurred simultaneously with those in the hippocampal cortex when the person fell on

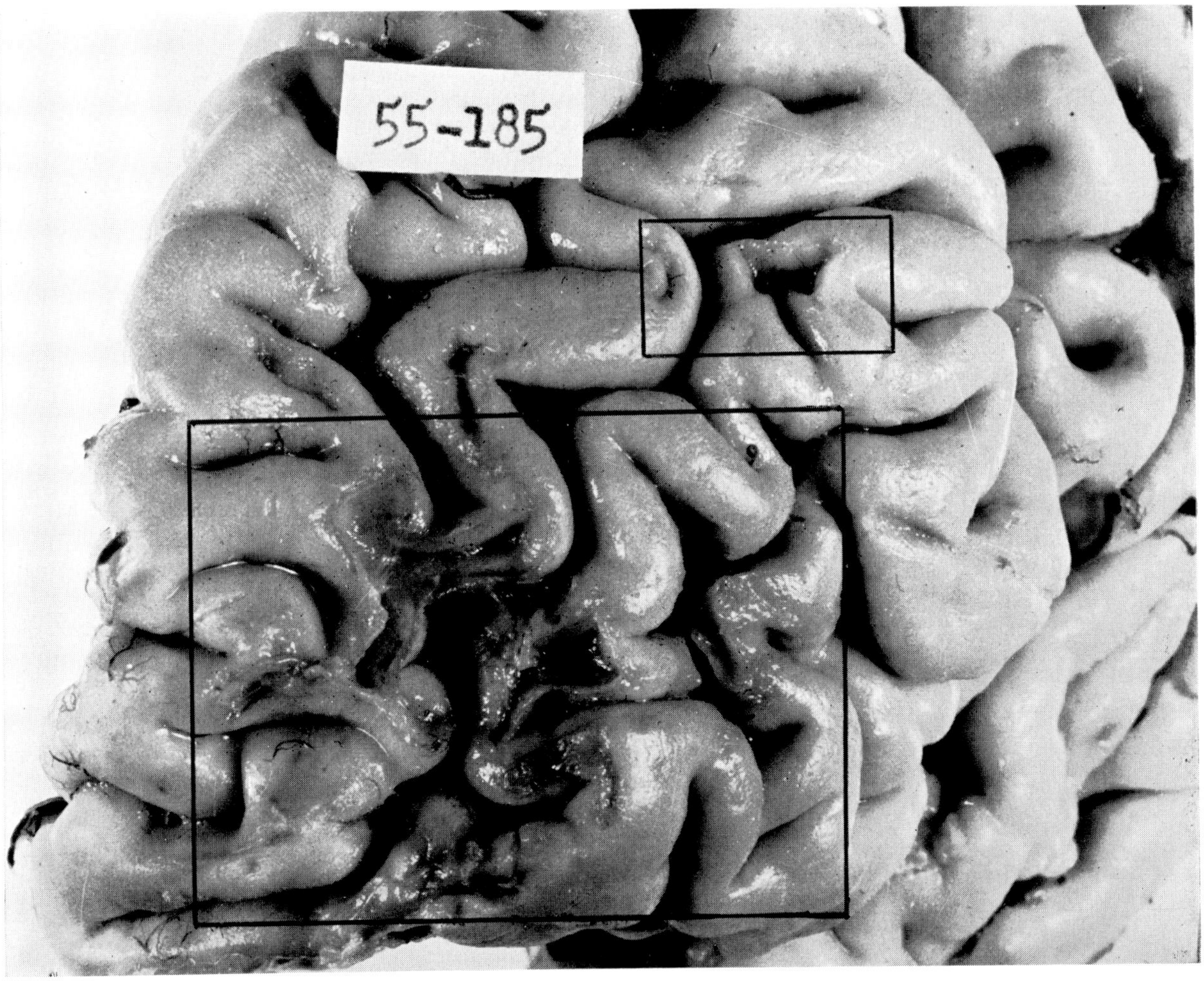


FIGURE XVII-14. Old cortical contusions typically located at the crests of convolutions (framed).

the top of his head and the corpus was shifted downwards and at the same time stretched to either side.

With longer survival, cortical hemorrhages often enlarge. They may form miniature hematomas or a larger hematoma by coalescence. This is not unusual in individuals with hypertension or in alcoholics, because they often have an abnormal coagulation mechanism. In rare instances a larger artery is damaged, and the hematoma may extend through the white matter and rupture into a lateral ventricle. Such a hematoma may be the only contusion throughout the entire brain if the head was struck by a small object producing a momentary localized depression of the skull that incidentally contused the artery. In falls on the head, frontal and temporal white matter are sites of predilection for the development of hematomas. They may be arterial in origin or result from coalescence of venous contusion hemorrhages. Temporal lobe hematomas often destroy the optic radiation. If the patient survives, this produces homonymous hemianopsia towards the opposite side from the injury. An air study may reveal that there is a free communication between the lateral ventricle and the subarachnoid space, called *traumatic porencephaly*.

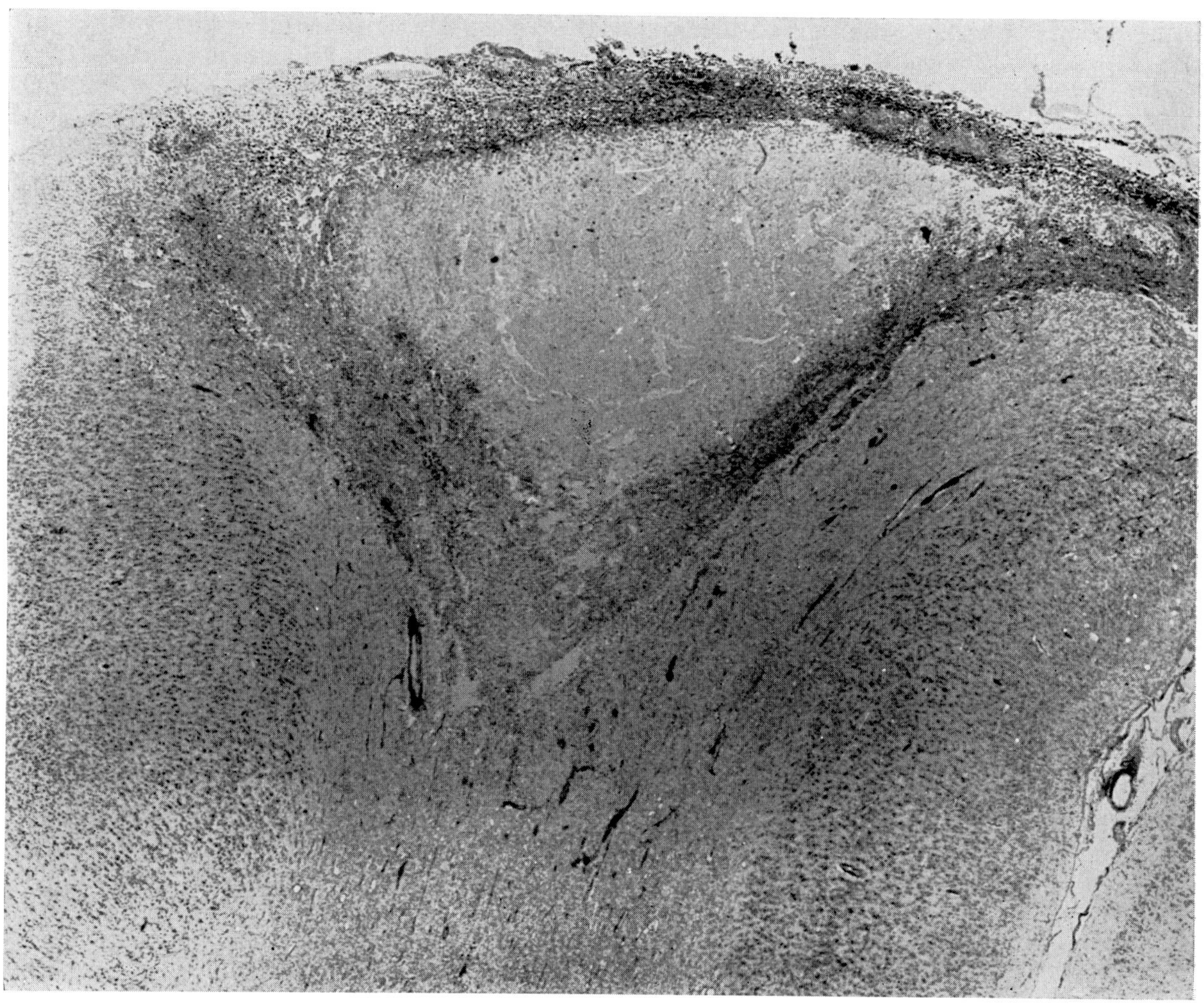

FIGURE XVII-15. Histologic section (Nissl's stain) of a cortical contusion necrosis survived for three months. Phagocytosis along the margin of a triangular coagulation necrosis. Destruction of the outer layer of the cortex.

### *Contusion Necroses*

It is not generally realized that contusion necroses constitute a separate entity among contusions. In their ultimate cystic phase they have been known for a long time and were called in the French literature *plaques jaunes* or *état vermoulu.* They were considered to be a variation of circulatory lesions, most likely due to arteriosclerosis. As can be seen in Figure XVII-14, they are essentially located at the crest of convolutions and form small clefts, irregularly shaped holes or trenches with sharply outlined walls. If they are not many years old, they are somewhat brown in color. If the leptomeninges are removed, as they were in this case, one finds that they openly communicate with the subarachnoid space and usually contain no network of residual blood vessels so frequently seen in cystic infarcts. On cut sections most necroses are triangular or wedgelike, the wedge pointing into the white matter. In contrast to most circulatory lesions of the same size, the margins of contusion necroses are surprisingly straight, as if cut by a knife. This can be recognized as early after injury as three to five hours. Phagocytosis of the necrotic tissue takes place from the margins of the contusion. The cellular reaction within these marginal areas permits assessment of the age of the lesion.[5] The necrotic core is only gradually broken down. In a three-month-old cortical contusion unaltered necrotic tissue may still persist in the center of the lesion, as is illustrated in Figure XVII-15.

Removal of the necrotic tissue also proceeds along the outer surface of the lesion by cells derived from the subarachnoid tissue network and the pia. This is another important criterion for differentiating contusion necrosis from a circulatory infarct of similar size. Such an infarct is covered towards the pia by a glial membrane, as most of the first cortical layer survives. Over contusion necroses, the first layer of the cortex is always destroyed, except for short stumps. This serves to illustrate that the necrosis of a cortical contusion is mechanically induced and not the result of a circulatory disorder secondary to thrombosis or spasm of blood vessels. Cortical contusion occurs at the moment of impact, when the crest of the convolution is flattened or depressed by striking against the dura.

Since this deformation of the crest spreads from the point of impact to the periphery of the convolution, the tissues at this point are pushed deepest towards the white matter, while displacement of the adjacent areas of the crest decreases in depth on either side. This explains the triangular shape of a cortical contusion and is diagrammatically illustrated in Figure XVII-16, which shows the deformation of the skull resulting from a blow. The same happens if the convolution is suddenly pushed against the stationary bone, as in a fall. In either case, this process of laterally spreading deformation produces shearing forces within a wedgelike area of tissue. Their action on submicroscopic structures is the cause of the necrosis. If several adjacent convolutions are involved, the lesions are characterized by the persistence of multiple U-shaped portions of cortex (a) around deeper parts of sulci and the absence of those portions that formerly formed the crest of the convolutions. This is illustrated in Figure XVII-17. Both orbital lobes are involved by old contusions. In addition to the horseshoe-like remnants of cortex (a), there is decreased density of the subcortical white matter on either side (b). This

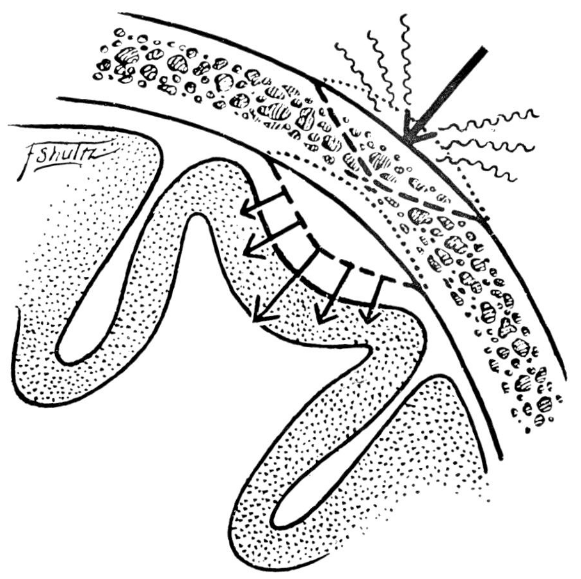

Figure XVII-16. Diagram showing distribution of forces caused by blunt impact to the skull.

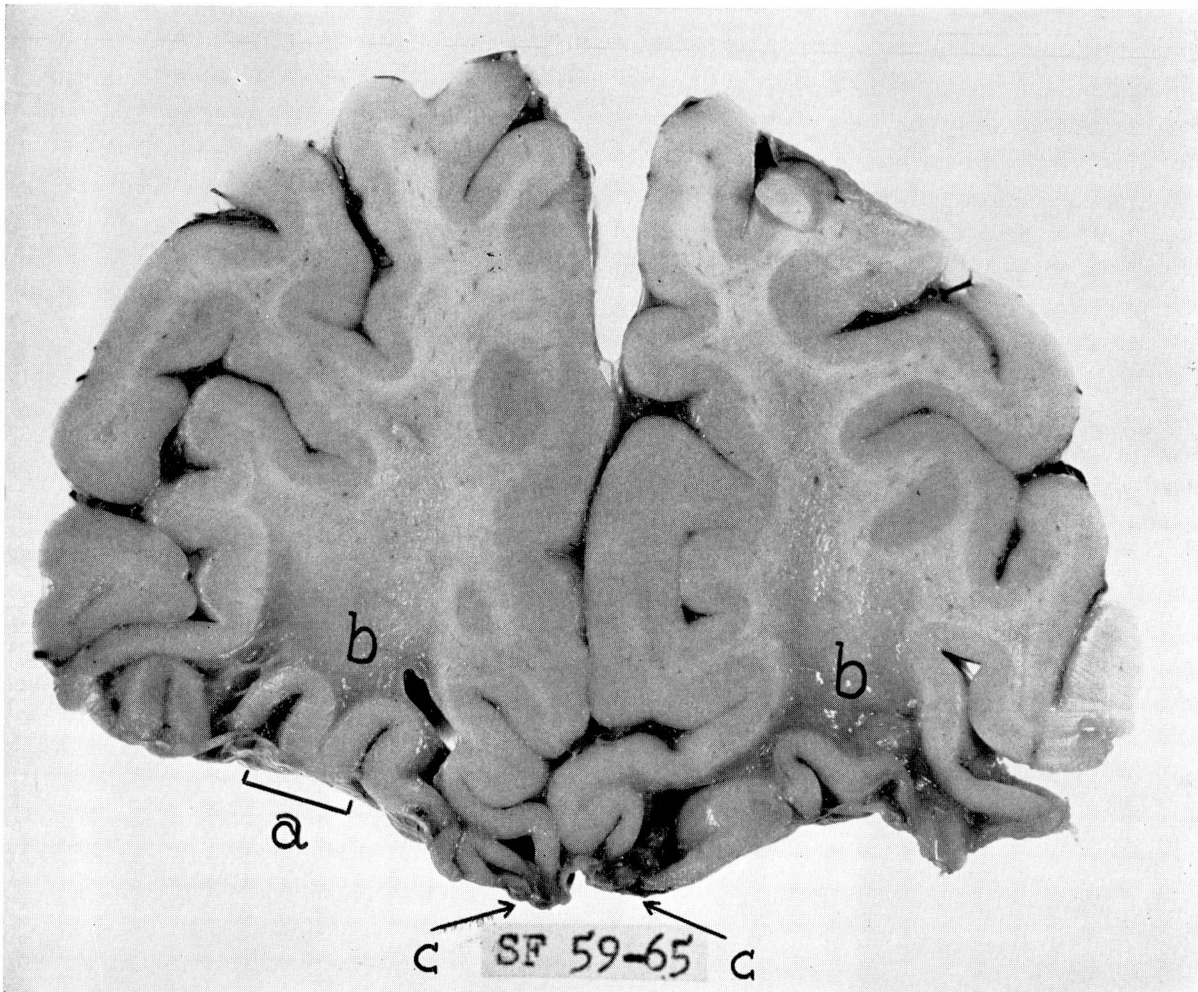


FIGURE XVII-17. Old cortical contusion necroses of the orbital lobe, showing loss of crests of the convolutions and persistence of U-shaped portions of the cortex (a) around the depths of the sulci. Decreased density of subcortical white matter (b) from former swelling and degeneration of nerve fibers. Destruction of the olfactory tracts (c).

is due in part to degeneration of fiber tracts and in part to former swelling.

### *Contusion Tears*

Contusion tears are caused by stretching and shearing forces within the tissues produced by blunt force. In infants up to the age of five months they are the dominant type of contusion. At this young age the skull is easily deformed, and the immature brain is quite soft. The tears usually involve the white matter of the upper frontal convolutions, orbital lobes and temporal lobes. These slitlike, sometimes irregularly shaped lesions often contain so little blood that they may be mistaken for artifacts.[6] Illustrations and further discussion are found in Chapter XVIII.

In the adult brain incomplete and sometimes complete tearing of the corpus callosum is not an unusual finding in falls on the forehead or the convexity of the skull, as will be discussed. Tears in other parts of the cerebral white and gray matter are extremely rare. In severe, instantly fatal injuries with extensive fractures of the skull, the midbrain or the lower medulla oblongata may be completely torn. Because of the absence of hemorrhage it is difficult to tell from this finding itself whether these tears are genuinely traumatic or postmortem artifacts.

Tearing of the pyramidal motor fibers at the junction of the pons and the medulla oblongata deserves special mention. These tears are often not artifacts but true traumatic lesions and as such are usually accompanied by very small perivascular hemorrhages, which tend to spread into the posterior base and the tegmentum of the lower pons (Fig. XVII-18). In some cases there is subarachnoid hemorrhage and sometimes a subarachnoid hematoma over the base of the brain. These tears with their associated findings constitute a traumatic entity. They are the result of a sudden overextension of the head.[7] Such severe overextension most often occurs in falls on the face accompanied by a somersault movement of the body in reverse, and in automobile collisions when the occupant is thrown forward and his head arrested by the dashboard or the steering wheel while his body continues to move beneath it. The case of a man who fell with his shoulder on the rim of a bathtub and received these tears was cited earlier. In most of these cases contusions in other portions of the brain are minor or absent.

### *Classification of Contusions According to Causative Mechanism*

It is customary to distinguish between coup and contrecoup contusions. The word *coup*

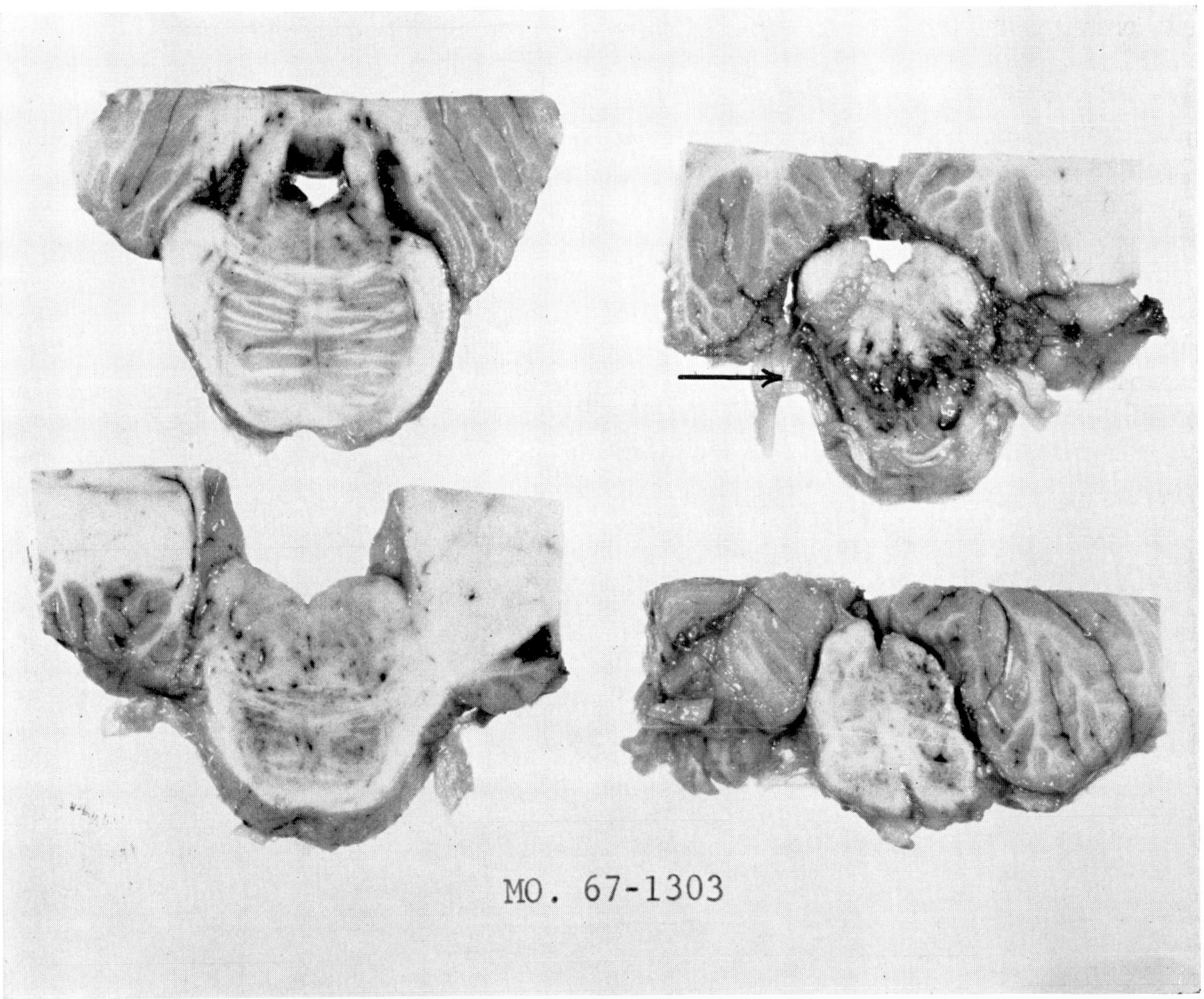


FIGURE XVII-18. Tear in the pyramids at the junctions of the pons and medulla oblongata (arrow) associated with punctate hemorrhages caused by hyperextension of the head in a pedestrian who was struck by a car. Death was instantaneous.

(impact) signifies that the contusions are located beneath the area of impact and were caused directly by the impacting force. The word *contrecoup* means that the lesions are located in an area opposite the side of impact. A line drawn between the centers of both areas corresponds to the direction of the impact relative to the head.

In many cases there are additional contusions noted in the brain that do not fit into either of these groups. Lindenberg and Freytag[8] introduced new names for these lesions, characterizing their particular causative mechanism. Lesions found in deeper structures of the brain along the line of impact are called *intermediary coup contusions*, the word *coup* signifying the relationship to the direction of impact. Contusions caused by fracture of the skull are called *fracture contusions*. Hemorrhages or individual hematomas in the cortex and white matter of the frontal and central convolutions near the upper margin of the hemispheres may be the only contusions throughout the brain and show no relationship to the area and direction of the impact. They are called *gliding contusions* and are attributed to stretching and shearing forces occurring in the region of the pacchionian granulations during a brief back-and-forth gliding of the brain within the skull in response to a moderately severe impact. Finally, contusions in the cerebellar tonsils and the medulla oblongata caused by a momentary shifting of the brain towards the foramen magnum are named *herniation contusions*. They have been discussed previously as distant contusions occurring in gunshot injuries (*see* Figs. XVII-9 and 10) and are also seen in injuries from a blow with a blunt object.

Identification of these types of contusions is important, since only bona fide coup, intermediary coup and contrecoup contusions can be used for reconstructing the direction of the impacting force, for estimating its relative magnitude and for determining whether the head was struck by an object (blow) or whether it struck an object in a fall or fall-like motion. The latter determination is often of greatest importance in cases of alleged homicide.

As is stated in Table XVII-II, a blow to the head produces coup contusions, while contrecoup contusions are either small or absent. Conversely, in a fall on the head, contrecoup contutions occur while coup contusions are small or absent. Only if a person falls on a sharp or pointed object, such as the sharp corner of a piece of furniture, may the findings be the same as those caused by a blow with a blunt instrument.

How can this phenomenon be explained? Since 1766, when the Royal Academy of Surgeons in Paris offered a prize for the best theoretical explanation of the mechanism of contrecoup, numerous investigators have devoted their efforts to solve the problem, but have

TABLE XVII-II

CONTUSIONS

| Dependent on Site and Direction of Impact | Independent of Site and Direction of Impact |
|---|---|
| COUP – INTERMEDIARY COUP – CONTRECOUP CONTUSIONS | FRACTURE – GLIDING – HERNIATION CONTUSIONS |
| ↓ BLOW to the Movable, Resting Head<br>Acceleration Simultaneous With Indentation of Skull | → FALL on the Head<br>Acceleration Preceding Indentation of Skull |
| COUP – no or small CONTRECOUP CONTUSIONS | CONTRECOUP – no or small COUP CONTUSIONS |

been unable to come up with a solution explaining all findings observed at autopsy.[9] On the basis of the findings in a number of selected cases, we attempted to retrace the physical events which take place.[8] The following represents our conclusions.

## PHYSICAL EVENTS IN IMPACTS BY BLUNT FORCE AND RELATED LESIONS

### Minor Impacts

The effects of a minor blow to the resting but movable head, as by a fist, will be considered first. Without deforming the skull, such a blow produces a momentary acceleration of the head. The acceleration is more or less rotational, since the head is eccentrically affixed to the spinal column and the neck. This abrupt acceleration reaches its peak shortly after the head is set in motion. The brain, as a large mass, is inert to such fast acceleration. This produces a positive pressure between the brain and the skull at the site of the impact and a negative pressure over the opposite surface of the brain. This is indicated in Figure XVII-19 by the white plus and minus signs. The white arrow signifies that the brain resists the pressure by the skull, which is moving in the direction of the black arrow. Since these intracranial pressures result from acceleration of the skull, they are called acceleration pressures. When the head returns to its normal position, the brain tends to continue in the direction of its motion. This reverses the pressures, and a rapidly subsiding rotational movement of the brain relative to the skull follows. This movement is possible because of the presence of the subdural space, permitting gliding of the arachnoid relative to the dura. Undoubtedly, the initial acceleration pressures are the greatest, but neither the positive acceleration pressure at the site of impact nor the negative pressure on the opposite side produce coup or contrecoup contusions. Instead, subdural and subarachnoid bleeding and, less commonly, gliding contusions in the upper marginal portions of the cerebral hemispheres may result, as was mentioned previously.

In a minor fall on the head the skull is suddenly decelerated, and the brain tends to *continue falling* because of its momentum. The brain is suddenly pressed against the skull at the site of impact, and a corresponding negative pressure is present on the opposite surface of the brain. These forces subside rapidly or become reversed with decreasing magnitude if the head bounces. They are too insignificant to produce coup or contrecoup contusions but may give rise to the same lesions as described for minor blows to the head.

### Major Impacts

Changes in the brain at the moment of a severe blow to the head that causes depression

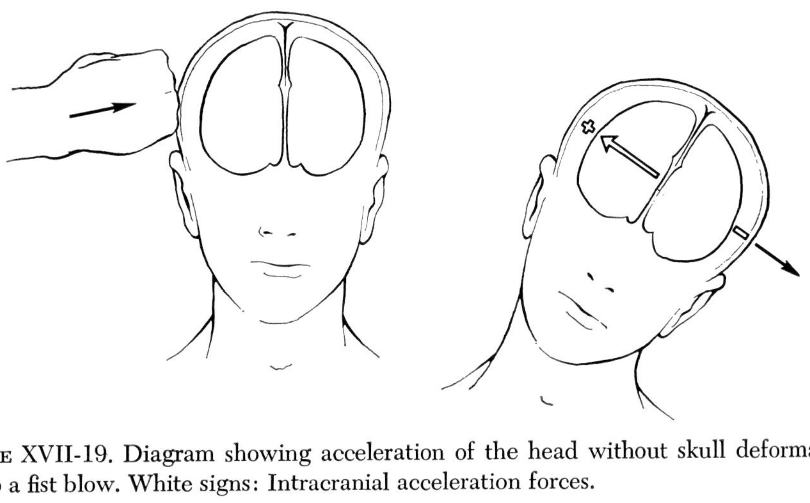

FIGURE XVII-19. Diagram showing acceleration of the head without skull deformation, due to a fist blow. White signs: Intracranial acceleration forces.

or flattening of the impact area are considered in the following pages. The depression of the skull acts as a momentary space-occupying lesion and initially creates only positive intracranial pressure lasting a few milliseconds. It is greatest at the site of impact where the deforming bone presses on the underlying hemisphere of the brain, forcing it to momentarily shift, mainly towards the opposite side. Since at the moment of this deformation the head is accelerated, two positive pressures act on the brain tissue subjacent to the site of depression. This is indicated in Figure XVII-20 by the two plus signs, the black one signifying deformation pressure. Since the pressure associated with the shifting of the brain (black arrow) is counteracted by the acceleration pressure (white arrow), which moves the brain to the opposite side, it may not reach the opposite surface of the brain, or if it does, it may be neutralized there by the simultaneously existing negative acceleration pressure. This explains why in a major skull-deforming blow coup contusions are always present. Only when the deformation at the site of impact is so great that at the opposite side the brain is pressed against the skull will contrecoup contusions develop also.

Much depends on the mass of tissue between the site of impact and the potential area for contrecoup. Thus, a blow of a certain force inflicted to the convexity of the forehead may produce contrecoup contusions in the orbital cortex but if applied to the side of the head may fail to do so. If the deformation pressure is not sufficiently severe to result in contrecoup contusions, the brain may shift towards the area of least resistance, the foramen magnum, producing momentary herniation of the tonsils of the cerebellum. Tonsillar herniation contusions are thus frequently observed not only in gunshot wounds but also in blows to the head, causing only coup contusions. However, if contrecoup contusions are produced, tonsillar herniation contusions are absent.

In general, deformation of the skull leads to fracture. If the fracture remains depressed, it is further evidence that coup and contrecoup contusions are caused by the initial positive pressure and not by a negative sucking force, which would have followed with the return of the normal contour of the skull.

In a more severe fall the head is accelerated prior to impact and deformation of the skull. Consequently, in a fall on the back of the head,

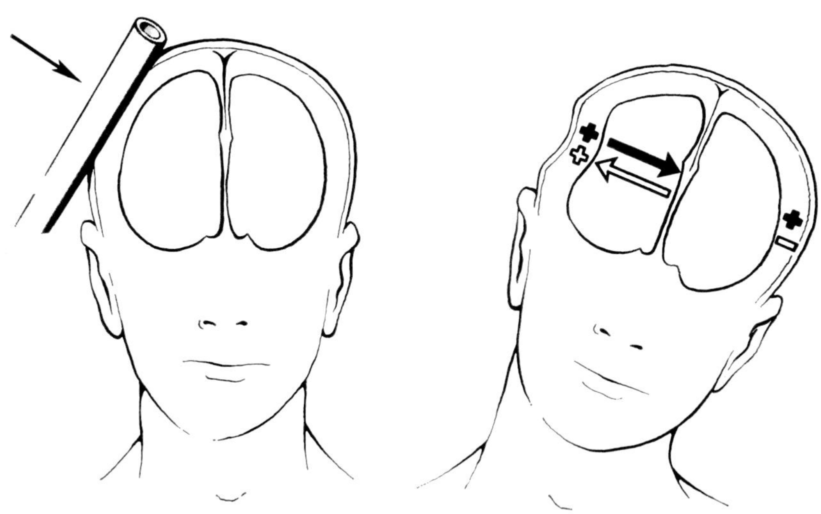

FIGURE XVII-20. Diagram showing the combination of acceleration and deformation of the head during a severe blow by a blunt instrument. White signs: Intercranial acceleration forces. Black signs: Deformation forces. Note the two positive forces at the site of the coup.

the inertia of the brain produces a positive acceleration pressure over the fronto-orbital region and negative acceleration pressure over the occipital and cerebellar regions of the brain. These pressures last until the deformation of the skull at the site of impact reaches its maximum. Since with the onset of this deformation the brain becomes displaced towards the opposite side, two positive forces act on the fronto-orbital cortex. At the site of impact, however, the positive force of deformation is diminished by the still-existing negative acceleration pressure. This mechanism explains the formation of contrecoup contusions in falls on the head (Fig. XVII-21). The rate of acceleration of the head prior to impact has an important bearing on the production of contrecoup contusions. It has practically no upper limit. The deformation, however, has a limit beyond which the bone absorbs the excess of the deformation force by fracturing. Thus, with faster acceleration, the contrecoup damage increases in extent. The degree of acceleration does not depend on the height of the fall. It may be greater and produce more damage in a fall from a sitting position than from a standing position. In a fall from a high building, brain and skull accelerate at the same rate, and no acceleration pressures develop within the skull prior to impact. This explains why the skull may be totally fractured in such cases while coup and contrecoup contusions are minimal. Thus, fractures of the skull cannot be taken as evidence of the severity of brain involvement. On the contrary, one often finds most severe contusions in the absence of a fracture.

Finally, contusion hemorrhages occur if the shearing force within the tissues exceeds the cohesive strength of the vessel walls. For the production of contusion necrosis, however, a much greater force is needed. If the contusion necrosis involves the entire cortex and the respective white matter of two convolutions to form a large triangular lesion, the force was even greater than that necessary for producing a contusion necrosis at the crest of one convolution.

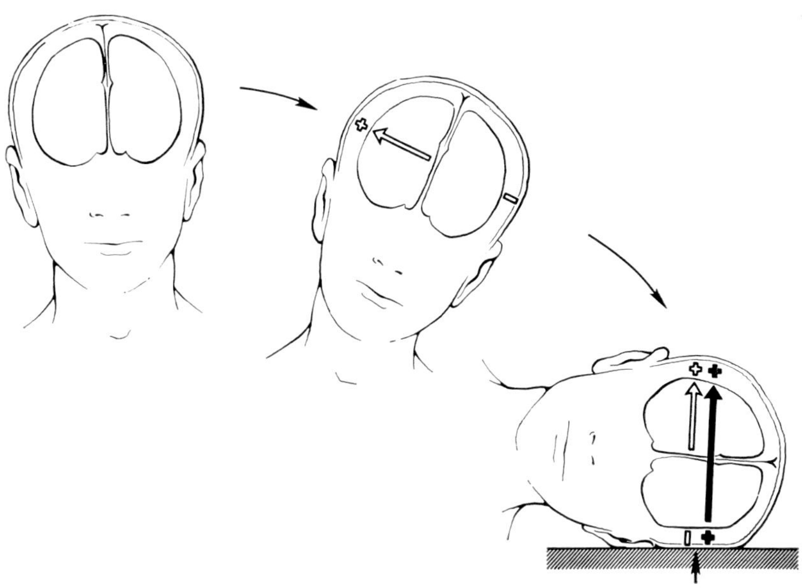

FIGURE XVII-21. Diagram showing acceleration during a fall prior to impact and the action of intracranial acceleration and deformation forces at the time of impact. White signs: Intracranial acceleration forces. Black signs: Deformation forces. Note the two positive forces at the site of the contrecoup.

## DISTRIBUTION PATTERNS OF CONTUSIONS CAUSED BY BLOW AND FALL

What has been stated about the mechanism and the respective patterns of distribution of coup and contrecoup lesions in blows to the head and in falls on the head is now illustrated by a few examples. Figure XVII-22 shows a large contusion in the left parietal lobe (a) as a result of a blow with a baseball bat. When a comminuted fracture in this area was lifted and partially removed during operation, the swollen, necrotic tissue interspersed by hemorrhages protruded against the unprotected dura. No contrecoup contusions are seen in the cortex of the right hemisphere. There are, however, herniation contusions in both cerebellar tonsils (arrows).

Another case (Fig. XVII-23) presented a multitude of fresh contusion hemorrhages in the cortex and white matter of almost the entire convexity of the right cerebral hemisphere (arrows) and even a few hemorrhages along the medial aspect of the hemisphere where it faces the falx (a). The left hemisphere shows not a single contrecoup contusion. The injury was caused by a horizontal blow to the right side of the skull with a heavy wooden board. The skull over the right hemisphere was fractured. The right hemisphere of the brain shown in Figure XVII-24 is equally damaged by a multitude of fresh contusion hemorrhages. However, these lesions are all contrecoup contusions

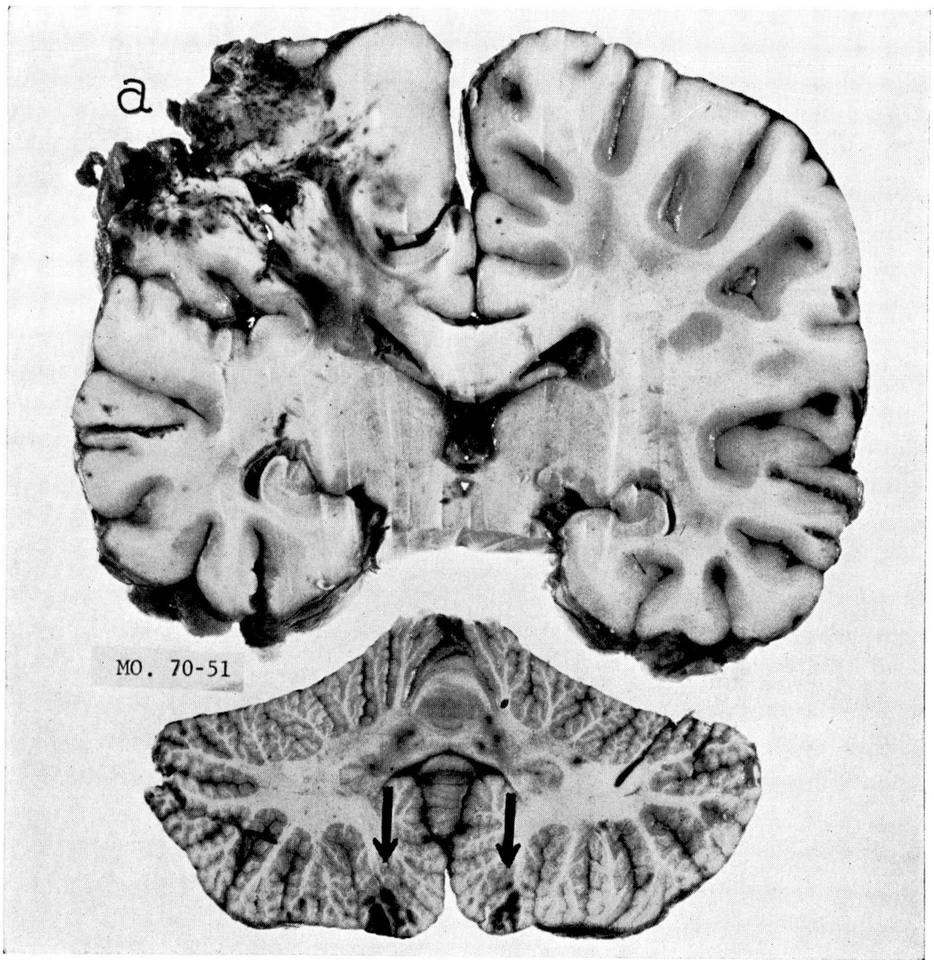


FIGURE XVII-22. Large coup contusion in the left parietal region (a) due to a blow with a baseball bat. Herniation contusions in both cerebellar tonsils (arrows). No contrecoup contusions. Survival one hour.

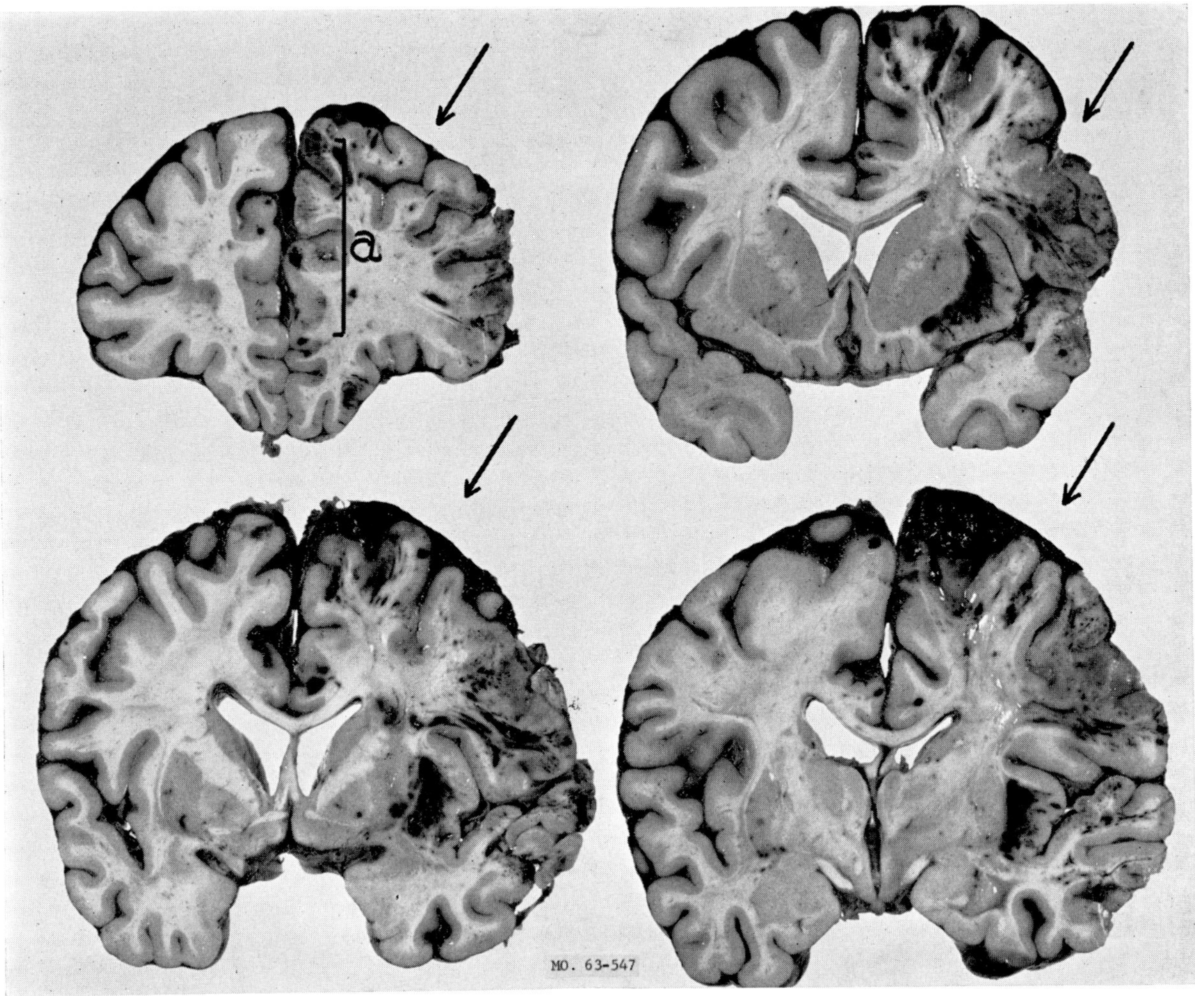


FIGURE XVII-23. Extensive coup contusions in the right cerebral hemisphere (arrows) caused by a blow to the right side of the head with a wooden board. Few contusion hemorrhages along the medial aspect of the right cerebral hemisphere (a). No contrecoup contusions. Found dead.

received in a fall on the left side of the head. The only coup contusion present involves the left temporal convolution near the pole (arrow). There was only a short linear fracture of the skull over the lateral portion of the left hemisphere.

Figure XVII-25 illustrates the classical location of contrecoup contusions (arrow) in the frontal pole, orbital lobe and temporal pole caused by a fall on the back of the head. No coup contusion is present. The final outcome of such lesions was shown in Figure XVII-17. It is of clinical interest that in this type of injury both olfactory nerves are often destroyed, resulting in total or one-sided loss of the sense of smell. The sense of smell should therefore be tested in every patient with posttraumatic complaints. A negative result does not preclude damage to other parts of the brain. If the patient is anosmic (cannot smell), other causes should be ruled out, such as congenital absence of the olfactory nerves, an olfactory groove meningioma or alterations of the nose, the upper nasopharynx and the ethmoidal sinuses.

Destruction of the orbital convolutions produces a change in personality. These persons

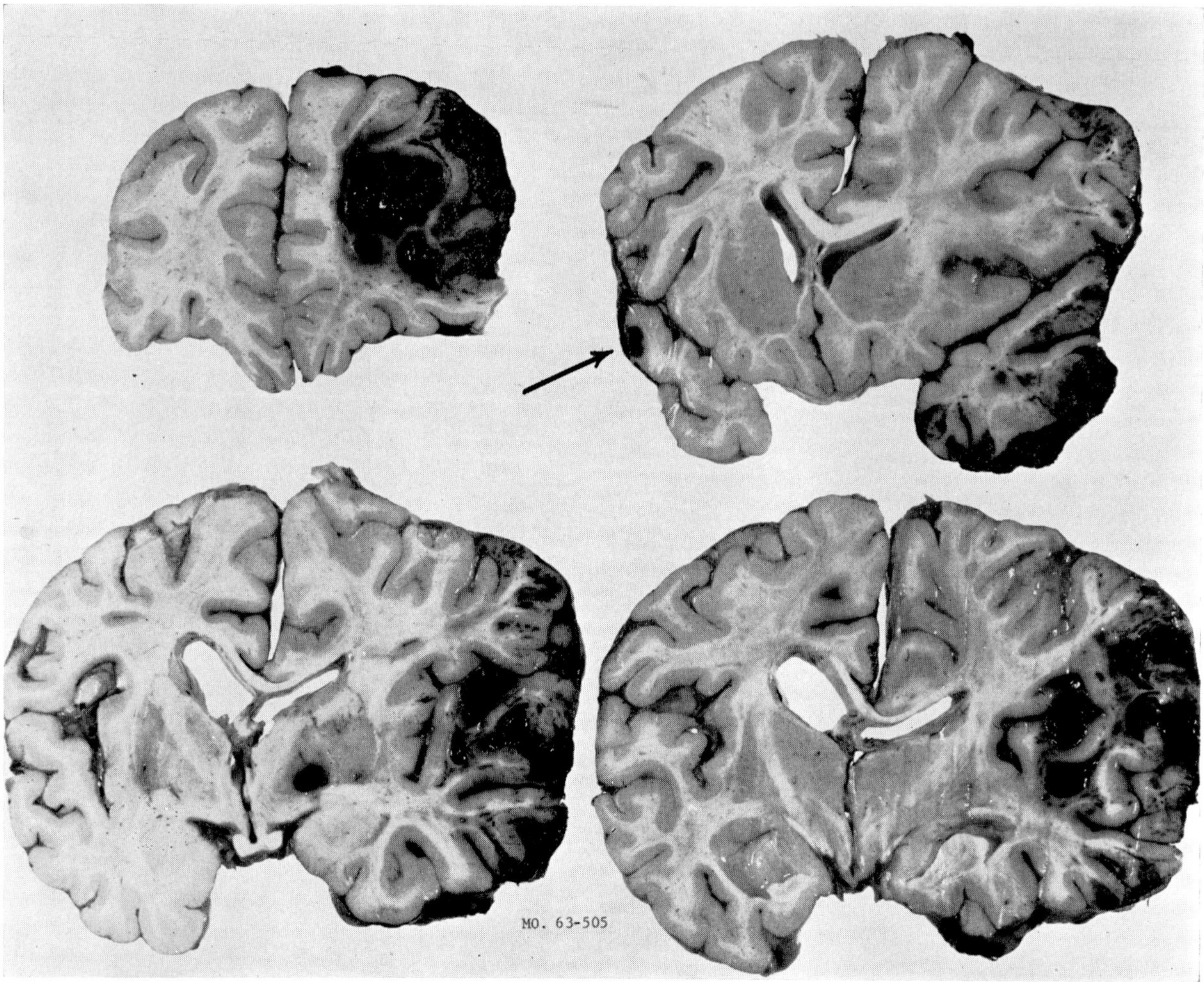


FIGURE XVII-24. Severe contrecoup contusions in the right cerebral hemisphere caused by a fall on the left side of the head. Small coup contusion near the left temporal pole (arrow). Survival fourteen hours.

usually become hypermanic and in their elevated mood care little about themselves and socially established customs or laws. They become uninhibited and ethically unrestrained, although they know the difference between right and wrong.

It would be wrong to assume that in a fall on the back of the head the orbital lobes are always damaged. The determining factor is the precise location of the impact on the back of the head and the direction of the impact relative to the head. In the case shown in Figure XVII-26, the deceased had fallen on the back of the head, but the impact area was off the midline to the left, as can be seen by the small coup contusion in the left cerebellar hemisphere (a). The direction of the impact was pointed towards the right lower central and precentral area. The orbital lobes and olfactory nerves remained largely intact. Instead, the contrecoup contusions involved the right frontal pole (b) and predominantly the precentral, central and adjacent temporal convolutions (c). If the patient had been genuinely left handed and had survived, he would have shown a motor weakness in the opposite side of the face and in the opposite arm as well as so-called motoric aphasia, characterized by inability to say words understandably and properly while understanding their meaning. One such patient personally ob-

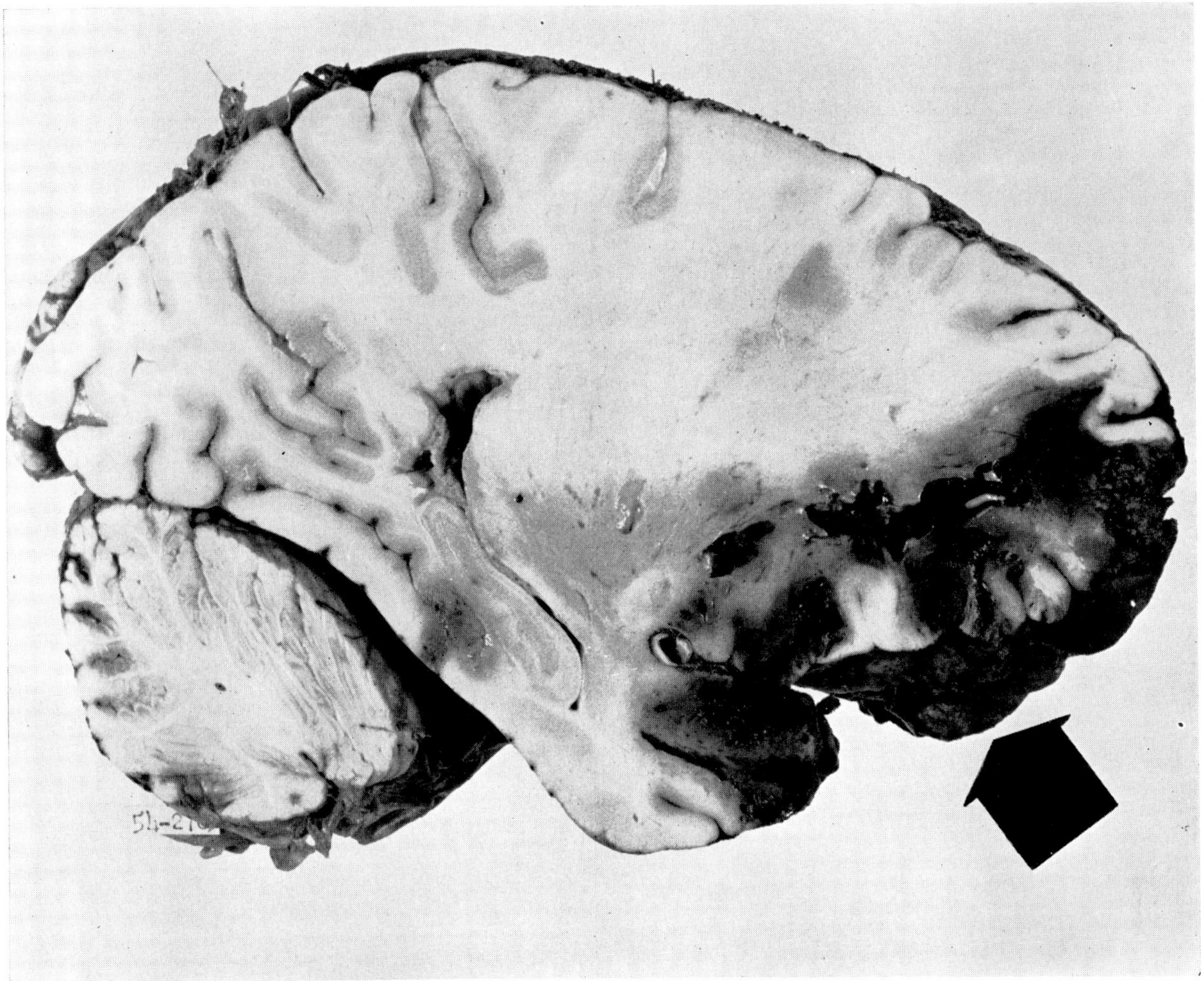

FIGURE XVII-25. Large contrecoup contusions in the right frontal pole, orbital lobe and temporal pole (arrow) due to a fall on the back of the head. No coup contusions. Survival nine hours.

served appeared to be intelligent according to his behavior and his actions. However, when asked a question, he answered with a jumble of words without coherent meaning.

The diagram in Figure XVII-27 shows five variations of a fall on the back of the head. Not only the impact area but also the direction of the injury as reconstructed from the findings differed. Case 1 fell on the right parieto-occipital region, and all contrecoup contusions were located in the left temporal lobe. Case 2 corresponds to the one shown in Figure XVII-25 and Case 3 to that shown in Figure XVII-26. Case 4 fell on the cerebellar region, and the force of impact traveled forward, causing contrecoup contusions in the pons and only a few small contrecoup contusions in one gyrus rectus. Case 5 fell on the lower surface of the occipital region and showed intermediary coup contusions in the tegmentum of the pons and in the cerebellum, contrecoup contusions in the lower temporal lobes and multiple hemorrhages in the thalami.

In general, falls on the back or on one side of the head seldom produce contusions in deeper structures of the brain. The same is true of blows to the head producing coup and contrecoup contusions. The situation is quite different, how-

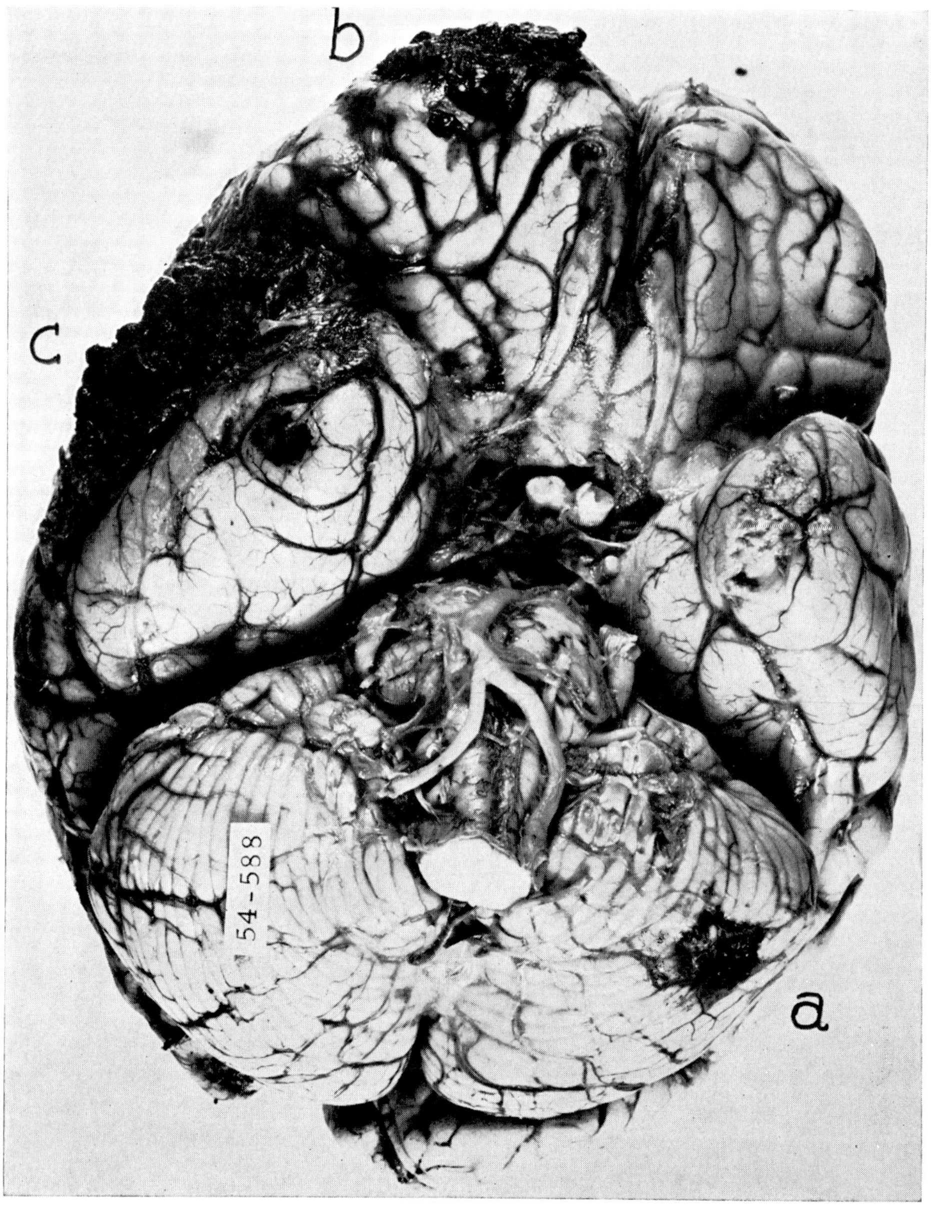


FIGURE XVII-26. Base of the brain. A fall on the left side of the back of the head resulted in a small coup contusion in the left cerebellum (a) and large contrecoup contusions in the right frontal pole (b) and frontotemporal convexity (c). Orbital lobes are not injured. Survival twelve days.

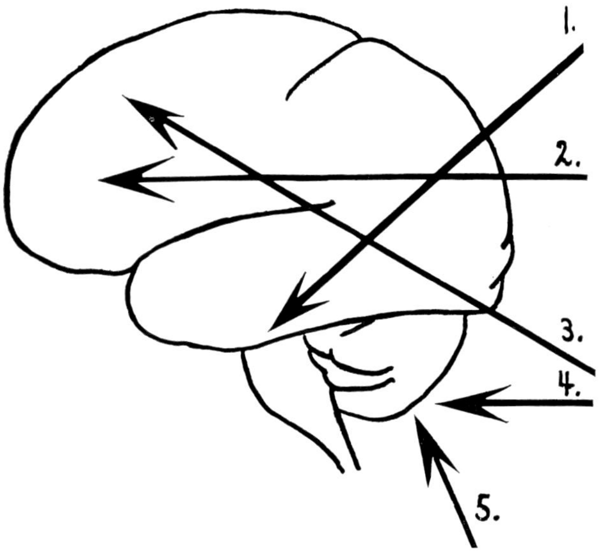


FIGURE XVII-27. Diagram showing various impact directions due to a fall on the back of the head.

ever, if the accelerated head strikes an unyielding object with the forehead or the convexity above the level of the corpus callosum. This occurs if a pedestrian who is struck by a motor vehicle is thrown through the air and lands on the forehead or the convexity of the head, or if in a collision an occupant of a vehicle is suddenly thrown forward, striking his head on the dashboard or the window frame. In these cases deformation of the forehead or convexity of the head shifts the brain along the line of the direction of the impact towards the tentorium and its opening. At the same time, elongation of the axis between both temples occurs, due to bulging of the temporal bones. The combined deformations often produce lesions in the corpus callosum ranging from hemorrhages to tears. Because of the shifting of the brain towards the tentorium, intermediary contusions may involve areas of the brain below the corpus callosum along the line of force (striate bodies, pallida, internal capsules and lower midbrain and pons).

Coup contusions may be seen in the first frontal or upper central convolutions, and contrecoup contusions commonly involve the unci and hippocampal gyri. Figure XVII-28 illustrates such a central pattern of lesions in the brain of a passenger of an automobile who was thrown forward in a collision, struck the top of his head against a firm structure and survived eight days. It is characteristic that cortical contusions take a subordinate role in such cases. They may be more pronounced if the face or forehead are the site of impact and the impact direction is parallel to the tentorial plane. In such injuries they may be found in the occipital lobes as contrecoup contusions.

The localization of the lesions in deeper structures can give rise to a variety of clinical signs and symptoms that may confuse the examining physician because it is usually believed that these structures are relatively well-protected against traumatic damage. A few examples are mentioned. Involvement of the pallidum and striate bodies may produce involuntary movements of the choreoathetotic type. Hemorrhages in the lower internal capsule may produce transient or permanent motor weakness in the face, arm or leg of the opposite side of the body. Lesions in the thalamus may influence the intellectual activity of the patient or produce a deficit in the perception of sensory stimuli in a portion of the body on the opposite side. Involvement of a lateral geniculate body, which receives visual impulses from the eye, may result in homonymous hemianopsia towards the opposite side. Lesions in the midbrain may involve the nuclei of the third and fourth cranial nerves with respective inabilities to move the eyes in certain directions. Damage of the substantia nigra may result in parkinsonism of the opposite side, with or without the characteristic involuntary shaking movements.

## SECONDARY ALTERATIONS

In many cases of head injury there are lesions in the brain that are neither wounds nor contusions. They develop after the injury took place and are called *secondary alterations.* Most of these are caused by circulatory disorders of various natures; others result from infection. Internal hydrocephalus belongs to this category. The changes as such are not specific for trauma

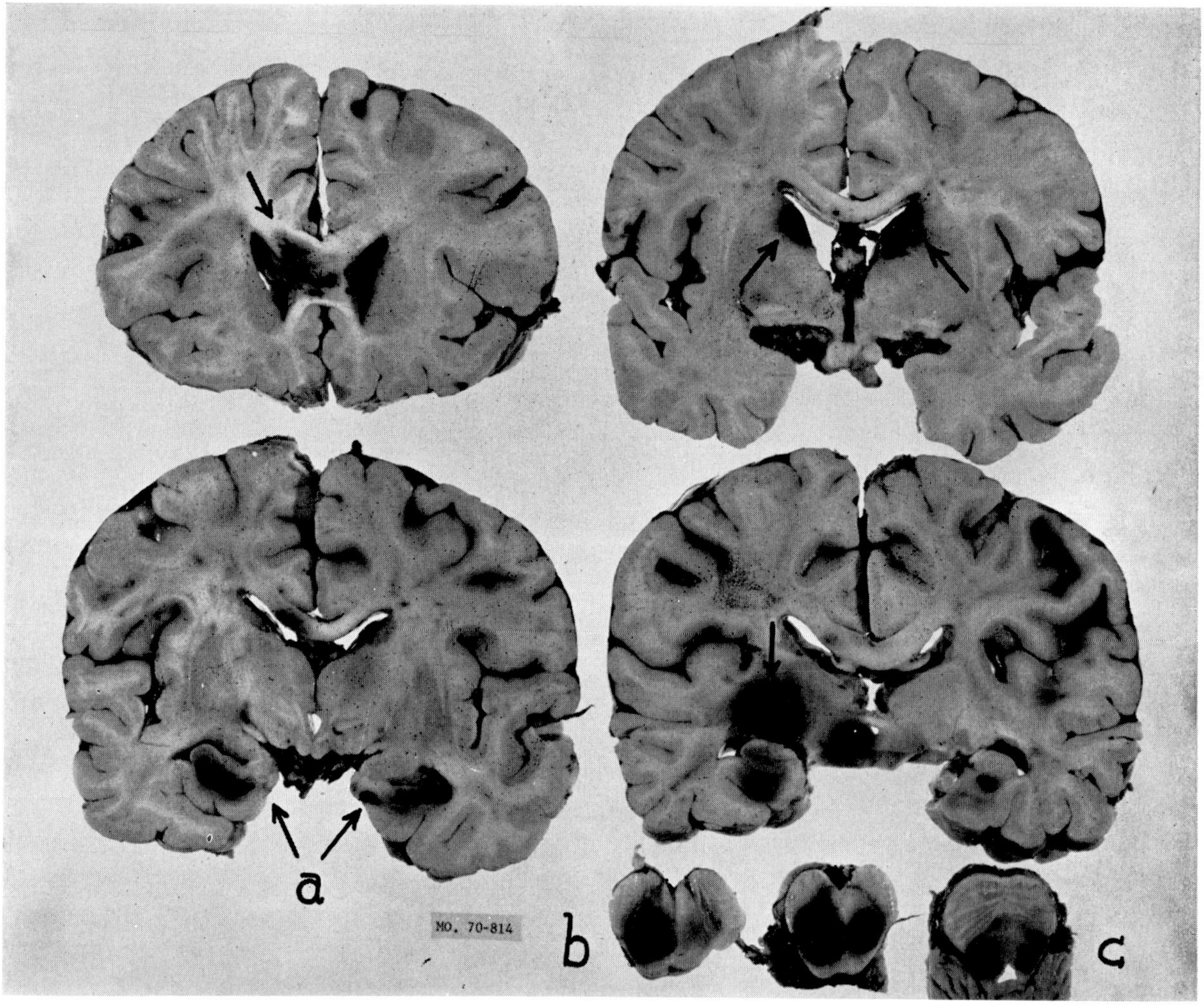


FIGURE XVII-28. Impact to the top of the head resulting in contrecoup contusions only in hippocampal gyri (a) and in intermediary coup contusions in the central structures of the cerebrum (arrows), midbrain (b) and pons (c). Survival eight days.

and may be observed in many nontraumatic situations. The circulatory alterations are the most frequent and important ones and are discussed first.

### Alterations Due to Circulatory Disorders

Circulatory disorders in the brain are manifested by swelling of the brain tissues, usually a reversible alteration, and by irreversible necrosis of cells, with or without hemorrhage.

The swelling may be perifocal and limited to the tissues surrounding a brain wound, a contusion hematoma or a contusion necrosis. It results from reduced perfusion with blood and contributes to the space-occupying effect of the respective lesion. On the other hand, the swelling may be generalized, involving both hemispheres of the brain and also the brain stem and the cerebellum. This overall swelling of the brain is usually referred to as posttraumatic brain swelling. It is one of the most important secondary changes, since it may develop very rapidly. By pressing on the midbrain and/or the medulla oblongata, it may cause death within twenty or thirty minutes, although the trauma may have produced only a bruise on the skin and no skull fracture or primary intracranial lesions. Posttraumatic brain swelling occurs more often in children than in adults. The swelling is not the direct result of the stress that acted on the brain at the moment of impact. Instead, it is a response to the acute shock that brings about acidosis and swelling of the network of cells supporting the brain (astrocytes and oligodendroglia). It commences in the deeper cerebral white matter. The swelling causes pressure on the capillaries and small blood vessels within the brain and thus further reduces the blood flow through the white matter to a degree that at autopsy it is not only swollen but also very pale as if anemic.

Any type of shock, be it from loss of blood, external burns or a toxic infection, may cause the same type of swelling. Space-occupying primary lesions already pressing on the vascular system of the brain usually promote swelling. In such cases a minor drop in the output of the heart, which would otherwise be considered inconsequential, may bring about significant swelling. In cases in which extra- or subdural hematomas are the only or prevalent space-occupying lesions, their size cannot always be considered responsible for the fatal outcome. It is generally agreed that a hematoma becomes dangerous to the brain when it exceeds 50 cc in mass. However, the brain can yield to a larger hematoma as long as it does not swell. As soon as swelling sets in, a vicious circle of events takes place that invariably ends in death. The same is true of a preexisting space-occupying lesion of nontraumatic nature, such as meningioma or pituitary gland adenoma. These tumors may have been clinically silent until the patient suffers a head injury. With the onset of posttraumatic brain swelling, signs and symptoms appear. These should not be interpreted as evidence of a traumatically induced faster growth of the tumor. This is exemplified by the following observation.

A captain in the merchant marine was struck on the top of the head with a blunt instrument and robbed in front of his house. He was briefly unconscious. During the subsequent hours he developed a scalp hematoma, increasing headaches and weakness of the left arm. At the hospital no skull fracture was found, and an exploratory operation revealed marked swelling of the brain but no extracerebral bleeding. After a few days of unconsciousness the patient recovered and was again able to use his fishing boat. After several weeks, weakness of the left arm and headaches recurred because of brain swelling. At this time it was found that he had a pulmonary carcinoma, inoperable because of its extent. He died three months after the injury. At autopsy a metastasis the size of a cherry was found near the motor area for the left arm in the right cerebral hemisphere. It must have been present at the time of posttraumatic swelling of the brain and was probably responsible for the weakness in the left arm by causing particularly severe swelling of the surrounding brain tissues. Since the metastasis was small at the time of autopsy, it does not seem that the trauma had influenced its growth.

In rare instances the swelling of the cerebrum is not from shock but from obstruction of the superior longitudinal sinus of the dura. Partial or total thrombosis of this sinus may be secondary to trauma if the sinus is injured by a foreign body or a fracture crossing the sinus. Thrombosis of the so-called straight sinus or the great vein of Galen may have the same effect because these channels drain the blood from most of the cerebral white matter and from the basal ganglia, which are the deep-seated gray structures of the cerebral hemispheres.

Swelling of only one cerebral hemisphere is not rare. It may develop in the unconscious patient as a result of pressure on one side of the neck by the sharp edge of an object that reduces the blood flow to the brain via the internal carotid artery; or a previously existing or traumatic or posttraumatic thrombotic obstruction of the artery in the neck may be the cause. If its intracranial portion is patent, there may be obstruction of its proximal section extending from the bifurcation of the common carotid artery to its S-shaped section within the cavernous sinus. If the petrous portion of the temporal bone is fractured, the artery may be obstructed within its bony canal. More frequently the obstruction is found in the neck region. Here the thrombosis is often caused by severe arteriosclerosis, but it may also be the result of a tear in the artery, although no significant hemorrhage may be present in the periarterial tissues. A tear and thrombosis of a carotid artery were found in a passenger of a motor vehicle who survived an accident for two days in coma. The corresponding cerebral hemisphere was severely swollen, in fact necrotic, and only a few contusion hemorrhages involved one temporal lobe. Swelling of one temporal lobe and its vicinity points to involvement of the adjacent transverse sinus. The thrombosis may be posttraumatic or develop from an infection of the middle ear.

### Necroses and Hemorrhages

Necrotic and hemorrhagic secondary lesions are caused by compression of blood vessels or similar mechanical stress, especially during a period of low blood pressure or by transient cardiac arrest. Necroses and hemorrhages caused by compression are most frequent and may occasionally be confused with contusions if the necrotic area is hemorrhagic.

The smallest lesions are found in the cortex of the cingulate and hippocampal gyri, where they are pressed against the margins of falx and tentorium, respectively. They occur after herniation of these gyri and are due to capillary compression in the area of notching. They can be differentiated from contusion hemorrhages,

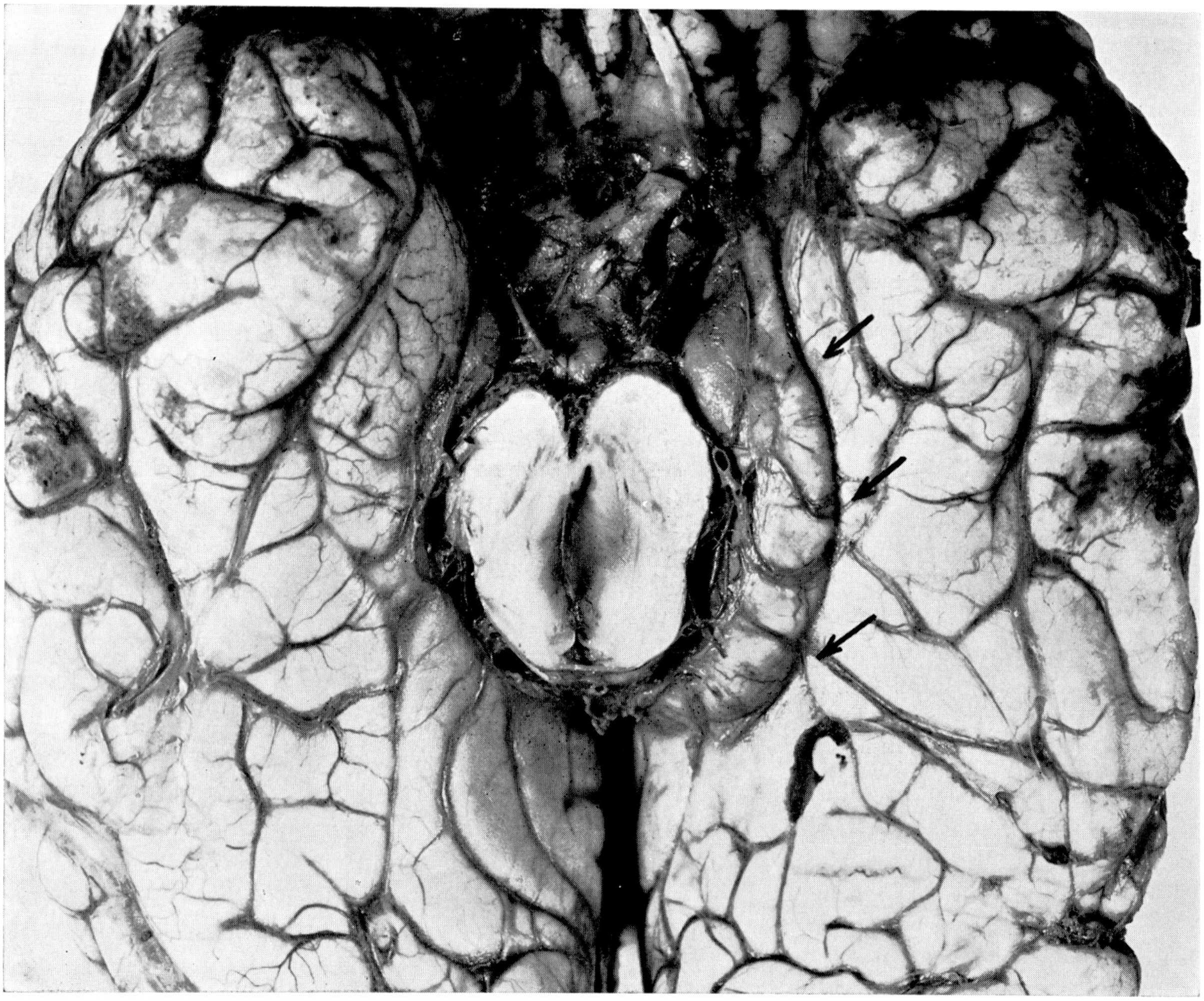

FIGURE XVII-29. Edema and secondary midline hemorrhage of the midbrain caused by compression of arteries in the interpeduncular fossa due to herniation of the left hippocampal gyrus (arrows). Extradural hematoma over the left hemisphere. Survival twenty-six hours.

as they are not usually hemorrhagic, and contusions herniate with the gyri as was shown in Figure XVII-13. Cerebellar tonsils that herniate into the foramen magnum may develop cortical necrosis leading to sclerosis.

Most of the lesions from vascular compression are large. Best known are the hemorrhages in the midbrain and pons. In the midbrain they usually occupy the lower half and extend from there into the tegmentum of the upper pons. They develop from uni- or bilateral pressure on the midbrain by the hippocampal gyri. In trauma this is usually seen with subdural and extradural hematomas pressing upon the brain. In such cases the interpeduncular fossa between the anteriorly located peduncles of the midbrain is narrowed. When the mammillary bodies shift into fossa, the blood supply of the midbrain becomes critical. Edema develops and is often associated with hemorrhages, which tend to commence in the midline. This is illustrated in Figure XVII-29, which presents an extradural hematoma over the left cerebral hemisphere received in a fall. During the twenty-six hours of survival the left hippocampal gyrus (right, indicated by arrows) herniated over the rim of the tentorium and shifted the midbrain towards the opposite side. Here it met with counterpressure from the nonherniated right hippocampal gyrus. The fossa between the peduncles became compressed, resulting in the lesions. The hemorrhages are sometimes of considerable size and may involve practically the entire tegmentum of the midbrain. This is seen on the left of Figure XVII-30. Here the lower midbrain (a) is almost totally destroyed by necrosis and extensive bleeding, which was formed by the confluence of several smaller hemorrhages. These hemorrhages have the tendency to spread into the tegmentum of the upper pons (b) because some of the arteries under pressure within the interpeduncular fossa supply the tegmentum. The involvement of the base of the pons is the result of kinking and compression of arteries that originate from the basilar artery and supply the base of the upper and lower pons and both base and tegmentum of the middle pons. Involvement of the midbrain and the pons by

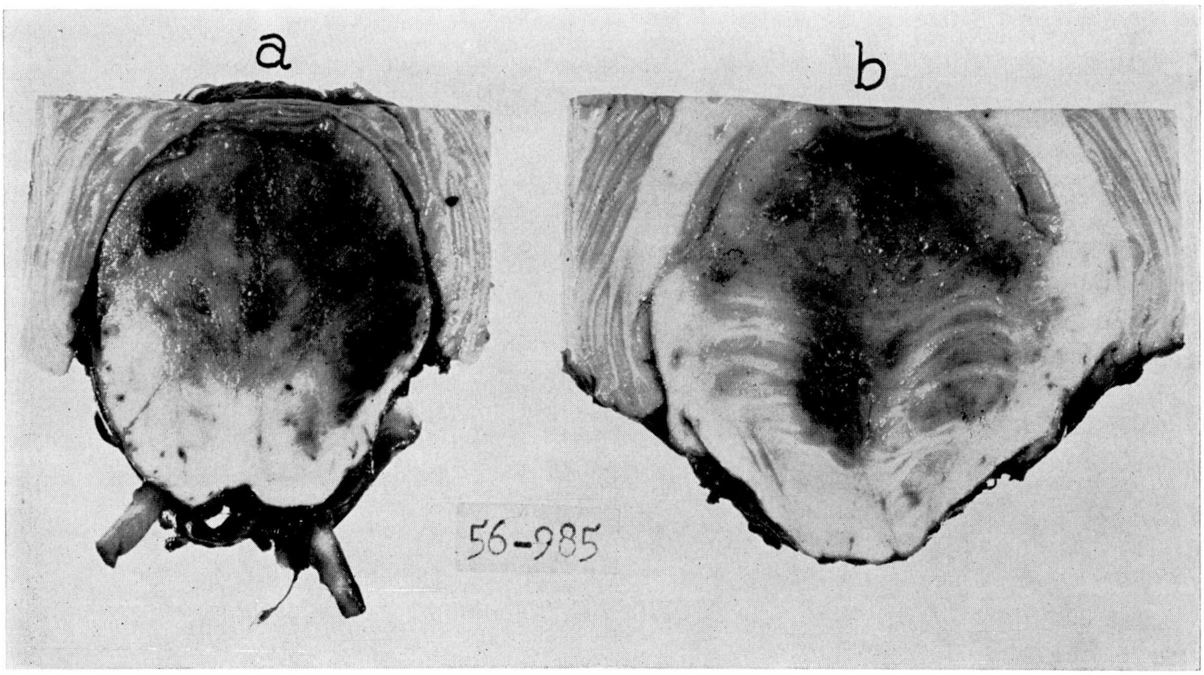


FIGURE XVII-30. Large secondary hemorrhage involving the entire tegmentum of the midbrain (a), extending into the tegmentum of the pons (b). Hemorrhage of the base of the pons. Subdural hematoma, survival five days.

these secondary changes is always associated with loss of consciousness, i.e. with coma, decerebrate rigidity and depression of respiration, which may be the cause of death. Freytag, in 1963,[2] found them in approximately 50 percent of all cases with brain injuries from blunt force, including those who died instantly. Secondary lesions were present in approximately 80 percent of the cases who survived the injury for some time.

If the supratentorial pressure on the midbrain develops more gradually, the regulation of respiration may be taken over by the medulla oblongata, and the patient, though only vegetating and unconscious, may survive for months or years, depending on care and the development of complications such as pneumonia. Figure XVII-31 shows extensive destruction of midbrain and pons, which was survived for two and one-half months. The patient fell on the back of the head and sustained a large subdural hematoma. In spite of its operative removal on two occasions, the secondary lesions developed and determined the fate of the patient. As was mentioned previously, these secondary alterations may appear within thirty minutes after injury from rapidly progressing extra- or subdural hematoma. Sometimes the hemorrhages

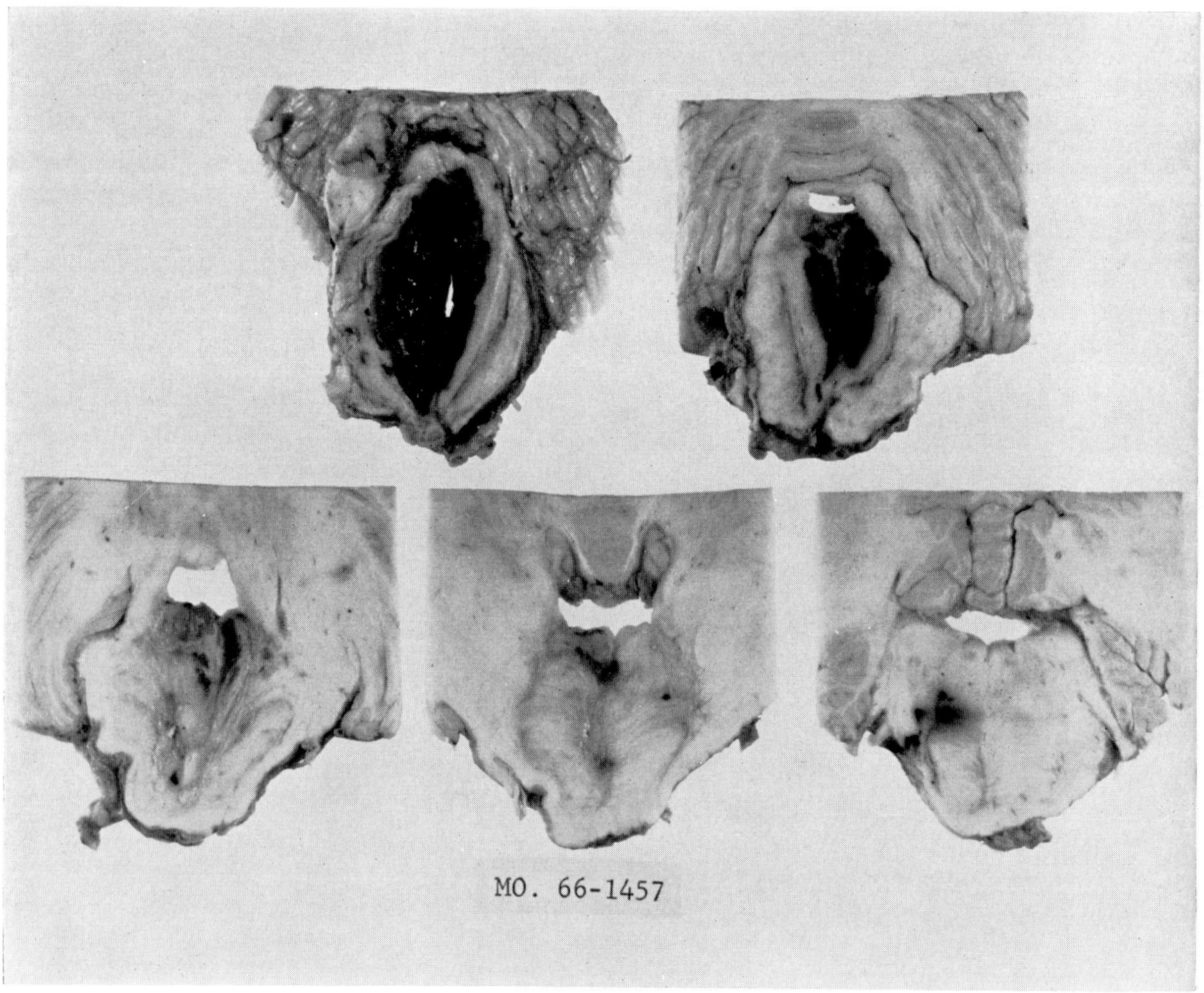


FIGURE XVII-31. Large old secondary lesions throughout the midbrain and pons due to a subdural hematoma. The victim survived for two and one-half months in an unconscious condition.

may be small or absent, whereas necroses of various midbrain structures and of the base of the pons dominate.

Other frequent locations of secondary lesions are the supply territories of the posterior cerebral arteries. Figure XVII-32 shows hemorrhagic softening of most of the cortex supplied by the left posterior cerebral artery (c). Branches of this artery were pressed against the tentorial margin by the herniating left hippocampal gyrus (arrow). Therefore, the softening starts at the point of compression and extends towards the periphery. The calcarine or visual cortex is often included in the lesion, as it is in this case, or it may be individually infarcted. If the lesion is survived, it produces a contralateral homonymous hemianopsia.

Another important part of the cortex supplied by branches of the posterior cerebral artery is the hippocampal gyrus with the Ammon's horn. If these arterial branches are compressed, the Ammon's horn (a) may lose neurons, terminating in sclerosis (Fig. XVII-33). Ammon's horn sclerosis is clinically of interest because it

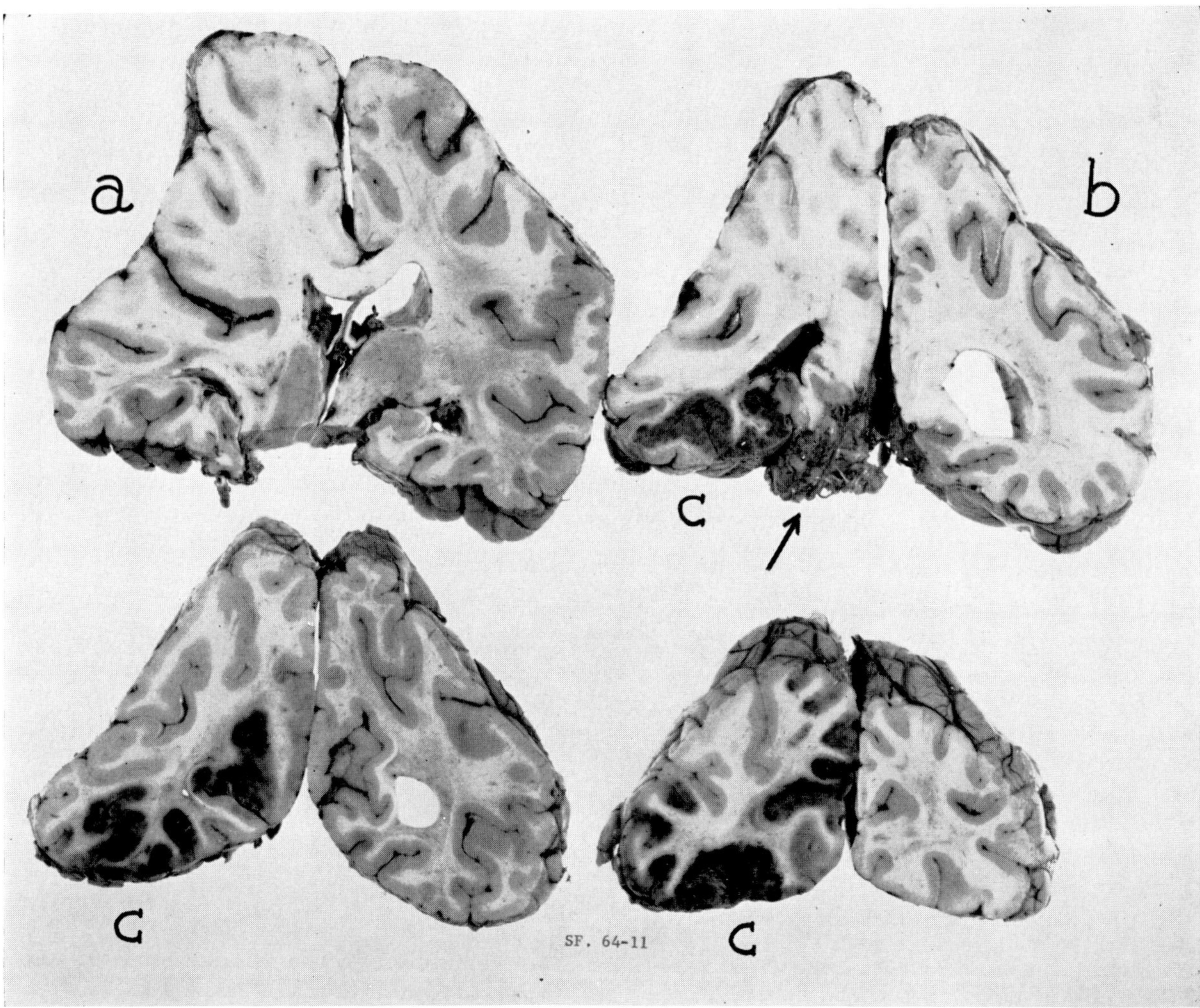


FIGURE XVII-32. Severe compression of the left cerebral hemisphere (a) by a former subdural hematoma, resulting in herniation of the left hippocampal gyrus (arrow) with hemorrhagic necrosis in the supply territory of the compressed branches of the left posterior cerebral artery (c). Small subdural hematoma (removed) over the right cerebral hemisphere (b). Survival three days.

often triggers attacks of psychomotor epilepsy. These attacks range from episodic emotional disorders with abnormal aggressiveness to generalized clonic-tonic seizures with loss of consciousness. Posttraumatic epilepsy may also be caused by sclerosis of other parts of the gray matter or by adhesions between the cortex and the dura. Involvement of both Ammon's horns in their entire length may cause epilepsy; however, the dominant clinical pattern is that of dementia because of the inability of the patient to remember even the most recent events or actions.

It may be of interest to note that approximately 30 percent of epileptics have no epileptogenic foci in the brain.[10]

Vascular compression is often responsible for lesions in the medial portions of the pallida. These are supplied by the pallidum branches of the anterior choroidal arteries, which also cross the tentorium and are thus vulnerable to pressure or distortion. The tissue damage ranges from loss of nerve cells to infarction and may involve one or both pallida. In cases without head injury, bilateral pallidum necrosis is often considered characteristic of carbon monoxide poisoning and is attributed to a particular vulnerability of the pallida to oxygen deficiency. Our experience indicates that pallidum necrosis may develop during a period of brain swelling from shock due to acute loss of blood, barbitu-

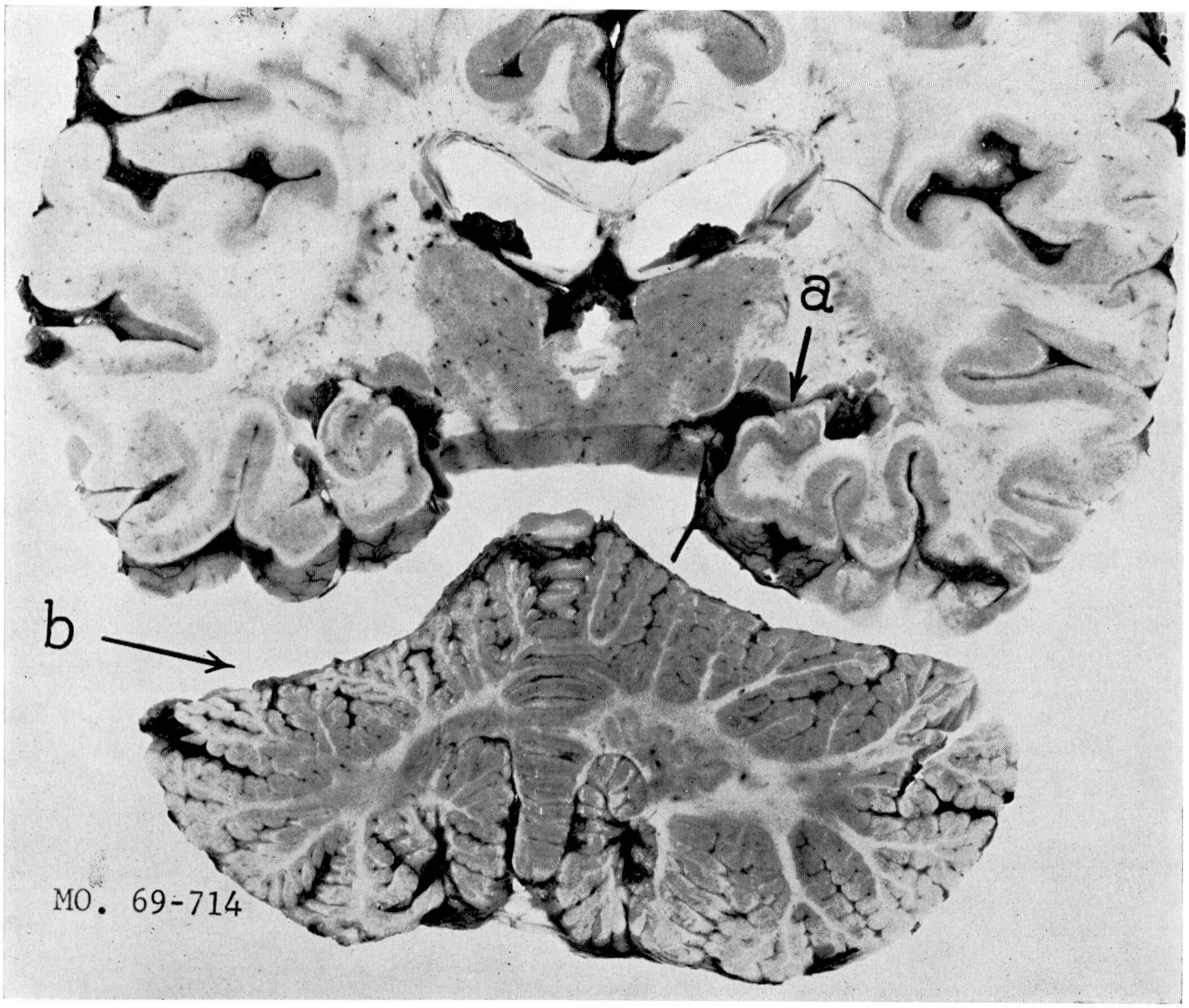


FIGURE XVII-33. Atrophy of right Ammon's horn (a) associated with atrophy of the left cerebellar hemisphere (b) due to a former subdural hematoma over the right cerebral hemisphere.

rate poisoning or hypoglycemia. Associated lesions may be found in the unci and in the central portions of the optic nerves, chiasm and tracts, ranging from atrophy with glial scarring to true necroses, all the result of pressure.[11]

The cerebral and cerebellar cortex along the depth of sulci may be damaged from compression of smaller blood vessels within the sulci. The cerebellum may also show other patterns of necrosis. One is seen in Figure XVII-33. It consists of atrophy of the cortex of the left hemisphere (b) and is located on the opposite side of a former subdural hematoma, which also caused atrophy of the right Ammon's horn (a). Such involvement of the peripheral cortex of the cerebellum is often clinically silent. However, if the vermis is affected, the patient shows a truncal ataxia. Ataxia is limited to the legs if only the upper vermis is involved. This has been observed in alcoholics. Some believe these changes result from nutritional deficiency.[12] In our opinion this lesion is of vascular nature, caused by temporary compression of the cerebellar arteries supplying the upper vermis and its vicinity by the tentorial margin during a period of brain swelling. Simultaneous involvement of the cortex of the cerebellar tonsils or of the area facing the margins of the foramen magnum supports this concept.

In concluding the description of some of the

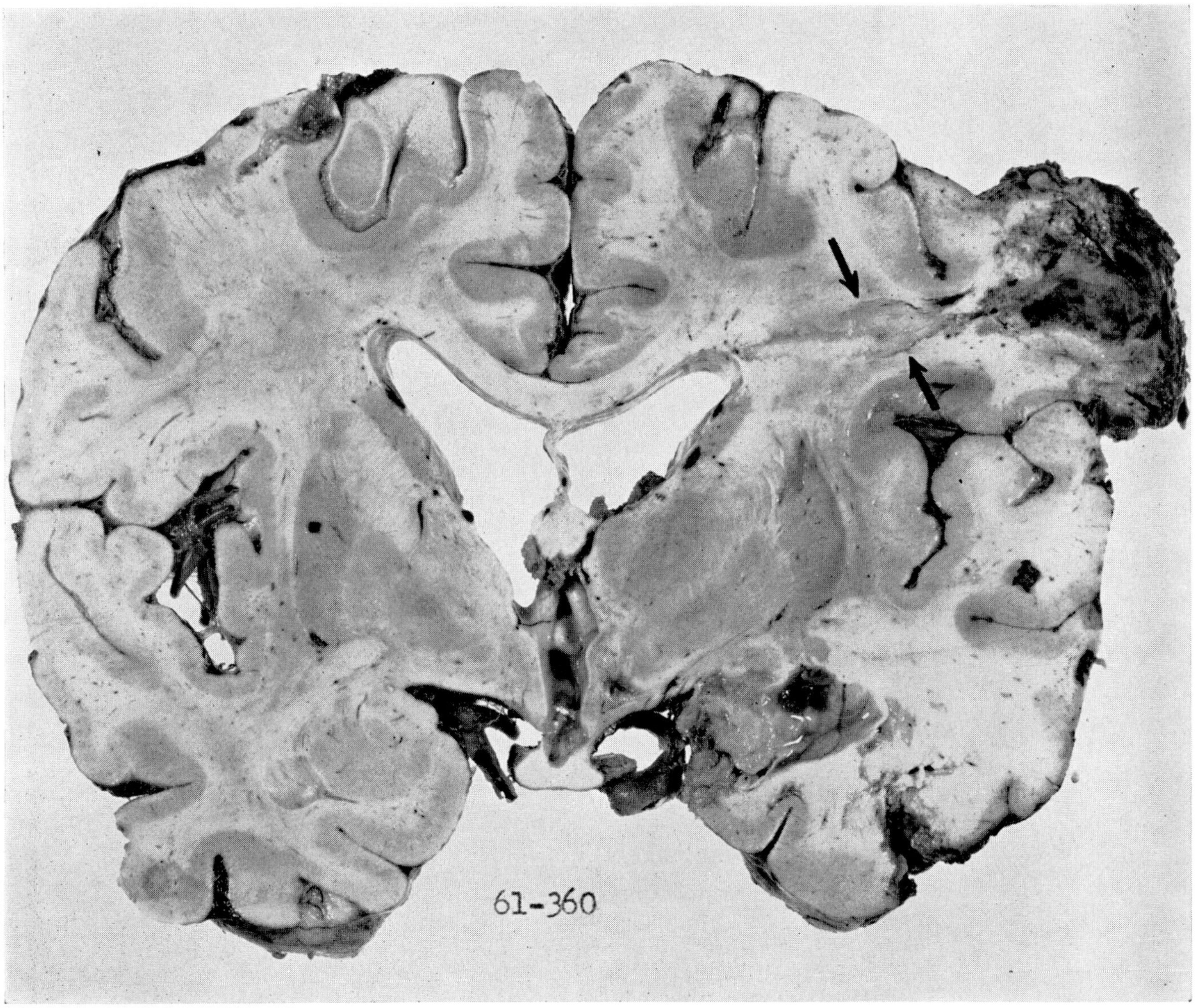


FIGURE XVII-34. Persistent brain fungus (right) due to swelling into a surgical opening of the skull associated with infarction of deeper white matter (arrows). Survival one month.

secondary lesions caused by circulatory disorders, mention must be made of alterations related to operative procedures, more precisely to trephination and incision of the dura. For exploratory purposes burr holes are made, and if no extradural hematoma is found, the dura is incised in search of a subdural hematoma. In the course of this procedure the cerebral cortex may be injured, or if the brain is swollen, the cortex may herniate into the burr hole. The herniated portion of the brain may *strangulate* its blood supply by pressing against the margins of the bone and thus become hemorrhagic and necrotic. The necrosis may extend into deeper tissues, and their swelling may in turn produce further herniation. Such growing mushroomlike protrusion of necrotic brain tissue is called *fungus*. An example is shown in Figure XVII-34.

### Posttraumatic Hydrocephalus

Local or diffuse enlargement of the ventricles is not uncommon in persons who survived a head injury. Local pouching is due to tissue loss from an old primary or secondary lesion. In rare cases the pouch may reach the surface of the brain, causing traumatic porencephaly,

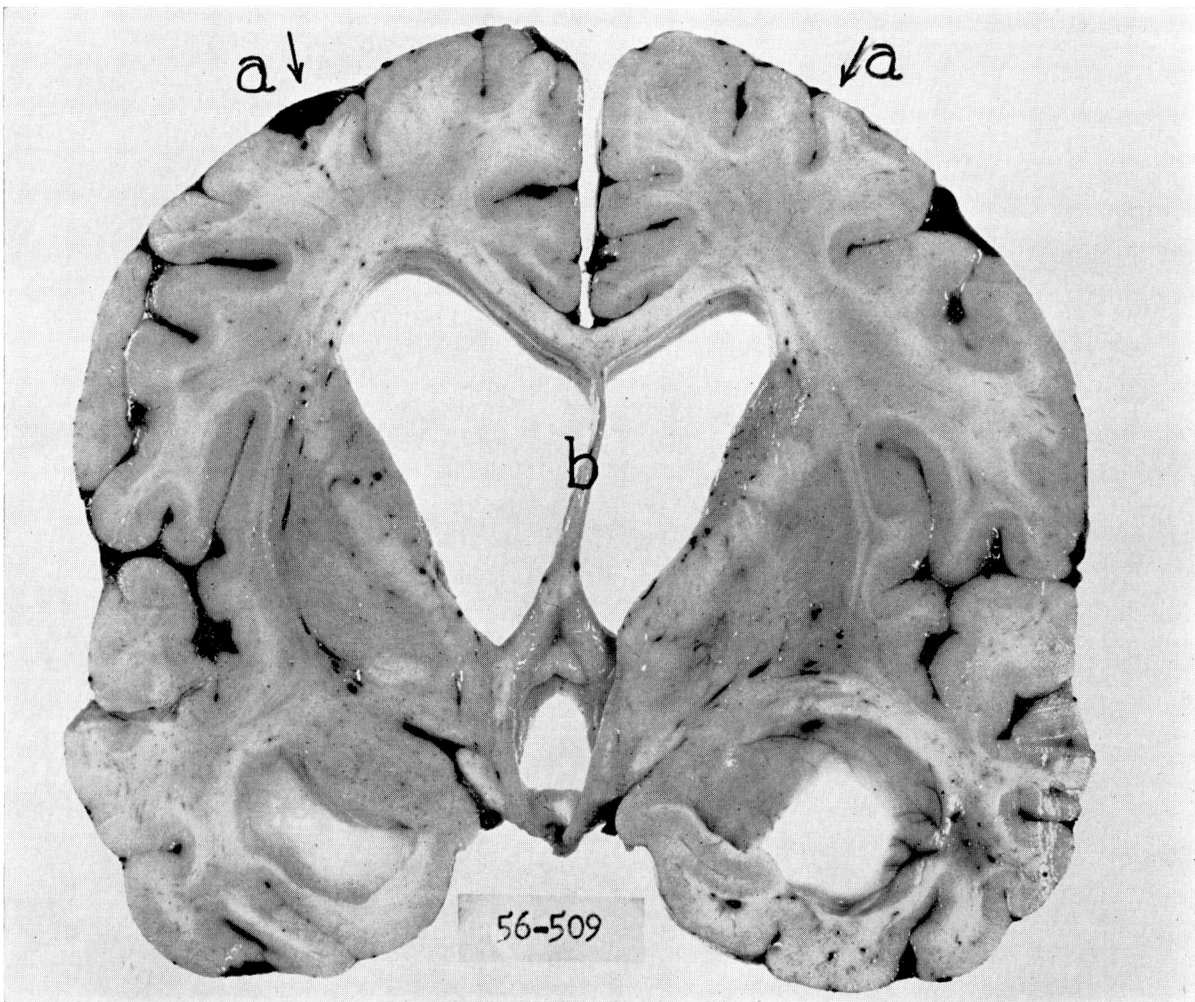


FIGURE XVII-35. Posttraumatic transient cardiac arrest survived for one year with quadriplegia and cortical blindness. Symmetrical atrophy in the border zones of the supply areas of the major cerebral arteries (a). Hydrocephalus *ex vacuo* due to shrinkage of the white matter. Preserved septum pellucidum (b).

with cysts or defects permitting communication between the subarachnoid space and the ventricular system.

Diffuse and more or less symmetrical enlargement of the ventricles may result from atrophy of the white matter following degeneration of myelinated axons. Such hydrocephalus *ex vacuo* is shown in Figure XVII-35. In other cases hydrocephalus is due to distension of the ventricles by elevated pressure of the cerebrospinal fluid. This occurs if the aqueduct or the exits of the fourth ventricle are narrowed or obstructed. In such case one speaks of an *obstructive internal hydrocephalus*. However, if the ventricular cavities are in continuity with the lumbar subarachnoid space, it is termed *communicating hydrocephalus*. Such high pressure hydrocephalus may develop within a few hours. If the pressure is not released within a few weeks, the ventricles often remain large in spite of treatment. Occasionally a communicating hydrocephalus is seen without scarring of the leptomeningeal spaces. In such case the cerebellar tonsils may show sclerosis of their cortex. This indicates that at one time swelling of the cerebellum forced the tonsils into the foramen magnum, temporarily obliterating the foramens of Magendi and Luschka. During this time the

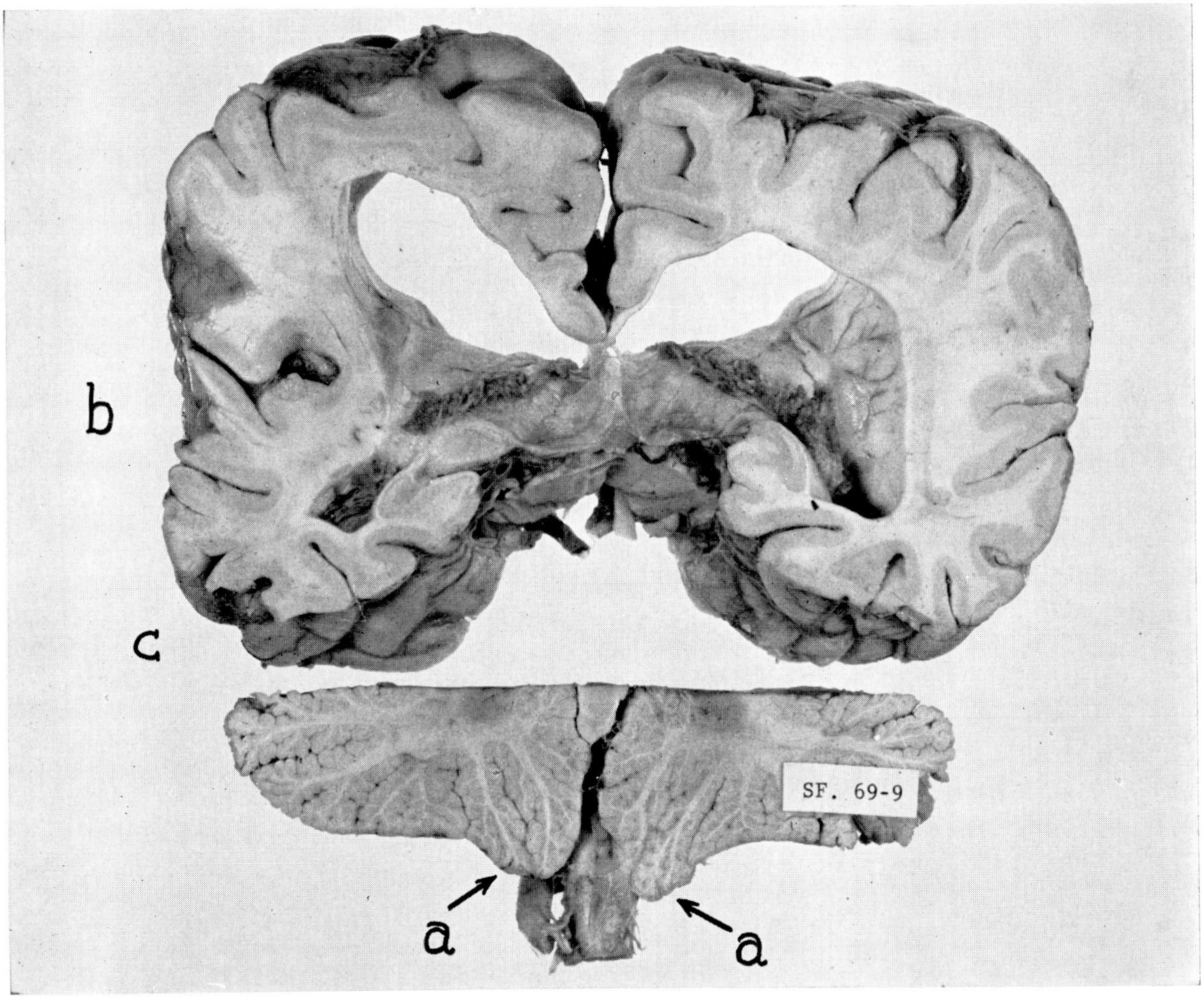


FIGURE XVII-36. Occlusive high pressure hydrocephalus of the lateral and third ventricles caused by former herniation of tonsils (a) due to brain swelling following a blow with a baseball against the left temporal region. Old contusions in the left lower parietal (b) and temporal lobes (c). Sclerosis of the tonsils. Survival forty-three years in a mental hospital.

hydrocephalus developed. The fourth ventricle is not dilated in such cases, as it too was compressed by the swollen cerebellum. The hydrocephalus illustrated in Figure XVII-36 developed in this manner after trauma.

A sixty-six-year-old patient of a mental hospital was struck by a baseball over the left temporal region when he was twenty-three years old. This impact caused a skull fracture and coup contusions in the left lower parietal lobe (b) and adjacent temporal convolutions (c). He was briefly unconscious and later unable to understand and use words properly (sensory aphasia). When this subsided, he was found to be psychotic and at times confused; as a result, he had to be institutionalized. At autopsy the lateral and third ventricles and aqueduct were markedly enlarged, whereas the fourth ventricle was normal and its exits patent. The cerebellar tonsils, however, showed chronic herniation and sclerosis (a). The hydrocephalus probably contributed to the development of the posttraumatic psychosis.

Forgetfulness, confusion and other mental changes are known to be produced by hydrocephalus. The intraventricular pressure need not be continuously elevated. Shunting of the enlarged ventricles may bring about remarkable recovery.

## Secondary Infections

In spite of the great advances made in the field of antibiotics, posttraumatic meningitis and intracerebral abscesses are still encountered.

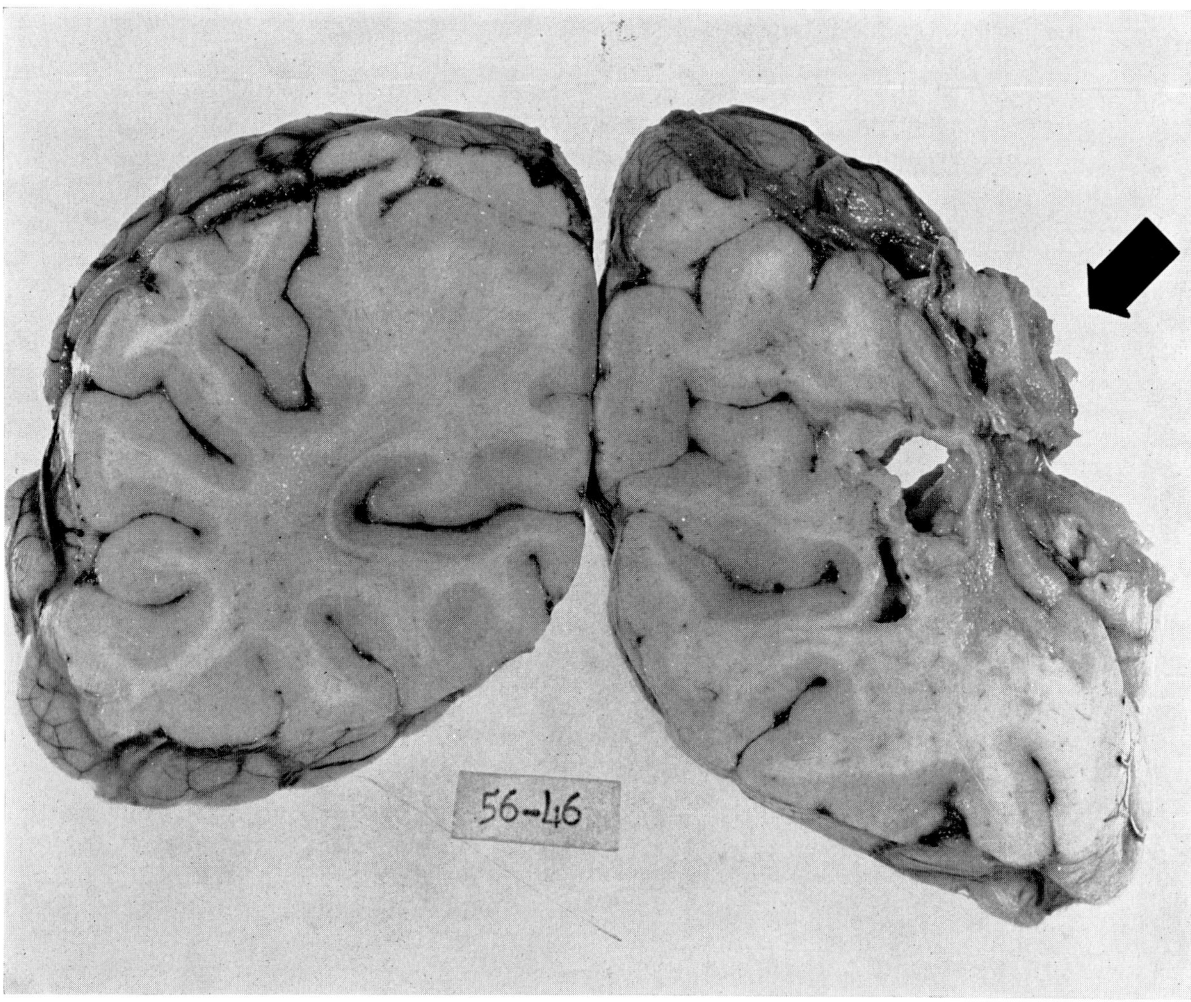


FIGURE XVII-37. Old abscess in the right parieto-occipital region (arrow) due to impact to this area resulting in an open injury from a depressed fracture. Survival forty-five days.

Meningitis may develop from an infected open injury caused by a foreign body or from fractures in the wall of one of the cranial sinuses associated with a tear in the dura and arachnoid. In rare instances it is derived from a poorly healing surgical wound. Even if clinically recognized, the bacteria causing it may be resistant to antibiotics. If meningitis is severe, the inflammation may proceed retrograde through the foramens of Magendi and Luschka into the ventricular system. It may directly penetrate into the third ventricle if the chiasm, the tuber cinereum or the pituitary stalk is injured.

Abscesses within the brain are usually seen in the vicinity of primary lesions responsible for the infection, i.e. near contusions of one or both orbital lobes that face fractures in the roofs of the ethmoidal sinuses. Concomitant meningitis is often limited to the area of injury. Figure XVII-37 shows a small round, empty abscess in the right parieto-occipital area beneath an adhesion between the thickened dura and the chronically inflamed leptomeninges (arrow). This person suffered a depressed fracture of this area, which he sustained in a traffic accident. He survived forty-five days. In spite of treatment with antibiotics, the abscess broke through the ventricle wall and filled the ventricle with pus, forming a pyencephalus. In such case it is characteristic that the choroid plexus is covered

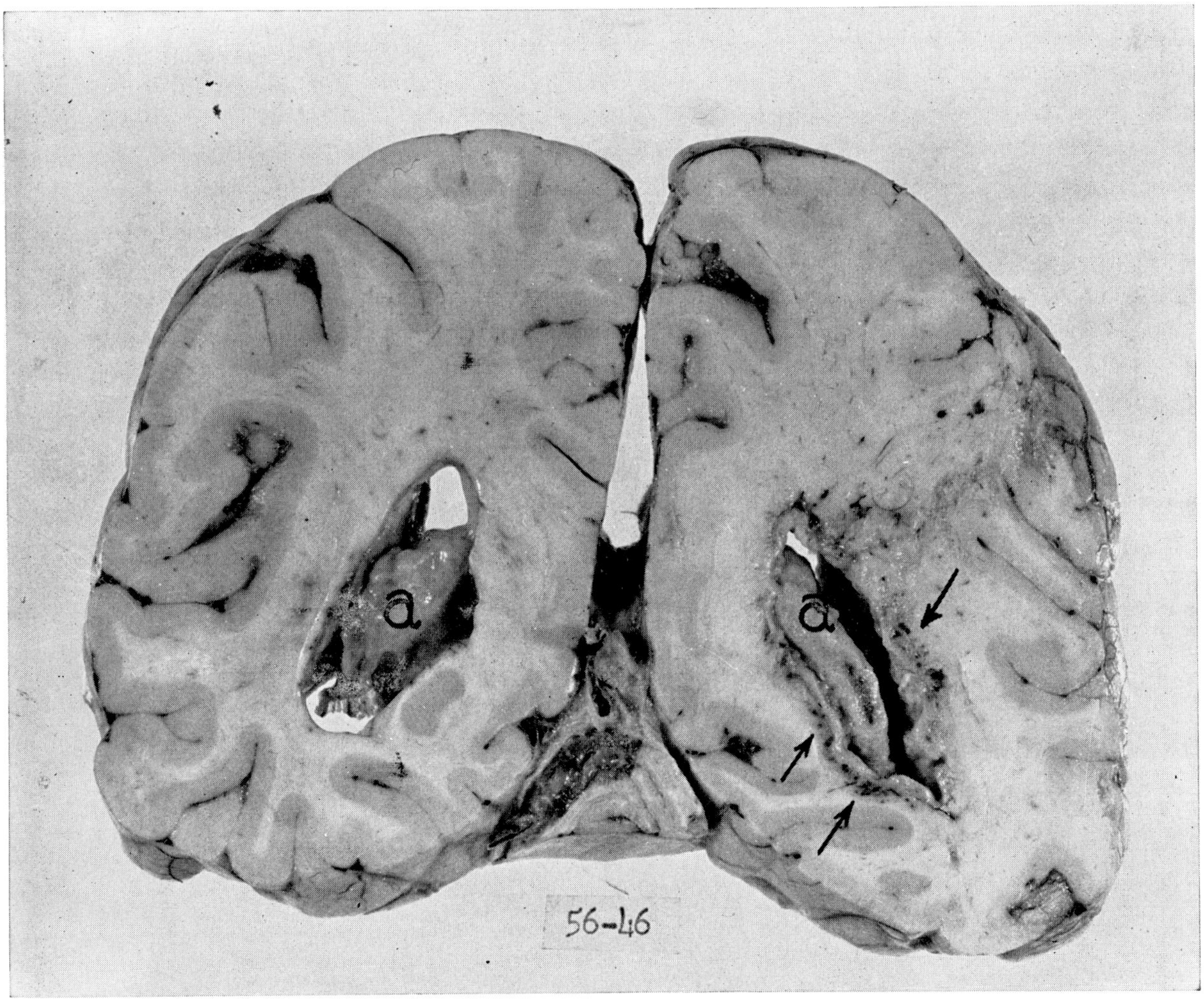


FIGURE XVII-38. Same case as in Figure XVII-37. Pyocephalus of the lateral ventricles with pus covering the choroid plexus (a). Subependymitis around the right lateral ventricle (arrows) extending upward into the white matter.

with pus, as if topped by icing. This is seen in Figure XVII-38, of the same case. The loose pus within the ventricles was easily removed, but the pus covering the choroid plexus (a) could not be washed away. Furthermore, this photograph shows a hemorrhagic reaction along the wall of the right ventricle (arrows), a subependymitis. Although the inflammatory reaction in the subependymal layer may be impressive, it usually does not extend into the deeper white matter. In the present case, however, it continued into the white matter along the upper portion of the lateral wall of the ventricle and caused a phlegmonous encephalitis. From the ventricles the infection spread into the subarachnoid space and gave rise to meningitis over the base of the brain, while the convexity of the brain showed practically no evidence of inflammation.

**Fat and Air Embolism**

Although neither fat and bone marrow embolism nor air embolism are complications secondary to craniocerebral injuries, they are mentioned here because they may be present in addition to primary and secondary lesions of the brain and may cause difficulties in the interpretation of the findings. In a significant percentage of cases fat embolism produces scattered hemorrhages that predominantly occupy the cerebral white matter (Fig. XVII-39). If present in gray structures, they may simulate small contusion hemorrhages.

In air embolism, hemorrhages are rare. Instead, more or less well demarcated miniature infarcts in gray and white matter are found. They are best identified if the patient survives one day or longer. The irregular distribution of these infarcts contradicts the assumption that

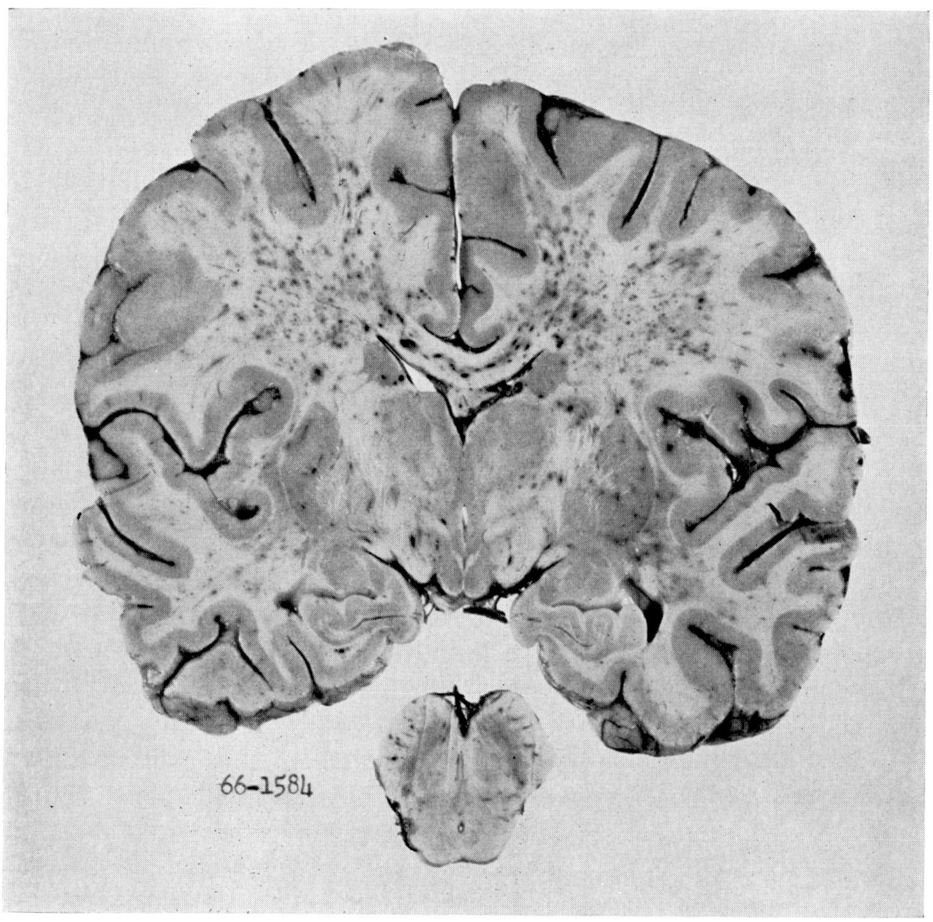


FIGURE XVII-39. Numerous punctate hemorrhages scattered in the white matter due to fat embolism. Survival four days.

they result from vascular compression. In rare instances of stab wounds of the neck that involve the carotid or vertebral artery, air and fat may be sucked into the peripheral portion of the respective artery, causing infarctions in which the involved gray matter is dotted with round-shaped, well-circumscribed hemorrhages. These infarctions are, of course, limited to the supply territory of the injured vessel.

## REFERENCES


1. Lindenberg, R.: Systemic oxygen deficiencies; Trauma of meninges and brain; forensic neuropathology. In Minckler, J. (Ed.): *Pathology of the Nervous System,* vols. II and III. New York, McGraw, 1971, 1972.
2. Freytag, E.: Autopsy findings in head injuries from blunt forces. Statistical evaluation of 1,367 cases. *Arch Pathol, 75:*74, 1963.
3. Pudenz, R. H., and Shelden, C. H.: The lucite calvarium. A method for direct observation of the brain. II. Cranial trauma and brain movement. *J Neurosurg, 3:*487, 1946.
4. Freytag, E.: Autopsy findings in head injuries from firearms. *Arch Pathol, 76:*215, 1963.
5. Lindenberg, R., and Freytag, E.: Morphology of cortical contusions. *Arch Pathol, 63:*23, 1957.
6. Lindenberg, R., and Freytag, E.: Morphology of brain lesions from blunt trauma in early infancy. *Arch Pathol, 87:*298, 1969.
7. Lindenberg, R., and Freytag, E.: Brainstem lesions characteristic of traumatic hyperextension of the head. *Arch Pathol, 90:*509, 1970.
8. Lindenberg, R., and Freytag, E.: The mechanism of cerebral contusions. A pathologic-anatomic study. *Arch Pathol, 69:*440, 1960.
9. Sellier, K., and Unterharnscheidt, F.: Mechanik und Pathomorphologie der Hirnschäden nach stumpfer Gewalteinwirkung auf den Schädel. *Hefte Unfallheilkd, 76,* 1963.
10. Freytag, E., and Lindenberg, R.: 294 medicolegal autopsies on epileptics. *Arch Pathol, 78:*274, 1964.
11. Lindenberg, R., and Walsh, F. B.: Vascular compression involving intracranial visual pathways. *Trans Am Acad Ophthalmol Otolaryngol,* July-August, 1964.
12. Victor, M., Adams, R. D., and Mancall, E. L.: A restricted form of cerebellar cortical degeneration occurring in alcoholic patients. *Arch Neurol, 1:*579, 1959.

*Chapter XVIII*

# INVESTIGATION OF DEATHS IN CHILDHOOD

*Part 1*

## INFANTICIDE

WERNER U. SPITZ

*Black's Law Dictionary* defines infanticide as *the murder or killing of an infant soon after its birth.* In the majority of instances infanticide is committed by the mother and is attributable to a disturbed state of mind following delivery and sometimes during the period of breast feeding (postpartum depression). With the liberalization of abortion laws in the United States, cases of infanticide have become quite rare. When it occurs, the murder of a newly born infant is usually especially gruesome and quite horrifying. Except in straightforward cases where infanticide is obvious, diagnosis requires experience and detailed information regarding

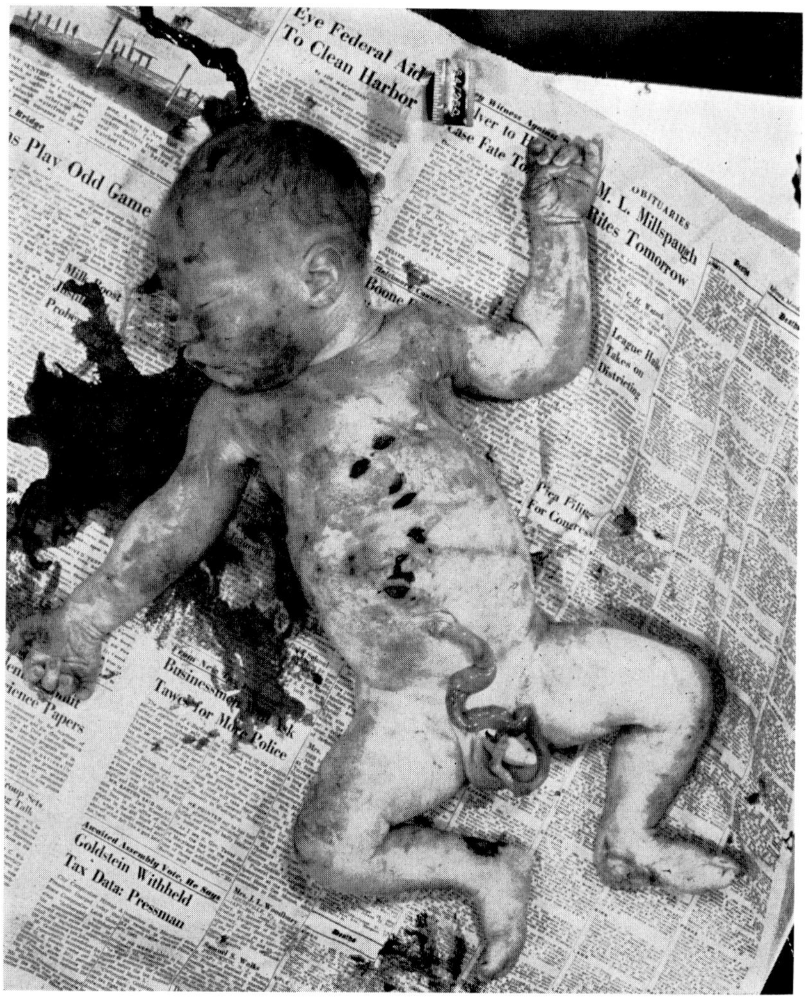


FIGURE XVIII-1. Newborn infant with multiple stab wounds found wrapped in newspapers in a trash can placed on the street for disposal.

the circumstances of birth (Figs. XVIII-1 and XVIII-2).

Smothering and strangulation are the most common methods of infanticide. In both, death is caused by anoxia due to interference with oxygen supply. Faint, often superficial bruises or scrapes may be found on the infant's cheeks and nose or lips and, less frequently, in the mucosa of the mouth as a result of pressure applied to shut the airway. Such injuries are of considerable significance, because anoxia due to birth trauma and other natural causes accounts for the largest loss of fetal and neonatal life before and during delivery.

Cerebral injury, with or without associated skull fracture, is the second most common cause of neonatal mortality and is often equally as difficult to interpret as is death by suffocation. A newborn's skull, being soft and pliable, fractures quite differently from that of an adult. Such a fracture in the thin membranous bone of a newborn's skull may be better characterized as a ragged tear.

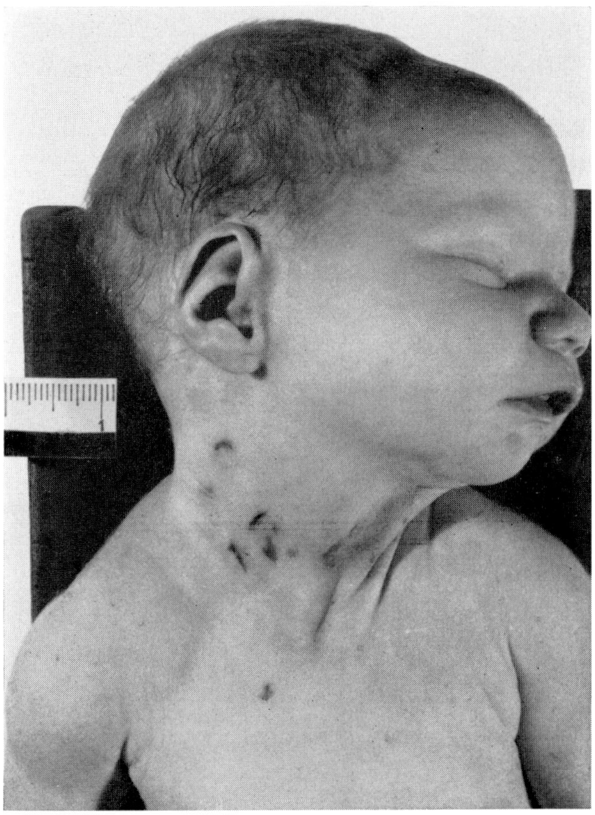

FIGURE XVIII-2. Fingernail marks on the neck of a newborn, suggestive of manual strangulation. The teenaged mother claimed that these were inflicted during her attempts to deliver the baby by herself.

A description of all the injuries that may occur in the course of delivery is considered beyond the scope of this chapter. Excellent texts are available that give detailed accounts of birth trauma and its sequelae.[1] It should, however, be emphasized that any well-founded conclusion of infanticide must be based on the correlation of the anatomical findings at autopsy with an account of the circumstances of the birth as related by the mother or a witness. This will enable the pathologist to determine whether in fact the injuries of the child are compatible with the manner in which they are said to have occurred. Physical examination of the mother by a gynecologist is often helpful, since it may establish conditions capable of explaining an abnormal delivery, which may be responsible for injury of the newborn.

Precipitous deliveries, in which the child is forcibly ejected from the uterus and is injured by falling on the ground or drowns by being born into a toilet bowl, sometimes occur in multiparous women, especially if the child is premature. A certain amount of skepticism is usually warranted under such circumstances. Swelling of the baby's scalp, indicating difficult and prolonged labor, refutes this type of allegation. Neglect of the newborn child and consequent death as a result of exposure must also be classified as infanticide.

Attempted disposal of the remains of a newborn child may strengthen the evidence of infanticide (Fig. XVIII-3). Occasionally, however, the death of the infant may be the result of natural or accidental causes, and disposal of the body follows for the purpose of concealing the birth because of fear of impending suspicion of foul play (Fig. XVIII-4). Inspection of the severed edges of the umbilical cord may provide information as to whether the latter was cut or torn. If drying has set in, soaking the umbilical stump in cold water may still permit a meaningful examination. Microscopic study of the severed edge may be helpful in determining

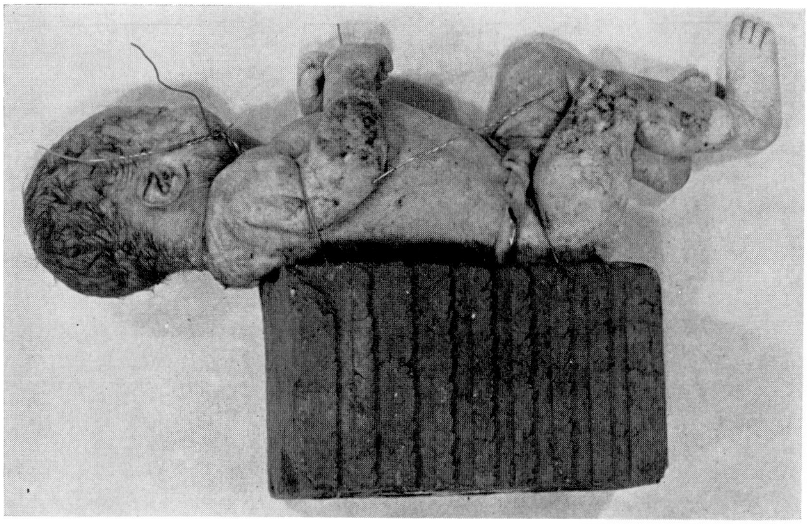

FIGURE XVIII-3. The body of a newborn infant wired to a building block recovered from the Baltimore harbor. Such bodies are occasionally recovered during dredging activities.

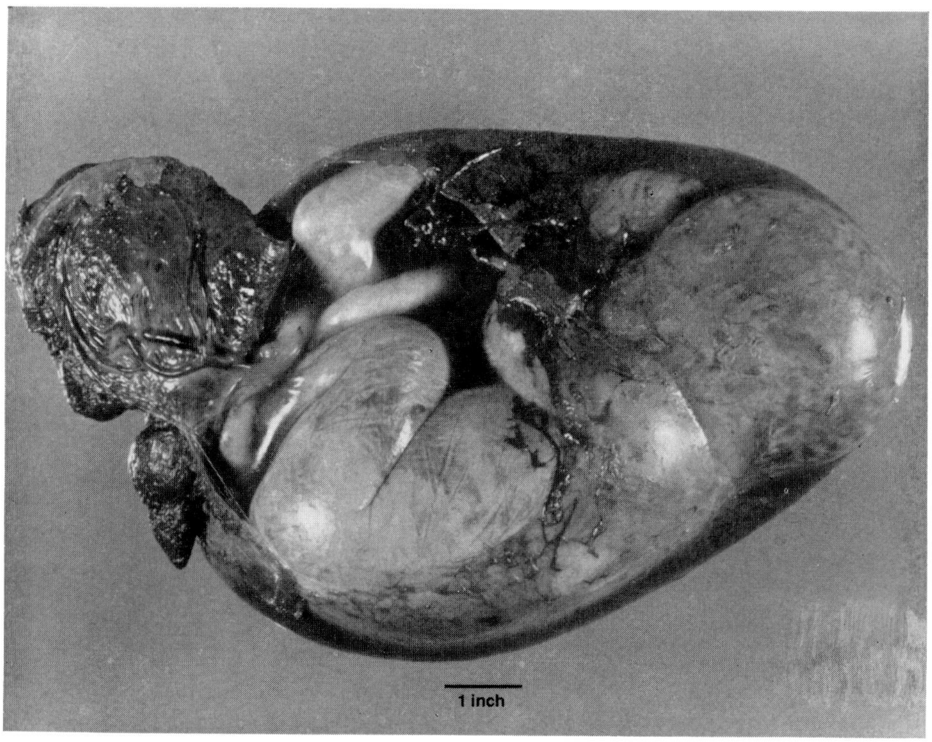


FIGURE XVIII-4. A traveling bag containing the body of a full-term well-developed baby enclosed in its intact amniotic sac (bag of waters) was found abandoned in a communal bathroom in a girls' college. The child died of asphyxia due to failure to rupture the amniotic membrane. This was considered to be a natural sequence in this case, since it could not be expected of the mother, if the delivery was unattended, to have the knowledge or the presence of mind to rupture the bag of waters immediately following the birth. The sac was opened at autopsy.

reactive changes, for example the time that has elapsed since severing occurred.

Two major criteria must be met before infanticide can be established: (a) that the child was born alive, (b) that the child was viable, i.e. able to sustain life independently.

### Was the Child Born Alive?

Determination of whether the child was born alive can be made on the basis of the presence of (a) air in the lungs, (b) air in the stomach and the intestine, (c) air in the middle ears, (d) food in the stomach.

A *lung that is expanded with air,* i.e. a lung that has breathed, is doughy, salmon pink in color and completely fills its pleural cavity. Probably many respirations are required before full expansion of the lung occurs; in the interim it has a mottled pink to dark red appearance due to the presence of areas that are unexpanded and airless. A lung that did not breathe is shrunken, dark purple-red and leathery-firm. Small portions from various parts of the lung, if immersed in water, sink if they are airless and float if the child has breathed. This test must not, however, be regarded as absolute, since postmortem gas formation due to decomposition will keep a piece of lung afloat even if breathing has not occurred. A small cube of liver may serve as a control. If the liver floats, the floating of the lung must be considered meaningless. Attempted resuscitation by artificial respiration and alcohol fixation of the lung will also give a false positive result.

Conversely, if the birth occurs into the toilet bowl or into a bucket containing liquid, the infant, if breathing, will inhale the liquid; consequently, death will be due to drowning, and the lung flotation test will be negative.

Microscopic examination of the lungs in such cases is often revealing, insofar as foreign particles contained in the drowning fluid may have been inhaled and may be found in the lungs. Such foreign particles may consist of cellulose and other undigestible substances often present in fecal matter. It must be emphasized in this regard that inhalation of amniotic fluid, such as may occur in the course of normal delivery, will also result in the presence of particulate material in the lungs. It is imperative, therefore, that particles of amniotic fluid be recognized and distinguished from elements of extraneous origin.

*The presence of air in the stomach and the intestine* of the newborn infant indicates that swallowing has occurred after delivery and consequently that the infant was born alive, provided postmortem gas formation has not occurred and no artificial respiration has been given. Before removal of the gut from the body, the gut is separated from the mesentery, and the lower end of the esophagus and the small intestine are tied. A ligature is also placed between the stomach and duodenum. The stomach is then placed in a water bath to determine flotation. Opening the stomach under water will release bubbles. The same procedure is carried out with the small intestine. In the case of intrauterine infection, the infant's gastrointestinal tract may contain gas from bacterial growth, thus giving a false positive finding.

*Air reaches the middle ears* by way of the Eustachian tubes as a result of swallowing. Consequently, in cases of stillbirth no air is present in the middle ears. For the purpose of carrying out this test, the middle ears must be opened under water, using a chisel or strong shears for removal of the tegmen tympani. A bubble of air will emerge from the middle ear if the test is positive. In the case of decomposition the test is meaningless.

Although the presence of air in the lungs, the bowel and the middle ears no doubt serves as a valuable confirmatory test of respiration, the limits of this method must also be recognized.

*The presence of food in the stomach,* by contrast, is absolute proof of live birth, there being no other way for food to reach the stomach besides swallowing.

### Was the Child Viable?

The determination of whether the child was viable, provided it was given adequate care, is based primarily on the developmental stage of the newborn and the exclusion of congenital abnormalities incompatible with life. A newborn is usually able to sustain life independently after a gestation period of twenty-eight weeks. Prematurity is by far the most common cause of death among newborns. It is generally agreed that a premature infant is one who weighs 5.5 lb. (2500 gm) or less at birth, regardless of the time of gestation. Microscopic examination of the lungs of premature infants often reveals only partial aeration, while most of the areas are collapsed and solid due to incomplete development.

As regards certification of a live birth or stillbirth, most jurisdictions dictate that—

"Irrespective of the length of the period of uterogestation, if the child shows any evidence of life after complete birth, even though it be momentary, the birth shall be registered as a live birth and a death certificate shall be filed. Birth is considered complete when the child is altogether (head, trunk and limbs) outside the body of the mother, even if the cord is uncut and the placenta is still attached.

Stillbirth or fetal death is death prior to complete expulsion or extraction from its mother of a product of conception which has advanced through the twentieth week of uterogestation; the death is indicated by the fact that after separation, the fetus does not breathe or show any other evidence of life such as beating of the heart, pulsation of the umbilical cord, or definite movement of the voluntary muscles. A stillbirth certificate must be filed under such circumstances."[2]

## REFERENCES

1. Potter, E. L.: *Pathology of the Fetus and the Newborn.* Chicago, Year Bk Med, 1953.
2. Michigan Vital Statistics Laws 326.15 (M.S.A. 14.235).

*Part 2*

# SUDDEN INFANT DEATH SYNDROME ("CRIB DEATH")

JOHN E. SMIALEK

IN THE PAST, inadequate medicolegal investigation of sudden infant deaths frequently resulted in the certification of these deaths as due to smothering. The continued existence of this theory is evidenced by the suspicions with which investigators often approach the scene of a sudden infant death.

Inadequate postmortem examinations of these infants, compounded by a lack of appreciation of the *normal findings* in autopsies in this age group, has resulted in a considerable lag in understanding the single most common cause of death in infants under one year of age. The *Sudden Infant Death Syndrome* (SIDS) is responsible for over 8,000 deaths per year in the United States. *Asphyxiation by bedclothes* or *regurgitated milk* are terms that continue to be found on death certificates, indicating, erroneously, that these deaths are accidental. However, bedclothing has been demonstrated to allow adequate access of air to preclude asphyxiation,[1] and regurgitation of milk often occurs due to contraction of the stomach at the time of death.

In order to establish a common terminology and eliminate many confusing and misleading diagnoses, the term *Sudden Infant Death Syndrome* was defined at the Second International Conference in Seattle, Washington, in 1969 as the death of an infant in apparent good health who dies suddenly and unexpectedly and in whose case an autopsy does not reveal a commonly accepted cause of death.[2]

This definition points out the necessity of autopsy in cases of sudden infant death to rule out other possible causes occurring in infants commonly described to the investigator as being previously well. It is important that the investigator at the scene of an infant death be cognizant of certain findings, which, if not properly interpreted, may lead to erroneous conclusions, including child abuse (Fig. XVIII-5).

Terminal pulmonary edema and congestion may cause bloody froth to accumulate at the nostrils and mouth of the infant, staining surrounding bedclothes. In addition, Negro and Mongolian infants sometimes have large patches of dark pigmentation in the buttock and sacral region, so-called *Mongolian spots,* which tend to diminish or disappear in the first year of life (Fig. XVIII-6). This prominent dark area may be mistaken for bruising, suggesting physical abuse. Incision of the area may be required to establish the nature of the discoloration. Intense postmortem lividity with pale zones caused by pressure may also give the erroneous impression of bruises. This is especially common when seen on the infant's face after he has been found in a facedown position. It is essential that the investigator, in compiling his basic data, determine the exact location where the baby was found and the position at the time of discovery. Examination of the sleeping area may reveal a

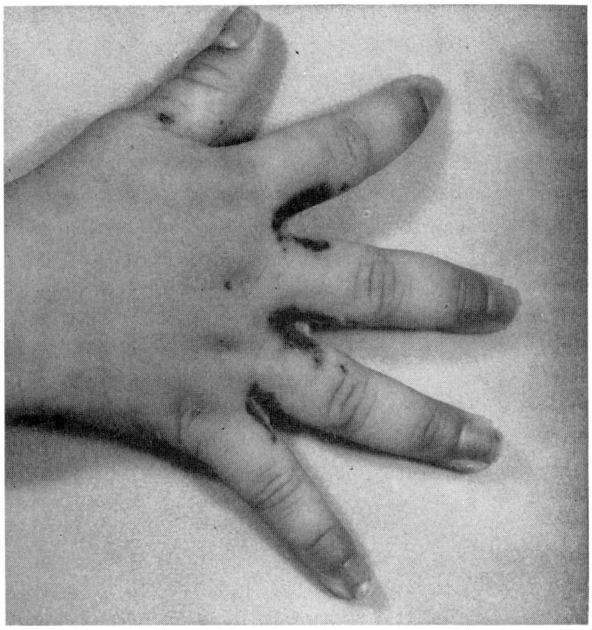

FIGURE XVIII-5. Postmortem roach bites in the webs of the fingers, as well as on the face and left arm of this infant, misinterpreted as scratches, led to the diagnosis of child abuse in the hospital emergency room. The cause of death was SIDS.

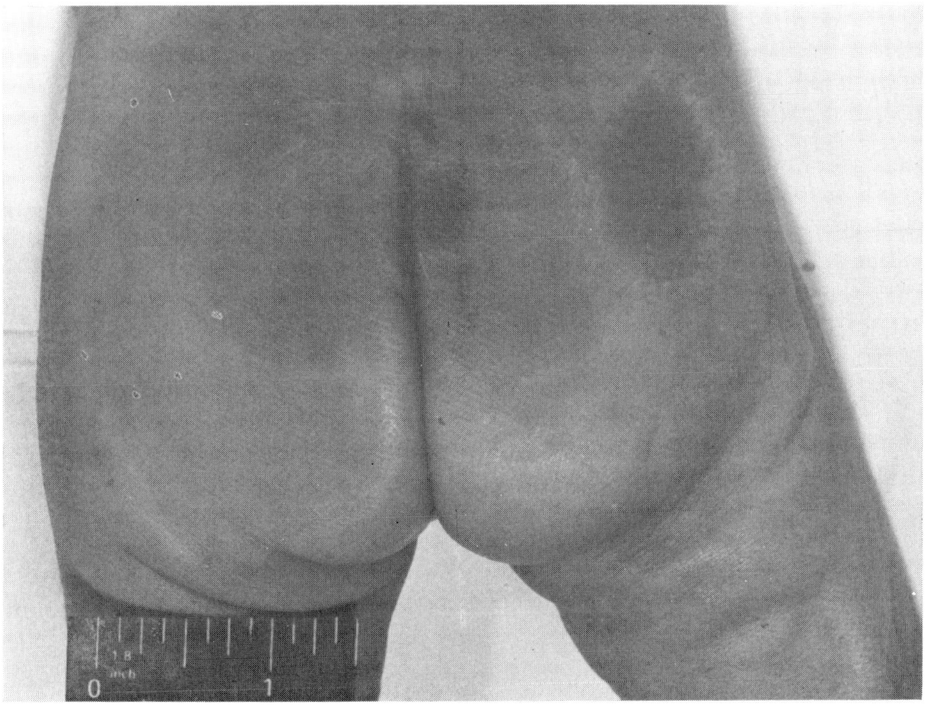

FIGURE XVIII-6. Large *Mongolian spot* on the buttocks and sacral region of a two-month-old Negro child. In some areas the pigmentation is more pronounced, resembling bruises.

faulty crib, which permitted the child to slip off of the mattress and remain suspended by the neck (as shown in Fig. XII-8). Autopsy examination in such cases reveals no characteristic findings to indicate the accidental nature of the death.[3] The investigator should also be aware that active infants can end up in unusual, often awkward positions in their cribs.

The previous health of the infant, including his birth history, must be documented, along with any treatment and medication received. Recent changes in the infant's behavior and activity are significant. Siblings and other members of the household may indicate an existing source of infection.

Postmortem findings in infants dying of SIDS are few and nonspecific. The infants are usually well developed; their size and state of nutrition are normal. Pinpoint hemorrhages are frequently found under the visceral pleura, pericardium and epicardium and under the capsule of the thymus gland. Pulmonary edema of varying degree is also a common finding. In conditions other than SIDS such hemorrhages are usually not so intense. Evidence of mild upper respiratory tract infection, including otitis media, is not unusual. Regurgitated milk may be present in the upper airway.

Endeavors to uncover the cause of SIDS have led investigators to explore the hypothesis of chronic oxygen lack occurring before or after birth. A possible malfunction or immaturity of the respiratory center in the brain has been considered. This theory would be supported by the fact that deaths due to SIDS very rarely occur after twelve months of age, at which time such centers presumably mature. Many of these children demonstrate periodic apneic spells, which are only revealed when a careful history is obtained. Other infants demonstrate no abnormalities with regard to their respiration.

One aspect common to most victims of SIDS is the history whereby the child was fed as usual, put to bed and found unresponsive just a few hours later.

Pathologic findings described by Naeye[4] supporting the hypothesis of a respiratory disorder include increased thickness of the walls of the blood vessels in the lungs and the right ventricle of the heart, retention of brown fat and hepatic erythropoieses, as well as an abnormal increase in astroglial fibers in the brain stem. We have noted an unusually large amount of fat in the liver cells of infants dying of SIDS. The cause of these changes awaits further elucidation.

Factors that have been identified in placing infants at high risk for SIDS include prematurity, low birth weight, maternal smoking and maternal drug addiction.[5] The incidence of SIDS in twins is significantly higher than in the general population.

Because of prevailing misconception on the part of the public with regard to SIDS, many parents develop a profound guilt complex thinking that they may have been able to prevent their infant's death. In this respect it is helpful if the coroner, medical examiner or pathologist ensures that the autopsy findings are relayed and explained to the parents as rapidly as possible. Notification of the public health department provides knowledgeable personnel able to support and counsel families as they attempt to understand and cope with their tragedy.

## REFERENCES


1. Wooley, P. V., Jr.: Mechanical suffocation during infancy. *J Pediatr, 26*:572-575, 1945.
2. Bergman, A. B., Beckwith, J. B., and Ray, C. G. (Eds.): *Sudden Infant Death Syndrome: Proceedings of the Second International Conference on Causes of Sudden Death in Infants.* Seattle, U of Wash Pr, 1970, p. 248.
3. Smialek, J. E., Smialek, P. Z., and Spitz, W. U.: Accidental bed deaths in infants. *Clin Pediatr, 17*:32, 1977.
4. Naeye, R.: The sudden infant death syndrome—A review of recent advances. *Arch Pathol Lab Med, 101*:156-167, 1977.
5. Valdez-Dapena, M.: The sudden infant death syndrome—1975—An update for pathologists. *Int Acad Pathol Bull, 16*:15-25, 1975.

*Part 3*

# THE BATTERED CHILD

JAMES T. WESTON

MAN'S INHUMANITY to man in its most extreme form—mistreatment and murder of his offspring—has been well documented throughout each era of recorded history. This mistreatment has been rationalized by virtually every justification known to man, including religious beliefs and practices, discipline and education and, to a large degree, economic gain. The reaction not only of those in influential positions but even of the general population has consistently oscillated between complete abandonment of physical punishment and its excessive use to the point of savagery. Tales of extreme physical abuse for economic gain were common during the period of the Industrial Revolution, both in Great Britain and in the early United States, with children as young as five to ten years of age frequently chained to industrial manufacturing devices for as long as twelve to sixteen hours in one period. This abuse to children throughout the ages has provoked periodic waves of sympathy, each arousing public indignation and then subsiding until the next period of provocation.[1]

The medical literature has made it clear that there is virtually no conceivable form of inhumanity to children that has not been documented. Newspaper accounts have described in vivid detail instances of closeting of children in lightless rooms for weeks and months; restraint of children to the top and underside of beds; suspension of children by their wrists from shower curtain rods and other wall hardware; prolonged exposure to extremes of temperature, including forcing of children to be seated unclad on blocks of ice for extended periods of time; and thermal punishment, varying from burning with cigarettes to forcing of children with wet pants to be seated on stoves and radiators or immersed in hot water until extensive burns result. Death caused by inhalation of pepper[2] administered for disciplinary reasons and death as a result of starvation for the same purpose have also been described.

Estimates of the number of children requiring protective services annually in the United States vary from 250,000 to 500,000.[3] It has also been said that, in the United States, one or possibly two children are being killed by their parents each day.

The distinguished pediatric radiologist Caffey[4] in 1946 initiated the most recent surge of interest by reporting his observation of a common association of subdural hematoma and abnormal x ray changes suggestive of trauma in the long bones. Similar observations were reported by Silverman[5] several years later, while in 1955 Woolley[6] revealed that the trauma noted, largely fractures in the long bones in these immature victims, was in many cases willfully inflicted by parents or siblings. In 1961 Dr. Henry Kempe,[7] at a symposium of the American Academy of Pediatrics, proposed the term *battered-child syndrome* in order to direct attention to the seriousness of the problem. Unfortunately, such a denotation did not initially include the case of the neglected child, which has subsequently been designated by many as the *failure to thrive syndrome*.[8, 9] More recent comprehensive considerations, which attempt to include all types of pathologic parent-child interaction, have added designations for *emotional neglect* and *emotional abuse*. These conditions are by far the most common form of abuse in all strata of today's society. They present no evidence of physical injury but are increasingly recognized as conditions that may set the stage for serious adolescent sociopathic

---

Some of the material in this chapter has been taken from the author's original contribution in *The Battered Child*, edited by R. E. Helfer and C. H. Kemp, University of Chicago Press, 1968.

behavior, provide the impetus for suicide or create a subsequent generation of emotional or physical abusers.

Child abuse as it is presented in this part will not deal with infanticide, the intentional killing of an infant, usually by its mother, in the newborn period. Neither will this chapter include intentional homicide, which differs from child abuse in that the latter is not expected to culminate in death. Instead, emphasis will be placed on the setting in which child abuse occurs and on the recognition of characteristic injuries that identify an abused child.

## THE INVESTIGATION OF SUSPECTED CHILD ABUSE

Whether in a metropolitan or rural locale, it is usually an arm of the law enforcement community that is first notified of unexpected or sudden deaths among infants or preschool children. After such notification, it is usually the responsibility of detectives, augmented by children's protective service caseworkers if they have been following the family, to conduct the necessary in-depth investigation into the family's living conditions and circumstances of the child's death. In each such death an orderly investigation should be conducted by an individual thoroughly familiar with all of the ramifications of child abuse.

The terminal position of the body and the findings surrounding the infant's death, whether or not they appear unusual at the time, are of considerable significance. Occasionally the terminal position of a baby in a crib may indicate a physical hazard and the mechanism of death while subsequent postmortem examination is inconclusive.

The investigator should note the geographic location of the home within the community, and a comparison should be made of this home and its state of repair with adjoining residences. The state of repair of sanitary accommodations, lavatory facilities, range, illumination, heating appliances and, in general, the degree of cleanliness, as well as any indication that the scene might have been modified to any degree prior to the officer's arrival, are pertinent data. Any observation of overt trash or the presence of fecal material, a urinous odor or numerous domestic animal droppings within the home should be recorded. Dangerous environmental conditions, such as exposed electric wires and inadequately ventilated or overcrowded rooms, are significant. Evidence of long-standing infestation by rodents or insects is similarly important. If the home is not considered satisfactory for human habitation, the appropriate public health agency should be immediately notified.

Documentation by photography, gathering of physical evidence and reporting have to be objective, outlining all observations in a way that will enable another individual to evaluate these findings and arrive at an independent conclusion concerning the *degree of care* for the children and *degree of maturity* of the parents as reflected within the home environment. It is not sufficient for an investigator to incorporate within his report or relay to the examining pathologist information that in his opinion the home was *filthy* or that the parents were *chronic alcoholics* just because the refrigerator was laden with beer rather than milk for the youngsters.

The individual most qualified to make the necessary detailed observations on the body of the deceased is the pathologist or, if he is unavailable, an individual trained to recognize and record accurately the body temperature, rigor mortis and other postmortem manifestations of earlier death. There is no substitute for the pathologist who observes the terminal surroundings and position of the child.

The investigator may call upon an experienced children's protective service worker, who in turn may point out hitherto unrecognized unusual features in the home environment and in the nature of the interrelationship between the deceased and the siblings or parents. The initial visit is usually not the appropriate time to delve in depth into the nature of the family structure. However, often candid observations concerning the reaction of the parents, siblings or even of the neighbors to the youngster's death cause sufficient suspicion in the officer or social worker to warrant review of the initial impression and immediate pursuit of the investigation in some depth.

The examination of the home is of more value if done as early as possible, but this opportunity may be lost as a result of delayed reporting and in cases where the child has been taken to the hospital for treatment. When it is necessary to conduct such delayed investigation of the home environment by arrangement or even by surprise, the findings must be weighed accordingly and very careful observation afforded to any recent changes there or to any allegations of parents passed on to neighbors, friends or relatives outside the home. Questioning of adults in the home is best conducted individually as well as together. Occasionally the interview of siblings conducted out of the parents' presence provides information of great value. Siblings presenting testimony that might be injurious to their general welfare if returned to the home should be offered permanent protective shelter. All of the findings of the investigation, when not conducted with the pathologist present, should be discussed with him as soon as possible. This affords the investigating officer the opportunity of thorough pursuit of all the possible evidential ramifications.

## MEDICAL EXAMINATION

Upon initial inspection of the body, the question often raised by physicians unaware of all aspects of child abuse is that of the necessity of internal examination. Recognizing the possibility of several variations in the syndrome of childhood abuse, the physician should proceed with a detailed medicolegal autopsy in every instance of infant or childhood death, with the possible exception of those who expire after a long-substantiated medical history of a natural condition. The absence of overt trauma on the body exterior is no contraindication for an autopsy, since this often bears no relationship to trauma in the interior of the body. Careful search of the body exterior for any type of trace evidence may afford a clue to the assailant or the nature of the weapon used. Trace evidence, such as semen, if found, should be carefully preserved, documented and submitted for appropriate laboratory examination in accordance with all the well-established patterns for handling such evidence, maintaining preservation of its chain. Initial documentation should include detailed photography of the child as he was originally received.

Inspection of the body should note the nature of the clothing, the degree of cleanliness and state of repair, as well as external characteristics of the child, including height, weight, appropriate circumferences, state of nutrition and any suggestions of apparent selective nutritional deficiency. If the body has not been seen by a physician at the time of death, observation of postmortem changes such as temperature, rigor and livor mortis, the presence of postmortem infestation by maggots or other insects and, if present, the degree of putrefactive changes should be correlated with information presented by the investigator. This may substantiate or negate the initial allegations of the family concerning their care of the child at or before the time of death. Discrepancies between the distribution of livor mortis and the terminal position of the body, body temperature and the alleged final care or the obvious state of nutrition or well-being of the infant or child and the apparent concern of the parents require follow-up investigation.

The state of nutrition as reflected by the subcutaneous fatty depots, the degree of diaper rash and any secondary manifestations of this, such as infection, scarring or loss of pigmentation, and insect infestation, including fresh bites or secondary infection in older bites, are important manifestations of neglect. Diligent search, not only of the external but of the internal portions of the body, may be necessary to rule out any specific chronic condition that may have contributed to or caused the *failure to thrive* syndrome.

Internal malformations and chronic dietary conditions characterized by exacerbations, remissions and often specific avitaminosis may play a role not only in the cause of the terminal episode, but also indirectly, by presenting the parents with a less-than-perfect anatomic specimen, specifically provoking neglect or abuse.

Whether or not the children appear to have been afforded the customary amenities of food, clothing and sanitation, the external examination should record any instance of trauma, either recent or old, noting size, shape, location, color and the degree of healing in specific objective terms. Injuries that suggest a pattern consistent with a weapon recovered at the scene should be photographed together with the weapon to better illustrate the mechanism of the injury. In the absence of photographic equipment, tracing of the injury may be considered. Special attention afforded the description of such pattern, with indication not only of the size and nature of each wound but also of its specific location with reference to other wounds within the pattern, is always rewarding. Wounds that resemble human bite marks, whether simple patterned contusions or accompanied by breaks in the skin, are best examined by a forensic odontologist if possible but in any event should be carefully photographed with a ruler in place. Bite marks on the upper extremities must be compared with impressions of the victim's teeth. A swab of the bite area may be used to determine the blood type of the saliva deposited on the skin.

Each wound should be specifically topographically located on the body with reference to known anatomic landmarks. Adjacent wounds may have been caused by a single blow that inflicted two separate wounds. The question is often asked, how many blows were dealt to the body? The experienced practitioner usually retains an adequate margin of error, being apprised of the fact that the irregular contours on the body exterior and the relationship of the soft tissues to the underlying bony structures may well produce a pattern wherein one blow produced two distinct wounds separated by apparently normal tissue. Such a phenomenon is frequently observed following a beating with a stick, whip or belt as outlined in Chapter VII.

Certain areas of the body are sometimes overlooked in hospital autopsies. These include the scalp, particularly posteriorly, and the nape of the neck, the back and abdomen, as well as those more obscure portions of the body that sometimes are intentionally subjected to physical trauma in order to conceal this from the other parent, physicians, social caseworkers or police officers. Parents, acquainted with the practices of *welfare doctors* within one community, knew that the busy practice of these physicians with inadequate paramedical assistance would limit the examination to the head and upper trunk. In one instance a child died the day following such examination, which was restricted to measure of oral temperature and inspection of the head and neck, while the lower portion of the body remained wrapped in the blanket within which it was presented.

Examination of the buttocks and the soles of the feet, followed by incision of the skin in these locations, may reveal fresh or resorbing subcutaneous hematomas not suspected by external examination. Deep bruises of the buttocks are invariably due to severe beating.

Examination of the body orifices may show mucosal tears of the mouth, laceration of the frenulum and tongue and chipped or dislocated teeth. The female genitals may disclose evidence of penetration which may not be only by a penis but by finger manipulation or insertion of a foreign object. Manifestations of earlier or repeated sexual penetration include relaxation and healed mucosal tears, venereal warts and infection. Upon suspicion of penetration of any of the body orifices by a penis, appropriate specimens for detection of seminal constituents, as described in Chapter XIX, should be collected.

Roentgenographic examination of the entire skeleton prior to autopsy is required whenever child abuse is suspected. If subtle changes are noted, another x ray examination conducted following removal of the organs may be more revealing. A radiologist may be of great assistance in establishing episodes of injury to the bony structures, since he is routinely called upon to evaluate the degree of healing of fractures.

### Internal Examination

A medicolegal examination includes a detailed objective observation and description of all internal findings related to disease or changes arising out of unnatural conditions or trauma. Color changes, adhesions or other evidence of healing may assist in dating a traumatic episode. Microscopic examination, including special stains, is of great importance for the aging of injuries in the skin and subcutaneous tissues as well as in the internal organs.

Routine histologic examination should be conducted of every organ system in the neglected infant to rule out the possibility of underlying obscure, constitutional, debilitating disease that might lead to progressive wasting. In evaluating the degree of healing of injuries, it is significant that preexisting natural disease be considered. Certain chronic conditions are likely to retard the process of wound healing.

Continuing contributions to the literature point out the importance of a general toxicologic examination to rule out the introduction of exogenous poisons or overdoses of therapeutic agents as contributing factors to the deaths of children.[10, 11] The toxicologic assay should be both qualitative and quantitative and as comprehensive as the scope of the toxicologic laboratory will allow. While most of these investigations are negative, the absence of such analyses could prove grounds for *reasonable doubt* during the course of criminal litigation. The postmortem toxicologic screen should rule out the role of lead as a primary or contributing factor in the death of these children. A defense attorney may legitimately inquire about the possibility of a craving for unnatural articles of food, which is known to occur in pica.

When a child is suspected to have expired as a result of neglect, examination should include the contents of the gastrointestinal tract and, when appropriate, photographic documentation of its contents. Postmortem bacteriological studies may assist in establishing the etiologic agent or agents causing or contributing to the death if of an infectious nature.

Upon completion of the postmortem examination and ideally after a period of twelve to twenty-four hours of refrigeration, it is of value to reexamine the exterior of the child's body. Drainage of the visceral blood in the course of the autopsy and continued settling of the peripheral blood frequently allow progressive blanching of the skin, which enables better delineation of superficial bruises and may reveal patterned injuries not noted on earlier examination. On at least three occasions in the author's experience, initial examination of a body revealed only obscure, minor swelling of the face associated with minimal discoloration consistent with artifactual trauma, possibly resulting from the placing of a resuscitation mask over the nose and mouth. Upon subsequent refrigeration and examination after autopsy, the detailed imprints of wounds caused by knuckles and fingertips were outlined. Thus an initial ambiguous but suspicious examination may evolve into one in which there is well-documented evidence of trauma. When such is the case, it is important that these findings be documented and that the prosecutor be advised of this progressive change in the examiner's observations. It is also important that the prosecutor be appraised of the fact that these do not represent a postmortem change in the wounds but rather a postmortem change in the background surrounding the wounds, allowing them to be exposed.

### Evaluation of Findings and Follow-up

As the pathologist completes his preliminary investigation and examination, he should acquaint the investigating officer or social worker with all of the possible alternatives of his observations in order to institute a prompt and thorough follow-up investigation. The experienced forensic pathologist who during his career has conducted a large number of postmortem examinations on maltreated infants and children may have less hesitation to unequivocally express an opinion of child abuse in a certain case than the hospital pathologist who is rarely called upon to conduct medicolegal examinations and whose experience may include only an occasional such examination on neglected or otherwise abused children.

Two studies presently in progress, one in Great Britain,[12] another by Helfer and associates in the United States,[13] provide information that may be of assistance in evaluating intentional injuries in children. This information was derived from studies of living children in whom the mechanism of injury was documented. In a preliminary report of the former, in which 9523 inspections were conducted on 481 children attending day nurseries, 1543 accidental injuries were recorded. None of these injuries was found to be bilaterally symmetrical about the long axis of the body—affecting both sides of the head or both arms. The second study is a review of 246 children under five years of age who fell out of beds or cribs or off examining tables, a height of 36 inches or less. None of these children suffered any serious life-threatening injuries from their falls. Eighty percent of these incidents resulted in no observable injuries; 17 percent were reported to have had bumps, lumps, bruises and scratches. Three children had identifiable skull fracture on x ray films, but none had sustained brain damage.

The authors of the study conclude that closed head injury with brain damage or injury of any type is extremely rare in children aged five and under who fall out of bed.

The hospital pathologist is often apt to be misled by information from an investigator concerning an innocent account of minor trauma. Whether forensic or hospital pathologist, when the order of magnitude of mistreatment, neglect or abuse is not in keeping with the preliminary investigative report relayed to him, he should request that the investigator pursue his investigation more aggressively.

When the suspected perpetrator is confronted with the news that the nature of the injury has led the pathologist to conclude that it was the result of abuse and not consistent with inadvertent accidental injury, an admission of inflicted minor physical abuse to the child as a result of momentary aggravation and rage may be evoked. Persistent interrogation after such an admission usually leads to ultimate unfolding of the entire sordid episode. Separate information gleaned by individual interrogation of the parents, when brought together, may provoke hostility between the parents and thereafter prompt admission or further implication.

In the absence of such an admission, physical injury may be of such magnitude as to allow the examining physician to conclude that it was purposefully inflicted. Dating of the injury may further place a certain perpetrator alone with the deceased child. Under such circumstances, prosecution may be successful based on postmortem findings.

When child abuse is suspected, consideration should be given to the welfare of the remaining siblings, irrespective of the ultimate outcome of criminal litigation.

---

→

FIGURE XVIII-7. (a): Six-month-old child, revealing loss of subcutaneous fatty depots associated with loss of skin turgor and accumulation of dirt. Note the absence of any specific changes of avitaminosis, such as rachitic rosary. (b): Back of the same infant, demonstrating peculiar wizened appearance of the trunk and extremities associated with marked atrophy of the extremities and concavity of the cheeks. There is no indication of severe diaper rash, but peculiar wrinkling of skin over the buttocks consistent with loss of skin turgor and chronic depletion of subcutaneous fat is present. (c): Closeup appearance of the lower abdomen and genitalia in the same infant, showing extensive depigmentation around the genitalia and thighs in the absence of secondary inflammation or dermatitis.

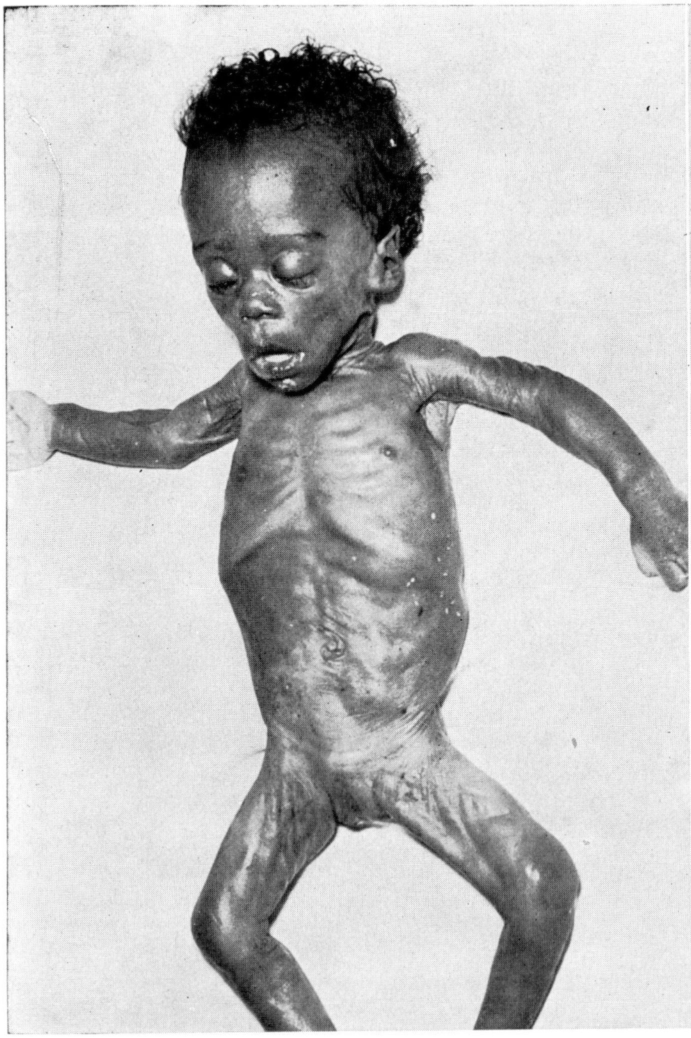

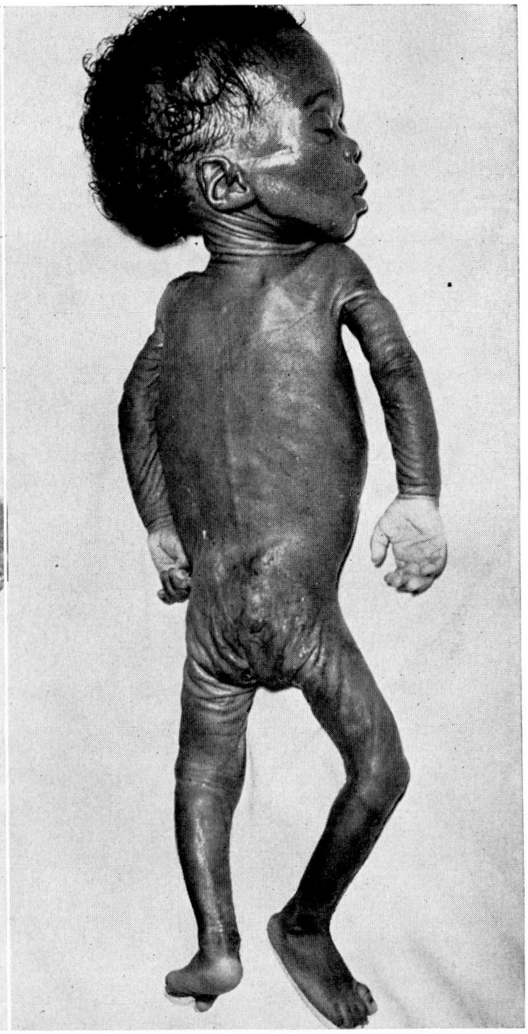

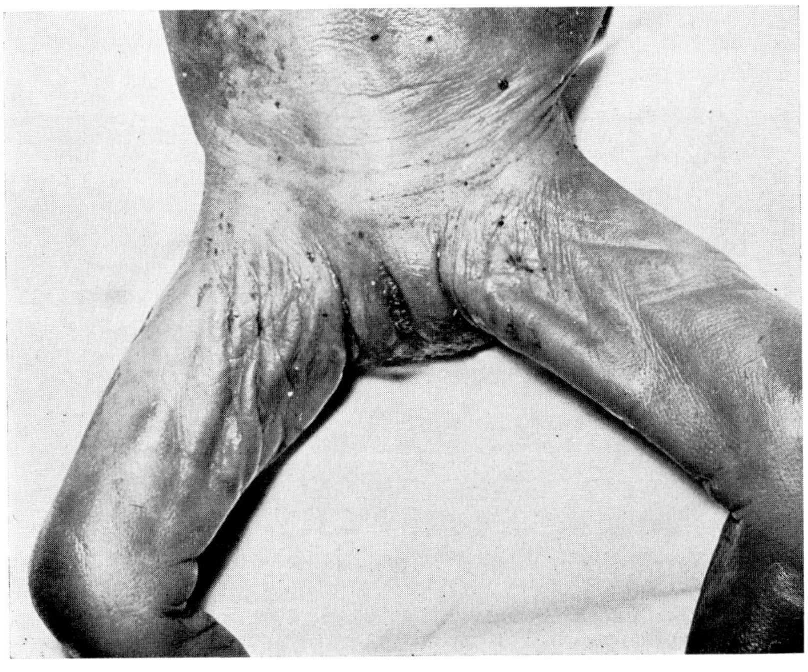

The external appearance of neglected children is that of dereliction of the necessary amenities of food, clothing and sanitation.

A six-month-old child was presented by the natural mother and a paramour to the emergency services of a large metropolitan hospital at 2:00 A.M., with a history of having been left alone for several hours while the parents were out at a party in the neighborhood. Physical examination revealed loss of subcutaneous fatty tissue, with the infant presenting a peculiar wizened appearance of the trunk and extremities, over which the excess skin was folded with excessive wrinkling (Fig. XVIII-7a, b).

Extensive deposition of urine, fecal matter and dirt were present about the lower abdomen, genitalia and thighs, associated with an extremely foul odor (Fig. XVIII-7c).

The paramour indicated no concern for the child. The mother, with a similar flat emotional response,

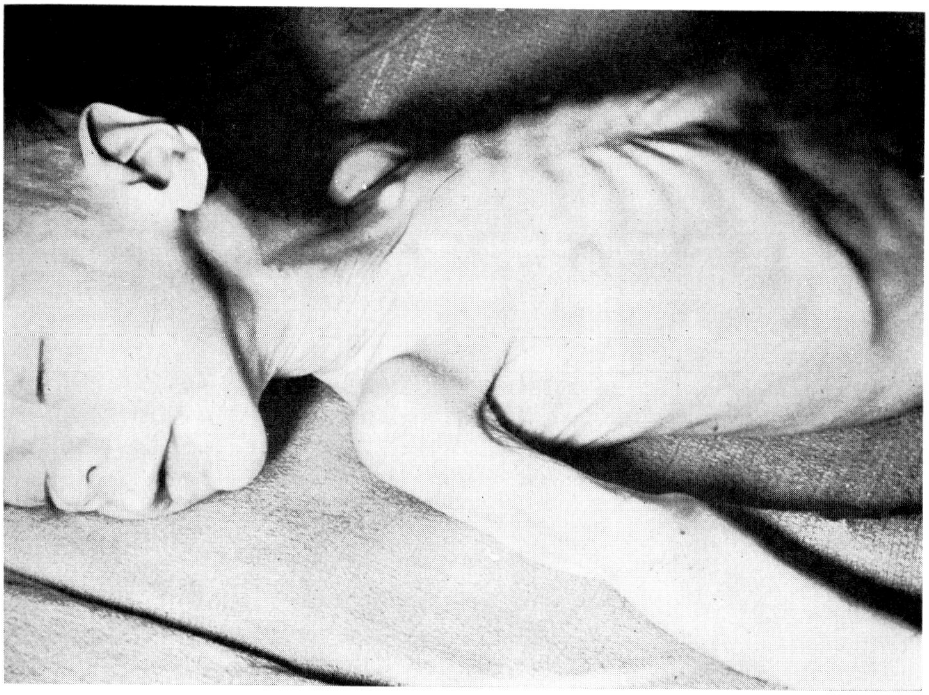

FIGURE XVIII-8. Four-month-old child with complete absence of fatty tissue on the face, neck and trunk and relative increase in the front-to-back diameter of the chest. Note the absence of rachitic rosary.

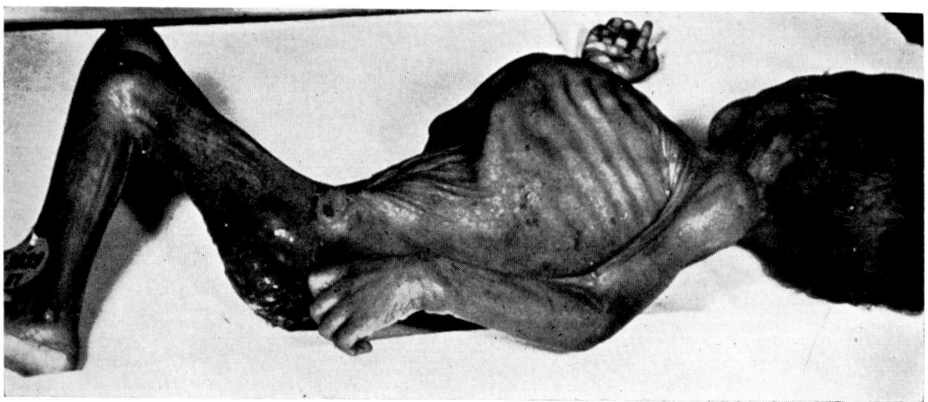

FIGURE XVIII-9. Extremely starved six-month-old child with complete absence of subcutaneous tissue and virtually all muscle in the extremities and trunk. There is a prominent increase in the front-to-back diameter of the chest associated with changes of avitaminosis-D and a prominent rachitic rosary. Also present are skin changes of the buttocks and lower extremities, consistent with infected diaper rash.

indicated this child to be the youngest of the six within her home, conceived by three different fathers. She explained to the pediatrician that the responsibility of caring for the younger children was that of the nine-year-old sibling of the deceased child. She thought her responsibility ended with making welfare-supplied food available to these children for their consumption.

The clothing is usually soiled, frequently caked with a mixture of dirt, urine and feces. This may have to be soaked from the body to avoid denudation of the skin while undressing.

These infants are usually devoid of subcutaneous fat, with complete loss of turgor. The skin hangs loosely over the bones of the extremities and is often depressed into the concavities of the face (Fig. XVIII-8). The abdomen is often markedly sunken with the ribs presenting an unusually prominent front-to-back diameter (Fig. XVIII-9).

A nine-month-old child in a moribund condition was presented to the welfare pediatrician in a large city with obvious clinical sepsis associated with extreme fever. Examination revealed extensive weeping diaper rash extending from the armpits to the soles of the feet, involving virtually the entire back of both thighs and lower legs. This was associated with denudation, weeping and infection of the subcutaneous fat tissue, precipitating the sepsis (Fig. XVIII-10).

Questioning of the mother revealed that she was in the habit of placing the child, one of five within the family who were largely unattended during the day, on a rubber sheet placed over a poorly constructed mattress. Urine and feces were allowed to accumulate within this cradle from week to week. The mother did, on Saturday afternoon, remove the baby and rinse it lightly under the tap water. She similarly rinsed the sheet. The baby was thereupon placed back in the crib, and a similar arrangement persisted for the following week.

Food was supplied by an older sibling and was delivered in a bottle held in place by a folded pillow. The mother claimed that the baby had not been bathed during its entire lifetime within the home, having been delivered at home by a midwife neighbor.

Infrequent changing of diapers and bedding is often manifested by severe diaper rash, frequently associated with weeping denudation of the skin of the genitalia and perineum. However, a neglected child may not have diaper rash, as diapers may not have been used. Diaper rash, when present over an extended duration, may cause extreme scarring, loss of pigmentation and often pockmark-type residua of sec-

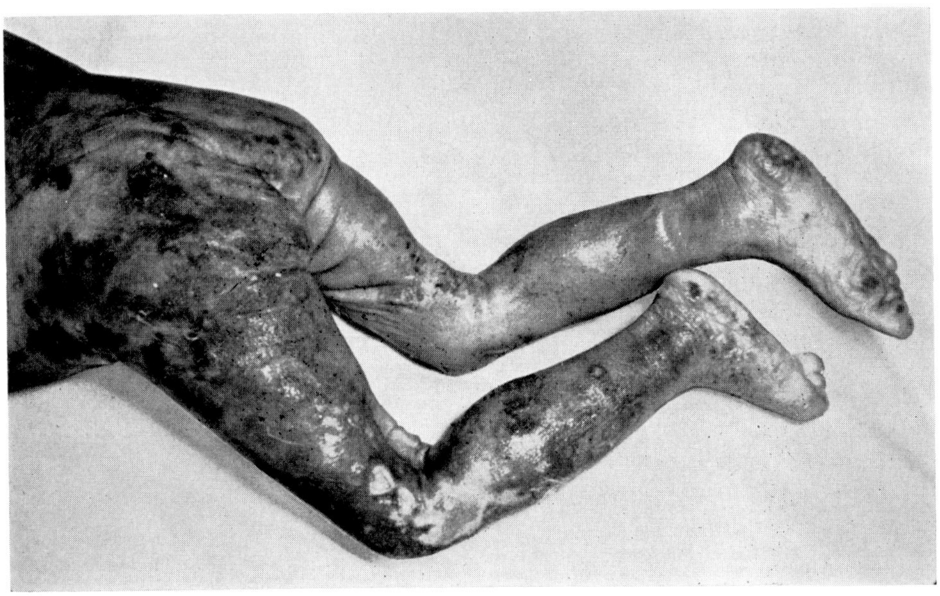

FIGURE XVIII-10. Nine-month-old child, delivered at home by a midwife. Microscopic examination confirmed the presence of residual vernix on the baby, who had never had a water or oil bath. The back, buttocks and lower extremities show severe infected diaper rash extending over the soles of the feet. (From Helfer and Kempe: *The Battered Child.* Chicago, U of Chicago Pr, 1972.)

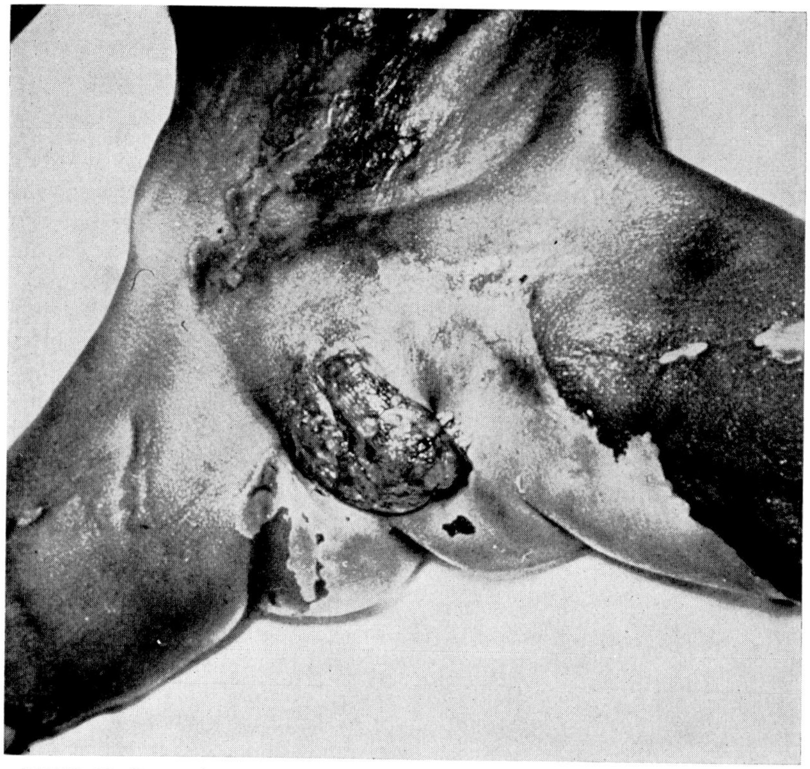

FIGURE XVIII-11. Loss of pigmentation in the area about the genitalia following severe diaper rash with persistent secondary infection in an eleven-month-old child.

ondarily infected sores, which commonly persist following treatment (Figs. XVIII-11, XVIII-12 and XVIII-13).

When such infants are seen by clinicians during the terminal period of their lives, the clinical manifestations are usually similar. The in-

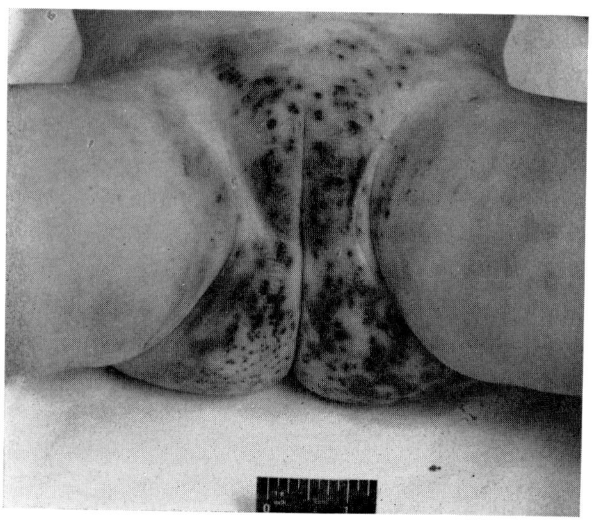

FIGURE XVIII-12. Ten-month-old child with a pocklike diaper rash. This extent of diaper rash is quite common and indicates neglect.

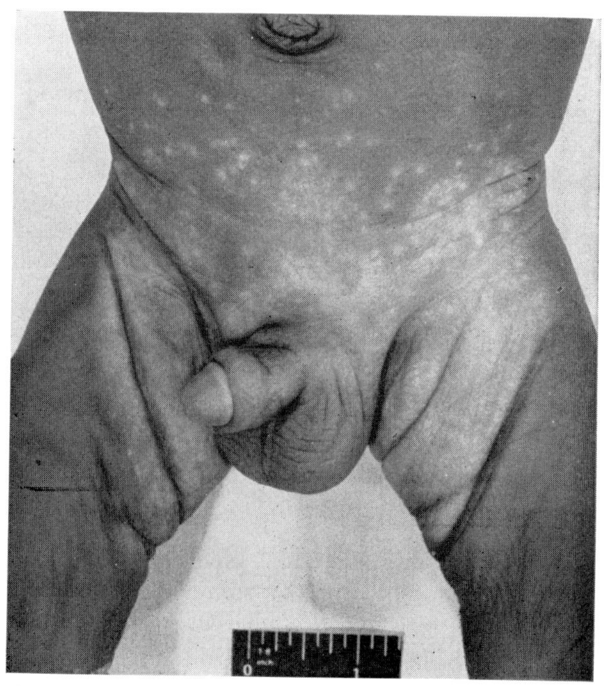

FIGURE XVIII-13. Punctate and confluent residual scars of earlier diaper rash.

fants present an extremely low state of metabolism associated with marked diminution in the respiratory rate and volume, low body temperature and often vascular collapse, which exist until death, in spite of administration of parenteral fluids, oxygen and steroids. These children often are presented with the story that *the baby was put to bed well the evening before and found extremely sick or dead for no explained reason in the morning.*

An eight-month-old child was admitted moribund to a metropolitan hospital with almost complete absence of fat and extensive secondarily infected diaper rash over the back and buttocks.

The child responded well to *intense mothering,* wherein he was afforded food, love, constant care and medication to correct his skin irritation. Seven weeks after admission he had regained the expected body weight and, although somewhat flat in his emotional response, physically was a normal infant marked only by scars (Fig. XVIII-14a). Although followed by caseworkers of a social service agency, the same infant was subsequently found dead within his residence, clad in oversized clothing with terminal milky vomitus about his nose and mouth.

Postmortem examination revealed complete depletion of fatty depots (Fig. XVIII-14b) externally and internally, extensive reinfection of severe diaper rash associated with the scars of preexisting ulcerations (Fig. XVIII-14c) and, within the gastrointestinal tract, no indication of feeding within twenty-four to forty-eight hours prior to death.

Parents often go to extreme measures to cover up their neglect. The clothing may be changed during the period immediately prior to or after the death and the skin denuded by extensive scrubbing.

A six and one-half-month-old male child was received cold with advanced rigor mortis in the emergency room of a metropolitan hospital at approximately 10:00 A.M. He was clad in a clean diaper and a sparkling clean christening gown, which had a persistent smell of mothballs and beneath which was an infant-type shirt still bearing the price tag. The parents initially alleged that they had placed the baby in this condition in the crib the evening before. They had been out of the home until approximately 1:00 A.M. and, upon returning, found the child apparently well. However, when they awakened in the morning, they found the child in a lifeless condition.

Subsequent interviews revealed that the parents had been grossly negligent in the child's care, and that, upon awakening following an early-morning return from a party, they had found their child cold and lifeless. The mother readily admitted that it took approximately thirty to forty minutes of soaking to remove the extremely soiled diaper from the infant without denuding the skin. They accomplished this and then scrubbed the deceased baby extensively with a vegetable brush, the residue of which was apparent on the body. The father, as soon as a local store opened, purchased the shirt and diaper. After placing the christening gown on the baby, the parents delivered him to the nearest emergency room.

Neglect of infants and children is not consistently associated with prolonged deprivation of food and sanitary amenities. The definition of childhood neglect and the basis for legal intervention may vary considerably from community to community. In some areas it includes the deprivation of medication necessary for survival. Similarly, in many communities prosecution for neglect may ensue following the death of unattended children in homes destroyed by fire.

Exasperation and preoccupation with other domestic situations may result in more extreme measures. In one instance a two and one-half-month-old child expired as a result of generalized sepsis and bronchopneumonia, complicating gangrene and paraphimosis following the placement of a rubber band ligature about the distal portion of the infant's penis. The mother complained that the washing of diapers for her single offspring at this early age demeaned her to a position wherein she could no longer command self-respect.

Other unusual circumstances, such as the extended absence of a spouse, may place emotional stress upon one or both parents who otherwise consistently cared for their offspring in a satisfactory manner.

A lifeless eight-month-old child, well developed, well nourished, clean and apparently well cared for, was brought to the emergency room of a local hospital in the early morning after the parents allegedly had put him to bed the evening before in good health. Initial external examination revealed the presence of skin changes consistent with maggot infestation. Interview with the parents indicated that the father, who was a sailor, had been absent from the home for approximately eight months. Upon his return, the parents charged a teenager within the apartment with the responsibility of the infant and were *out on the town*

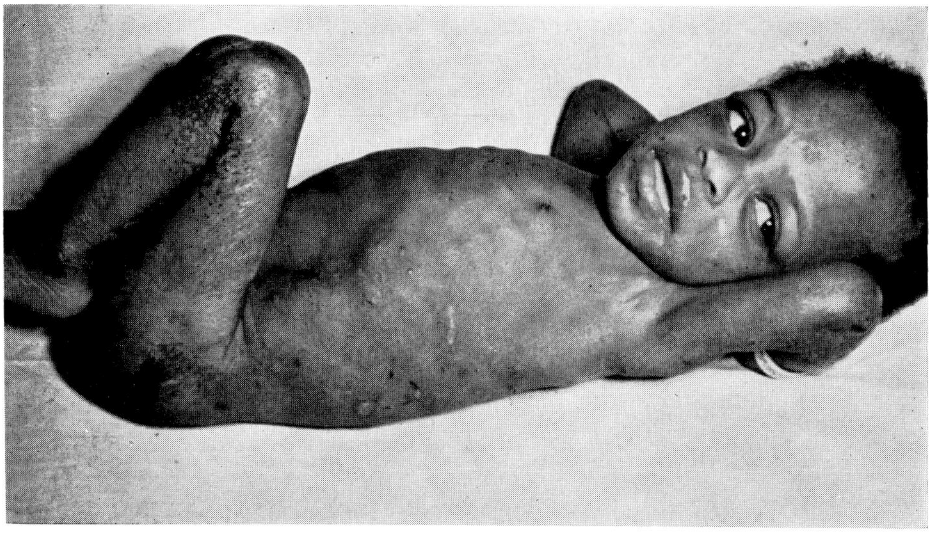

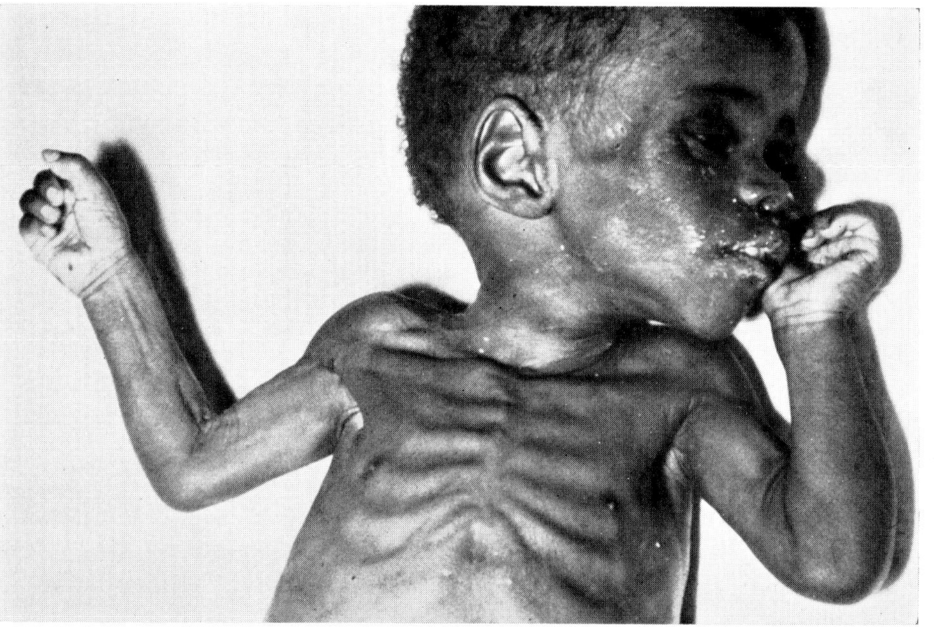

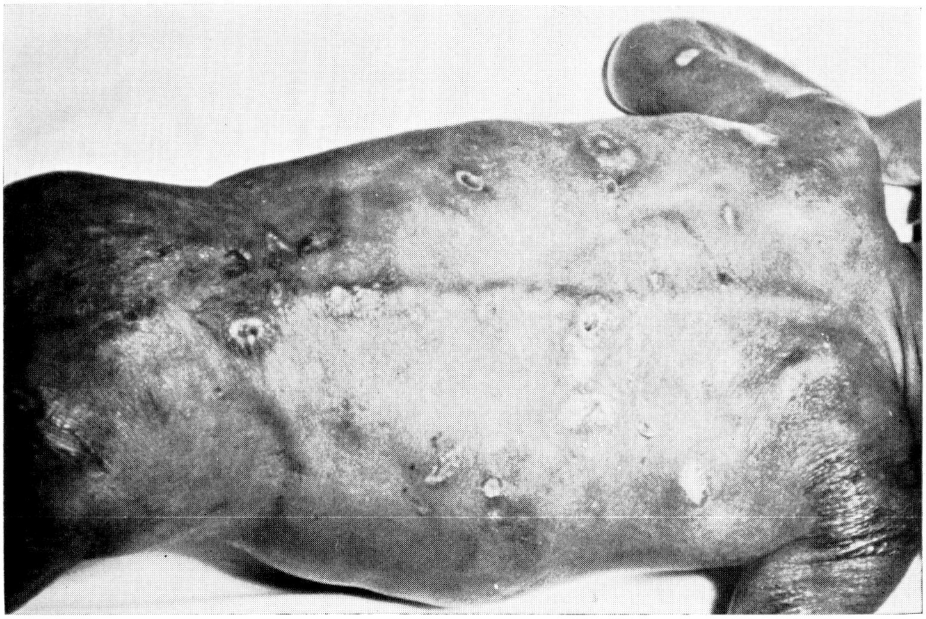

in excess of forty-eight hours. The exact mechanism of the child's death was not identified. Presence of the *maggot tracks* served only to indicate absence of care for an extended period.

Autopsy reveals depletion of fat, not only within the subcutaneous tissue but within the internal fatty depots. The stomach and intestine usually contain little or no recently digested food, although there may be terminal fecal impaction.

The poor general state of health of such infants represents a significant predisposing factor for the development of complications that eventually lead to death. Most common among these are bronchopneumonia, sepsis associated with cellulitis, otitis media, laryngotracheobronchitis and urinary bladder infection. Unrecognized underlying constitutional conditions, congenital or acquired, that could have contributed to the starvation and emaciation are quite rare. Nevertheless, cystic fibrosis, celiac disease or possibly other, more obscure pancreatic exocrine disorders must be excluded.

Exhaustive chemical analyses in neglected infants have failed to reveal any evidence of lead or other exogenous poisons or drugs, except for two known instances of methemoglobinemia associated with exposure to sodium nitrate as a sedative. Within the literature are reported instances of children maintained in clinical semicoma or coma by extended use of tranquilizers or barbiturates, which, in several instances following exposure at relatively high levels for long periods, resulted in convulsions with permanent brain damage.[14]

The weights of neglected infants at the time of death may vary from as low as 35 percent to 90 percent of the expected weight, except for isolated instances in which death results from neglect apart from food deprivation.

Initial confrontation of the parents usually elicits a story readily contradicted by the presenting physical appearance, one of a child *put to bed the evening before and found dead in bed the next morning*. Repeated interrogation and confrontation by the obvious disparity between this allegation and the findings on the infant usually provokes an assertion that the child would not take his feeding, may have suffered with a mild diarrhea or upper respiratory infection, may have fallen or suffered other minor trauma on a day or two prior to his demise or, occasionally, that *the child never did well after birth* or had always *failed to thrive.* The attempted postmortem cleaning of a number of the children associated with redressing reflects either concern by the parents about possible retribution by authorities or a conscious or subconscious sense of guilt following the infant's death.

Review of the family background and home conditions usually reveals that a child expiring as a result of overt neglect is the last-born of a family averaging six to seven children. Birth out-of-wedlock is common, and the socioeconomic level of the parent(s) is usually quite low (Fig. XVIII-15).

In general it might be said that the mother, unable to provide proper nutrition and hygienic care, is likewise either uninformed or otherwise incapable of providing an acceptable state of cleanliness or repair within her home. Occasional exceptions were reflected among *proud parents,* who find it necessary for mother and father to seek employment in order to provide food and shelter and who were unwilling to accept

FIGURE XVIII-14. (a): Eight-month-old child after seven week hospitalization, in which he virtually completely regained expected body weight. Hygienic care resulted also in the healing of severe secondarily infected sores associated with diaper rash about the genitalia, over the buttocks and on the back. (b): Same infant at thirteen months of age, revealing complete depletion of fatty depots on the extremities, trunk and face. (From Helfer and Kempe: *The Battered Child*. Chicago, U of Chicago Pr, 1972.) (c): Back view of the same infant, illustrating secondary infection resulting from diaper rash. Note pocklike scars of healed ulcerations.

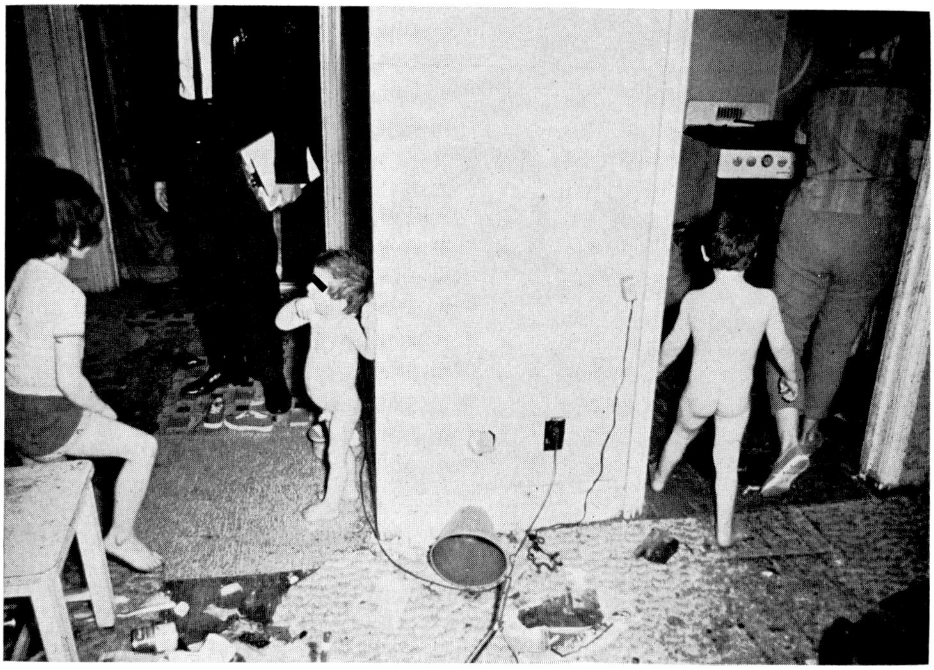

FIGURE XVIII-15. Typical home environment of a neglected child. Note absence of clothing on preschool children, presence of soiled food containers, fecal matter, papers, etc. on the floor, and state of disrepair of the home and furniture.

public contributions. Mothers of these children often have offspring by more than one father, frequently from as many as three or four paramours whose whereabouts are unknown. The mother is often young (eighteen to twenty-two years), often marrying before graduation from high school and abandoned by the young husband following mutual dissatisfaction with their teenage romance.

Trained social workers and investigators frequently make reference in their reports to *filthy homes,* wherein they describe the odor of urine, feces—both human and animal—and wherein they make repeated references to infestation by insects, particularly roaches and flies. Observation of the food supplies often reveals only sparse quantities of the necessities in refrigerators and kitchens. In some instances the homes are considered not fit for human habitation. Interviews of the neighbors of these families often indicate a pattern of long-standing dereliction with no apparent regard for the children's welfare.

Another reasonably valid indication of lack of parental concern for the offspring may be found in examination of available medical records. Frequently, well-baby appointments are not kept, and the infants are not afforded medical treatment when ill.

Occasionally, the infant expiring in the first year of life as the result of neglect either may have associated traumatic changes of a repetitive nature, with roentgenographic examination revealing multiple healed fractures, or he may have expired of acute trauma following a violent emotional outburst. If a child, particularly in an urban area, survives through the first year of life in a family situation as described, his physical appearance, emotional forlornness and the apparent disregard shown him by the parents often results in neighbors and friends affording the necessary care for such a child to survive when he is capable of venturing abroad. It has been said, and perhaps rightly so, that once an infant in this group is capable of even crawling into the hallway adjacent to his residence or reaching the sidewalk in front of his home, his pathetic appearance almost invariably results in attention, which often is of a lifesaving nature.

## PHYSICALLY ABUSED CHILDREN

### Children with No Previous Injury

Some physically abused children present no external or internal indication of previous injury. However, after physical examination, internal examination, medical history, roentgenographic examination or subsequent investigation with confession, evidence of previous trauma is apparent in approximately one-half of the cases in this group. These children vary in age from one month to six years, and approximately one-half are under one year of age. There is a slight male preponderance.

The socioeconomic and educational backgrounds of parents in this group are substantially different from those of the majority of parents of children expiring as a result of neglect or repetitive abuse. Virtually all of the homes are middle or upper middle class and could be described as clean and well maintained.

Included among these cases are children whose death or injury was unintentional (Table XVIII-I). As indicated in the table, upon initially presenting these infants and children for medical attendance, a small number of the parents readily accounted for the injuries resulting in their offspring's demise. In the majority of instances no premeditation was apparent, and the hand or fist served as the sole weapon. Mostly, however, the parents initially denied any knowledge of how the injury occurred. In a substantial number of the group postmortem findings were incontrovertible, and upon confrontation with these findings, the parents usually slowly unraveled a tale of physical trauma. The first confession was often that of a minor reprimand, while follow-up interview and repeated confrontation with the extent of the injuries elicited the story of extended trauma. A busy man after a hard day's work returns home to his favorite comfortable chair and attempts to find refuge with a cocktail and the evening paper. On occasion he has been nagged or climbed upon by the attention-seeking child to the point of such exasperation that he has inflicted physical injury upon the child, occasionally resulting in death. Such incidents include children whose heads strike the floor or baseboard or children deliberately pushed out of a father's lap, resulting in inadvertent injury to a vital portion of the body.

A six and one-half-year-old female child was presented to the emergency room of a metropolitan hospital in the early evening with a story of having been found dead in bed following her nap. Physical examination revealed no indication of trauma or other apparent disease. Postmortem examination revealed a fracture dislocation of the cervical spine associated with adjacent spinal cord contusion and hemorrhage, readily explaining the child's death. Subsequent interview of the father and confrontation with the anatomic findings elicited a story of his having been left with the child while the mother was out of the home for a few minutes securing groceries for dinner. The father became aggravated by the child's crying and nagging and shook her violently, a situation readily explaining the internal injuries.

Another rather typical setting for children expiring with this pathological syndrome is that

TABLE XVIII-I

CONTRAST BETWEEN THE ALLEGED AND CONFESSED METHODS OF INJURY IN CHILDREN WITH ONLY ONE EPISODE OF INJURY

| *Alleged Method of Injury (number)* | | *Confessed Method of Injury (number)* | |
|---|---|---|---|
| Fell from crib, lap or down stairs | 7 | Struck with hand | 8 |
| Found dead in crib | 5 | Struck with object (plastic toy, vacuum cleaner, hairbrush) | 3 |
| I hit baby | 2 | Threw or pushed | 2 |
| Beat up by brother | 1 | Threw object at baby (plastic milk bottle) | 1 |
| Overturned hot water | 1 | Immersed in hot water | 1 |
| Baby disappeared | 1 | Unknown | 1 |
| | | Elbowed by baby-sitters watching TV | 1 |

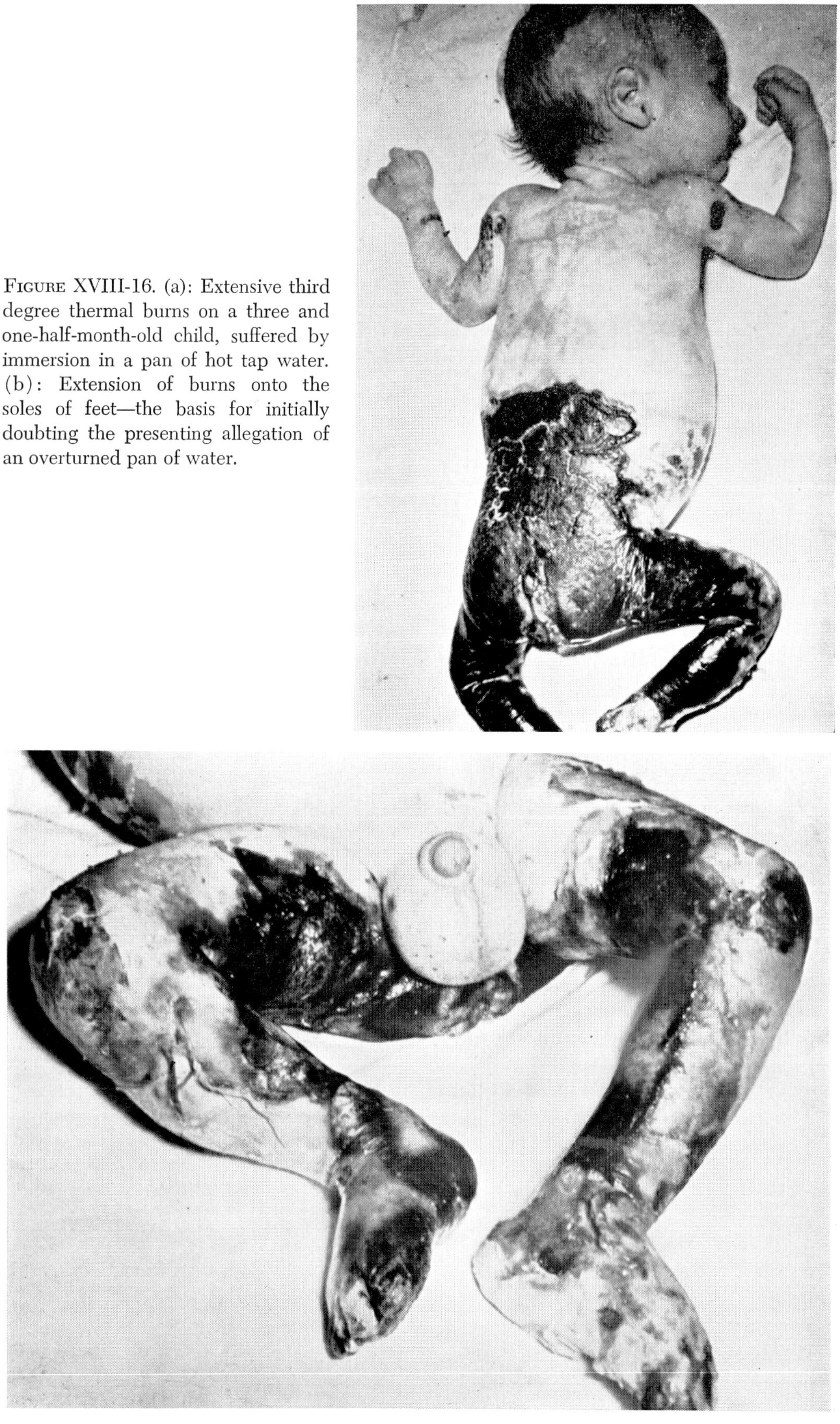

FIGURE XVIII-16. (a): Extensive third degree thermal burns on a three and one-half-month-old child, suffered by immersion in a pan of hot tap water. (b): Extension of burns onto the soles of feet—the basis for initially doubting the presenting allegation of an overturned pan of water.

of a father left to baby-sit for a somewhat extended period of time, which may be inconvenient to his other plans and somewhat repugnant to his male ego. The situation is often aggravated to some degree by prolonged minimal to moderate consumption of alcohol. These children, often severely pummeled by fists through bedclothing, may present little or no external evidence of trauma to indicate the magnitude of abuse received during the short outburst of the parent. Internal examination, however, may indicate such severe disruption as to completely rule out the possibility of an inadvertent accident. Internal examination of children pummeled over the chest and abdomen often reveals tears of the capsules of the liver, spleen and mesentery and occasional hematomas in the anterior mediastinum, which sometimes are associated with rib fractures.

A four-year-old female child was presented by both parents to a metropolitan hospital with a history of having been found dead in bed in the morning. Physical examination revealed no indication of external trauma or disease. Postmortem examination revealed multiple lacerations of the liver, spleen, mesentery and stomach without recognizable contusion in the thoracic or abdominal wall. When the parents were confronted with the anatomic findings, the father, who was from a middle-class family, readily admitted that in the course of the previous afternoon he had attempted to observe a major sports event on television, during which time he had imbibed approximately six cans of beer. He was repeatedly disturbed by the crying and whining of this child, who was suffering from a minor respiratory infection. At the point of exasperation, he approached the child and, with the bedclothing in place, punched the child over the thorax and abdomen like a punching bag. He felt immediate remorse; however, he did not seek medical attention, and the child expired as a result of internal hemorrhage.

Occasionally internal examination may reveal subcutaneous and intramuscular hemorrhages of a nature and pattern that allow positive identification of knuckle imprints and measurement of the knuckle size, even in the absence of conspicuous external trauma.

The most common injuries encountered externally are bruises, which over bony prominences may be associated with lacerations. If the violence is severe, there may be fractures, most commonly of the skull, ribs and extremities. Where the rib cage is concerned, the age of the infant often allows severe compression and trauma without necessarily causing fractures.

In addition to the bruises on the chest and abdomen due to pummeling, there may be similar bruises on the back incident to fist blows or kicks or on the upper arms incident to firm grasping or wrenching. Bruises on the scalp may not be apparent until reflection at autopsy. Reflection must be far enough downward to permit noting the lower occipital and upper cervical areas. Bruises over the bony prominences may be incident to banging of the head inadvertently when forcefully restraining or positioning the child during beating on the trunk.

The finding of symmetrical bruises in the skin of the lower abdominal area in association with dislocation or fracture of the cervical spine or intracranial subdural hematoma may occur if the child was violently shaken when grasped at the hips or flanks. The neck injury is due to the backward thrust of the head and represents a whiplash-type injury. Tears of the liver and

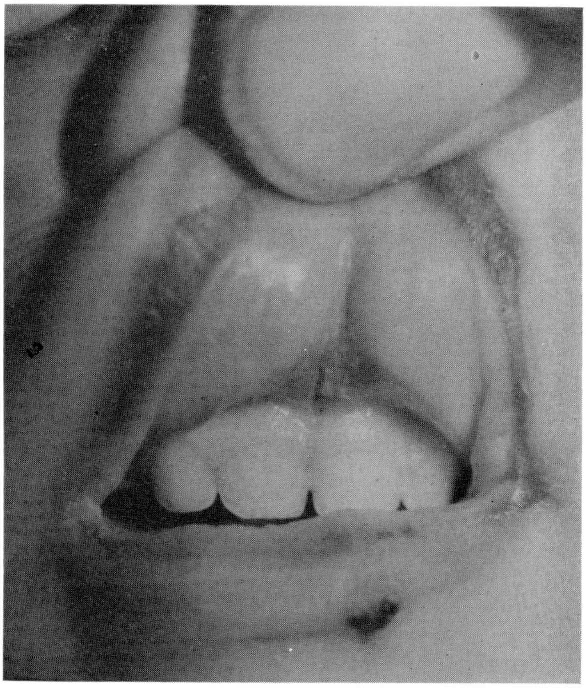

FIGURE XVIII-17. Laceration of the frenulum, a common finding in physically abused children.

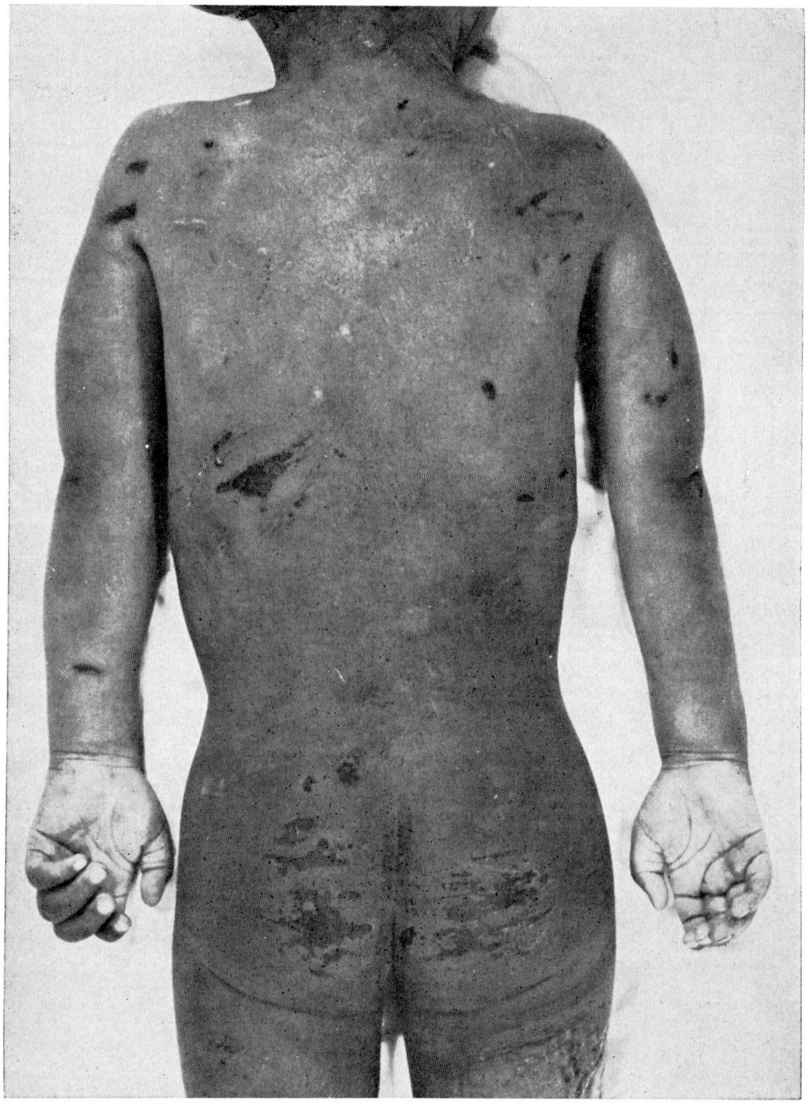

FIGURE XVIII-18a. Back view of a battered two-year-old child. Note injuries in various stages of healing on the back and denudation on the buttocks associated with repetitive beating.

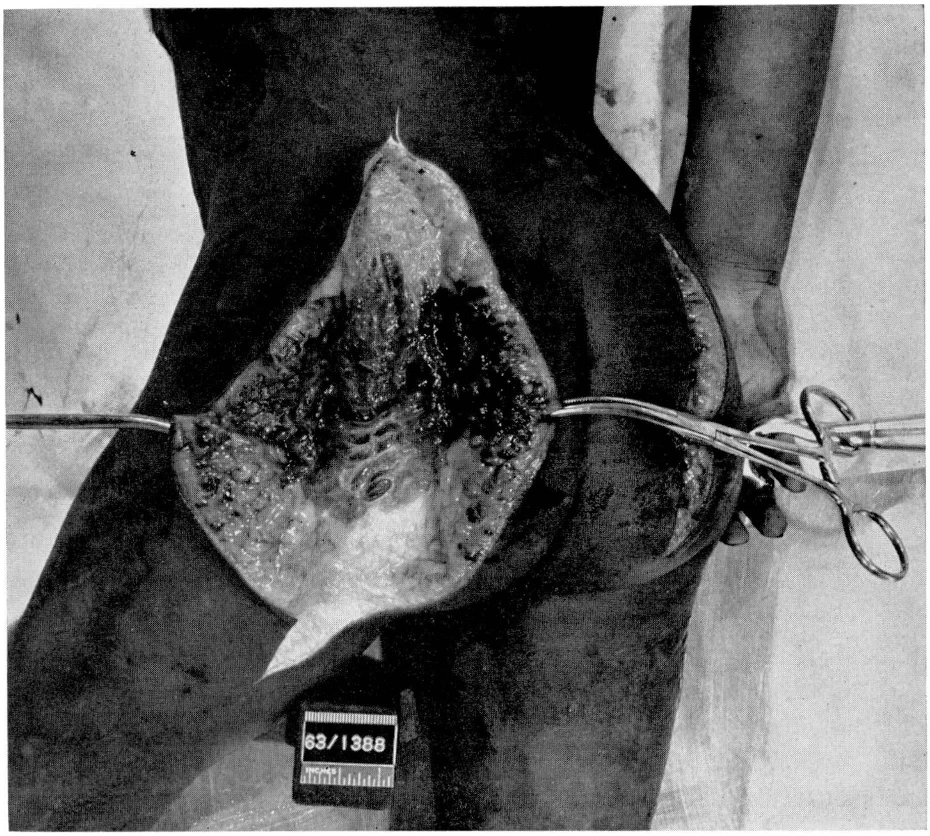

FIGURE XVIII-18b. Closeup appearance of the thighs and buttocks of the same child. Only incision of the wounds of the buttocks enabled adequate examination, which showed extensive deep fresh hemorrhage as well as deep scarring. The latter indicates prolonged mistreatment during several months of the child's life.

spleen, and sometimes retroperitoneal or mesenteric hemorrhages, may occur as a result of such shaking. Other possible injuries include hemorrhage into spinal ligaments, and subsequent calcification may be demonstrable on x ray films. Violent shaking has also been described as being associated with retinal hemorrhage in 50 percent of cases.[15] Other eye injuries incident to such trauma have also been reported.[16] Since fundoscopic examination is often impossible because of postmortem corneal clouding, removal of the eyes for examination may be necessary.

The entire body surface should be *carefully* inspected, both before and after autopsy, for evidence of injury. When internal findings indicate blunt force was applied to the body, incisions into the subcutaneous tissue and musculature of the area may indicate location of bruises and possibly the number of impacts.

Deep injury of the abdomen, including laceration of the small intestine and pancreas associated with delayed death, has been observed as a result of fist blows and kicks to the back. This may be caused by forward pushing of the spine, which compresses these structures while the body is resting on a firm surface.

Children suffering abuse in a single episode of injury sometimes fall victim to inexperienced or callous baby-sitters.

A thirteen-month-old baby, left in the care of two teenage baby-sitters, both of alleged previous high character, was found in a moribund condition by the middle-class parents upon their return from the theater. The child was dead on arrival at a local hospital, presenting no perceptible evidence of trauma or disease.

Postmortem examination revealed extensive lacerations of the mediastinum, liver, spleen and mesentery associated with extensive intra-abdominal hemorrhage and a small laceration of the intrapericardial portion of the inferior vena cava associated with hemorrhage. Initial confrontation of the baby-sitters elicited no history of trauma, even after elaboration of the anatomic findings, but subsequent interrogation elicited a story that the child had *fallen against a coffee table.* The pathologist's refusal to acknowledge this mechanism of trauma, even under some duress on the part of a senior law enforcement officer, ultimately resulted in more aggressive investigation. An older sibling in the family related the story of the child who was on the sofa between the two teenagers engaged in watching television. He was crawling from lap to lap, interfering with their viewing. In exasperation the two girls began alternately elbowing him. Subsequent confrontation of the two girls with this information elicited a confession of abuse consistent with the internal injuries.

The final group of circumstances that may account for severe injury or death in a child without evidence of preexisting trauma, again throughout virtually the entire socioeconomic and social range, is found among the offspring of the psychologically deranged or the mentally retarded. In this group, a review of medical examiner records in any major city will elicit instances of the severely upset sociopathologic or borderline-psychotic mother literally exterminating her offspring by design.

A young mother, remarried, had adorable twin children within her home who were progeny of her first marriage. She was preparing for a joint birthday party and had issued invitations to a number of neighbors' children. She had also procured a number of gifts, which were already carefully wrapped in anticipation of the party. When the children returned from nursery school on the day of the party, the mother hastily drowned each of the seven-year-old boys in a previously prepared tub of water, placed them on their beds and notified the parents of their friends that they were ill and that there would be no party. She then completed the unwrapping and return of the gifts to the local merchants before calling the law enforcement agency and advising them of her act. Previous psychatric examination revealed a state of extreme psychoneurosis, aggravated by identification of the offspring of her first marriage with her previous husband.

Resentment of the offspring and the attention afforded it by a natural parent, when the paramour or other parent is emotionally immature or retarded, may result in similar dire consequences irrespective of the child's age.

A three and one-half-month-old child, whose mother was a registered nurse and whose father was sufficiently mentally retarded to make employment impossible, suffered extensive thermal burns over the back and buttocks, genitalia and lower extremities when immersed in a pan of hot tap water (Fig. XVIII-16).

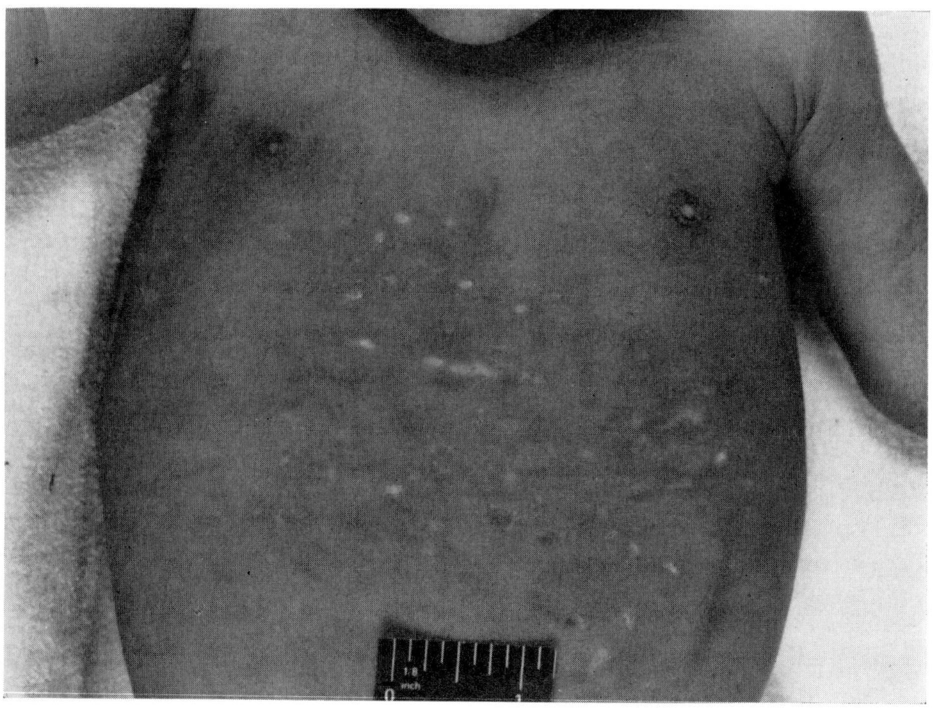

FIGURE XVIII-19. Residual scars from previous beatings in a six-month-old child.

The father alleged that the burns were suffered as a result of the child's overturning a glass container of hot water. Postmortem examination, however, revealed that the burns extended onto the soles of the feet. Irrespective of the setting, which was carefully staged to give the appearance of an accidental injury, interviews of neighbors within the apartment building indicated that the child had cried incessantly on the morning of his death (probably because of minor upper respiratory infection), ultimately exasperating the father to this point of abuse.

### Children with Repetitive Injury

Often a clear delineation between children dying of neglect and deprivation and those expiring as a result of repetitive injury is not apparent. It is not unusual for the repetitively mistreated, scarred youngster to be within the lower percentiles of weight and stature and, when seen clinically, to present evidence of psychologic withdrawal or organic dysfunction of the brain.

Inconceivable as it may be to most parents, this repetitive pattern of injury, acknowledged by other siblings within the family and certainly evident to the opposite partner of the marriage, may continue for a period of months and years before resulting in the child's death.

Often the event precipitating the trauma, such as crying or discharge of urine, may be aggravated following the trauma. This leads ultimately to a state of exasperation with extreme terminal violence, similar to that noted in the earlier group of cases, superimposed upon evident injuries of a repetitively mistreated youngster.

A six-year-old handsome male child, well liked by his friends in the neighborhood, suffered incessant punishment at the hands of both parents from the age of fourteen months, when he was expected to be completely toilet trained. This included slaps and blows to the face and head, which resulted in marked swelling and extensive bruising. Sticks, coiled ropes, belts, switches and electric light cords were used to inflict similar punishment over the remaining torso and extremities, no portion of which in excess of three square inches was spared some nature of abrasion scar or bruise.

The parents on several occasions had punished the child by forcing him to sit on heating appliances in order to dry out his wet pants. This was evident at postmortem examination by concentric scars on the

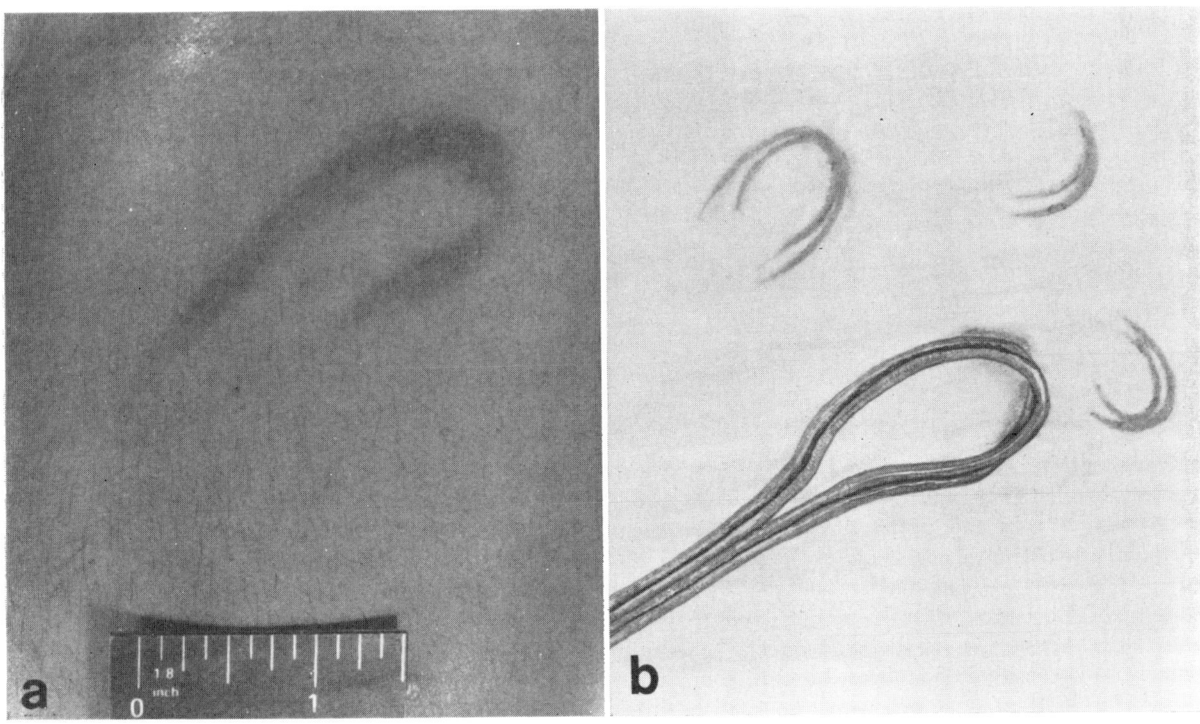


FIGURE XVIII-20. (a): Closeup of a bruise produced with a looped extension cord. (b): Diagram showing the mechanism of the same.

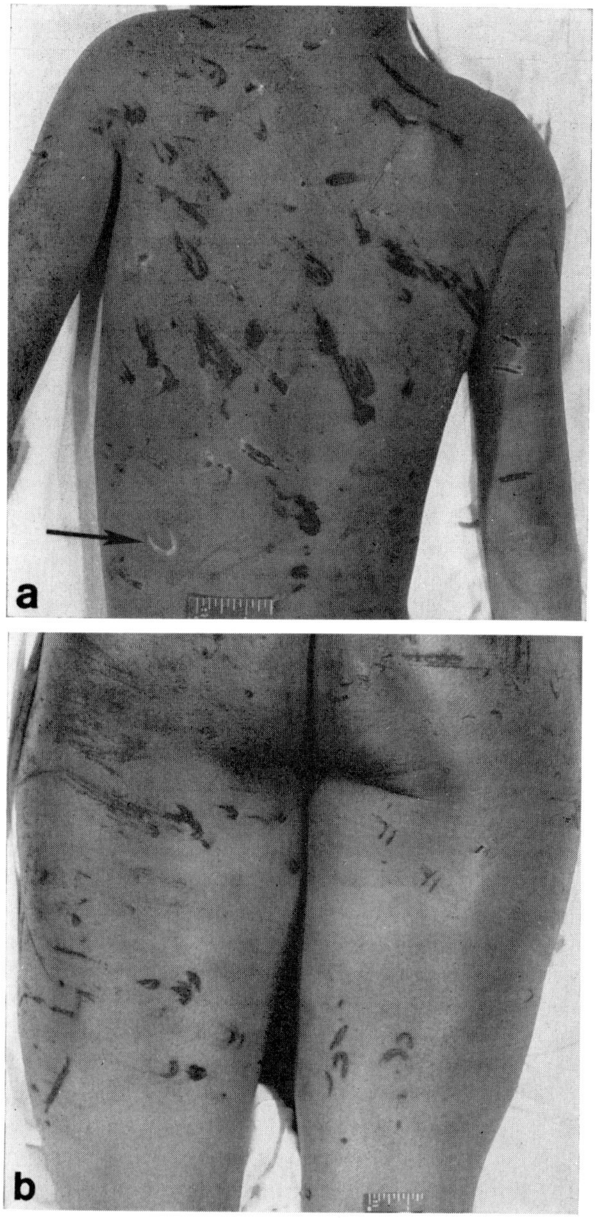


FIGURE XVIII-21. Multiple looped bruises and abrasions produced by repetitive beating with an extension cord. The arrow shows a residual looped scar.

buttocks, residua of burns suffered while sitting on a gas hot plate in the basement, and more recent burns on the lower buttocks and upper thighs, resulting from forced placement on a gas steam radiator in his bedroom as his enuresis continued. The terminal episode in this child occurred after he urinated on a newly purchased floor rug in the living room of the family apartment; it consisted of prolonged excessive pummeling of the chest and abdomen with associated tears of the liver and mesentery.

This syndrome of abuse, unlike that described with a single episode of trauma, occurs predominantly in the lowest socioeconomic and educational levels of the community. The exception is the obviously psychotic parent who, by superficial psychiatric examination, might be determined to be of a sadistic nature. However only 10 percent of battering and neglectful parents are considered to be psychotic or to have mental illness. Most children in this category are males, and their ages range from several months to ten or eleven years. The majority are in an age in which parents anticipate toilet training and cessation of repetitive crying. A very frequent explanation offered by the parents is that of a fall down stairs or from a crib, bed or toy. Rarely have parents acknowledged beating the children in punishment they considered appropriate.

External observation of children in this group poses no difficult diagnostic problems, either for the clinician or the pathologist. Every recognizable type of injury may be found in a large series, often in virtually every phase of repair. It is not uncommon to find repetitive injury of the frontal regions of the head, probably occurring as a result of attempted withdrawal when injury is inflicted elsewhere on the body. Blows with the palm or back of the hand over the face and mouth may be so extensive as to cause cracks and tears of the lips and frenulum (Fig. XVIII-17) and subcutaneous hematomas of the scalp, which may undergo organization and sometimes calcification. In association with these there may be patterned injuries over the chest and abdomen in various stages of healing (Figs. XVIII-18 and XVIII-19).

Patterned abrasions and bruises on the body exterior may afford positive identification of the weapon used to inflict the injury. Belt buckles are commonly used. It is sometimes possible to measure or overlay the buckle for matching with a curved design on the body surface. Occasionally the imprint of a chain where the pattern reflects the nature and size of the coil can be identified.

A common patterned injury is the characteristic loop welt inflicted by a coiled rope or elec-

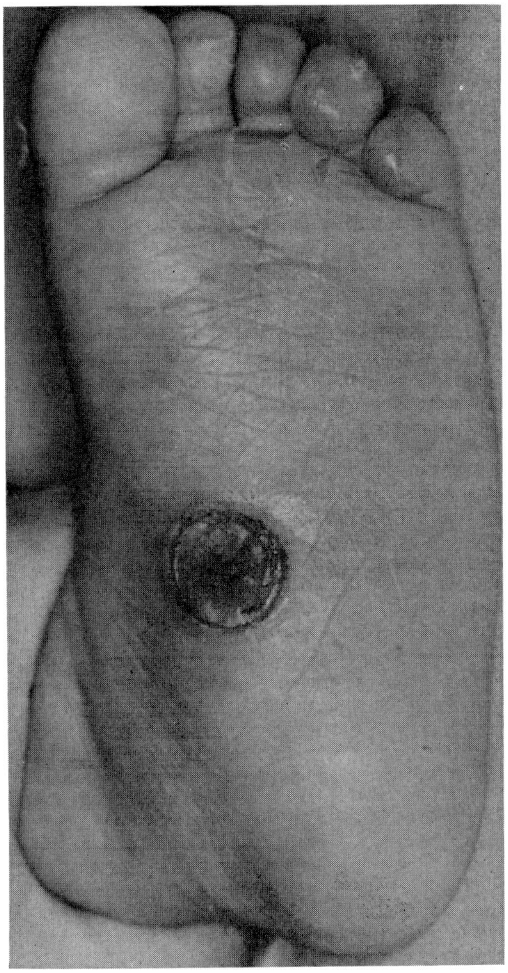

FIGURE XVIII-22. Cigarette burn two days after infliction.

trical cord (Figs. XVIII-20 and XVIII-21). Rings on the assailant's fingers may also produce a patterned imprint on the victim. Occasionally fragments of the instrument used for the beating are deposited on or beneath the skin, enabling matching with the weapon.

Other commonly mentioned injuries, perhaps more because of their sadistic nature than their frequency, are burns inflicted with a lighted cigarette (Fig. XVIII-22). Burns present in a *stocking distribution* are sometimes present as a result of immersion in hot water or chemicals such as liquid bleach. An analysis of the depth, configuration and distribution of burns produced by liquids, with particular reference to areas around joints that have been spared due to bending, assist in determining the child's position when burned.

Defense injuries on the hands and arms result from attempts to ward off blows to other portions of the body and may be in the same stages of healing as the principal injuries (Fig. XVIII-23).

Bite marks (Fig. XVIII-24) are often reported on abused children.[17] Although in many instances bite marks are inflicted by the parents, they may have been produced by the child himself, especially on the hands or arms, to avoid crying out.[18]

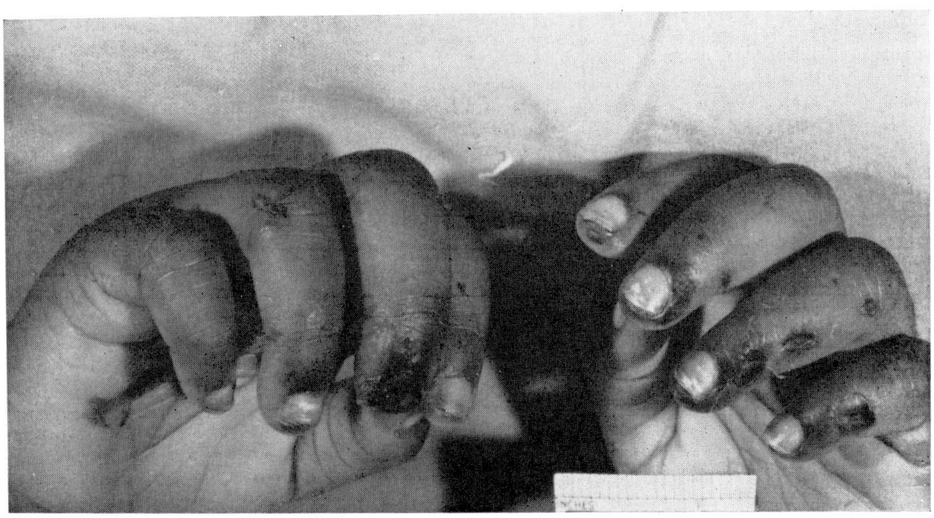

FIGURE XVIII-23. Necrosis of the fingertips of a child sustained in an effort to protect himself when repeatedly beaten on the head.

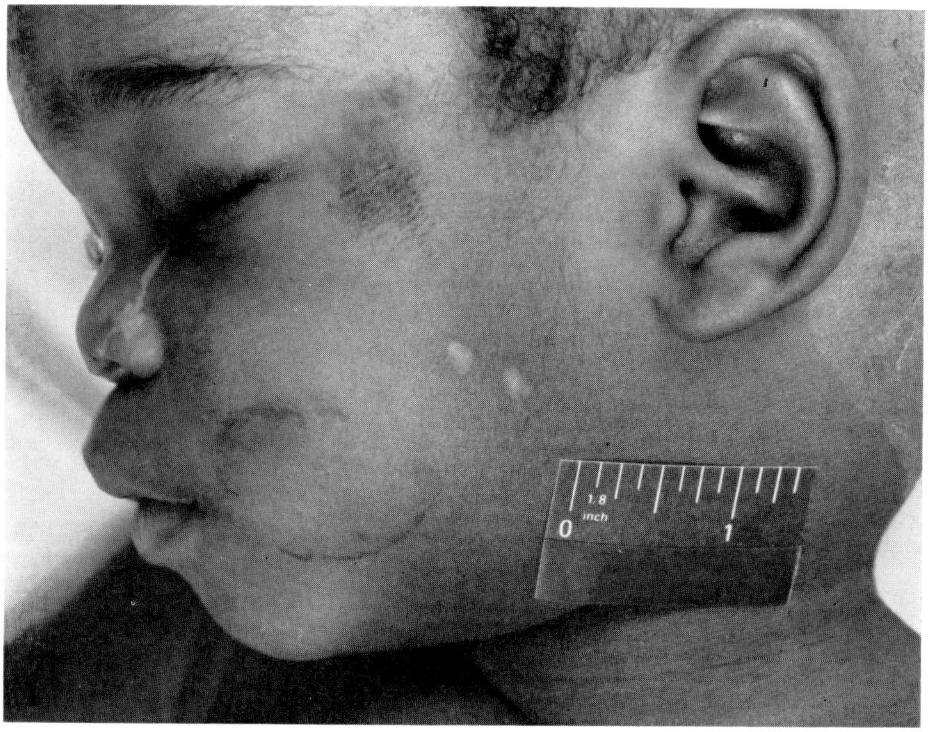


FIGURE XVIII-24. Abrasions, scars and a bite mark on the cheek of a fourteen-month-old child.

## ARTIFACTS AND POSTMORTEM FINDINGS THAT MAY BE CONFUSED WITH CHILD ABUSE

Certain conditions that occur naturally may be confusing and lead to suspicion of child abuse.

As the body cools after death and the subcutaneous fat congeals, tight clothing may cause indentations in the skin, and on the neck these may simulate ligature strangulation or hanging (Fig. XVIII-25). Examination of the clothing by the pathologist for the purpose of matching with patterns on the skin is necessary in order to verify the nature of the marks. Similar depressions may occur on the upper thighs due to elastic bands on plastic pants. When such pants are exceptionally tight, the skin may be abraded as a result of pressure and slight rubbing, and the dark discoloration of the abraded areas, a result of drying, may resemble bruising. Genuine superficial bruising may occur as a result of the same mechanism in children with capillary fragility (Fig. XVIII-26). Chemical irritation by urine is usually more pronounced in areas of tight pressure.

Dark blue or gray areas of pigmentation, such as Mongolian spots, on the sacral region of the back may resemble bruises (*see* Fig. XVIII-6). Mongolian spots are commonly small and discrete, or large and poorly defined, often asymmetrical. They often disappear spontaneously by the fourth year of life. They may be readily distinguished from bruises by incision of the skin into the underlying fat.

Positive-pressure breathing may cause superficial bruising and scraping of the skin about the nose and mouth. Bruises on the chest due to mechanical resuscitation attempts are usually symmetrical and readily identifiable, as are the ringlike linear superficial burns caused by defibrillation. Other injuries attributable to recent hospitalization may also be perplexing to the nonmedical investigator (Fig. XVIII-27).

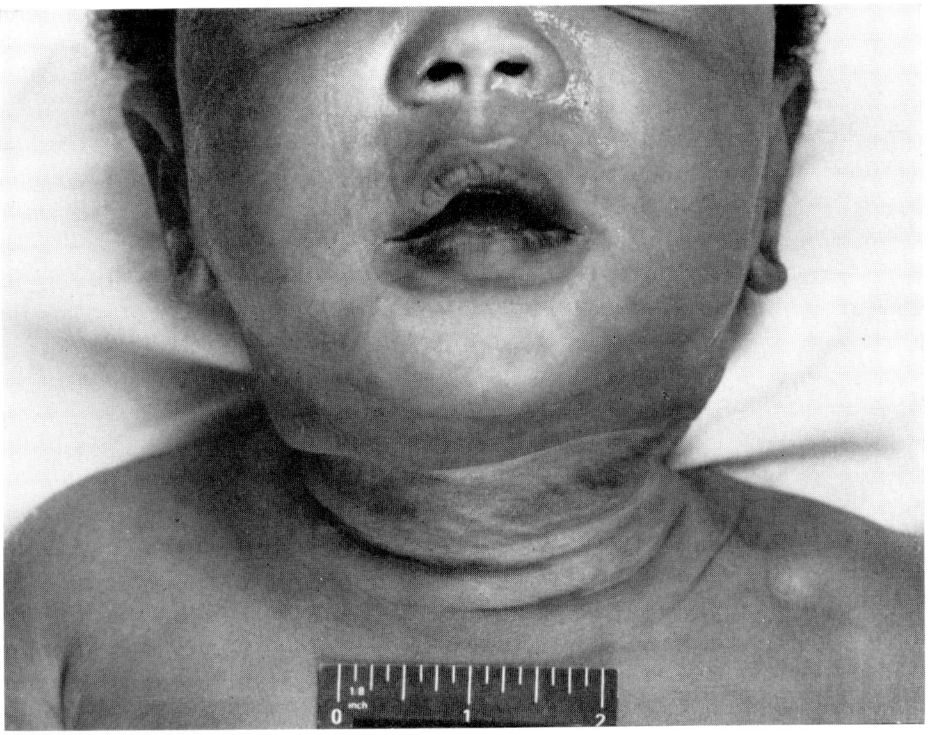

FIGURE XVIII-25. Congealing of subcutaneous fat may cause indentation of the skin to resemble an imprint of a noose or ligature.

Cutdowns in the chest for drainage may be mistaken for stab wounds. Radiographic evidence of certain healed skeletal fractures may have to be ascertained as not having resulted from birth trauma.

Careful evaluation of the extent of injury, as well as information from the emergency medical service and hospital personnel or the parents as to the alleged cause of the injuries, is necessary to determine the actual nature of areas believed to be traumatized.

Subdural and subarachnoid hemorrhage associated with brain swelling, with or without skull fracture, accounts for most deaths from child abuse. Intercranial findings are sometimes inconsistent with the clinical manifestation in the last few hours of life. A blow inflicted with the open hand on the face or head may cause subdural hemorrhage, but even in the absence of such injury, minimal subarachnoid hemorrhage and brain swelling caused by edema may give rise to loss of consciousness as a result of concussion. Brain swelling may be difficult to quantitate in an infant under one year of age due to the soft consistency of the brain. Lindenberg[19]

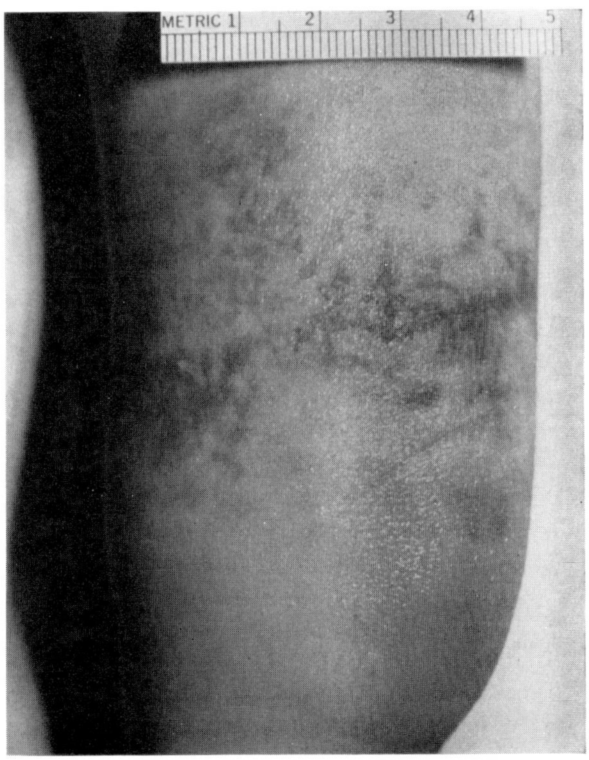

FIGURE XVIII-26. Bruises on the legs from overly tight elastic bands on plastic pants may occur in children with capillary fragility. This may be mistaken as evidence of restraints.

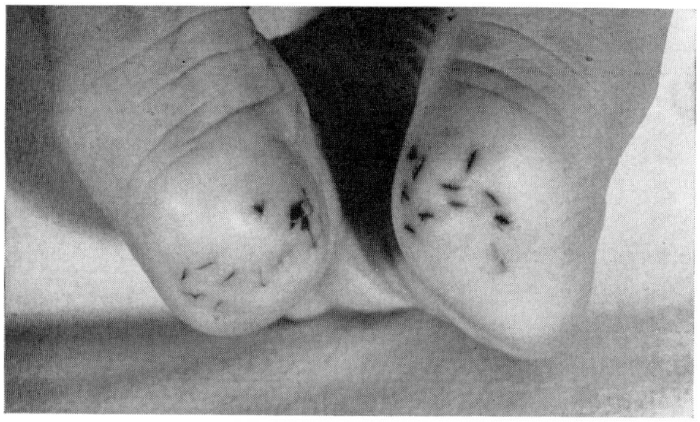

FIGURE XVIII-27. Lancet stabs in a baby's heels inflicted to obtain blood samples for laboratory analyses in earlier hospitalization.

points out the value of detailed neuropathological examination of the brain. The microscopic study of tears of the white matter of the cerebral cortex may separate different episodes of injury (Fig. XVIII-28).

Infrequent findings in abused children include hemorrhages beneath the scalp attributed to hair pulling. This may cause separation of the soft tissues between the skin and subcutaneous tissues and the underlying bone.

Hemorrhages within the wall of the small bowel have been described due to blunt abdominal injury.[20, 21] Intussusception with ob-

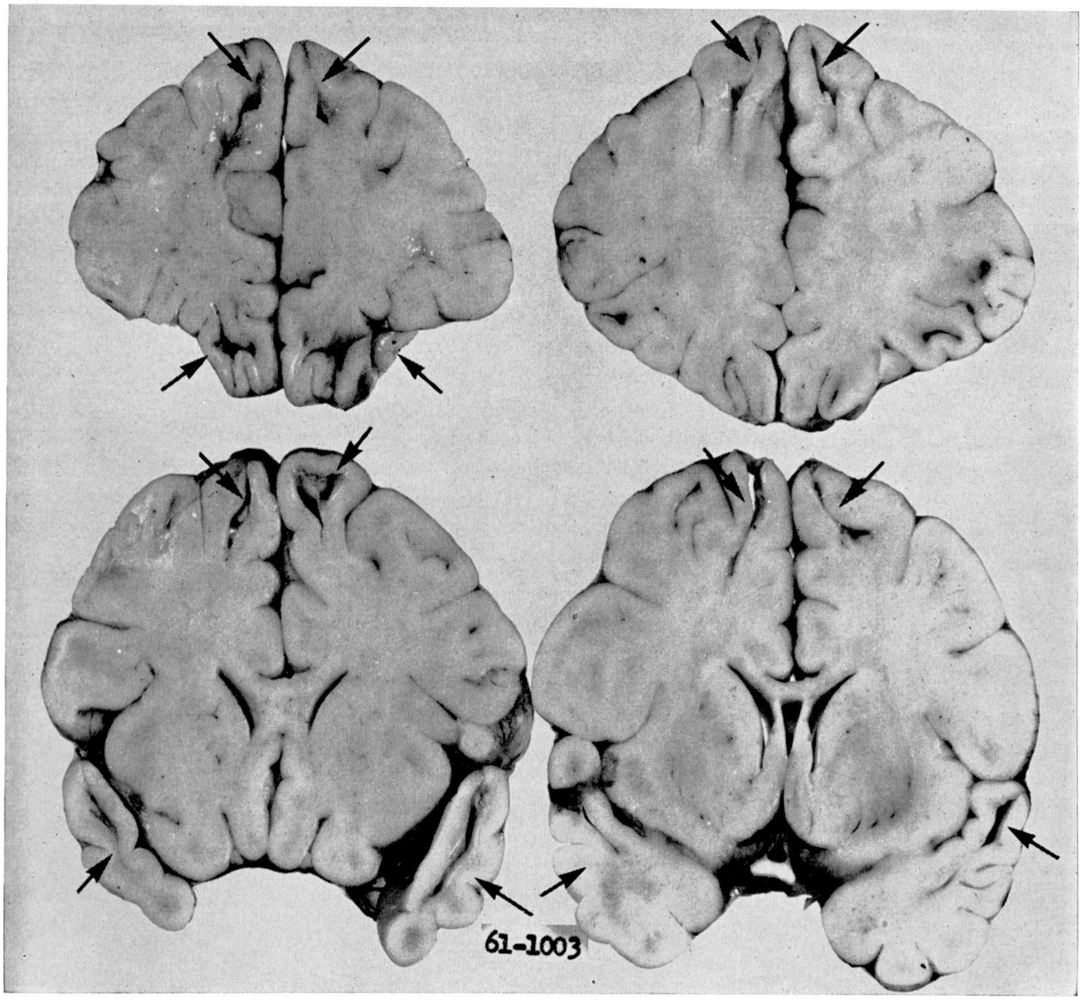


FIGURE XVIII-28. Recent tears (arrows) in the white matter of the orbital lobes and two-week-old tears (arrows) in the white matter of the anterior temporal lobes and first frontal convolutions. Impact fracture through both parieto-occipital regions. (Photo courtesy of Dr. Richard Lindenberg. From *Arch Pathol, 87*:298, 1969, reprinted with permission.)

struction and infarction of the bowel may occur at an extended interval after such injury, leading to confusion concerning the time of the assault. Microscopic examination may reveal a distinction between the initial hemorrhage and that associated with the infarction. Other intra-abdominal findings that have been reported include pancreatitis and pseudocyst of the pancreas.[22, 23]

### Allegations of Parents

Table XVIII-II indicates again the contrast between the initial allegation of the parents and the ultimate confession following extended interview or confrontation with the anatomic findings. Although bed-wetting and excessive crying were the most common explanations for the trauma, one group of parents acknowledged pleasure at inflicting bodily harm on their offspring. One parent acknowledged that she felt that the infant derived pleasure from attention of any sort, including this type of punishment. Another parent acknowledged ritualistic orgies wherein she beat the child to a point of semi-consciousness on three occasions following abandonment by her husband. Repetitive torture has been identified by the author in three instances; in one of these, cigarette burns produced extensive scarring on the soles of the feet and the back of the hands.

The significance of trauma in the background of a parent may be reflected by the fact that in a group of nine mothers who were proven assailants, two admitted that they had been beaten not only during childhood but in the weeks and months immediately prior to the death of their offspring. Among those five children upon whom an older sibling inflicted the fatal injury, in each instance physical abuse had been inflicted upon them by their parents, in one case to the point of constituting torture by immersion in cold water.

The experienced investigator who is carrying a family on his records for a follow-up from week to week, even in the absence of significant external or internal trauma, may assist in accounting for the terminal episode of some of these children. One child in the group, age five, was presented moribund with a severe upper respiratory infection and bilateral broncho-pneumonia from which she died shortly thereafter. The parents were not confronted concerning the possibility of trauma but rather queried concerning the reason for their delay in seeking medical attendance, inasmuch as both were college educated and in the higher socio-economic group. Even initial interview by the psychologist attached to the investigating team created the impression of psychological or psychiatric derangement in the mother. Follow-up psychiatric therapy eventually led to the unfolding of the grotesque tale leading to the child's death. She was forced nightly to sit unclad on a cake of ice in the kitchen of the residence, often falling asleep and remaining on the linoleum kitchen floor through the night. Such was

TABLE XVIII-II

CONTRAST BETWEEN THE ALLEGED AND CONFESSED METHODS OF INJURY IN A SERIES OF REPETITIVELY ABUSED CHILDREN

| *Alleged Method of Injury (number)* | | *Confessed Method of Injury (number)* | |
|---|---|---|---|
| Fell from furniture | 9 | Struck with fists | 15 |
| Fell down stairs | 7 | Struck with hands | 11 |
| Found dead | 4 | Struck with weapon (belt, cord, switch, ruler, wire coat hanger, strap) | 10 |
| Beat child | 4 | Banged head in attempted withdrawal | 1 |
| Banged head in attempted withdrawal | 2 | Burned on gas burner | 1 |
| Fell down | 1 | Burned on radiator | 1 |
| Overturned bottle of hot water on baby | 1 | Burned by immersion in hot water | 1 |
| Car bed collapsed on baby | 1 | Unknown | 1 |
| Drowned in bathtub | 1 | Struck with hands and neglected | 1 |

the circumstance on the evening prior to the child's death. None of this was elicited in the presenting story to the physician.

Examination of children in this category should include careful inspection for evidences of restraints. One child had extensive scars over the back of both wrists, and by overlaying the right hand on the left, the actual pattern of restraint could be identified, including the location of the knots. Similar evidences of restraint about the ankles were apparent.

Follow-up investigation and interrogation of witnesses pursued as a matter of routine with suspected child abuse may, on occasion, reveal a story of accidental, completely unpremeditated violence leading to the child's death, by parents who have only the deepest concern for their offspring. In the presence of only subarachnoid or subdural hemorrhage or minimal contusion of the brain, the pathologist should beware of reaching a definitive conclusion of parental violence irrespective of other findings on the body.

An eighteen-month-old female child, found deceased lying on a sofa on the first floor of a well-kept middle-class apartment, was suffering from a minimal bruise on the face, a single loop-type welt mark on the anterior thigh and healing burns on the palm and the back of the hand. Initially considered a rather classical instance of child abuse, internal examination revealed a single subcutaneous and intragaleal hemorrhage in the back of the scalp. Extended investigation, much of it documented by interrogation of witnesses, revealed that this child had a habit of feces stomping, whereby excreta were dropped from her pants onto the crib mattress and tracked about the crib, aggravating the mother occasionally to the point of slapping the child. Punishment inflicted occasionally included a belt, which produced the loop on the thigh, while a witnessed episode of upsetting a pan when playing about the stove accounted for the burns on the hand of the child.

The description of the terminal episode by the mother, which was substantiated by the father, was as follows: the child had bumped the back of her head on a hard kitchen floor, which produced the subcutaneous hematoma and subdural hematoma. She had messed her bed and was being cleansed and spanked by the aggravated mother. The remaining siblings within the family were cared for by the grandparents. Both parents were of a religious affiliation that did not recognize medical treatment. However, they had read that a child losing consciousness should be kept alert and therefore walked their offspring about the apartment until she completely lost consciousness. Thereupon they placed her on the sofa where she was found postmortem. The parents spent the entire evening in prayer for the welfare of the child. The next morning, upon reaching the conclusion that the infant was deceased, the father called the appropriate law enforcement agency and described in detail all of the circumstances of the previous twenty-four hours.

Other incidents of trauma in children who are afforded minimal physical punishment reflected by scars on the outside of the body may mislead even the experienced investigator. A review of the children in the neighborhood of the aforementioned deceased child indicated that it was the practice of the average parent to punish his child by use of a belt, and in a substantial percentage of those examined even casually, there was evidence of contusion resulting from this punishment.

## SEXUAL ABUSE

Increasingly there are reports of sexual activity in association with child abuse. The propensity of abusing parents to inflict physical injury to or around the genitals suggests that sexual preoccupation, either conscious or subconscious, plays a greater role in the pathogenesis of child abuse than some recognize.

Although incest, usually unreported, is the most common form of sexual abuse,[24] one now notices a significant increase in cases of vaginal and anal penetration in youngsters expiring from child abuse. This may be associated with the finding of semen in the orifices, dilatation suggestive of repeated penetration or laceration and hemorrhage incident to an attack where there was marked disproportion between the instrument, penis or otherwise, and the orifice. Repetitive sexual activity may be associated with transmission of venereal disease to the child or venereal warts (condyloma acuminata).

A one-year-old Indian boy was found dead on the sofa in his trailer home. The twenty-three-year-old illiterate father and weeping mother told of a *fall* by the baby down two steps the day before and of the baby vomiting "green mucus" on two occasions since that time.

Upon questioning, the father initially admitted only spanking with his hand *on the baby's bottom,* then acknowledged slapping the baby's ribs, neck and stomach *to play.* He subsequently admitted striking the baby with the butt of his hand and *massaging the baby's neck.* He stated that he struck the child out of jealousy, indicating his wife ignored him and paid attention only to the child. He further stated that he was on probation and had been in and out of jail since age eighteen. He repeatedly stated that he *never meant to hurt the baby.*

Examination of the child revealed bruises and abrasions over the face, trunk and extremities. None of the injuries indicated microscopic evidence of breakdown to hemosiderin. On the back was a circumscribed injury suggesting a shoe imprint. On the pubis, penis and scrotum were symmetrical tears resembling bite marks. The anus was dilated, with multiple bleeding tears. Internal examination revealed bilateral subdural hematomas and laceration of the duodenum, with spilling of the contents intraperitoneally. Within the testes was subcapsular and interstitial hemorrhage. In the wall of the rectum was a healing, nonperforating tear. Impressions of the father's mouth matched the bite marks on the genitals. Laboratory examination of the rectal contents indicated no seminal constituents at the time of death.

## THE RADIOLOGIST AND THE BATTERED CHILD

In life, as documented in the historic observations of the classical descriptions of the battered child, the radiologist may be the first to call attention to preexisting trauma in a child suffering from acute violence. Numerous contributions have been made by radiologists throughout the years to the understanding of this problem. Not only is the radiologist often able to date and serialize bone injuries more accurately than the pathologist, but in those portions of the body that the pathologist may be reluctant for aesthetic reasons to examine, he may document injuries hitherto unsuspected.

Multiple skeletal injuries in different stages of healing, as commonly encountered in abused children, include separation of the metaphyses of long bones due to rough handling and violent shaking (Fig. XVIII-29*). This is observed more frequently in children under one year of age. Destruction of the adjacent end of the bone can usually be seen in about two weeks and, if not immobilized, may continue. Injuries of the metaphyses are probably the most typical among the skeletal manifestations of child abuse. Another commonly encountered radiographic finding is separation of the periosteum from the underlying bone to which, in the very young, it is loosely adherent. Resulting subperiosteal hemorrhages may be apparent radiographically even before they calcify. Calcium deposits may be identified radiographically within two to three weeks following the injury. Subperiosteal hemorrhages are usually the consequence of twisting or wringing of the soft tissues and are seen most commonly on the arms and thighs (Fig. XVIII-30).

Skeletal injuries routinely seen by radiologists are either quite fresh or have been subjected to medical care. Such injuries may present a quite different degree of healing when compared to injuries that have been neglected. Care must be exercised in aging of bony injuries from which treatment has been withheld. A rare entity that must be considered in the differential diagnosis of skeletal injuries is the kinky hair syndrome,[25] associated with copper deficiency, wherein epiphyseal spurring and metaphyseal fragility on x ray may simulate bony injuries of child abuse. The multiple fracture associated with osteogenesis imperfecta and certain skeletal changes due to avitaminoses, such as a deficiency of D and C, may also be confused with child abuse.

* The author is indebted to Dr. Frederic N. Silverman, Director of the Division of Roentgenology, The Children's Hospital, and Professor of Pediatrics and Radiology, Departments of Pediatrics and Radiology, University of Cincinnati College of Medicine, Cincinnati, Ohio, for his assistance in providing radiographs of typical injuries noted among battered children (Fig. XVIII-29), and to Dr. Patrick D. Lester, Assistant Professor, Department of Radiology, University of Utah College of Medicine, for his assistance in interpreting them.

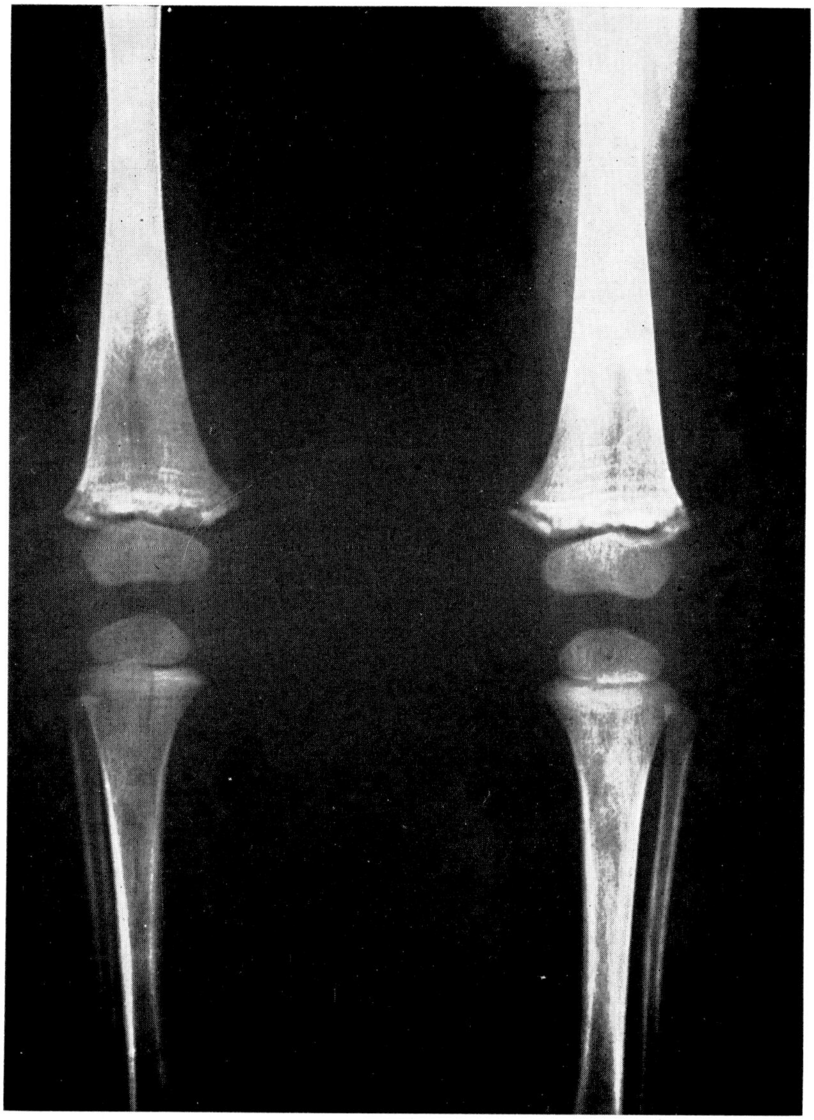

FIGURE XVIII-29a. AP radiographic view of the knees in a child, demonstrating metaphyseal fragmentation of the distal end of each femur, most prominent at the margins. Incomplete *bucket handle* appearance, a rather specific sign of trauma, is present at these metaphyses. There are transverse dense lines in the distal ends, indicating previous growth disturbance. New subperiosteal bone formation is present in the left proximal femur, indicating trauma of recent origin. Cortical thickening is present in the other long bones, especially the left tibia, evidence of more remote injury. Other metaphyseal fractures were present in this patient. (Courtesy, Dr. Frederic N. Silverman, University of Cincinnati College of Medicine.)

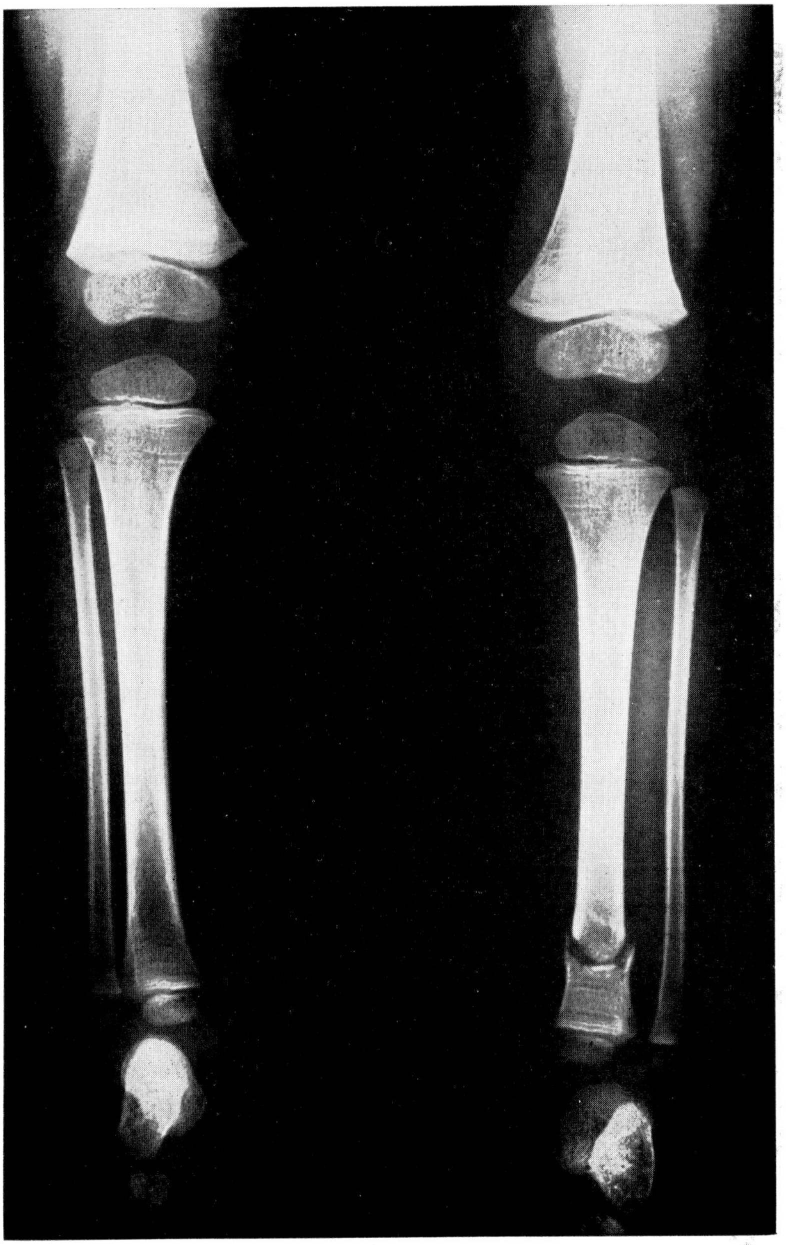

FIGURE XVIII-29b. AP radiographic view of the lower legs in a child, revealing an old fracture of the distal left tibia, with bone resorption and shortening. No medical attention was sought; hence, no immobilization or other therapy was afforded. (Courtesy Dr. Frederic N. Silverman, University of Cincinnati College of Medicine.)

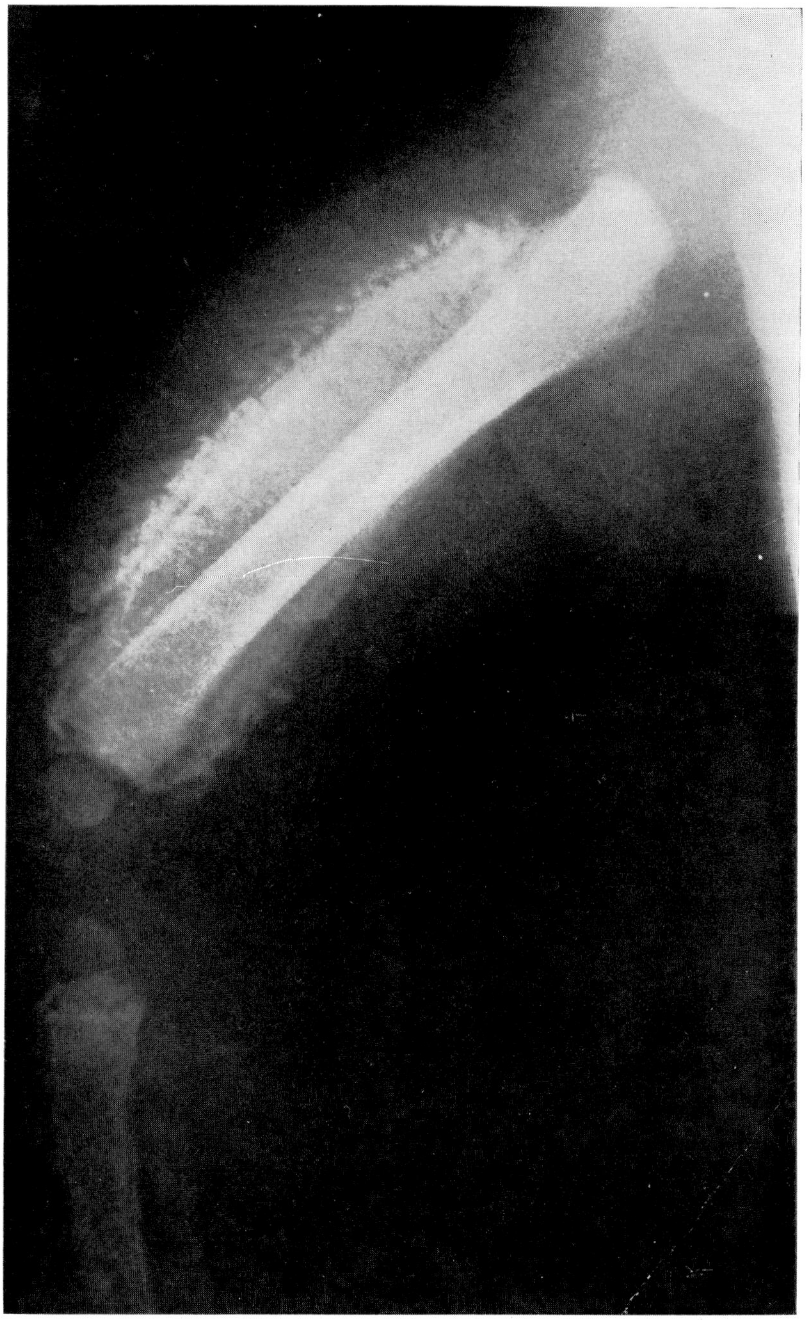

FIGURE XVIII-30. X ray of a large ossified subperiosteal hematoma of the left femur in an eighteen-month-old child. This type of injury is usually due to *wringing* of the extremity, which causes separation of the periosteum from the bone and bleeding. It is noted especially in children, where the periosteum is somewhat more loose than in adults. (Courtesy Office of the Chief Medical Examiner, Baltimore, Maryland.)

## CHILD ABUSE AND DRUG ABUSE

Ethanol, the most common drug problem in the United States, probably is also the most significant drug factor in childhood maltreatment. It is estimated after survey[26] that alcohol is involved in 54 percent of all reported child abuse incidents and 67 percent of those associated with sexual attack.

Likewise, no contemporary discussion of child abuse would be complete without commenting on the impact of the drug culture and illicit drug traffic upon the next generation of teenagers. Illegitimate children born in a transient commune type of domestic situation are much more prone to suffer from any of the previously discussed patterns of childhood maltreatment. This is not limited to abandonment, deprivation of food and hygienic amenities often similarly neglected by the parents, but may include, while the parents are under the influence of certain drugs, sadistic treatment and punishment with long-lasting scars or death to the offspring. Similarly, among those afflicted with habitual addiction, the possibility of a newborn addicted child has been repeatedly described within the literature. This should be suspected and treatment afforded if brought to the attention of an attending physician.

## THE LAW AND CHILD ABUSE

Each of the states has enacted appropriate legislation that in some measure requires the reporting of incidents of child abuse, known or suspected, to the proper authority. Such responsibility also rests with the pathologist who conducts an autopsy on the body of a child with features of child abuse, whether or not such abuse was the cause of the child's death. The physician should be aware of the party or parties to whom such reports should be made in his community; it may be more than one agency. Many states now have criminal statutes making child abuse a felony offense with penalty comparable to that of homicide. Under the provisions of such a law, it may not be necessary for the pathologist to unequivocally state that the injury responsible for the child's death was a consequence of abuse but rather only that abuse occurred.

Some of the states also have a provision within their child abuse statutes whereby if one parent is considered guilty of childhood maltreatment, the other parent, if living with the family, may also be considered culpably negligent in not reporting such occurrence. The constitutionality of such a provision has been recently tested and supported by the New Mexico Supreme Court.[27]

Failure to report such suspicions of maltreatment following examination by the pathologist is considered a misdemeanor in most states. Further, if the pathologist should fail to report such findings to proper authorities and there is subsequent injury or death to another child in the same family, he can be considered liable for civil damages arising out of the injury to the subsequent child. The instability of such families and the hostility of one parent that may develop against the other following such abuse may set the stage for such civil action.[28]

The pathologist experienced in the examination of fatal child abuse cases may be called upon to examine living children and subsequently testify in civil custody proceedings. He should be familiar with the distinctions in the quantum of proof imposed on him in such litigation in contrast to that imposed in a criminal trial.

## REFERENCES

1. Radbill, S. X.: History of child abuse and infanticide. In Helfer, R. E., and Kempe, C. H. (Eds.): *The Battered Child,* 2nd ed. Chicago, U of Chicago Pr, 1974.
2. Adelson, L.: Homicide by pepper. *J Forensic Sci,* 9:391, 1964.

3. Zalba, S. R.: The abused child. I. A survey of the problem. *Soc Work, 11:*3, 1966.
4. Caffey, J.: Multiple fractures in the long bones of infants suffering from chronic subdural hematoma. *Am J Roentgenol Radium Ther Nucl Med, 56:*163, 1946.
5. Silverman, F. N.: Roentgen manifestations of unrecognized skeletal trauma in infants. *Am J Roentgenol Radium Ther Nucl Med, 69:*413, 1953.
6. Woolley, P. V., Jr., and Evans, W. A.: Significance of skeletal lesions in infants resembling those of traumatic origin. *JAMA, 158:*539, 1955.
7. Kempe, C. H., Silverman, F. N., Steele, B. F., Droegemueller, W., and Silver, H.: The battered child syndrome. *JAMA, 181:*17, 1962.
8. Adelson, L.: Homicide by starvation. *JAMA, 186:* 458, 1963.
9. Goldson, E., Cadol, R. V., Fitch, M. J., et al.: Nonaccidental trauma and failure to thrive. *Am J Dis Child, 130:*490, 1976.
10. Pickering, D.: Salicylate poisoning as a manifestation of the battered child syndrome. *Am J Dis Child, 130:*675, 1976.
11. Smialek, J. E., Monforte, J. R., Aronow, R., and Spitz, W. U.: Methadone deaths in children: A continuing problem. *JAMA, 238:*2516, 1977.
12. Lasing, S. A., and Buchan, A. R.: Bilateral injuries in childhood: An altering sign? *Br Med J, 2:*940, 1976.
13. Helfer, R. E.: Injuries resulting when small children fall out of bed. *Pediatrics, 60:*533, 1977.
14. Olson, R. J.: Index of suspicion. Screening for child abusers. *Am J Nurs, 76:*108, 1976.
15. Harcourt, B., and Hopkins, D.: Permanent chorioretinal lesions in childhood of suspected traumatic origin. *Trans Ophthalmol Soc, 93:*199, 1973.
16. Tomasi, L., and Rosman, N.: Purtscher retinopathy in the battered child syndrome. *Am J Dis Child, 129:*1335, 1975.
17. Sims, B., and Cameron, J.: Bite-marks in the "Battered Baby Syndrome." *Med Sci Law, 13:*207, 1973.
18. Anderson, W., and Hudson, R.: Self-inflicted bite marks in battered child syndrome. *For Sci, 7:*71, 1976.
19. Lindenberg, R., and Freytag, E.: Morphology of brain lesions from blunt trauma in early infancy. *Arch Pathol, 87:*298, 1969.
20. Eisenstein, E. M., Delta, B. G., and Clifford, J. H.: Jejunal hematoma: An unusual manifestation of the battered-child syndrome. *Clin Pediatr, 4:* 436, 1965.
21. Bratu, M., Dower, J. C., Siegel, B., et al.: Jejunal hematoma, child abuse and Felson's sign. *Conn Med, 34:*261, 1970.
22. Kim, T., and Jenkins, M.: Pseudocyst of the pancreas as a manifestation of the battered-child syndrome. *Med Ann DC, 36:*664, 1967.
23. Slovis, T. L., Berdon, W. E., Haller, J. O., et al.: Pancreatitis and the battered child syndrome. *Am J Roentgenol Radium Ther Nucl Med, 125:* 456, 1975.
24. Jaffe, A. C., Dynneson, L., and ten Bensel, R. W.: Sexual abuse of children. *Am J Dis Child, 129:* 689, 1975.
25. Adams, P. C., Strand, R. D., Bresnan, M. J., et al.: Kinky hair syndrome. Serial study of radiological findings with emphasis on the similarity to the battered child syndrome. *Pediatr Radiol, 112:*401, 1974.
26. Bennett, M. D.: Mental health and accident-violence problems in New Mexico: A benefit/cost perspective. Report to New Mexico Health and Social Services Department, 1977.
27. State v. Adams, 89 N.M. 737.
28. Curran, W.: Law-medicine notes. Failure to diagnose battered-child syndrome. *Med Intell, 296:* 795, 1977.

*Chapter XIX*

# SEX CRIMES

William F. Enos and James C. Beyer

A death resulting from a deviate sexual act can present unique and sometimes bizarre findings, both at the scene of the death (Fig. XIX-1) and in the pattern and type of injuries to the deceased. Law enforcement personnel or hospital pathologists who lack experience and knowledge in the details of the various deviate practices can misinterpret evidence. In some of these cases the manner of death is natural, in others accidental with a possible underlying desire for self-destruction, while certain cases are obvious homicides.

In the investigation of these cases it is essential that a very close working relationship be established between the investigators of the law enforcement agency and the pathologist. It is frequently necessary that the pathologist have information additional to that which is readily apparent in the examination of the deceased on the autopsy table. In many cases the pathologist should be notified shortly after the police have responded to their call so that he can visit the scene and conduct a preliminary examination prior to the time the remains are removed to the morgue. This on-site examination may facilitate the medical investigation and permit a more accurate interpretation of patterns of injury, determination of cause of death and collection of pertinent specimens for subsequent analyses. In addition, the pathologist may be able to alert

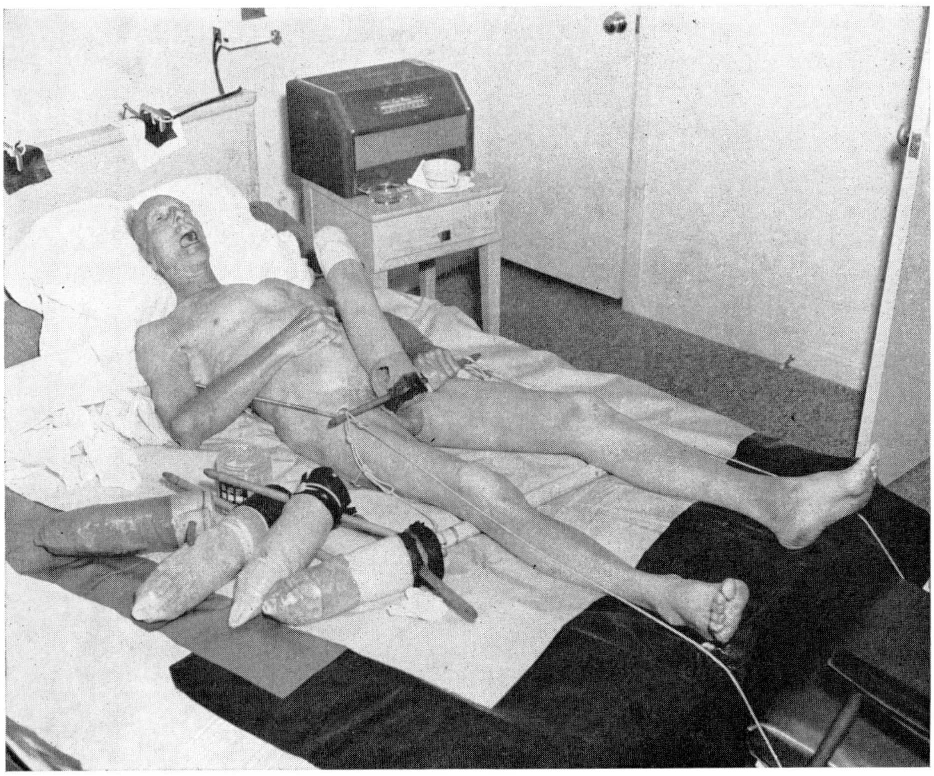

Figure XIX-1. Extreme case of sadomasochism. This man inserted large dildos into his anus and with the trapeze-like contraption could produce in-and-out movements by flexing his knees. The cause of death was a heart attack.

police early in their investigative efforts in regard to certain psychosexual abnormalities of both the deceased and possible assailant. This could facilitate the location and screening of suspects.

When an attempt is made to develop a restrictive definition of normal sexual behavior, there is great difficulty in encompassing traditional, racial and social variations, especially in today's rapidly changing mores. This difficulty is also augmented by statements from some of our psychiatric colleagues, proclaiming that homosexuality among consenting adults is within the realm of normal sexual behavior. Based on the experience of forensic pathologists, such statements are difficult to accept as being entirely factual. However, normal sexual activity may be defined as an adult expressing his or her sexual desires with an adult partner of the opposite sex with mutual respect, tenderness and love.[1] Deviation from normal sexual practices may cause injury and even death. The variety and ingenuity of deviant sexual practices include many methods and devices, among which are sodomy, bondage with ropes, handcuffs or chains, flagellation with whips or belts and the use of fetishes and dildos. Death can result from the psychological desire for destruction or from accidental asphyxiation due to the use of ropes, ligatures or even manual strangulation to produce a hypoxic state.

A schematic diagram of the various major abnormal sexual practices that may result in death is shown in Figure XIX-2. These groups rarely present themselves in a pure form, and the overlapping and interrelationship of the major groups are represented by the interconnecting lines and arrows of the inner circle. If one starts at the uppermost position on the *Sex Wheel,* one may become involved with deaths that result from *normal* sexual activities. These deaths include natural death, such as a

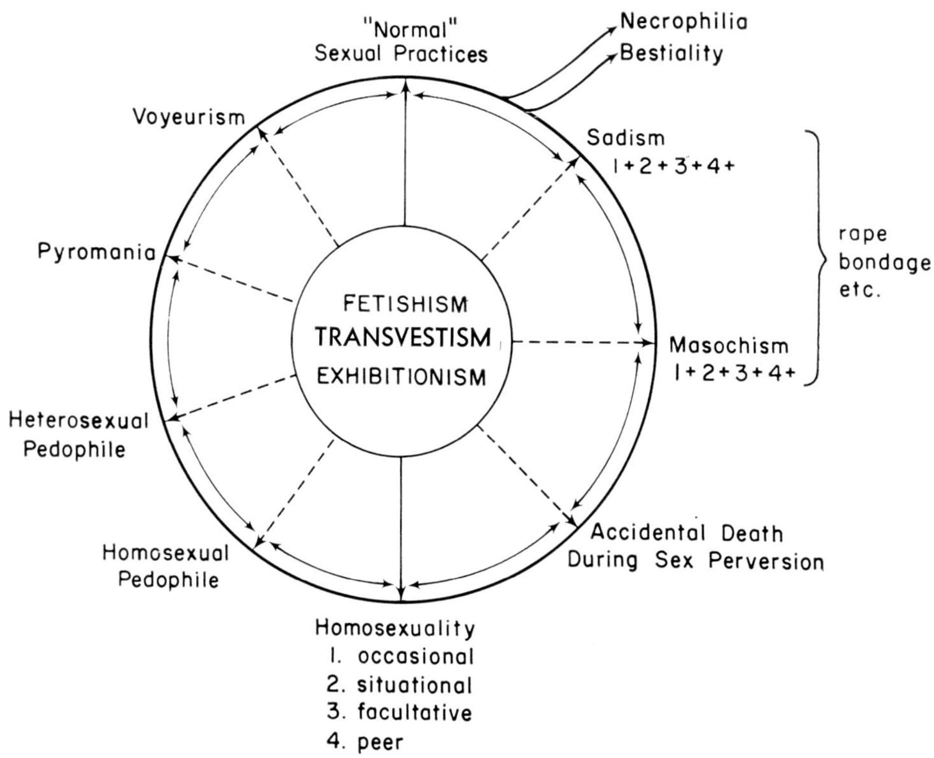


FIGURE XIX-2. *Sex Wheel:* Schematic presentation of major deviate sexual practices. These are presented in a clockwise configuration, with indication of overlapping and intermingling of the various types.

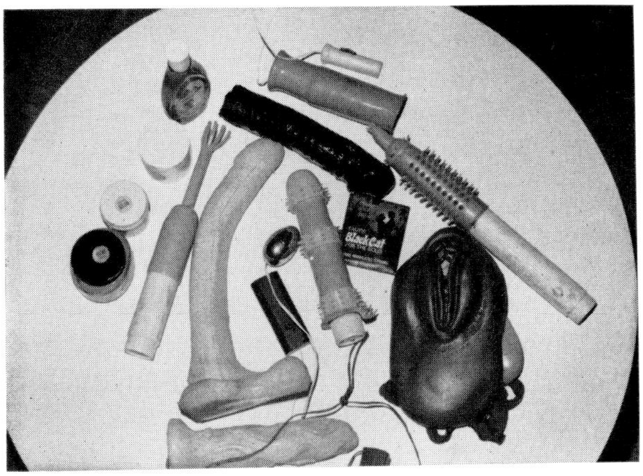

FIGURE XIX-3. Various types of dildos, vibrators and lotions found in the apartment of a homosexual.

heart attack, murders resulting from jealousy or potential loss of a sexual partner, revenge killings caused by unfaithful sex partners and, finally, murders resulting from incestuous relationships. Alcohol is frequently a precipitating factor in these cases. The method of inflicting death in these categories ranges from a single gunshot or stab wound to numerous wounds of various types manifesting sudden, unpredictable sadistic behavior. Frequently the identity of the killer is readily apparent and no major problems are encountered in the investigation of the crime or performance and interpretation of the postmortem examination.

One must also be aware that natural deaths can occur during normal and deviate sexual practices, and the police investigation is of considerable importance in developing the sequence of events leading to the death. The majority of these deaths are related to acute coronary artery insufficiency in the male during or following sexual intercourse. A typical case involves a man who is found dead in an apartment or hotel room with a history of recent extramarital intercourse. At autopsy there is evidence of severe coronary artery disease and possible myocardial scarring. Many times there is no documented medical history of chest pains or a previous myocardial infarction.[2] Likewise, a man may have been engaging in sodomy, as noted by dilatation of the anal canal and rectum, and suffer a bout of acute coronary insufficiency and death as a result of this exertion. Irregularities of the heartbeat have been observed during prostatic massage as well as during sigmoidoscopy and barium enema.[3] Male homosexuals engaging in oral intercourse may also have bouts of coronary artery insufficiency and die. The cause of death is generally readily discernible at autopsy, but the circumstances surrounding the death are not apparent unless the pathologist performing the autopsy routinely collects oral and anal material for examination for sperm or has been alerted by the law enforcement officer that such acts might have occurred. Smears from the anal canal and oral cavity should be a routine part of autopsy procedures of all men found dead without documentation of the circumstances surrounding their deaths. Thorough investigation of the scene of death is essential to document the presence of homosexual literature and devices (Fig. XIX-3). Dilatation of the anus in a body with advanced putrefactive changes may result from increased intra-abdominal pressure due to buildup of gases. This should not be construed as evidence of sodomy or homosexuality.

## SADISM-MASOCHISM

*Sadism* is the attaining of sexual pleasure from acts of cruelty or infliction of pain upon one's partner. *Masochism* is a desire to receive pain for purposes of sexual gratification.[4] These are very complicated and involved conditions, rarely found in a pure state and usually present as a blending of deviate practices with one type dominant over the other. In our society the combining of these practices is called *bondage*. The practice of bondage is found in all age groups and is present throughout all socioeconomic levels. The participants generally include one or more pairs of members of the opposite sex, with the engagement ranging from simple observation to acts involving the sharing of partners. These individuals utilize very complicated and unique methods of tying each other up through the use of chains, ropes and belts. Ropes may also be placed around the neck, but the underlying skin is generally protected by an intervening pad or towel; frequently, gags are placed in the mouth. *Flagellation* is usually accomplished through the use of belts, straps or whips. These acts of cruelty generally furnish stimulation for eventual engagement in the act of vaginal intercourse or sodomy. The acts of masochism are frequently associated with a desire to be humiliated or dominated, and the usual depiction in the erotic literature is that of a commanding female figure clothed in high black boots, black pants, brassiere and long black gloves, brandishing a whip over the submissive male figure. It would appear that heterosexual masochism is more common in the male than in the female. Deaths occurring during bondage can be accidental, resulting from an overaggressive act or failure to recognize signs of asphyxiation. Other deaths may be natural, resulting from heart attacks caused by rectal stimulation.

The acts of cruelty or pain associated with sadomasochism can serve either as a stimulant for or as a complete substitute for sexual intercourse. The gradation of these acts can be arbitrarily assessed as ranging from 1 to 4, depending on the increasing severity of the inflicted trauma. Utilizing a graded scale such as this, one would not expect to see deaths resulting from level 1 acts. This group would include enthusiastic forms of physical contact, such as sucking (hickeys), bites, scratches and bruises secondary to palpation. At level 2 there is a greater degree of divergence from normal practices, with a real need for some form of pain acting as a stimulation so that erection, intercourse and ejaculation or climax can take place. If this occurs during a depressed state following the use of alcohol or drugs, it is possible that an accidental death can occur. This is particularly true if the deviate form requires cerebral hypoxia through the use of a ligature or manual compression of the neck. The resultant death is not intended.

A prostitute was found dead in bed with an electric appliance cord around her neck. Death was due to strangulation. The man with whom she had been living gave a history of being previously married, and his wife stated that the only way he could accomplish orgasm was by choking her during intercourse. This represents a type of sadism where the male partner must inflict some form of trauma or pain on his partner before he can accomplish orgasm.

Even though this would appear to be a homicide, it probably represents an example of accidental death during deviate sexual practice. The average jury, however, finds this a difficult explanation to accept.

An unusual subdivision in this category is *weapon worship,* in which a handgun serves as a phallic symbol. The gun, which is usually loaded and cocked, is placed in the mouth, and fellatio is simulated while intercourse or sodomy is practiced by one or more participants.

A young female was found dead with a penetrating gunshot wound of her mouth. Police investigation revealed that she was participating in a sexual orgy in which "weapon worship" was practiced. The deceased was simulating fellatio with a gun barrel while other members fondled her external genitalia. The gun accidentally discharged.

In pure masochistic practices it is very uncommon to have high levels of injury unless the participating party has sadistic tendencies. At the two higher levels of sadism, death of the recipient sexual partner frequently occurs and is considered a requirement for attainment of satisfaction at level 4. At this stage, the infliction of pain is generally a prerequisite for attaining any sexual stimulation and pleasurable satisfaction, with actual performance of sex acts frequently being secondary in nature or not required. It is in these forms of sadism that the deceased's body is frequently extensively mutilated. Multiple injuries are inflicted to many body areas, but particular emphasis is placed upon the breasts and external genitalia.

A prostitute was found murdered. During the investigation the defendant stated that his mother had been a prostitute, and during his childhood he had frequently witnessed her in the company of male partners. Following this, he had developed a deep hatred for women and desired only to inflict pain upon them.

### Prostitution

The practice of prostitution frequently involves sadomasochistic tendencies on the part of both the participating partners. Both male and female prostitutes fall into this category. Male prostitutes engaging in homosexual acts can express a conscious or subconscious desire for subjugation and self-humiliation, or they may receive partial or complete sexual gratification from the humiliation of their male partners. Others allow themselves to be participants in normal or deviate sexual practices with considerable masochistic overtones. In most areas there are call girls who are specialists in acts of bondage and discipline, and they generally receive referrals from other prostitutes when a client expresses a wish for such activities. Death can occur in the prostitutes either accidentally during deviate sexual practices involving some form of upper airway obstruction and resultant asphyxiation, or at the hands of a sadistic partner who escalates beyond his customary practices. Many massage parlors maintain private rooms completely equipped for all practices of bondage and discipline and have girls who will make house calls on demand.

In the investigation of deaths resulting from acts of bondage, the police should notify the pathologist, and he should visit the scene prior to the time when any attempt is made to release the victim from the suspension halters or ligatures. In addition to the body, the pathologist can also view the surroundings, with particular references to bondage paraphernalia, pictures, books and magazines dealing with sadomasochism and possible weapons (Fig. XIX-4). Once the body has been released to the pathologist, materials should be collected for identification of seminal contents, as outlined later in this chapter. Collection of this material is to be accomplished at the earliest opportunity, rather than waiting for the time of the general postmortem examination, which might involve a delay. If the victim is male, the material should be collected from both the oral and anal cavities. The latter site should not be overlooked, since anal intercourse among sexual deviates is far more common than is generally appreciated.

If the victim is female, material should be collected from the oral, anal and vaginal cavities. At the postmortem examination, a detailed written report with anatomic diagram should include a description of distribution, location and type of ligature marks, with a photographic record, if possible, before and after removal of all restraining devices. Blood and other body fluids and organs should be preserved for complete toxicologic analyses.

### Sexual Asphyxia

A subdivision of bondage includes those accidental deaths that occur during acts of sexual perversion practiced by one individual. While these victims are generally young males, predominantly Caucasian and usually in an age range between twelve and thirty years, sexual asphyxia has been observed during senility. These cases encompass in one individual a blending of various aspects of masochism, fetish-

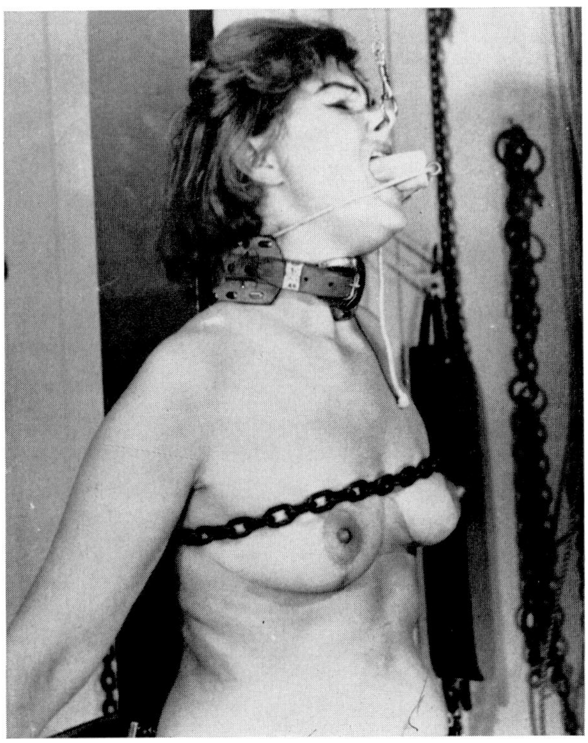

FIGURE XIX-4. *Professional model* demonstrating the use of a gag, collar, ligatures and chains. This photograph was found at the scene of a sadomasochistic death.

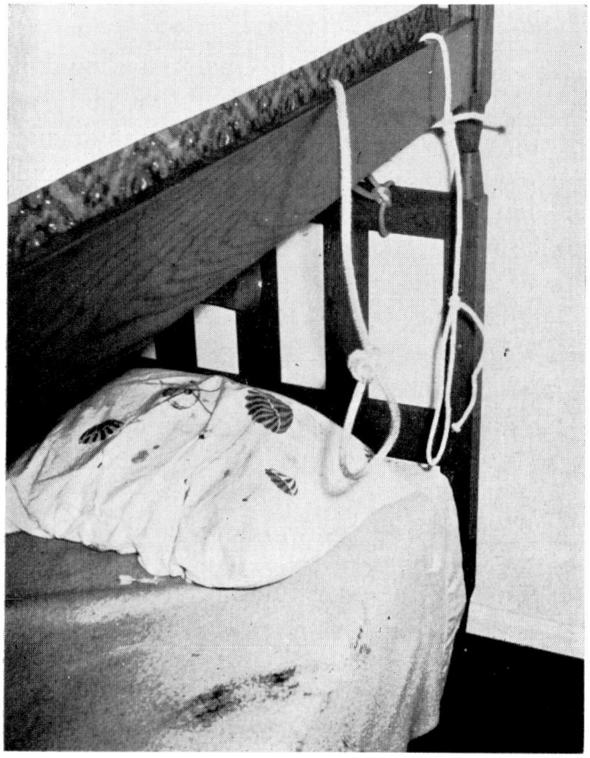

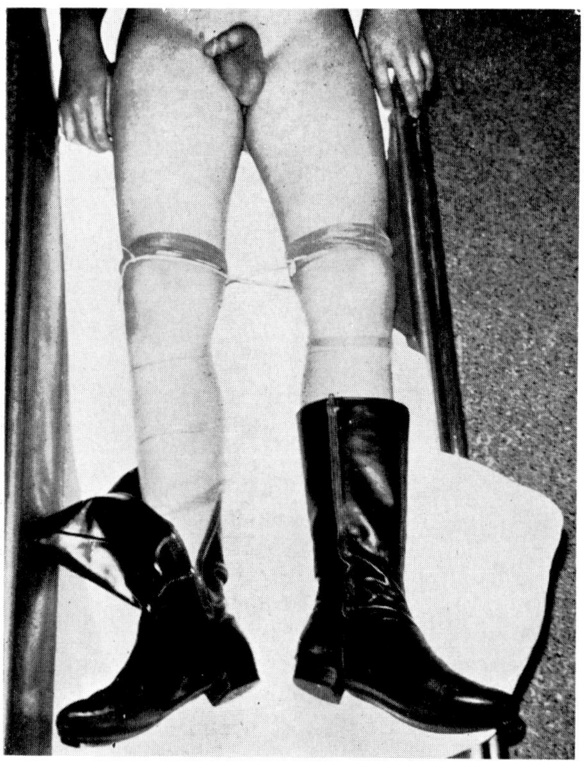

FIGURE XIX-5. Fifteen-year-old boy found hanging from a bunk bed wearing his mother's bra, silk stockings and high boots (female), with his knees tied together.

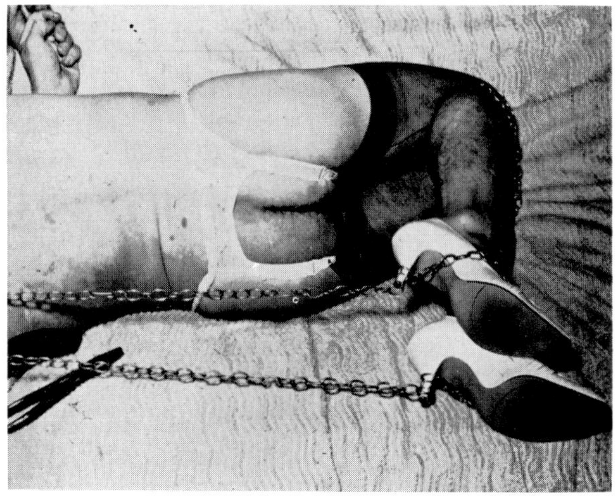

FIGURE XIX-6. Accidental death during an act of sex-perversion. The deceased was attired in a female garter belt, silk stockings and high-heeled shoes. A complicated restraining device of chains extends from the feet to around the neck. Pliers were present to release the individual from his restraints.

ism and transvestism. They involve the most complicated and bizarre utilization of ropes, chains, straps or belts gathered about the neck, external genitalia and upper and lower extremities (Figs. XIX-5 and XIX-6). The one constant feature of these acts appears to be the desire of the deceased to produce a degree of cerebral hypoxia by means of a ligature placed around the neck. A suicidal desire is apparently not present, because the region of the neck is often protected by a towel or some other soft cloth padding. The victim may be nude (Fig. XIX-7) or, more characteristically, be partially clothed in various forms of female apparel such as brassiere, underpants and panty hose. The ligature around the neck can be attached to the posteriorly flexed lower extremities, or there may be suspension from a piece of furniture, a doorknob or a specifically located hook or bolt. Mirrors, as well as erotic literature, are sometimes located near the body. Rarely, there is evidence that the deceased was either attempting or had completed masturbation.

The initial impression upon viewing the victim at the scene is that the death represents an unusual variant of suicide or even murder. However, the protection of the neck beneath the ligature and the presence of an escape tool support the concept of an accidental death. The escape tool, such as pliers, can be used to release the critical restraining device prior to the loss of consciousness. The notched top of a door or the localized polishing of beams in the ceiling may point out the repetitive nature of this activity and thus the accidental manner of death, even if the body has been cut down to disguise any sexual implications. The restraining device around the neck is used to produce a degree of cerebral hypoxia that apparently enhances the erotic sexual aura. However, if the individual slips beyond the last stages of consciousness, the nonresisting weight of the body causes death through strangulation.

Related to sexual asphyxia is death occurring while an individual has a plastic bag over his head. Some of these cases are further complicated by the use of aerosol sprays containing fluorohydrocarbons to produce a *high.* These chemicals are known to cause cardiac arrhythmias.[5]

Sexual asphyxia in females is quite rare. To our knowledge only two cases have been described.[6, 7]

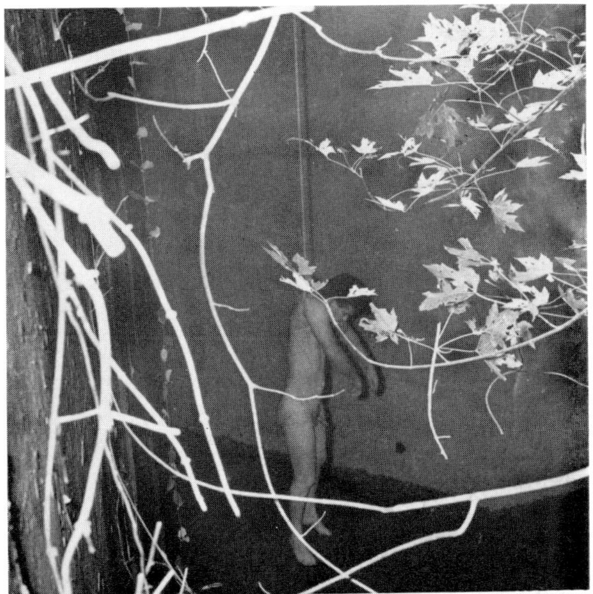

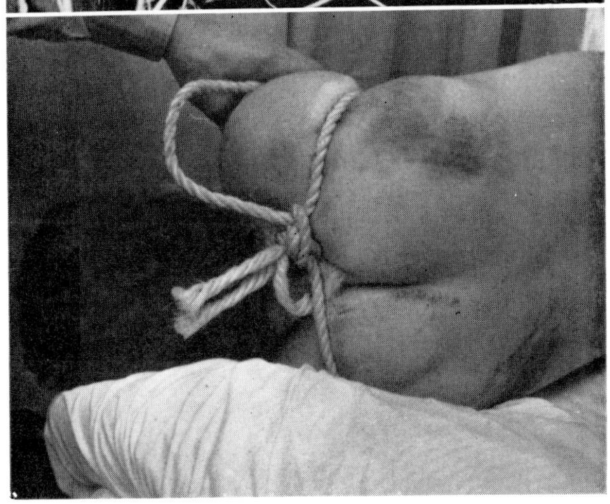

FIGURE XIX-7. Unusual type of sexual asphyxia with a rope around the upper chest. Death resulted from exhaustion of the intercostal muscles with respiratory depression and cardiac arrest.

## RAPE

Although the incidence of rape in the United States is increasing, the number of murdered rape victims remains relatively small. When they occur, there is usually a series of murders of a similar type perpetrated by the same individual.

While it has been shown that physical and laboratory examination of a rape victim may be entirely negative,[8] successful prosecution in a case of suspected rape requires proof of sexual assault with penetration. It is therefore necessary that the postmortem examination of the victim include a search for such evidence whenever rape is suspected.

The pathologist should make a detailed description of the genitalia, the thighs and the pubic region (including pertinent negative points), and vaginal mucus should be subjected to microscopic examination to determine the presence of spermatozoa. A drop of fluid from the vaginal pool can be examined for sperm motility. The duration of sperm motility in the vagina has been variously described as ranging from thirty minutes to sixty hours, but usually sperm become nonmotile in three to four hours.

A thorough search for spermatozoa is best conducted in a number of smears. Smears should be prepared as soon as the victim's body is available for examination by the pathologist. A cotton swab is used to prepare a smear. The material may be taken from anywhere in the vagina, but the cervical canal appears to give the best results. Smears of the oral and rectal mucosa should also be examined. In interpreting the latter, consideration must be given to contamination by vaginal contents. The smears are stained with any of the conventional methods, but, while the Papanicolaou stain is used by most hospital cytology laboratories, hematoxylin and eosin seem to provide better differentiation of cytoplasmic and nuclear elements. This is especially important when the tail of the sperm cell is absent.* Methylene blue has not given very satisfactory results in that particular difficulties are encountered with this stain in distinguishing between sperm cells and artifacts.

Decomposition of the body does not preclude the possibility of finding identifiable spermatozoa, and embalming of the body helps preserve them. Intact spermatozoa, i.e. with tails, *are rarely found* in the vagina later than seventy-two hours after coitus. As a general rule, if the lining cells of the vaginal or oral cavities are preserved, the probability of identifying spermatozoa is reasonably good. We were able to identify spermatozoa obtained from the cervical canal in a partially frozen victim who had been dead one and one-half months. The vaginal vault was filled with ice. Wilson identified spermatozoa in a body sixteen days after rape and murder.[9]

It should be mentioned that centrifuging of vaginal aspirate creates artifacts that render identification of spermatozoa more difficult. Loss of tails occurs commonly due to centrifugation. Mucus and cell debris (especially in rectal smears) as well as fungus and pollen can also be quite misleading (Fig. XIX-8). Identification of spermatozoa follows an *all-or-none* law, and reports are *positive* or *negative*. The terms *suspicious of* or *consistent with* are strictly avoided.

* Dr. Charles Petty of the Southwestern Institute of Forensic Sciences in Dallas, Texas, uses picroindigocarmine, which stains sperm heads red and the tails green and red. The procedure is easy and fairly foolproof.

Vaginal secretions should also be obtained for acid phosphatase determination. The specimen is collected with a pipette attached to a rubber bulb using 25 to 30 cc of saline. A positive test is not necessarily proof of the presence of seminal fluid, but a high value of this enzyme is most suggestive, since it does indicate the presence of prostatic secretions. The concentration of acid phosphatase gradually falls with time. Thus, in cases of alleged sexual assault, a quantitative acid phosphatase determination may indicate not only the presence of seminal fluid but also the approximate time of coitus, even in the absence of spermatozoa.[10] The length of time acid phosphatase remains positive in the vaginal canal depends primarily on the postmortem condition of the body.[11] Values as high as 30 Bodansky units (BU) have been obtained up to forty-eight hours after death. Cooling of the body preserves acid phosphatase activity over an extended period. Values ranging from 10 to 30 BU suggest rape shortly before death rather than consentual intercourse five to ten hours earlier. The determination of acid phosphatase is of considerable significance, since vasectomy has been growing in popularity and atrophy of the seminiferous tubules in the testicles is frequently found in middle-aged alcoholics with cirrhosis.

If the presence of seminal fluid is established in the vaginal, oral or rectal cavity, a smear from that site should be subjected to blood type determination. A stain suspected of being semen on clothing or hair may be extracted with physiologic saline and the fluid from this washing treated in the same fashion. Well-preserved spermatozoa can be identified in even old and dry stains. The same is true of acid phosphatase determination. Approximately 80 percent of men secrete water-soluble blood group substances in their seminal fluid. The identification of A, B or H blood group substances is based on the ability of seminal fluid to at least partially neutralize the agglutinating activity of the specific antiserum. This may be used to show that the seminal fluid found in the victim is of

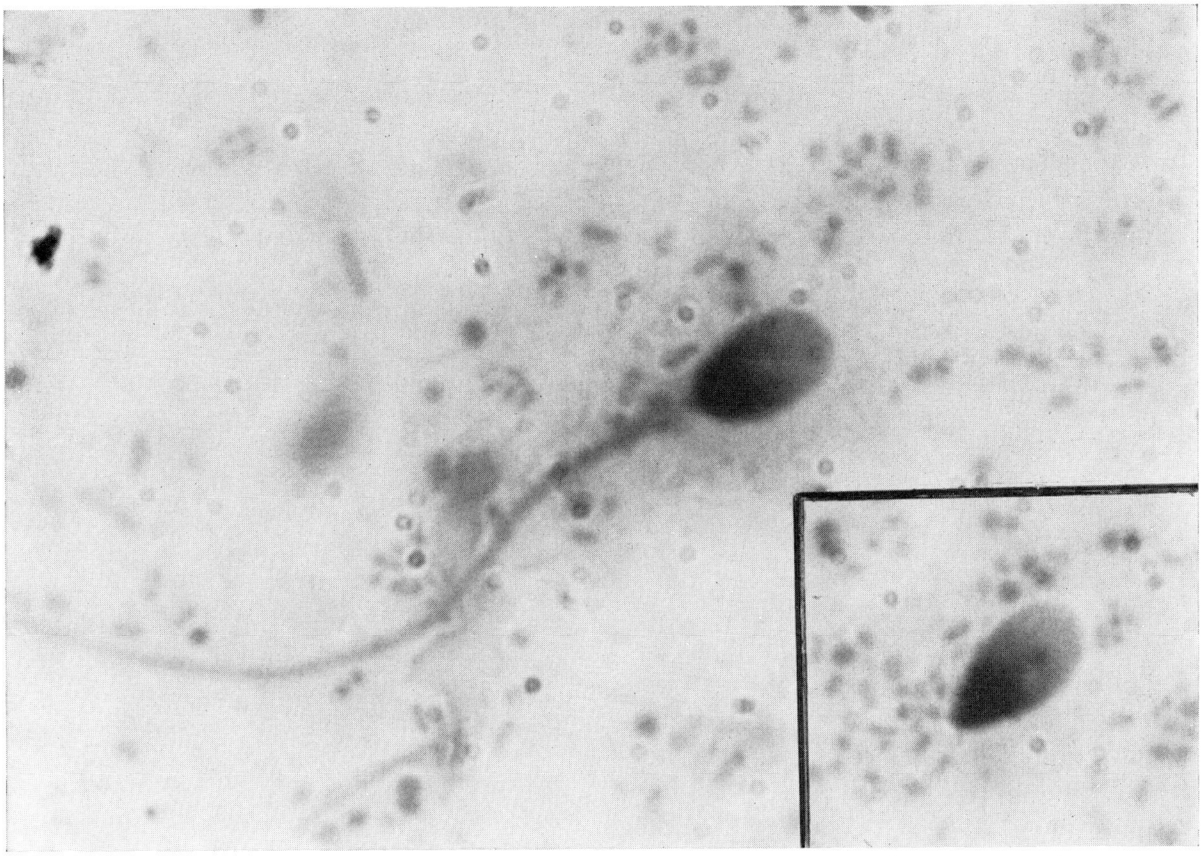

FIGURE XIX-8a. Intact sperm cell. Insert: Tailless sperm. (Both ×1500, H&E stain.)

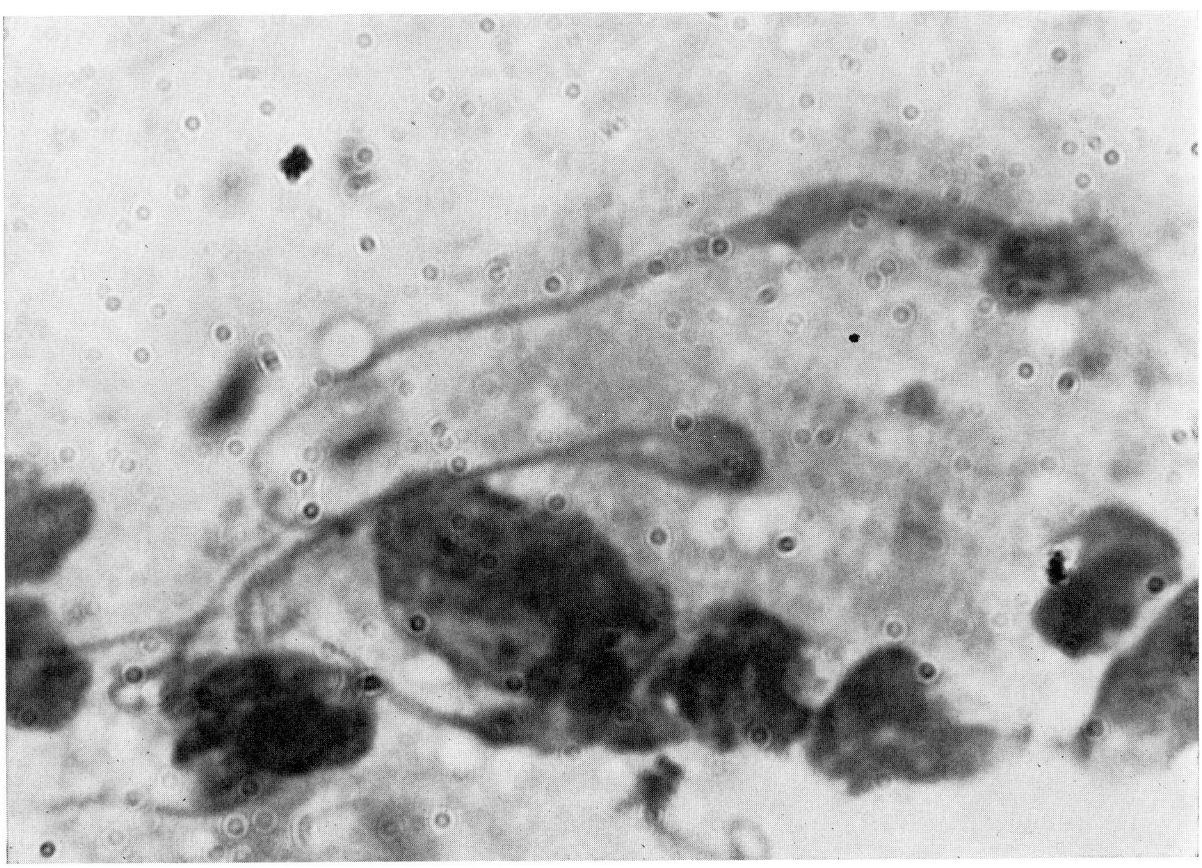

FIGURE XIX-8b. Mucus threads. (×1500, H&E stain.)

a different blood type than that of the suspected assailant.[12]

Additional evidence to be collected by the pathologist from a suspected rape victim should include fingernail clippings and hair samples from the pubic area and scalp. These specimens are usually examined by the police crime laboratory.

In some cases with definite sexual overtones, semen cannot be identified by any of the methods that have been described. Information gained from police investigation indicates that many of these men are impotent and, because of underlying psychopathology, harbor a deep hostility toward females. Such individuals are unable to accomplish penile penetration in any of the body orifices, although premature ejaculation may occur to contaminate the skin, clothing or surrounding environment. There is frequently a history obtained of manual manipulation of the breasts and external genitalia as well as cunnilinguism. In such cases, swabs moistened with saline applied to the external genitalia may be used for subsequent serologic typing.

## HOMOSEXUALITY

*Homosexuality* indicates a sexual attraction between members of the same sex with attainment of sexual gratification. The subjects of etiology and psychopathology of homosexuality are beyond the scope of this discussion. Classification of types of homosexuals is also controversial, but at least four general groups can be identified.[13, 14]

1. The *occasional* or *exploratory* homosexual. This is an individual who for a variety of reasons will engage in a rare or even single homosexual act with no further evidence of an abnormality.
2. The *situational* or *deprivation* homosexual. These individuals are seemingly forced into homosexual acts when they are deprived of any contact with members of the opposite sex. This is most typically seen in prisons, and frequently the individuals refrain from any further evidence of homosexuality once they are released from incarceration.
3. The *facultative* or *latent* homosexual. These individuals frequently evidence an option in their selection of sexual partners and will maintain a relatively normal heterosexual behavior pattern with an accompanying desire to have periodic sexual contacts with members of their own sex. In recent years it has become apparent that members of prominent motorcycle gangs fall into this category.
4. The *peer* or *compulsive* homosexual. These individuals have a continuing irresistible desire for performing sex acts with partners of the same sex. The quantity of sex acts attempted frequently surpasses those ascribed to the most active of heterosexual practices. Only a small percentage of these individuals assume the manner of dress, walk, voice or body movements of the opposite sex. When they do, they are generally considered as *going in drag.*

The incidence of homosexuality is certainly much higher than one would deduce from the review of emergency room and hospital records or a collection of cases from medical examiners' files. The homosexual is frequently exposed to assault, robbery and blackmail. The *fairy hawk* who haunts the gay bars or *fairy flats* or other meeting areas, such as parks, waiting for a pickup will permit a homosexual act but is primarily interested in robbing the peer or compulsive homosexual of his money or clothes or acquiring the use of his automobile. Orgasm may not occur during such a clandestine meeting due to the lack of emotional attachment of the *fairy hawk* to the peer homosexual. Also, the inserting partner may have used a condom if anal sodomy was performed. The finding of such condoms, sometimes contaminated with lubricant and feces, in proximity of a body with multiple wounds, is suggestive of a homosexual motive for the killing. This underscores the need for adequate investigation and preservation of the crime scene. If the peer homosexual survives the assault, he prefers to allow the incident to go unreported, and only in dire necessity will he present himself to an emergency room for treatment.

If such a visit is necessary, there is usually falsification as to etiology of the trauma. Deaths among homosexuals occur most often to the male peer homosexual who, following a cruise in a gay bar or a gay crowd looking for a *dreamboat,* becomes involved with a *fairy hawk* or *dirt* or *gay dirt.* These male prostitutes will submit to homosexual acts either as oral or anal inserters or recipients and will even perform intercourse in the armpits.

The *straight world* is generally unaware, and certainly unappreciative, that anal intercourse *(buggery)* is probably the more acceptable and predominant sex act among male homosexuals.

Deaths among *dykes* or lesbians or female homosexuals are not as common as among their male counterparts. When deaths do occur in association with female homosexuals, they more often involve the intruding male who attempts to convert one member of the homosexual marriage over to heterosexual practices. This frequently incites the husband or *butch,* who sees a threatening influence on the continuation of their homosexual life and proceeds to kill the male invader. This form of homicide is generally routine and involves the use of a knife, gun or at times even strangulation.

Deaths resulting from male homosexual practices usually have a characteristic pattern both in the findings at the scene of the crime and in the injuries resulting in the death (Fig. XIX-9). The pathologist should visit the scene prior to any removal of evidence or of the deceased. Frequently, furniture, artwork and literature permit an immediate assessment as to the exact circumstances leading to the death. The literature not only includes commercially prepared and published stories and pictures but frequently involves a large number of photographs of previous guests.

Smears from the oral and anal cavities or axillae should be obtained as soon as possible for identification of sperm and acid phosphatase. In the majority of these cases, the pattern of injuries is characteristic in that it involves a large number of wounds representing *overkill*—wounding far beyond that required to cause death (Fig. XIX-10). The wounds are often scattered over different body regions. A wide range of weapons can be involved, generally representing those that are most readily available. Knives, scissors, guns, bottles and hammers are commonly used. This wound pattern reflects the psychopathology of the murderer at the time the act was committed.

A peer homosexual picked up a *fairy hawk* and brought him back to his apartment. After performing an act of oral intercourse, the deceased resisted attempts at robbery and sustained a total of forty-three wounds. These consisted of multiple lacerations of the scalp with fractures of the skull, numerous contusions, lacerations and abrasions of the face with fractures of

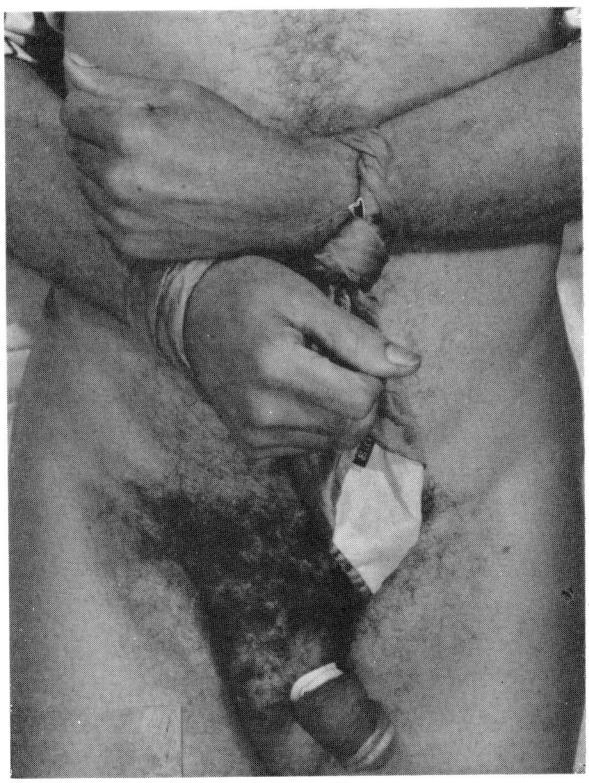

FIGURE XIX-9. Married homosexual found tied, gagged and beaten to death at a local homosexual meeting place. Note the *cock ring* at the base of the penis, sometimes used to maintain an erection.

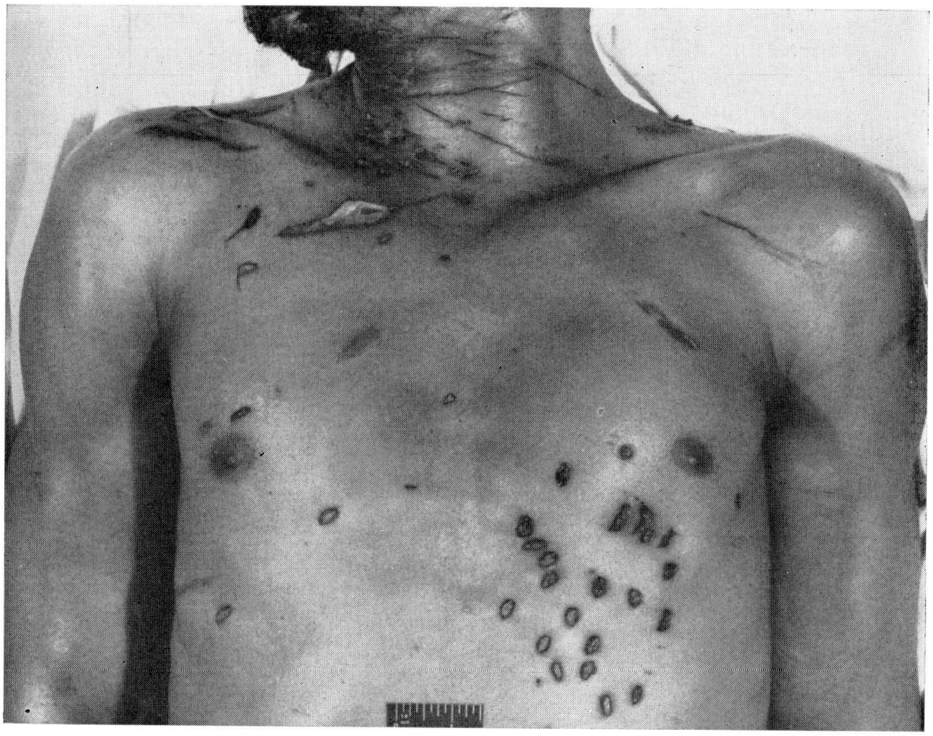

FIGURE XIX-10. Homosexual killed by his jealous partner. The head was crushed and battered with a hatchet, and the neck was cut with a blade. Aftershave lotion and table salt were sprinkled over the entire body. Death was due to multiple stab wounds of the chest. Spermatozoa were found in the mouth and rectum.

the facial bones, multiple small lacerations of the neck and nine stab wounds of the chest.

The *fairy hawk* is faced with a threat of exposure that he has been involved in homosexual acts, which embroils him in an inner conflict between his homosexual and heterosexual tendencies. This emotional conflict explodes in a panic phase, and the individual then attempts to destroy this challenge to his heterosexual identity and existence. In those cases where robbery is the predominant feature, the robbery motive is frequently overshadowed by a guilt complex generated by indulgence in the homosexual act and accentuates the amount and degree of trauma inflicted on the victim.

A unique group of deaths having a conglomerate of features relating to sadism, masochism and homosexuality is found in deaths among members of motorcycle gangs. The pattern of injuries is very similar to that seen in deaths among the more usual homosexual practices in that there are a large number of wounds dispersed over many body regions and frequently produced by multiple weapons. These cases present a stimulating challenge to the pathologist in an attempt to identify the various types of injury. Generally, there will be evidence of beating, particularly around the head and face. In addition, both gunshot and knife wounds may be present. The knife wounds frequently follow a pattern of cuts in the neck and stab wounds throughout the chest and abdomen. In a number of cases, the most prominent stab wound has been one placed in the area of the epigastrium and inflicted by a knife of rather large dimension. The gunshot wounds are also multiple, frequently involving the head and chest, and quite often a *coup de grace*-type gunshot wound is present in the back of the head or neck. Rectal and oral smears may show presence of sperm cells. When arrested, the assailants frequently indicate that the use of drugs produced personality changes leading to their deviate behavior.

Occasionally there are cases in which the police investigation and the pattern and types of wounds strongly indicate a homicide with homosexual implications. However, smears from the oral and anal canal are negative for sperm. These generally involve assailants who manifest a strong sense of *machismo*. When they find themselves in a situation where their exaggerated male awareness is challenged, they pass into a homicidal frenzy and kill the offending male.

A sixty-year-old white male picked up a young hitchhiker who was a kung fu expert. He was also interested in body building and similar endeavors. The older male made homosexual advances toward the younger man, who responded by beating him. At autopsy the larynx was found to be fractured, and a portion of broken denture was lodged at the base of the tongue, obstructing the upper airway. No semen was found in this case.

## HOMOSEXUAL PEDOPHILIA—HETEROSEXUAL PEDOPHILIA

*Pedophilia* involves a sexual act occurring between an older individual of either teen age or adulthood and an individual of preadolescent age. The homosexual pedophile is attracted to and may attempt to have either oral or anal intercourse with his victim, but the usual preference is sodomy. The heterosexual pedophile may attempt oral, vaginal, anal or intercrural intercourse, as well as cunnilingus, but attempts at vaginal penetration are the most common. The assailants range in age from the teens to old age, and their victims are most often under the age of ten. Often the victims are enticed to accompany the pedophile through promises of candy, money, etc.

After enticing a young boy into his shop with offers of candy, a male pharmacist would perform fellatio and then prepare a plaster cast of the boy's penis. These casts were found initialed with the dates and the first names of the boys.

Trauma inflicted upon the victim can range from attempted vaginal or anal penetration to more extensive injury involving contusions, abrasions and biting of breasts and external genitalia. In cases of curious teenagers or dirty old men, shame or fear of exposure often will escalate the act and result in the death of the victim.

The mode of death generally involves head injury or strangulation. In some instances, the panic state of the assailant results in extensive mutilation of the victim's body.

A twelve-year-old boy was lured into a wooded area by a twenty-seven-year-old homosexual pedophile who had a long record of homosexual attacks on prepubertal boys. The victim apparently struggled to avoid sodomy. There was a small laceration of the rectal verge, but no sperm was found in the anorectal canal. The attacker apparently became enraged, strangled the victim and enucleated the eyes.

The pathologist's report should include examination of oral, anal and vaginal cavities for spermatozoa as well as determination of acid phosphatase levels. A search of the body surface and any available clothes for foreign materials is of considerable significance. Frequently, the victim's body is hidden or disposed of at a place distant from the scene of death, and recovered foreign material could lead to identification of the scene of death or possible suspects. Dried residues on the body or stains from the clothes should be examined for seminal fluid and possible blood typing. Plant material found under the body should also be noted. Larval forms of insects on the body may furnish rough guidelines as to the time of death. Maggots can be preserved in 70% alcohol for later transmittal to an entomologist for examination.

## GERONTOPHILIA

*Gerontophilia* is the deviate practice of male sexual attraction to older persons of the opposite sex for sexual gratification. These cases generally involve young male rapists who select their victims from females of relatively advanced age, that is, over sixty-five years of age. The victims generally sustain considerable injuries, with bruises, lacerations and facial bone fractures. Fellatio and cunnilingus are also attempted as preliminaries to vaginal intercourse. Because of the age and possible frail physical condition of the victims, there is a very strong possibility of their deaths. Trauma to the genital organs frequently accompanies vaginal intercourse or manipulation due to postmenopausal involution of these anatomic sites.

## VOYEURISM (PEEPING TOMS)

The usual case of *voyeurism* produces alarm and discomfort among its victims, but this form of psychopathology is not usually associated with death. The Peeping Tom may present a far more advanced sexual and emotional instability than is readily apparent from a superficial examination of his acts. Since the act of observation almost invariably involves a male attempting to observe an unwitting female, this can be preparatory to selection of a victim for a rape attack. Rape can proceed to higher levels of sadism, serious injury to the victim or death. Observation can also result in attempts at exhibitionism or masturbation. In the latter two instances, the Peeping Tom can be forced into a panic due to fear of exposure and possible capture and will kill or injure anyone attempting to restrain him.

## PYROMANIA

*Pyromaniacs* exhibit an underlying psychosexual disorder, which lies at the root of their desire to set fires. Some of these individuals may be exhibiting a latent form of sadism, while others obtain sexual stimulation or gratification while viewing the flames and destruction of a building. Another form of pyromania is exhibited among homosexuals where there has been infidelity among the sexual partners. The feelings of jealousy and desire to attain revenge can be exhibited by the setting of a fire within the apartment or house of the transgressing partner. If the latter individual happens to be caught within the confines of the fire, severe injury or death may result. An immediate on-the-scene investigation as well as a careful autopsy may facilitate the exposure of events surrounding the origin of the fire.

## EXHIBITIONISM

It is extremely uncommon for death to result from the usual forms of exhibitionism. These usually involve male subjects who are attempting to expose themselves to female children or adults. This produces great shock and alarm among the victims, but rarely is there any physical contact or violence.

## BESTIALITY

*Bestiality* involves the transference of the object of sexuality from a human to an animal, with the subsequent attainment of sexual gratification by some form of sexual contact with the animal or mutilation of it. One level of this practice appears to occur among individuals of lower levels of intelligence or in areas of restricted contact with members of the opposite sex, such as in isolated rural areas, or when individuals are under the influence of alcohol or drugs. These individuals, usually men or boys, attempt some form of sexual contact with animals including cats, dogs, sheep, cows and even chickens. Bestiality among women generally involves cunnilinguism or vaginal intercourse with dogs. Another category of bestiality involves acts of sadism perpetrated by young boys on various animals, usually dogs, cats or birds. In the latter group there is generally no attempt at any form of sexual contact with the animals. This form of deviate practice generally does not result in death, except occasionally that of the offended animal. The transgressing human can sustain injuries when he is unable to restrain a large animal upon whom he is making sexual advances.

## OTHER OBSCURE CAUSES OF DEATH DURING SEXUAL ACTIVITY

Most forensic pathologists have seen cases of air embolism resulting from vigorous cunnilingus accompanied by blowing of air into the vagina during pregnancy. A large volume of air is blown into the vagina, causing the fetal membranes to separate and expose venous sinuses, with air entering the circulation. According to gynecologists who have counselled pregnant females concerning the danger of this phenomenon, this procedure in the pregnant female stimulates a marked erotic sensation, thus accounting for acceptance or request of this type of deviate sexual behavior.

Other rare causes of death include aspiration of semen occurring during homosexual activity. Rupp[15] discusses a death in homosexuals performing fellatio with the erect penis impinging on and injuring the soft tissues of the posterior pharynx and aspiration of semen. We autopsied a male homosexual who was found nude in bed in a fetal position. He had apparently engaged in sodomy, since rectal smears were positive for sperm. The cause of death was marked bilateral pneumothorax secondary to ruptured emphysemous bullae of the lungs. Ruptured ectopic pregnancies have also been observed. Other cases have been reported in which varied types of articles inserted into the rectum have resulted in perforation of the rectum, peritonitis and occasional death.

## NECROPHILIA

*Necrophilia* involves the desire for and use of a dead body for sexual purposes. This may take the form of a fetish, where portions of the dead body, such as the breasts of a female, are removed and either worn by the male offender in a female fashion or retained in his possession for observation or physical contact.

Other individuals exhibit a far greater degree of sadistic tendencies with the desire to mutilate bodies of dead women stolen from funeral parlors or removed from graves in a cemetery. In addition to the extensive mutilation, particularly of the genitalia, there is frequently removal of portions of the body, most often breasts or genitalia, for later fetishes.

A third category involves either the utilization of a dead body for sexual purposes and satisfaction, such as cunnilingus or vaginal intercourse, or the murder of an individual in order to have sexual contact after he or she is dead. This type of deviate practice is extremely rare and in most instances involves desecration of a dead body rather than homicide. However, it should be borne in mind whenever a sadistic murder has occurred and portions of the body are missing.

## REFERENCES

1. Keneflick, D. P.: Medical Legal Conference Series. Boston University, April, 1964, pp. 44-112.
2. Malck, M. O. A.: Emotional stress as a precipitating factor in sudden death due to coronary insufficiency. *J Forensic Sci, 8:*47, 1973.
3. Beyer, J. C., and Enos, W. F.: Obscure causes of death during sexual activity. *Med Aspects Hum Sexuality, 11:*81-94, 1977.
4. Allen, C.: *A Textbook of Psychosexual Disorders,* 2nd ed. New York, Oxford UP, 1969, pp. 117-173.
5. Flowers, N. C., and Horan, L. G.: Nonanoxic aerosol arrhythmias. *JAMA, 219:*33, 1972.
6. Henry, R. D.: *Medico-Legal Bulletin, 20(2):* Bulletin 214. Richmond, Virginia, Office of the Chief Medical Examiner, 1971.
7. Sass, F. A.: Sexual asphyxia in the female. *J Forensic Sci, 20:*181, 1975.
8. Groth, A. N., and Burgess, A. W.: Sexual dysfunction during rape. *N Engl J Med, 297:*764-766, 1977.
9. Wilson, E. T.: Sperm morphologic survival after 16 days in the vagina of a dead body. *J Forensic Sci, 19:*561-564, 1974.
10. Findley, T. P.: Quantitation of vaginal acid phosphatase and its relationship to time of coitus. *Am J Clin Pathol, 68:*238-242, 1977.
11. Standefer, J. C., and Street, E. W.: Postmortem stability of prostatic acid phosphatase. *J Forensic Sci, 22:*163, 1973.
12. Cannon, Donald C.: Examination of seminal fluid. In Davidsohn, I., and Henry, J. B. (Eds.):

*Todd-Sanford Clinical Diagnosis by Laboratory Methods,* 15th ed. Philadelphia, Saunders, 1974, pp. 1300-1306.

13. Oliver, J. F.: *Sexual Hygiene and Pathology,* 2nd ed. Philadelphia, Lippincott, 1965, p. 549.

14. Willis, S. E., II: *Understanding and Counselling the Male Homosexual.* Boston, Little, 1967, pp. 25-35.

15. Rupp, J. C.: Sudden death in the gay world. *Forensic Sci Gazette, 1:*4, 1965.

*Chapter XX*

# INVESTIGATION OF DEATHS FROM DRUG ABUSE

MICHAEL M. BADEN

WIDESPREAD USE of drugs during the past two decades has been attended by a conspicuous increase in deaths related to such drug use. Heroin and methadone abuse have become the leading causes of death between the ages of fifteen and thirty-five in New York City. No other type of death is more often obscured or inadvertently made to appear homicidal. The body often has been moved from the place of death. Injuries may have been caused by futile resuscitation attempts and during movement of the body, and drug paraphernalia usually have been removed. Thorough investigation of all fatalities in which illicit drugs may be involved is essential to establish accurate cause of death. Such investigation is also necessary to determine the medical effects drugs have on body organs and the epidemiological patterns of drug abuse in a community, information that is important for development of effective drug abuse prevention programs.

## DEFINITIONS

Substance abuse refers to the socially proscribed or nonmedical taking into the body of any chemical for purposes of producing change in mood, usually some degree of euphoria. The term encompasses improper use of common products, such as glue or paint thinner; excessive use of a permissible substance, such as alcohol; and drug abuse, which includes any use of an illegal drug, such as heroin, or the use of legal drugs, such as barbiturates or amphetamines, in a nonmedical manner. Although many drugs are abused, the narcotic drugs are of most concern to law enforcement because of a high association with criminal activity.

*Narcotic* derives from the Greek *narkosis*, meaning a *benumbing*, and pharmacologically refers to drugs that induce a state of *analgesia*, obtunded perception of pain and *stupor*. However, in recent years legal definitions have superseded and expanded the medical one in international conventions and national laws to include drugs that do not produce narcosis, such as cocaine, which is a stimulant, and marijuana, which is a mild hallucinogen.

The first narcotic drug, opium, was the single most important medication during the many centuries in which relief of pain was the chief end of medicine. The collection of opium was a large industry in Asia Minor well before the birth of Christ; writings from that time describe the manner in which the immature head of the poppy *(Papaver somniferum)* should be incised and the milky juice collected. This juice (opium) was the principal active ingredient of many medicinal preparations for more than 2,000 years.

In 1803, Sertürner, a pharmacist in Germany, isolated morphine (named for Morpheus, the Greek god of dreams) from opium. Codeine was isolated in 1832. None of the more than a score of other naturally occurring structurally similar alkaloidal drugs subsequently separated from opium presently enjoy wide clinical use. The effects of opium are primarily due to its content of morphine, which is the alkaloid present in largest amount and constitutes 10 percent by weight of raw opium. Dreser in 1898 added acetic acid to morphine and synthesized heroin (diacetylmorphine), which is a more potent analgesic and is more euphorogenic than the parent compound. Dilaudid®, apomorphine, Numorphan® and metopon are also *semisynthetic narcotic* drugs derived from morphine.

All narcotic and analgesic drugs effective against severe pain thus far have proven to be addicting—all produce physical and/or psychological dependence. Much research is still devoted to developing a nonaddicting pain reliever. Meperidine (pethidine, Demerol®) and methadone (Dolophine®) are synthetic narcotic drugs, not derived from opium and having no structural similarity to morphine, which were initially erroneously thought not to be addicting. The term *opiate* by common usage has come to refer not only to any natural or semisynthetic derivate of opium but also to any chemically unrelated synthetic analgesic drug with narcotic properties.

One characteristic of repeated opiate use is the development of *tolerance,* which refers to the need to increase the amount of a drug to maintain a given response. Continued use of opiates and of various other drugs can lead to *physiological dependence* manifest, when use of the drug is stopped, by *physical withdrawal,* also termed the *abstinence syndrome.* The symptoms include restlessness, runny eyes and nose, abdominal pains, sweating, nausea and vomiting, which subside within a few days and in themselves constitute no danger to the individual. There has never been a death of an addict in New York City demonstrated to be due to withdrawal from heroin. In contrast, convulsive seizures and death have occurred as a result of withdrawal from barbiturates and other hypnotics, and deaths have occurred from administration of methadone to prevent heroin withdrawal symptoms, most commonly of persons while in official custody.

During the past few decades the public has remained fascinated by the seemingly justifiable retribution of the addict enduring *cold turkey*—physical withdrawal not eased by medication—which is a dramatic but unimportant aspect of drug addiction; the much more clinical medical aspects have been largely neglected. The *psychological dependence* associated with addiction is not as directly produced by the drug as is the physical dependence. Psychiatric disturbances, avoidance of problem solving and inability and unwillingness to function and mature as a non-self-destructive member of society often precede the abuse of drugs. Drug abuse then reinforces the underlying emotional deficits and creates additional psychological problems. This mental component that initially leads to the addiction is a major factor in the very high relapse rate among addicts freed of any physical dependence while in prison or following detoxification.[1]

The term *addiction* has been used in many ways but presently implies a life-style in addition to the mental or physical drug dependence: the development of a pattern of compulsive drug use wherein the obtaining of the drug supersedes all other activities to the detriment of the individual or of society. The continued injection of a drug such as heroin, despite constant awareness of the risk of sudden death and despite repeated infections and the continued production of mutilating scars, attests to the basic self-destructive nature of this life-style. The ritualistic aspect of parenteral drug taking is also a significant component of the addiction process: for many addicts the preparation of the drug for injection, often a group activity, and the actual needle puncture are almost as significant as the drug itself.

## HISTORY

Initial abuse of opium in this country was by means of oral preparations. Thomas DeQuincey's *Confessions of an English Opium-Eater* in 1822 did much to encourage and popularize the nonmedical use of tincture of opium (laudanum) for purposes of pleasure and euphoria; this tragic masterpiece also called attention to the potential for addiction, which was largely ignored. The introduction of the hypodermic syringe to the United States in 1856, just prior to the Civil War, and the medical profession's rather uncritical belief that morphine was nonaddicting, encouraged the rapid creation of so many subcutaneous morphine addicts that this condition became known as *army disease.* Morphine was widely dispensed by physicians as the cure for opium addiction and alcoholism, and patients were maintained for many years on morphine.

The burgeoning patent medicine industry during the last third of the nineteenth century, with opium the active component of many of the more popular preparations, competed with doctors in creating and maintaining narcotic addicts. By 1900 there were estimated to be between 100,000 and 1,000,000 opium and morphine addicts throughout the country, the majority middle-aged white women who legally obtained oral preparations from pharmacies and who remained an integral part of the community.[2]

Heroin, introduced in 1898, was immediately hailed by medical articles in Europe and America as the most effective analgesic known, as nonaddictive and as the treatment of choice for opium, morphine and codeine addictions. A small but increasing number of heroin addicts, many from antisocial and criminal subcultures, was not initially recognized. These heroinists obtained the drug legally by physician prescriptions. Addiction to heroin or other narcotics was not considered a cause of criminal activity. The potential for and severity of physical addiction to heroin was not recognized until about 1910. Popular revulsion to magazine and newspaper descriptions of the *enslavement* of the heroinist and the horrors of withdrawal, not evidences of criminality, in 1914 prompted enactment of narcotics control legislation, the Harrison Narcotic Act, which made heroin prescription and use illegal. Uncertainties created by subsequent court decisions also effectively stopped physicians from treating or maintaining opiate addicts with morphine. There was an immediate marked decrease in the number of narcotic addicts, especially among the noncriminal and older drugstore addicts. However, heroin became the narcotic most readily available in the illicit market, particularly among those already criminal or emotionally marginal, and there was rapid conversion of previously legal opium and morphine addicts to illegal subcutaneous heroinists. The price of heroin rose, and now increase in criminal activity began to be attributed to addicts.

Because of humanitarian interest and as a hoped-for crime preventive, forty cities across the country opened outpatient clinics where diminishing doses of morphine and sometimes heroin were officially dispensed to addicts. These clinics were closed in 1920 by the Commissioner of Internal Revenue for being in violation of the Harrison Act. During its nine months of existence 7464 narcotic addicts registered in the New York City clinic: 96.5 percent were addicted to heroin, 79 percent were male and the average age was 23.7 years; almost all were white. The change in the addict population from the socialized female oral opium abuser and older morphinist to the younger, antisocial and criminal male needle heroinist was established. The intravenous use of heroin became the route of choice for most addicts during the 1930s.

Kolb's[1] psychiatric studies of addicted prisoners during the 1920s demonstrated, as others had previously maintained, that the vast majority of addicts were criminal prior to drug use and that underlying psychopathology produced a susceptibility to opiate abuse. The updated Gluecks' studies[3] of antisocial adolescent behavior, begun in 1925 and now spanning more than five decades, strongly demonstrate that criminal activity, including abuse of drugs, is a symptom of and not a cause of delinquency; that the causes of delinquency often lie in deep emotional disturbances, which may be apparent even prior to adolescence.

The number of addicts in this country decreased during World War II as the heroin supply diminished. However, addicts unable to obtain heroin did not become productive members of society; rather, they turned to alcohol and barbiturates. Population dislocations during the war, as workers were drawn from rural areas to jobs in urban defense plants and navy yards, contributed to the creation of black ghetto areas such as Harlem that proved receptive to heroin trafficking when postwar travel resumed.

Between 1920 and 1940 the median age at

death from narcotism in New York City had increased from twenty-eight to forty-five. The addicts did not mature out; rather, they grew older and had longer histories of addiction. There is no indication that significant numbers of addicts outgrow their addiction and concomitant emotional immaturity to become functioning, contributing members of society unless there is definite therapeutic intervention. Older addicts, unable to obtain sufficient monies for narcotics, may switch to alcohol or cheaper drugs. The median age at death decreased following the war because of increase in the number of young addicts. In 1950, 50 percent of addicts who died were thirty-four or younger; in 1960 this median age had dropped to twenty-nine, and in 1969 it was twenty-three, reflecting the marked increase in adolescent addicts in that year.[4]

Thus the opium eater of the early nineteenth century was superseded by the Civil War medical morphinist and the drugstore addict of 1900; they were in turn replaced by the criminal subcutaneous addict of the 1920s and the intravenous heroinist of the 1930s, who have been joined by the postwar ghetto addict and the more recent high-school addict.

Vaillant's conclusion[5] in a recent follow-up study of heroin addicts treated at the federal hospital in Lexington, Kentucky, are similar to those of Kolb four decades earlier:

> The choice of drug—be it heroin, morphine or alcohol—is a function of the culture, but abuse of that drug is a function of man. Long-term follow-up suggests that what is wrong with the addict is not that he is addicted to a drug—heroin. Rather, he is an intelligent person unable to sustain employment; he is a suicidal person unable to admit depression; he is a lonely person who inadvertently substitutes drugs for people; he is a person with a paucity of gratifying alternatives rather than a man whose instinctual needs are readily answered by heroin.

## EPIDEMIOLOGY

The persistence of heroin use during the 1950s and 1960s permitted and perhaps encouraged its spread in increasingly wider circles: from the criminal and antisocial to the noncriminal psychiatrically and emotionally marginal individual and, strikingly manifest in 1969, to the young, apparently normal teenager who used heroin much like prior generations of rebellious identity-seeking adolescents had used beer and marijuana. There were 1000 deaths from narcotics abuse in New York City in 1969, which included the first deaths due to heroin use in persons under fifteen years of age. The proportion of teenaged narcotic deaths had increased markedly to 25 percent; 55 percent were black, 25 percent were white and 20 percent Puerto Rican; six times as many males died as females. The majority had antisocial records, including juvenile delinquency, truancy and arrests, prior to onset of heroin use.

During the early 1970s deaths from heroin use were noted among returned war veterans. The high incidence of heroin use documented among soldiers while in Vietnam was in large measure due to local environmental conditions: easy and cheap availability of relatively pure heroin, boredom, conditions of war—not to basic psychological deficits. When these individuals returned, the great majority stopped using heroin and thereby demonstrated that heroin use itself did not produce a permanent biochemical defect in the brain, resulting in continuous need for heroin. (The latter theory had been a major basis for development of methadone maintenance treatment programs.) Many of those veterans who died from continued heroin addiction had had life-styles associated with civilian heroin use prior to the military experience.

The increase in deaths directly due to narcotism since 1918 is apparent in Table XX-I. The figures indicate primarily acute deaths following injection of the heroin mixture (often mistakenly referred to as overdose) plus infectious deaths directly resulting from unsterile procedure *(dirty needles)*: hepatitis, tetanus and infective endocarditis. Since 1969 the number of persons dying from drug abuse in New York City has remained about 1000 per year. How-

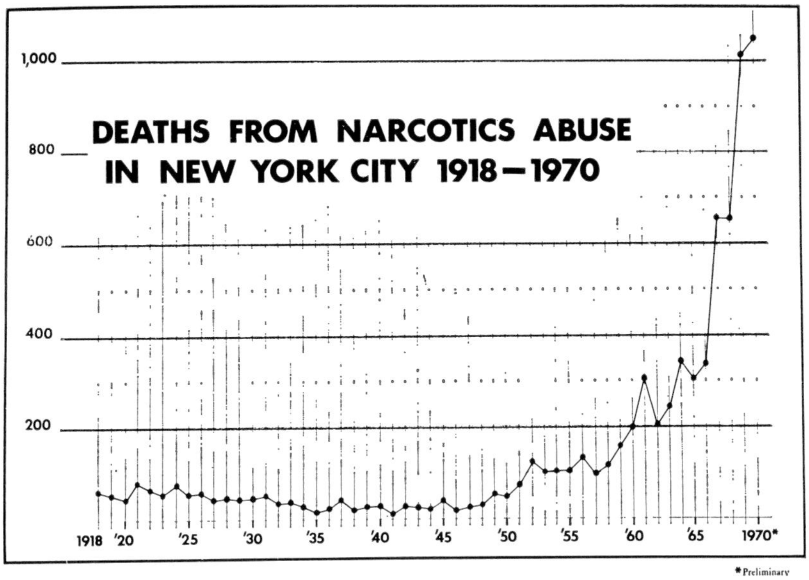


TABLE XX-I

ever, precise classification of these deaths has been complicated by a great increase in abuse of multiple drugs. The number of deaths directly due to heroin alone or with other drugs has decreased to about 350 yearly, but the number of deaths due to methadone alone or with other drugs has increased to more than twice as many as those due to heroin.

The rise in the number of deaths caused by methadone reflects its increasing illicit use by nontolerant persons for purposes of euphoria; also, the relatively large amounts in which it is taken: about 100 mg of methadone in a bottle of juice as compared to 5 mg of heroin present in a *street bag*. Since methadone and heroin are of approximately equal potency milligram for milligram, a therapeutic maintenance dose of 100 mg of methadone is equivalent to more than 20 bags of heroin. This is a pharmacologically lethal dose for the nontolerant user. In New York City illicit methadone is commonly obtained from a methadone maintenance patient who has take-home privileges.

## TRAUMATIC DEATH

In addition to deaths directly due to the injection of the heroin mixture, violent deaths such as homicide, vehicular accidents and suicide also are in high incidence in the addict population. In 1977 more than 300 addicts died as a result of homicide in New York City, most in arguments among addicts and pushers, some shot by storekeepers or police during commission of crimes.*

Many narcotic dealers or pushers are not users and show no needle marks. There is a very high incidence of homicidal deaths in this group. Heroin addiction in many ways can be considered a suicidal equivalent, and overt suicides are not uncommon. Suicides in custody have attracted particular notice because of their preventability and because of community concerns about possible police brutality. Most suicides occur in the first three days of incarceration.[7] It is prudent that all deaths in prison be autopsied and toxicological analyses done, not only to ascertain the cause of death but also in anticipation of questions that may arise later.

* A study conducted in Detroit in 1973 indicates that the percentage of homicide victims associated with the narcotic traffic could be as high as 60 or 70 percent.[6]—ED.

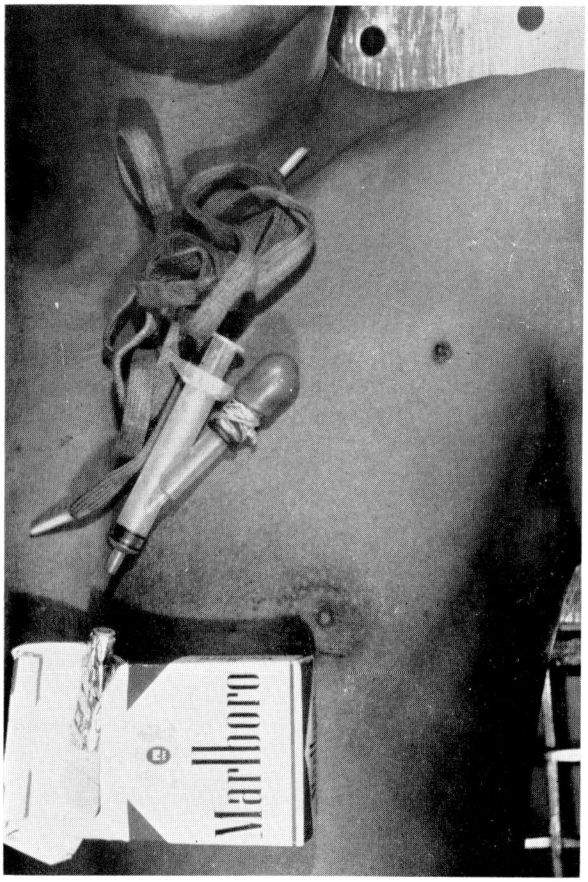


FIGURE XX-1. Homicide: Fifteen-year-old heroin addict shot during an argument about the quality of heroin. *Works* were found in a pocket in a cigarette box. Note the gunshot wound of entrance in the left upper chest. A .22 caliber bullet was recovered from the heart.

A fifteen-year-old addict was shot to death in a youth recreation center. Heroin *works* were in his pocket. The boy's friends indicated that the deceased had been an addict for three years and had often purchased heroin at the center. He was shot after he accused the pusher of having sold him poor quality heroin and demanded his money back (Fig. XX-1).

A nineteen-year-old heroin addict was found hanged in his prison cell twenty hours after confinement. He had fashioned a ligature from torn bedsheet strips. In some cities belts and shoelaces are routinely removed from imprisoned addicts because of the potential for suicide, but hangings have been accomplished using sheets, blankets and clothing. Autopsy showed morphine, the breakdown product of heroin, in urine and bile.

The *battered-child syndrome* is not uncommon in children of addicted mothers, who are also usually prostitutes; repeated beatings are often inflicted by the mother's customers or friends. Children of addicts are poorly supervised, and inadvertent deaths may occur due to falls from open windows, drowning in bathtubs or malnutrition. There is a high mortality rate among babies born to addicted mothers, due in part to poor prenatal care, poor living conditions and prematurity. In addition, the babies are born addicted and may exhibit abstinence symptoms, such as increased irritability and dehydration, if not detoxified by gradual withdrawal. There is no evidence that being born addicted itself predisposes to future addiction. Rather, it is probably the psychologically damaging environment within which the child develops that is now producing second- and third-generation addicts.

A ten-month-old female was dead on arrival at a local hospital. Multiple fresh and old bruises and bite marks were present on the body. Autopsy revealed old rib fractures, fresh lacerations of the liver and internal hemorrhage. The mother was an addict-prostitute, and her current boyfriend admitted to having beaten the child on a number of occasions.

An eleven-month-old child was suffocated beneath a mattress when his addict mother, while *high,* inadvertently put the mattress over him and then slept on it. She did not hear any cries or feel anything unusual; on awakening six hours later, she found the baby dead (Fig. XX-2).

## THE WORKS

Heroin addicts die because of the manner in which the heroin is taken: in unknown and varying quantities with unknown diluents and without sterile precautions. Physician and nurse morphine and meperidine addicts who take known amounts of the unadulterated drugs sterilely rarely die or have infectious complications.

Figure XX-3 illustrates the *works,* which is the intravenous apparatus used by narcotic addicts. The heroin bag in New York City presently contains about 100 mg of white or brownish

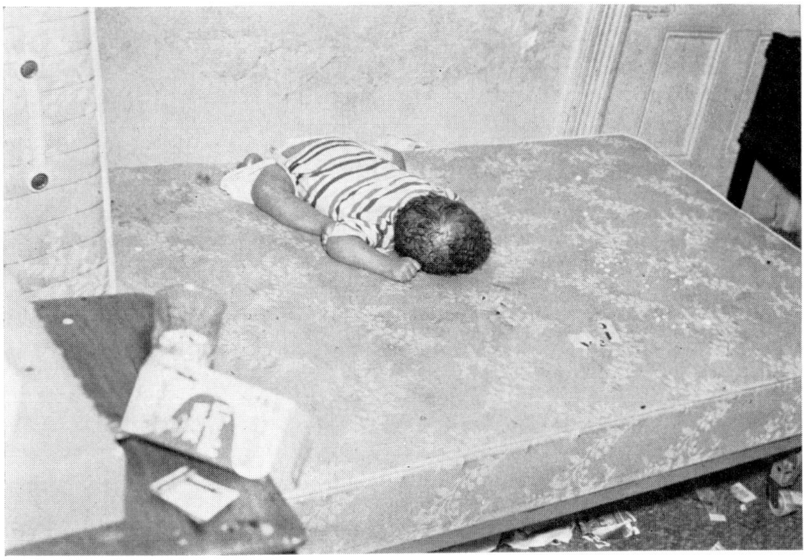

FIGURE XX-2. Child neglect: Mother, while *high* on heroin, lowered the mattress on the left onto the box springs, suffocating the baby. She was unaware of the baby's presence.

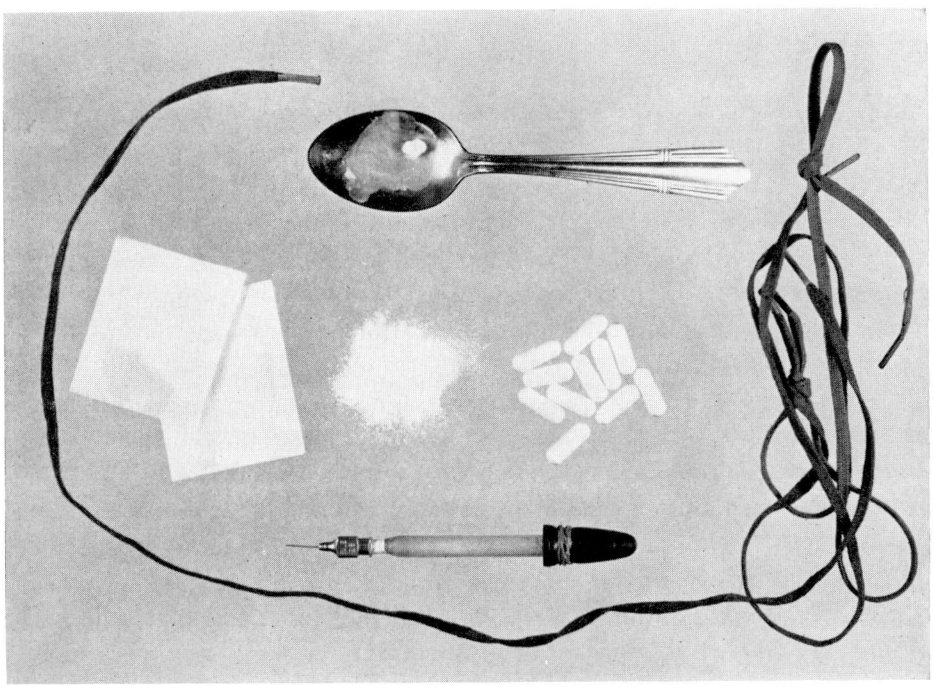

FIGURE XX-3. The *works:* Homemade eyedropper syringe, teaspoon *cooker* with adherent cotton intended to remove impurities, and shoelace tourniquet. The *street* heroin mixture is usually sold in folded stamp-collector-type glassine envelopes or aluminum foil and occasionally in gelatin capsules.

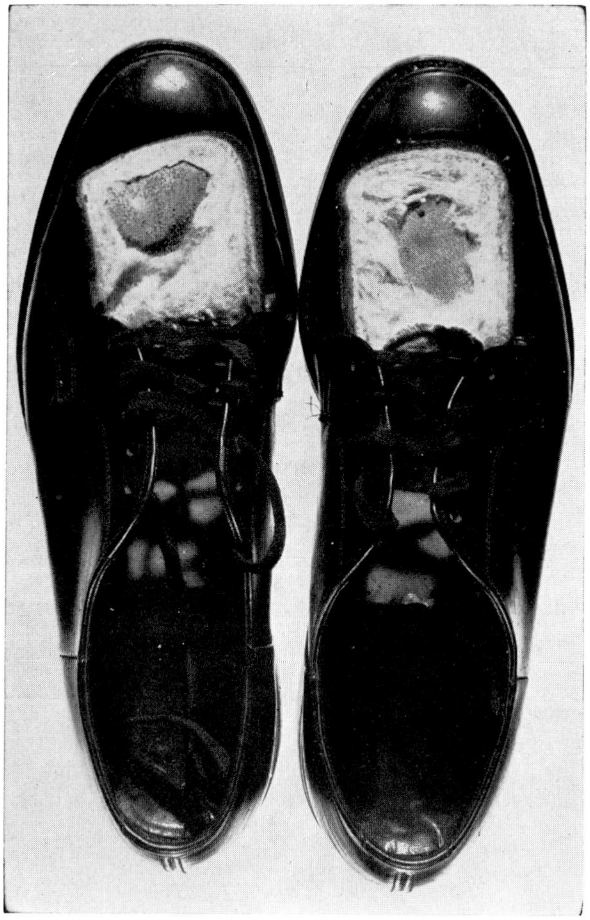

FIGURE XX-4. Addict's shoes: Removed from a thirty-year-old heroin addict who died following an intravenous injection of heroin. Note that fragments of cotton have been removed from the undersurface of the tongues of the shoes for use in the *cooker*.

powder, of which from 1 to 15 mg are heroin, 0 to 40 mg are quinine and the rest various sugars or other diluents. The amount of heroin in the *average bag* has diminished during the past few years and presently contains not more than 2 to 5 mg of heroin—thus, 95 percent or more of the contents is made up of non-heroin substances. The envelope is emptied into a bottle top or spoon *(cooker);* water is added and heated by a match, and the solution is drawn through a piece of cotton, which may be obtained from the tongue of a shoe (Fig. XX-4), into a syringe. The cotton is believed by the addict to remove impurities and germs. The forearm veins, made prominent by a belt, rope or shoelace tourniquet, are most commonly used for intravenous injections. Syringes found at the scene of death often contain blood, a result of the *booting* technique most addicts utilize of repeatedly injecting the contents of the syringe and then aspirating blood. The homemade eyedropper syringe is preferred by most addicts to the traditional medicinal syringe because it is more easily manipulated with one hand. Soot is present on the undersurface of the *cooker.*

Quinine, an antimalarial drug, was first added to the heroin mixture in the early 1940s because of the many deaths then occurring from malaria among needle-sharing addicts in New York City. There have been no deaths of addicts from malaria since; however, recently cases of malaria have been reported from the West Coast, where quinine is not commonly used as a diluent. Many addicts mistakenly attribute the bitter taste of quinine to heroin. Recently a pusher was found shot to death in Harlem with many hundreds of newly packaged heroin bags alongside, thought by taste by the perpetrators to be *duds* or devoid of heroin. Analysis revealed 25 mg of heroin per bag and no quinine.

Very rarely is an overt poison such as strychnine found in the heroin bag, and when present, usually in trace amounts, it is intended to add a pleasant sensation and not to cause death. Rarely is death due to a *hot shot,* an injection meant to cause death by means of a poison or a very large concentration of heroin. Since the addict does not know what is in the bag, the potential for many deaths to result from overt poisoning always exists, and constant official alertness is required for clustering of cases that might be the first indication of such an occurrence.

## CAUSE OF DEATH

Death may result a few minutes or even a few hours following the intravenous injection of the heroin-quinine-sugar mixture and is often erroneously termed *overdose*. However, the death is not due to a true pharmacologic overdose of heroin in the great majority of instances, as determined by toxicologic comparison of the packets, syringes and urine from living and dead addicts, which reveal no qualitative or quantitative differences.[8]

Although addicts commonly inject heroin obtained from the same source in groups, rarely does more than one addict die at a time, which suggests that the amount of drugs in the packets is not necessarily the critical factor in causing death. There is no suggestion at autopsy of an allergic or anaphylactic reaction, i.e. that the decedent was unusually sensitive or susceptible to heroin or other substances, which might be indicated by severe obstructing laryngeal edema as is found in fatalities due to allergy to penicillin, fish or bee sting. Usually the addict collapses soon after the fatal injection and dies at the place of using. However, he may go to another location or home before collapsing and be found with a fresh needle puncture in his arm, confusing subsequent investigation. Sometimes the addict is found with the needle and syringe still in the vein. Although this implies loss of consciousness very shortly after the injection, it does not necessarily mean that death occurred immediately. The addict may have remained unconscious for many hours prior to death, unable to remove the needle. Secondary aspiration bronchopneumonia is commonly found at autopsy, and sometimes the death is mistakenly attributed to the pneumonia.

The conclusion that a death is due to narcotism is based on an examination of the scene where the body is found, investigation of circumstances, history obtained from relatives and friends, autopsy examination that demonstrates drug use and excludes other causes of death and toxicologic analysis. In New York City the acute narcotic death apparently occurring in the course of drug abuse is left unclassified as to mode. Death is not accidental in the sense of being unexpected and by unforeseen chance, since the addict deliberately took the drug knowing that he risked death. Should an addict intentionally take too much heroin, or should a pusher deliberately package too much heroin, or should another person administer the fatal injection, the postmortem findings alone would not be distinguishable from the inadvertent self-administered acute reaction death. Rarely, a suicide note or a homicide confession permits classification as to mode.

In many jurisdictions, however, inadvertent death due to self-administration of a narcotic drug for purposes of euphoria is classified as accidental in that the death is unexpected and unintentional; some jurisdictions classify this same type of death as suicidal because of the inherent self-destructive nature of the drug taking and the known risks involved; and others classify the same death as natural, considering it akin to death from chronic alcoholism, which most jurisdictions classify as a natural disease.

A twenty-year-old female heroin addict and police informer was found dead in the ladies' room of a bus station with a needle and syringe still in her arm. Further investigation and statements from friends revealed that she had been sold highly concentrated *(uncut)* heroin intentionally to cause her death. The seller was not apprehended. The anatomic autopsy findings were not distinguishable from the usual unintentional death following heroin use.

## SCENE INVESTIGATION

Heroin is usually taken by addicts in places where they are not likely to be disturbed or discovered: in a friend's apartment, in a common tenement bathroom, in an abandoned building or in an infrequently trafficked area such as a rooftop or a roof landing. Should death occur, the body may be left where it is and the heroin and *works* taken, often for later use. If, however, the place of death is someone's apartment, the body may be removed and *dumped* in a non-incriminating place.

A fourteen-year-old boy was found dead on a rooftop landing in a tenement building. Many old and fresh glassine envelopes and scattered burned matches on the landing indicated that this area was used as a *shooting gallery* by many addicts. Needle track spurs were pres-

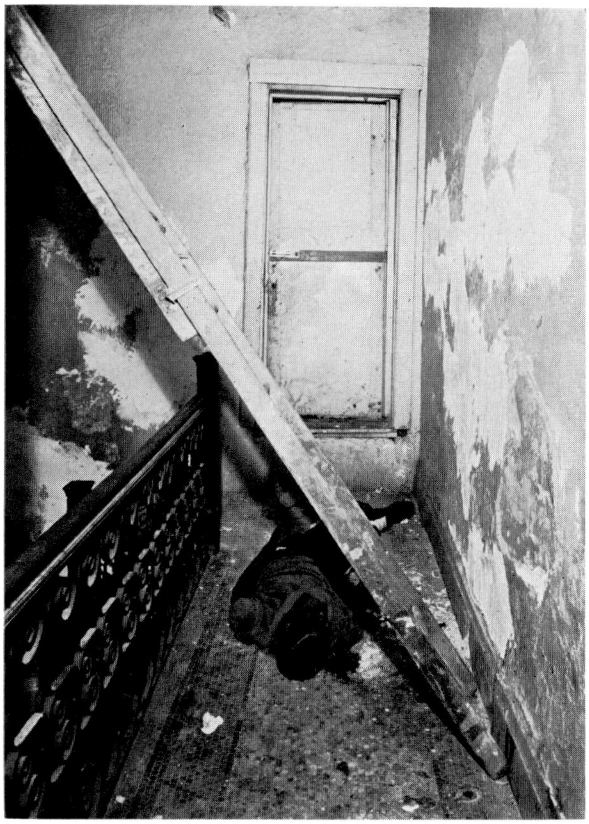

FIGURE XX-5. Scene of death: Fourteen-year-old heroin addict found on a tenement roof landing used as a *shooting gallery*.

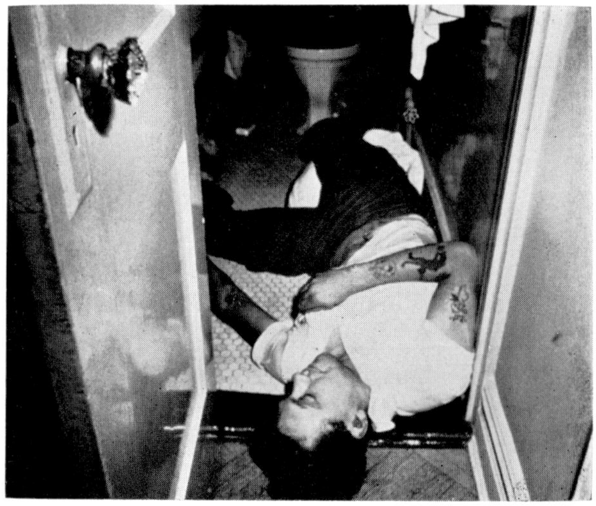

FIGURE XX-6. Scene of death: Twenty-three-year-old addict in a bathroom. Note tattooing on the arms, which is common in addicts.

ent on the forearms, and a fresh needle puncture was apparent in the left elbow fossa. The needle and syringe were not present (Fig. XX-5).

A twenty-three-year-old male was found dead in a bathroom at home. His parents were vacationing abroad. The *works* and an unopened heroin bag still present and the apartment door locked from the inside indicated that the deceased had been alone when taking the heroin (Fig. XX-6).

Initial examination of the dead addict may suggest homicide if the scene of death has been tampered with, if the body has been moved after death or if there are marks on the body secondary to attempted resuscitation. Scraping abrasions and bruising may occur during the moving of the dead body. It is not uncommon for the decedent to be removed to a park, a wooded area, an empty lot, a roadway or, when in an apartment house, into the common hallway or stairway. *Dumping* is suggested when the body is found in a frequently trafficked area in a building. If the body is moved more than a few hours after death, inappropriate rigor mortis or lividity may be apparent. Sometimes the dead person is not moved until after decomposition has begun, thus threatening detection because of the odor. The decedent's clothing and identifying papers are often left with the body, and no attempt is made to conceal identity.

Two male cousins were found dead—one an addict just released from prison and the other an occasional narcotic user. Inappropriate rigor mortis and lividity were evident in the former, who apparently had been turned over by a friend who had found them dead and who then called the police anonymously. Analysis of two heroin packets from the scene revealed 70 mg of heroin in each, sufficient to cause a true pharmacological overdose (Fig. XX-7). The rarity of multiple deaths despite frequent group use of heroin bags from the same source suggests that true pharmacological overdose due to highly concentrated heroin or poisoning due to an improper diluent is uncommon.

A young unknown girl was found at 4 A.M. dead between two parked cars in a roadway, her dress pulled above the hips. The possibility of murder during an attempted rape was immediately considered. However, identification of old and fresh needle marks on the arm at the scene suggested an acute heroin reaction with dumping of the body. Immediate search identified an apartment used by heroin addicts in the building across the street; the occupant, who was packing

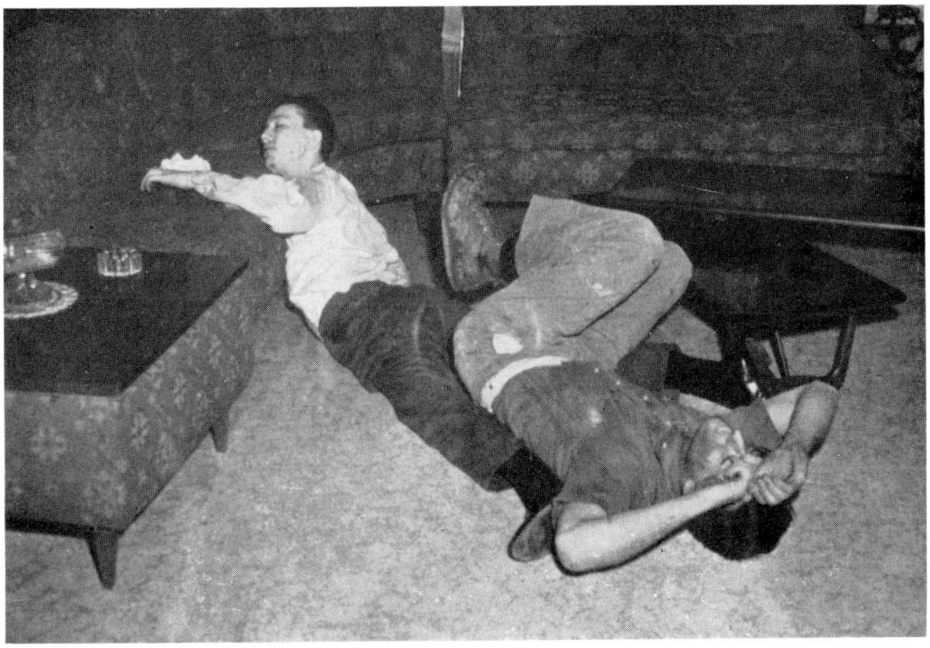

FIGURE XX-7. Disturbed scene of death: Two cousins dead of true pharmacologic overdose of injected heroin. Inappropriate rigor mortis of the extremities indicates that the body on the right was turned over a few hours after death.

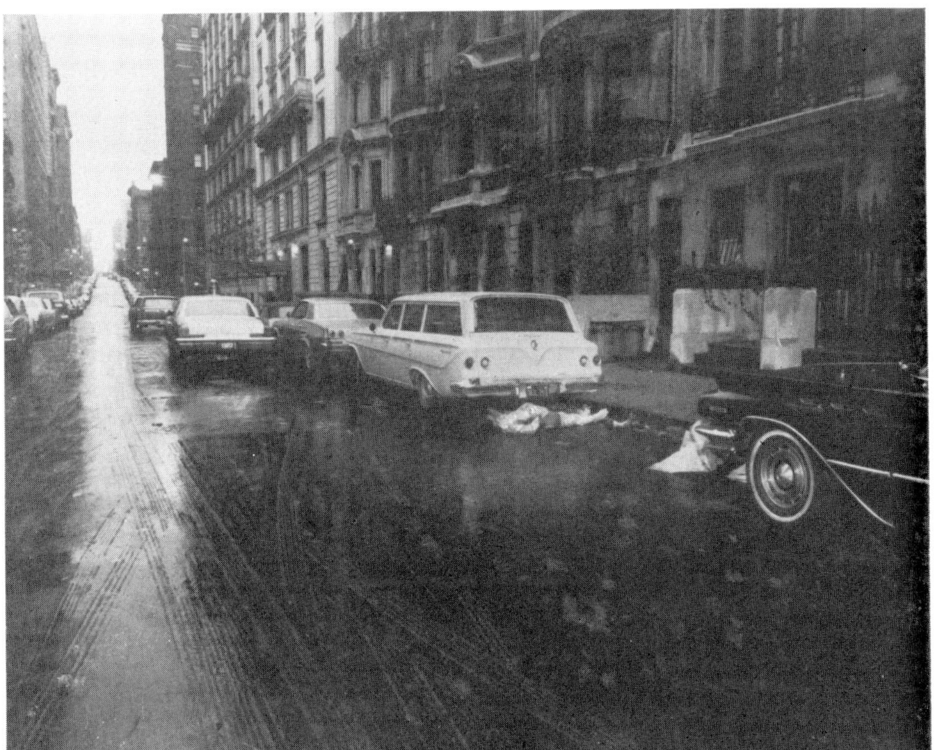

FIGURE XX-8. Dumped: The body of a young female addict that was moved from a nearby apartment into the street following death from intravenous heroin injection.

and about to leave the city, admitted to moving the body after the girl died following heroin use there (Fig. XX-8). If the police had had to wait for the autopsy results before investigating, the only witness would not have been found.

A nineteen-year-old college girl was found in a partly wooded area in Baltimore eighteen hours after having been reported missing; panty hose were tied over the face, scratch marks were present on the neck and homicide was initially suspected. College friends admitted to having given her four capsules of heroin to sniff during a twenty-minute period at a party, where she suddenly collapsed and died. The body was then taken in a car and dumped, with panty hose wrapped around the face to prevent oozing of secretions. No old or fresh needle marks were identified, but morphine and quinine were demonstrated in the bile. The marks on the neck were self-inflicted during terminal difficulty in breathing.

The body of a nineteen-year-old girl was found in a steamer trunk in an abandoned building. Old and fresh needle marks were evident on the forearms and hands, and autopsy indicated that death was due to intravenous narcotism. The police located a woman in the building next door who had seen two men carry the trunk from a car a few hours before police were anonymously called (Fig. XX-9).

The partially decomposed body of a twenty-two-year-old member of a motorcycle gang was found in a metal oil drum washed ashore in Chesapeake Bay. Cut marks were present on the body that corresponded to punctures in the metal drum. Fresh injection sites were identified in the antecubital fossae. Further investigation indicated that death had occurred following use of heroin at the gang's headquarters. Attempt was made to dispose of the body in the drum; holes were made in it with an axe in the mistaken belief that this would cause the drum to sink (Fig. XX-10).

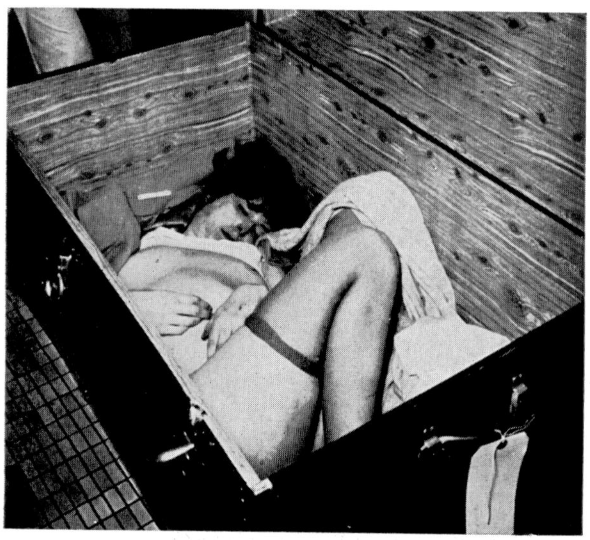

FIGURE XX-9. Dumped: Nineteen-year-old girl placed in a trunk and removed to an abandoned building following death from intravenous narcotism. Note the fresh injection site on the back of the left hand and the clothing disposed of with the body.

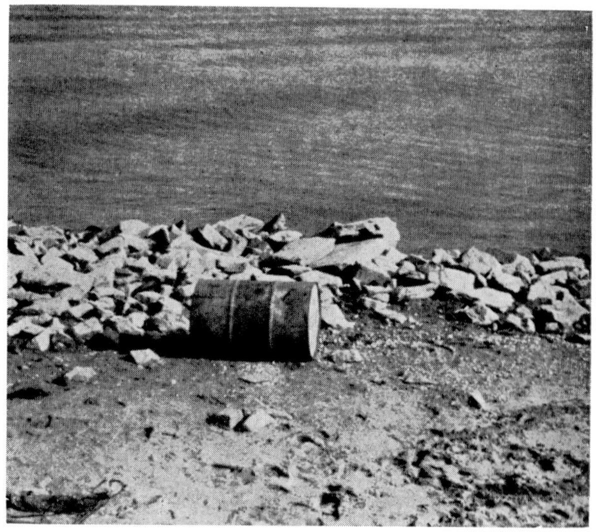

FIGURE XX-10. Dumped: Punctured oil drum found washed ashore. The drum contained the partially decomposed body of an addict who died of narcotism.

The decomposing body of a twenty-four-year-old girl was found protruding from between two mattresses dumped on a busy Manhattan highway at about 6 A.M. Identification papers and psychiatric clinic cards were present on the body. History was obtained of long-term multiple drug abuse, including narcotics, amphetamines and L.S.D. Autopsy revealed large amounts of barbiturates in the stomach and tissues. Subsequent investigation revealed that death had occurred about five days earlier in a friend's apartment, where the body had remained until the odor forced him to move it (Fig. XX-11).

Addicts employ many folklore remedies in attempting to revive someone who loses consciousness following use of heroin. They may inject saline, amphetamine, water or even milk into the arms, back of hands or buttocks. The unconscious addict may be immersed in a cold shower or tub of water, where the body may be found later should he die (*see* Fig. XIII-2). Other methods of attempted resuscitation include putting ice on the genitalia or pouring

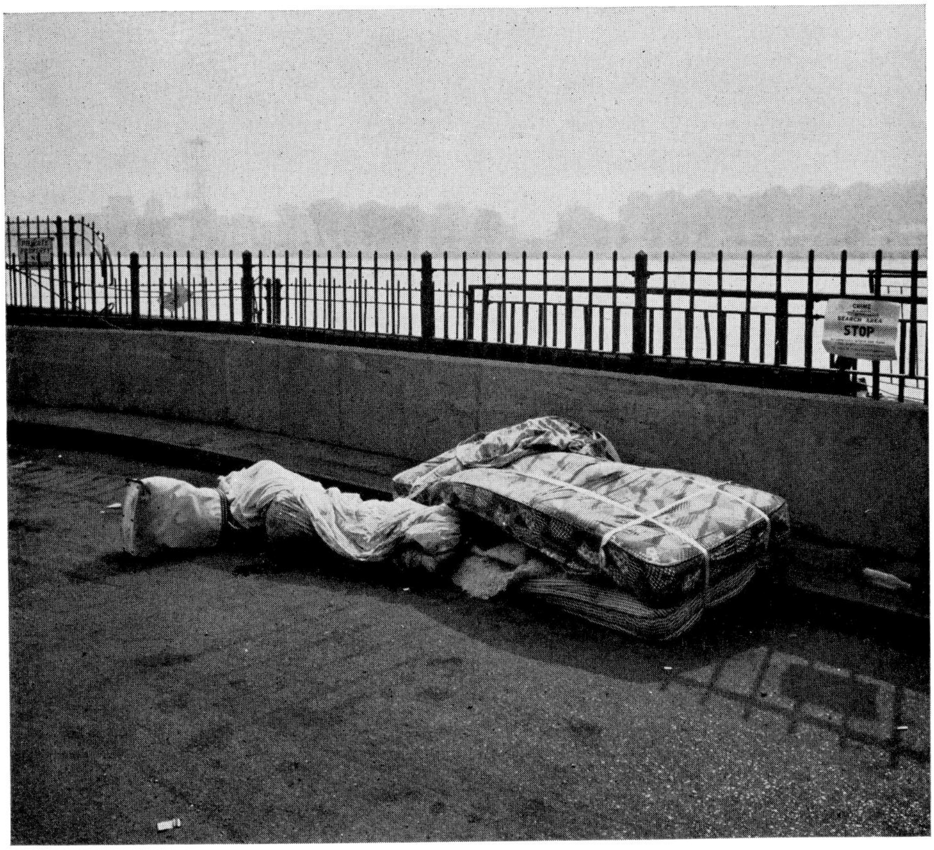


FIGURE XX-11. Dumped: The decomposing body of a twenty-four-year-old female who had died at a friend's house as a result of drug abuse was wrapped with sheets, placed between two mattresses to absorb putrefaction fluids and dropped on a highway.

milk into the mouth, often with aspiration of the milk into the lungs and resultant severe bronchopneumonia if the addict should survive the initial loss of consciousness.

A twenty-three-year-old male was found dead on a staircase with a paper towel protruding from his mouth. Autopsy revealed evidences of chronic addiction and fresh needle puncture marks. The paper wadding, probably inserted to keep the mouth open, had completely occluded the air passages, causing suffocation. Although this probably represented a resuscitative attempt, deliberate homicide could not be excluded. Witnesses were not found (Fig. XX-12).

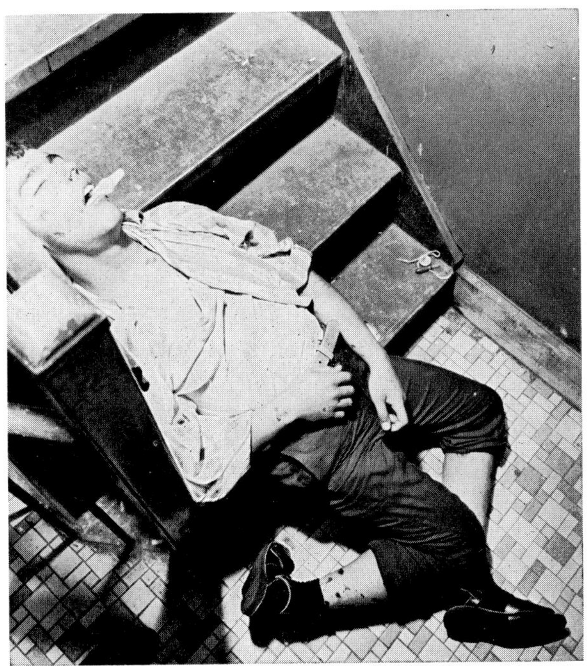

FIGURE XX-12. Folklore remedy: Protruding paper wadding that had been forced into the mouth of an addict who lost consciousness after an intravenous injection, presumably to help him breathe, caused suffocation instead.

An eighteen-year-old girl was found dead in her boyfriend's apartment with extensive needle track scars and a fresh discrete needle puncture mark in the right elbow fossa. There was a large blotchy fresh ecchymosis and needle puncture on the dorsum of the hand; morphine and quinine were found in the bile, and amphetamines were demonstrated in the injection site on the hand. The boyfriend subsequently admitted to injecting amphetamines in an attempt to resuscitate her after she lost consciousness following an injection of heroin. Perimortem injections often produce subcutaneous hemorrhages, resulting from difficulty in finding collapsed veins.

Occasionally a death that appears to be due to narcotism is found at autopsy to be homicidal or to be caused by occult trauma or natural disease, thus emphasizing the necessity of performing autopsies in all suspected addiction deaths.

A twenty-one-year-old female was found dead on a rooftop with prominent needle track scars on the forearms and fresh needle puncture marks. She was initially thought to have died of an injection of heroin. At autopsy a small bullet perforation was found in the posterior occipial bone, and a .22 caliber bullet was recovered from the brain. The contact entrance wound in the back of the scalp, which was covered by abundant thick hair, had not been noted on external examination.

The frozen and partially skeletonized body of a twenty-two-year-old drug user and heroin pusher was found in a wooded area in Baltimore in winter. He had been missing for three months. The soft tissues of exposed portions of the head and hands had been removed by small animals prior to the onset of cold weather and freezing of the body. The initial impression was that the body had been dumped after *overdose* death. Three bullet holes were found in the back, and three .22 caliber bullets were recovered from the body. Identification of the deceased was made by clothes and teeth.

A thirty-two-year-old female heroin addict was found dead in bed at home with the *works* on a bedside table. There were old needle track scars and fresh injection sites on the forearms. Autopsy revealed massive subarachnoid hemorrhage from a spontaneous rupture of a saccular (berry) aneurysm of the middle cerebral artery.

A death that initially appears to be due to narcotism in the course of drug abuse may prove to be homicidal if subsequent investigation indicates that the fatal injection was administered by someone else.

A thirty-two-year-old female heroin addict with needle track scars and a fresh puncture mark in the forearm was found dead in her brother's apartment. The brother admitted to having administered heroin to her at her request and that he had given her the fatal injection. He was indicted for manslaughter, pleaded guilty to criminally negligent homicide and received a three-year prison sentence.

Addicts in general hospitals often have little difficulty in obtaining heroin from visitors, hospital employees or other patients, and death may occasionally result from surreptitious heroin use in the hospital. Acute fatalities due to narcotism have occurred in legal custody when the addict was able to smuggle in the *works* and drugs either by inserting them in the rectum or by swallowing them, often wrapped in a condom, and waiting until they passed in the stool. An addict may swallow a needle while attempting to hide it in his mouth from examining police, or he may accidentally aspirate it into the trachea while attempting to clean it by sucking on it while euphoric. X rays will reveal the internal presence of the needle, either in the stomach, intestine, rectum, trachea or bronchus.

A twenty-two-year-old drug addict was found dead in his prison cell two days after arrest. A fresh needle mark was noted in the left arm, but no *works* were present. The prisoner across the way said he saw the deceased remove the *works* wrapped in a condom from the toilet in his cell after defecating; he injected himself, then flushed the condom and *works* down the toilet. A few minutes later he collapsed.

Unconsciousness and death need not immediately follow an injection of heroin but may occur hours after injection when the addict has gone elsewhere.

A twenty-one-year-old army private on leave was found dead in his bed by his mother. A fresh needle mark was present in the left arm. No narcotic paraphernalia were present. The mother stated that she thought he was slightly drunk when he returned home about midnight and that he went right to sleep with his clothes on; she could not arouse him in the morning. The deceased's friend stated that they had gone to a party that night and that about 11:30 P.M. the deceased had taken an injection of heroin and had then gone home. Morphine and quinine were found in the bile, liver and urine.

A twenty-two-year-old heroin addict was brought to a local hospital by a friend because he appeared groggy after just having taken a shot of heroin. Physical examination and x rays were negative, and he was kept under observation. One hour later he lost consciousness; examination and chest x ray now showed evidences of severe pulmonary edema.

## AUTOPSY FINDINGS

### External

The intravenous addict *(mainliner)* can be identified by typical linear needle track scars, which are most common overlying the veins of the antecubital fossae, forearms and dorsal aspect of the hands (Fig. XX-13), and by recent needle punctures (Fig. XX-14). The scars, sometimes pigmented or hypertrophied, result from multiple nonsterile injections and can be present any place where there are veins, including the neck, lower extremities and penis (Fig. XX-15). A single fresh needle puncture may be difficult to identify on the skin of a recent addict or of an occasional user. However, incision through the skin may reveal a prominent perivenous hemorrhagic track.

A twenty-one-year-old prostitute nonaddict collapsed at a party after taking an injection of heroin. A single fresh needle puncture was noted in the left elbow fossa. The deceased was also a lesbian. The triad of prostitution, lesbianism and addiction is common, with the addiction often developing last.

A twenty-seven-year-old woman was found dead in a Baltimore apartment used by a number of heroin addicts. There were no needle marks present on the arms, but there were fresh needle punctures just below the left breast, with underlying focal fresh hemorrhagic tracks apparent at autopsy. A friend said that she had attempted to inject heroin subcutaneously in that area and collapsed and expired shortly thereafter.

The subcutaneous heroin user *(skin popper)* enjoys a less rapid and intense feeling *(rush)* of euphoria and well-being *(high)* than the intravenous addict, but the pleasurable sensation is

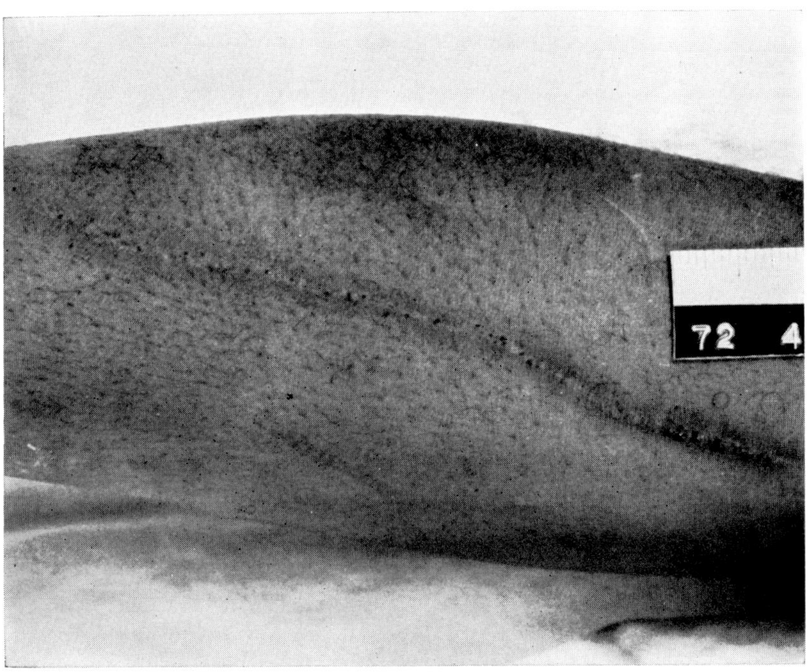

FIGURE XX-13. Intravenous *(mainline)* track. Linear pigmented scars overlying veins extending from the elbow fossa to the wrist.

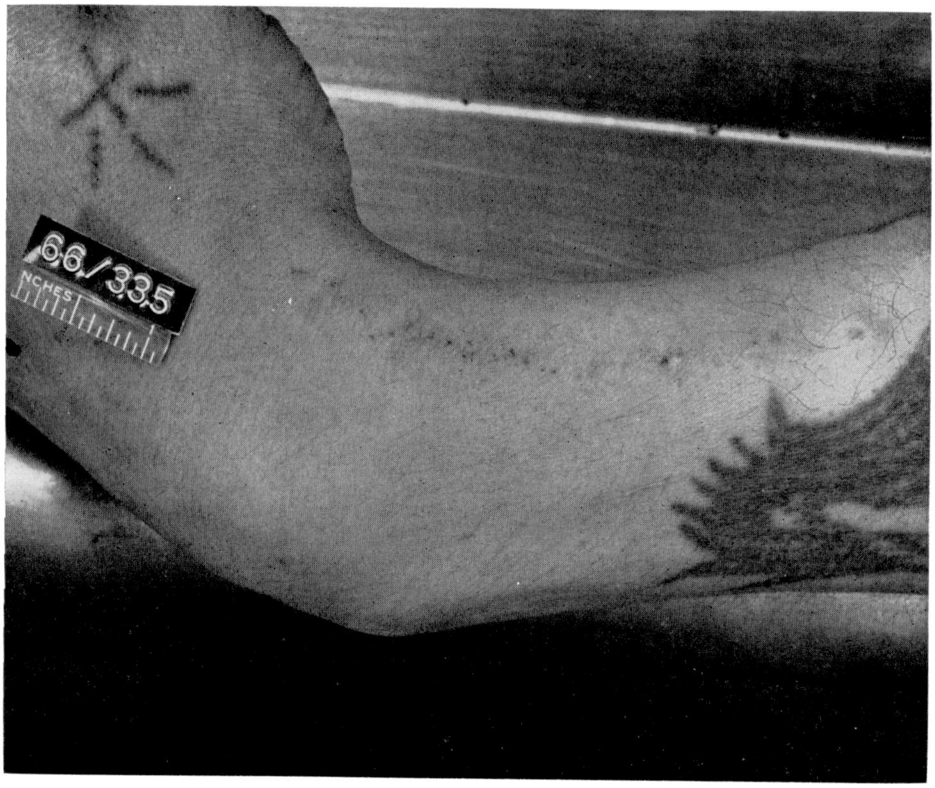


Figure XX-14. Intravenous track on the wrist. Note the crusted pinhead-size fresh needle punctures and the typical homemade addict-type tattoo of a pachuco cross with lines above it at the base of the thumb.

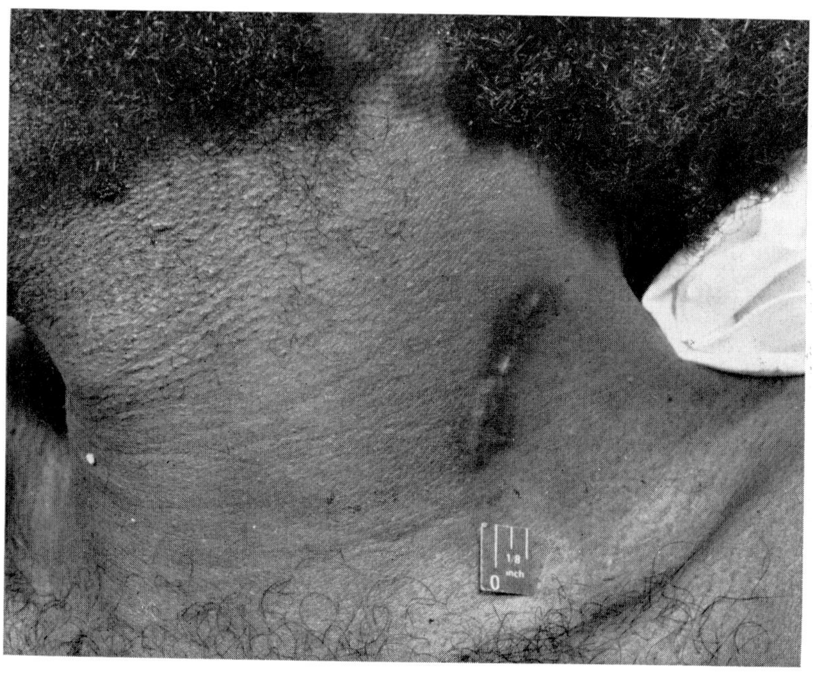

FIGURE XX-15. Intravenous *(mainline)* track on the neck.

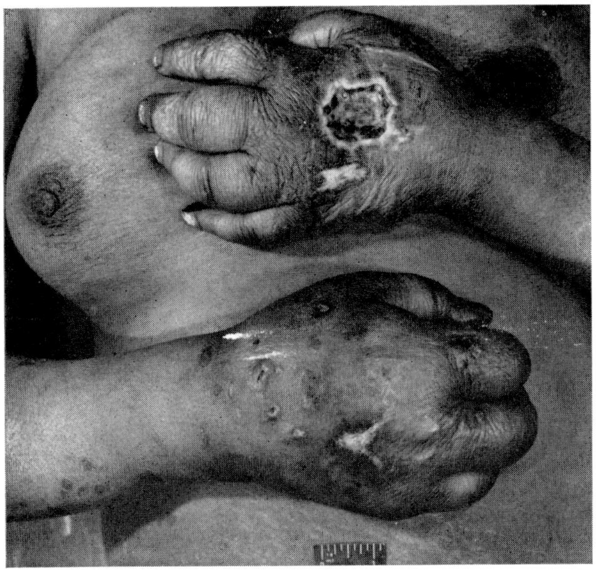

FIGURE XX-16. Subcutaneous narcotism: Old and healing *skin-popping* ulcerations.

more prolonged. There is much less risk of an acute fatal reaction when heroin is administered by this route compared to the intravenous route, but this group exhibits a higher incidence of abscesses and tetanus, which in New York City is now limited almost exclusively to narcotic addicts. Figures XX-16, XX-17 and XX-18 show the typical depressed circular and geographic atrophic scars and ulcerations that are the sequelae of abscesses at sites of subcutaneous injection.

Heroin and cocaine can also be taken by inhalation or insufflation (*snorting* or *sniffing*), which causes irritation, congestion and atrophy of the nasal mucosa and can result in perforation of the nasal septum. Heroin is not taken orally because it is rapidly hydrolyzed in the stomach. However, if opium is taken by mouth, the morphine content is readily absorbed and can cause death.

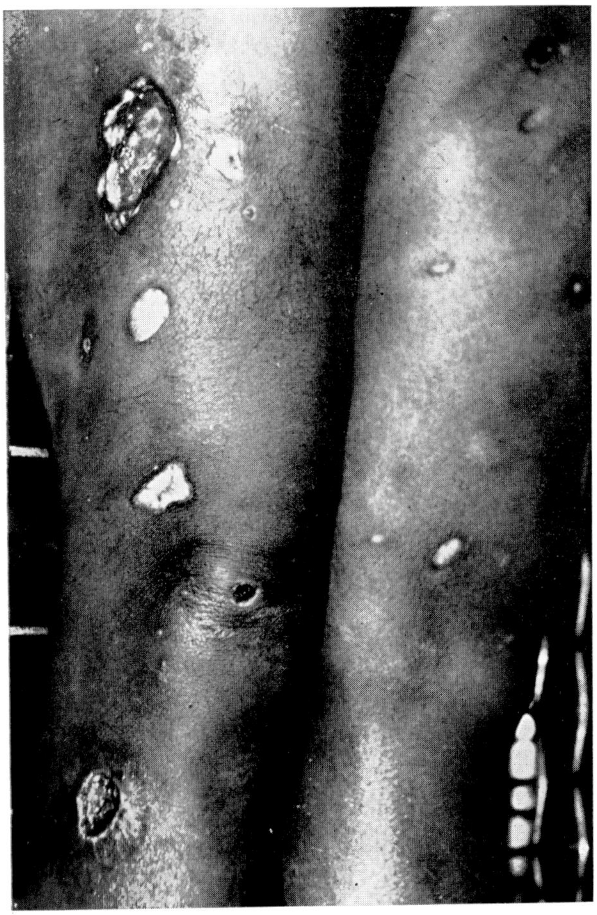

FIGURE XX-17. Subcutaneous narcotism: Note the recent ulcerations and old scars. Cause of death was tetanus.

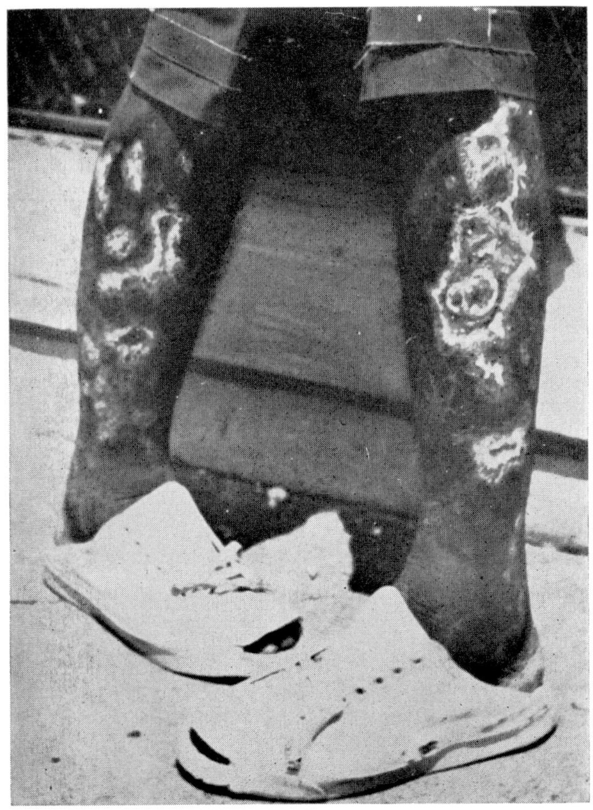

FIGURE XX-18. Subcutaneous narcotism: Living addict with extensive geographic scarring and ulcerations. (Courtesy Baltimore City Police Department.)

A twenty-nine-year-old college student ate a large quantity of opium while on an L.S.D. *trip,* collapsed and was dead on arrival at a nearby hospital. Recognizable fragments of opium were found in the stomach. Large quantities of morphine, as well as thebaine and codeine, which are also present in opium, were recovered from the bile, blood, urine and stomach.

The smoking of heroin has recently been reported to have been widespread among American soldiers in Vietnam, but it is not at all common in the United States. There is relatively little heroin absorbed using this technique.

Tattooing is common among addicts, sometimes to conceal old scars or fresh injection sites (Fig. XX-19), but often manifesting psychiatric significance: *Born to lose, Love is hate, I do not believe in friends* (Fig. XX-20). The *pachuco* tattoo, a cross and three lines often placed at the base of the thumb, is popular in certain criminal and antisocial subcultures (*see* Fig. XX-14). *Mother* is common.

Family interviews often reveal a strong maternal influence and an absent, distant or weak father figure.

### Internal

Characteristic scarring, fresh needle puncture marks and toxicologic demonstration of morphine and quinine indicate that the deceased was a long-term addict who had recently taken heroin. However, these same findings are also present in living addicts. A heroin injection can be a competent cause of death, but it does not have to produce death. In fact, in New York City probably less than one death occurs for well over 200,000 injections of the unsterile *street* heroin mixture: approximately 100,000 addicts take three or four injections a day, which result in about one acute reaction death

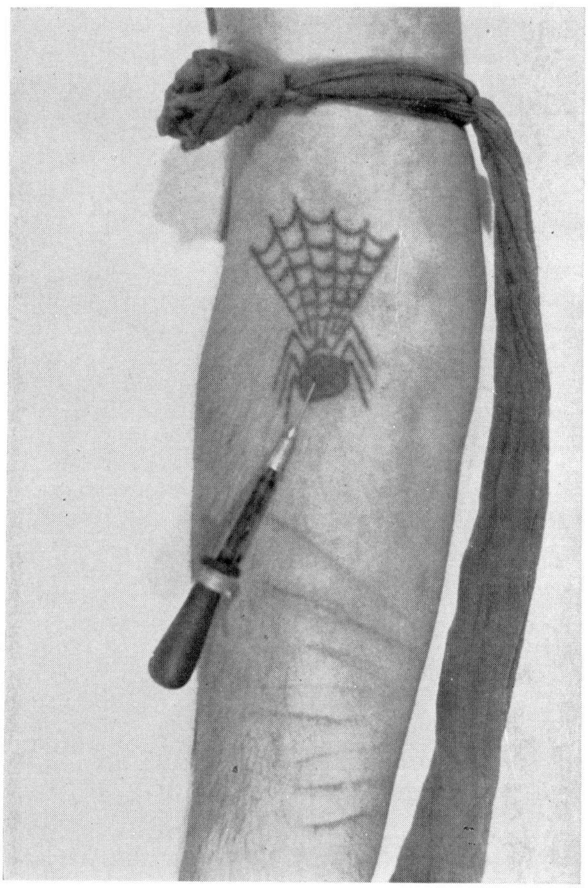

FIGURE XX-19. Addict-type tattoo used to conceal injection sites. Note the multiple scars due to incised wounds typical of self-mutilation.

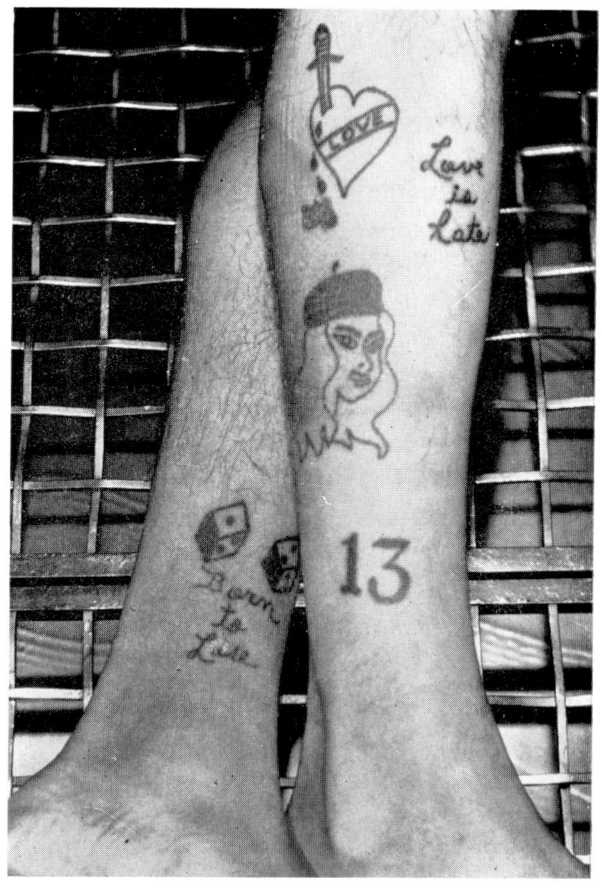


FIGURE XX-20. Addict-type tattoos manifesting psychiatric significance.

daily. A greater incidence of deaths occurs from reaction to penicillin given sterilely by physicians. A critical factor in attributing death to injection of a narcotic is the exclusion of other causes of death, natural or unnatural, such as spontaneous intracerebral hemorrhage, occult subdural hematoma or overdose of a nonnarcotic drug, which also occur in this population group.

Internal abnormalities due to narcotism are not prominent at autopsy. Examination of the needle scars will reveal perivenous fibrosis in the intravenous addict and acute or chronic abscesses or diffuse subcutaneous scarring in the *skin popper.* Small streaks of black carbon may be present in subcutaneous scar tissue, deposited by needle tips heated by a match in a naive attempt to achieve sterility. Microscopic examination often reveals foreign materials in the scar tissues, such as fragments of cloth, cotton, talc or unidentifiable matter, inadvertently injected with the heroin mixture. These are most prominent in the *skin poppers,* with surrounding foreign body giant cell reactions (Fig. XX-21). In *mainliners* the veins may show old or recent partial or complete thrombosis. A fresh puncture may be manifest as a discreet focal maroon perivenous hemorrhage that can be aged microscopically from the inflammatory response.

The long-term use of heroin itself causes no damage to the body organs that can be identified at autopsy. There are subtle chronic asymptomatic changes in the reticuloendothelial system that probably result from persistent antigenic stimulation by unsterile injection of foreign material many times a day for many years. These changes include enlargement of lymph nodes near the liver and pancreas, prominence of the thymus gland, mononuclear cell infiltrates in the portal triads of the liver and increased gamma globulin levels, which can be demonstrated in serum obtained at autopsy.[4, 7]

The history given by an eighty-two-year-old sailor that he had been a heroin addict for more than fifty years was not initially believed when he was admitted to a hospital for evaluation of a lung mass. The following day he exhibited severe withdrawal symptoms that required treatment with methadone until his death one week later. At autopsy long pale, faint linear

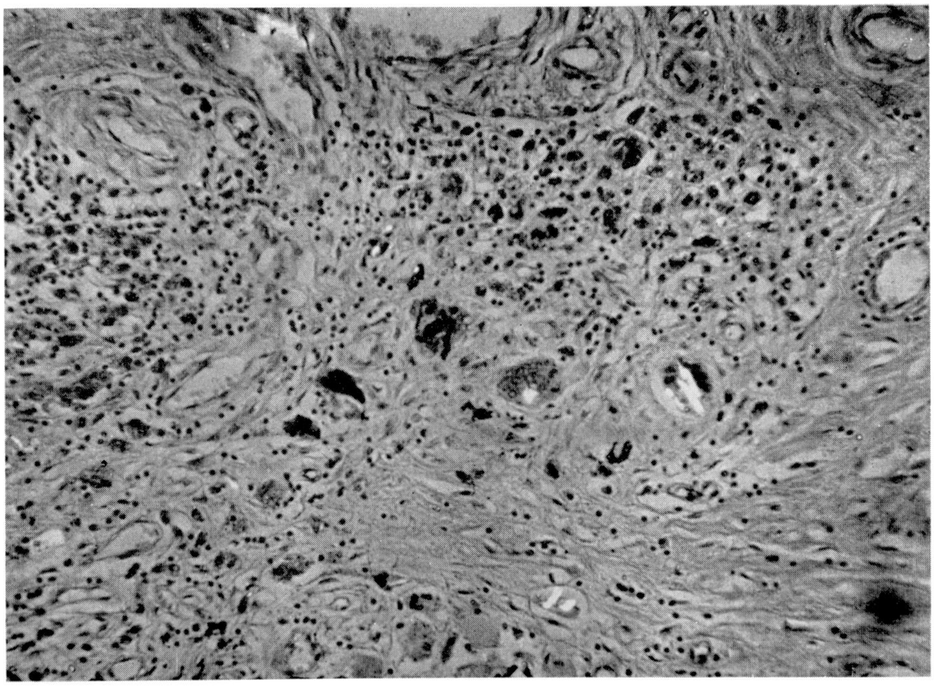

FIGURE XX-21. Microscopic examination: Subcutaneous scarring and foreign body reaction in a *skin popper,* with some foreign materials made prominent by polarized light (×200).

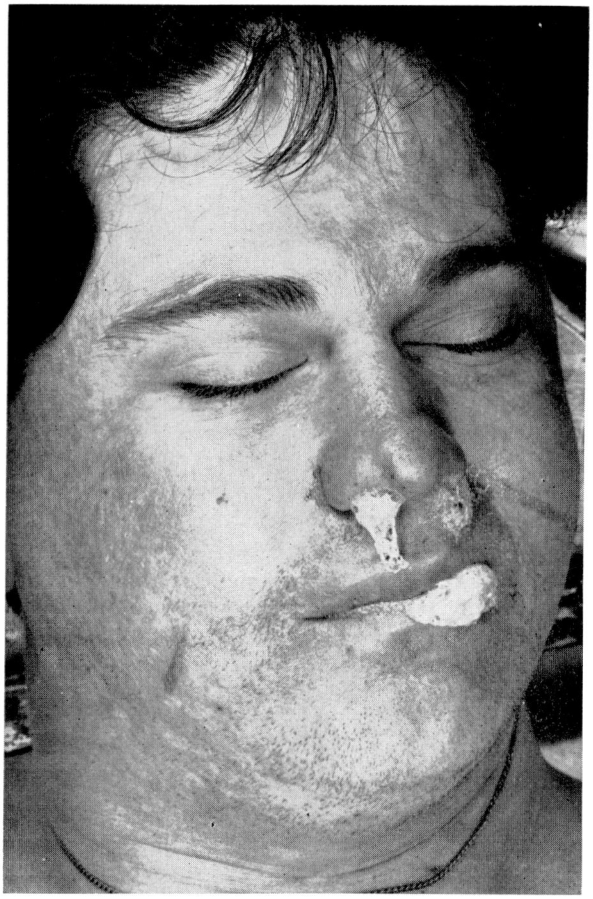

FIGURE XX-22. *Shaving cream froth* often exudes from the mouth and nose of addicts in mushroom fashion following death from intravenous narcotism as a result of severe pulmonary edema. Initially this froth is gray-white, but it may become blood tinged as tissue autolysis progresses.

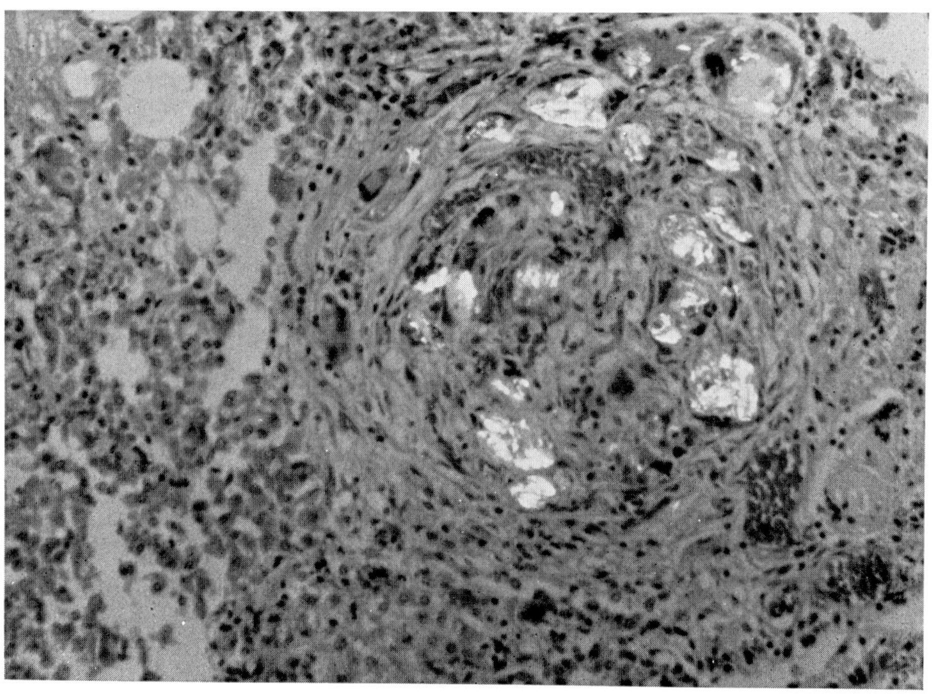

FIGURE XX-23. Microscopic examination: Foreign body reaction to insoluble crystals trapped in the lung of heroin addict who had dissolved and injected methadone pills meant for oral use (×200 under polarized light).

needle track scars were identified on both arms. The lymph nodes in the portal areas adjacent to the liver were markedly enlarged. Otherwise, the organs of the body, including the brain, where a detailed examination was made, were surprisingly unremarkable except for a cancer of the lung, which caused death. The long history of addiction was confirmed by relatives.

The most striking change following a fatal narcotic injection is severe congestion and edema of the lungs, with abundant gray froth filling the bronchi and trachea and protruding from the nose and mouth in *shaving cream* fashion (Fig. XX-22). This is also prominent in deaths following overdosage of methadone. Initially the froth is usually gray-white, but post-mortem autolysis of tissues of the nose and mouth may impart a red-maroon color to the froth. Bronchopneumonia often develops, in addicts who lose consciousness but then survive, because of aspiration, while comatose, of gastric contents or of milk administered by well-meaning friends. If drugs intended for oral use are injected intravenously (barbiturates, antihistamines, pentazocine, methadone), foreign body granulomata may be found on microscopic examination of the lungs, where poorly soluble filler materials such as talc are filtered out in the capillaries (Fig. XX-23).

Viral hepatitis is the most common of the infectious diseases associated with addiction and is a result of the unsterile technique and sharing of needles. Australia antigen associated with serum hepatitis can occasionally be demonstrated at autopsy. Bacterial and fungal endocarditis, caused by *Candida* species, and tetanus are very special complications, and endocarditis should be suspected whenever an addict has an unexplained fever. Infectious complications seen occasionally are meningitis and brain and pulmonary abscesses. A variety of neurological abnormalities have been reported in addicts, including bilateral symmetrical necrosis of the globus pallidus and transverse myelitis, which may be secondary to prior episodes of coma and hypoxia in the course of drug taking. Occasionally an addict who becomes comatose following a heroin injection is revived after irreversible brain damage has occurred, and he may then live in coma for weeks or months until death occurs, usually from a secondary infection. Acute muscle necrosis with myoglobinuria and renal failure also occasionally occurs in addicts.[9]

## TOXICOLOGY

Heroin is rapidly metabolized in the body to morphine, so that the taking of either heroin or morphine results in the finding of morphine toxicologically. Blood, urine and bile are good specimens for morphine recovery. In the absence of urine and bile, kidney and liver should be retained for analysis. In the United States very little morphine is sold in the street as compared to heroin. Recovery of quinine from the tissues with morphine suggests that heroin was the narcotic used, because morphine is not usually diluted with quinine. However, quinine may also derive from other sources, particularly tonic water. Inability to find evidence of heroin toxicologically may occur for any one of the following reasons: Because a very small amount was injected (many *bags* contain less than 5 mg of heroin, and death often is not related to the amount of heroin taken); appropriate tissues may not have been examined, e.g. in a very rapid death the drug may be in the blood but not in sufficient amount elsewhere (the needle and syringe may still be present in the arm, and bile and urine may be negative); laboratory techniques may be deficient, e.g. up to 90 percent of morphine may be bound as glucuronide and not recoverable by most techniques that do not include hydrolysis; pneumonia or brain damage caused by a narcotic injection may result in death days or weeks later, with no drug recoverable at autopsy. However, even when the morphine is found in tissues, it may derive from the drug taken six or eight hours earlier and not from the last fatal injection.

Sometimes chemical analysis may detect morphine and permit the diagnosis of acute narcotism when a fresh needle puncture is not demonstrated: in the occasional or beginning user, where a single puncture may be difficult to find; when the injection site is in an unusual location, such as beneath the tongue or in the perineal region; or because the drug has been sniffed rather than injected. Heroin, morphine, quinine or cocaine can be readily identified in swabs or extracts of the nasal septum after *snorting;* this should be considered when circumstances and autopsy findings suggest drug use but a fresh injection site is not apparent.

Quantitation of the amount of narcotic present must be cautiously interpreted, since the extent of tolerance cannot be determined from the autopsy. Further, the distribution of drug in the body and the manner and rate of metabolism vary from person to person. The same amount of drug can be fatal for one addict and insufficient to prevent withdrawal for another, depending on level of tolerance. Also, death following heroin use usually cannot be directly correlated with the amount of heroin taken.

Any paraphernalia found at the scene should be preserved for analysis. Heroin often can be identified in the needle or syringe, in the dried residue in the *cooker* and in the emptied glassine envelope.

Toxicologic examination is also essential to determine presence of drugs other than narcotics: alcohol is present in about 40 percent of the deaths due to heroin use in New York City; in 15 percent other drugs are also demonstrated, such as barbiturates, amphetamines, propoxyphene (Darvon®), ethchlorvynol (Placidyl®), glutethimide (Doriden®) and tranquilizers.

Intravenous methamphetamine *(speed)* and barbiturate addicts may develop needle track scars similar to those of the heroin addict. The relatively large amounts of these drugs used in the course of addiction, up to many grams a day, permit a higher incidence of toxicologic confirmation than is possible with the milligram amounts used by the heroin addict.

There is much current interest in urine testing as a means of detecting drug abusers.[9] This testing is necessary to identify oral users who do not develop physical stigmata. Most addicts who inject drugs will show scars and needle punctures that are apparent on a routine physical examination; however, once this addict begins a treatment program, urine testing becomes necessary to detect surreptitious drug use.

## METHADONE

Methadone, a narcotic synthesized by the Germans during World War II because of unavailability of morphine and named Dolophine® after Adolph Hitler (hence the street name *dollys*), was later used to minimize the discomforts of heroin withdrawal by being administered in doses for about ten days—a process termed *detoxification.* An entirely different use of methadone, which has become the major treatment method for addicts in this country in the last decade, is long-term maintenance treatment of heroin addicts. It has long been known that a person made tolerant to a large dose of one narcotic will also be made cross-tolerant to many of the effects of another narcotic. This was the reason, unappreciated at the time, that heroin was able to "cure" morphine and codeine addictions in 1900; the physicians did not realize initially that they were converting their patients to heroin addiction. The proponents of methadone maintenance contend that if a heroin addict is made tolerant to large doses of methadone and stabilized at 40 to 120 mg per day, as compared to the usual 8 to 10 mg medicinal dose for analgesia, he not only will no longer experience euphoria from the methadone use but he will also not get *high* when he injects heroin. He will therefore stop using heroin and will not have to steal to obtain funds to purchase it. Any other narcotic drug in sufficiently high doses would provide a similar blockade. The advantages of methadone, however, are that it can be taken by mouth without losing effect and that it is long lasting, requiring only one dose a day. Critics have argued that methadone maintenance merely substitutes one addicting narcotic arbitrarily made legal and free for another that has been made illegal and expensive; that doses given to maintain tolerant addicts can be fatal for nontolerant persons; that take-home methadone provokes illicit diversion of the drug; that the program is more oriented to protecting property than rehabilitating people; that a methadone program indicates to other members of the community that drug taking in general is a viable and acceptable life-style; that multiple drug abuse is becoming increasingly more common, and methadone maintenance does not discourage, and may encourage, abuse of alcohol, barbiturates, amphetamines, cocaine, tranquilizers and other nonnarcotic drugs to which it does not produce cross-tolerance.

Deaths related to methadone have increased prominently as methadone use has increased, and they can be divided into tolerant and nontolerant categories. Investigation of the first 100 deaths of addicts on methadone maintenance programs in New York City showed that more than one-half died as a result of abuse of alcohol, barbiturates, amphetamines or heroin. Homicide, accidental death and suicide were also in high incidence. The nontolerant group includes persons not on maintenance—often multiple drug abusers—who obtain methadone illicitly, usually to get *high*, not realizing that the same 100 mg dose to which a friend has gradually been made tolerant can be fatal for the nontolerant.

Similarly, deaths have occurred when someone misrepresents that he is a heroin addict or that he is on methadone maintenance in order to obtain methadone to get *high*, and the physician, without confirming the story, prescribes a maintenance dose of 40 mg or more, which has proven fatal for many nontolerant individuals. This type of death is most likely to occur in situations where the doctor is pressed to rely on the history from the patient, as when someone is just admitted to a hospital or a prison or when someone is seen for the first time by a private doctor. A number of accidental deaths have occurred in children who have ingested small amounts of their parents' methadone, which is sometimes distributed in an attractive orange-juice-like solution.

Complete toxicologic examination is necessary in a suspected methadone-related death. The examination must be performed not only to determine what drugs are present, but also because the absence of methadone in a maintenance patient indicates that he did not take his medication, often because he sold it illicitly or did not want it to interfere with his using heroin. Since methadone is taken orally, the stomach contents should be examined. Methadone is constantly present in blood and tissues of methadone maintenance patients if a therapeutic dose is taken every twenty-four hours.

Methadone abuse presently causes more than twice as many deaths as heroin abuse in New York City. This reflects a trend of diminishing number of deaths from heroin abuse that has been evident for the last two years. During a thirty-one-month period from 1973 to 1975, more than 1500 persons died in New York City directly as a result of taking methadone alone (one-third) or with other drugs (two-thirds); in an additional 600 persons who died violently, most commonly from gunshot homicide, methadone was found at autopsy.

The recognition of problems associated with methadone treatment has stimulated investigation of other drugs that might be useful in treatment of heroin addiction. These include a variety of long-acting methadonelike preparations and narcotic antagonists such as naloxone (Narcan®).

A forty-seven-year-old male addict who had been on methadone maintenance for two years, receiving 100 mg daily, was found dead at home with the needle and syringe in a leg vein, the *cooker* alongside. Heroin was identified in the syringe and *cooker;* methadone, morphine and quinine were identified in bile and urine. His wife said that he often injected heroin in the leg because the doctors at the methadone clinic only examined his arms for needle marks.

A nineteen-year-old male was brought comatose to a city hospital with a history of having ingested methadone two hours earlier. He responded initially to an injection of nalorphine, a narcotic antagonist, but lapsed into coma six hours later and died. Subsequent history indicated that the deceased had stolen 1 oz. of a solution containing between 80 and 160 mg of methadone from a maintenance program where he worked as a janitor. He and two friends each took one-third of the liquid to get *high;* they then became sleepy, and each went home. The two friends *walked off* their drowsiness at home, but the deceased could not be roused by his family and was rushed to the hospital. At autopsy methadone was demonstrated in the stomach, brain, bile and urine; nalorphine was also identified.

A number of potentially unavoidable fatalities have occurred because doctors did not realize that nalorphine lasts only four to six hours. This is sufficient to counteract the effects of heroin, which is similarly short acting; however, methadone is long acting, so that the patient must remain under medical observation and antagonists must be given repeatedly for twenty-four to forty-eight hours.

A thirty-five-month-old girl drank between 20 and 40 mg of methadone that had been distributed in a grape-juice-type solution and had been illicitly purchased by the parents, who were addicts, from an addict on a methadone maintenance program. One-half hour later she lapsed into coma, and irreversible brain damage was already present when the child reached a hospital one-half hour later. She died shortly thereafter, despite heroic efforts at resuscitation.

## NONNARCOTIC DRUG ABUSE

Abuse of nonnarcotic drugs, often referred to by the somewhat misleading term *soft drugs* to distinguish them from the *hard* narcotics, is much more extensive than opiate abuse. These drugs are associated with many less direct deaths, however, because they are usually taken by mouth, in known amounts and unadulterated:

1. *Hypnotics or downers:* barbiturates, glutethimide (Doriden®), methyprylon (Noludar®), ethchlorvynol (Placidyl®).
2. *Stimulants or uppers:* oral amphetamines, injectable methamphetamine (*speed* or *meth.*), methylphenidate (Ritalin®), phenmetrazine (Preludin®), cocaine.
3. *Nonnarcotic analgesics:* propoxyphene (Darvon®), pentazocine (Talwin®).
4. *Tranquilizers:* diazepam (Valium®), chlordiazepoxide (Librium®) and others.
5. *Hallucinogens:* marijuana, L.S.D. (lysergic acid diethylamide), S.T.P., D.M.T. (dimethyltryptamine), peyote, phencyclidine *(PCP, hog, angel dust)* and various hydrocarbon preparations that are inhaled: glue, cleaning fluid, paint thinner, fluorocarbons (Freon®) and other inhalants (e.g. nitrous oxide).

When deaths do occur from illicit use of these drugs, they are usually traumatic, consequent to clouding of the sensorium, transient impairment of judgment and faulty perceptions caused by the drugs that may result in vehicular accidents, falls from heights, suicide and inadvertent taking of other drugs in too great quantities. If the drugs are injected, infections may result due to lack of sterile precautions: hepatitis, skin abscesses and ulcerations. At autopsy no specific anatomic changes caused by these drugs are identifiable in any organs. When fatalities occur, complete toxicologic examination is necessary to determine which drug has been taken: stomach contents, bile, urine, brain and liver are most valuable, and the lungs should be examined if an inhalant is suspected. Similarly, urine toxicology has proven most valuable in determining abuse of most of these drugs in living patients.

### Barbiturates

Barbiturates are usually taken by mouth but can also be taken by injection. When injected, they may induce large sterile subcutaneous abscesses because of the irritant effect of the alkaline solution produced by the combination of the weak barbituric acid and a strong base, $Na^+$.

The nude body of a seventeen-year-old girl was found in a trunk floating in the Hudson River. Autopsy revealed no anatomic cause of death, but needle puncture marks were noted in the right buttock. Toxicologic examination revealed large amounts of secobarbital in the stomach, liver, bile and brain and amphetamines in the soft tissues of the buttock. Her friends later admitted that while she was at a *pill party* she got *high* and inadvertently took a few handfuls of barbiturates, then collapsed and died. The friends attempted resuscitation by injecting amphetamine into the buttock. Then, in panic, they purchased the trunk, put the body into it and dumped it in the river six days before it was found. The coldness of the water preserved the body.

Overtly suicidal deaths due to deliberate barbiturate overdosage by a nonabuser of drugs are common and should be distinguished from inadvertent death of a drug abuser.

### Amphetamines

Amphetamines are widely used as an appetite depressant in diet pills. The intravenous preparation (methamphetamine) is referred to as *speed* or *meth*. Death from true overdose occasionally occurs.

A fifty-year-old male was found dead in his luxury apartment. Fresh and old needle tracks were noted on the forearms. Autopsy was otherwise not remarkable. Toxicology revealed a large amount of amphetamines in the brain, liver and urine. Further investigation disclosed that the deceased had been maintained on intravenous amphetamines and vitamins for twenty-five years by a private physician and that he had taken an injection of amphetamines and had engaged in strenuous sexual activity just prior to death.

### Cocaine

Cocaine is obtained from the leaves of a South American shrub, *Erythoxylon coca*, commonly found in Peru and Bolivia. The coca leaves have been chewed by Indians in the Andes Mountains for centuries. The use of the purified alkaloid, cocaine, for medical and recreational purposes was popularized by Freud, Sherlock Holmes and others in the late nineteenth century and by Coca-Cola® until prohibited by the Pure Food and Drug Act of 1906.

Cocaine is a physical and mental stimulant and is effective when taken by mouth, intravenously, or when sniffed. There has been a marked increase in illicit cocaine use in the United States during the past decade, with development of a middle-class mystique that includes use of specific paraphernalia or a long

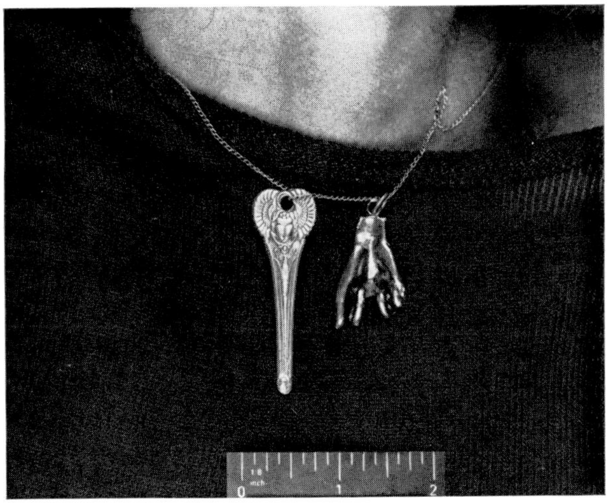

FIGURE XX-24. *Coke spoon* worn next to a medallion around the neck suggests that the deceased was a cocaine user. This was an *execution-type* death, with a contact gunshot wound in the back of the head. The victim was bound and gagged.

pinky fingernail for measuring and sniffing purposes (Fig. XX-24). This reputation is enhanced by its greater cost requirements than for heroin because cocaine is consumed in greater quantities at each use than is heroin.

The drug is associated with psychological dependence and development of tolerance, but it produces little physical addiction or withdrawal symptoms. It can cause death. Twelve fatalites from acute cocaine poisoning have been documented in New York City during the past five years. Half of these deaths resulted directly from sniffing or intravenous use and half from swallowing cocaine for purposes of hiding evidence or smuggling. Taken by mouth, 1.2 grams or more of cocaine can cause death.

A twenty-eight-year-old woman injected cocaine intravenously, as she had done many times previously, in the presence of her husband. Within a few minutes he observed her to develop convulsions, become comatose and stop breathing. Autopsy revealed cocaine at the injection site and in the blood and no other cause of death.

A twenty-one-year-old student en route to Toronto from Venezuela was found dead on arrival at John F. Kennedy Airport. Autopsy revealed more than 100 small plastic bags within the stomach and small and large intestines that had been fashioned from condoms and glove fingertips, each filled with approximately 5 gm

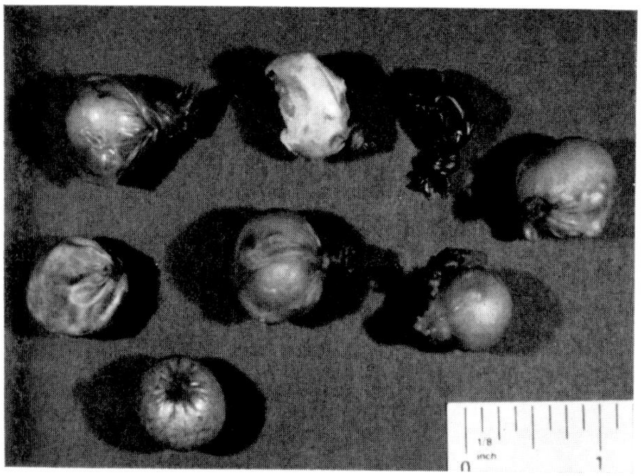

FIGURE XX-25. Some of more than 100 homemade bags containing cocaine that had been swallowed in a smuggling attempt and recovered from the stomach and intestinal track at autopsy. Some of the bags had burst. Lethal levels of cocaine and benzoylecgonine were identified at autopsy.

of 50% pure cocaine. Some of the bags had burst, and some were filled with gastric fluid that had osmosed into the intact bags, with dissolved cocaine osmosing out. Further investigation revealed that he had swallowed the bags in Venezuela with the intention of recovering them after arrival in Canada. Cocaine (benzoylmethylecgonine) was identified in the stomach and blood, and benzoylecgonine, a cocaine metabolite, was identified in the urine and bile (Fig. XX-25).

## L.S.D.

There are conflicting reports as to whether L.S.D. causes more chromosomal damage than other drugs and whether, if it does, such damage is harmful to the individual or to his offspring. L.S.D. has been associated with suicide attempts, but in the majority of the successful suicides, histories of significant psychiatric disturbance or suicide attempts prior to L.S.D. use are obtainable.

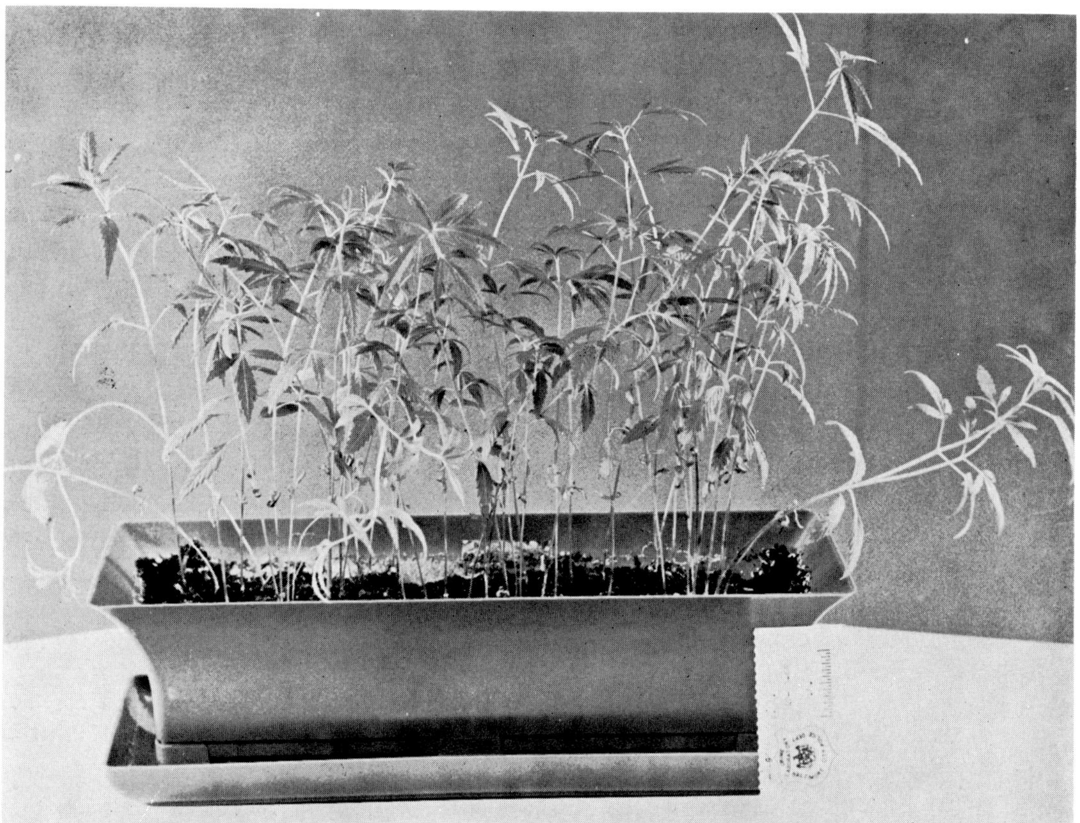

FIGURE XX-26. Young marijuana plants growing in a window box. Under proper conditions, plants may grow many feet in height. The leaves are compound and characteristically consist of an uneven number of serrated slender leaflets or lobules 2 to 6 in. long, pointed at both ends.

A twenty-five-year-old folksinger electrocuted himself in a bathtub, where he was found in a few inches of water, the torn end of a plugged-in electric cord adjacent to his bared left chest, where a small electric skin burn was apparent. He had a history of emotional problems and had developed marked evidences of paranoia, supposedly after drinking a soda six months prior to his death to which L.S.D. had been surreptitiously added.

### Marijuana *(Cannabis sativa)*

No specific organic changes in the body are detectable at autopsy following prolonged use of marijuana, but accidental deaths do result from falls or vehicular accidents while the user is euphoric.

A twenty-year-old male struck a pole while driving his car, and he and a passenger were killed. A history was obtained that they had just left a party at which marijuana was smoked. Chloroform swabs of the fingers and lingual aspects of the teeth revealed marijuana components to be present.

Metabolized marijuana, like metabolized L.S.D., cannot be identified reliably in body tissues. However, unmetabolized marijuana components (tetrahydrocannabinol, cannabinol and cannabidiol) can be detected on the fingers and teeth for a few hours after the last use.[10]

The marijuana plant is easily grown (Fig. XX-26), and the leaves, stems and seeds are ground together for distribution (Fig. XX-27). Hashish is a solid resin extract of marijuana with higher concentration of the active cannabinols.

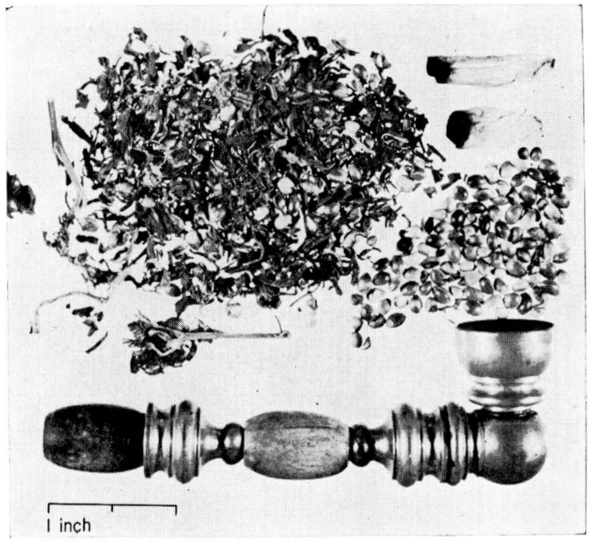


FIGURE XX-27. Upper left: Dried marijuana; stems, leaves and seeds ground together. Upper right: Marijuana cigarettes that have been smoked almost to the end *(roaches)*. Middle right: Characteristic marijuana seeds. Bottom: Pipe for marijuana smoking.

### Phencyclidine

*PCP, hog, angel dust, peace pill, DOA, crystal, animal tranquilizers* are among the street names for phencyclidine. It was originally introduced in 1958 as Sernyl® for use as a general anesthetic, but it was withdrawn from human use because of a high incidence of adverse effects. It has hallucinogenic and hypnotic properties and is presently available only as a veterinary tranquilizer, Sernylan®. However, it can be manufactured illicitly rather easily.

Its first street use was noted in San Francisco in 1967, and it is now used illicitly by oral ingestion, intravenous and intramuscular injection, inhalation and smoking, often on parsley or marijuana. Sudden deaths have been reported after each of these routes of administration. Phencyclidine has become widely abused during the past few years. It can rapidly produce a confused state, agitation, increase in blood pressure, irregular involuntary eye movements (nystagmus) and stupor, often with the eyes remaining open. A definite clinical diagnosis is established by toxicological analysis of the urine.

### Analgesics

Pentazocine (Talwin®) was introduced as a nonaddictive strong analgesic. Unfortunately, all strong analgesics thus far developed are also addicting: morphine, codeine, heroin, meperidine and methadone have each in turn been introduced as a nonaddicting painkiller.

A forty-three-year-old prominent physician was found dead at a friend's residence with a needle and syringe still in his forearm. There was extensive confluent ulceration and eschar formation on the forearms. History revealed addiction to pentazocine for one and one-half years. Pentazocine was found in the brain and stomach and in the syringe (Fig. XX-28).

If the oral pentazocine is injected intrave-

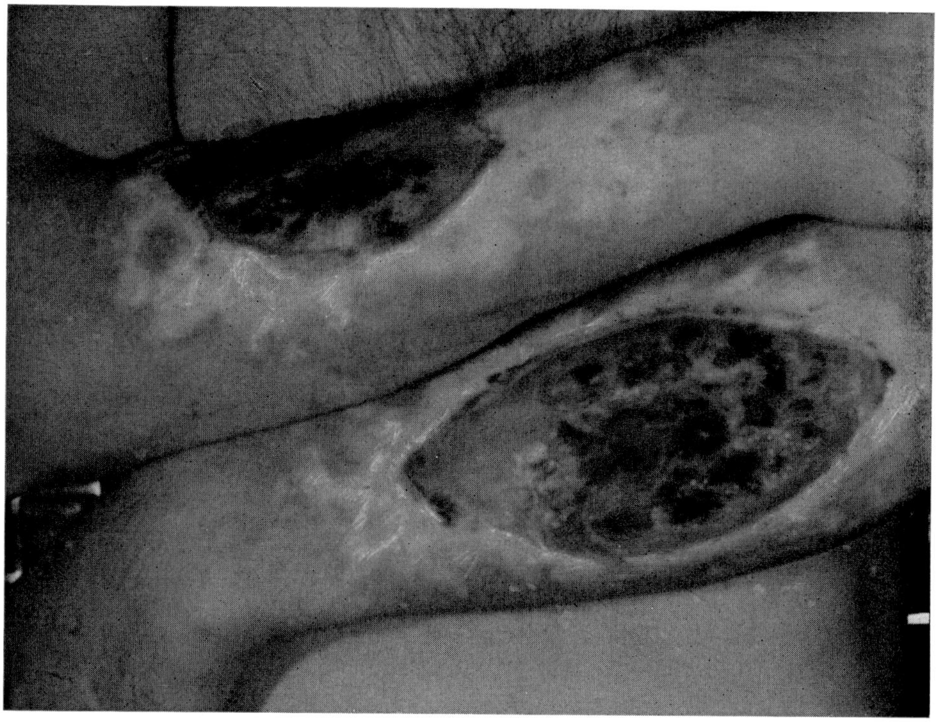

FIGURE XX-28. Ulcerations and eschar formation on the forearms due to prolonged injection of Talwin®.

nously, polarizable crystalline filler materials with foreign body giant cell reactions may be seen in the lungs.

### Inhalants

Many substances containing hydrogenated hydrocarbons, such as glue, paint, gasoline and cleaning fluids, will cause euphoria when inhaled.

A fifteen-year-old boy was found dead with a plastic bag collapsed over his head and a bottle of cleaning fluid nearby. Death was initially thought to be suicidal. Investigation into the circumstances and history, however, indicated that the deceased attempted to emulate friends who sniffed glue, but he mistakenly used a plastic bag instead of a paper bag, not realizing that should he lose consciousness the plastic bag would collapse and cause suffocation. Trichloroethylene and trichloroethane were recovered from the lungs and brain.

Occasionally when such deaths occur, the plastic bag is removed by friends or relatives and the reason for death is obscured; toxicologic analysis is critical in establishing the correct diagnosis. Freon® can cause death during inhalation by directly inducing a cardiac arrhythmia and can be readily identified in lung and other tissues.

A fourteen-year-old boy was observed walking in the street, inhaling the contents of a balloon held in his mouth. He suddenly collapsed and was pronounced dead a few minutes later. At autopsy a can of a Freon®-containing compound was found in a coat pocket, and the same compound was recovered from within the balloon and from the tissues on toxicological analyses. His brother indicated that he had inhaled Freon® and other volatile compounds from balloons in the past after filling the balloon with the chemical.

Recent government bans on aerosol products that contain fluorocarbons were enacted because of concerns that these chemicals may damage the atmospheric ozone layer. These new regulations should decrease the abuse of such aerosols for euphoric purposes.

## CONCLUSION

Thorough investigation of all potential drug abuse related deaths, including scene examination, autopsy and toxicologic analysis, is necessary to determine an accurate cause of death. Often the scene of death has been tampered with, and a fatality following a self-administered heroin injection may appear homicidal. On the contrary, there is a high incidence of obvious and unsuspected violence among drug users, and a death that initially appears to be due to heroin use may at autopsy prove to be homicidal. Investigation of drug-related deaths also provides a unique opportunity to obtain information concerning patterns of drug abuse and effects of drugs on the body that can contribute to the prevention of these deaths.

## REFERENCES


1. Kolb, L.: *Drug Addiction: A Medical Problem.* Springfield, Thomas, 1962.
2. Terry, C. E., and Pellens, M.: *The Opium Problem.* New York, N.Y., for the Committee on Drug Addiction in Collaboration with the Bureau of Social Hygiene, 1928.
3. Glueck, S., and Glueck, E.: *Delinquents and Non-delinquents in Perspective.* Cambridge, Harvard U Pr, 1968.
4. Baden, M.: Narcotic abuse—A medical examiner's view. In Wecht, C. H. (Eds.): *Legal Medicine Annual 1971.* New York, Appleton, 1971.
5. Vaillant, G. E.: The natural history of narcotic drug addiction. *Semin Psychiatry, 2:*486, 1970.
6. Baden, M.: Homicide, suicide, and accidental death among narcotic addicts. *Hum Pathol, 3:*91, 1972.
7. Monforte, J. R., and Spitz, W. U.: Narcotic abuse among homicide victims in Detroit. *J Forensic Sci, 20:*189, 1975.
8. Helpern, M., and Rho, Y.: Deaths from narcotism in New York City. *NY State J Med, 66:*2391, 1966.
9. Richter, R. W. (Ed.): *Medical Aspects of Drug Abuse.* New York, Har Row, 1975.
10. Baden, M., Valanju, N. N., Verma, S. K., and Valanju, S. N.: Confirmed identification of biotransformed drugs of abuse in urine. *Am J Clin Pathol, 57:*43, 1972.

*Chapter XXI*

# GUIDELINES FOR PRESERVATION OF TOXICOLOGIC EVIDENCE

Henry C. Freimuth

Defined in its broadest possible sense, toxicology is the science involving the study of poisons. In a more restricted sense one might say that toxicology is concerned with chemical and physical properties of toxic substances, their effects upon the body, their identification and quantitation in biologic and nonbiologic material, as well as methods of treatment of poisonings, including specific antidotes.

When one attempts to set forth a definition of a poison that would fit all cases, some difficulty is encountered. However, a working definition of a poison is any substance that will cause ill health or death in a healthy person when that substance is introduced into the body in a soluble form and in sufficient quantity. The term *solubility* here refers to solubility outside the body as well as to solubility in gastrointestinal juice. Hence, *white arsenic,* or arsenic trioxide, becomes a toxic substance because it is soluble in the hydrochloric acid found in the stomach, although it is relatively insoluble in water. In order to determine whether a given substance is a poison, one must also know the amount of that substance with which one is concerned. Many substances in low dosage are used therapeutically, while larger amounts of the same substances would, at the very least, produce clinical intoxication and possibly cause death. The last qualifying phrase in the definition indicates the action of the substance in a healthy person. Many persons, however, may be adversely affected by a so-called nontoxic dose of a given substance. For example, a person suffering from a debilitating disease is more adversely affected by a given dose than a person in good health. Conversely, a person addicted or habituated to a given drug can tolerate much larger doses of that drug than the normal individual.

Poisonings may be suicidal, accidental or homicidal, with the majority of cases falling into the first two categories. As a matter of fact, homicidal poisonings are of such comparative rarity that they generally attract considerable attention from the public press. However, if the discovery of homicidal poisonings is to be ensured, it is necessary to assume that all poisonings are homicides until proven otherwise. Only by the exercise of an acute index of suspicion will such homicides be made apparent. Proof that poisoning has occurred is based upon several factors, taken singly or in combination:

1. Evidence of signs and symptoms associated with a specific toxic substance.
2. Demonstration, by chemical analysis, of the presence of a poison in some food or drug product taken by the deceased.
3. Demonstration, by chemical analysis, of the presence of a particular toxic substance in the tissues and body fluids of the deceased.
4. Demonstration of gross or histologic pathological findings associated with a toxic substance in the tissues of the deceased.
5. A history of exposure of the deceased to a specific toxic substance.

## ANALYSIS OF GASTRIC CONTENTS

Many persons labor under the mistaken impression that the only criterion needed to establish whether poisoning has occurred is the identification by chemical analysis of a poison in the gastric contents. However, such a chemical analysis, whether resulting in positive or negative findings, neither establishes nor eliminates poisoning as a factor in a given death. Negative findings may be due to the fact that the individual took a poison orally and survived more than six hours until death. During this time interval the poison will have passed out of the stomach and would not be present in identifiable amounts. Another possible cause of negative findings in analysis of gastric contents, even though poisoning may have been responsible for the death, would be the fact that the poison had been introduced into the body by some means other than an oral route. Poisons that have been inhaled, injected, absorbed through the skin or introduced into the vagina or rectum are not demonstrable in gastric contents.

Positive findings resulting from the analysis of gastric contents, on the other hand, do not necessarily demonstrate that poisoning has occurred.

Analysis of gastric contents in one case showed the presence of phenol. No phenol could be demonstrated, however, in any of the other tissues or body fluids. Since it is known that phenol is extremely rapidly absorbed upon oral ingestion, the absence of the compound in the organs and body fluids suggested that the phenol had to have been introduced into the stomach postmortem. As subsequent investigation showed, the victim had been smothered with a pillow and the phenol had been introduced into the stomach by means of a stomach tube in order to make the death appear suicidal.

## ANALYSIS OF BODY FLUIDS AND TISSUES

Proof that poisoning has occurred rests only with demonstration of absorption of the toxic substance. The most direct evidence of such absorption is obtained by identifying the substance, through chemical analysis, in tissues or body fluids, followed by quantitative analysis in order to assess the effects upon the individual.

In some fatal poisonings none of the poison is found upon chemical analysis, since death may not occur until several days after absorption of the poison. During the period of survival the poison is either excreted or is completely metabolized to products that are no longer demonstrable. In many of these cases, pathological changes in the organs will have occurred that are demonstrable by gross and/or microscopic examination. For example, carbon tetrachloride poisoning frequently does not result in death until a week to ten days after exposure. At the end of such a time interval, there is no carbon tetrachloride detectable by chemical analysis. However, the poison causes a central necrosis of the liver and a lower nephron nephrosis, which can be observed grossly and microscopically. Although such findings are not specific for carbon tetrachloride poisoning, if the investigation discloses this pathologic picture and an exposure to carbon tetrachloride within a reasonable time prior to death, one could logically ascribe the death as being due to the action of this toxic agent.

An exception to the general rule requiring demonstration of absorption of a toxic agent occurs in those cases involving ingestion of a corrosive acid or alkali, such as concentrated sulfuric acid or lye. Such corrosives can be identified only in gastrointestinal contents because they are converted to substances normally present in the body after absorption, and the latter does not significantly alter the concentrations of these ions normally found.

## COLLECTION AND PRESERVATION OF EVIDENCE

A pathologist who performs a medicolegal autopsy has the primary responsibility for the collection and preservation of proper samples for toxicologic examination. All too frequently, inadequate samples are obtained (Fig. XXI-1). It is generally impossible to obtain additional samples if the initial sample collection has been inadequate. It is suggested that the following samples be retained for analytical purposes: as large a sample of heart blood as possible, all urine present in the bladder, gastric contents, duodenal contents, all bile present in

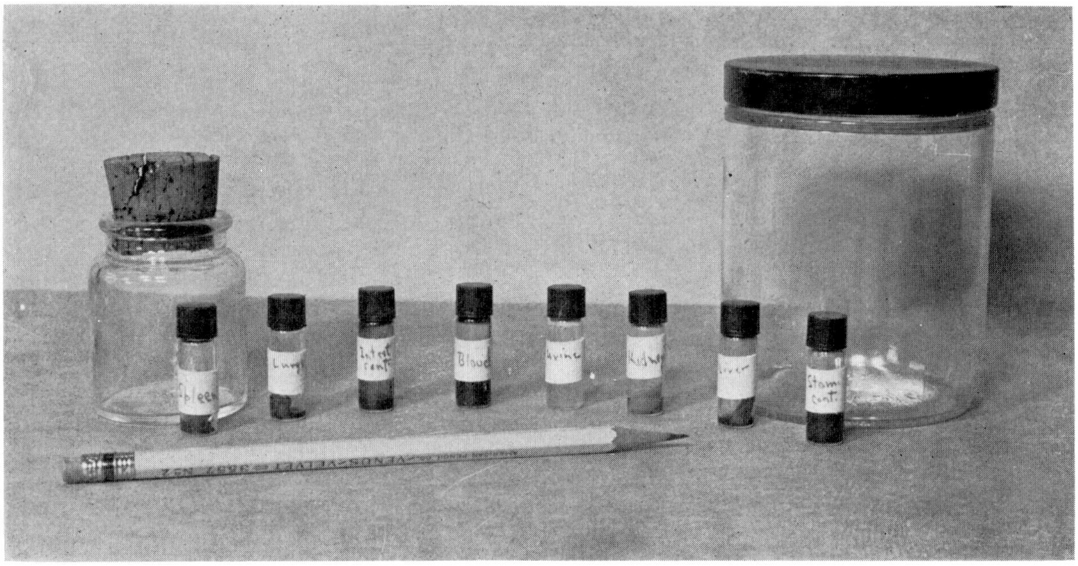

FIGURE XXI-1. Inadequate samples submitted for toxicologic analysis. The large containers shown in the photograph are the type to be used for transmittal of samples.

the gall bladder (many drugs are concentrated here), one kidney, one half of the liver, one half of the brain, a sample of body fat, one lung, samples of bone and hair (in suspected chronic poisoning due to metallic compounds).

Each of the samples itemized should be placed in a separate container, which is sealed as promptly as possible in order to avoid loss of volatile substances as well as to prevent possible contamination by extraneous materials that might be in the area of the autopsy room. Glass jars that have been chemically cleaned serve quite well in most instances. In addition, plastic bags make excellent containers and are preferred if the samples are to be frozen, since such containers do not break during freezing or thawing. Each container should be labelled immediately, and the identification should bear the date and time of the autopsy, the name of the decedent, the identity of the tissue sample and the signature of the pathologist. Preservation is accomplished by refrigeration or freezing, and no chemical preservatives should be added to any of the samples. In the absence of a mechanical freezer, freezing can be accomplished by packing the containers in dry ice. Samples that have been frozen and packed in this way can be transported to a laboratory even though a considerable distance or time delay might be involved. An adequate chain of custody of the specimens submitted for analysis must be maintained.

The sealed containers, when they are delivered to the laboratory, should be received by the toxicologist, who then makes a record of the identities and nature of the specimens submitted, together with the date and time of their receipt and the name of the person delivering them. In the laboratory, the specimens are to be stored in a locked refrigerator or freezer. In most laboratories the specimens in a case are given an accession number when they are received, and thereafter they are handled under this number. When the analysis is being conducted, it is important for the analyst to make a record of the weights or volumes of any samples used in the various steps in the procedure. It is also important that the date of the analysis be recorded and that one-third of the original sample be preserved for possible use by another toxicologist. Especially in criminal cases, the defense might challenge the original findings and wish to have the samples analyzed by an expert of their own choice.

## CHOICE OF METHOD BY THE TOXICOLOGIST

In the majority of cases that involve poisoning as a cause of death, a specific substance is suspected as the causative agent and a direct analysis for such a substance can be made. Factors that may indicate a specific agent are the information obtained during the investigation at the scene of the death and the clinical history resulting from the general investigation of factors surrounding the death. Leads that often shorten the time involved in completing an analysis may be obtained from empty or partially filled containers of medications found at the scene. The failure to find such containers from which the poison may have been taken suggests the need for a more thorough police investigation. This may develop information leading to proof of homicide rather than suicide.

A case of homicidal poisoning with potassium cyanide developed on the basis of such an investigation, and the case might have gone undiscovered had this routine check for a container not been made. It involved the death of a woman in her seventh month of pregnancy, and it was believed that her death had resulted from suicidal ingestion of potassium cyanide. This was supported, in part, by the finding at the scene of an unmailed letter in the handwriting of the deceased. Although this letter did not contain direct statements that the woman was going to take her own life, the general tenor of the writing suggested that the woman was in a state of agitated depression. The police were requested to search the scene for empty or partially filled containers from which the potassium cyanide may have been taken. Such a container could be expected to be present, since most persons who commit suicide with a poison, particularly with a cyanide, have neither the time nor the interest to dispose of the container. The result of this search of the scene was the finding only of some empty gelatin capsules and similar gelatin capsules that had been filled with quinine sulfate. No potassium cyanide was found in the home.

The police then began a more thorough investigation, which ultimately disclosed that the woman and her husband had been having serious marital difficulties, even to the point of physical violence perpetrated by the latter. A routine background check among employees of the Municipal Department of Public Works, where the husband was employed, disclosed that he had been making inquiries of a chemist in the department concerning *good poisons.* He had been told that potassium cyanide was such a substance. The police obtained the bottle of potassium cyanide reagent from the laboratory shelf and were able to develop a thumb and forefinger impression of the husband. Since the man was not employed in the laboratory, this suggested the probability of his having stolen some potassium cyanide from the bottle.

When confronted with this information, the man admitted the theft, although he claimed that he had done this because it was his intent to commit suicide to get away from his unhappy domestic situation. He claimed that he had filled two capsules with potassium cyanide and had placed these in a dresser drawer, where there were also present the similar capsules containing quinine sulfate that his wife was in the habit of taking for colds and muscle aches. His wife must have mistakenly taken the potassium cyanide capsules and thereby met her death. The man was ultimately convicted of manslaughter.

Poisoning as a possible cause of death is usually indicated by the history of the case or by gross or microscopic pathologic findings or the lack thereof. Just as the pathologist should not approach an autopsy without some preliminary background investigation, so, too, should the toxicologist not begin an analysis without having available as complete a history as possible. Toxicological analyses, at best, are quite time-consuming, and any information or aid that might shorten the procedure is most desirable. The history should generally include the following information:

1. A clinical history, obtainable either from an attending physician or from members of the family or friends of the decedent.
2. The occupation of the decedent, with a detailed description of the duties performed in this occupation.
3. Any treatment administered either as an antidote for a suspected poison or for some illness prior to death.
4. The nature of the food or drink last taken.
5. A description of the gross autopsy findings.
6. Time relationships involved between the onset of symptoms, if any, and death.

Such a history will frequently suggest or rule out specific toxic agents. As an illustration, it would be futile to do any analyses for volatile toxic substances or for most organic drugs in a case in which an individual had been hospitalized for several weeks prior to death. During such an interval substances of this type would have been completely metabolized and eliminated by the body. The only toxic substances that might be detectable in such cases would be metallic poisons.

In some cases there may be no anatomic cause of death discoverable as the result of an autopsy and no information concerning the background of the deceased and the factors surrounding the death. Such cases become what the toxicologist describes as *a general unknown.* The individual toxicologist's approach to such a problem will vary and will be modified by the geographic area in which the death has occurred. The availability and prevalence of use of certain substances in a particular location would make it necessary to include such substances in the general search procedure, while these same substances might not even be considered as possibilities in other areas. For example, in a highly agricultural environment organic phosphate insecticides are of major importance, whereas these same compounds are not considered a problem in most urban areas. Similarly, narcotic drugs present a major problem only in the cities.

The most informative autopsy is one that is performed on an unembalmed body, and this is especially true when dealing with cases involving possible poisoning. The embalming process will interfere with both the qualitative identification of poisons and their quantitation. The latter will materially affect the interpretation of any positive findings. As typical examples, cyanides react chemically with the formalin in the embalming fluid so that they are no longer identifiable. Also, most embalming fluids contain ethyl or methyl alcohol, or both, rendering analyses for these substances meaningless. Fixation of the tissues by formalin makes extraction procedures with organic solvents less efficient. Since such extraction is involved in the separation of many organic drugs, no or low recoveries of such substances will result. However, in cases involving investigation of death after disinterment, it is impossible to avoid the embalming process. In such cases, it is imperative that a sample of any embalming fluids used in preparing the body for burial be used as controls should any positive chemical findings be obtained.

Another complicating problem in toxicological analysis is that which is encountered when dealing with putrefied bodies. During the putrefactive process many substances that might be present in the tissues undergo chemical changes, so that the parent substance is no longer identifiable by chemical tests. Further, the putrefactive process may result in the production of substances from normal tissue components that give chemical reactions quite similar to those obtained from toxic compounds. The majority of volatile toxic substances would be lost as the result of putrefaction, while some, such as ethyl alcohol and cyanide, may be produced from normal tissue components. Although the amount of cyanide so produced is only in trace quantities, alcohol produced by advanced putrefaction may be as high as 0.20%. Such factors may obviously lead to serious difficulties in interpretation of analytical results.

Despite the limitations placed upon the analyst by the embalming process or by putrefaction, many toxic substances are still detectable. These include carbon monoxide, fluoride, relatively stable organic compounds such as strychnine and some barbiturates, yellow phosphorus and heavy metals such as arsenic, lead, mercury and thallium.

The use of vitreous humor as a sample for analysis for alcohol in cases that involve embalming or putrefaction prior to autopsy is mentioned in Chapter XXII. It has also been demonstrated[1] that vitreous humor, in such cases, may be used for analysis for a number of substances of toxicological importance, such as barbiturates, meprobamate, propoxyphene, pentazocine, amphetamines, digoxin and others.

From the analytical standpoint, poisons are grouped according to the method used to isolate these substances from the tissues or body fluids. This is in contrast to the usual type of chemical analytic schemes, which are, in general, based upon similarities in the chemical structures and properties or the substances encountered. In analytical toxicology there are five major groups, which are described in the following pages.

### Group I—Noxious Gases

Gases may be separated from body fluids or tissues by simple aeration procedures followed by specific tests for individual compounds. The samples used for these purposes are blood and lungs. However, the majority of gases having toxicologic significance are not readily detected in tissue samples, and analytic procedures are usually restricted to air samples collected at the scene of exposure.

### Group II—Steam Volatile Substances

Group II includes organic and inorganic chemical compounds that may be isolated from the biological material by the simple process of steam distillation. Such distillation may be from either an acidic or basic medium. Included in the group of substances distillable from an acidic medium are alcohol, cyanides, yellow phosphorus, chlorinated hydrocarbons, benzol, phenols and similar substances. The group of basic steam volatile substances includes nicotine, aniline, amphetamines, Demerol® and others.

### Group III—Metallic Poisons

Metallic poisons may be separated from tissue by oxidizing or burning off the organic matter comprising the tissue, leaving the metallic substances in the tissue ash. The tissue destruction, or ashing, may be accomplished either by a dry process at 450° C or by a wet ashing method involving the use of an oxidizing mixture of nitric, sulphuric and perchloric acids. In either event the tissue ash is then used for qualitative detection and subsequent quantitation of metals.

### Group IV—Nonvolatile Organic Poisons

The compounds included in Group IV consist of the majority of drug products that may be encountered either as the result of therapeutic use or as the result of overdosage. The isolation and identification procedures for these substances are the most difficult of all those encountered in analytic toxicology. The problem involves the separation of a comparatively small amount of an organic compound, in a state of purity that makes identification possible, from the relatively huge amount of other organic compounds that make up the tissue matrix. The method used to separate these compounds is based upon selective extraction with organic solvents under varying conditions of acidity. Employing such techniques, it is possible to classify the substances further into three subgroups:

1. Organic acids and organic neutral compounds, including such substances as barbiturates, salicylates, caffeine, hydantoins, glutethimide, acetanilid, phenacetin and others.
2. Organic bases, which would include such substances as cocaine, quinine, strychnine, amphetamines, phenothiazines, nicotine, Demerol®, codeine and many others.
3. Amphoteric organic compounds: The principal compounds of concern are morphine, dionine and Dilaudid®.

### Group V

Group V includes all other substances that are not classifiable in any of the other groups. The substances included here are, in general, inorganic anions as well as organic compounds insoluble in water or alcohol. In general, some specific procedures must be employed for the identification and quantitation of each of these substances.

It is beyond the scope of this book to present details of the analytical procedures used in toxicology. However, a typical separation scheme is indicated in Table XXI-I. After the various groups of poisons have been separated, their identification and quantitation is achieved by a variety of techniques, which include color reactions, crystal tests, ultraviolet and infrared spectrophotometry, thin-layer chromatography, gas chromatography, mass spectrometry, fluores-

## TABLE XXI-I
## SCHEMA FOR ISOLATION OF POISONS*

**TISSUE SAMPLE (Minced)**

- **100g.** — Acidify and steam-distill
  - Distillate: Test for acidic volatile substances, e.g. alcohols, cyanide, phosphorus, phenols, etc.
  - Residue: Make alkaline with NaOH or MgO and redistill.
    - Distillate: Test for alkaline volatile substances, e.g. nicotine, aniline, amphetamine, etc.
    - Residue: Evaporate to dryness and wet ash. Use for *METALS*
- 50 g. for Reinsch test for As, Hg, Sb, Bi.
- 500 g. for non-volatile organic poisons. Heat at 60° C with 500 ml. 1.0 N HCl. After 30 min. filter.
  - Residue: Repeat HC1 treatment. Filter and combine filtrate with filtrate 1.
  - Filtrate 1: Extract in continuous liquid-liquid extractor for two hours with $CHCl_3$
    - Organic phase: Evaporate. Take up residue with 50 ml. $CHC1_3$. Shake with 10 ml. phosphate buffer pH 7.4.
      - Aqueous phase: Make acid with HCl and re-extract with 3×30 ml $CHCL_3$. Dry $CHCl_3$ with anhydrous sodium sulfate
        - Organic phase: Evaporate to dryness. *STRONG ACID FRACTION*
        - Aqueous phase: Discard
      - Organic phase: Filter and shake with 10 ml. 0.45N NaOh
        - Aqueous phase: Acidify with HCL and re-extract with 3 × 30 ml $CHCl_3$. Dry latter with $Na_2SO_4$ and evaporate to dryness. *WEAK ACID FRACTION*
        - Organic phase: Wash with $H_2O$, dry with $Na_2SO_4$ evaporate to dryness *"NEUTRALS"*
    - Aqueous phase: Make alkaline with NaOH to pH 10. Re-extract in continuous liquid-liquid extractor with $CHC1_3$ for two hours.
      - Organic phase: Evaporate solvent *ALKALOIDS AND ORGANIC BASE FRACTION*
      - Aqueous phase: Make acid with HCl and then neutralize by addition of solid $NaHCO_3$. Re-extract in continuous liquid-liquid extractor with chloroform-ethanol mixture (9:1) for two hours.
        - Organic phase: Evaporate solvent *MORPHINE FRACTION*
        - Aqueous phase: Discard
- **1/3** — Reserve for future use.

* Reproduced by permission of Warren H. Green, Inc., St. Louis, from *Laboratory Diagnosis of Diseases Caused by Toxic Agents*, p. 88.

cence spectrometry and immunoassay. A considerable amount of literature is available giving details of such procedures.[2-7]

The procedure outlined in Table XXI-I is designed for a large sample of tissue and is quite time-consuming. The high sensitivity of many of the newer instrumental analytical techniques makes it possible to achieve the same results using much smaller samples, such as 3 to 10 ml of blood, 20 to 25 gm of liver, 20 to 25 ml of urine or 2 to 10 ml of bile in the analysis for nonvolatile organic substances. Volatile compounds may be looked for in 0.5 to 1.0 ml of blood using a head space sample injected into a gas chromatograph similar to the technique used for the analysis for alcohol mentioned in Chapter XXII. Similarly, atomic absorption spectrophotometric techniques makes it possible to use 10 to 25 gm samples for the analysis for metallic substances.

In medicolegal work exact identification of any toxic substance is absolutely essential. Hence, the analyst should not rely upon a single qualitative criterion when making such an identification. The quantum of proof required for an identification will, of course, vary with the experience and knowledge of the analyst, but in no case should fewer than two qualitative characteristics be used to make a positive statement concerning the identity of a substance involved in a death.

## TOXICOLOGY IN NARCOTIC CASES

A major problem in most areas today is concerned with deaths due to narcotism. Many of these deaths occur minutes after administration of an intravenous dose of the narcotic, and in some instances the victim is even found with the needle, with syringe attached, still in the vein. In many of these cases, for some as yet unexplained reason, it is not possible to identify any of the narcotic in the tissues analyzed. Such negative results obviously do not rule out narcotism as the cause of death.

The most commonly used narcotic among the addict population is heroin, which is diacetyl morphine. The drug itself is not usually demonstrable in the tissues, but metabolic processes in the body degrade the compound to morphine, and the latter substance is found upon analyses of liver, bile and urine. If at autopsy a fresh needle puncture mark can be observed, the injection site should be excised and submitted for analysis. It is frequently possible to demonstrate the presence of heroin in such an injection site. This, coupled with the finding of morphine in the tissue, would be sufficient to say that the latter was derived from usage of heroin.

Codeine is methyl morphine, and it, too, is converted metabolically to morphine. However, only a small part of absorbed codeine is converted in this manner. Hence, the finding of a high concentration of codeine with small amounts of morphine suggests that the origin of the latter was probably codeine. Conversely, the finding of a high concentration of morphine and only small amounts of codeine indicates that the former was due to the use of either morphine or heroin along with the codeine.

A frequent finding in narcotic deaths is quinine, which is commonly used as an adulterant in street samples of heroin. Its presence in bile and/or urine of persons having relatively fresh and old needle marks suggests the possibility of heroin addiction, even though no narcotic may be demonstrable in the same fluids.

It was mentioned earlier that bile and urine should be retained for chemical analysis. This is suggested since narcotic drugs, as well as many other organic drugs, are excreted in the bile and urine as conjugates and are present in these fluids in much higher concentrations than they are in other parts of the body. Hence, they are more readily detectable in these fluids.

## REPORT AND INTERPRETATION OF RESULTS

The toxicologist will, in general, submit a final report of his analyses, which will state only those substances that have been found and their concentrations. However, it is important for him to maintain a detailed record of all this work, including the techniques that were employed and the substances for which negative results were obtained.

Although it is the responsibility of the pathologist, rather than the toxicologist, to determine the cause of death, ideally there should be close liaison between these two individuals. Mutual discussion of findings, both anatomic and analytic, will frequently resolve problems of interpretation of results.

A gangland figure died in a hospital some time after being shot. The cause of death was obviously the gunshot wound, but material collection at autopsy was submitted for toxicologic examination. In the course of the analysis, the toxicologist found mercury in the tissues and thereupon stated to the press that the man had died of mercury poisoning, despite the fact that the pathologist had found none of the pathologic indications of mercury poisoning. Had the toxicologist bothered to check, he would have found that the source of his mercury was an organic mercurial compound (Merthiolate®) used as a preservative in the blood plasma that had been given as transfusions during this man's hospitalization.

Proper interpretation of any analytical results requires that the analyst be familiar with the percentage of error inherent in any procedure and also with the range of concentration of the toxic substance that can be expected in the particular tissue analyzed. This includes knowledge of various concentrations that might be found under extremes of therapeutic administration and variations in concentration that might be dependent on time between exposure to the toxic substance and death, age, weight, prior state of health, sex, etc.

Should a given case require court testimony of either civil or criminal nature, the toxicologist should thoroughly familiarize himself with all aspects of the case before his court appearance. Also, as is true in any situation involving expert testimony, the expert should confer with the trial counsel before going into court. At such a conference, which may be quite lengthy in some cases, both counsel and expert will become familiar with the questions and answers concerned in the points at issue. Counsel will learn how best to phrase his questions to elicit the information he wishes to establish, and the expert will learn how to answer the question in language that is understandable to a lay jury and not obscured by technical terminology.

## REFERENCES

1. Coe, J. I.: Postmortem chemistry: Practical considerations and a review of the literature. *J Forensic Sci, 42*:529, 1951.
2. Gonzalez, T. A., Vance, B., Helpern, M., and Umberger, C. J.: *Legal Medicine, Pathology and Toxicology*, 2nd ed. New York, Appleton, 1954.
3. Curry, A. S.: *Poison Detection in Human Organs*, 3rd ed. Springfield, Thomas, 1976.
4. Stewart, C. P., and Stolman, A.: *Toxicology, Mechanisms and Analytical Methods*, vols. I and II. New York, Acad Pr, 1960, 1961.
5. Clarke, E. G. C.: *Isolation and Identification of Drugs*, vols. I and II. London, Pharmaceutical Pr, 1969, 1975.
6. Stolman, A.: *Progress in Chemical Toxicology*, vols. I, II, III, and IV. New York, Acad Pr, 1963, 1965, 1967, 1969.
7. Sunshine, I.: *Handbook of Analytical Toxicology*. Cleveland, Chemical Rubber Co., 1969.

*Chapter XXII*

# FORENSIC ASPECTS OF ALCOHOL

HENRY C. FREIMUTH

THE MOST COMMON single substance encountered in toxicologic analyses is alcohol. From the standpoint of the chemist, the word alcohol refers to a large group of chemical compounds characterized by the possession of a functional –OH group. In common usage, however, the word alcohol has been accepted as indicating a specific compound, i.e. ethanol, having the molecular formula $C_2H_5OH$. For the purposes of this chapter, the word alcohol will be used to designate the compound ethanol, present in various fermented and distilled beverages.

From the medicolegal standpoint, there is perhaps no other chemical compound more frequently encountered as a contributing or causative factor in violent or natural deaths. Alcohol is also involved in many nonfatal incidents that ultimately come under the scrutiny of law enforcement agents. Because of this ubiquity, it is well to consider the various facts involved in the consumption, absorption, distribution and elimination of alcohol by the body.

Alcohol almost invariably enters the body by ingestion of an alcoholic beverage. The alcohol in such beverages is the result of fermentation of sugar by yeast. Fermentation of barley with added hops results in the production of beers and ales, while fermentation of fruits results in the formation of wines. Fermentation of grains and fruits followed by distillation results in the production of whiskey, gin, brandy and vodka. The sole purpose of the distillation process is to increase the concentration of alcohol in the finished product. This is necessary because fermentation ceases when the alcohol concentration is approximately 12% to 14% by volume. Alcoholic beverages are primarily a mixture of water and alcohol with small amounts of other substances, which impart the characteristic odors and tastes to the various beverages. These substances are referred to as congeners, since they are simultaneously produced during the fermentation process. The congeners consist of organic acids and esters and, in the case of wine and brandy, methyl alcohol. The latter is responsible for the common finding of trace amounts of wood alcohol in body fluids and tissues of persons who have consumed large quantities of wine or brandy, particularly cheaper brands, prior to death. The so-called *odor of alcohol* frequently detected at autopsy is not due to alcohol but to the aforementioned congeners. This odor may persist in the tissues for several hours after all alcohol has been metabolized. Hence, the conclusion that alcohol is present based upon odor may be erroneous. Such a conclusion is valid only if founded upon a chemical analysis.

The concentration of alcohol in fermented beverages is expressed as percent by volume, while the term *proof* is used to express concentration of alcohol in distilled beverages. In the United States the term proof refers to twice the percentage of alcohol by volume. Thus, the common 86 proof whiskey sold in this country contains 43% alcohol by volume.

Alcohol requires no preliminary digestion and, unlike foods and most drugs, is readily absorbed from the stomach. It is possible that almost half of the total absorption occurs by this route. The remainder of the absorption occurs by way of the small intestine. The rate and relative percentage of absorption from the stomach and the intestine are affected by several factors, such as the amount and kind of food present; the amount, kind and dilution of the alcoholic beverage consumed; possible presence of pylorospasm; and variation in the permeability of the gastric and intestinal mucosa, which may differ from person to person. It is because of these variables that complete absorption of alcohol from the gastrointestinal tract may require a time interval varying from forty-five minutes to three hours. The longer the total time required for complete absorption to occur, the lower will be the peak blood alcohol concentration. Maximum blood alcohol concentrations are usually reached within forty-five to ninety minutes after ingestion of alcohol, with the majority of individuals reaching their maximum one hour after ingestion.

Alcohol is poorly absorbed through intact skin. Also, inhalation of air containing high concentrations of alcohol in the vapor state does not produce significant blood alcohol levels, even after prolonged exposure.

Absorbed alcohol is carried from the gastrointestinal tract via the portal vein to the liver. It is for this reason that, during the period of active absorption, the alcohol concentration in the blood of the portal vein exceeds that in the blood elsewhere in the body. Later the portal vein blood alcohol level decreases because of loss of alcohol to the liver, metabolism of alcohol by the liver and mixing with blood from the hepatic artery. Ultimately, the blood containing alcohol reaches the right atrium, whence it begins its circulation through the body. As the arterial blood passes through the lungs, some alcohol is lost by diffusion into the alveolar air. The concentration of alcohol in the arterial blood further diminishes as the result of passage through the capillary network. Alcohol is lost from the blood to the tissues in proportion to the water content of the tissues with which it comes in contact. Eventually a condition of storage equilibrium is reached between the blood and the tissues. However, during a period of very rapid absorption, there may be a considerable difference between the concentration of alcohol in the arterial blood and that in the venous blood. This accounts for the difference sometimes observed in the determination of blood alcohol concentration by analysis of alveolar breath compared with direct analysis of a sample of venous blood. The former result is sometimes higher than the latter, but it more truly represents the concentration of alcohol in the blood reaching the brain and therefore more accurately reveals the effects of the alcohol upon the individual. The difference in the concentration of alcohol in the arterial and venous systems is at its maximum during a period of active absorption and disappears when a state of equilibrium between blood and tissues occurs.

During the period of active absorption the blood alcohol concentration rises quite rapidly and then continues to increase at a slower rate until the maximal concentration is reached. After this maximal blood alcohol concentration has been attained, the alcohol level in the blood decreases at a linear rate during the postabsorptive period until a zero level is again reached.

When equilibrium has been reached, the distribution of alcohol in the various tissues and body fluids would be of the order shown in Table XXII-I.

The major part of the alcohol that has been absorbed is eliminated from the body as the result of oxidation effected only in the liver, which contains the enzyme alcohol dehydrogenase. More than 90 percent of the absorbed alcohol is eliminated by this oxidative route.

In addition to oxidation, alcohol may be eliminated unchanged by way of the kidneys, lungs, sweat glands and colon. Of these, excretion by way of the feces is relatively insignificant. Normally, excretion by way of sweat occurs at about one-half the rate of elimination by way of urine, and this is related to the fact that the volume of sweat is approximately one-half the urinary volume. However, in excessively hot climates, or with unusual exertion accompanied by excessive perspiration, the loss of body water by way of the skin may increase five- to tenfold. This would result in a corresponding five- to tenfold increase in the loss of alcohol by way of the skin.

TABLE XXII-I

RELATIVE CONCENTRATION OF ALCOHOL AT EQUILIBRIUM

| *Sample* | *Relative Concentration* |
|---|---|
| Whole blood | 1.00 |
| Plasma or serum | 1.12-1.20 |
| Brain | 0.85 |
| Spinal fluid | 1.10-1.27 |
| Urine (ureteral) | 1.3 |
| Alveolar air | 1/2100 |
| Liver | 0.85 |

The ureteral urine alcohol concentration is 1.3 times that of the blood. This ratio is restricted to urine as it is being formed and does not apply to the concentration of alcohol in bladder urine.

The loss of alcohol by way of the breath occurs at a rate approximately equal to that of the urinary loss. The concentration of alcohol in alveolar breath is less than that in the blood. In accordance with Henry's law, alcohol distributes between pulmonary blood and alveolar air in a ratio of 2100 to 1. In other words, 2100 cc of alveolar air contain the same weight of alcohol as 1 cc of blood.

The question is frequently raised as to the existence of a normal alcohol content of human tissue and blood. The general consensus, as the result of analyses employing specific techniques, is that the normal concentration of alcohol does not exceed 0.001%.

Primary factors involved in the interpretation of postmortem results are the method of collection of samples, the choice of sample for analysis and the preservation of the sample.

In most jurisdictions blood is the sample chosen for analysis. However, it is necessary to observe certain precautions when blood samples are collected. If an autopsy has not been performed, it is common practice to obtain a sample by puncture of the chest wall, with the needle ideally entering the heart. This can lead to considerable error, since it is possible to nick the esophagus while performing this procedure, thus contaminating the sample with esophageal contents. Another possible source of contamination is internal injury giving rise to rupture of the stomach and diaphragm, resulting in bathing of the thoracic cavity with gastric contents. If the latter contains any alcohol, an erroneously high blood alcohol level will result. For example, the writer recently analyzed a blood sample, collected in the above-described way, that contained in excess of 1% ethyl alcohol! When an autopsy is not performed, it is better to obtain a sample of cerebrospinal fluid taken from the cisterna magna. Even if such fluid is contaminated with blood, the determined ethyl alcohol concentration is less subject to doubt than the result of an analysis of a sample collected through the intact chest wall.

When blood is obtained from the heart, it should be collected using a clean, dry syringe and needle. It is advisable to massage the heart gently before taking the sample in order to promote mixing of the blood contained in the chambers. This is to avoid the possibility of obtaining a sample with either a high or low hematocrit, which could lead to falsely achieved high or low alcohol results. Such results would be caused by the fact that serum or plasma alcohol concentration is 12% to 20% higher than that of whole blood.

Blood samples that are not to be analyzed immediately should be preserved by the addition of approximately 5 mg of sodium fluoride per ml, followed by thorough shaking. This will prevent loss of alcohol and production of alcohol as the result of bacterial action. Samples that have been preserved in this manner will maintain their alcohol concentration for several weeks even at room temperature. Refrigeration or freezing coupled with such fluoride treatment will maintain the alcohol concentration of a sample for an almost indefinite period of time.

Since the analysis of blood is carried out in order to obtain information concerning the concentration of alcohol in the brain, it is obvious that a direct analysis of brain tissue may also be performed. As a matter of fact, analysis of such tissue is preferable, since there is less chance for contamination of the brain in the course of performing an autopsy. It is not necessary to preserve the entire brain for this purpose, since the writer has shown that samples of tissue taken from different parts of the brain do not vary significantly in their alcohol concentration.[1]

If an individual has been embalmed prior to autopsy, it is useless to determine the alcohol concentration in blood or tissue, since most embalming fluids contain ethyl alcohol in addition to the other components in such mixtures.

When putrefaction has occurred, one must exercise extreme caution in interpreting blood or tissue alcohol levels obtained by analysis of such putrid samples. This is due to the fact that alcohol may be lost or produced by bacterial action during the putrefactive process. The latter is by far the more serious problem, since it may lead to the conclusion that alcohol consumption was a contributing factor in causing the death. It is, nevertheless, worthwhile to do an alcohol analysis on such putrid samples, despite the fact that it will not give a true picture of the state of intoxication of the deceased at the time of death. Alcohol concentrations in excess of 0.20% would indicate alcohol consumption prior to death, while levels below 0.20% may be ascribed to possible putrefactive alcohol production.

More accurate information concerning the antemortem alcoholic status of a deceased person may be obtained, even in cases involving prior embalming or putrefaction, by using vitreous humor as the sample for analysis. Felby and Olsen[2] have shown that the alcohol concentration in vitreous humor, unlike that of blood, remains quite constant, even over a postmortem interval up to 99 hours, while Scott et al.[3] showed that vitreous humor alcohol remains essentially unchanged after embalming. Coe and Sherman,[4] in a study involving 174 cases, the largest series reported in the literature, state that the ratio of blood alcohol concentration to that of vitreous humor is $0.89 \pm 0.02$.

There may be some cases of death due to trauma resulting in the production of a subdural hematoma. Such individuals frequently survive many hours after sustaining the fatal injury. Analysis of a blood sample obtained postmortem would not give any indication of the state of intoxication, if any, at the time of injury. However, the subdural blood clot will contain alcohol in a concentration essentially the same as that in the blood at the time of the fatal injury. Such clots should therefore be retained for analysis for alcohol.

In some cases, severe internal injury may cause gastric contents, possibly containing some alcohol, to collect in the thoracic cavity. This may give rise to the possibility of diffusion of alcohol into the heart blood, resulting in an erroneously high blood alcohol concentration when the fluid is analyzed. It may also be impossible, due to head injuries, to obtain adequate samples of brain or spinal fluid for analysis instead of heart blood. In such cases the blood sample for analysis should be obtained from the femoral vein.

A common erroneous technique employed in the collection of blood samples involves scooping up a sample of blood from that which has pooled in the chest cavity after severance of the blood vessels leading to and from the heart. This practice can only give rise to contamination of the blood sample and a corresponding erroneous blood alcohol concentration.

There are three major methods by means of which the alcohol concentration in body fluids and tissues may be determined:[5, 6]

1. Distillation (or microdiffusion) of the alcohol and subsequent reaction with potassium dichromate and sulfuric acid. The potassium dichromate solution is so prepared that a given volume represents a known weight of ethyl alcohol in the sample analyzed. By determination of the amount of potassium dichromate remaining unreacted in the mixture and knowing the amount of potassium dichromate initially used, one can, by difference, calculate the amount of potassium dichromate that has reacted with the alcohol in the sample. By simple arithmetic calculation one can thus compute the percentage of alcohol in the sample analyzed. This method is relatively nonspecific, and before one can state that the sample contained ethyl alcohol, one must eliminate by qualitative chemical tests the presence of formaldehyde, acetaldehyde, wood alcohol and isopropyl alcohol, which are commonly encountered interfering substances that will react with the potassium dichromate.

   When putrefied samples are analyzed by this method, it is necessary to redistill the original distillate from an alkaline mercuric cyanide solution (Scott-Wilson's reagent) in order to eliminate or minimize any error resulting from the production of volatile reducing substances, other than alcohol, during the putrefactive process.

2. A more specific procedure involves the enzymatic determination of alcohol using the enzyme alcohol dehydrogenase. The disadvantage of this method is that it becomes somewhat costly when large numbers of alcohol determinations are being performed.
3. In more recent years the gas chromatographic method of analyzing samples for ethyl alcohol has become quite commonly used, since it is reasonably specific and will permit the simultaneous detection and quantitation of the commonly encountered interfering alcohols—methyl and isopropyl alcohol. The technique involves analysis of the head space (vapor phase) of an equilibrated blood sample and is adaptable to automation. This is most useful in situations where large numbers of samples must be analyzed routinely. Such an automated procedure has been described by Machata.[7]

The relationship of various blood alcohol concentrations to clinical signs and symptoms is shown in Table XXII-II.

In most medicolegal situations involving death, the important point at issue is the condition of the individual at the time of an injury. If the death results essentially instantaneously subsequent to trauma, then a postmortem blood alcohol determination will give a true picture of the condition of the individual at such time. No significant change in blood alcohol concentration occurs after death until putrefaction begins. However, should some time elapse between the time of injury and the time of death, the postmortem blood alcohol concentration would not necessarily reflect the condition of the individual at the time of injury. It is generally agreed that blood alcohol concentration decreases by 0.015% per hour, although it has been the writer's experience that this rate of decrease may be considerably higher in many individuals. This is particularly true in heavy drinkers and chronic alcoholics without liver damage and may be at as high a rate as 0.04% per hour. If one can establish that a given individual was in the postabsorptive state at the time of sustaining a fatal injury, one can, based upon the above factors, estimate the probable range of alcohol concentration at the time of injury. Such estimation would be based upon the postmortem blood alcohol concentration and the time interval between injury and death. However, should there be any information indicating that alcohol consumption had occurred within one to one and one-half hours prior to the injury, there would remain the possibility of continued absorption of alcohol from the gastrointestinal tract subsequent to the injury, and one could not, therefore, be certain when the maximal blood alcohol concentration may have been reached in relationship to the time of injury. Hence, under these circumstances, any back calculation from a given postmortem blood alcohol

TABLE XXII-II

PHYSIOLOGICAL EFFECTS OF ALCOHOL

| *Blood Alcohol Concentration* | *Effects* |
|---|---|
| 0 -0.04% | Varies from no significant effect to mild euphoria. |
| 0.05-0.09% | Decreased inhibitions, increased self-confidence, decreased attention span, alteration of judgement. Many European countries have adopted this range of concentration to indicate impaired ability to operate a motor vehicle. |
| 0.10-0.14% | Some mental confusion, emotional instability, loss of critical judgement, memory impairment, sleepiness, slowed reaction time. In this range most motor vehicle laws in the U.S. place prima facie evidence of drunken or impaired driving. |
| 0.15-0.29% | Loss of muscular coordination, staggering gait, marked mental confusion, exaggeration of emotions, dizziness, decreased pain response, disorientation and thickened speech. |
| 0.30-0.39% | Stupor, marked incoordination, marked decrease in responses to stimuli, possibly coma. |
| 0.40% and above | Anesthesia, depression of responses, deep coma, death. |

concentration would be subject to considerable doubt.[4, 5]

Death due to acute alcoholic intoxication with blood alcohol concentrations below 0.40% occurs with some frequency in individuals with chronic debilitating diseases, particularly severe arteriosclerotic heart disease and pulmonary emphysema. Other chronic lung diseases and conditions associated with varying degrees of hypoxia may also contribute to death in the presence of relatively low levels of alcohol. Prolonged coma due to alcohol consumption sometimes leads to irreversible hypoxic brain damage, which in turn may cause death. The blood alcohol level in such cases is commonly low, as would be expected after survival of several hours.

In instances such as the aforementioned, one can frequently obtain additional information concerning the degree of intoxication of the decedent at some time prior to death by analyzing both blood and urine obtained at autopsy. Based upon the ratio of blood alcohol concentration to ureteral urine alcohol concentration of 1 to 1.3, a given bladder urine alcohol analysis would show that at some time the blood alcohol concentration would have to have been at least 77% as high as that of the urine. However, one must also bear in mind the fact that such alcohol as may have been present in the ureteral urine may have been diluted by preexisting alcohol-free urine in the bladder.

A fact that further complicates interpretation of alcohol findings is the simultaneous presence of another drug. Most depressants and sedative drugs will, at the very least, have an additive effect. Some drugs will, in addition, have a potentiating effect. Perhaps the most common group of drugs in the latter category would be barbiturates, which are mutually potentiating in the presence of alcohol. Among other drugs that are dangerous in combination with alcohol are narcotics, tranquilizing agents, antihistaminics and hypnotic drugs.

## REFERENCES


1. Freimuth, H. C., Volatile, M., and Fisher, R. S.: The results of studies on the determination of ethyl alcohol in tissues. *J Crim Law Crim Pol Pol Sci, 42*:529, 1951.
2. Felby, S., and Olson, J.: Comparative studies of postmortem ethyl alcohol in vitreous humor, blood, and muscle. *J Forensic Sci, 14*:93, 1969.
3. Scott, W., Root, I., and Sanborn, B.: The use of vitreous humor for determination of ethyl alcohol in previously embalmed bodies. *J Forensic Sci, 19*:913, 1974.
4. Coe, J. I., and Sherman, R. E.: Comparative study of postmortem vitreous humor and blood alcohol. *J Forensic Sci, 15*:185, 1970.
5. Stewart, C. P., and Stolman, A.: *Toxicology, Mechanisms and Analytical Methods,* vol. II. New York, Acad Pr, 1961.
6. Stolman, A.: *Progress in Chemical Toxicology,* vol. III. New York, Acad Pr, 1967.
7. Machata, G.: Determination of alcohol in blood by gas chromatographic head space analysis. *Clin Chem Newsletter, 4*:29, 1972.
8. Fox, B., and Fox, J.: *Alcohol and Traffic Safety.* USPHS Publication #1043. Washington, D.C., U.S. Govt. Print. Office, 1963.
9. Committee on Medicolegal Problems: *Alcohol and the Impaired Driver.* Chicago, American Medical Association, 1968.

*Chapter XXIII*

# METHODOLOGY AND INTERPRETATION OF TOXICOLOGICAL PROCEDURES

JOSEPH R. MONFORTE

## SAMPLES FOR TOXICOLOGICAL ANALYSIS

THE CONCEPT of obtaining adequate samples for toxicological analysis has been discussed elsewhere in this book (*see* Chapter XXI), but it may be useful to review the particular attributes of the various samples available to the toxicologist. In any analysis the procurement of a representative sample is the most critical step in the procedure. No matter how competent the analyst or sophisticated the instrumentation, if the sample is not carefully and adequately obtained, the analytical result will be meaningless.

Blood, either whole blood or plasma, is the sample that in most instances reflects the clinical condition of an individual. Reliable postmortem blood samples are obtainable from either the femoral vein or artery or directly from the heart. Heart blood samples should be procured after the chest cavity has been opened and the heart exposed, not prior to autopsy. A blood sample obtained through the chest wall may be contaminated with esophageal contents.

The entire stomach contents should be submitted for toxicological analysis. In an acute poisoning, large quantities of substances may be present in the stomach contents. The odor of the stomach contents is sometimes helpful; the odor of cyanide resembles bitter almonds, and the odor of Placidyl® is reminiscent of carrots. Certain solvents have characteristic odors, and insecticides of the organophosphate group, such as parathion, strongly suggest garlic. Another advantage of stomach contents is that, with only a few exceptions, the drug may be recovered in unmetabolized form. This simplifies interpretation of procedures, because complications arising from the presence of metabolites are minimized. In cases where a substance may be ingested in relatively small quantities—LSD, for example—the stomach contents may be the only sample where a detectable amount of drug remains.

Most drugs are metabolized in the liver and therefore are usually present in this organ in high quantities. Analysis of a large sample of liver tissue considerably increases the likelihood of detecting an exogenous substance. Liver/blood ratios have been employed to estimate survival times in fatal barbiturate poisoning; however, many drugs accumulate in the liver during therapy, and it is not always possible to relate the concentration of drug in the liver to an acute fatal episode.

Urine, if available, is an important specimen. Many drugs are excreted in the urine in high concentrations, even at very low or nondetectable blood concentrations. Amphetamine is a good example, for a concentration as high as 1 mg/dl can occur in the urine after ingestion of 10 mg of Dexedrine®. Urine is therefore a good sample for general screening purposes, but meaningful quantitative data cannot usually be derived from urine analysis. Many drugs, such as quinine, Librium®, Placidyl® and the phenothiazines, are excreted over a period of days, and it is therefore difficult to relate a quantitative urine analysis to a fatal drug exposure. The presence of a drug in urine means that exposure to the drug has occurred, and quantitative analysis of other biological samples is indicated. Kidney samples are useful for analysis if no urine is present. Under such circumstances at least one entire kidney should be submitted to the laboratory.

Lung samples are valuable if an inhalation or sniffing death is suspected. Acute inhalation deaths due to exposure to aerosol sprays or to cocaine or heroin *snorting* result in high concentrations of these materials in the lung, while their concentration in other organs or fluids may be undetectable.

Central nervous system depressant drugs, such as barbiturates and narcotics, are the most common substances detected in deaths due to drug overdose. Since barbiturates and narcotics act directly on the brain, this tissue is a good sample for the detection of these drugs. Data relating fatal concentrations of drugs in the brain are scant, but due to the fact that a blood-brain barrier exists for most drugs, it is expected that, in most instances, the brain concentration will be slightly lower than that of the blood.

The spleen contains a high concentration of red blood cells and is an excellent sample for the detection of compounds that bind to hemoglobin. Substances such as cyanide and carbon monoxide appear in high concentrations in the spleen.

In recent years the vitreous humor has assumed some toxicological significance when blood and spinal fluid are unobtainable or when putrefaction has rendered them unsuitable for analysis. This sample has been reported to be reliable for ethanol determinations, even if it is procured after embalming.

(An observation was recently made at the Wayne County Medical Examiner's Office in Detroit: Pentobarbital (Nembutal®) was identified in a small quantity of ashlike material found within the skull of an individual who had been buried in the southern California desert sand for three and one-half years, then for five months in a Michigan cemetery. The remains were entirely skeletonized. The material submitted for analysis is believed to represent the final breakdown products of the soft tissues within the skull—Ed.)

## SEPARATION METHODS

Separation methods remove drugs from a biological specimen such as blood, bile, urine, cerebrospinal fluid, vitreous humor or tissue, thereby permitting tests to be performed on the separated drugs so that its identity may be ascertained. Several comparable separation methods are known, and the choice of which procedure to use depends upon the number of samples to be analyzed and the speed with which a result is required.

Distillation methods are used for separating substances with low boiling points. Volatile alcohols may be separated in this fashion. The sample is heated in a flask, and volatile compounds are removed due to their conversion to the gaseous state. The gaseous compounds then pass through a condenser, which is a water-cooled tube, and in so doing return to the liquid state. The presence of alcohols in the distillate can be determined enzymatically, colorimetrically or by gas chromatography, but the distillate is generally suitable for any type of analysis. Since many substances that naturally occur in biological specimens are not present in the distillate, any test performed is considerably less subject to interference.

Microdiffusion resembles distillation in that it separates volatile substances from biological samples. A special apparatus (Conway Microdiffusion Cell) is usually employed, and typically this consists of a circular porcelain unit containing a center well separated from an outer well. A square piece of glass is used to cover the unit (Figure XXIII-1).

The sample containing the volatile to be analyzed is placed in the outer well, along with a reagent that releases the volatile from the biological sample. The inner well contains a reagent that will either dissolve the volatile substance or chemically react with it, producing a nonvolatile compound that remains soluble in the contents of the inner well. The process of the volatile travelling from the outer well into the inner well is called diffusion and takes place after the Conway Cell has been sealed with the cover glass. After diffusion is complete,

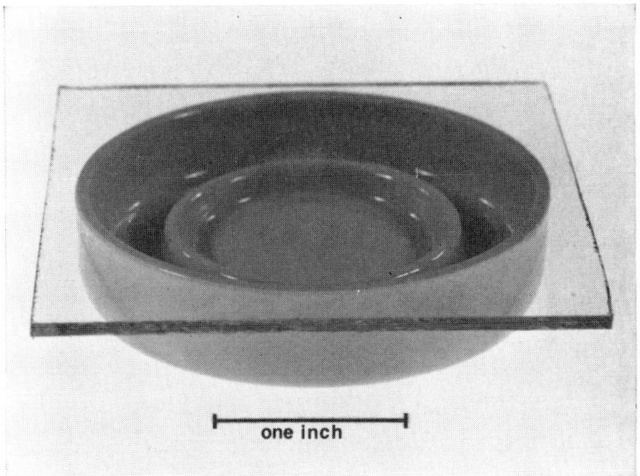


FIGURE XXIII-1. Conway microdiffusion cell.

the contents of the inner well are subsequently analyzed.

This technique is commonly employed for the detection of substances such as volatile alcohols and carbon monoxide. For such alcohol analysis, sodium carbonate is the releasing reagent added to the outer well and potassium dichromate is added to the inner well. After diffusion, any volatile alcohols in the sample chemically react with the potassium dichromate, causing it to change color. In the case of carbon monoxide, sulfuric acid is added to a blood sample in the outer well and palladium chloride is added to the inner well. After diffusion, the appearance of a shiny film (elemental palladium) in the palladium chloride compartment is indicative of a volatile substance, which chemically reduces palladium ions to elemental palladium.

Another separation method is solvent extraction. This is an efficient technique for separating a wide variety of drugs from biological specimens. This method transfers the drugs from the original sample into an organic solvent. Commonly employed organic solvents are ether and chloroform. If the sample is made acidic, only acidic compounds, such as salicylate and barbiturates, are extracted, while an alkaline sample permits basic compounds, such as amphetamines and most narcotics, to be separated. Chemically neutral compounds, such as meprobamate (Equinal®), diazepam (Valium®), etc., appear either in the acidic or the alkaline fractions, and it is usually desirable to further separate these compounds. Details of these additional extraction procedures are described in Chapter XXI.

To complete the analysis, the organic solvent is evaporated to dryness and the residue is dissolved in 100 $\mu$l to 200 $\mu$l of an appropriate solvent. The concentrated sample may now be subjected to analysis such as gas or thin-layer chromatography.

Since the amount of solvent is usually in the range of 50 to 100 ml, evaporation of the organic solvent is the most time-consuming step in the analysis. To expedite the procedure, microextraction methods have been developed. For example, 2 ml of urine can be extracted with 50 $\mu$l of chloroform and the chloroform layer injected directly into a gas chromatograph. Sample preparation time is usually less than five minutes.

Ion-exchange paper may also be used to separate drugs from biological samples and is particularly suited for urine. In this procedure drugs are removed from the specimen and absorbed onto a strip of the paper. Acids, bases and neutral drugs are adsorbed, then selectively removed from the paper prior to analysis. Ion-exchange paper was first employed to separate drugs from urine samples obtained from patients in methadone programs. Its objective was to enable processing of a large number of samples concurrently.

The method is simple and rapid and permits methadone clinics to perform the separation, then wash and dry the papers and submit them to a laboratory for analysis. A disadvantage of this technique is that recovery of some drugs is quite low; therefore, their presence may not be detected.

A similar technique, which has found wide applicability, is a form of column chromatography employing a non-ionic resin.* The biological sample is poured onto a glass or plastic column filled with the resin. Drugs in the sample adhere to the column, while all other compo-

* Amberlite XAD-2®, Rhom and Hass Company, Philadelphia, Pennsylvania.

nents of the sample pass through the column and are discarded. After the column is washed with water to remove water-soluble contaminants, the drugs are removed from the column by an organic solvent, which is collected and evaporated prior to analysis. All classes of drugs appear in the evaporated residue. In contrast to ion-exchange paper, this technique lends itself to analysis of all different types of biological samples—blood, bile, urine and tissue homogenates.

Activated charcoal has been used to separate drugs from serum and urine samples. This material is capable of adsorbing many classes of drugs in a ratio much greater than its weight. Clinically, if administered to an overdose victim, further absorption of the drug from the stomach is prevented due to adherence of the drug to the charcoal. This same principle is utilized in the laboratory; the sample to be analyzed is mixed with approximately 0.5 gm of activated charcoal. After appropriate manipulations, the drugs are removed from the charcoal into an organic solvent, which is subsequently evaporated and the residue subjected to analysis.

This technique is relatively rapid and removes most drugs from the specimen with adequate recovery. However, several manipulations are required to achieve an analysis by this method.

## METHODOLOGY

For many substances there exists more than one method of analysis. The choice of method depends upon the instrumentation available and the sensitivity, specificity and precision required in a particular instance.

The methods and associated instrumentation may be categorized as follows:

1. Spectrophotometry (ultraviolet, visible, fluorescence).
2. Chromatographic methods (thin-layer, gas, liquid).
3. Immunologic methods (radioactive, nonradioactive).
4. Gas chromatography-mass spectrometry.
5. Methods for metal analysis (atomic absorption spectroscopy, anodic stripping voltammetry).

The principles of each method will be discussed and some of the more common applications presented.

### Ultraviolet Spectrophotometry

Ultraviolet spectrophotometry is one of the most common physical methods employed for drug analysis. An ultraviolet spectrum is the energy absorption pattern obtained when a substance is subjected to radiation in the ultraviolet region of the electromagnetic spectrum. The resulting absorption spectrum is dependent upon the electronic structure of the molecule under investigation and therefore offers significant qualitative information. This is achieved by comparing the spectrum of the sample with those of other known substances. Many excellent references of ultraviolet spectra are available for comparison. Quantitative information is obtainable as well, provided the compound adheres to the mathematical relationship known as Beer's Law.

In comparison with other methods, ultraviolet spectrophotometry is usually regarded as one of the less sensitive techniques for analysis of drugs in biological fluids. In most cases, a relatively large concentration of drug is necessary to obtain a satisfactory ultraviolet spectrum, but this is dependent upon the molecular structure of the compound in question. For example, in terms of sensitivity, ultraviolet spectrophotometry competes favorably with gas chromatography for the analysis of barbiturates in blood but is approximately 100 times less sensitive for diazepam (Valium®) than an available fluorometric method. Salicylate (aspirin) is a compound that is well suited to ultraviolet spectrophotometric analysis, both at therapeutic and toxic blood concentrations.

An excellent application of ultraviolet spectrophotometry is the analysis of stomach contents for organic bases (codeine, phenothiazines, antihistamines). These compounds are usually present in milligram quantities, which is sufficient to obtain a satisfactory ultraviolet absorption. The total amount of drug recovered from the stomach contents should be calculated. This may be helpful in establishing the manner of death, i.e. accident versus suicide, in an overdose victim.

Ultraviolet spectrophotometry enables easy detection of organic bases, such as quinine, methapyrilene and most phenothiazines, in bile and urine. This is due to the relatively high concentration of these compounds in these samples and the high absorbance properties of these drugs. By contrast, drugs such as methadone (Dolophine®) have much lower absorbance properties, and a more sensitive technique is required for analysis of these compounds.

A disadvantage of ultraviolet spectrophotometry is that it does not permit separation of compounds if a mixture is present. Thus, two or more substances in a specimen give an ultraviolet spectrum that is a combination of all components. This renders interpretation difficult and may eliminate the possibility of obtaining quantitative data.

Another disadvantage is that several compounds may exhibit the same ultraviolet spectrum. A common example is a group of antidepressant drugs, amitriptyline (Elavil®), nortriptyline (Aventyl®), and protriptyline (Vivactil®). These compounds vary only slightly in chemical structure, and consequently an ultraviolet spectrum must be supplemented by an additional technique to distinguish these compounds in a biological extract.

### Visible Spectrophotometry

Visible spectrophotometry involves measuring the color intensity of a chemical reaction after introduction of a reagent to the sample to be tested. The color produced is in the visible region, and its intensity is proportional to the quantity of drug present. Quantitative analysis is achieved by measuring the absorbance of the resulting reaction mixture with a spectrophotometer and comparing the result with suitable standards.

Visible spectrophotometric procedures generally fall into two categories.

**A.** The reagent employed combines with the drug under suitable reaction conditions. This principle is employed for the analysis of drugs such as ethchlorvynol (Placidyl®) and chlordiazepoxide (Librium®). Placidyl® combines with diphenylamine to produce a red color. Librium® is hydrolyzed to a benzophenone, which undergoes diazotization with napthylenediamine to produce a purple color.

**B.** The chemical reagent is allowed to react with the substance of interest. The amount of reagent remaining is measured by adding a second reagent, which reacts with the excess reagent from the first reaction. The color produced in this instance is *indirectly* related to the amount of drug present in the sample. This approach has been employed in the analysis of alcohol. One procedure is to permit the alcohol to react with potassium dichromate. The amount of potassium dichromate remaining after the reaction is measured by observing the color produced after the addition of brucine.

Visible spectrophotometric methods are subject to interferences of varying degrees, depending on the procedure employed. In the procedure described for Librium®, any compound containing a diazotizable amino group on a basic compound can interfere. The most common drugs with this structure are the sulfonamides. In the procedure described for alcohol, any compound capable of reducing potassium dichromate solution will interfere. Therefore, substances such as methanol and isopropanol must be excluded by other techniques.

Visible spectrophotometric procedures are designed to measure the presence of a specific substance and are not usually of much assistance in the analysis for a general unknown. Frequently, these procedures are employed to quantitate a drug that has either been identified by some other method or was known to have been available to the individual in question.

### Fluorometry

Fluorometry (fluorimetry, spectrophotofluorometry) measures a compound's ability to emit light in the visible range of the electromagnetic spectrum after having absorbed light in the ultraviolet region.

Spectrophotofluorometers are instruments that record the excitation and emission spectra of a compound. The excitation spectrum is a plot of absorption as a function of wavelength. The wavelength at which maximum absorption occurs is referred to as the excitation wavelength, and the instrument is set at this wavelength for irradiation of the sample. The wavelength at which emission is most intense is known as the emission maximum, and the magnitude of this peak may be used for quantitative analysis.

Instrumentation for fluorometry consists of a light source, sample compartment, light filters or monochromators and a detector. The light source is a mercury or xenon lamp, which is used to excite the sample, and either filters or monochromators are employed to distinguish the excitation wavelength from the fluorescence wavelength. The detector is a photomultiplier tube, which responds to light emitted by the sample.

Fluorometry is a very sensitive technique. Typically, it can detect nanogram quantities of fluorescing material. Its inherent sensitivity is due to instrument design, since the detector responds primarily to light which is produced by the fluorescing sample, rather than light generated by the light source (mercury or xenon lamp).

Some compounds have the proper electronic structure and fluoresce inherently. This is sometimes referred to as native fluorescence. An example of such a compound is quinine, which is highly fluorescent in dilute sulfuric acid. This is exceptional, however. Most drugs do not have this property, and if a fluorescence measurement is desired, the substance must be chemically converted to a fluorescent compound (fluorophor). Several reagents are available for this purpose, and procedures have been described for many drugs, including the amphetamines, Darvon® and several phenothiazines.

## Chromatographic Methods

Chromatographic methods are basically separation methods but are also used for identification and, in some cases, quantitation. Chromatographic analyses operate under the principle whereby a compound is distributed between a mobile and stationary phase. The mobile phase, which may be a gas or solvent, carries the compound through the stationary phase, which may be a thin-layer plate, packed column or paper. The different chromatographic techniques are characterized by their mobile and stationary components and derive their names accordingly.

### *Thin-Layer Chromatography*

Thin-layer chromatography (TLC) is a commonly employed technique. The equipment necessary is simple and relatively inexpensive. The essential components include a glass or plastic plate coated with an appropriate adsorbent material such as silica gel (stationary phase), a chamber or jar to contain the plate, and a solvent system (mobile phase).

An extract of a biological sample is applied to the thin-layer plate. The plate is then placed in the chamber containing the solvent, and the latter is allowed to migrate up the plate for a predetermined distance, usually 10 to 15 cm. Different drugs migrate to different levels; thus, a drug can be tentatively identified by its migration distance divided by that of the solvent. This is referred to as the *Rf* value of the compound. After the plate is removed from the solvent and dried, most drugs are not visible, but they are made visible by chemical reaction when appropriate reagents are sprayed on the plate. Colored spots indicate the presence of drugs. The color and migration distance are compared with standards.

Many spray reagents are available, depending on the analysis desired. Mercury sulfate plus diphenylcarbazone is used for barbiturates, ninhydrin for primary amines such as amphetamine, potassium iodoplatinate for tertiary amines such as morphine and Dragendorff's reagent for any nitrogenous base.

### *Gas Chromatography*

Gas chromatography has the advantages of

chromatographic techniques in general and the added attribute of providing precise quantitative information.

Many commercial instruments are available. They all contain an injection port, column and detector. The function of the injection port, which is generally heated to 200° to 300° C, is to convert the sample from a liquid or solid state to a gas. A carrier gas, usually nitrogen or helium, conveys the vaporized sample from the injection port onto the column. The column, contained in a heated oven, is the most important part of the instrument, since its function is to separate the components of a mixture. Different substances are retained by the column packing to different extents. Substances that are retained poorly travel through the column more rapidly than those retained more strongly. The *retention time* necessary for a drug to travel through the column is a qualitative parameter used for identification purposes.

Periodically, retention times of substances subjected to analysis on the same instrument may differ, causing variations in results. Introduction of a stable substance known to be absent from the sample helps alleviate the problem. This compound serves as an *internal standard.* Division of the retention time of the internal standard into that of the unknown compound yields the *relative* retention time of the substance. The relative retention time is reproducible and can be used as a reliable means of identification of different compounds in the sample.

After the compound has travelled through the column, it proceeds to the detector. The purpose of the detector is to sense that a substance has emerged from the column and to produce a signal that can be amplified and recorded. Typically, this is achieved by a recorder, which registers a plot of detector response as a function of time. The magnitude of the signal is dependent on the amount of material in the sample.

Many applications of gas chromatography to forensic toxicology have been developed in the last ten to fifteen years. Two frequent examples illustrate some of the more important aspects of this technique.

The determination of ethyl alcohol is the most common analysis performed in the toxicologic laboratory. The presence of alcohol in a large percentage of motor vehicle, homicide and drug overdose victims necessitates a method that has both qualitative and quantitative capabilities.

Figure XXIII-2 represents a recording of a gas chromatogram of the more common volatile compounds found in biological samples. Each component requires a unique amount of time to travel through the column to the detector; therefore, each retention time is characteristic of a particular component. The area under each peak represents a quantitative parameter, since its size depends upon the amount of material present in the sample.

The importance of identifying each component becomes evident when one considers the

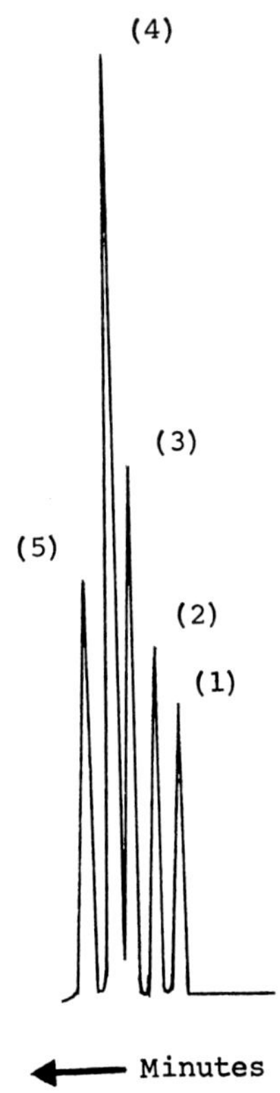


FIGURE XXIII-2. Gas chromatograms of volatile alcohols: (1) methanol, (2) ethanol, (3) acetone, (4) isopropanol and (5) *n*-propanol.

metabolic processes of the more common alcohols. Ethyl alcohol is the compound present in all alcoholic beverages sold for human consumption. These include beers, whiskeys and wines. Methyl or wood alcohol is not sold for human consumption but is occasionally ingested by the desperate alcoholic in search of a cheap substitute for ethanol. Methyl alcohol is extremely toxic, and acute exposure results in respiratory acidosis and acetone formation. Isopropyl or rubbing alcohol is also occasionally ingested by the alcoholic and metabolically is also transformed to acetone.

An effective method for alcohol analysis must distinguish these compounds so that the identity of the material consumed can be ascertained.

The alcohols represent compounds that can be directly analyzed by gas chromatography, but not all compounds have this property. Some substances are retained on the column for such a long time that analysis is unduly delayed and the shape of the eluted peak is too poor to permit reliable quantitative analysis. A technique that alleviates this problem is conversion of the compound to a different substance, which has more favorable gas chromatographic properties. This technique is used in the analysis of morphine, in which case the trimethyl silyl derivative is produced, enabling quantitation of morphine in blood.

Barbiturates constitute the class of drugs most commonly prescribed as sedatives, and gas chromatography is an effective method for the analysis of these compounds in blood. For both therapeutic and diagnostic purposes it is important to identify the particular barbiturate involved. For example, a therapeutic concentration of phenobarbital, which is long acting, may well be a toxic concentration of short-acting secobarbital. In addition, amobarbital and pentobarbital are difficult to separate using conventional thin-layer chromatographic solvent systems, but gas chromatography can effectively distinguish these drugs. Figure XXIII-3 illustrates the gas chromatographic separation of the more common barbiturates after conversion with a methylating reagent.

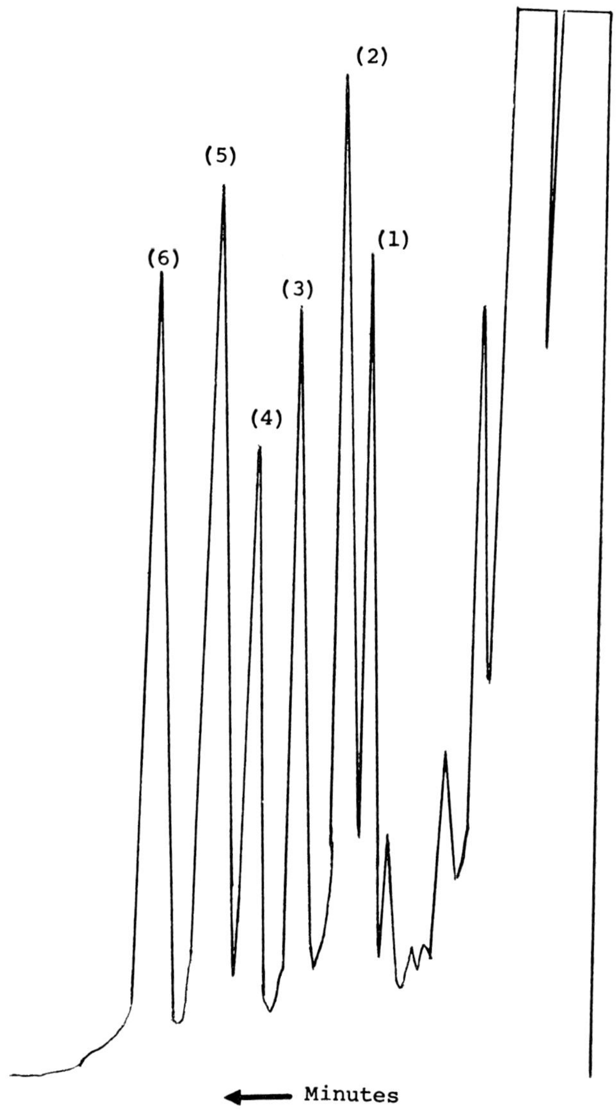


FIGURE XXIII-3. Gas chromatogram of methylated barbiturates: (1) phenobarbital, (2) aprobarbital, (3) butabarbital, (4) amobarbital, (5) pentobarbital and (6) secobarbital.

### *Liquid Chromatography*

Liquid chromatography (LC) is one of the oldest and best analytical techniques, but, ironically, it has not found widespread application until recently. The analysis time was prohibitive in many instances, but improvements in instrumentation have reduced this from several hours to a few minutes.

The principle of this technique is as follows. A dilute solution of the sample is passed through a tube or column packed with solid particles, which may or may not be coated with another liquid. These techniques are referred to as liquid/solid chromatography (LSC) and liquid/liquid chromatography (LLC), respectively. A solvent (mobile phase) is passed through the column (stationary phase), and the substances in the sample are carried through the column, continuously being extracted by the solvent and adsorbed by the column. Separation is achieved by the relative affinity of a particular substance for the stationary and mobile phases.

Initially, liquid chromatography was a slow separation process because the solvent flowed through the column only by gravity. Reduction in analysis time has been made possible by pumping the solvent through the column at pressures up to and occasionally exceeding 1000 psi. This technique is presently referred to as high pressure liquid chromatography (HPLC).

Several high pressure liquid chromatographs are presently commercially available. The major components in all instances include a solvent reservoir, pump, injector, packed column and a detector. The solvent reservoir contains the solvent (mobile phase), which is continuously pumped through the packed column (stationary phase). The sample is injected onto the column by means of a syringe and is carried through the column by the solvent. The detector responds to any compound eluted from the column and typically detects fluorescence or ultraviolet absorption.

Similarly to gas chromatography, the signal from the detector is recorded as a deviation from a baseline. The peak position along the curve denotes the particular component, once its elution characteristics have been determined for a given set of operating conditions. With appropriate calibration, the height of the peak is a measurement of the amount of the component present in the sample. As in gas chromatography, internal standards can be employed, and derivative formation to improve the sensitivity for detecting a given compound also has been utilized.

Applications of liquid chromatography to the analysis of drugs in plasma or serum include the determination of cyclocytidine (Cyclo-C), an anticancer agent; theophylline, an antiasthmatic; and phenobarbital-diphenylhydantoin (Dilantin®) combinations, which are used as anticonvulsants. Several drugs of abuse have been determined in urine, but significant improvements and a greater number of applications are likely to appear in the future.

## IMMUNOLOGIC METHODS

Immunologic techniques are based on the binding of a specific, labelled drug to an antibody. The analysis depends on the competitive displacement of the labelled drug from the antibody complex by the unlabelled drug in the sample. The amount of labelled drug displaced is related to the amount of unlabelled drug in the sample. High sensitivity and specificity give immunologic techniques the ability to assay virtually any biologic sample without prior separation of the drug from it. However, cross-reaction by structurally similar drugs may produce an erroneous result.

There are currently four immunologic assay systems on the market, and these differ only in the way the drug is labelled and in the method by which the displaced labelled drug is observed and quantitated.

Radioimmunoassay (RIA) was the first immunologic technique developed for drug analysis, and it employs a radioactive isotope to label the drug. After the bound and free forms of labelled drug are separated, the amount of displaced (free) labelled drug present is measured by liquid scintillation spectrometry or gamma counting. The amount of drug present in an unknown sample is obtained by comparing the radioactivity released by the unknown to a standard curve prepared by measuring the amount of radioactivity released by a series of solutions of known concentrations of the drug.

The EMIT® System* is a nonradioactive immunoassay technique that utilizes an enzyme (lysozyme) to label the drug. The reaction of the liberated enzyme on a bacterial suspension is observed spectrophotometrically by measuring the rate of clearing of a turbid solution. Instrumentation is available that automates the procedure by calculating the change in optical density over a period of time. The magnitude of this change is related to the quantity of drug present. The system can analyze urine samples for specific drugs or their metabolites (methadone, cocaine, propoxyphene) or for classes of drugs (barbiturates, opiates, benzodiazepines). A few drugs (digoxin, phenobarbital, diphenylhydantoin) may be quantitated in serum as well but require a different enzyme system.

The value of the EMIT System is the speed with which an analysis may be completed. This is on the order of minutes, which competes favorably with any other technique available. Some precautions must be exercised, however, particularly since the reaction depends upon the presence of an enzyme that may be endogenously present in urine, giving a false positive result. The quantity of endogenous lysozyme present is generally small and would give rise to a corresponding low concentration of drug.

The free-radical assay technique (FRAT) is a nonradioactive immunoassay technique that uses a stable free radical (such as nitroxide) attached to the drug. A positive test results in the liberation of the free radical, whose presence is measured by an electron spin resonance (ESR) spectrometer.

The FRAT system permits an analysis for morphine in about one minute. It is particularly applicable for mass screening of urine samples, since a single operator can perform several hundred analyses per day. A serious limitation of this technique is that the response for codeine, a common component of cough medication, exceeds that for morphine, the major metabolite of heroin. Consequently, it is imperative that an additional test be used to substantiate that a positive FRAT result is due to morphine rather than codeine.

Hemagglutination inhibition (HI) is a nonradioactive immunologic method that employs a red blood cell (RBC) as the label. Several molecules of drug are attached to the label, and stabilization is achieved by treatment with formaldehyde. All antibodies have two binding sites per molecule, so each may bind to two different red blood cells and agglutination (clumping) may occur. If the sample to be tested contains sufficient free drug to saturate the antibody binding sites, the red cells will not be agglutinated. This effect appears as a sharp pellet of cells at the bottom of a tiny conical well in which the reaction takes place. A negative result (agglutinated cells) forms a diffuse red-brown background without a clear pellet. The advantage of this technique is its low cost, since no major equipment is required.

Hemagglutination inhibition is a relatively slow technique, since the cells in each sample must be allowed to settle for up to three hours. Many samples can be processed simultaneously, however. In the analysis for morphine, cross-reactivity with codeine and dextromethorphan (a component of some cough medications) may occur.

### *Gas Chromatography-Mass Spectrometry*

Gas chromatography-mass spectrometry is the most sophisticated analytical technique currently available. It combines the capabilities of separating components in a complex mixture and enables identification of each component with utmost accuracy.

The principles of gas chromatography have been discussed. The mass spectrometer bombards the eluent from the gas chromatograph with an electron beam. This results in fragmentation of the molecules in the sample, and a record is made of the mass of each fragment produced. The exact chemical structure of a compound may be determined from the masses of these fragments. No two substances produce identical fragmentation patterns; thus, identi-

* Syva, Palo Alto, California.

fication of an unknown drug is achieved by matching its mass spectrum with that of a known substance. This has been greatly simplified by the availability of computers.

Sample preparation prior to a gas chromatograph-mass spectrometer analysis could be any of the separation methods outlined earlier. The instrument is applicable to the analysis of either extracts of biological specimens or of confiscated drug materials, such as pills, powders and syringe residues.

## METHODS FOR METAL ANALYSIS

Industrial and public education programs have kept deaths due to exposure to metals an infrequent occurrence.

Basically, there are three methods available for analysis of metals. The oldest technique is the Reinsch test. This is a wet-chemical method, details of which are outlined in the procedure section of this chapter. The two remaining methods are atomic absorption spectroscopy and anodic stripping voltammetry.

### *Atomic Absorption Spectroscopy*

Atomic absorption spectroscopy involves the absorption of light by atoms. After suitable preparation, a sample is introduced into a flame, which converts the element present to its atomic state. A light of the same wavelength as that of the element to be analyzed (for example, lead) is passed through the flame in the instrument. The atoms (lead) present in the sample absorb this light in proportion to their concentration.

Atomic absorption spectroscopy depends upon the absorption of light and is classified as a spectrophotometric method. Instrumentation differs from other spectrophotometers in that a flame and a special light source supplement the usual monochromators, detector and recorder. The light source is a lamp consisting of the element to be analyzed. It emits light at a wavelength characteristic of the element in question, thereby allowing atoms of the same element in the sample to absorb this radiation. Lamps consisting of different elements may be exchanged in the instrument, depending on the particular analysis desired. Multi-element lamps are available for analyzing several metals.

Sample preparation time differs, depending on the element involved and the nature of the sample. Serum analysis for lithium is performed by diluting the sample with distilled water and introducing it into the flame. Lead in blood is frequently analyzed by first combining it with an organic compound, then extracting the resulting chelate with an organic solvent. Tissue samples require acid digestion prior to analysis.

Atomic absorption spectroscopy is the most versatile technique for metal analysis. Metals routinely determined by this method are lead, copper, zinc, cadmium, arsenic, antimony, bismuth, thallium, cobalt, nickel and iron. Mercury is usually determined by a special technique known as flameless atomic absorption.

### *Anodic Stripping Voltammetry*

Anodic stripping voltammetry (ASV) is the most recent technique for analyzing metals in biological specimens. It is an electrochemical technique involving two steps: (1) depositing (plating) the metal onto an electrode under controlled potential and (2) removing (stripping) the plated metal from the electrode. When the metal is removed from the electrode, a current is generated, the intensity of which is dependent upon the amount of metal present. This current is measured and recorded. The peak on the recording is employed for quantitative analysis. The position of the peak on the recording is a qualitative parameter.

Instruments are commercially available or may be constructed in the laboratory. An electrode unit for controlling the plating and stripping potentials, electrodes and a cell compartment are required. The commercially available electrode is composed of mercury impregnated onto graphite.

All metals cannot be deposited onto a mercury-graphite electrode. Consequently, ASV is more limited than atomic absorption spectroscopy. Lead, copper, bismuth, antimony, zinc, cadmium and thallium may be analyzed by this technique with adequate sensitivity and specificity. Acid digestion usually is necessary to prepare a biological sample for analysis by ASV.

## INTERPRETATION OF TOXICOLOGICAL PROCEDURES

The interpretation of toxicological procedures involves the interpretation of qualitative and quantitative data. The qualitative data enable the toxicologist to conclude which substance was involved in a particular poisoning. Knowledge of metabolic transformations is invaluable in allowing correct identification of the substance to which the individual was exposed. Some of the more common biochemical transformations are isopropanol to acetone, Primidone® to phenobarbital, methamphetamine to amphetamine, imipramine to desipramine, and codeine and heroin to morphine.

Quantitative data enable the determination of the relevance of a drug to the clinical appearance of toxic symptoms or to a fatality. Many individuals ingest prescription and over-the-counter medications daily, so the mere fact that a drug is detected and identified in a fatality may or may not be relevant. Quantitative data are required, but even these should be evaluated together with the medical history, circumstances surrounding the death and the gross and microscopic autopsy findings. All of these are of equal importance and together contribute to the final decision determining the cause and manner of death.

Therapeutic and potentially toxic blood con-

TABLE XXIII-I

THERAPEUTIC AND TOXIC BLOOD CONCENTRATIONS OF COMMON DRUGS AND POISONS FOUND IN FATALITIES

| *Substance* | *Therapeutic Concentration (mg/dl)* | *Toxic Concentration (mg/dl)* | *Methodology*[1] |
|---|---|---|---|
| Amitriptyline | 0.1 | 1.0 | G.C. |
| Barbiturates | | | |
| Slow-acting (Phenobarbital) | 1-3 | 8.0 | G.C. |
| Intermediate-acting (Amobarbital) | 0.5 | 3.5 | G.C. |
| Rapid-acting (Secobarbital) | 0.2 | 1.0 | G.C. |
| Carbon Monoxide | — | 40* | C. |
| Chlorpromazine | 0.2 | 1.0 | UV |
| Codeine | 0.01 | 0.5 | G.C. |
| Cyanide | — | 0.4 | C. |
| Diphenhydramine | 0.1 | 1.0 | G.C. |
| Ethchlorvynol | 0.5 | 5.0 | C. |
| Glutethimide | 0.5 | 1.5 | G.C. |
| Imipramine | 0.1 | 0.5 | UV |
| Meriperidine | 0.1 | 1.0 | G.C. |
| Meprobamate | 1-5 | 10 | G.C. |
| Methaqualone | 0.5 | 2.0 | UV |
| Methyprylon | 0.5-1.0 | 5.0 | C. |
| Pentazocine | 0.05 | 0.8 | G.C. |
| Propoxyphene | 0.05 | 0.3 | UV |
| Quinidine | 0.1-0.5 | 1.5 | UV |
| Salicylate | 5-20 | 50 | UV |
| Thioridazine | 0.5 | 1.0 | UV |

G.C. = Gas Chromatography—measures only parent drug.
C. = Colorimetry—measures parent drug plus metabolite(s).
UV = Ultraviolet Spectrophotometry—measures parent drug plus metabolite(s).

* Percent hemoglobin saturation. May be as low as 20% or 25% in elderly individuals with advanced arteriosclerotic heart disease and/or emphysema.

centrations of drugs are variable, depending on the nature of the drug, the presence of alcohol and/or other drugs and the tolerance developed by a particular individual. With few exceptions, tolerance is virtually impossible to assess postmortem.

Data relating the concentration of a drug in blood to the death of an individual have been abundantly tabulated in the toxicologic literature. These data are important and contributory, but they should be considered only a guideline, giving the analyst a frame of reference upon which he can compare his findings in a suspected drug fatality. The figures published usually represent the personal experiences of workers in the field and are dependent upon factors such as the methodology employed, pathological state of the deceased, previous exposure to the drug and the time interval between exposure to the drug and death. Blood morphine concentrations in deceased narcotic addicts exemplify the variability that can occur, for the morphine concentration can be from a nondetectable quantity to greater than 200 μg/dl of blood.

Table XXIII-I summarizes therapeutic and potentially toxic blood concentrations of several drugs and poisons. The values are based on personal experiences, and the numbers have been rounded off for convenience. The method used to measure the drug concentration is also indicated, since some methods only measure the parent drug while others measure the parent drug as well as one or more major metabolites.

## TESTS ON BIOLOGICAL SAMPLES

Most United States pathologists who perform medicolegal autopsies do not have available rapid toxicological services. This often results in delays in diagnosis and probably in some unnecessary autopsies.

The following analyses are simple, office-type procedures requiring a minimum of reagents and equipment. However, considerable experience and expertise with these tests are required. These analyses may be used in some cases to provide qualitative information to indicate if additional, more elaborate testing is required. The fact that these tests are exclusionary must be emphasized, as well as the fact that in many instances a negative test result may be as significant as a positive one.

Each section of a drug or class of drugs includes the procedure, interpretation of the results, reagents required and references. The latter indicate primarily from where the procedure was obtained.

### Barbiturates[1]

#### *Procedure*

1. Place 5.0 ml of the sample (blood, urine, stomach contents, positive control aqueous blank) into a screw-capped culture tube and add 5.0 ml of pH 7.0 buffer and 5.0 ml of dichloromethane.
2. Cap the tube and gently mix for 1 minute. Centrifuge, discard the aqueous (upper) layer and filter the dichloromethane into a clean screw-capped culture tube.
3. Add 2.0 ml of the dilute mercuric chloride solution and mix gently for 1 minute. Centrifuge and discard the aqueous (upper) layer.
4. Add 10 ml of distilled water, mix gently for 1 minute, centrifuge and discard all of the aqueous (upper) layer.
5. Filter the dichloromethane into a clean test tube and add 2.0 ml of the diphenylcarbazone solution.
6. After mixing, observe the color.

#### *Interpretation*

A pale amber to orange color will result if the barbiturate concentration is greater than 0.2 mg/dl. Negative samples produce no color change in the diphenylcarbazone solution. Any residual mercuric chloride solution (from step 3) will produce a false positive result. Other drugs will interfere, and it is essential to confirm any positive result by another technique.

*Reagents*

1. Dichloromethane.
2. pH 7.0 Buffer.
   Any nonbarbiturate pH 7.0 buffer.
3. Mercuric Chloride, 20 mg/100 ml.
   Dissolve 0.50 gm of mercuric chloride in distilled water, add 3 drops of concentrated nitric acid and dilute to 50 ml. Take 1 ml of this solution and add it to a 50 ml volumetric flask containing 0.4 gm of sodium bicarbonate dissolved in distilled water. Dilute to the mark with distilled water.
4. Diphenylcarbazone (Dithizon®), 1 mg/100 ml.
   Dissolve 10 mg of diphenylcarbazone in 1 liter of dichloromethane. Store in a dark bottle at 4° C.

### Bromide[2]

*Procedure*

1. To three drops of the sample (urine or stomach contents) in a porcelain spot dish add two drops of reagent (glacial acetic acid-hydrogen peroxide) and two drops of fluorescein reagent.
2. Immediately observe the color formed. Heat the sample to dryness on a steam bath.

*Interpretation*

If bromide ions are present, a deep yellow color will form upon the addition of the glacial acetic acid-hydrogen peroxide reagent, and a rose pink color appears when the sample is heated to dryness.

*Reagents*

1. Glacial Acetic Acid-Hydrogen Peroxide.
   To 10 ml of glacial acetic acid add 10 ml of 30% hydrogen peroxide. This reagent should be refrigerated and not stored for a period greater than two weeks.
2. Fluorescein Reagent.
   To 100 ml of 95% ethanol add 200 mg of fluorescein.

### Carbon Monoxide[3]

*Procedure*

1. Pipet 3.0 ml of palladium chloride into the center well of a Conway microdiffusion cell* and 1.0 ml of 3.6N sulfuric acid into the outer well.
2. Add 0.5 ml of whole blood to the outer well and seal the cell. Mix the contents of the outer well by gentle rotation. Allow the cell to stand at room temperature for two hours.

*Interpretation*

The appearance of a shiny film of metallic palladium in the center well of the Conway cell indicates the presence of carbon monoxide. The detection limit is approximately 10% carboxyhemoglobin. At this point the procedure is semiquantitative, but it may be quantitative, provided an ultraviolet spectrophotometer is available and a hemoglobin determination is performed on the blood sample. If the blood sample is putrified, the lead acetate-acetic acid solution should be substituted for the 3.6N sulfuric acid, since sulfides resulting from the putrefaction process will react with the palladium chloride.

A commercial instrument dedicated to carboxyhemoglobin analysis is presently available.† The instrument employs automated differential spectrophotometry, and the percent carboxyhemoglobin present in the sample is automatically computed and digitally displayed. Total analysis time is less than five minutes.

*Reagents*

1. Hydrochloric Acid, 0.1N.
   Dilute 8.3 ml of concentrated hydrochloric acid to 1 liter with distilled water.
2. Palladium Chloride, 0.005N.
   Dissolve 0.44 gm of palladium chloride in 500 ml of 0.1N hydrochloric acid in a 1 liter volumetric flask. Mix the solution, allow it to stand overnight, then dilute it to 1 liter with 0.1N hydrochloric acid.
3. Sulfuric Acid, 3.6N.
   Dilute 10.0 ml of concentrated sulfuric acid to 100 ml with distilled water.

---

* Scientific Products, Div. Amer. Hospital Supply Co., McGaw, Illinois, catalog number 01815-1.

† Co-Oximeter®, Instrumentation Laboratory, Lexington, Massachusetts.

4. Lead Acetate-Acetic Acid Solution.
   Dilute 10.0 ml of glacial acetic acid to 100 ml with distilled water. Saturate this solution with lead acetate.

## Chloral Hydrate[4]

***Procedure***

1. To 2 ml of the sample (urine or stomach contents) in a test tube add 2 ml of 6N NaOH and 2 ml of pyridine.
2. Heat in a boiling water bath for approximately two minutes.
3. Observe the color of the pyridine (upper) layer.

***Interpretation***

A pink to red color indicates the presence of a trichlorinated compound. Chloral hydrate and/or its metabolite, trichloroethanol, will produce a positive test. This test is fairly sensitive but nonspecific; therefore, positive and negative controls must be included with the samples. Chloroform, a reagent commonly found in the laboratory, will produce a positive result.

***Reagents***

1. NaOH, 6N.
   Dissolve 240 gm of NaOH in distilled water and dilute to 1 liter with distilled water.
2. Pyridine.
   Analytical grade.

## Cyanide[5]

***Procedure***

STOMACH CONTENTS

1. Place 3 ml of the sample into a test tube that contains a layer of solid ferrous sulfate ($FeSO_4$) covering the bottom of the test tube.
2. Add 3 ml of 6N NaOH and heat on a boiling water bath for thirty seconds.
3. Cool the solution and add approximately 0.5 ml of 6N HCl. Look for a deep blue (Prussian blue) color.

BLOOD

1. Place 2 ml of blood and 1 ml of 10% $H_2SO_4$ into the outer well of a Conway microdiffusion cell.
2. Place 2 ml of 0.1N NaOH into the inner well of the same cell.
3. Seal and cover the cell, and allow it to stand at room temperature for two hours.
4. Add several drops of freshly prepared 10% ferrous sulfate until a brown precipitate forms. Add 6N HCl dropwise until the brown precipitate disappears and a deep blue (Prussian blue) color forms.

***Interpretation***

Good evidence of an acute episode of cyanide poisoning is the very characteristic bitter almond odor that is observable during examination of the stomach contents. A strongly positive Prussian blue reaction will confirm this observation. In a fatal case, the test described for blood will also produce a positive result. In any case of cyanide poisoning, accurate quantitative analyses of blood and tissue samples are essential. Since small amounts of cyanide may be formed postmortem, the blood and tissue analyses should be performed as soon as possible. Blood and spleen samples will contain the highest concentrations of cyanide, due to the high amounts of erythrocytes in these samples. For this same reason, urine is a poor sample to submit for cyanide analysis.

***Reagents***

1. NaOH, 6N.
   Dissolve 240 gm of NaOH in distilled water and dilute to 1 liter with distilled water.
2. HCl, 6N.
   Mix equal volumes of concentrated HCl and distilled water.
3. $H_2SO_4$, 10%.
   Add 10 ml of concentrated $H_2SO_4$ to 90 ml of distilled water.
4. $FeSO_4$, 10%.
   Dissolve 10 gm of ferrous sulfate in 90 ml of distilled water.

## Desipramine, Imipramine, Trimipramine[6]

***Procedure***

1. To two drops of urine in a spot plate add two drops of Forrest reagent. Promptly observe the color produced.

*Interpretation*

Absence of a *green* color indicates a negative result. Presence of a green color is an indication that desipramine (Pertofrane®) and/or imipramine (Tofranil®) and/or trimipramine (Sumontil®) may be present in the specimen. Development of a purple color may indicate the presence of phenothiazine derivatives.

*Reagents*

1. Potassium Dichromate, 200 mg/100 ml of water.
   Dissolve 200 mg of potassium dichromate in 100 ml of water.
2. Sulfuric Acid, 12N.
   Dilute 30 ml of concentrated sulfuric acid to 100 ml with water.
3. Perchloric Acid, 20 ml/100 ml.
   Dilute 20 ml of concentrated perchloric acid to 100 ml with water.
4. Nitric Acid, 8N.
   Dilute 50 ml of concentrated nitric acid to 100 ml with water.
5. Forrest Reagent.
   Mix equal volumes of the above four reagents.

## Ethanol[7, 8]

*Procedure*

1. Place 2 ml of sodium dichromate solution in the center well of a Conway microdiffusion cell.
2. Place 1 ml of the sample (blood or urine) and 2 ml of 20% $Na_2CO_3$ solution in the outer well. Cover the cell and carefully mix the contents of the outer well.
3. Place the cell in a water bath (37° C) for one hour or allow to stand at room temperature for several hours.
4. Observe any change in the color of the sodium dichromate solution (inner well).

*Interpretation*

If a volatile alcohol is present, the dichromate solution will change from yellow to green or blue. The reaction is not specific, since ethanol, methanol, isopropanol or diethyl ether will produce an identical color change. The procedure can detect 0.02% (w/v) of ethanol and is an excellent method for excluding the presence of this substance.

*Reagents*

1. Sodium Dichromate, 1.667 gm/liter.
   Place 1.667 gm of sodium dichromate in a 1 liter volumetric flask and dissolve in approximately 200 ml of distilled water. Cool in an ice bath, slowly adding 500 ml of concentrated sulfuric acid. Dilute to 1 liter with distilled water.
2. Sodium Carbonate, 20% w/v.
   Place 100 gm of sodium carbonate ($Na_2CO_3$) in a 500 ml volumetric flask and dilute to the mark with distilled water.

## Ethchlorvynol (Placidyl®)[9, 10]

*Procedure*

1. To 0.5 ml of urine in a spot plate add 0.4 ml of 5% diphenylamine and 0.2 ml of 80% (v/v) sulfuric acid.
2. Immediately observe the color produced in the chloroform layer.

*Interpretation*

The immediate formation of a red color indicates the presence of ethchlorvynol (Placidyl®).

*Reagents*

1. Diphenylamine, 5% in Chloroform.
   Add 5 gm of diphenylamine to a 100 ml volumetric flask and dilute to the mark with chloroform.
2. Sulfuric Acid, 80% v/v.
   Carefully add 80 ml of sulfuric acid to 20 ml of distilled water as the water is cooling in an ice bath.

## Ferrous Ion[11]

*Procedure*

1. Centrifuge the stomach contents to separate the fluid from the solid material.
2. Transfer 4 to 5 ml of the fluid to a test tube and add a spatula tip of solid potassium ferricyanide.

3. Observe the formation of a dark blue color.

*Interpretation*

This test is designed as a rapid one to preclude the possibility of poisoning by a ferrous salt. Other confirmatory tests should be performed to corroborate a positive result from this test. In addition, an accurate method for the determination of serum iron should be included once the presence of ferrous ions in the stomach contents is substantiated.

*Reagents*

1. Potassium Ferricyanide ($K_3Fe_3(CN)_6$), solid.

**Paranitrophenol (Metabolite of Parathion)**[12]

*Procedure*

1. To 5 drops of urine add 5 drops of saturated sodium hydroxide.

*Interpretation*

A deep yellow or orange color indicates the presence of paranitrophenol.

*Reagents*

1. Sodium Hydroxide, saturated.

**Phenothiazines**[13]

*Procedure*

1. Add 2 drops of FPN reagent to 1 drop of urine.
2. Observe the intensity and color produced in ten seconds. Discard any change that takes place after ten seconds.

*Interpretation*

If a blue, purple or red color forms within ten seconds, this may be an indication that phenothiazines are present. The color and intensity vary with the particular phenothiazine involved.

*Reagents*

1. Ferric chloride, 5 gm/100 ml.
   Dissolve 5 gm of ferric chloride in 100 ml of water.
2. Perchloric acid, 20% v/v.
   Dilute 20.0 ml of 70% perchloric acid to 100 ml with water.
3. Nitric acid, 7.5N.
   Dilute 50 ml of concentrated nitric acid to 100 ml with water.
4. FPN Reagent.
   Mix 5 ml of the ferric chloride solution with 45 ml of 20% perchloric acid and 50 ml of 7.5N nitric acid.

**Salicylate**[14]

*Procedure*

STOMACH CONTENTS OR URINE

1. To a few drops of the sample (fluid from stomach contents or urine) in a porcelain spot plate add several drops of ferric nitrate reagent.
2. Look for the immediate formation of a purple color, indicating the presence of salicylate.
3. Add a few drops of concentrated sulfuric acid. If the purple color in the above step is due to salicylate, it will fade upon the addition of this strong acid.

BLOOD

1. To a 15 ml centrifuge tube containing 5.0 ml of water and 0.5 ml of blood add 5.0 ml of Trinder's reagent.
2. Mix the contents of the tube well, allow it to stand for five minutes, then centrifuge it.
3. Look for the appearance of a purple color in the supernatant.

*Interpretation*

STOMACH CONTENTS OR URINE

A positive test in the stomach contents indicates a recent ingestion of a compound containing salicylate. This may be due to aspirin (acetyl salicylic acid), salicylamide or methyl salicylate. A positive test from the urine indicates exposure to a compound containing salicylate but may or may not be significant in terms of an acute toxic episode. In either case, quantitative analysis of the blood is indicated. If present in high concentrations, phenothiazines may interfere with the aforementioned test. This possibility is minimized, however, by the addition of concentrated sulfuric acid. The purple color will deepen upon the addition of this reagent if phenothiazines are present but will disappear in the presence of a salicylate compound.

BLOOD

This procedure may be used quantitatively if a salicylate solution of known concentration and water as a reference blank are analyzed simultaneously with the blood sample. An instrument (for example a Coleman Jr.® capable of measuring absorbance at 540 nm is required for quantitative analysis. This procedure is designed to detect elevated salicylate concentrations and is accurate within ± 5%. Fatal concentrations in the blood are usually greater than 50 mg/dl and may exceed 100 mg/dl. In fatal cases of poisoning with Darvon® Compound, blood salicylate concentrations are usually in the area of 15 to 25 mg/dl.

***Reagents***

1. Hydrochloric acid, 1N.
   Dilute 8.3 ml of concentrated hydrochloric acid to 100 ml with water.
2. Trinder's Reagent.
   Place 4 gm of ferric nitrate $(FE(NO_3)_3 \cdot 9 H_2O)$ and 4 gm of mercuric chloride in a 100 ml volumetric flask. Add 12.0 ml of 1N HCl. Dissolve the salts, dilute to 100 ml with water and filter.

### Thiocyanate[14]

***Procedure***

1. To 5 drops of urine add 1 drop of ferric chloride solution. Immediately observe the color produced.

***Interpretation***

Thiocyanate produces an orange color, and salicylate produces a purple color. Phenothiazines in high concentrations may produce a purple color.

***Reagents***

1. Hydrochloric acid, 5N.
   Dilute 42 ml of concentrated hydrochloric acid 100 ml with water.
2. Ferric chloride, 5% in 5N HCl.
   Dilute 5 gm of ferric chloride to 100 ml with 5N HCl.

## TESTS ON NONBIOLOGICAL SAMPLES

Many tests not applicable to biological samples are employed by forensic chemists for identification of suspected illicit drugs. Among the most popular are the Duquenois test for marijuana and the Marquis test for narcotics.

### The Duquenois-Levine Test[15, 16]

***Procedure***

1. Extract 5 mg of the plant with 2 ml of petroleum ether.
2. Recover the petroleum ether and evaporate to dryness in a test tube.
3. Dissolve the residue in 5 drops of Duquenois reagent.
4. Add 10 drops of concentrated hydrochloric acid and mix.
5. If a blue-violet color appears within ten minutes, add 15 drops chloroform and shake the entire contents of the tube. Observe the color of the chloroform (lower) layer.

***Interpretation***

A blue-violet color appearing after the addition of concentrated hydrochloric acid indicates the presence of cannabinoids, the physiologically active constituents of marijuana and hashish. The specificity of the test is improved by extracting the test mixture with chloroform. If a positive test result is due to the presence of cannabinoids, the blue-violet color is transferred into the chloroform layer upon shaking the reaction mixture. Any positive result may be confirmed by other (thin-layer chromatography, gas chromatography, gas chromatography-mass spectrometry) more specific techniques.

***Reagents***

1. Duquenois Reagent.

To 0.4 gm of vanillin add 5 drops of acetaldehyde and 20 ml of 95% ethanol.

## The Marquis Test[17]

### *Procedure*

1. Add a few drops of Marquis reagent to the substance (powder, solution) to be tested.
2. Observe the color formed.

### *Interpretation*

Many compounds react with the Marquis reagent, producing a variety of colors. Both heroin and morphine produce a purple color, while amphetamine produces an orange color that turns to brown. Since several compounds may produce the same color, the test is not specific.

### *Reagents*

1. Marquis Reagent.
   Add 5 drops of 40% formalin (formaldehyde) to 5 ml of concentrated sulfuric acid. This reagent must be prepared immediately before use.

## REFERENCES


1. Helman, E. Z.: Emergency screening of urine, plasma or gastric contents for barbiturates. *Clin Chem, 16:*797, 1970.
2. Fiegl, F.: *Qualitative Analysis by Spot Tests,* 3rd ed. Amsterdam, Elsevier, 1946, p. 195.
3. Williams, L. A., Linn, R. A., and Zak, B.: Ultraviolet absorptiometry of palladium for determination of carbon monoxide hemoglobin. *Am J Clin Pathol, 34:*334, 1960.
4. Kaye, S.: *Handbook of Emergency Toxicology,* 3rd ed. Springfield, Thomas, 1973, pp. 196-197.
5. Gettler, A. D., and Goldbaum, L.: Detection and estimation of microquantities of cyanide. *Anal Chem, 19:*270, 1947.
6. Forrest, I. S., Forrest, F. M., and Mason, A. S.: A rapid urine color test for imipramine. *Am J Psychiatry, 116:*1021, 1960.
7. Kozelka, F. A., and Hine, C. H.: Method for the determination of ethyl alcohol for medicolegal purposes. *Ind Eng Anal Ed, 13:*905, 1941.
8. McBay, A.: Ethanol. In Sunshine, I. (Ed.): *Methodology for Analytical Toxicology.* Cleveland, CRC Pr, 1975, pp. 145-146.
9. Andryauskas, A., Matusiak, W., and Dal Cortivo, L. A.: Ethchlorvynol in toxicological analysis. *Int Microfilm J Legal Med, 2:* card 4, 1967.
10. Finkle, B. S., and Bath, R.: Ethchlorvynol. In Sunshine, I. (Ed.): *Methodology for Analytical Toxicology.* Cleveland, CRC Pr, 1975, pp. 155-156.
11. Kaye, S.: *Handbook of Emergency Toxicology.* 3rd ed. Springfield, Thomas, 1973, p. 263.
12. Kaye, S.: *Handbook of Emergency Toxicology.* 3rd ed. Springfield, Thomas, 1973, p. 248.
13. Forrest, I. S., and Forerst, F. M.: Urine color test for the detection of phenothiazine compounds. *Clin Chem, 6:*11, 1960.
14. Trinder, P.: Rapid determination of salicylates in biological materials. *Biochem J, 57:*301, 1954.
15. Butler, W. P.: Duquenois-Levine test for marijuana. *J Assoc Off Agr Chem, 45:*597, 599, 1962.
16. Pitt, C. G., Hendron, R. W., and Hsai, R. S.: The specificity of the Duquenois color test for marijuana and hashish. *J Forensic Sci, 17:*693-700, 1972.
17. Clarke, E. G. C.: *Isolation and Identification of Drugs,* vol. 1. London, The Pharmaceutical Press, 1969.

*Chapter XXIV*

# SELECTED PROCEDURES AT AUTOPSY

WERNER U. SPITZ

A MEDICOLEGAL AUTOPSY differs from a hospital autopsy in both objective and significance. Consequently, certain procedures that are of little or no use in the hospital practice of pathology are applied routinely by the forensic pathologist. Several of these procedures are described in conventional autopsy manuals. The aim of this chapter is to collate such selected autopsy procedures and techniques that we have found to be helpful in the routine performance of medicolegal postmortem examinations.

## AIR EMBOLISM

Every autopsy in a case of suspected abortion or an open wound of the neck area should begin with a check for air embolism. An interrupted blood column, i.e. fragmentation of the blood line in the coronary arteries, the arteries of the meninges or elsewhere in the body, is usually artifactual and must not be mistaken for air embolism.

The presence of air in the vascular system can be demonstrated by the use of an easy and accurate method. A T-shaped incision is made over the heart area. Extension of the *T* will later constitute the regular autopsy incision through which the organs are removed. The skin and muscles are flapped back, and the precordial part of the sternum and ribs are removed. The aim at this stage is to disturb the tissues as little as possible, and care must be taken to avoid pulling these parts at the time of resection. This is to avoid creating negative pressure in the tissues, which may result in aspiration of air into the vessels. The pericardial sac is incised anteriorly, and the edges are grasped with hemostats on each side. It is helpful to have an attendant hold the hemostats. The pericardial sac is filled with water, and the heart is submerged. The right side of the heart is then stabbed with a scalpel under the water level. The scalpel should be twisted a few times when in the heart to ensure that the wound is open. If air is present, bubbles will rise; otherwise blood will be seen to emerge from the wound.

It is recommended that the amount of air be measured. For this purpose an inverted water-filled graduated glass cylinder (preferably over 300 cc) is placed over the heart, with the mouth of the cylinder in the pericardial water. When the heart is stabbed, the gas will escape into the cylinder displacing the water. A stopper then placed on the mouth of the cylinder will ensure retention of its contents for chemical analyses if such are indicated. Aluminum foil secured with a tight rubber band will equally serve the purpose (Fig. XXIV-1).

## PNEUMOTHORAX

Pure pneumothorax is rare. It is usually associated with injury to the lung, resulting in the presence of blood in the pleural cavity (hemopneumothorax). The pleural cavities should be checked for the presence of air in every case involving injury to the chest.

Incision of the body is as outlined in the discussion of air embolism. The skin and muscles on the injured side of the chest are reflected and dissected to form a *pocket.* This is filled with water. A scalpel is introduced under the water level through an intercostal space into the costodiaphragmatic sinus. The scalpel should be twisted a few times to ensure that the wound is open. An inverted graduated cylinder filled with

The cooperation of Commander Frank O. Raasch, MC, USN, Armed Forces Institute of Pathology, in preparing the original drawings for this chapter is gratefully acknowledged.

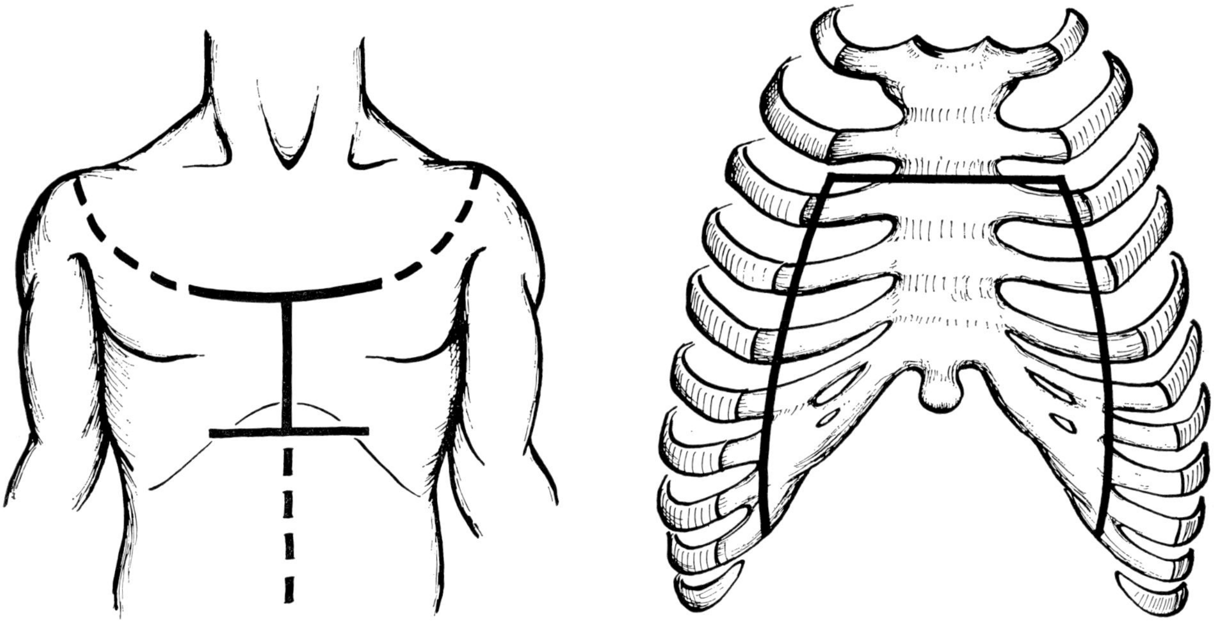

FIGURE XXIV-1. (a): *Step 1*—Incision of the skin for exposure of the heart. The dotted line indicates the subsequent extension of the incision for the regular autopsy. (b): *Step 2*—Indicated area represents the section of the rib cage and sternum to be removed.

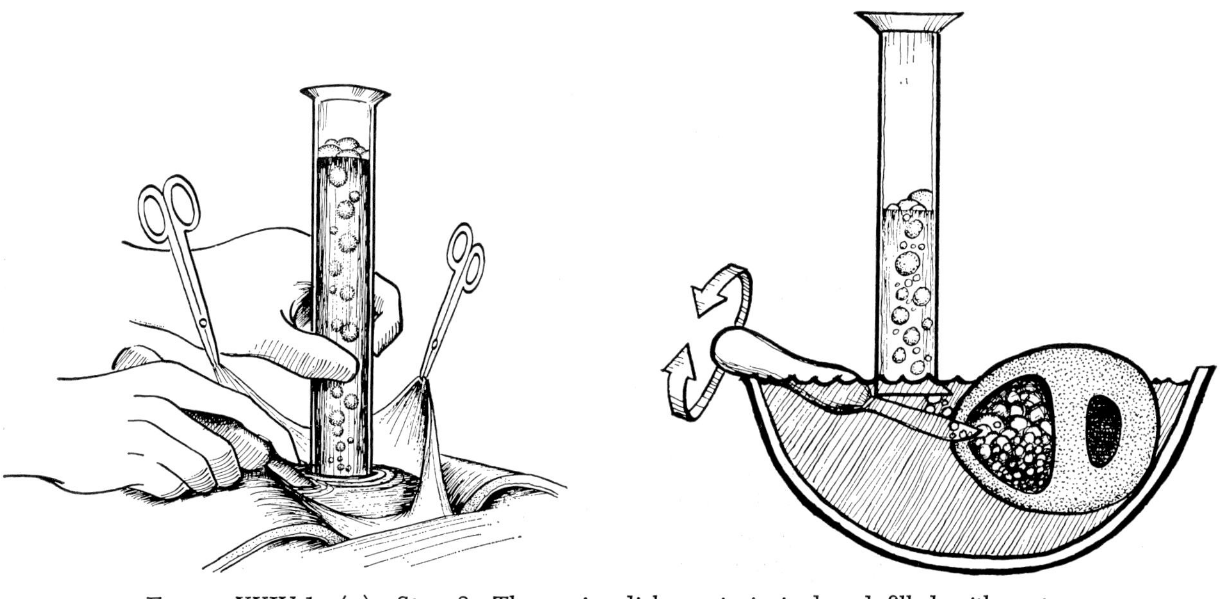

FIGURE XXIV-1. (c): *Step 3*—The pericardial sac is incised and filled with water. Hemostats can be used to elevate the pericardium, and an inverted graduated cylinder containing water is placed over the right side of the heart, while the latter is punctured with a scalpel to permit the escape of gas into the cylinder. (d): Cross-sectional view, showing detail of the scalpel puncturing the heart. The escaping gas replaces the water in the cylinder. It is advisable to twist the scalpel to ensure adequate opening of the puncture site.

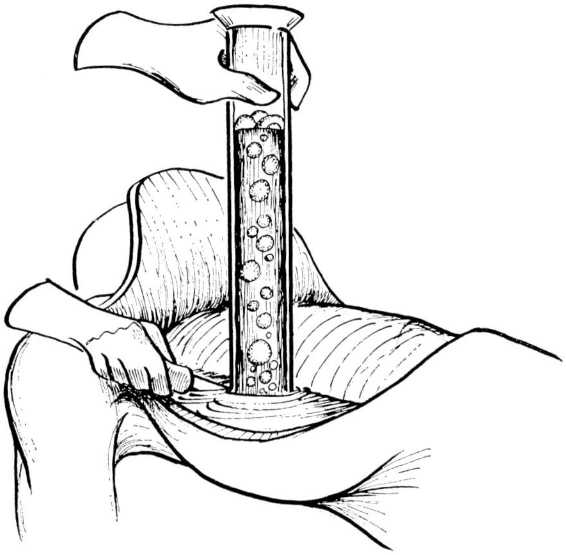

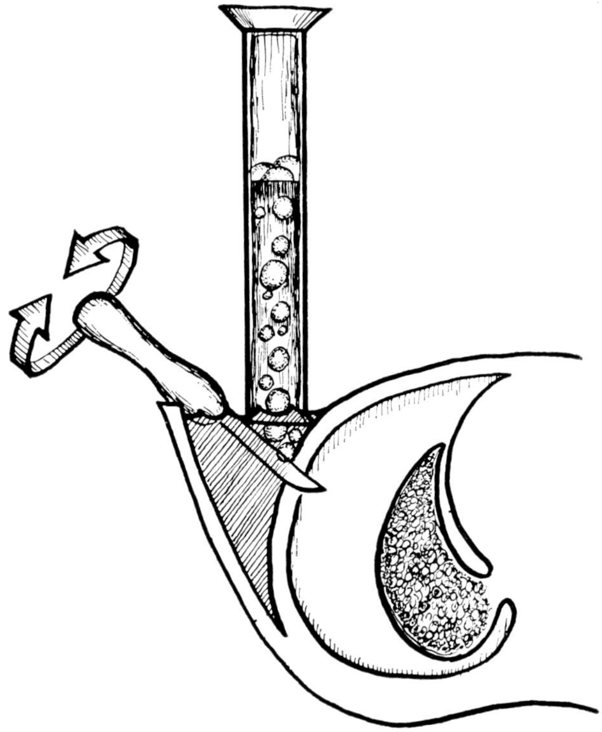

FIGURE XXIV-2. (a): Inverted graduated glass cylinder is held over the water-containing *pocket* in the side of the chest, while an intercostal space is stabbed with a scalpel below the water level to permit the escape of air into the cylinder. The scalpel should be twisted to ensure adequate opening of the puncture site. (b): Side view, showing scalpel puncturing the intercostal space and gas bubbles replacing the water in the cylinder.

water held over the pocket may be used to collect and measure the amount of air in the pleural cavity (Fig. XXIV-2).

## DEMONSTRATION OF THROMBI IN THE CALVES

Formation of thrombi in the calves is a frequent complication of prolonged bed rest and may occasionally follow direct trauma to the legs. Dislodging of a leg vein thrombus may cause fatal pulmonary embolism. It is impossible to determine the source of an embolus in the lung by direct examination, but its origin is likely to be the calf if other thrombi are found in that area. It is often difficult, using conventional methods of dissection, to distinguish a fresh thrombus in an intramuscular leg vein from a postmortem artifact. The following technique has proven to be a satisfactory alternative to other common methods used to demonstrate calf vein thrombi. The calf is incised from the heel to the popliteal fossa, and the skin is reflected. The tendon of Achilles is divided. With a long knife, the calf musculature is then separated from the bones from the heel upward. Excessive traction and handling of the muscles should be avoided.

Transverse sections about 1 in. apart are then placed in the calf musculature. Thrombi, if present, will *pop out* as firm, solidly structured *sausages*, which cannot be mistaken for postmortem artifacts. The major arteries of the calf pass between the tibia and the fibula. They remain intact if this procedure is properly carried out. Interference with subsequent injection of embalming fluid into the limb is thereby avoided (Fig. XXIV-3).

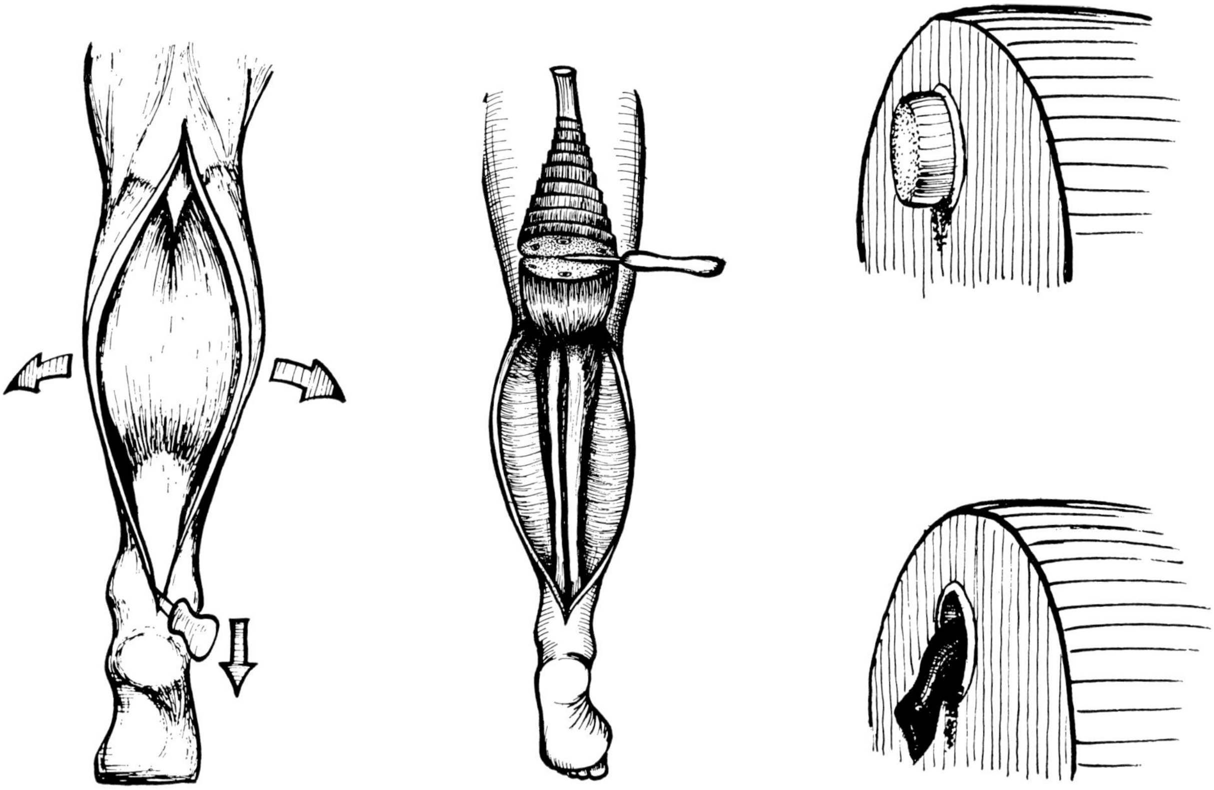

FIGURE XXIV-3. (a): *Step 1*—Extent of the cutaneous incision for exposure of the calf musculature. (b): *Step 2*—Using a long knife, the calf musculature is separated from the bones and is reflected upward. Transverse incisions of the reflected muscles will disclose the presence of thrombi. c: Firm, solidly structured thrombi *pop out* as *sausages* from the transected vein (above). The postmortem clot is flabby in comparison and does not *pop* (below).

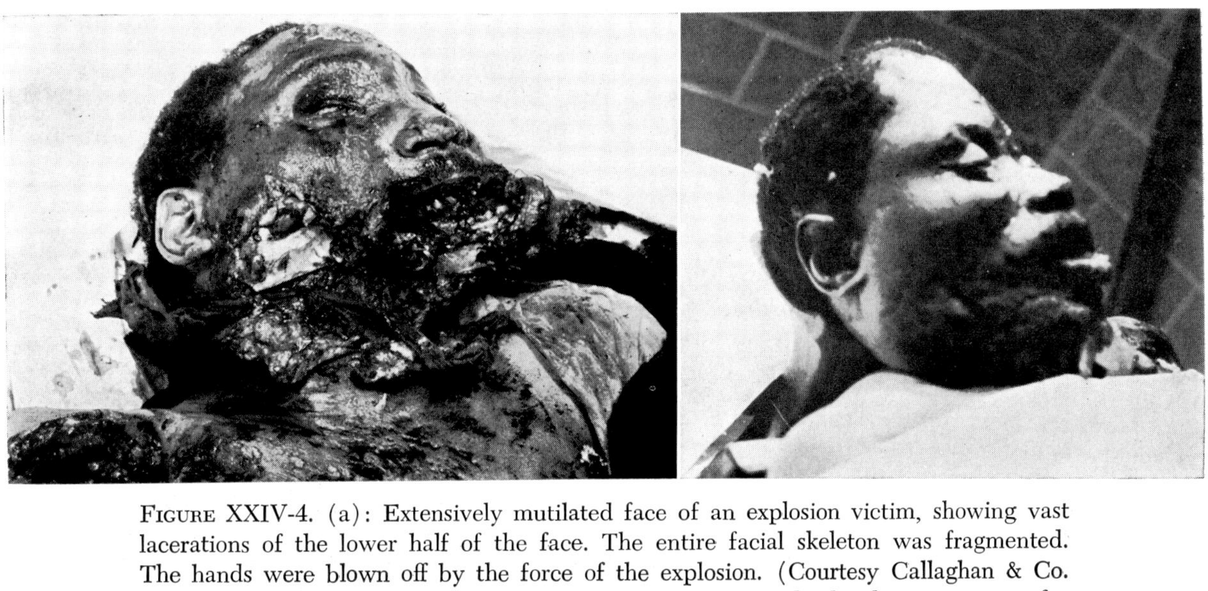

FIGURE XXIV-4. (a): Extensively mutilated face of an explosion victim, showing vast lacerations of the lower half of the face. The entire facial skeleton was fragmented. The hands were blown off by the force of the explosion. (Courtesy Callaghan & Co. From Spitz, W. U., Sopher, I. M., and DiMaio, V. J. M.: Medicolegal investigation of a bomb explosion in an automobile. *J Forensic Sci, 15*:537-552, 1970.) (b): Polaroid photograph of the same victim as shown in Figure XXIV-4a after reconstruction of the facial skeleton using copper wire and an electric drill. This was followed by *redressing* of the face with the *repaired skin*. Where bone fragments were missing, wet paper towels were used to *mold* the contour. Finally, the lower half of the face was shaded for the purpose of taking this photograph. Relatives of the deceased were shown this photograph and identified the victim without hesitation. (Courtesy Callaghan & Co. From Spitz, W. U., Sopher, I. M., and DiMaio, V. J. M.: Medicolegal investigation of a bomb explosion in an automobile. *J Forensic Sci, 15*:537-552, 1970.)

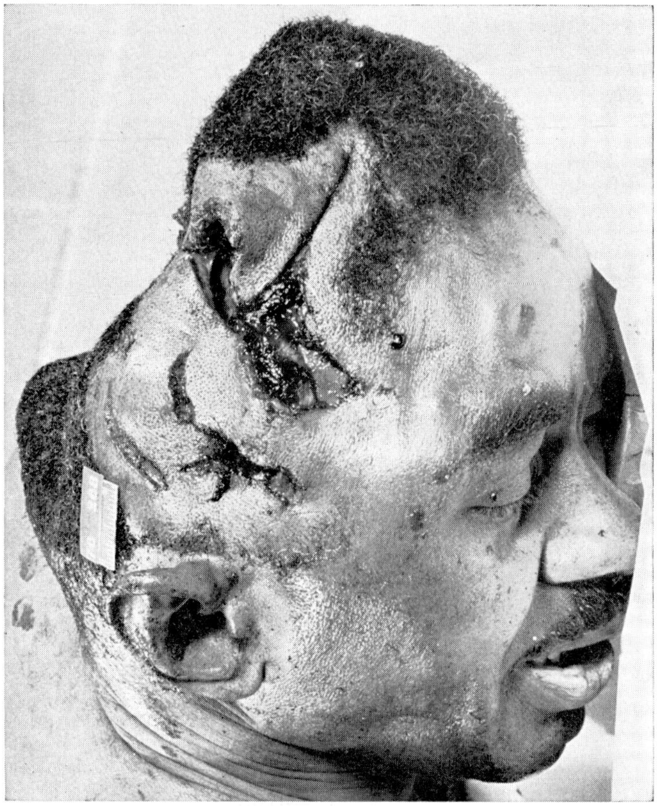

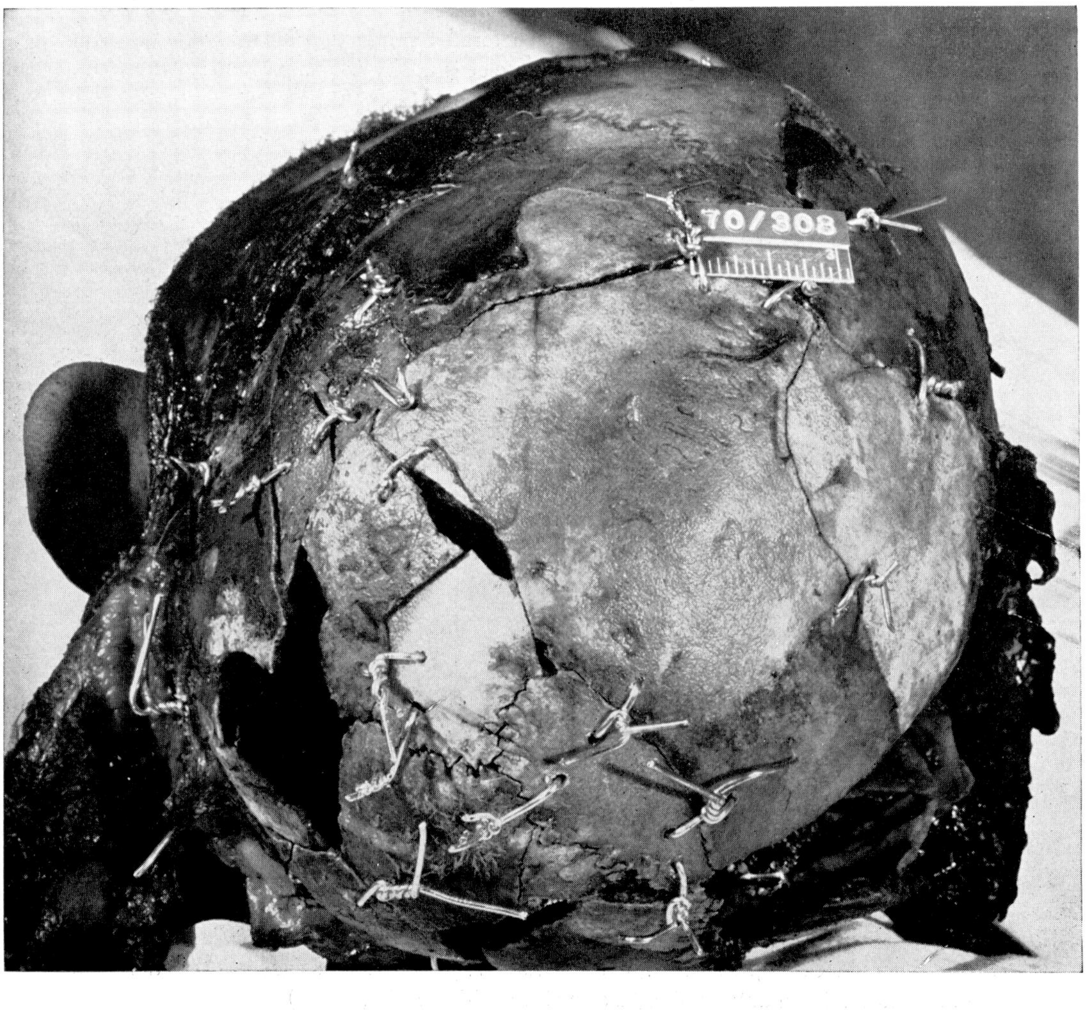


FIGURE XXIV-5 (a): Victim, showing extensive tears of scalp and fractures of the skull at first attributed to blunt impacts. (b): Alignment of the skull fragments using copper wire and an electric drill. This reveals a circular defect behind the left ear, presumably caused by a rifled slug.

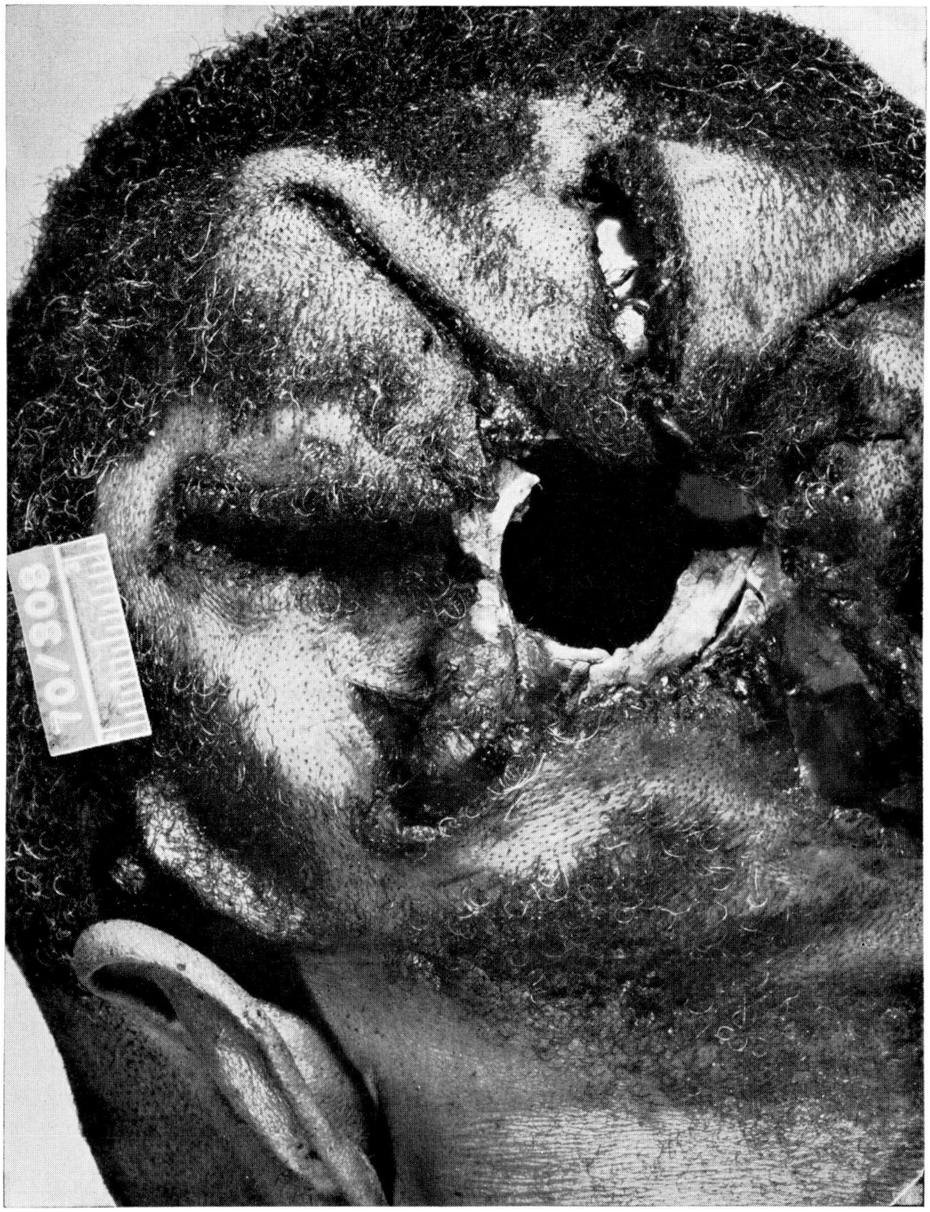


FIGURE XXIV-5c. The *redressed* scalp over the circular defect in the bone shows what is now a typical wound of entrance.

## RECONSTRUCTION OF THE SKULL FOR PERSONAL IDENTIFICATION AND DETERMINATION OF TYPE OF VIOLENCE

Occasionally the skull is fractured to the extent that facial features are not recognizable and the type of violence responsible for the mutilation cannot be ascertained. Restoration of the contour of the skull frequently provides the answer to these questions. Replacement and fixation of the bone fragments may be carried out by using an electric drill and copper wire.

The fragmented skull and badly mutilated face of an explosion victim were reconstructed in this fashion.[1] The victim was then photographed, and identification of the Polaroid® picture was made by three members of his family. An artist's sketch and Identikit® reproductions were not recognized as being consistent with the features of the deceased (Fig. XXIV-4).

In another case, the body of a bound and gagged man was found in the trunk of an automobile that was parked alongside the road. The head was crushed, suggesting multiple blows with a blunt object, and beating was thought to be the mode of homicide. Subsequent alignment of the bone fragments and redressing of the scalp clearly indicated a circular bullet wound of entrance in the back of the head. The size of the wound and the hole in the skull, as well as the absence of shotgun pellets within the skull, suggested a single large missile, probably a rifled slug. The secondary tears in the skin, at first ascribed to blunt impacts, resulted from bone fragmentation through the scalp. A gaping exit wound was located in the right side of the forehead (Fig. XXIV-5).

## REMOVAL OF THE JAWS FOR DENTAL IDENTIFICATION

Identification of a dead person by dental comparison is often the only alternative in cases of extensive mutilation of the body or advanced putrefaction. Disarticulation of the mandible and excision of the upper jaw may be necessary under such circumstances to enable adequate examination and possible preservation as evidence (Fig. XXIV-6). Using an electric or manual bone saw, the upper jaw is excised by means of a horizontal cut placed above the hard palate. We have found this procedure useful in many instances. Due to the extent of disfigurement already present before removal of the jaws, funeral directors commonly cooperate fully when this procedure is indicated.

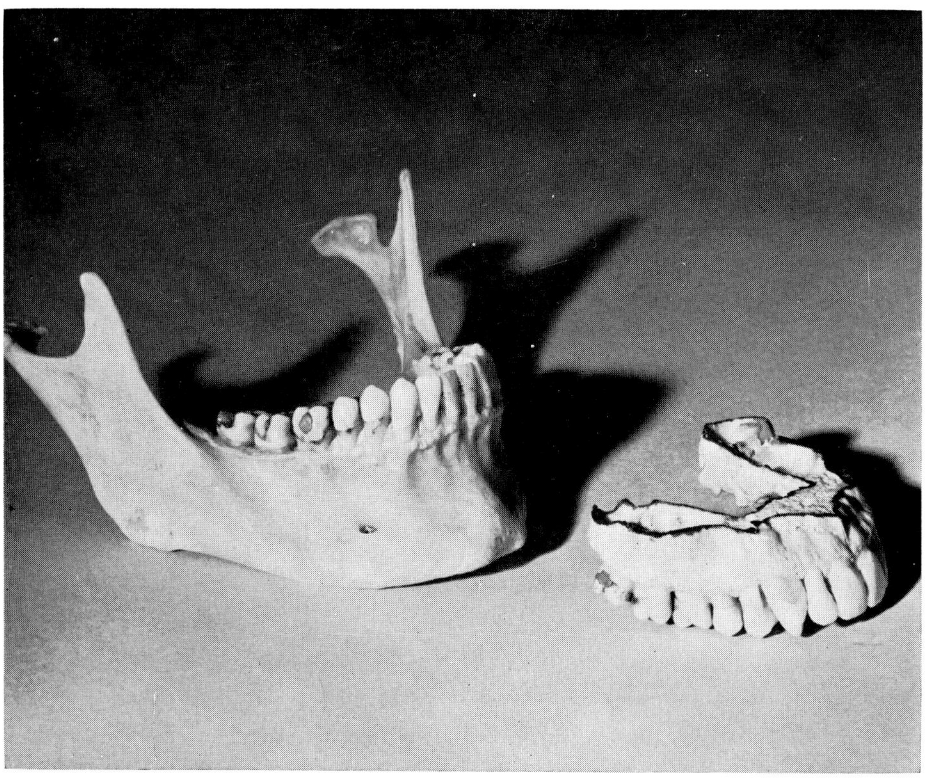

FIGURE XXIV-6. Upper and lower jaws removed for the purpose of identification from an unknown victim. The victim was later identified by dental charts. The maxilla was resected along the black line (inked for better contrast).

## EXAMINATION OF THE CERVICAL SPINE FOR WHIPLASH INJURY

An autopsy of a traffic death or of the victim of a fall is incomplete without a thorough examination of the cervical spine. Clinically, so-called whiplash injuries have been described as most often located in the level of C-4 to C-6. In our experience at autopsy, C-1 and C-2 are involved more frequently. Injuries to this area range from severe fractures and dislocations to a few deep hemorrhages in the musculature. The latter probably result from tears of individual muscle fibers. Most frequently encountered injuries in the level of the first two vertebrae are tears of the articular capsules and ligaments associated with intraarticular or periarticular hemorrhage.

Even in the presence of another well-documented cause of death, the significance of whiplash injury as a component of a certain mechanism of injury cannot be overlooked. The search for whiplash injuries is greatly facilitated by the following technique. The body is placed face down. A wooden block is placed under the chest, and the head is bent downward. This stretches the cervical spine. Through a midline incision, the musculature is dissected layerwise down to the vertebral column. The atlantooccipital joint capsules are then incised and the articular surfaces examined. Subsequently, the atlas is disarticulated and removed. Laminectomy is now performed on the remainder of the cervical spine; the dura mater is incised, and the spinal cord is inspected *in situ* and then removed. The underside of the base of the skull can now be inspected as far forward as the pharynx. Replacement of the atlas and tight suture of the incision in the skin permit good reconstruction with fair stability of the head.

## REMOVAL OF THE TONGUE

The tongue should be examined routinely. The presence of a fresh bite mark in the tongue lends support to the probability that a seizure preceded death. In an epileptic a bite mark in the tongue may be the only anatomical evidence to suggest that death occurred during an epileptic attack. As bite marks in the tongue are not usually noted on external examination, the tongue should be incised. A single horizontal cut starting at the tip of the tongue is recommended. *Bread-loaf-type* incisions would miss small injuries. Bite marks are mostly located along the sides of the tongue, less frequently at the tip. A small hemorrhage under an intact mucosa is usually all that is seen.

Removal of the tongue is best done with a double-edged knife. Following the usual Y-shaped incision, the skin of the chest and neck is reflected and the knife is inserted under the chin through the floor of the mouth. The tip of the blade will emerge under the tongue. A cut is then made along the sides of the mandible to the angle of the mandible. At this point, the blade is turned inward to avoid severing the carotid artery. With the index and midde fingers, the tongue is now pushed down under the mandibular arch. The soft palate is then cut to include the uvula and tonsils with the tongue and neck organs to be removed (Fig. XXIV-7). Should the carotid artery be accidentally damaged during removal of the tongue and neck organs, this can be rectified by the use of a polyethylene tube firmly tied into the vessel. This will enable subsequent injection of embalming fluid to the head.

## CHECK OF STOMACH CONTENTS FOR CRYSTALLINE MATERIAL

Inspection of the stomach contents is part of every autopsy, and the results should be recorded. The nature of the contents indicates the type of food ingested at the last meal. The amount of stomach contents and the extent of their digestion may be helpful in approximating

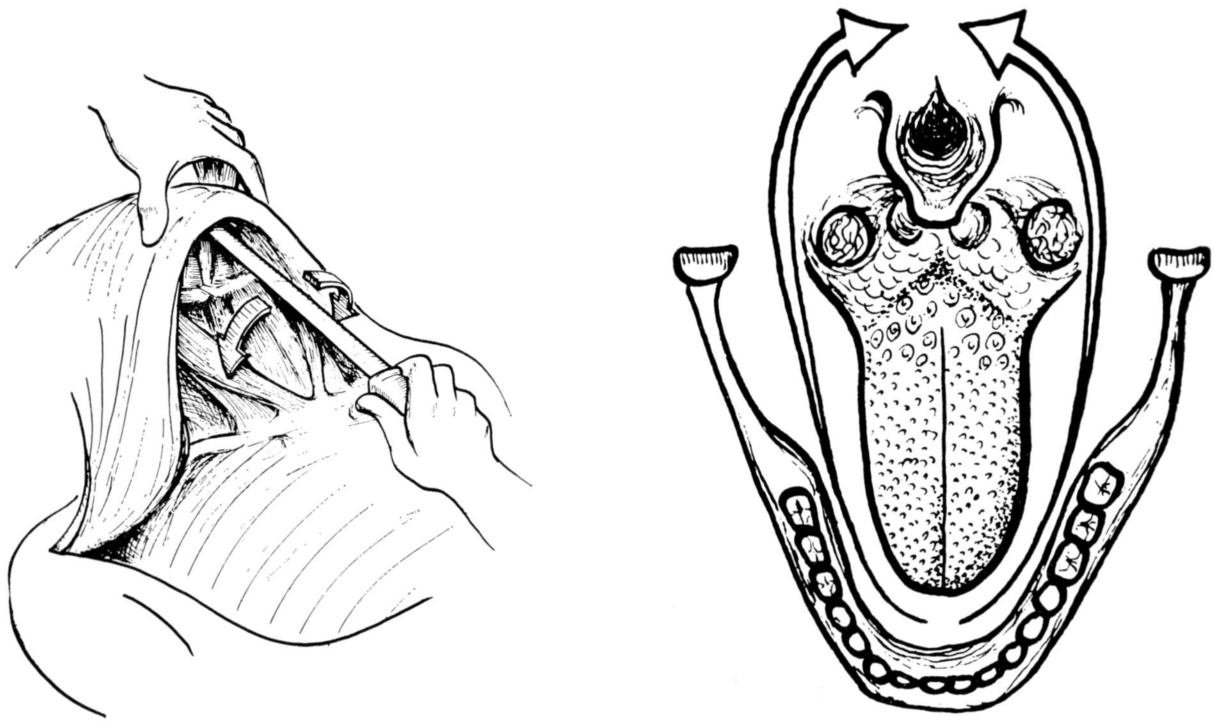

FIGURE XXIV-7. (a): Technique of removal of the tongue. In case of suspected strangulation, layerwise dissection of the neck musculature and detailed examination of each muscle prior to removal of the tongue is advisable. (b): The arrows on both sides of the tongue indicate the movement and direction of the blade to include the tonsils and the uvula but avoid the large vessels on either side.

the time of death. It should be noted, however, that digestion of the stomach contents continues after death for a considerable length of time. Preservation of the stomach contents for subsequent chemical analyses is recommended in every case in which ingestion of a poison is suspected. During the autopsy the liquid part of the stomach contents is placed in a glass funnel, the outlet of which has been sealed. Any crystalline material intermixed with the stomach contents will settle to the bottom of the container (Fig. XXIV-8). The supernatant fluid is removed, and the crystalline fraction may be examined microscopically. Occasionally, the presence of crystals of familiar shape and color may direct the chemist to a specific analysis. Additional information regarding the probability of suicide versus accident may be derived from the amount of crystalline material that has settled to the bottom of the funnel. A large quantity of crystalline material tends to favor the assumption of suicidal poisoning, since it is unlikely that a large number of tablets could be ingested accidentally.

Fats in normal stomach contents sometimes convert to soaps, which settle in a manner similar to that of crystalline material. Microscopic examination of the sediment may be required to distinguish between such soaps and crystals.

## REMOVAL OF THE SPINAL CORD BY ANTERIOR APPROACH

The spinal cord is probably the most neglected organ at autopsy. Unless a definite history requires that it be examined, the cord usually remains untouched and unobserved. The main cause of this apparent lack of interest is that removal of the cord from the body is both laborious and time-consuming. Yet over forty years ago, Kernohan, at the Mayo Clinic, de-

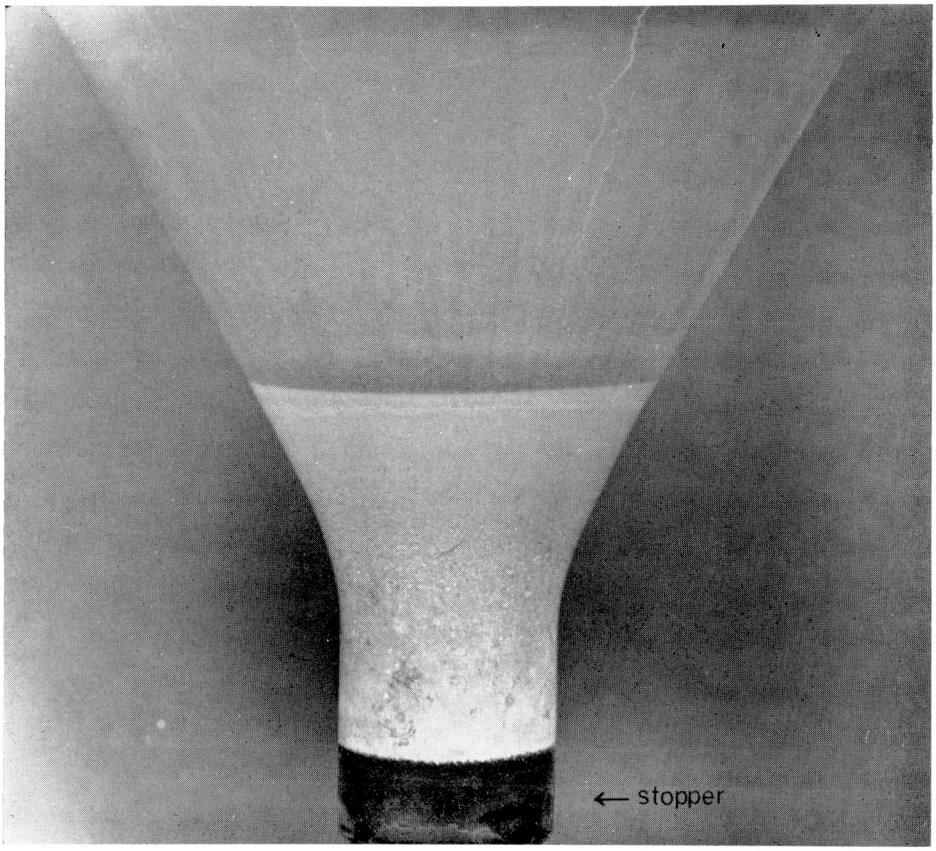


FIGURE XXIV-8. Glass funnel containing stomach contents from a person who ingested an overdose of assorted pills and capsules. The crystalline material has settled to the bottom of the container. The large amount of crystalline material is suggestive of suicide.

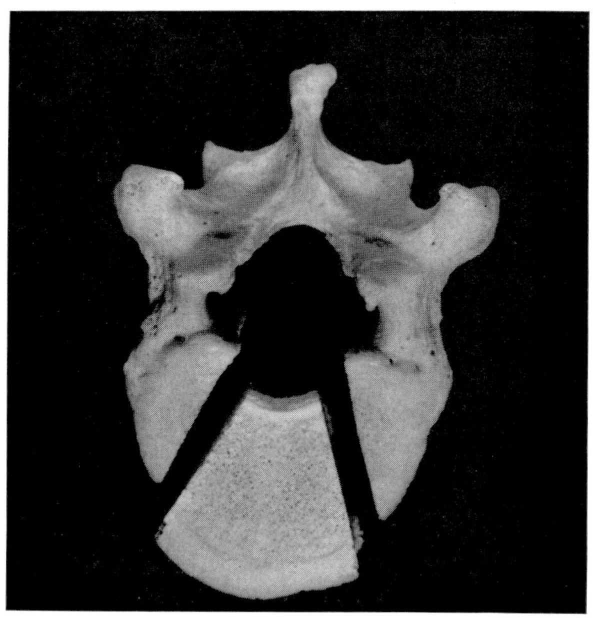

FIGURE XXIV-9. Vertebra, showing the wedge removed for exposure of the cord.

veloped a method that permits removal of the entire spinal cord without major effort and in no more than two to three minutes.[2]

This method requires no special instruments; in fact, a sturdy knife, a Stryker saw, a chisel and a hammer are likely to be all the instruments that will be needed. The cord is retrieved intact and suitable for gross and microscopic examination. Incision of the back is avoided, which eliminates turning the body and unnecessary work for the funeral director.

The autopsy is performed in the usual way. The brain is removed from the body, and the nerve roots in the cervical area are severed through the foramen magnum. After the chest and abdominal cavities have been evacuated, removal of the spinal cord is continued as follows. An intervertebral disc anywhere in the upper lumbar spine is transected, and another disc is cut in the lower thoracic area. A Stryker saw is then used to cut out the segment of vertebral bodies between the two separated discs (Fig. XXIV-9). Prying with a chisel may be necessary to facilitate removal of the bony wedge. This will expose 2 to 2½ in. of the terminal dural disc, which should be slit vertically and reflected sideways. At this stage, the lowest portion of the spinal cord, or the cauda, is cut and a moist cloth or paper towel is placed around the proximal segment. Gentle and slow traction downward (toward the feet) applied to the exposed part of the cord permits retrieval of the cord in its entirety from within its dural encasement.

We have employed this procedure routinely and have found the cord to be in an excellent state of preservation. There were no artifactual tears, nor was the histologic appearance distorted.

## FIXATION OF THE BRAIN

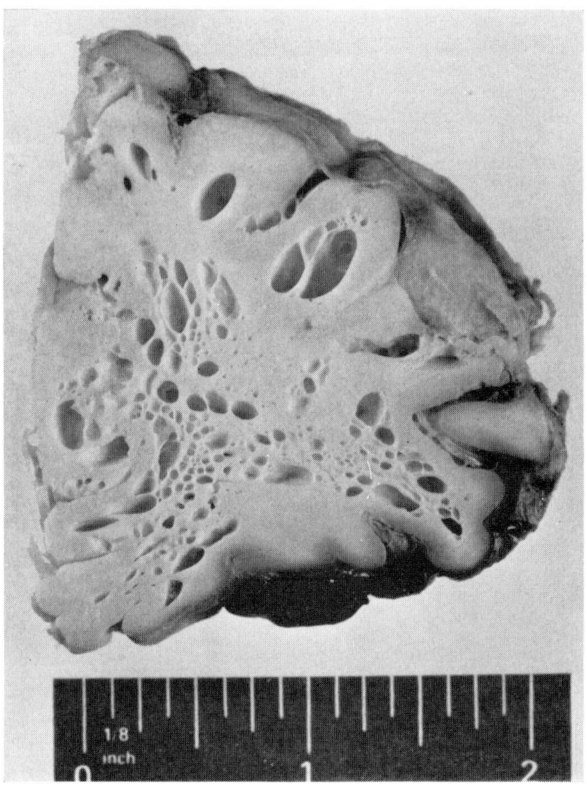


FIGURE XXIV-10. Brain with gas bubbles from decomposition.

To permit a meaningful examination, the brain should be fixed in formalin for at least four to five days before being sectioned, unless fixation is accomplished by vascular injection. It is customary in many institutions that the brain be suspended in a bucket of formalin, using a string through the circle of Willis to avoid flattening of the surface in touch with the bottom of the container.

Especially in a warm environment and certain infectious cases, rapid growth of anaerobic bacteria in the brain occurs if it is handled as described above, and gas bubbles throughout the brain tissue often render it useless for subsequent examination (Fig. XXIV-10). This can be avoided by placing the brain into chilled formalin. A supply of buckets containing formalin can be maintained in the body refrigerator. The bucket with the brain is then returned to the refrigerator for fixation under refrigeration. A handful of kitchen salt dissolved in the formalin provides for flotation of the brain in the solution and obviates the necessity of tying a string through the basilar vessels. Drying of a small area of tissue extending above the fluid level can be avoided by covering the area with a paper towel, which will soak up the solution and keep the area wet. Shrinkage of tissue resulting from the addition of salt is so minimal as to cause no detectable microscopic changes.

## AUTOPSY ROOM PHOTOGRAPHY

It is unfortunate that, in spite of the growing popularity of amateur photography in pathology departments, photographs, though often in color and of generous size, fail to relate the desired information. The following are thought to be useful suggestions for the pathologist who documents his pertinent findings at postmortem examination. It may seem that these principles are to a large extent self-evident; however, experience has shown that they are not commonly adhered to.

1. Photographs of the victim are often unsuitable because the camera is held at an incorrect angle to the body. For instance, a photograph taken from the foot end or sideways of the prone body on the autopsy table shows big feet and a small head and is of no real value for documentation of the upper half of the body. This is often referred to as *perspective distortion,* even though it is not a true distortion.

This fault can be readily remedied by taking the photograph from above, at right angles to the body (Fig. XXIV-11). Adequate results may be obtained, for example, by using a freestanding 6 ft. ladder and a 35 mm camera. A single-lens reflex camera is recommended, since it affords an exact image, avoiding paralax.

2. Photographs of the victim must not be too gory, especially when in color. Photographs showing abundant blood on the body or in the background are often considered offensive and are not admitted in evidence in the courts, as they may tend to prejudice the jury and preclude dispassionate judgment. A clean sheet of

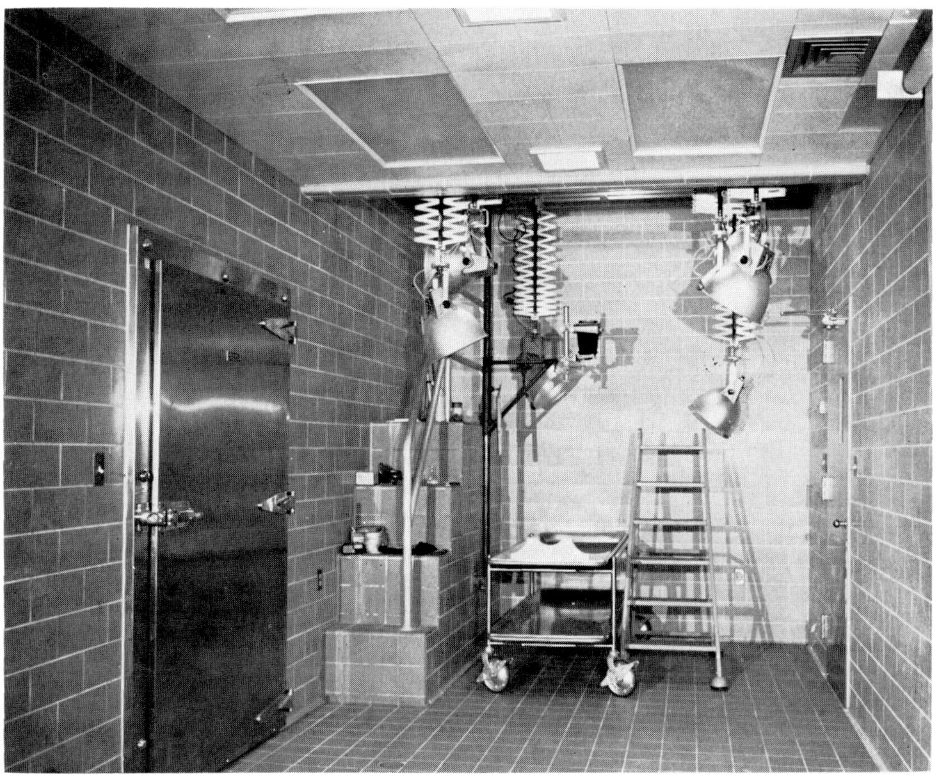

FIGURE XXIV-11. Photography area of the Medical Examiner's Office of Maryland in Baltimore. This setup has been found most advantageous over a period of many years.

material or paper used as a background for the body will be less distracting and will also help obtain a clearer and less gruesome picture. All extraneous objects, such as scalpels and scissors, must be rigorously excluded in case the photographs may be submitted in evidence.

Hospital bandages and wrappings should be taken off, the body must be wiped and dry blood adherent to the surface removed to show all particulars. Care must be taken not to remove evidence of close-range gunfire when the body is thus prepared. The case number or date and a scale of size suitable for the subject being photographed should be included in every photograph. These should be clearly legible and positioned in the same plane as the principal points of interest. The case number is best placed in a corner or along one edge of the photograph, enabling its removal should this become necessary. Suitable scales are available commercially or can be manufactured as required. A pointer, such as a narrow triangle of thin cardboard, may be used where a lesion is not readily discernible.

3. In cases of violent death, front and back views of the uncleaned body with its clothes and in the nude are recommended. It is often important to show the condition of the body when first viewed by the pathologist.

Two shots are mandatory of the nude body: (a) distant shot to indicate the location of the injuries; (b) closeup shot of major wounds to show details. The closeup photograph must enable the viewer to get a clear concept of position with reference to the area of the body.

4. Personal identification of the victim is often made possible by a photograph of the face. Repair of facial injuries and possibly application of makeup by a well-qualified mortician are frequently helpful in such cases.

Any identification photograph of a face should be taken with a lens of longer focal length than normal (e.g. 105 to 135 mm lens on 35 mm camera) to obtain correct representation. Many of the close-up lenses used in laboratories for specimen photographs are of short length, and significant distortion of features occurs whenever the camera is moved nearer in order to fill the frame. It is noteworthy that all professional

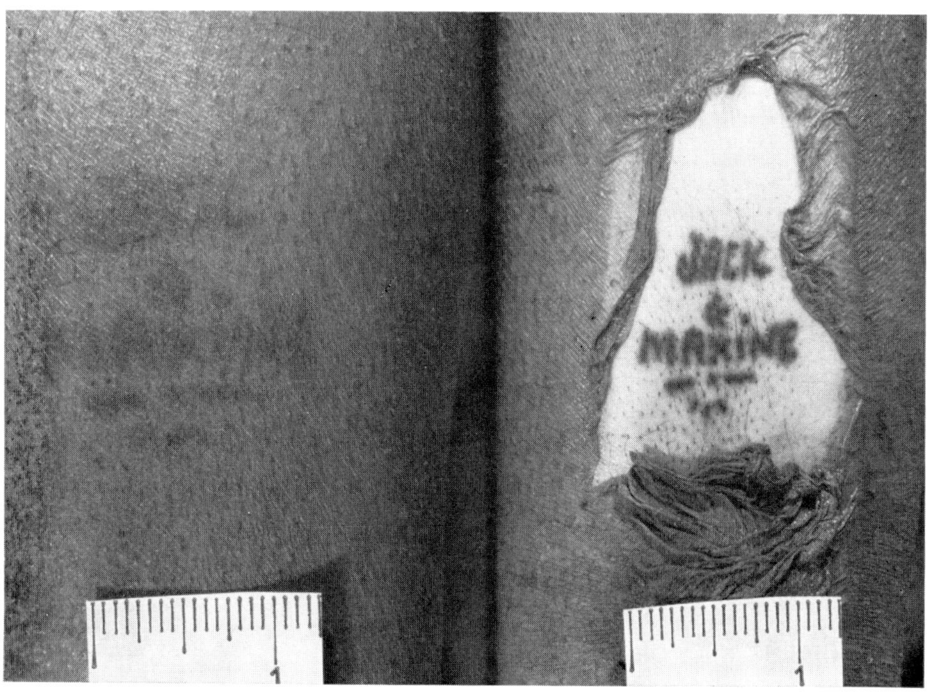


FIGURE XXIV-12. Forearm of a Negro male. Left: Illegible tattoo. Right: Same tattoo after removal of the epidermis, made possible by application of heat to the skin using a 1000 w lamp for five minutes from a distance of 12 in.

portrait photographers use longer focal length in order to obtain a satisfactory representation of the features.

5. Tattoos are frequently important in the identification of an unknown victim. Excessive pigmentation of the skin may obscure a tattoo so as to render it barely recognizable. The same holds true for an old tattoo. Removal of the superficial layers of the skin has proven to be advantageous to enhance the tattooed image and enable superior documentation photographically. This is best done by producing a second degree burn of the area and subsequently wiping off the detached epidermis. Placement of the tattooed area 2 or 3 in. under a hot lamp will produce the desired effect in several minutes (Fig. XXIV-12).

An incidental observation is that tattoos frequently fade considerably and may with time even disappear entirely. This particularly applies to *homemade tattoos,* as are often produced in jails. In such tattoos the amount of pigment in the skin is usually much less than in those professionally made. Thus, a tattoo described by relatives that is absent at the time of autopsy could lead to a mistaken identification unless it is realized that the pigment may have been removed to the regional lymph nodes, in which it can be detected microscopically.

6. Photography of the palmar surface of the victim's hand is often necessary to show electrical burns, defense cuts, bullet wounds or discoloration of the skin due to handling of certain drugs, such as red by Seconal® and Placidyl® or green by Tuinal®, etc. Such photographs are often neglected, or they are rendered unsightly by strings tied to the fingers to overcome rigor mortis.

Severing the flexor tendons of the fingers can be easily performed through a ¼ to ½ in. horizontal incision at the wrist. This procedure will allow complete opening of the hand and good exposure for adequate lighting and photography. We have been practicing this method for many years without complaints from relatives or funeral directors.

## REFERENCES


1. Spitz, W. U., Sopher, I. M., and DiMaio, V. J. M.: Medicolegal investigation of a bomb explosion in an automobile. *J Forensic Sci, 15:*537, 1970.
2. Kernohan, J. W.: Removal of the spinal cord by the anterior route: A new post mortem method. *Am J Clin Pathol, 3:*455, 1933.

*Chapter XXV*

# THE MEDICOLEGAL AUTOPSY REPORT

WERNER U. SPITZ

MOST MEDICOLEGAL autopsies in the United States are performed by hospital pathologists with little or no medicolegal training or experience. Consequently, considerable disparity exists in the quality of these autopsies and in the documentation of postmortem findings.

Several medicolegal textbooks have been published in the United States in recent years, but the space devoted to autopsy techniques and to the formulation and preparation of a medicolegal autopsy report is woefully inadequate. A medicolegal autopsy differs from a hospital autopsy in both objective and significance. Whereas a hospital autopsy is conducted pursuant to the wishes of the next-of-kin, an autopsy conducted by a medicolegal investigative system is pursuant to statute. Contrary to popular belief, a medicolegal autopsy is by no means solely concerned with establishing the cause of death. In fact, in many cases the cause of death is already evident at the scene, and the junior police officer present has a fair idea of what it is. The *manner* and *mechanism* of death are not usually so obvious. Furthermore, a medicolegal autopsy places special emphasis on identification of the deceased, the time of death, proper handling of evidence and the recognition of any injuries or pathological conditions that may be relevant to the judicial handling of the case.

All the pertinent findings have to be properly recorded and adequately described to facilitate retrieval when necessary, because legal implications of a death may arise soon after the autopsy, or months or even years later. It is, therefore, imperative that certain specific and basic information be included in every autopsy report. A case that appears to be straightforward at the time of postmortem examination may subsequently become complicated by unforeseen ramifications.

The basic medicolegal autopsy report, like a standard hospital autopsy report or any other medical evaluation or opinion, corresponds in essence to an established format. Yet certain differences exist, depending upon the type of case. The following provides suggestions on how to arrange and phrase a medicolegal autopsy report. Directions are given to discern which findings need specific mention because of their presence and which are significant because of their absence. Emphasis is placed on formulation of an opinion as to cause, manner and mechanism of death. Finally, brief mention is made of special autopsy techniques to complement those in Chapter XXIV. These added procedures are considered fundamental in establishing certain findings that might otherwise be overlooked.

## PRELIMINARY INVESTIGATION

The individual who is charged with determining the cause and manner of death in cases that require official investigation must be furnished a detailed account of the circumstances surrounding the death and of the scene where the body was found. This is usually obtained from the police. It must be understood, however, that police interest in a case usually prevails only for as long as the question of prosecution remains undecided. Once the decision is made that there will be no criminal charges, police interest in a case rapidly wanes. This deficiency must be promptly corrected. Whereas it would certainly be valuable if the medical examiner, and preferably the pathologist who will conduct the postmortem examination, were to examine every scene of death, this is by no means practical in all cases and probably is not essential.

A phone call or two by him or a trained investigator to elicit the pertinent information are often all that is required.

For example, in the case of an apparent nonviolent death or a suspected drug overdose, inquiry should be made into the medical background of the deceased, including old or recent surgery, recent state of mind, previous suicide attempts, alcohol consumption habits, drugs to which the individual may have had access, etc. Such information, commonly obtained from family physicians, hospitals, relatives, neighbors and friends, frequently eliminates unnecessary autopsies and the need for an open-ended search for drugs by the toxicologist.

An individual found dead in the garage of his home may have died of carbon monoxide poisoning as a result of being overcome by exhaust fumes of the automobile he was trying to repair. In this case, the manner of death would have been accidental. Sometimes, however, a hose is found connected to the vehicle exhaust pipe, leading to the car interior, or all openings around the doors and windows of the garage may have been carefully sealed with tape to prevent leakage of fumes; both are indications of a suicidal manner of death. Of course, death may also have been due to natural causes such as a heart attack or spontaneous cerebral hemorrhage. Questions as to whether the garage door was open or shut, whether the door was operated manually or electrically, evidence of work being done on the car, keys in the ignition, ignition turned on or off, amount of fuel in the gas tank, location and position of the deceased's body in relation to the automobile and the muffler and the deceased's state of health, should be answered prior to autopsy.

In a traffic collision, references regarding whether the deceased was a pedestrian, driver or passenger and the type, year, make and model of vehicles involved in the crash are essential. A sketch placing all involved parties and objects and indicating directions of travel is helpful in explaining the mechanism of certain injuries. It also serves to corroborate anatomical findings in the victims with observations made at the scene.

Homicide scenes are frequently very informative where the medical examiner is concerned. Estimation of the time of death, for example, is considerably more meaningful if done on site before the body is handled. Correlation of patterned injuries and other manifestations on the body surface with evidence at the scene can often be done only by viewing the place where the body was found. On the other hand, in a witnessed incident such as a barroom shooting or a family dispute, the medical examiner's presence at the scene will contribute little to the police investigation unless specific questions need to be answered.

## EXTERNAL EXAMINATION

### Clothing

The external examination of a body in a medicolegal case should begin with a description of the clothing. In most instances of death from seemingly natural causes, a cursory statement relative to the clothes usually suffices. The body may then be undressed for further examination. In cases where death is caused by violence, or if foul play is suspected, the external examination should begin with front and back view photographs of the body as it was received. This is followed by closeup photographs of pertinent details. Hairy areas of the body must be shaved to afford an unobstructed view of all details (Fig. XXV-1). Much of the controversy surrounding the assassination of President Kennedy could probably have been avoided had the wound in the back of his head been shaved and adequately prepared for photography.

Sometimes the value of a detailed examination of the clothing may exceed that of the autopsy. For example, in an automobile collision, a single, minute fragment of lacquer discovered hidden in the clothing of a hit-and-run victim may shed light on the make, model and year of the car involved. Tire marks imprinted on the clothing

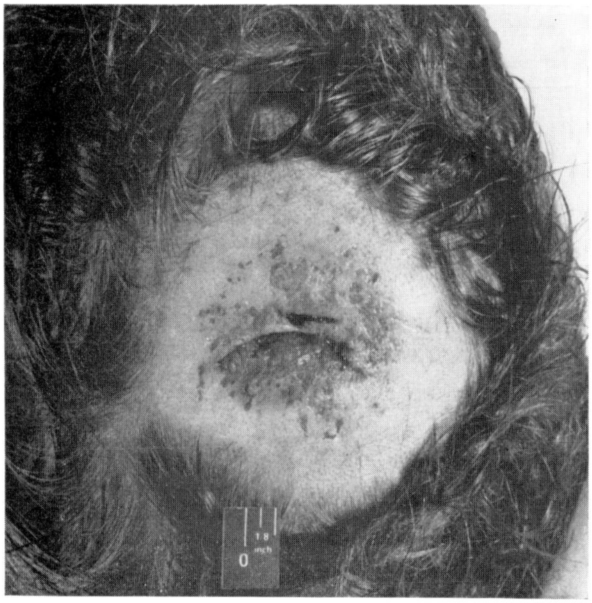

FIGURE XXV-1. Laceration of the back of the head sustained in a fall. The edges of the injury are abraded and show the imprint of gravel. The area was shaved for the purpose of examination and photography.

may assist the police in identifying the offending vehicle and enlighten the pathologist regarding certain findings subsequently found at autopsy. In a shooting death, the frayed fibers of a coat may point out the direction of a shot, and soot or gunpowder deposits on a garment may indicate the distance from which a weapon was fired.

Clothes that early in the postmortem examination are believed to be of subsequent evidentiary significance should be removed from the body with care and as little mutilation as possible. Such clothes should not be cut unless it is unavoidable. Under such circumstances, the cuts are made through undamaged parts of the clothes and a notation to this effect is made in the file. After the body is undressed, the clothes are handed to the police for further examination by the crime laboratory.

A useful method for preserving possible trace evidence in clothing is to undress the body on a clean white sheet on the floor. After the nude body is placed back on the tray or autopsy table, a pouch is made of the sheet by knotting its four corners. Now the sheet with its contents is tagged for identification and can be handed to the police. Wet clothes, such as from a drowning victim, or clothes soaked in blood should be thoroughly line dried at room temperature before being folded. Drying at high temperatures may destroy substances that could otherwise subsequently be used for blood grouping. Folding or packaging of wet clothes causes soiling of previously clean areas and renders subsequent examination more difficult or impossible.

The chain of custody of clothing, as with all evidence, must be maintained at all times. A signed receipt listing each item should be obtained from the police officer who takes the clothes to the crime laboratory.

An adequate description of this part of the postmortem examination may be worded as in the following examples.

### *Natural Death*

The body is that of a well-developed, well nourished, fully clothed elderly white male, weighing 170 lbs. and measuring 5 ft. 10 in. in length. The clothes worn by the deceased are unremarkable. The deceased appears to be the stated age of 72 years.

### *Gunshot Wounds*

The body is that of a . . . fully clothed white male. . . . Examination of the clothes shows a bullet hole of entrance measuring ¼ in. in diameter located in the back of the cream-colored shirt, 1 in. from the shoulder seam and 2 in. to the left of the midline. The fibers of the fabric at the edge of the tear are frayed inward. The tear is surrounded by densely distributed particles of gunpowder extending over a diameter of about 1½ in. In the front of the shirt on the right side, 6 in. below the shoulder seam, there is noted a tear apparently produced by the exiting slug. The fabric fibers at the edge of this tear are frayed outward. The T-shirt worn by the deceased has holes in locations corresponding to those seen in the shirt. No additional bullet holes are noted in the clothing. All clothing items are listed and turned over to the police. (The signed receipt for the clothing is enclosed with the file.)

### *Pedestrian Struck by an Automobile*

The body is that of a well-nourished, well-developed elderly white male. . . . The body is fully clothed except for the right shoe, which is obtained separately. Examination of the clothes shows the trousers to be extensively torn, and a patterned imprint of what is believed to be tire marks is seen in the left thigh area. The clothes are all soiled with road dirt, and the shirt is soiled with blood. (All the clothes are listed and turned over to the police.)

It is advisable to mention the amount of blood present in the clothing (soaked, streaked, spotted) and describe in general terms the areas that are soiled (e.g. left sleeve and back of shirt, etc.). In the case of a shooting or stabbing victim who died at the hospital, it is a good practice for the police to have the clothes viewed by the pathologist before delivering them to the crime laboratory. For example, when the clothes have filtered out soot or gunpowder deposits and the entrance wound in the skin is devoid of evidence of close-range firing, examination of the clothes by the pathologist is required to enable him to formulate an opinion regarding the manner of death. Suicidal gunshots are usually fired at contact or at very close range (Fig. XXV-2).

To verify whether a shooting was accidental, the circumstances of the incident must be reconstructed and correlated with the findings on the body. Examination of the clothes in such a case is essential. The presence or absence of soot and/or gunpowder will assist the pathologist in estimating the range of fire.

A cut in an article of clothing may enlighten the examiner regarding the shape of the blade that caused the stab wound and help in identifying whether an injury was due to one or more thrusts of the weapon. Due to the relatively low elasticity of certain materials such as leather and synthetics, the shape of the blade is often far better maintained in these than in skin or other tissues.

Clothes may be of considerable significance in cases of unknown identity. Mutilation of the face by injury or advanced postmortem deterioration of the body may render conventional identification methods unsuitable. Under such circumstances, the clothes should be retained for later viewing by a potential identifier. Certain institutions, such as psychiatric hospitals and homes for the elderly, etc., often mark patients' clothing so that it is easily identifiable.

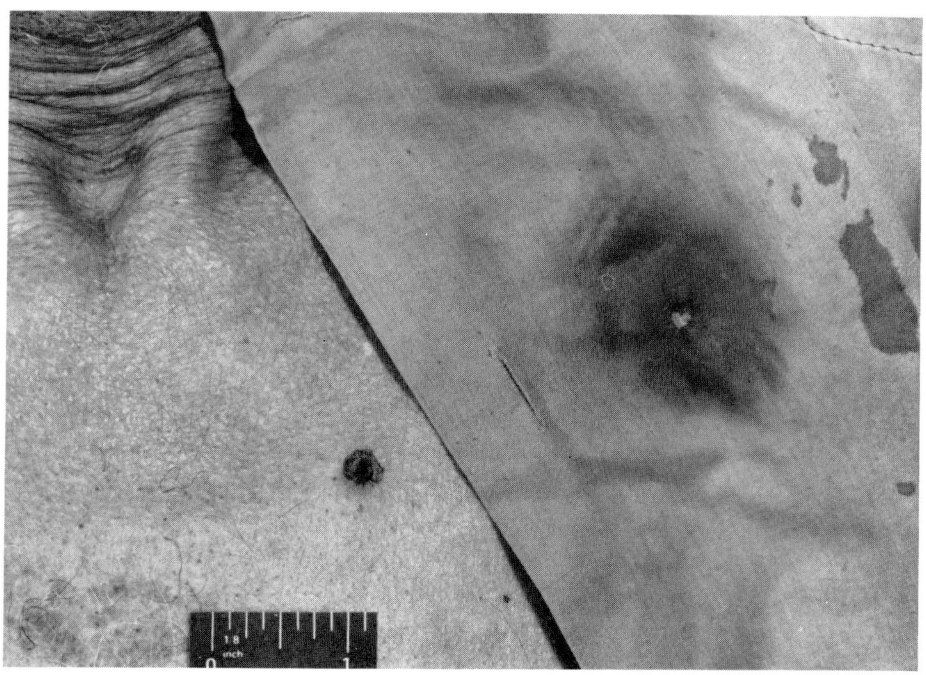

FIGURE XXV-2. Suicidal near-contact shot of the chest. Abundant soot is deposited around the bullet hole in the shirt. The wound in the skin is devoid of evidence of close-range firing. Without the shirt, this wound would be interpreted as a distant shot—unlikely to have been self-inflicted.

### The Body

The postmortem examination of a body, in particular the external examination, is essential for understanding the mechanism of injury in all cases of violent death. Therefore, injuries should not be listed as merely tears or lacerations, abrasions and bruises, but characteristic injuries that are recognized from past experience as being caused in a certain way should not only be described but also named accordingly, e.g. brush burns, tire marks, stab wounds, bullet wounds of entrance or exit, contact shot, gunpowder stippling, etc. This provides for conciseness of the record and enhances understanding of the report. In this way injuries produced by dragging on the ground should be described as *brush burns;* the imprint of the automobile steering column on a driver's chest should be noted, and pedestrian injuries believed to be caused by an automobile bumper may be described as *bumper injuries.* The same holds true for *dicing* produced by broken tempered glass, *dashboard injuries,* the imprint or indentation of the skin produced by the noose in a hanging victim, needle tracks in a narcotic addict, etc.

The external examination of the body lists the age, race, sex, length and weight of the deceased, as well as the state of nourishment and any congenital abnormalities. The presence and distribution of rigor and livor mortis are important, as is body temperature, although in most cases it may suffice to state whether the body is warm or cold to the touch. In cases where estimation of the time of death is important, liver or rectal temperature measurement may be of value, provided the body has not been refrigerated.

The degree of corneal clouding is significant if the eyes are shut, otherwise corneal clouding and drying set in very rapidly. The conjunctivae may be congested or pale. Conjunctival hemorrhages, petechial or otherwise, should be noted. The presence of pinpoint-sized hemorrhages in the eyelids must be recorded. Such hemorrhages are especially significant if strangulation is suspected. It is often necessary to slightly stretch the upper eyelids to identify these faint and very delicate reddish dots. The presence of cataracts or artificial eyes may have special significance in the case of a traffic collision. The description should also include the oral cavity. Bruises and tears of the lining membrane caused by pressure against the teeth are sometimes noted in cases of manual smothering. Such injuries are more often located opposite the molars.

In cases of questionable identity, all details that may be pertinent to the identification of the deceased are mentioned in the report. Thus, hair and eye color, moles, tattoos and all scars on the body are important. Under such circumstances, identification photographs and fingerprints should be taken by police technicians. Good sets of fingerprints are often obtainable even in the presence of advanced decomposition. Postmortem dental charts and roentgenograms of both jaws, as well as other skeletal x rays, are invaluable if antemortem data are available for comparison.

If the face is badly mutilated or decomposition has advanced to the extent that the body cannot be displayed, it is often advantageous to remove the jaws from the body to facilitate a more accurate examination and possible consultation with a dentist. The technique is discussed in Chapter XXIV.

Tattoos in areas where the skin is darkened by smoke or old tattoos that have become difficult to recognize may be identified by removal of the epidermis. In a fire victim, or in the case of slippage of the skin due to decomposition, the epidermis can be removed simply by wiping the area. Otherwise, a second degree burn produced by a regular light bulb held close to the skin for a few minutes will have the same effect.

The external genitalia must be examined and described. If sexual assault is suspected, vaginal, oral and rectal specimens in females and oral and rectal specimens in males should be obtained in triplicate. One set of specimens is used for the preparation of smears. These are stained with any conventional cytological stain, including hematoxylin and eosin, and scanned microscopically for the presence of spermatozoa. A second set is subjected to a determination of acid phosphatase activity, and a third set is typed. The presence of what appears to be dry semen on the thighs, abdomen or pubic area of a body should be noted. The material may be scraped gently with a scalpel blade and placed in a test tube containing saline for later identification. Dry semen on the thigh of a man in close proximity of the genital area has no significance. It is usually the result of *expulsion* of semen due to postmortem rigidity of the seminal vesicles.

In every case of suspected sexual assault, pubic and scalp hair and finger nail clippings are retained, placed in separate envelopes, properly labeled and sent to the crime laboratory. The hair should be plucked rather than cut and the area from which it is obtained noted. Scalp hair and fingernail clippings or scrapings should be retained in any type of assault in which there was body contact between the parties. In such cases, the hands should be carefully inspected for foreign materials. Hairs adhering to the victim's fingers may be most significant.

Gags, ligatures and bindings that have been used to immobilize the victim should be photographed before removal from the body. Removal of any of these, or a noose, from the body is done by cutting the item away from the knot and tying the cut ends with string or wire. This assures adequate preservation, although it may sometimes be necessary to secure the knot independently.

## Evidence of Injury

All injuries are described, both externally and internally. Bullet wounds, stab wounds and certain other injuries should be precisely located on the body. For purposes of testimony, it is desirable to always use three parameters in accurately locating an injury on the body:

1. Number of inches from the top of the head or above the sole of the foot.
2. Number of inches to the right or left of the anterior or posterior midline of the body.
3. Number of inches from a well-established landmark, such as the nipple in the male, below the collarbone, or from the naval, the groin, etc.

A wound in an extremity should be described with the limb in the anatomic position using the joints, i.e., shoulders, wrists, elbows, knees, ankles, as points of reference.

### *Gunshot Wounds*

In the case of *gunshot wounds,* aligning a wound in a shoulder or an upper extremity with a possible reentry wound in the trunk, neck or head helps ascertain the total number of shots that struck the victim.

This description is not only accurate, but it facilitates the demonstration of an injury on one's own body if asked to do so for the benefit of the jury at the time of a trial: "Doctor, would you please show the jury on your own body where this wound that you have just described to us was situated?" Thus, in the case of a *gunshot wound:*

> On the front of the chest, 18 in. from the top of the head, 5 in. to the left of the midline and 2 in. below the left nipple, there is noted a gunshot wound of entrance. The wound measures ¼ in. in diameter, and its edges are abraded. There is no evidence of soot deposit or gunpowder stippling on the skin surrounding this gunshot wound.

Note in the description of the bullet wound of entrance the mention of marginal abrasion, soot and gunpowder. As described in Chapter X, the marginal abrasion of an entrance wound indicates the angle at which the bullet struck the body. It is therefore important that an eccentric marginal abrasion be accurately noted in the report. The *o'clock* system is best used for this purpose. Twelve o'clock is oriented superiorly. For example:

> The edges of the bullet wound are abraded. The widest point of the abrasion is at three o'clock, tapering off toward one o'clock.

Similarly, if the gun sight or extractor rod is imprinted on the skin, the description may be worded using the same system:

> A ¼ in. diameter semicircular abrasion and bruise are

situated between two and four o'clock of the gunshot wound of entrance. . . .

If the shot was inflicted at close range, the exact diameter of the gunpowder stippling around the wound must be recorded:

Gunpowder stippling is noted scattered over a diameter of 3 in. around the entrance wound.

After all pertinent information relative to the external description of the wound has been recorded, the description may proceed with an account of the wound track in anatomical order. Regardless of the type of violence, the entire extent of the injury, beginning with the external appearance and followed by the internal findings, should be described together in one paragraph. In this way the injury is outlined in a natural sequence, and with almost no effort one can visualize the entire wound complex. Such description significantly simplifies retrieval of this information at the time of courtroom testimony.

. . . Subsequent autopsy shows the bullet to graze the upper edge of the fifth rib and pass through the lower lobe of the left lung. A deformed small caliber, nonjacketed lead slug is recovered from the left side of the back, 25 in. below the top of the head and 2 in. to the left of the midline, and retained. Massive bleeding (1500 cc of liquid and clotted blood) is noted within the left chest cavity and along the entire wound track. The wound path is from front to back, downward and slightly inward.

The description of the slug should be noted with respect to location and type: lead, jacketed or nonjacketed; caliber if specifically known, otherwise described as small, medium or large caliber; and condition—intact, deformed or fragmented.

In the case of a through-and-through bullet wound of an upper extremity and reentry into the body, the text should be worded accordingly:

Manipulation of the right upper extremity permits the through-and-through gunshot wound in the right hand to be aligned with an atypical gunshot wound

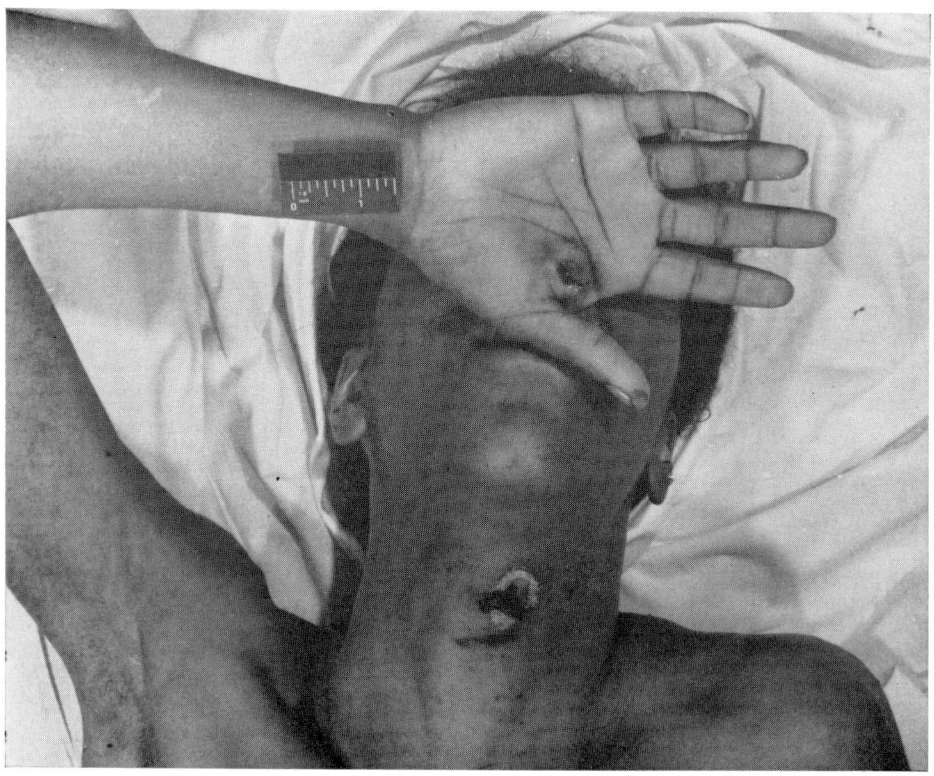

FIGURE XXV-3. Through-and-through close-range entrance bullet wound of the right hand and reentry of the same slug into the neck. The pattern of injury suggests that the wound in the hand may have been a *defense-type* wound.

in the front of the neck, suggesting that the two injuries were caused by the same slug (Fig. XXV-3).

The bullet wound in the hand may well be a *defense-type* injury, and a sentence to that effect should be included in either the descriptive text of the autopsy report or, preferably, in the *opinion* at the end.

In cases of multiple gunshot wounds, it is often advisable to number each wound. The wounds may be numbered consecutively from top to bottom, regardless of whether they are entrance or exit wounds. To avoid possible misunderstanding that the wound labeled #1 was necessarily the first shot inflicted, an explanatory sentence should be added to the opinion at the end of the report: "The sequence of the shots cannot be ascertained." The description of the injuries has now been completed, and there is no need to repeat this outline when detailing the individual organ systems, except for a short reference to this paragraph.

The base of a bullet recovered during autopsy should be marked for identification. If the slug is mutilated, markings may be placed in a suitable location, ensuring that rifling marks are not tampered with. The markings should be recorded in the pathologist's notes, so that the slug can be identified when needed. Each bullet recovered is placed in a separate envelope or other secure container to prevent damage to the bullet surface by scratching. The container states the name of the victim, the medicolegal examiner's case number, date of the autopsy, name of the prosector, the part of the body where the slug was found and the individual to whom the slug was given.

### *Stab Wounds*

In the case of *stab wounds,* the injury in the skin should be measured and this measurement recorded in the report. Then, after adjusting the wound edges in accordance with the lines of cleavage to the skin, a second measurement of wound length and its width (representing the blunt edge of the blade) is made and also recorded. Thus, a report of the external examination of a stab wound might read as follows:

On the left chest, 18 in. from the top of the head, 5 in. to the left of the midline and 2 in. below the left nipple, there is noted a vertical stab wound, which measures ⅞ in. in length and gapes to a width of ⅜ in. Approximation of the sides of the wound changes its dimensions and shape. Following alignment of the wound, it becomes triangular, the upper edge representing the base of the triangle, measuring ⅛ in. in length. The sides of the triangle each measure 1 in. in length. The apex of the triangle points downward.

Adjacent to the upper edge of the stab wound there is a rectangular abrasion having approximately the same length as the *base* of the triangle; this may have been caused by the hilt of the knife (*see* Figs. VIII-6, VIII-7 and VIII-8).

Subsequent autopsy indicates the stab wound to sever the left fifth rib cartilage and proceed into the lower lobe of the left lung to a depth of 4 in. with the chest in a normal state of expansion.

It is important to record the dimensions of a stab wound in any serosal surface such as the liver capsule, the pleura or in bone. Often these measurements more closely approximate those of the blade than the dimensions of the wound in the skin.

The entire wound track is infiltrated with a large amount of blood, and there are 1500 cc of liquid and clotted blood in the left chest cavity. The entire length of the stab wound is approximately 5½ in. The wound track passes from front to back, downward and inward.

Multiple stab wounds in a given area of the body may be described together:

Around the left nipple, over a diameter of 7 in., there are twelve stab wounds. Most are vertical, but some are slightly slanted. They range in length from ¾ in. to ⅛ in.

The pathologist should then proceed to describe one typical stab wound and ascertain how many penetrate the pleural cavity and the lung, ribs involved, extent of hemorrhage, etc.

Similar grouping of injuries for the purpose of description may be done with other types of trauma. In a case of manual strangulation, for example, the following type of description may be used:

On the neck there are fingernail marks, multiple semilunar and straight linear abrasions up to ½ in. in length, which are especially numerous on the left side.

Hammer injuries to the scalp may also be described as one entity, noting the number of wounds and their locations. Several typical wounds should be chosen for more detailed description of their shape, diameter, underlying involvement of the skull, etc.

## INTERNAL EXAMINATIONS

The description of the internal examination in a medicolegal autopsy report does not materially differ from that of any regular hospital autopsy. Findings that were described under the heading Evidence of Injury need not be repeated with the description of each organ system, except possibly for a general statement such as *the following observations are limited to changes other than injuries that were described above.*

Injuries that were not found on external examination, such as contusions of the scalp, are described in detail. Their location and extent may indicate the site and severity of impacts. A fracture of the skull should be described as to size and shape, depressed, comminuted, etc. A close-up photograph of the fracture, after removal of all external periosteal tissues by scraping with the sharp edge of a scalpel, may be helpful for identification of a weapon. A subdural hematoma is best weighed or its volume determined in a graduated cylinder. In a patient who survived the incident twenty-four hours or less, the subdural blood should be analyzed for alcohol content. A traumatic clot from within the brain should be handled in the same way. Alcohol in the peripheral blood may have been metabolized during this time period.

Dissection of the cervical spine by posterior approach as outlined in Chapter XXIV is necessary in certain cases. This procedure is best carried out at the end of the postmortem examination when the tissues have been drained by removal of the organs. Whiplash injuries of the upper part of the spine are not necessarily associated with fractures. In automobile drivers they are far more frequent than is commonly acknowledged. In other cases, injury of the cervical cord may have caused paraplegia, thus immediate collapse. Injury of the medulla oblongata is likely to cause instantaneous death. This finding in the autopsy report would immediately exclude any chance of recovery in a subsequent claim for pain and suffering.

A description of the degree of calcification or porosis of certain bones provides an assessment of their fragility. Osteoporosis is common in the elderly, in whom fractures can occur with relatively little trauma. At autopsy ribs with advanced osteoporosis fracture upon minor inward bending with a sound reminiscent of breaking cardboard. Artifactual fracture during autopsy of an osteoporotic spine occurs occasionally above the edge of the wood block placed across the shoulders to facilitate the Rokitansky technique of organ removal. The hyoid bone and laryngeal cartilages, of particular importance in cases of suspected strangulation, should be evaluated for their fragility and reference to this effect made in the autopsy description. Sectioning of the thyrohyoid ligaments between the greater cornua of the hyoid bone and the superior cornua of the thyroid cartilage permits manipulation of both structures independently and inspection for possible fractures and deep hemorrhages.

*In situ* examination of the larynx or removal of the neck organs is meaningful only after the brain and chest organs have been removed from the body to provide for a bloodless dissection field in the neck area. This technique excludes artifactual hemorrhages. In a fire victim incision of the trachea prior to evisceration is advantageous to ascertain that soot present in the airway was inhaled rather than due to contamination as a result of handling of the body.

Inspection of the organs *in situ* is also required in gunshot and stabbing cases, where evisceration upsets normal anatomic relationships and distorts wound tracks. X ray examination of the body to locate foreign objects does not outline the path of hemorrhage.

Injuries that result from attempts at resuscitation should be described accordingly. These may include fractures of the ribs and sternum, bruising and laceration of the lungs with interstitial emphysema, and even tears of the heart, due to pounding of the precordial area. Tears of the liver, especially at the ligamentum teres, are frequently noted. Only a small amount of bleeding is usually associated with these injuries, but occasionally, if the heart was reactivated, a beat or two would suffice to cause extensive hemorrhage into the tissues and body cavities.

Areas of aspirated blood in the lungs indicate that breathing continued for an indeterminable period of time. The origin of the inhaled blood can be anywhere in the respiratory system or the oropharynx. A possible origin of the bleeding is the base of the skull, where fracture of the area of the sella turcica opens the pharyngeal vault, exposing the airway.

Appearance of the esophageal, gastric and intestinal mucosa is of particular significance in poisoning cases. The stomach may contain powder and remnants of pills. Stomach contents should be described as to amount, quality, color and odor. The amount of bile in the gall bladder is significant, as is the amount of urine in the bladder. A markedly distended bladder suggests an extended period of unconsciousness preceding the death.

## OPINION

Like its clinical counterpart, a medicolegal report of a postmortem examination should be concluded with a well-rounded *opinion,* tying together all salient points of the case. We have found that a properly worded explanatory note at the end of the report appreciably cuts down the necessity of live courtroom testimony by the prosector.

The medicolegal opinion relates the cause and manner of death, based not only on the results of the postmortem examination and laboratory analyses, but on all available pertinent information that has been collected relative to the case. The scene where the body was found, circumstances surrounding the death, records of recent hospitalization and other medical history are some important considerations in the formulation of a medicolegal opinion. The opinion should be concise and factual. Depending on the type of case and the manner of death, the opinion can be limited to a single short paragraph or encompass a page or two. It is the only part of the report that is sure to be read by anyone with interest in the case, including law enforcement agencies, defense attorneys, judges, juries, the deceased's family and the public at large, as well as physicians. Thus, this part of the report must be worded plainly, to be understandable and leave no room for speculation. A list of technical diagnoses, in order of significance, may be included in a separate paragraph following the descriptive text of the report or as an explanatory adjunct, in parentheses, in the opinion. In a death due to arteriosclerotic heart disease the opinion might read as follows:

> This fifty-seven-year-old white male, JOHN DOE, died of a heart attack (arteriosclerotic heart disease or acute myocardial infarction with a fresh thrombus in the left anterior descending coronary artery, as the case may be). The manner of death is natural.

To be effective as a comprehensive summary of the report, the opinion should provide answers to certain anticipated questions, including negative statements, where appropriate, to enlighten the reader.

> This twenty-eight-year-old black male, JAMES DOE, died of injuries sustained in an automobile collision. The deceased had not consumed alcoholic beverages.

> This nineteen-year-old black male, JOHN DOE, died of what is believed to be a self-inflicted gunshot wound of the right temple. The bullet wound of entrance showed evidence of contact-range firing. A bullet wound of exit was noted in the left temple, and no fragments of metal were found along the wound track. The wrists showed horizontal scars suggestive of a previous suicide attempt. The deceased had a blood alcohol level of 0.18% at the time of his death. Needle tracks on the forearms suggest chronic narcotic use.

> This forty-nine-year-old black female, MARY JONES, died of gunshot wounds that involved the left hand,

right forearm and the forehead. The skin around the gunshot wound of the left hand showed evidence of close-range firing. The other bullet wounds showed no evidence of close-range firing. One medium caliber, nonjacketed lead slug was recovered from the back of the head and was retained. The wounds of the left hand and right forearm may not have been immediately fatal. It is conceivable that a single shot inflicted all three wound tracks, if the forearms were crossed in front of the head. Fingernail marks on the left wrist suggest an altercation. The deceased had not consumed alcoholic beverages shortly preceding her death.

This thirty-eight-year-old white male, JOHN DOE, died of an acute heart attack (acute coronary occlusion) while swimming. It cannot be excluded that he inhaled water during the attack, thus that the death was due to drowning. The death, therefore, is considered to be accidental.

This forty-nine-year-old white male, JOHN SMITH, died of suicidal hanging. No malignant or other tumors were found at autopsy. The deceased had a blood alcohol level of 0.05%.

This fifty-eight-year-old white male, JOHN SMITH, died of head injuries (subdural hematoma) sustained as a result of a fall. An incidental finding at autopsy was cirrhosis of the liver, as is commonly found in cases of chronic alcoholism. Blood alcohol level could not be determined due to prolonged hospitalization following the injury.

This fifty-six-year-old white female, MARY DOE, died of a heart attack (acute coronary thrombosis). The automobile crash in which she was involved is believed to have been the result of her death at the wheel. Blood alcohol level was negative.

It is not imperative that the manner of death be spelled out in each instance if it is implied. Thus, if the bullet wound of entrance shows no evidence of close-range firing, it would be highly improbable that the injury was self-inflicted. Similarly, stab wounds in the back would probably exclude suicide.

This eighteen-year-old white male, JOHN DOE, died of massive internal bleeding due to a gunshot wound of the chest involving the left lung and heart. A small caliber, nonjacketed lead slug was recovered from the spine and retained. The bullet wound of entrance showed no evidence of close-range firing on the skin. The deceased had not been consuming alcoholic beverages.

This twenty-one-year-old white male, JOHN DOE, died of a gunshot wound of the abdomen that perforated the bowel, causing spillage of the bowel contents into the abdominal cavity and subsequent infection (peritonitis). . . .

Occasionally no absolute statements can be made relative to some of the postmortem findings. Under such circumstances, the prosector should elaborate on his uncertainties and convey his impressions rather than avoid the issue and leave the questions open for subsequent debate by other interested parties. The pathologist is certainly the most qualified to express an opinion relative to his findings and conclusions.

Keith Simpson, quoting Voltaire, once said, "We can none of us be certain we are right—'*Only an charlatan is certain.*' But we can try to come as near the truth as the evidence allows, and we can put it in words that are understandable, not only by the lawyers, but by jury men and women also."

# INDEX

## N



## O



## P



## Q



## R